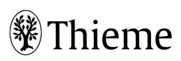

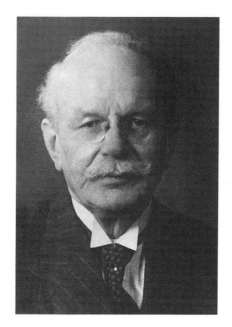

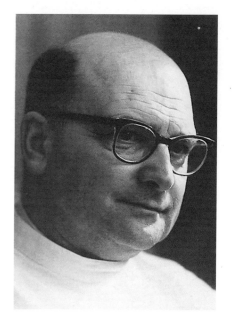

Alban Köhler
1874–1947

Emil-Alfred Zimmer
1908–1981

Freyschmidt's "Koehler/Zimmer"

Borderlands of Normal and Early Pathological Findings in Skeletal Radiography

Fifth revised edition

Juergen Freyschmidt, M.D.
Professor and Director
Division of Diagnostic Radiology
and Nuclear Medicine
Zentralkrankenhaus Sankt-Juergen-Strasse
Bremen, Germany

Juergen Wiens, M.D.
Division of Diagnostic Radiology
and Nuclear Medicine
Zentralkrankenhaus Sankt-Juergen-Strasse
Bremen, Germany

Joachim Brossmann, M.D.
Professor
Division of Diagnostic Radiology
Hospital of the University of Kiel
Kiel, Germany

Andreas Sternberg, M.D.
Division of Diagnostic Radiology
and Nuclear Medicine
Zentralkrankenhaus Sankt-Juergen-Strasse
Bremen, Germany

Foreword by Donald Resnick, M.D.

4206 Illustrations
74 Tables

Thieme
Stuttgart · New York

Library of Congress Cataloging-in-Publication Data
is available from the publisher

1st German edition, 1910	1st English edition, 1956
2nd German edition, 1915	2nd English edition, 1961
3rd German edition, 1920	3rd English edition, 1968
4th German edition, 1924	4th English edition, 1993
5th German edition, 1928	
6th German edition, 1931	1st French edition, 1930
7th German edition, 1939	2nd French edition, 1936
8th German edition, 1943	3rd French edition, 1956
9th German edition, 1953	1st Italian edition, 1955
10th German edition, 1956	2nd Italian edition, 1967
11th German edition, 1967	3rd Italian edition, 1986
12th German edition, 1982	
13th German edition, 1989	1st Spanish edition, 1933
14th German edition, 2001	2nd Spanish edition, 1959

This book is an authorized and revised translation of the 14th German edition published and copyrighted 1910, 2001 by Georg Thieme Verlag, Stuttgart, Germany. Title of the German edition: Freyschmidt's „Köhler/Zimmer": Grenzen des Normalen und Anfänge des Pathologischen in der Radiologie des kindlichen und erwachsenen Skeletts

Translated by Terry C. Telger, Fort Worth, TX, USA

Important Note: Medicine is an ever-changing science undergoing continual development. Research and clinical experience are continually expanding our knowledge, in particular our knowledge of proper treatment and drug therapy. Insofar as this book mentions any dosage or application, readers may rest assured that the authors, editors, and publishers have made every effort to ensure that such references are in accordance with **the state of knowledge at the time of production of the book**.

Nevertheless, this does not involve, imply, or express any guarantee or responsibility on the part of the publishers in respect to any dosage instructions and forms of applications stated in the book. **Every user is requested to examine carefully** the manufacturers' leaflets accompanying each drug and to check, if necessary in consultation with a physician or specialist, whether the dosage schedules mentioned therein or the contraindications stated by the manufacturers differ from the statements made in the present book. Such examination is particularly important with drugs that are either rarely used or have been newly released on the market. Every dosage schedule or every form of application used is entirely at the user's own risk and responsibility. The authors and publishers request every user to report to the publishers any discrepancies or inaccuracies noticed.

© 1956, 2003 Georg Thieme Verlag,
Rüdigerstraße 14, D-70469 Stuttgart, Germany
http://www.thieme.de
Thieme New York, 333 Seventh Avenue,
New York, N.Y. 10001 U.S.A.
http://www.thieme.com

Cover design: Thieme Marketing
Typesetting by Druckhaus Götz, Ludwigsburg
Printed in Germany by Druckhaus Götz, Ludwigsburg

ISBN 3-13-784105-4 (GTV)
ISBN 1-58890-150-5 (TNY)   1 2 3 4 5

For our children
Fritz-Maximilian, Johannes, Benedikt, Christina
and grandchildren
Carla, Felix, and Robert

Foreword

Once again, I have the honor to prepare the foreword for the monumental text *Borderlands of Normal and Early Pathological Findings in Skeletal Radiography*, edited by Drs. Juergen Freyschmidt, Joachim Brossmann, Juergen Wiens, and Andreas Sternberg. This latest edition is true to the tradition of excellence that was readily apparent in the previous version. It again emphasizes the interface between what should be considered normal and what is pathologic, an interface that is encountered every day on multiple occasions by any physician who is involved in the interpretation or review of imaging studies, whether they appear on the viewbox or, with increasing frequency, on the computer screen.

As would be expected, much has transpired since the publication of the last edition of this work. Old concepts have been clarified, have changed considerably, or have even been discarded, and new concepts have emerged. Dr. Freyschmidt and colleagues have addressed these modified or new ideas through the use of important alterations in the text and a dramatic increase in the number of illustrations, all well chosen to display the findings in as vivid a fashion as possible. A new emphasis on advanced imaging methods, such as computed tomography and magnetic resonance imaging, is apparent throughout and certainly justified, but the importance of conventional radiographic analysis remains central. The organization of the book has also been updated, with new reliance on the assessment of five basic pathologic processes: dysplasia, trauma, necrosis, inflammation, and tumor.

Why purchase and read this book? Simply, because the knowledge that one would gain by doing so would clearly lead to a marked improvement in accurate assessment of skeletal images. More specifically, one's ability to differentiate between clinically significant and insignificant findings would improve dramatically, resulting in more appropriate patient care. Yes, there are other available books on this subject, and some are quite good. *Borderlands* is unique and my favorite, however, because of its organization, completeness, and focus. The previous edition was situated in a prominent place in my office—I referred to it often (some of its pages are now folded or torn) as did our residents and fellows. This new addition will sit alongside it and I expect its fate will be the same. In short, this is not a book to be placed on the shelf and forgotten but one to use on a regular basis.

Dr. Freyschmidt and colleagues are to be congratulated for once again providing the rest of us with an invaluable reference source. To complete such a work is no easy task, and the authors have my deep admiration. It is a privilege for me to provide this foreword, and I congratulate the editors on a job well done.

Donald Resnick, M.D.
Chief, Osteoradiology
Professor of Radiology
University of California, San Diego

Preface

With the increasing use of cross-sectional imaging modalities in skeletal radiology, our knowledge of the true anatomic relationships of many normal variants and borderline findings has grown considerably. Meanwhile, concepts regarding the clinical importance of some variants and borderline findings have changed, especially in sports-related conditions.

Faced with these facts, we felt that a new approach was needed in organizing our material.

This fifth edition of *Borderlands* is based on a new didactic approach, which is intended to give the book an unprecedented logical consistency throughout. The material is organized according to the basic diagnostic questions that are raised by the primary clinical findings, the primary radiographic findings, or both. As in other organ systems, key diagnostic issues are based on several broad pathologic categories:

- Anomaly
- Trauma
- Necrosis
- Inflammation
- Tumor

When faced with a skeletal finding that may be a normal variant or one of the basic types of pathology listed above, the reader can turn to a specific portion of the book to decide whether the finding is normal or definitely pathologic.

Borderline findings are difficult to collect for publication, either because they were missed or because the first radiographic examination was performed too late. Also, borderline findings can be difficult to portray in an illustration, as it is not possible to bring out certain relevant details by changing the viewing conditions (e.g. by using an iris diaphragm with a halogen source for reading a plain film or by adjusting the computer screen). For these reasons, the book also deals with pathological conditions in their fully established forms. By knowing the fully developed presentation, the radiologist can easily picture earlier forms that occupy the "borderland" range.

We have maintained the tradition of including some rare entities among the illustrations. This has been done to uphold the reputation of the book as an "all-in-one" reference source.

We suggest that the reader study Chapter 1, as it covers methods and stratagems for separating the wheat from the chaff, i.e., differentiating normal and still normal findings (variants) from findings that are definitely pathological.

Bremen, Kiel
Autumn, 2002

J. Freyschmidt
J. Brossmann
J. Wiens
A. Sternberg

Contents

1 Introduction to the Radiological Evaluation of Normal Variants   1

J. Freyschmidt

References   5

Appendix   6

2 Upper Extremity   15

J. Freyschmidt

The Hand   16

Metacarpus and Phalanges   16
General Aspects   16
  Normal Findings   16
  Pathological Finding?   22
    Normal Variant or Anomaly?   22
    Fracture?   52
    Necrosis?   52
    Inflammation?   57
    Tumor?   63
    Degenerative Changes?   69
    Soft-Tissue Calcifications   71
Specific Bones of the Hand   76
Distal Phalanges   76
  Normal Findings   76
  Pathological Finding?   77
    Normal Variant or Anomaly?   77
    Fracture? Dislocation?   78
    Necrosis?   80
    Inflammation?   83
    Tumor?   84
Middle Phalanges   85
  Normal Findings   85
  Pathological Finding?   85
    Normal Variant or Anomaly?   85
    Fracture?   87
    Necrosis?   87
    Inflammation, Tumor?   88
    Other Changes?   88
Proximal Phalanges   89
  Normal Findings   89
  Pathological Finding?   89
    Normal Variant or Anomaly?   89
    Fracture?   90
    Inflammation?   90
    Tumor?   91

Thumb   91
  Normal Findings   91
  Pathological Finding?   91
    Normal Variant or Anomaly?   91
    Fracture?   93
    Necrosis?   93
    Inflammation?   93
    Other Changes?   94
Metacarpus   94
  Normal Findings   94
  Pathological Finding?   96
    Normal Variant or Anomaly?   96
    Fracture?   97
    Necrosis?   98
    Inflammation? 100
    Tumor? 100
References 102

Carpus (wrist) 104
General Aspects 104
  Normal Findings 104
  Pathological Finding? 117
    Normal Variant or Anomaly? 117
    Fracture, Subluxation, or Dislocation? 125
    Necrosis? 130
    Inflammation? 130
    Tumor? 131
Specific Bones of the Carpus 132
Trapezium 132
  Normal Findings 132
    Normal Variant or Anomaly? 132
    Fracture or Dislocation? 132
    Necrosis? 136
    Tumor? 137

Trapezoid 137
   Normal Findings 137
   Pathological Finding? 137
     Normal Variant or Anomaly? 137
     Fracture or Dislocation? 138
Capitate 140
   Normal Findings 140
   Pathological Finding? 140
     Normal Variant or Anomaly? 140
     Fracture or Dislocation? 141
     Necrosis? 141
Hamate 144
   Normal Findings 144
   Pathological Finding? 144
     Normal Variant or Anomaly? 144
     Fracture or Dislocation? 144
     Necrosis? 148
     Inflammation? Tumor? 148
Scaphoid 148
   Normal Findings 148
   Pathological Finding? 150
     Normal Variant or Anomaly? 150
     Fracture or Dislocation? 152
     Necrosis? 159

Inflammation? 162
   Tumor? 162
Lunate 164
   Normal Findings 164
   Pathological Finding? 165
     Normal Variant or Anomaly? 165
     Fracture or Dislocation? 167
     Necrosis? 169
     Inflammation? 173
     Tumor? 173
Triquetrum 174
   Normal Findings 174
   Pathological Finding? 174
     Normal Variant or Anomaly? 174
     Fracture or Dislocation? 174
     Necrosis? 180
Pisiform 180
   Normal Findings 180
   Pathological Finding? 180
     Normal Variant or Anomaly? 180
     Fracture or Dislocation? 182
     Necrosis? 183
     Inflammation? 183
References 184

Forearm   **186**

Distal Radius and Ulna 186
   Normal Findings 186
   Pathological Finding? 189
     Normal Variant or Anomaly? 189
     Fracture, Subluxation, or Dislocation? 194
     Necrosis? 197
     Inflammation? 198
     Tumor? 198
     Other Changes? 200
References 201

Diaphysis of the Forearm 202
   Normal Findings 202
   Pathological Finding? 204
     Normal Variant or Anomaly? 204
     Fracture, Subluxation, or Dislocation? 205
     Necrosis? 206
     Inflammation? 206
     Tumor? 208
References 209

Elbow Region   **210**

   Normal Findings 210
   Pathological Finding? 218
     Normal Variant or Anomaly? 218
     Fracture, Subluxation, or Dislocation? 227
     Necrosis? 229

     Tumor? 232
     Inflammation? 234
     Soft-Tissue Calcifications and Ossifications,
     Changes at the Fibro-osseous Junction 234
References 236

Upper Arm   **238**

Diaphysis 238
   Normal Findings 238
   Pathological Finding? 242
     Fracture 242
     Inflammation, Tumor? 242
     Soft-Tissue Calcifications 242
References 244

Proximal Humerus 245
   Normal Findings 245
   Pathological Finding? 253
     Normal Variant or Anomaly? 253
     Fracture, Subluxation, or Dislocation? 254
     Necrosis? 256
     Tumor? 258
     Inflammation? 259
References 260

3 Shoulder Girdle and Thorax   261

J. Freyschmidt

Scapula   262

Normal Findings 262
Pathological Finding? 271
   Normal Variant or Anomaly? 271
   Fracture, Subluxation, or Dislocation? 276

Necrosis? 281
Inflammation? 281
Tumor? 282
References 285

Acromioclavicular Joint   287

Normal Findings 287
Pathological Finding? 287
   Normal Variant or Anomaly? 287
   Fracture, Subluxation, or Dislocation? 288
   Necrosis? 289

Inflammation? 290
Tumor? 290
Other Changes? 290
References 291

The Shoulder Joint as a Whole   292

Soft-Tissue Anatomy of the Shoulder Joint 292
Shoulder Impingement and Rotator Cuff Tears 296
Shoulder Dislocation and Shoulder Instability 297

*Calcifications and Ossifications in the Soft Tissues of
the Shoulder* 299
References 304

Clavicle and Sternoclavicular Joint   305

Normal Findings 305
Pathological Finding? 309
   Normal Variant or Anomaly? 309
   Fracture, Subluxation, or Dislocation? 310
   Necrosis? 311

Inflammation? 312
Tumor? 317
Other Changes? 318
References 318

Sternum   320

Normal Findings 320
Pathological Finding? 326
   Normal Variant or Anomaly? 326
   Fracture, Subluxation, or Dislocation? 334
   Necrosis? 334

Inflammation? 335
Tumor? 337
Other Changes? 338
References 339

Ribs   340

Normal Findings 340
Pathological Finding? 342
   Normal Variant or Anomaly? 342
   Fracture, Subluxation, or Dislocation? 348
   Necrosis? 350

Inflammation? 350
Tumor? 350
Other Changes? 354
References 355

4 Skull   357

J. Wiens, A. Sternberg

General Aspects 358
References 366

Cranial Vault   367

Normal Findings 367
Pathological Finding? 375
  Normal Variant/Anomaly? 375
  Fracture? 392
  Necrosis? 397
  Inflammation? 397
  Tumor? 398

Special Aspects 405
  Frontal Bone 405
  Parietal Bone 407
  Squamous Temporal Bone 411
  Occipital Bone 414
References 419

Skull Base   421

Anterior, Middle, and Posterior Cranial Fossae 421
  Normal Findings 421
  Pathological Finding? 428
    Normal Variant/Anomaly? 428
    Fracture? 440
    Necrosis? 441
    Inflammation? 441
    Tumor? 442
Sella Turcica 445
  Normal Findings 446
  Pathological Finding? 449
    Normal Variant/Anomaly? 449
    Fracture? 453
    Tumor? 454
Temporal Bone 457
Middle Ear, Air Cells, and External Auditory Canal . 464
  Normal Findings 464
  Pathological Finding? 466
    Normal Variant/Anomaly? 466
    Fracture? 469

Necrosis? 470
Inflammation? 471
Tumor? 475
Petrous Temporal Bone and Inner Ear 477
  Normal Findings 478
  Pathological Finding? 482
    Normal Variant/Anomaly? 482
    Fracture? 486
    Necrosis? 486
    Inflammation? 486
    Tumor? 488
Styloid Process, Hyoid Bone, Larynx 490
  Normal Findings 490
  Pathological Finding? 495
    Normal Variant/Anomaly? 495
    Fracture? 497
    Necrosis? 497
    Inflammation? 497
    Tumor? 498
    Other Changes? 498
References 499

Facial Skeleton   502

Orbit 502
  Normal Findings 502
  Pathological Finding? 506
    Normal Variant/Anomaly? 506
    Fracture? 508
    Inflammation? 509
    Tumor? 510
    Other Changes? 510
Nose: Nasal Bone, Cartilaginous Nasal Skeleton, and
Nasal Cavity 511
  Normal Findings 511
  Pathological Finding? 512
    Normal Variant/Anomaly? 512
    Fracture? 514
    Necrosis? 514
    Inflammation? 514
    Tumor? 516
    Other Changes? 517
Paranasal Sinuses 517
  During Growth 517
Maxillary Sinus 519
  Normal Findings 519
  Pathological Finding? 523

Normal Variant/Anomaly? 523
Fracture? 524
Inflammation? 525
Tumor? 527
Frontal Sinus 528
  Normal Findings 528
  Pathological Finding? 528
    Normal Variant/Anomaly? 528
    Fracture? 530
    Inflammation? 530
    Tumor? 531
Ethmoid Cells 531
  Normal Findings 531
  Pathological Finding? 533
    Normal Variant/Anomaly? 533
    Fracture? 533
    Inflammation? 533
    Tumor? 534
Sphenoid Sinus 534
  Normal Findings 534
  Pathological Finding? 535
    Normal Variant/Anomaly? 535
    Fracture? 537

Inflammation? 537
Tumor? 538
Zygomatic Arch 538
Normal Findings 538
Pathological Finding? 538
Normal Variant/Anomaly? 538
Fracture? 538
Inflammation? 539
Tumor? 539
Mandible 539
Normal Findings 539
Pathological Finding? 541
Normal Variant/Anomaly? 541
Fracture? 543

Necrosis? 544
Inflammation? 544
Tumor? 545
Other Changes? 547
Temporomandibular Joint 548
Normal Findings 548
Pathological Finding? 549
Normal Variant/Anomaly? 549
Fracture, Subluxation, or Dislocation? 550
Necrosis? 551
Inflammation? 551
Tumor? 551
Other Changes? 552
References 552

5 Spinal Column   557

J. Brossmann

Introduction 558

Atlas and Axis   564

Normal Findings 564
Pathological Finding? 575
Normal Variant or Anomaly? 575
Fracture, Subluxation, or Dislocation? 592
Necrosis? 598

Inflammation? 598
Tumor? 600
Other Changes? 601
References 604

Midcervical and Lower Cervical Spine   608

Normal Findings 608
Pathological Finding? 615
Normal Variant or Anomaly? 615
Fracture, Subluxation, or Dislocation? 624
Necrosis? 628

Inflammation? 628
Tumor? 632
Other Changes? 634
References 641

Thoracic Spine   645

Normal Findings 645
Pathological Finding? 653
Normal Variant or Anomaly? 653
Fracture, Subluxation, or Dislocation? 658
Necrosis? 662

Inflammation? 662
Tumor? 663
Other Changes? 663
References 669

Lumbar Spine   671

Normal Findings 671
Pathological Finding? 677
Normal Variant or Anomaly? 677
Fracture, Subluxation, or Dislocation? 699
Necrosis? 700

Inflammation? 700
Tumor? 706
Other Changes? 713
References 726

Sacrum and Coccyx   731

Normal Findings 731
Pathological Finding? 736
Normal Variant or Anomaly? 736
Fracture, Subluxation, or Dislocation? 741
Necrosis? 743

Inflammation? 743
Tumor? 743
Other Changes? 745
References 747

Sacroiliac Joints 749

Normal Findings 749
Pathological Finding? 750
Normal Variant or Anomaly? 750
Fracture, Subluxation, or Dislocation? 751

Necrosis? 752
Inflammation? 752
Other Changes? 758
References 760

6 Pelvis 763

J. Freyschmidt

General Aspects 764
Normal Anatomy 764
Examination Technique 764
Trauma 767
Osteonecrosis of the Acetabulum, Femoral
Head, and Femoral Neck 768
Ossification and Calcification of Soft-Tissue
Structures 768
Anomalies and Deformities 773
Structural Changes 773
References 777
Pelvis, Specific Section 778
Ilium 778
Normal Findings 778
Pathological Finding? 780
Normal Variant or Anomaly? 780
Fracture? 781
Necrosis? 785
Inflammation? 785
Tumor? 787
Other Changes? 787
References 789

Pubis, Pubic Symphysis, and Ischium 789
Normal Findings 789
Pathological Finding? 791
Normal Variant or Anomaly? 791
Fracture, Subluxation, or Dislocation? 796
Necrosis? 798
Inflammation? 799
Tumor? 801
Other Changes? 801
References 803
Hip Joint 804
Normal Findings 804
Pathological Finding? 821
Normal Variant or Anomaly? 821
Fracture, Subluxation, or Dislocation? 829
Necrosis? 836
Inflammation? 843
Tumor? 845
Other Changes? 849
References 856

7 Lower Extremity 859

J. Freyschmidt

Femur 860

Femoral Shaft 860

Normal Findings 860
Pathological Finding? 860
Normal Variant or Anomaly? 860
Fracture, Subluxation, or Dislocation? 868
Necrosis? 868
Inflammation? Tumor? 868
Other Changes? 871
References 875

Distal Femur 875

Normal Findings 875
Pathological Finding? 879
Normal Variant or Anomaly? 879
Fracture? 880
Necrosis? 880
Inflammation? 887
Tumor? 888
Other Changes? 895
References 899

Patella 900

Normal Findings 900
Pathological Finding? 904
Normal Variant or Anomaly? 904
Fracture, Subluxation, or Dislocation? 908

Necrosis? 910
Inflammation? Tumor? 911
Other Changes? 912
References 913

Proximal Tibia and Fibula   **914**

Normal Findings 914
Pathological Finding? 921
   Normal Variant or Anomaly? 921
   Fracture, Subluxation, or Dislocation? 924

Necrosis? 927
Inflammation? Tumor? 929
Other Changes? 935
References 936

Knee Joint as a Whole   **937**

Normal Findings, Variants, Early Pathological
Changes 937
Pathological Findings? 945

Other Changes? 950
References 952

Shaft of the Tibia and Fibula   **953**

Normal Findings 953
Pathological Finding? 958
   Normal Variant or Anomaly? 958
   Fracture? 961

Necrosis? 965
Inflammation? 965
Tumor? 965
References 970

Distal Tibia and Fibula   **971**

Normal Findings 971
Pathological Finding? 975
   Normal Variant or Anomaly? 975
   Fracture, Subluxation, or Dislocation? 980

Inflammation? 986
Tumor? 986
Other Changes? 986
References 988

Foot   **989**

General Aspects 989
Normal Findings 989
Pathological Finding? 993
   Variants? 993
   Anomalies? 997
   Soft-Tissue Variants 1001
References 1001
Specific Bones of the Foot 1002
Normal Findings 1002
Pathological Finding? 1005
   Normal Variant or Anomaly? 1005
   Fracture, Subluxation, or Dislocation? 1013
   Necrosis? 1015
   Inflammation? Tumor? 1018
References 1019
Calcaneus 1020
Normal Findings 1020
Pathological Finding? 1025
   Normal Variant or Anomaly? 1025
   Fracture, Subluxation, or Dislocation? 1033
   Necrosis? 1034
   Inflammation? 1035
   Tumor? 1035
   Other Changes? 1036
References 1040
Navicular Bone 1040
Normal Findings 1040
Pathological Finding? 1044
   Normal Variant or Anomaly? 1044
   Fracture, Subluxation, or Dislocation? 1051
   Necrosis? 1051
   Inflammation? Tumor? 1053
   Other Changes? 1054
References 1054
Cuboid Bone 1055

Normal Findings 1055
Pathological Finding? 1055
   Normal Variant or Anomaly? 1055
   Fracture, Subluxation, or Dislocation? 1057
   Necrosis? 1057
   Inflammation? Tumor? 1058
References 1059
Medial Cuneiform Bone 1060
Normal Findings 1060
Pathological Finding? 1062
   Normal Variant or Anomaly? 1062
   Fracture, Subluxation, or Dislocation? 1065
   Necrosis? 1065
   Other Changes? 1065
References 1065
Intermediate and Lateral Cuneiform Bones 1066
Normal Findings 1066
Pathological Finding? 1066
   Normal Variant or Anomaly? 1066
   Fracture, Subluxation, or Dislocation? 1067
   Necrosis? 1067
References 1068
Metatarsal Bones 1069
Normal Findings 1069
Pathological Finding? 1071
   Normal Variant or Anomaly? 1071
   Fracture, Subluxation, or Dislocation? 1074
   Necrosis? 1079
   Inflammation? 1082
   Tumor? 1084
   Other Changes? 1084
References 1086
Sesamoid Bones 1087
Normal Findings 1087
Pathological Finding? 1088

Variant or Anomaly/Deformity? 1088
Fracture, Subluxation, or Dislocation? 1089
Necrosis? 1090
Inflammation? 1091
Other Changes? 1091
References 1093

Toes 1094
Normal Findings 1094
Pathological Finding? 1096
Normal Variant or Anomaly? 1096
Fracture, Subluxation, or Dislocation? 1101
Necrosis? 1101
Inflammation? Tumor? 1102
References 1104

Index **1105**

1 Introduction to the Radiological Evaluation of Normal Variants

J. Freyschmidt

The differentiation of a normal anatomic variant from a skeletal abnormality based on empirical visual assessment is not the real problem in the diagnostic radiology of borderline findings between normal and early pathology.

 This problem arises only when a patient's clinical symptoms may have something to do with the radiological variant, or when the variant itself may harbor pathological changes (e.g., necrosis), or when a pathological process mimics a normal anatomic variant (Table 1.**1**).

The problems in this situation cannot be solved by visual assessment alone. The solution, rather, lies in the true art of medicine, which includes the interpretation of pain and neurological symptoms and the selection of further diagnostic procedures (such as radionuclide scanning or MRI). It may also include recommending an appropriate treatment.

We know from experience that routine radiographic examinations in hospital and office settings most often demonstrate normal findings along with more or less harmless normal variants. Unless the radiologist is familiar with this type of finding, there are likely to be numerous false-positive studies leading to unnecessary additional (and costly) diagnostic and therapeutic measures.

At the same time, the prevalence of normal findings and harmless normal variants in routine practice can engender a kind of complacency that makes it hard for radiologists to recognize a symptomatic normal variant or even a definite abnormality that is mimicking a normal variant.

In any given case, therefore, the following question should be added to the standard checklist or algorithm for radiographic interpretation: Is it possible that the normal variant is clinically significant, or is a supposed normal variant actually a pathological process?

How Can These Pitfalls Be Avoided?

The basic approach to radiological interpretation follows the principles of pattern recognition.

The basic criteria for image interpretation in **conventional radiography** and **computed tomography** (CT) are as follows:

- Shape
- Size
- Position relative to surrounding structures (topography)
- Symmetry
- Density

In a **radionuclide bone scan**, the regional degree of tracer uptake is evaluated in addition to the basic interpretive elements of shape, size, topography, and symmetry.

 Most of the skeletal disorders discussed are associated with an increase in radiotracer uptake.

An increase in uptake means only that bone turnover or metabolism in a given area is increased or that the radiotracer has a greater affinity for the pathological process than for surrounding tissues. The cause of the increased uptake may be a traumatic, neoplastic, necrotic, or inflam-

matory process. Nevertheless, a radiologist with some experience in osteology and the recognition of radionuclide patterns can often establish the identity of a lesion.

 A whole-body scintigram should always be obtained, if necessary using SPECT (single-photon emission computed tomography) and a pinhole collimator.

In **magnetic resonance imaging** (MRI), the *signal intensity* in various sequences replaces density as a basic criterion for image interpretation.

In **projection radiography** (plain film or digital), which still accounts for more than 80% of all radiological studies, projection geometry and the superimposition effect are additional key elements in interpreting radiographic films.

Projection geometry influences shape, size, and topography, while the superimposition effect mainly influences density. Superimposition refers not only to the superimposed projection of several bones or bony elements but also to the summation of internal or substructures contained within a single bone. Thus, while a bony ridge produces a linear density in an orthograde projection, a bony groove or canal appears as a linear lucency. Plain radiographs of a cancellous bone area are never identical, because the slightest rotation of the bone relative to the film plane (even by 1° or 2°) will significantly alter the projection of the individual bony trabeculae and may cause them to appear thickened. If two bony elements of different density are superimposed, an effect called the **Mach band phenomenon** occurs, creating a line of apparent radiolucency that is comparable to an optical illusion. In zones of contrasting radiographic densities, areas of higher density are perceived as being darker while areas of lower density appear lighter.

The various changes of the individual elements of pattern recognition and their combination ultimately determine how a particular skeletal abnormality will be classified. The basic categories of skeletal abnormality that are encountered in radiological practice are listed below:

- Anomaly (malformation, deformity)
- Fracture, subluxation, or dislocation
- Necrosis
- Inflammation
- Tumor

Of course, changes in pattern recognition criteria do not create a pathological entity—the reverse is true. Nevertheless, the process of radiological interpretation always follows this "reverse path." So whenever a radiograph shows what appears to be a variant, it is important to ask whether the questionable feature might possibly be a component or manifestation of a fracture, necrosis, inflammation, etc.

The following cases will help to illustrate these points.

- An **isolated bony element at the end of the acromion** (Fig. 3.**34**) raises various diagnostic possibilities. It may be an acute or old nonunited fracture or a persistent apophysis with no clinical significance, or its shape and position may be such that it predisposes to rotator cuff impingement. In making this differentiation, it is important to consider the history and clinical findings. An isolated bony element found distal to the acromion after shoulder trauma should be interpreted as a fresh fracture if the patient reports isolated tenderness over the site, perhaps accompanied by crepitation. But if

Table 1.**1**   Some important "normal variants" that may become symptomatic (after J. P. Lawson, ISS Refresher Course, Dublin 1998; see also References at the end of the chapter)

	Name and location	Possible pathogenesis	Clinical manifestations	Further tests and treatment
A Variants based on chronic stress-induced chondro-osseous disruption	• Bipartite patella (~. 1–2% of all patients), superolateral pole of patella	Chronic, stress-induced structural changes in the cartilaginous attachment	Pain, swelling	Bone scan or MRI/CT → surgery (resection)
	• Dorsal defect of the patella (~ 1% of all patients), superolateral joint contour	Patellar subluxation with chronic traction stress at the insertion of the vastus lateralis muscle	Pain	Bone scan or MRI → surgery (patellar stabilization)
	• Os subfibulare Ossicle below tip of lateral malleolus between malleolus and talus	Chronic avulsion fracture of anterior talofibular ligament due to ankle instability	Pain, ankle instability	Bone scan → surgery (reattachment)
B Variants that predispose to traumatic or degenerative changes in a congenital synchondrosis	• Type II accessory navicular bone[1], triangular or heart-shaped ossicle located 1–2 mm from the navicular; is an accessory ossification center for the navicular	Chronic trauma to the synchondrosis between accessory and navicular	Pain, swelling on medial aspect of foot	Bone scan → surgery (resection)
	• Os trigonum on the posterior aspect of the talus (in 14–25% of patients)	Chronic stress from forced plantar flexion, especially in soccer players and ballet dancers	Pain, swelling	Bone scan or MRI → surgery (resection)
C Variants that predispose to premature local degenerative changes	• Os styloideum between capitate, trapezoid, and bases of second and third metacarpals (found in 1–3% of all normal wrists)	Early osteoarthritic changes in third carpometacarpal joint due to unphysiological motion	Carpal bossing with pain and swelling on dorsal side of wrist	Bone scan, CT → surgery (resection) Ultrasound or MRI
	• Acromial variants including os acromiale	Impingement of supraspinatus outlet	Rotator cuff tear and/ or tendinitis	→ surgery Bone scan, CT
	• Os intermetatarseum between bases of first and second metatarsals (1.25% of all foot radiographs); may be incorporated into first or second metatarsal or into cuneiform in form of exostosis-like process	Can lead to degenerative changes due to varus deformity of first metatarsal and hallux valgus	Pain, swelling, metacarpophalangeal joint	→ surgery (resection)

[1] Type I (os tibiale externum, naviculare secundarium) is round or oval, 2–3 mm in diameter, completely separate from the navicular and represents a sesamoid in the posterior tibial tendon. Generally it is not symptomatic.

these circumscribed signs are absent, it should be assumed that the feature is an incidental finding based on an anatomic variant. If radiographs were ordered for unexplained shoulder pain not related to trauma, the radiologist should decide whether the shape and position of the accessory bony element are sufficient to narrow the subacromial space and cause an impingement injury with a partial or full tear of the supraspinatus tendon in the case of hyperextension. This question is most easily resolved by ultrasonography or MRI, depending on availability and examiner experience.

• A 50-year-old woman complains of **pain in the metatarsophalangeal joint of the right big toe** after prolonged walking. She gives no history of trauma. A radiograph shows a **relatively dense "bipartite" lateral sesamoid** and mild hallux valgus deformity of the toe. *Question*: Is the lateral sesamoid a normal anatomic variant (duplication), does the bone exhibit necrotic fragmentation, or is the pain caused by metatarsophalangeal osteoarthritis that is not yet visible on radiographs? Clinical examination is not helpful in this case because both extreme flexion and hyperextension elicit pain throughout the metatarsophalangeal joint, and the pain is very poorly localized on palpation of the plantar side. Further evaluation by radionuclide bone scan is indicated (Fig. 7.**440**). Increased uptake in the lateral "bipartite" sesamoid would indicate necrotic fragmentation, necessitating surgical removal. Increased uptake in the subchondral portion of the bone would be more suggestive of osteoarthritis.

- A 5-year-old child presents with **nonspecific pain in the right knee**. Radiographs show rarefaction and irregularity of the distal medial metaphyseal cortex. *Differential diagnosis*: inflammation, malignant tumor, or cortical irregularity?

The region is completely normal to palpation and ultrasound scanning. The opposite knee has the same radiographic appearance. The finding can now be confidently interpreted as a transient cortical irregularity (normal variant), and there is no need for follow-ups (Fig. 7.**45**). It should be added, however, that highly typical radiographic findings in a bone do not always require a "confirmatory" view of the opposite side. Also, the absence of a corresponding finding on the opposite side does not preclude a normal variant, since many such variants occur on one side only. But if the area is tender to pressure and also shows slight swelling, the case warrants further investigation by bone scanning or modern sectional imaging techniques.

Rules for Correctly Identifying Variants

➤ Accessory bone element:

An accessory bone element arises from an isolated ossification center that is independent of the adjacent "established" bone, or it may result from a failure of fusion of a second ossification center at the margin of the established bone. In the last case generally a synchondrosis persists between the accessory element and the established bone. Painful regressive changes may develop in a synchondrosis that is exposed to adverse mechanical stresses (Table 1.**1**). The accessory bone element is entirely surrounded by cortical bone and does not "complete" the other bone (Figs. 2.**205** and 2.**151 b**). The **main differential diagnosis** is a **detached bone fragment**, which is generally distinguished by irregular fracture margins and by the absence of a cortical boundary in acute cases. This is not the case in nonunions (Fig. 2.**129 d**). Displaced fragments geometrically "complete" the adjacent bone from which they were fractured. Theoretically they could be fitted back into the defect in the parent bone, just as a surgeon does when performing an internal fixation. When a posttraumatic radiograph is obtained in an acute situation, clinical palpation and a knowledge of the possible fracture mechanism are helpful if the diagnosis is in question. When a patient is examined weeks or months later for purposes of disability assessment, the examiner should not only consider the morphological criteria listed above but also decide whether the accessory bone element seen in the radiograph corresponds to one of the known accessory bones that have been named and described. This problem is discussed more fully elsewhere in the text (p. 117 ff.).

With regard to the **naming of accessory bones**, most of these bones have been given Latin names based on their first describer or their anatomic location. Given the wealth of detailed knowledge that today's medical practitioners must have, we do not feel it is necessary to know the names of every accessory bone that may be encountered.

 It is not the name of an accessory bone that is important, but its correct identification as such.

Instead of using the term "os subfibulare," for example, it is quite acceptable to write: "accessory bone element located below the tip of the fibula."

The next entity requiring differentiation from an accessory bone element is a **fragmented osteonecrosis**. Generally the necrotic bone is denser than normal bone and lacks internal structural features. The radionuclide bone scan (see above) is definitive in terms of differential diagnosis.

A final differential diagnosis is an **ossified tissue matrix**, as illustrated by circumscribed myositis ossificans (Fig. 2.**235**) or paraosseous cartilaginous formations. The late stage of myositis ossificans is indistinguishable from an accessory bone by its morphological features alone, because the lesion has an internal structure and a cortical boundary (Fig. 2.**235**), contrasting with the ill-defined ossification seen in earlier stages. Cartilaginous calcification patterns usually show some kind of lobulation, and geometric figures (e.g., rings, arcs, stars) that come from a superposition of ossified interlobular septa.

➤ An unusual or extraneous-appearing density within a bone:

The density may result from a different overlapping bone, due either to an atypical projection or atypical relative positions of the bones. It can also have other causes such as an exceptionally well-developed bony ridge (e.g., linea aspera), which usually appears as a linear density (Fig. 7.**3 a**). Finally, it may represent a pathological bony structure on or within the bone. The best solution to this problem is to obtain a contralateral film or, when dealing with an unpaired element such as a vertebral body, to compare the left and right halves on the same film. Spot films can also be obtained to resolve projection-related issues. CT may be necessary in selected cases.

➤ An unusual or extraneous-appearing lucency within a bone:

If the lucency is linear, differentiation is required between a fracture and a Mach band phenomenon. If the lucency is not linear, it may represent a circumscribed area of rarefied cancellous bone, thinned cortical bone, or a deep groove or cleft in the outer surface of the bone. A familiar example is the greater tuberosity of the humerus, which appears as an elliptical lucency (Fig. 2.**431**). This feature can vary markedly among different individuals and is due simply to a diminution of cancellous trabeculae combined with an increased proportion of fatty marrow. In questionable cases, especially when symptoms are vague, doubts can be resolved by examining the opposite side or proceeding with CT or MRI. As a rule, though, the reader should know the typical skeletal sites at which such lucencies typically occur. The same applies, of course, to normally occurring densities.

 Beginners in particular should avoid ordering costly tests just because they lack the knowledge to interpret these phenomena correctly.

It is equally important, especially in symptomatic patients, to avoid the temptation to classify radiographic densities as normal, even if they appear to blend harmoniously with surrounding features.

The following two phenomena should be familiar to anyone who interprets radiographs:

- **Gray cortex:** The "gray cortex" is a result of circumscribed resorptive changes in normal cortical bone caused by focal osteoclastic activity induced, say, by an inflammatory or neoplastic bone lesion (Figs. 7.**10**, 7.**14a**, 7.**20a**).
- **Loss of differentiation between the cortex and marrow cavity, especially in tubular bones:** This occurs when the radiographic density of the bone marrow is increased due to a pathological process (matrix ossification due to osteosarcoma, bone necrosis, deposition of calcium phosphate or calcium carbonate compounds, etc.). Normally the marrow or medullary cavity of a tubular bone contains fat. Replacement of the fat by nonmineralized tumor tissue is not detectable on conventional radiographs unless the tumor tissue causes circumscribed, lacuna-like resorptive changes (scalloping) in the endosteal cortical margin.

➤ **A bony structure appears too large or too small or has an unusual shape:**

This finding may represent a normal variant, bone dysplasia, or an aquired deformity. Again, it is helpful to obtain contralateral radiographs for comparison. If the same changes are seen, they may result from a systemic pathological process. "Gamut lists" (like those of Reeder and Felson) are very often helpful for identifying morphological variants, and several chapters in this book list differential diagnoses based on morphological criteria. Otherwise the history and clinical findings should be used to aid interpretation. A detailed description of congenital skeletal dysplasias, dysostoses, and acquired deformities is beyond our present scope but may be found in the specialized literature.

The **1992 International Classification of Osteochondrodysplasias** is presented without commentary at the end of this chapter (Appendix, Table 1.**2**). Published by J. Spranger (*European Journal of Pediatrics* 51 [1992] 407–415), this classification was compiled by an international panel of experts on bone dysplasias at a conference in Bad Honnef (26–28 June 1991). Unlike the older Parisian Nomenclature for the classification of constitutional skeletal diseases, the International Classification is based solely on radiological criteria, with diseases grouped on the basis of similar morphological features. It was the opinion of the expert panel that the former "mixing" of clinical, pathogenetic, and radiological criteria led to inconsistencies and was too imprecise. Clinical criteria, such as age at disease onset and course, are no longer used because they are too variable and depend too much on the diagnostic experience and therapeutic activities of the reader. Spranger notes that, despite major advances in the fields of biochemistry and molecular biology, our knowledge of etiology and pathogenesis is still too sketchy to attempt a causal type of classification. But the table does provide information on gene locations, protein defects, and modes of inheritance. The classification pertains exclusively to osteochondrodysplasias, i.e., developmental disturbances of chondro-osseous tissue. The new classification does not include dysostoses, which are defined as developmental disturbances of individual bones.

Spranger also points out that the work done to date is still rudimentary and that further revision is needed. This prompted us to include the unabridged 1986 version of the Parisian Nomenclature, which does include dysostoses (Appendix, Table 1.**3**).

References

Berg, E. E.: The symptomatic os subfibulare: avulsion fracture of the fibula associated with recurrent instability of the ankle. J Bone Jt Surg. 73-A (1991) 1251

Cuono, C. B., H. K. Watson: the carpal boss: surgical treatment and etiological considerations. Plast. reconstr. Surg. 63 (1979) 88

Henderson, R. S.: Os intermetatarseum and a possible relationship to hallux valgus. J Bone Jt Surg. 45-B (1963) 117

Johnson, R. P., B. D. Collier, G. F. Carrera: The os trigonum syndrome: use of bone scan in the diagnosis. J. Trauma 24 (1984) 761

Keats, T. E.: Atlas of Normal Roentgen Variants That May Simulate Disease, 6th ed. Mosby-Year Book, Chicago 1996

Lawson, J. P.: Clinically significant radiologic anatomic variants of the skeleton. Amer. J. Roentgenol. 163 (1994) 249

Lawson, J. P., J. A. Ogden, E. Sella et al.: The painful accessory navicular. Skelet. Radiol 12 (1984) 250

Ogden, J. A., S. M. McCarthy, P. Jokl: The painful bipartite patella. J. pediat. Orthop. 2 (1982) 263

Reeder, M. R.: Reeder and Felson's Gamut's in Bone, Joint and Spine Radiology. Springer, Berlin 1993

Spranger, J.: International classification of osteochondrodysplasias. Europ. J. Pediat. 151 (1992) 407

Van Holsbeeck, M., B. Vandamme, G. Marchal et al.: Dorsal defect of the patella: concepts of its origin and relationship with bipartite and multipartite patella. Skelet. Radiol. 16 (1987) 304

Appendix

Table 1.**2**   International Classification of Osteochondrodysplasias (from Spranger, I.: *European Journal of Pediatrics* **51** [1992] 407–415). See text p. 5 for more details

Osteochondrodysplasias	Inheri-tance	Chromosome	Gene	Protein	MIM
A. Defects of the tubular (and flat) bones and/or axial skeleton					
1. Achondroplasia group					
Thanatophoric dysplasia	AD				187.600
Thanatophoric dysplasia-straight femur/ cloverleaf skull type	AD				187.600
Achondroplasia	AD				100.800
Hypochondroplasia	AD				146.000
2. Achondrogenesis					
Type IA	AR				200.600
Type IB	AR				200.600
3. Spondylodysplastic group (Perinatally lethal)					
San Diego type	Sp				151.210
Torrance type	Sp				151.210
Luton type	Sp				151.210
4. Metatropic dysplasia group					
Fibrochondrogenesis	AR				228.520
Schneckenbecken dysplasia	AR				269.250
Metatropic dysplasia	AD				156.530
					250.600
5. Short rib dysplasia group (with/without polydactyly)					
SR(P) Type I Saldino Noonan	AR				263.530
SR(P) Type II Majewski	AR				263.520
SR(P) Type III Verma-Naumoff	AR				263.510
SR(P) Type IV Beemer-Langer	AR				269.860
Asphyxiating Thoracic Dysplasia	AR				208.500
Ellis-van Creveld Dysplasia	AR				225.500
6. Atelosteogenesis/Diastrophic dysplasia group					
Boomerang dysplasia	Sp				–
Atelosteogenesis type 1	Sp				108.720
Atelosteogenesis type 2 (de la Chapelle)	AR				256.050
Omodysplasia I (Maroteaux)	AD				–
Omodysplasia II (Borochowitz)	AR				–
Oto-palato-digital syndrome type 2	XLR				304.120
Diastrophic dysplasia	AR	5q31–q34			222.600
Pseudodiastrophic dysplasia	AR				264.180
7. Kniest-Stickler dysplasia group					
Dyssegmental dysplasia-Silverman Handmaker type	AR				224.410
Dyssegmental dysplasia-Rolland-Desbuquois type	AR				224.400
Kniest dysplasia	AD				156.550
Oto-spondylo-megaepiphyseal dysplasia	AR				215.150
Stickler dysplasia (heterogeneous, some not linked to Coll CoL2 A1)	AD	12q13.1–q13.3	CoL2A1	Type II Collagen	108.300

→

Osteochondrodysplasias	Inheritance	Chromosome	Gene	Protein	MIM
8. Spondyloepiphyseal dysplasia congenita group					
Langer-Saldino Dysplasia					200.610
(Achondrogenesis type II)	AD	12q13.1–q13.3	CoL2A1	Type II Collagen	120.140.02
Hypochondrogenesis	AD	12q13.1–q13.3	CoL2A1	Type II Collagen	120.140.02
Spondyloepiphyseal dysplasia congenita	AD	12q13.1–q13.3	CoL2A1	Type II Collagen	183.900
					120.140.01
9. Other spondylo epi-(meta)-physeal dysplasias					
X-linked Spondyloepiphyseal dysplasia tarda	XLD	Xp22	SEDL		313.400
Other late onset Spondyloepi-(meta)-physeal dysplasias (ie. Namaqualand d., Irapa D.)					
Progressive pseudorheumatoid dysplasia	AR				208.230
Dyggve-Melchior-Clausen dysplasia	AR				223.800
Wolcott-Rallison dysplasia	AR				226.980
Immunoosseous Dysplasia	AR				–
Pseudachondroplasia	AD				177.150
Opsismodysplasia	AR				258.480
10. Dysostosis multiplex group					
Mucopolysaccharidosis I-H	AR	4p16.3	IDA	α-Iduronidase	252.800
Mucopolysaccharidosis I-S	AR	4q16.3	IDA	α-Iduronidase	252.800
Mucopolysaccharidosis II	XLR	Xq27.3–q28	IDS	Iduronate-2-sulfatase	309.900
Mucopolysaccharidosis III-A	AR			Heparan sulfate sulfatase	
III-B	AR			N-Ac-α-D-glucosami-nidase	
III-C	AR			Ac-CoA : α-glucosamini-dase-N-acetyltrans-ferase	
III-D	AR	12q14	GNS	N-Ac-glucosamine-6-sulfate-sulfatase	252.940
Mucopolysaccharidosis IV-A	AR			Galactosamine-6-sulfatase	
Mucopolysaccharidosis IV-B	AR	3p21–p14.2	GLBI	β-Galactosidase	230.500
Mucopolysaccharidosis VI	AR	5q13.3	ARSB	Arylsulfatase B	253.200
Mucopolysaccharidosis VII	AR	7q21.11	GUSB	β-Glucoronidase	253.220
Fucosidosis	AR	1p34	FUCA	α-Fucosidase	230.000
α-Mannosidosis	AR	19p13.2–q12	MANB	α-Mannosidase	248.500
β-Mannosidosis	AR	4	MNB	β-Mannosidase	248.510
Aspartylglucosaminuria	AR	4q23–q27	AgA	Aspartylglucosami-nidase	208.400
g$_{M1}$ Gangliosidosis, several forms	AR	3p21–p14.2	GLB1	β-Galactosidase	230.500
Sialidosis, several forms	AR	6p21.3	NEU	α-Neuraminidase	256.550
Sialic storage disease	AR				269.920
Galactosialidosis, several forms	AR	20	NgBE	Neur/Gal expressive protein	256.540
Mucosulfatidosis	AR			Multiple sulfatases	272.200
Mucolipidosis II	AR			N-Ac-Gluc-Phospho-transferase	252.500
Mucolipidosis III	AR			N-Ac-Gluc-Phospho-transferase	252.600
Mucolipidosis IV	AR				252.650
11. Spondylometaphyseal dysplasias					
Spondylometaphyseal dysplasia-Kozlowski type	AD				271.660
Spondylometaphyseal dysplasia-corner fracture type (Sutcliffe)	AD				–
Spondyloenchondrodysplasia	AR				271.550
12. Epiphyseal dysplasias					
Multiple epiphyseal dysplasia Fairbanks/ Ribbing	AD				132.400

→

Osteochondrodysplasias	Inheritance	Chromosome	Gene	Protein	MIM
13. Chondrodysplasia punctata (Stippled epiphyses) group					
Rhizomelic type	AR			Peroxisome	215.100
Conradi-Hünermann type	XLD	Xq28	CPXD		302.950
X-linked recessive type	XLR	Xpter–p22.32	CPXR		302.940
MT-type	Sp				–
Others including CHILD syndrome; Zellweger syndrome; Warfarin embryopathy, Chromosomal abnormalities; Fetal alcohol syndrome					
14. Metaphyseal dysplasias					
Jansen type	AD				156.400
Schmid type	AD				156.500
Spahr type	AR				250.400
McKusick type (CHH)	AR				250.250
Metaphyseal Anadysplasia	XLR?				–
Shwachman type	AR				260.400
Adenosine deaminase deficiency	AR	20 q13.11	ADA		102.700
15. Brachyrachia (Short spine dysplasia)					
Brachyolmia, several types					113.500
					271.530
16. Mesomelic dysplasias					
Dyschondrosteosis	AD				127.300
Langer type	AR				249.700
Nievergelt type	AD				163.400
Robinow type	AD				180.700
17. Acro/acro-mesomelic dysplasias					
Acromicric dysplasia	Sp				102.370
Geleophysic dysplasia	AR				231.050
Acrodysostosis	AD				101.800
Tricho-rhino-phalangeal dysplasia type 1	AD	8q24.12	TQPS1		190.350
Tricho-rhino-phalangeal dysplasia type 2	AD	8q24.11–q24.13	TQPS2		150.230
Saldino-Mainzer dysplasia	AR				266.920
Pseudohypoparathyroidism several types	AD				103.580
	AR?				139.320
	XLD?				203.330
					300.800
Cranioectodermal dysplasia	AR				218.330
Acromesomelic dysplasia	AR				201.250
Grebe dysplasia	AR				200.700
18. Dysplasias with significant (but not exclusive) **membraneous bone involvement**					
Cleidocranial dysplasia	AD				119.600
Osteodysplasty, Melnick-Needles	XLD				309.350
19. Bent bone dysplasia group					
Campomelic dysplasia	AR		CMD1,		211.970
Kyphomelic dysplasia	AR		SOX9		211.350
Stüve-Wiedemann dysplasia	AR				–
20. Multiple dislocations with dysplasias					
Larsen syndrome	AD				150.250
Desbuquois syndrome	AR				215.200
Spondylo-epi-metaphyseal dysplasia with joint laxity	AR				271.640
21. Osteodysplastic primordial dwarfism group					
Type 1	AR				210.710
Type 2	AR				210.720

→

Osteochondrodysplasias	Inheritance	Chromosome	Gene	Protein	MIM
22. Dysplasias with decreased bone density					
Osteogenesis Imperfecta (several types)	AD	17q21.31–q22.05	CoL1A1	Collagen type I	120.150
	AD	7q21.3–22.1	CoL1A2	Collagen type I	120.160
					166.210–60
	AR				259.110
					259.420
Osteoporosis with Pseudoglioma	AR				259.770
Idiopathic Juvenile Osteoporosis	Sp				259.750
Bruck syndrome	AR				259.450
Homocystinuria	AR	21q22.3	CBS	Cystathionine-β-Synthase	236.200
Singleton-Merten-syndrome	Sp				182.250
Geroderma Osteodysplastica	AR				231.070
Menkes syndrome	XLR	Xq12–q13	MNK		309.400
23. Dysplasias with defective mineralization					
Hypophosphatasia	AD	1p36.1p34	ALPL	Alkaline phosphatase	146.300
					171.760
					241.500
					241.510
Hypophosphatemic Rickets	XR				370.800
Pseudodeficiency rickets, several types	AR				264.700
					277.420
					277.440
Neonatal hyperparathyroidism	AR				239.200
24. Dysplasias with increased bone density					
Osteopetrosis					
a) precocious type	AR				259.700
b) delayed type	AD				166.600
c) intermediate type	AR				259.710
d) with renal tubular acidosis	AR	8q22	CA2	Carbonic anhydrase II	259.730
Dysosteosclerosis	AR				224.300
Pycnodysostosis	AR				265.800
Osteosclerosis–Stanescu type	AD				122.900
Axial osteosclerosis including					
a) Osteomesopycnosis	AD				166.450
b) with Bamboo hair (Netherton Syndrome)	AR				256.500
c) Tricho-thiodystrophy	AR				242.170
Osteopoikilosis	AD				166.700
Melorheostosis	Sp				155.950
Osteopathia Striata	Sp				–
Osteopathia Striata with cranial sclerosis	AD				166.500
Diaphyseal dysplasia, Carmurati-Engelmann	AD				131.300
Craniodiaphyseal dysplasia	AD				122.860
	AR				218.300
Lenz-Majewski dysplasia	Sp				151.050
Craniometadiaphyseal dysplasia	Sp				–
Endosteal hyperostoses					
a) van Buchem disease	AR				239.100
b) Sclerosteosis	AR				269.500
c) Worth disease	AD				144.750
d) with cerebellar hypoplasia	AR				–
Pachydermoperiostosis	AD				167.100
Fronto-metaphyseal dysplasia	XLR				305.620
Craniometaphyseal dysplasia					
a) severe type	AR				218.400
b) mild type	AD				123.000
Pyle (disease) dysplasia	AR				265.900
Osteoectasia with hyperphosphatasia	AR				239.000
Oculo-dento-osseous dysplasia					
a) severe type	AR				257.850
b) mild type	AD				164.200
Familial infantile cortical hyperostosis-Caffey	AD				114.000

→

Osteochondrodysplasias	Inheri-tance	Chromosome	Gene	Protein	MIM
B. Disorganized development of cartilagenous and fibrous components of the skeleton					
Dysplasia epiphysealis hemimelica	Sp				127.800
Multiple cartilaginous exostoses	AD	8q23–q24.1			133.700
Echondromatosis (Ollier)	Sp				166.000
Echondromatosis with hemangiomata (Maffucci)	Sp				166.000
Metachondromatosis	AD				156.250
Osteoglophonic dysplasia	Sp				166.250
Fibrous dysplasia (Jaffe-Lichtenstein)	Sp				174.800
Fibrous dysplasia with pigmentary skin changes and precocious puberty (McCune-Albright)	Sp				174.800
Cherubism	AD				118.400
Myofibromatosis (Generalized fibromatosis)	AR				228.550
C. Idiopathic Osteolyses					
1. Predominantly phalangeal					
Hereditary acrosteolysis, several forms					102.400
Hajdu-Cheney type	AD				102.500
2. Predominantly carpal/tarsal					
Carpal-tarsal osteolysis with nephropathy	AD				166.300
Francois Syndrome (Dermo-chondro-corneal dystrophy)	AR				221.800
3. Multicentric					
Winchester Syndrome	AR				277.950
Torg type	AR				259.600
Mandibulo-acral dysplasia	AR				248.370
4. Other					
Familial Expansile Osteolysis	AD				174.810

AD   autosomal dominant
AR   autosomal recessive
MIM   Mendelian inheritance in man (Mc Kusick catalogue)
Sp   sporadic
XLD   X-linked dominant
XLR   X-linked recessive

Table 1.**3** Parisian Nomenclature of constitutional bone diseases (1986 revision)

I. Osteochondrodysplasias
(Growth and developmental disturbances of cartilage and/or bone)

1. Growth and developmental disturbances of tubular bones and/or the spinal column

(A) Manifested at birth

(a) Usually lethal before or shortly after birth	Inheritance
1. Type I achondrogenesis (Parenti–Fraccaro)	AR
2. Type II achondrogenesis (Langer–Saldino)	
3. Hypochondrogenesis	
4. Fibrochondrogenesis	AR
5. Thanatophoric dysplasia	
6. Thanatophoric dysplasia with cloverleaf skull	
7. Atelosteogenesis	
8. Short-rib syndromes (with or without polydactyly)	
(a) Type I (Saldino–Noonan)	AR
(b) Type II (Majewski)	AR
(c) Type III (lethal thoracic dysplasia)	AR

(b) Usually nonlethal dysplasias	
9. Chondrodysplasia punctata	
(a) Rhizomelic form, autosomal recessive	AR
(b) X-linked dominant form	XLD, lethal in males
(c) Common, mild form (Sheffield); exclude: symptomatic forms, chromosome abnormalities	
10. Camptomelic dysplasia	
11. Kyphomelic dysplasia	AR
12. Achondroplasia	AD
13. Diastrophic dysplasia	AR
14. Metatropic dysplasia (several forms)	AR, AD
15. Chondroectodermal dysplasia (Ellis–van Creveld)	AR
16. Asphyxiating thoracic dysplasia (Jeune)	
17. Spondyloepiphyseal dysplasia congenita	
(a) Autosomal dominant form	AD
(b) Autosomal recessive form	AR
18. Kniest dysplasia	AD
19. Dyssegmental dysplasia	AR
20. Mesomelic dysplasia	
(a) Nievergelt type	AD
(b) Langer type (probably homozygous dyschondrosteosis)	
(c) Robinow type	AD, AR
(d) Reinhardt type	AD
(e) Other	
21. Acromesomelic dysplasia	AR
22. Cleidocranial dysplasia	AD
23. Otopalatodigital syndrome	
(a) Type I (Langer)	XLD
(b) Type II (André)	XLR
24. Larsen syndrome	AR, AD
25. Other syndromes with multiple joint dislocations (Desbuquois, etc.)	

(B) Manifested in later life

1. Hypochondroplasia	AD
2. Dyschondrosteosis	AD
3. Metaphyseal chondrodysplasia, Jansen type	AD
4. Metaphyseal chondrodysplasia, Schmid type	AD
5. Metaphyseal chondrodysplasia, McKusick type	AR
6. Metaphyseal chondrodysplasia with exocrine pancreatic insufficiency and cyclic neutropenia	AR
7. Spondylometaphyseal dysplasia	
(a) Kozlowski type	AD
(b) Other forms	
8. Multiple epiphyseal dysplasia	
(a) Fairbank type	AD
(b) Other forms	
9. Multiple epiphyseal dysplasia with early diabetes (Wolcott–Rallison)	AR
10. Arthro-ophthalmopathy (Stickler)	AR
11. Pseudoachondroplasia	
(a) Dominant	AD
(b) Recessive	AR
12. Spondyloepiphyseal dysplasia, tarda (X-linked recessive)	XLR
13. Progressive pseudorheumatoid chondrodysplasia	AR
14. Spondyloepiphyseal dysplasia, other forms	
15. Brachyolmia	
(a) Autosomal recessive	AR
(b) Autosomal dominant	AD
16. Dyggve–Melchior–Clausen dysplasia	AR
17. Spondyloepimetaphyseal dysplasia (various forms)	
18. Spondyloepimetaphyseal dysplasia with loose joints	AR
19. Otospondylometaepiphyseal dysplasia (OSMED)	AR
20. Myotonic chondrodysplasia (Catel–Schwartz–Jampel)	AR
21. Parastremmatic dysplasia	AD
22. Trichorhinophalangeal dysplasia	AD
23. Acrodysplasia with retinitis pigmentosa and nephropathy (Saldino–Mainzer)	AR

2. Anarchic development of cartilage and fibrous tissue

1. Dysplasia epiphysealis hemimelica	
2. Multiple cartilaginous exostoses	AD
3. Acrodysplasia with exostoses (Giedion–Langer)	
4. Enchondromatosis (Ollier)	
5. Enchondromatosis with hemangiomas (Maffucci)	
6. Metachondromatosis	AD
7. Spondyloenchondroplasia	AR
8. Osteoglophonic dysplasia	
9. Fibrous dysplasia (Jaffe–Lichtenstein)	
10. Fibrous dysplasia with skin pigmentation and precocious puberty (McCune–Albright)	
11. Cherubism (familial fibrous dysplasia of the jaw)	AD

3.   Anomalies of bone density, cortical structure, and/ or metaphyseal modeling defects

1. Osteogenesis imperfecta (several forms)	AR, AD
2. Juvenile idiopathic osteoporosis	
3. Osteoporosis with pseudoglioma	AR
4. Osteopctrosis	
(a) Autosomal recessive lethal	AR
(b) Intermediate recessive	AR
(c) Autosomal dominant	AD
(d) Recessive with tubular acidosis	AR
5. Pyknodysostosis	AR
6. Dominant osteosclerosis, Stanescu type	AD
7. Osteomesopyknosis	AD
8. Osteopoikilosis	AD
9. Osteopathia striata	AD
10. Osteopathia striata with cranial sclerosis	AD
11. Melorheostosis	
12. Diaphyseal dysplasia (Camurati–Engelmann)	AD
13. Craniodiaphyseal dysplasia	AR
14. Endosteal hyperostosis	
(a) Autosomal dominant (Worth)	AD
(b) Autosomal recessive (van Buchem)	AR
(c) Autosomal recessive (sclerosteosis)	AR
15. Tubular stenosis (Kenny–Caffey)	AD
16. Pachydermoperiostosis	AD
17. Osteodysplasia (Melnick–Needles)	AD
18. Frontometaphyseal dysplasia	XLR
19. Craniometaphyseal dysplasia (several forms)	AD
20. Metaphyseal dysplasia (Pyle)	AR or AD
21. Dysosteosclerosis	AR or XLR
22. Osteoectasia with hyperphosphatasia	AR
23. Oculodento-osseous dysplasia	
(a) Mild type	AD
(b) Severe type	AR
24. Infantile cortical hyperostosis (Caffey disease, familial type)	AD

II. Dysostoses
(Malformations of individual bones, isolated or combined)

1.   Craniofacial dysostoses

1. Craniosynostosis (various forms)	
2. Craniofacial dysostosis (Crouzon)	
3. Acrocephalosyndactyly	
(a) Apert type	AD
(b) Chotzen type	AD
(c) Other types	AD
4. Acrocephalopolysyndactyly (Carpenter, etc.)	AR
5. Cephalopolysyndactyly (Greig)	AD
6. Syndromes of the first and second branchial arches	
(a) Mandibulofacial dysostosis (Treacher–Collins, Franceschetti)	AD
(b) Acrofacial dysostosis (Nager)	
(c) Oculoauriculovertebral dysostosis (Goldenhar)	AR
(d) Hemifacial microsomia	
(e) Other (probably parts of a broad spectrum)	
7. Oculomandibulofacial syndrome (Hallermann–Streiff–Francois)	

2.   Dysostoses with predominant involvement of the axial skeleton

1. Vertebral segmentation defects (including Klippel–Feil)	
2. Cervico-oculoacoustic syndrome (Wildervanck)	
3. Sprengel deformity	
4. Spondylocostal dysostosis	
(a) Dominant form	AD
(b) Recessive form	AR
5. Oculovertebral syndrome (Weyers)	
6. Osteo-onychodysostosis	AD
7. Cerebrocostomandibular syndrome	AR

3.   Dysostoses with predominant involvement of the extremities

1. Acheiria	
2. Apodia	
3. Tetraphocomelia (Roberts) (SC pseudothalidomide syndrome)	AR
4. Ectrodactyly	
(a) Isolated	
(b) Ectrodactyly, ectodermal dysplasia (cleft palate syndrome)	AD
(c) Ectrodactyly with scalp defects	
5. Oroacral syndrome (aglossia syndrome, Hanhart syndrome)	
6. Familial radioulnar synostosis	
7. Brachydactyly types A, B, C, D, E (Bell's classification)	AD
8. Symphalangia	AD
9. Polydactyly (several forms)	
10. Syndactyly (several forms)	
11. Polysyndactyly (several forms)	
12. Camptodactyly	
13. Manzke syndrome	
14. Poland syndrome	
15. Rubenstein–Taybi syndrome	
16. Coffin–Siris syndrome	
17. Pancytopenia-dysmelia syndrome (Fanconi)	AR
18. Blackfan–Diamond anemia with thumb malformations (Aase syndrome)	AR
19. Thrombocytopenia-radial aplasia syndrome	AR
20. Orodigitofacial syndrome	
(a) Papillon–Leage type	XLD, lethal in males
(b) Mohr type	AR
21. Cardiomelic syndrome (Holt–Oram and others)	AD
22. Femoral focal defect (with or without facial anomalies)	
23. Multiple synostoses (including several forms of symphalangia)	AD
24. Scapuloiliac dysostosis (Kosenow–Sinios)	AD
25. Hand-foot-genital syndrome	AD
26. Focal dermal hypoplasia (Goltz)	XLD, lethal in males

III. Idiopathic osteolyses

1. Phalangeal (several forms)
2. Tarsocarpal
   (a) Including Francois type and others   AR
   (b) With nephropathy   AD
3. Multicentric
   (a) Hajdu–Cheney type   AD
   (b) Winchester type   AR
   (c) Torg type   AR
   (d) Other types

IV. Miscellaneous diseases with osseous involvement

1. Acceleration of skeletal maturity in young children
   (a) Marshall–Smith syndrome
   (b) Weaver syndrome
   (c) Other types
2. Marfan syndrome   AD
3. Congenital arachnodactyly with contractures   AD
4. Cerebrohepatorenal syndrome (Zellweger)
5. Coffin–Lowry syndrome   XLD
6. Cockayne syndrome   AR
7. Fibrodysplasia ossificans congenita   AD
8. Epidermal nevus syndrome (Solomon)
9. Nevoid basal cell carcinoma syndrome
10. Multiple congenital fibromatosis
11. Neurofibromatosis (several types)   AD

V. Chromosome abnormalities

VI. Primary metabolic disorders

AD   Autosomal dominant
AR   Autosomal recessive
XLD   X-linked dominant
XLR   X-linked recessive

2 Upper Extremity

J. Freyschmidt

The Hand

The skeleton of the hand (carpus, metacarpus, phalanges) contains an average of 31 bones including the more common sesamoids. The number of joints in the hand is variable, ranging from 25 to 28 depending on carpal joint anatomy. The metacarpals and phalanges (except for the sesamoids) are tubular bones, while the carpus is composed of small, irregular, nontubular bones. This abundance of bony elements and joints correlates with an almost overwhelming number of variants in terms of number, size, structure, and density and with a great variety of pathological changes due to trauma, necrosis, inflammation, etc.

The hand causes very little x-ray scattering, making its skeleton an ideal object for radiography. Some features, such as early structural bone changes and early inflammatory joint changes, are best displayed by using mammo-graphic technique and reading the film with a magnifying lens or by performing direct geometric magnification radiography using a microfocus tube.

> A good way to deal with equivocal findings is to obtain a radiograph of the opposite side and, when interpreting the films, examine each individual bony element for unusual or abnormal features.

The favorable imaging conditions in the hand are one reason why the hand is used as a radiological test region for many systemic disease processes (e.g., renal osteodystrophy, acromegaly, polyarticular joint diseases such as rheumatoid arthritis, psoriatic arthritis, etc.).

Metacarpus and Phalanges

General Aspects

We start with a discussion of the general radiographic aspects of the metacarpus and phalanges because numerous variants and pathological changes can exist in multiple bones simultaneously and in varying degrees, and a general perspective is needed to interpret and classify them correctly. Another purpose of this general introduction is to highlight certain anatomic and pathoanatomic features that the different bones have in common, and to show how certain pathological changes in one bone can also involve adjacent metacarpals or phalanges. By addressing these general issues now, we can avoid the repetitiveness of listing them in later sections that deal with specific bones in the hand.

Normal Findings

 During Growth

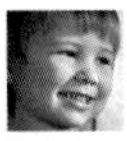

The ossification processes in the metacarpals and phalanges are subject to interindividual, sex-specific, and ethnic variations, especially with regard to the times at which the ossification centers appear and the growth plates become fused. These variations are beyond our scope, but Fig. 2.**1** shows the most common sequence for the development of the ossification centers in the hand.

For questions pertaining to skeletal age, including the prediction of adult height (growth prediction), we refer the reader to radiographic atlases of skeletal development (e.g., Greulich and Pyle, Tanner and Whitehouse).

 In Adulthood

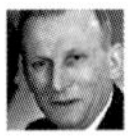

Figure 2.**2** shows the normal radiographic appearance of the adult hand, including the anatomic terms that will be used in the rest of the chapter.

All the metacarpals and phalanges are classified as small tubular bones, and they articulate via synovial joints. The size of the bones of the hand (length and width) depends chiefly on constitutional factors. The shape of the bones is determined mainly by the nature and extent of mechanical stresses. This is most evident at sites of tendon attachment: the stronger and more sustained the muscular traction, the larger and more prominent the bones appear. The bones of a manual laborer have a heavier, "stockier" appearance than those of an office worker (Fig. 2.**3a, b**).

In the normal hand, a line drawn tangent to the heads of the fourth and fifth metacarpals passes just above the head of the third metacarpal (Fig. 2.**4**). If the line intersects the head of the third metacarpal, this is a sign that a pathological condition (e.g., pseudohypoparathyroidism) is present. A tangent that just touches the articular surface of the third metacarpal is considered borderline.

Fig. 2.**1** Typical progression of the radiographic appearance of epiphyseal ossification centers in the carpus, metacarpus, and phalanges.

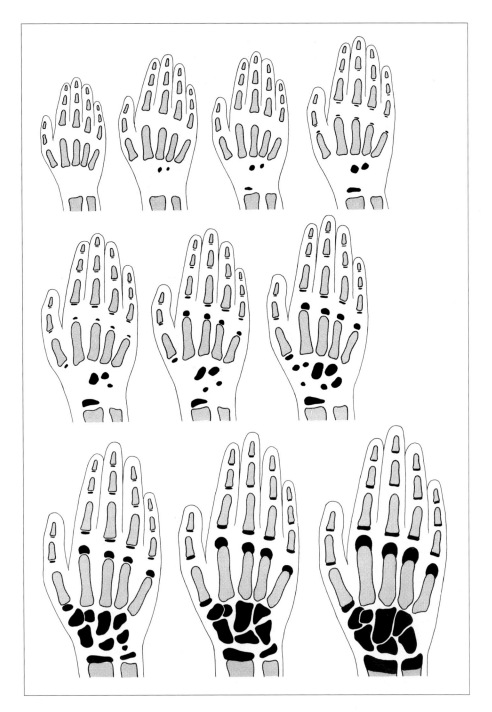

The sum of the lengths of the proximal and distal phalanges should approximately equal the length of the associated metacarpal bone (the "phalangeal sign" of Kosowicz 1965, Fig. 2.**4**). An analysis of measurements of phalangeal lengths with metacarpophalangeal pattern profile plots (Poznanski and Holt 1971) has been extended by correlating the measurements with the total length of the phalanges to obtain a single mean-value and standard-deviation table for all ages from 3 years to adult. This table can be used to compare published pictures with actual radiographic images (Dijkstra 1983). The many possible causes of disproportionately short or long metacarpals and phalanges are discussed fully in the section on Specific Bones of the Hand.

Normally the thumb has three tubular bones and the other fingers have four. There are several reasons why fewer than the normal number may be encountered in one or more fingers:

- Absence of a joint (congenital: symphalangia; acquired: postarthritic ankylosis)
- Congenital absence of one or more phalanges
- Loss of one or more phalanges (e.g., loss of a distal phalanx due to neoplastic or inflammatory destruction)

Two sesamoid bones are found at the base of the proximal phalanx of the thumb in virtually 100% of the population, one occurring more toward the radial side of the thumb and one toward the ulnar side. These sesamoids become radiographically visible between 12 and 14 years of age. Another sesamoid occurs at the interphalangeal joint of the thumb in approximately 70–75% of the population and at the head of the fifth metacarpal in 82.5% (Fig. 2.**5**).

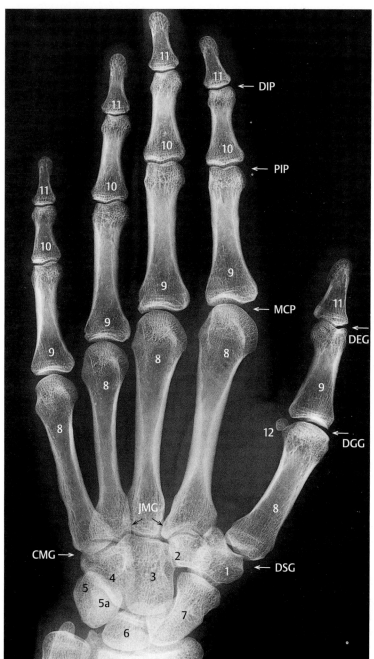

Fig. 2.**2**   Normal radiographic appearance of the adult hand, with anatomic nomenclature.

1	Trapezium
2	Trapezoid
3	Capitate
4	Hamate
5, 5 a	Triquetrum and pisiform, superimposed
6	Lunate
7	Scaphoid
8	Metacarpal bones
9	Proximal phalanges
10	Middle phalanges
11	Distal phalanges
12	Sesamoid
CMG	Carpometacarpal joint
DEG	Interphalangeal joint of thumb
DGG	Metacarpophalangeal joint of thumb
DSG	Carpometacarpal joint of thumb
DIP	Distal interphalangeal joint
IMG	Intermetacarpal joint
MCP	Metacarpophalangeal joint
PIP	Proximal interphalangeal joint

Fig. 2.**3 a–d**   The diverse radiographic anatomy of the hand.

a, b Mechanical stresses influence the size and shape of the hand bones. Film **a** is from an office worker, film **b** is from a manual laborer. In **b**, note the protuberant ligament and capsular attachments and the prominent nutrient canals, especially in the proximal phalanges.

c, d Radiographs from a healthy 37-year-old woman show very dense, thick cortical bone in the metacarpals and osteosclerosis of the distal phalanges (the patient had no clinical signs of Morgagni syndrome).

Supernumerary sesamoid bones may be encountered. They have no pathological significance (Figs. 2.**5**–2.**7**).

In principle, single or multiple sesamoid bones can occur at various metacarpophalangeal and interphalangeal joints and may even be found dorsal to the metacarpophalangeal joint of the thumb. When a sesamoid is found at an unusual location and is symptomatic, the differential diagnosis should include a fragment from an adjacent bone, heterotopic bone formation, and the ossification of a soft-tissue tumor (e.g., chondroma, soft-tissue osteoma). The presence of differentiated cancellous bone structures with a cortical margin generally identifies the bone as a sesamoid. A sesamoid that completely overlaps a bony structure such as the head of a metacarpal is indistinguishable from an in-

nocuous bone island (endosteoma), but neither one has pathological significance.

The radiographic density of the bones of the hand depends on the thickness of the cortical bone and the thickness and density of the cancellous trabeculae. Rarefaction of the cancellous trabeculae and thinning of the cortical bone are important signs of osteopenia. The Barnett–Nordin index, formerly used to diagnose osteoporosis, is a useful guide for determining the normal thickness of the cortical bone.

Barnett–Nordin index
➤ Ratio of cortical thickness to total transverse diameter at the midpoint of the second metacarpal bone.

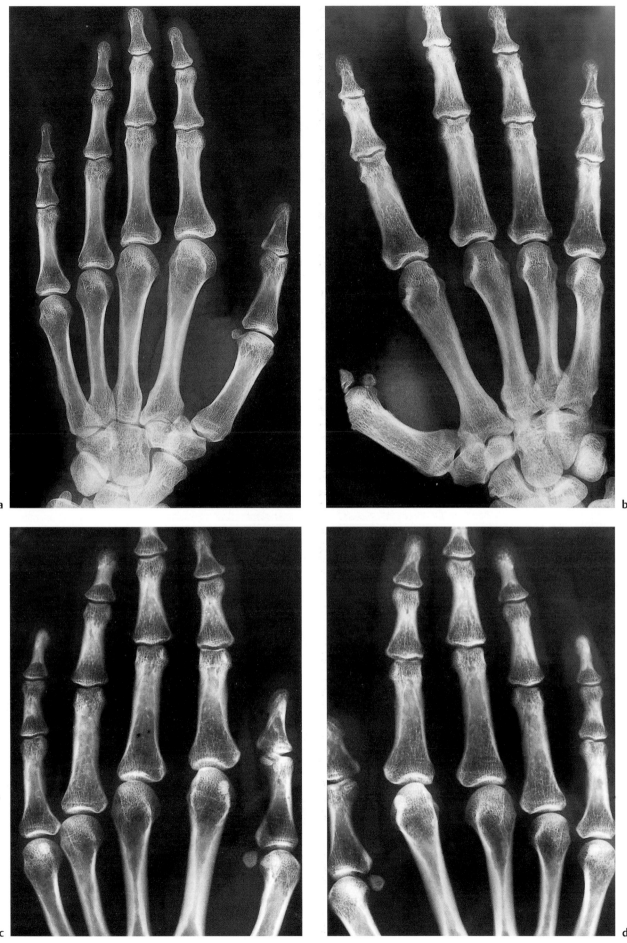

a

b

c

d

Fig. 2.**3 a–d**   (Legend p. 18)

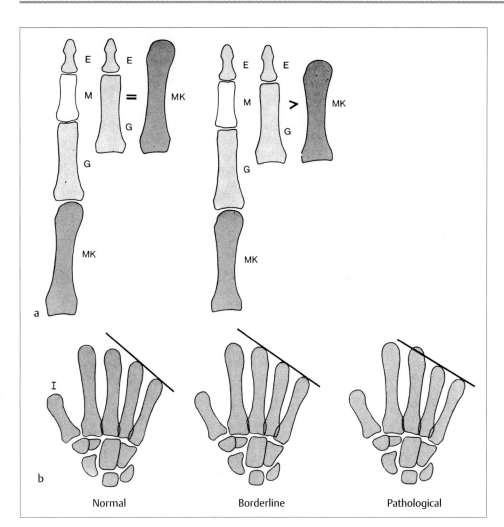

Fig. 2.**4a,b** Biometry of the metacarpals and phalanges.
a Phalangeal sign of Kosowicz.
b Metacarpal sign.
E   Distal phalanx
G   Proximal phalanx
M   Middle phalanx
MK Metacarpal

Normal   Borderline   Pathological

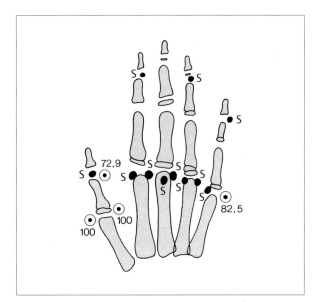

Fig. 2.**5** Sesamoid bones that have been described in the adult human hand (after Degen). Sesamoids are always found at the metacarpophalangeal joint of the thumb. The prevalence of the more common sesamoids is shown. The less common sesamoids are marked with the letter S (sporadic occurrence). Only one case has been observed and described for each of the distal interphalangeal sesamoids.

This index expresses the thickness of the cortex as a percentage of the total bone diameter and should average at least 43–44% in healthy adolescents and adults. The cortical thickness of all the metacarpals and phalanges declines slowly and steadily with aging, decreasing earlier in women than in men. Meanwhile, the cancellous bone undergoes a progressive rarefaction that is especially pronounced near joints. As a result, the bones become more radiolucent. Normally the cortex of the metacarpals and phalanges appears very solid and uniformly dense. The endosteal margin of the cortex may show slight undulations, but these have no pathological significance. The cortex of the metacarpals is sometimes very thick and dense and may greatly narrow the marrow space without pathological implications (Fig. 2.**3c, d**). Similarly, osteosclerosis of the distal phalanges and cortical thickening of individual phalanges do not necessarily have pathological significance (Fig. 2.**3c, d**). Occasionally, however, these hyperostotic changes may be associated with hyperostosis frontalis interna and endocrine disorders, especially in women 40 to 50 years of age (Morgagni syndrome). They may also be a manifestation of skeletal sarcoidosis or other diseases. "Roughening" of the cortical boundary and intracortical bone resorption always signify an abnormal structural change that may result from a metabolic disorder (e.g., hyperparathyroidism) or a regional increase in blood flow due to a pathological process. Fraying of the

Fig. 2.**6**   Multiple sesamoids.

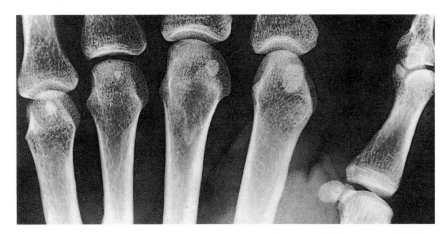

cortex or intracortical channels can result from dilation of the normally invisible Haversian canals (Figs. 2.**43**, 2.**44**). If this process occurs at a circumscribed site in the cortical bone, it produces a "gray cortex" sign like that seen with stress fractures, for example. If the inner cortical margin becomes poorly demarcated from the medullary canal, this may result from an incipient sclerotic process within the medullary cavity.

Linear Lucencies

Linear radiolucencies in the tubular bones of the hand can have two causes:

- Nutrient canals
- Projection-related lucencies

Nutrient canals in the metacarpal bones (Figs. 2.**8b**, 2.**9c**) run obliquely from the cortex to the medullary cavity in a distal-to-proximal direction. The nutrient canals in the phalanges show an opposite orientation, running in an oblique proximal-to-distal direction (Figs. 2.**3b**, 2.**8b**). This disparity results from differences in the longitudinal growth of the bone and of the vessels that traverse the canals. Longitudinal growth of the metacarpals occurs mainly in the distal portion of the bone, causing the metacarpal head to grow distally away from the proximal nutrient canals. By contrast, longitudinal growth of the phalanges occurs in their proximal portion, causing the bone to grow in a proximal direction away from the distal, more slowly developing vessels. A nutrient canal projected end-on appears as a small round lucency that, when viewed with a magnifier, is frequently surrounded by a dense rim (Figs. 2.**8a**, 2.**10**).

Projection-related linear lucencies are commonly found at sites where tendons attach to bony prominences. The grooves that flank the prominence and separate it from the adjacent cortex create a translucent effect (Fig. 2.**9a–c**).

Small, irregular densities ("calcium specks") found in areas of the metacarpals and phalanges with abundant cancellous bone are a summation effect caused by superimposed cancellous trabeculae and have no pathological significance (Fig. 2.**10**). Often they can be eliminated by changing the angle of the projection by a few degrees.

Fig. 2.**7**   Two normal and two rudimentary sesamoids at the metacarpophalangeal joint of the thumb.

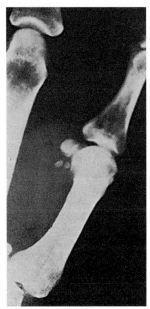

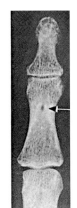

a

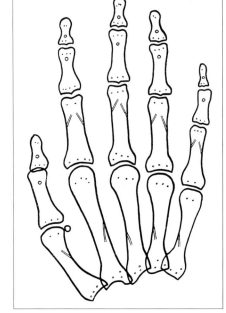

b

Fig. 2.**8a, b**   Nutrient canals in the metacarpals and phalanges.
a End-on projection of a nutrient canal (arrow).
b Course of the nutrient canals. Note how the orientation of the metacarpal canals differs from that in the proximal phalanges.

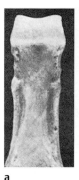

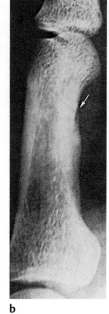

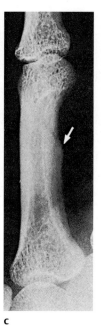

a

b   **c**

Fig. 2.**9 a–c**   Causes of linear lucencies on the phalanges: nutrient canals and bony prominences.
a Palmar aspect of a phalanx shows a bony prominence (for tendon attachment) flanked by groovelike depressions on each side.
b Clear projection of a bony prominence with a slight peripheral overhang (arrow) that mimics a fracture line.
c Lucency created by the base of a groove flanking a bony prominence and by a nutrient canal (arrow: point where the vessel enters the cortex).

Pathological Finding?

 Normal Variant or Anomaly?

While we cannot detail the many complex and diverse skeletal malformations and deformities that can occur in the hand, we can discuss variants, including extreme ones, and illustrate clear-cut malformations that are encountered in radiological practice. Table 2.**1** shows the classification and relative frequency of skeletal malformations of the hand according to Swanson (1976) and Lister (1993).

The tubular bones of the hand are normally mono-epiphyseal. Usually the epiphyses are somewhat narrower than the adjacent metaphyses, but they may also be of equal width or even slightly broader (Fig. 2.**11**).

Epiphyses that are large and cone-shaped and have irregular margins may reflect an enchondral epiphyseal ossification disturbance (Fig. 2.**12**), but in these cases they are generally associated with epiphyseal abnormalities in the long tubular bones and in the skeleton of the foot.

Table 2.**1**   Skeletal malformations of the hand

Malformations	Frequency (%)
Failure of formation of parts	12.2
Failure of differentiation of parts	31.3
Duplication	35.9
Overdevelopment	0.5
Underdevelopment	4.3
Ring constriction complex	6.5
Malformation syndromes	Variable

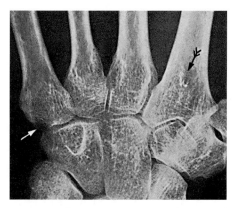

Fig. 2.**10**   The arrow points to a "calcium speck" caused by superimposed trabecular lines. It happens to be adjacent to a nutrient canal projected end-on. The white arrow points to a normal area of "thin bone" that should not be mistaken for cortical erosion.

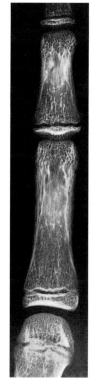

Fig. 2.**11**   Broad epiphyses in a 14-year-old boy.

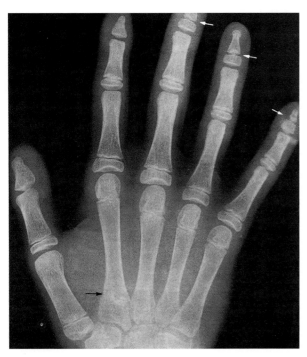

Fig. 2.**12**   Very stout, broad epiphyses in cleidocranial dysostosis. Note the pseudoepiphysis in the second metacarpal.

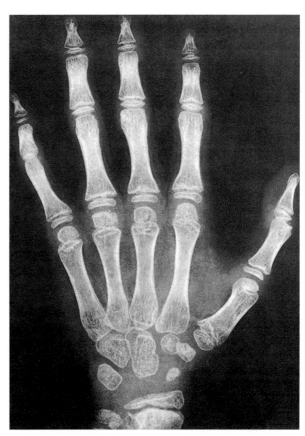

Fig. 2.**13**   These epiphyses appear small in relation to the metaphyses, especially in the phalanges.

Metaphyses that are broader than the epiphyses and diaphyses are illustrated in Fig. 2.**13** as an anatomic variant.

The epiphyseal plates usually show slight distal convexity in the phalanges and slight proximal convexity in the metacarpals, but this pattern is subject to variation (Fig. 2.**14**) without pathological significance.

The course of the epiphyseal plates changes during skeletal growth.

Extra epiphyses are known as **pseudoepiphyses**, apparently because they do not contribute significantly to the longitudinal growth of the tubular bone (Figs. 2.**15**–2.**17**). One or more pseudoepiphyses may be found in normal children and adolescents, but they may also reflect a systemic disturbance of skeletal growth (e.g., in hypothyroidism or Down syndrome). Three basic histological patterns of pseudoepiphysis formation and development are listed below in chronological order (Ogden et al. 1994).

- A central osseous bridge extends from the metaphysis into the epiphysis, where it appears as a centrifugally expanding, mushroomlike ossification center. The remaining intact epiphyseal plate does not have the hypertrophic cartilage cell columns that are otherwise typical of the growth plate.
- A peripheral osseous bridge is formed, creating either an osseous ring or an eccentric bridge between the metaphysis and the epiphysis. Centrally, the physis is preserved.
- Multiple bridging occurs. As in the first and second patterns, the nonossified portions of the physis lack typical columns of cartilage cells.

These bridging phenomena cannot always be seen on radiographs, but the pathoanatomic and histological studies of Ogden et al. (1994) indicate that, visible or not, they probably exist.

Pseudoepiphyses are most commonly found between 5 and 10 years of age. They close years earlier than the normal epiphyseal growth plate in the same bone. As mentioned, they do not contribute to longitudinal bone growth.

Pseudoepiphyses are found in the proximal second metacarpal of 20–60% of normal children and in the distal first metacarpal of up to 65% of normal children.

Schäfer (1952) ranked the bones of the hand in the following order with regard to the frequency of pseudoepiphyses:

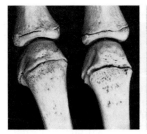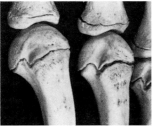

Fig. 2.**14**   Variants of epiphyseal lines in the metacarpals: transverse (left) and distally convex (right).

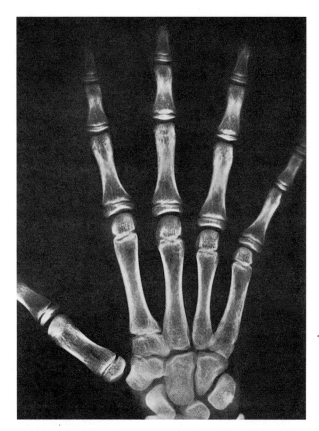

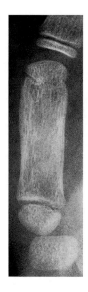

Fig. 2.**16**   Pseudoepiphysis in the distal portion of the first metacarpal.

◁ Fig. 2.**15**   Pseudoepiphysis in the second metacarpal bone. It is unusual that this bone is slightly too long relative to the third metacarpal, but this apparently has to do with the hypoplastic thumb (missing proximal phalanx) and the extra epiphysis on the first metacarpal. Also, the scaphoid appears somewhat small. Note also the relatively dense epiphyses of the middle phalanges (ivory epiphyses, see p. 52).

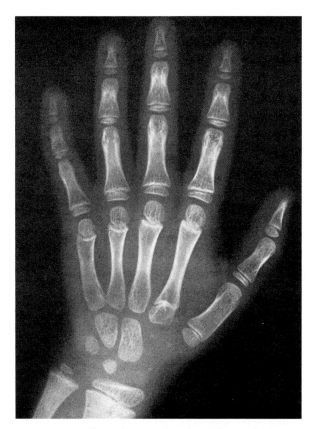

Fig. 2.**17**   Pseudoepiphysis in the proximal second metacarpal with the formation of an osseous bridge.

Relative frequency of pseudoepiphyses according to Schäfer
➤ First metacarpal > second metacarpal > fifth metacarpal > fifth middle phalanx > third metacarpal > fourth middle phalanx > first proximal phalanx > fourth metacarpal.

Rochels and Schmidt (1980) found pseudoepiphyses in 82.4% of patients with Down syndrome. Significant sex differences were not observed. The frequency of involvement is different from that in normal individuals:

Relative frequency of pseudoepiphyses in Down syndrome
➤ Second metacarpal > first metacarpal > fifth middle phalanx > fourth proximal phalanx.

The authors counted an average of 3.1 pseudoepiphyses per hand in children with Down syndrome. Brachymesophalangia was found in 67% of cases, dysmesophalangia in 4.6%, and clinodactyly in 56.4%.

The **cone-shaped epiphysis** (cone epiphysis) is a special morphological variant (Fig. 2.**18a–c**). Cone-shaped epiphyses are more commonly found in the skeleton of the foot in otherwise healthy individuals (Giedion 1968). It has been suggested that the condition is based on a disturbance in the timing and coordination of bone development. While the central portions of the bone become arrested in their growth, the peripheral portions continue to grow. Occasionally, though, cone-shaped epiphyses may be associated with clinical symptoms as illustrated by the case in Fig. 2.**18d, e**. Apparently, the cone-shaped epi-

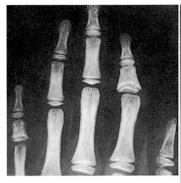

a

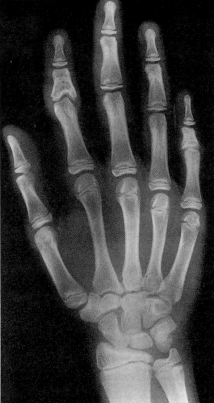

b

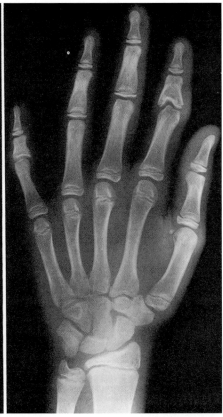

c

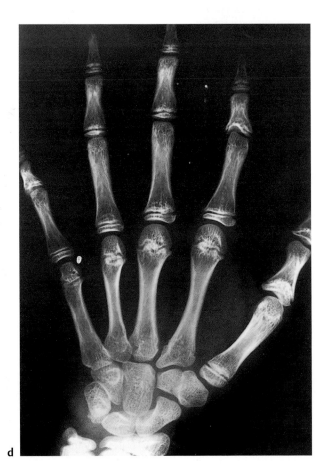

d

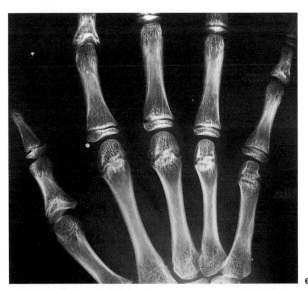

e

Fig. 2.**18 a–e**   Cone-shaped epiphyses.
a Cone-shaped epiphyses of the second and fifth middle phalanges on both sides (right side not shown).
b Cone-shaped epiphyses of the second and fifth middle phalanges on both sides (left side not shown).
c Pronounced cone-shaped epiphyses of all middle phalanges. The opposite hand showed the same changes with an otherwise normal appearance in a healthy 11-year-old child.
d,e Cone-shaped epiphyses on the proximal phalanx of the thumbs and the second and third middle phalanges of both hands. Also relatively dense epiphyses, especially on the third and fourth proximal phalanges of the right hand. This 14-year-old Arabic boy presented clinically with visible swellings (and mild pain) affecting the thumbs and the proximal interphalangeal joints of the index and small fingers.

physes in such cases signal a true deformity or trophic disturbance.

Very dense epiphyses occurring as a normal variant are discussed in the section on necrosis (p. 52).

In contrast to cone-shaped epiphyses, the presence of a **delta phalanx**, known also as a **longitudinally bracketed diaphysis** (Fig. 2.19), represents a pathological condition of the metacarpals (and metatarsals) and phalanges, most commonly involving the proximal phalanges of the hands and feet (Theander and Carstan 1974, Ogden et al. 1981, Theander et al. 1982).

In the literature to date, delta phalanges have been described in the following skeletal dysplasias and syndromes:

- All forms of microphalangia, polydactyly, and syndactyly
- Trisomy 21 (fifth middle phalanx)
- Acrocephalosyndactyly (Apert and Pfeiffer type)
- Rubinstein–Taiby syndrome (thumb)
- Catel–Manzke syndrome (second and third fingers)
- Holt–Oram syndrome

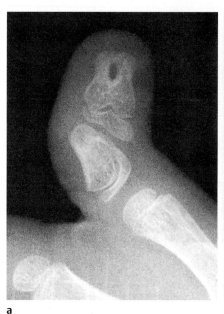
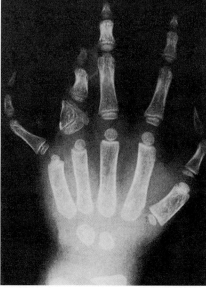

a   b

Fig. 2.**19 a, b**   Delta phalanges.
a Delta-shaped proximal phalanx of the thumb and duplication of the distal phalanx in a 3-year-old girl. Note the distal epiphysis on the first metacarpal.
b Delta-shaped proximal phalanx of the fourth finger of the left hand in a 3-year-old boy, resulting in shortening of that ray. Clinically, the patient had syndactyly of the third and fourth fingers and consequent or associated clinodactyly of the small finger.

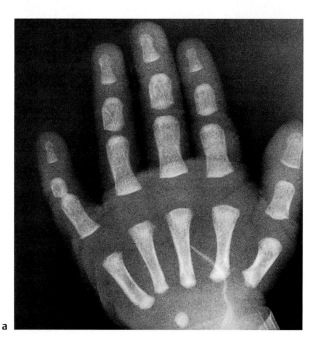
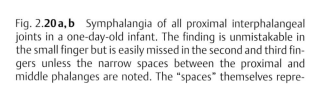

a

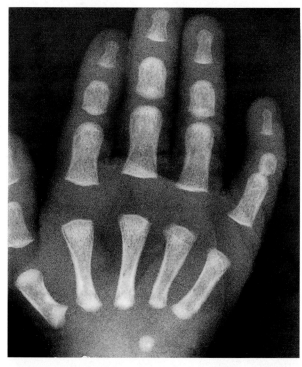

b

Fig. 2.**20 a, b**   Symphalangia of all proximal interphalangeal joints in a one-day-old infant. The finding is unmistakable in the small finger but is easily missed in the second and third fingers unless the narrow spaces between the proximal and middle phalanges are noted. The "spaces" themselves represent the proximal epiphyseal growth plates and the still-unossified epiphyses. The child's mother (Fig. 2.**21**) had the same changes (case courtesy of Professor Dr. D. Buck-Gramcko, Hamburg).

- Otopalatodigital syndrome
- Otofaciogenital syndrome
- Diastrophic dwarfism
- Nievergelt syndrome
- Hand–foot–genital syndrome (Giedion)

Symphalangia refers to the absence of the interphalangeal joints with resultant end-to-end fusion of the phalanges (Figs. 2.**20**, 2.**21**). This condition is classified as a hereditary dysplasia. In **adults**, it is easy to diagnose hereditary aplasia and hypoplasia of the interphalangeal joints: usually an absence of skin folds is noted over the aplastic joint, and the radiograph shows continuous bony trabeculation across the site of the synostosis, which may show a very slight fusiform expansion. Clinically, the affected finger is held in a position of extension or slight flexion, and hyperextension is occasionally seen. The ulnar digits are more commonly affected than the radial digits. Frequently, symphalangia affects both sides symmetrically and is as-

sociated with other skeletal anomalies in the hand. The spectrum of radiographic appearances of joint aplasias and hypoplasias is shown in Fig. 2.**22**.

Interphalangeal joint aplasias (symphalangia) and hypoplasias in the **growing skeleton** are more difficult to diagnose than in adults. The "synchondrotic" interphalangeal connections still show some springiness on clinical examination, and on radiographs they are indistinguishable from a normal joint space. The drawing by Dihlmann in Fig. 2.**23** clearly illustrates the potential for diagnostic errors.

An acquired bony ankylosis can also mimic symphalangia. The main cause of bony ankylosis in children is an antecedent articular cartilage injury or inflammatory joint disease. This cannot always be clearly determined from the history, as many of these patients will have forgotten the causal event. Acquired ankyloses are generally distinguished from congenital aplasias and hypoplasias by the presence of transverse skin folds over the ankylosed joint.

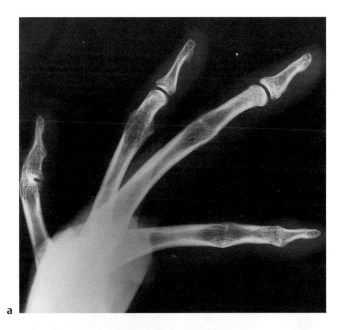
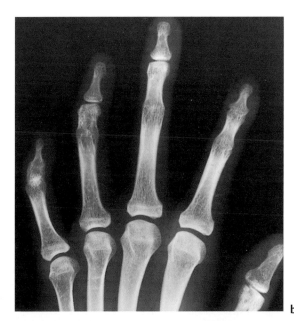
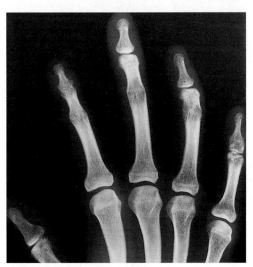
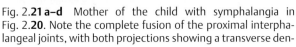
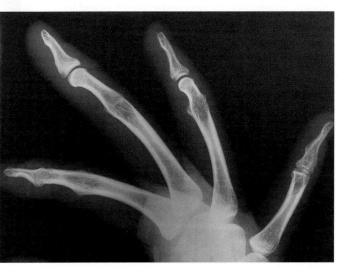

Fig. 2.**21 a–d** Mother of the child with symphalangia in Fig. 2.**20**. Note the complete fusion of the proximal interphalangeal joints, with both projections showing a transverse den-

sity where the joints should be. The periarticular cancellous bone structures are also typical of a joint anlage (case courtesy of Professor Dr. D. Buck-Gramcko, Hamburg).

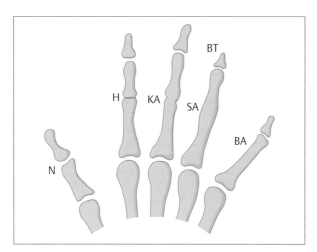

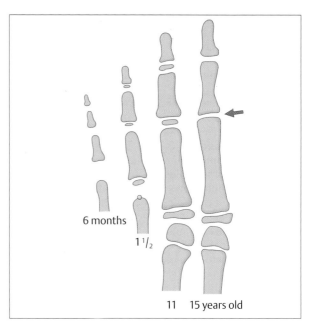

Fig. 2.**22** Anomalies of the phalangeal joints (after Dihlmann). Joint aplasias and hypoplasias in adults (illustrated for the proximal interphalangeal joints). The outlines of the phalanges are still visible but the joint is ankylosed.
BA Aplasia with brachymesophalangia, also cylindrical broadening of the synostosed proximal and middle phalanges
BT Incidental finding: brachytelephalangia (differentiate from acro-osteolysis)
H Hypoplasia
KA Aplasia with slight notching in the boundary zone
N Normal appearance
SA Aplasia with slight fusiform expansion of the boundary zone

Fig. 2.**23** Aplasia of the proximal interphalangeal joint in the growing skeleton (after Dihlmann). By 15 years of age, the "synchondrosis" has been transformed to a synostosis. This may also occur at an earlier age. The still-open epiphyseal growth plate in the middle phalanx (arrow) mimics a joint line. The growth plate in the distal phalanx has already closed in age-appropriate fashion. The space between the distal and middle phalanx represents the articular cartilage of the normally developed distal interphalangeal joint.

Remnants of the former joint contours or structural irregularities are usually found in the area of the ankylosis. Also, these changes are unilateral or at least asymmetrical.

Syndactyly most commonly occurs as a hereditary anomaly between the distal phalanges of two fingers (Fig. 2.**24**).

Axial deviations of the fingers occur as a congenital anomaly in the form of **camptodactyly** or **clinodactyly**. Camptodactyly (Fig. 2.**25**) refers to a congenital (sporadic or autosomal dominant) flexion contracture of individual phalangeal joints. Initially it is not accompanied by detectable bone changes. It usually affects the fifth finger and less commonly the fourth finger. Over time, the base of the middle phalanx becomes broadened and a notch develops in the neck of the proximal phalanx on the palmar side (Fig. 2.**25 b**). The pathoanatomic basis for the deformity is an anomalous insertion of the lumbricalis muscles or of the superficial digital flexors.

Clinodactyly with axial deviation of the distal phalanx is usually caused by a trapezoid-shaped middle phalanx (Fig. 2.**26**) or a delta phalanx (Fig. 2.**19**).

Other axial deviations are observed in the following diseases:

- Achondroplasia (spreading between the third and fourth rays, trident hand)
- Trisomy 17/18 (spreading between the second and third fingers)

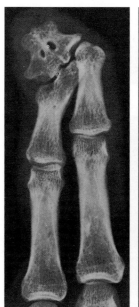
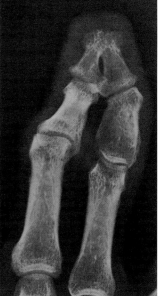

Fig. 2.**24 a, b** Syndactyly of the third and fourth fingers of each hand. Note the fused distal phalanges and the anomalous development of the third middle phalanx in **a**. The patient, a 42-year-old man, also had polydactyly of the fifth toe of each foot (not shown).

Fig. 2.**25 a, b** Camptodactyly.
a In a child. Initially the congenital flexion contracture is not accompanied by bone changes.
b In an adult. Note the broadened base of the proximal phalanx and the palmar notch in the neck of the proximal phalanx. The fifth digit is most commonly affected, followed by the fourth digit (with kind permission of Professor Dr. D. Buck-Gramcko, Hamburg).

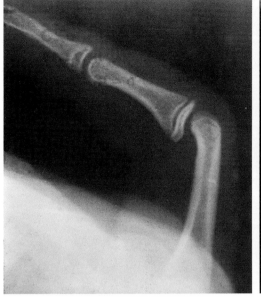
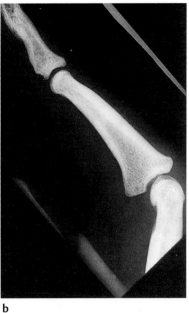

a   b

Fig. 2.**26** Clinodactyly.

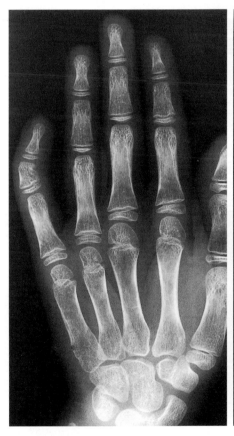
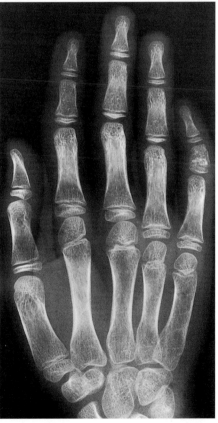

- Chondroectodermal dysplasia (Ellis–van Creveld syndrome) (usually combined with polydactyly, polycarpia, often with spreading between the fifth and sixth rays or between other rays)
- Metaphyseal dysplasia (Pyle disease) (spreading of all metacarpals and fingers).

Polydactyly (ulnar and/or radial sided multiplication) (Fig. 2.**27**) refers to the presence of more than five fingers and/or tubular bones in the metacarpal region. The super-numerary elements may be identical to the original bones, or they may be rudimentary (Fig. 2.**27 b**). In most cases polydactyly is combined with other anomalies. It very often involves duplication or triplication of the thumb, duplication of the fifth ray, simultaneous polydactyly of the thumb and small finger, or duplication of the middle ray.

Polydactyly can be classified as being of the **radial** (Fig. 2.**27 i, j, m**), **ulnar** (Fig. 2.**27 k, n**) or **central type** (second through fourth rays).

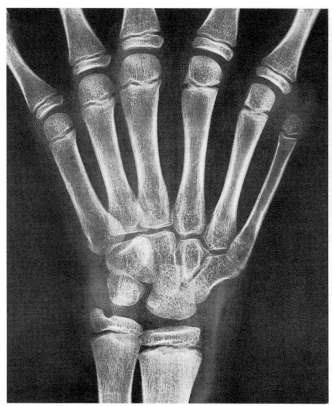
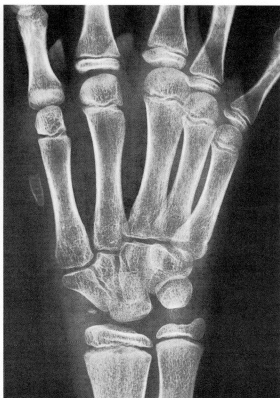

a

b

Fig. 2.**27 a–n**   Polydactyly.
a, b Bilateral polydactyly. Panel **a** (left hand) shows a supernumerary ray with a hypoplastic metacarpal bone and a stubby appendage distal to it (rudimentary type, see panel **g**). The adjacent metacarpal bone looks like a second metacarpal rather than a first metacarpal (which normally has a proximal epiphyseal plate). There is an associated carpal anomaly in which a scaphoidlike bone articulates with the supernumerary digit.

There is also an atypical enlarged, bulky lunate bone. The distal radius is underdeveloped, lacking a styloid process. In panel **b** (right hand), the supernumerary ray consists only of two rudimentary bony elements next to the adjacent metacarpal. The distal element is barely visible. The carpal anomalies are similar to those on the left side, with an additional small bony element interposed between the scaphoidlike bone and the radial styloid process.

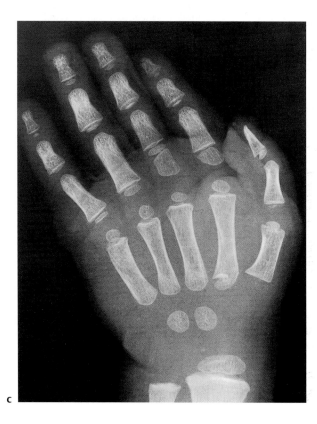

c

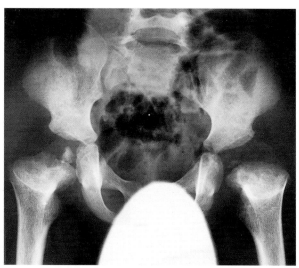

d

Fig. 2.**27 c, d**   Surgically corrected polydactyly in a patient with cretinism (preoperative films were unavailable). This case is distinguished by an unusual polyphalangia (hyperphalangia) of the third ray with an additional, undefined bony element at the base of the third proximal phalanx. A similar but smaller bony element occurs at the base of the proximal phalanx of the index finger; it may represent an oversized epiphysis. Panel **d** shows a typical absence of ossification centers about the hips.

Type	Diagram	Description
DIST type		**Distal phalangeal type:** incomplete duplication of the distal phalanges (1–5)
DIP type		**Distal interphalangeal joint type:** complete duplication of the distal phalanx (1–5) distal to the distal interphalangeal joint
MI type		**Middle phalangeal type:** incomplete duplication of the middle phalanx and complete duplication of the distal phalanx (2–5)
PIP type		**Proximal interphalangeal joint type:** complete duplication of the middle and distal phalanges (2–5) distal to the proximal interphalangeal joint
PROX type		**Proximal phalanx type:** incomplete duplication of the proximal phalanx and complete duplication of the middle (not first ray) and distal phalanges (2–5)

e

Type	Diagram	Description
MP type		**Metacarpo- or metatarsophalangeal joint type:** complete duplication of proximal, middle (not first ray) and distal phalanges (1–5) distal to the metacarpo- or metatarsophalangeal joint
MET type		**Metacarpal or metatarsal type:** incomplete duplication of the metacarpals or metatarsals and complete duplication of the proximal, middle (not first ray) and distal phalanges (1–5)
CM/TM type		**Carpometacarpal or tarsometatarsal joint type:** complete duplication of the metacarpals or metatarsals and of the proximal, middle (not first ray) and distal phalanges (1–5) distal to the carpometacarpal or tarsometatarsal joint
C/T type		**Carpal or tarsal type:** incomplete duplication of the carpals or tarsals and complete duplication of the metacarpals or metatarsals and the proximal, middle (not first ray) and distal phalanges (1–5)
IC/IT type		**Intercarpal or intertarsal joint type:** Complete duplication of the carpals or tarsals, metacarpals or metatarsals, and the proximal, middle (not first ray) and distal phalanges (1–5) distal to the intercarpal or intertarsal joint

f

Fig. 2.**27 e–h**   Classification of polydactyly based on radiographic criteria. (After Buck-Gramcko and Behrens 1989.)

Type	Diagram	Description	Type	Diagram	Description
RUD type	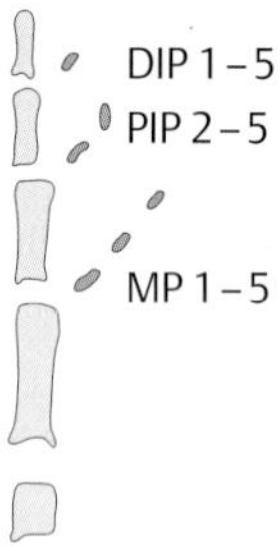 DIP 1–5 PIP 2–5 MP 1–5	**Rudimentary type:** supernumerary ray with or without rudimentary duplication of bones, also free-floating hypoplastic rays named for the corresponding joint levels (DIP, PIP, MP) (1–5)	(illustrated for the first ray) CM$_{Tr}$ type	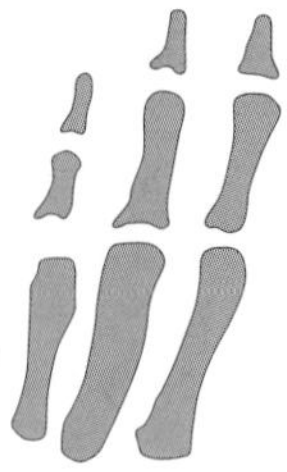	**Triple ray of the CM type:** completely separate, triple metacarpals/metatarsals, proximal, middle (not first ray) and distal phalanges (1–5) distal to the carpometacarpal or tarsometatarsal joint
MP type$^+$		**Metacarpophalangeal or metatarsophalangeal joint type+:** single triphalangism; complete duplication of the proximal and distal phalanges with an extra phalanx distal to the metacarpophalangeal or metatarsophalangeal joint	CM$_{Tr}$ type$^+$	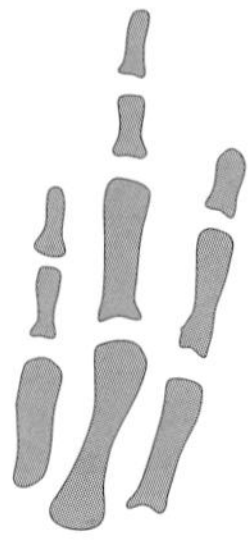	**Triple ray of the CM type+:** completely separate, triple metacarpals/metatarsals, proximal and distal phalanges with an extra distal phalanx (first ray) distal to the carpometacarpal or tarsometatarsal joint
MP type^{++}		**Metacarpophalangeal or metatarsophalangeal joint type++:** double triphalangism; complete duplication of the proximal and distal phalanges with two extra phalanges distal to the metacarpophalangeal or metatarsophalangeal joint	CM$_{Tr}$ type^{++}	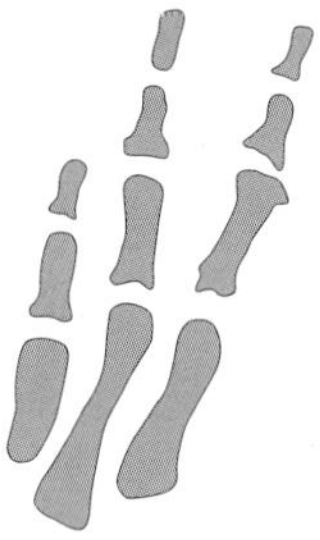	**Triple ray of the CM type++:** same as above, but with two extra distal phalanges (first ray)
CM type$^+$ TM type$^+$		**Carpometacarpal or tarsometatarsal joint type+:** single triphalangism	CM$_{Tr}$ type^{-++}	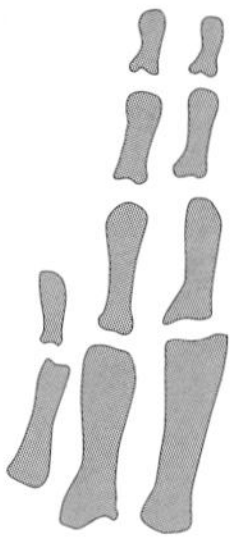	**Triple ray of the CM type-++:** same as above, but with two extra phalanges and concomitant aplasia of one phalanx (first ray)
CM type^{++} TM type^{++}		**Carpometacarpal or tarsometatarsal joint type++:** double triphalangism			
g			h		

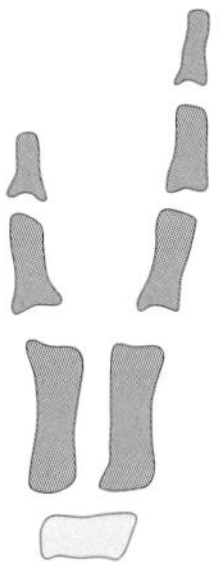

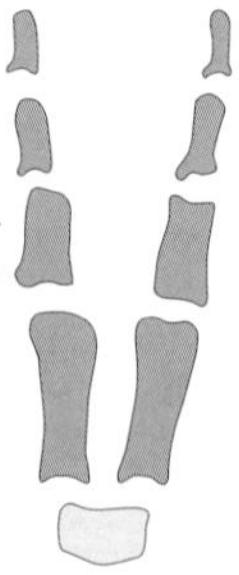

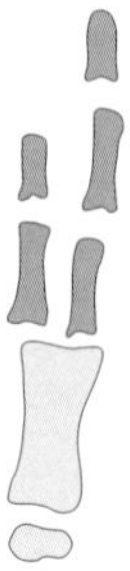

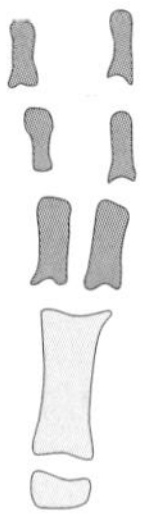

Fig. 2.**27 g–h**

Fig. 2.**27 i**   Radial polydactyly with two tri-phalangeal thumbs (CM type++), the radial of which is hypoplastic (5-month-old child). (Panels **i–n** with kind permission of Professor Dr. D. Buck-Gramcko, Hamburg.)
j Radial polydactyly (MP type+) with double biphalangism of the thumb distal to the first metacarpophalangeal joint (18-month-old child).

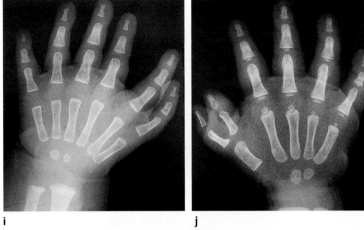

Fig. 2.**27 k, l**   Ulnar and fibular polydactyly in a 7-month-old child. Two triphalangeal small fingers (MP type), duplicated small toes, probably MET type. Also metatarsal synostosis or bifurcation.

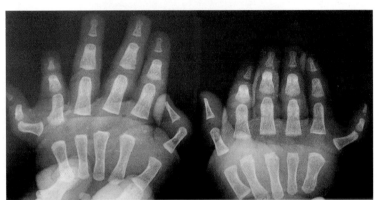

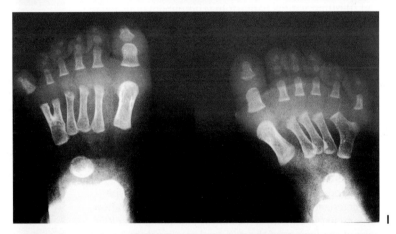

Fig. 2.**27 m**   Unilateral radial duplication (right hand) with a well-developed radial metacarpal topped on the radial side by a hypoplastic proximal phalanx without a distal phalanx. Ulnar to the radial metacarpal is a hypoplastic or rudimentary metacarpal associated with a hypoplastic proximal and distal phalanx (3-year-old child).

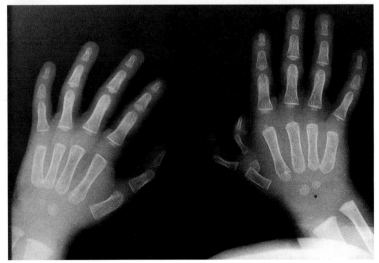

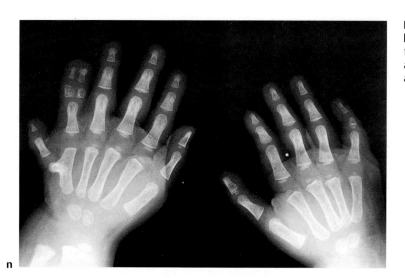

Fig. 2.**27 n**   Unusual case of ulnar polydactyly: A supernumerary biphalangeal ray arises from the fifth metacarpal. Also, the middle and distal phalanges of the true small finger are duplicated.

n

Polyphalangia (hyperphylangia) is an extremely rare anomaly in which one or more phalanges are duplicated in one digit (Fig. 2.**27 c, d**).

Disproportionately long fingers occur mainly in **arachnodactyly** (Marfan syndrome). The bones of the hand are elongated, and the fingers are abnormally long and thin. Premature ossification is also seen. The thumb is particularly long, and when the fingers are closed over the thumb, its tip protrudes out of the fist (Steinberg sign). Disproportionately long fingers are also found in **gigantism** and **fibrolipomatous hamartoma** (fibrolipomatous nerve enlargement, macrodactylia lipomatosa, lipofibroma, fibrofatty overgrowth, fatty infiltration of nerve, neurolipoma). The dominant feature of the latter condition is macrodactyly combined with heavy subcutaneous fat deposition and fat depots in tendons, muscles, and nerve (Fig. 2.**28**) (de Maeseneer et al. 1997).

Weber-type angiodysplasia is characterized by **unilateral proportional enlargement** of the bones of the hand. Accompanying arteriovenous malformations with the formation of arteriovenous shunts result in a lacunar cancellous bone structure and lacunar cortical defects (Fig. 2.**29 a–c**).

Angiodysplasia of the **Klippel–Trenaunay type** is characterized by a more **disproportional unilateral enlargement** (gigantism) of the bones of the hand. The difference in the lengths of the rays can be as much as 3.5 cm (Langer and Langer 1982, 1985; Langer et al. 1981). Cancellous and cortical bone changes are not often seen. There may be expansion of the nutrient canals. The condition is probably based on unilateral venous malformations (ectasia, displacement, absence of valves, tortuous veins, cutaneous hemangiomas) of the upper (and lower) extremity.

Proportionately short fingers (brachydactyly) are seen primarily in **endocrine disorders**. If the cause is a pituitary disorder with deficient hormone production (STH, TSH, pituitary dwarfism), the bones of the hand will be small but well-proportioned. If the endocrine disorder is due to thyroid disease with deficient production of T_3 and T_4 (cretinism), the fingers usually show normal relative proportions but there is an abnormal relationship between the width of the hand and the size of the carpal bones (exception: Fig. 2.**27 c, d**). With a parathyroid endocrine disorder (Fig. 2.**30**) in which the osseous and renal receptors

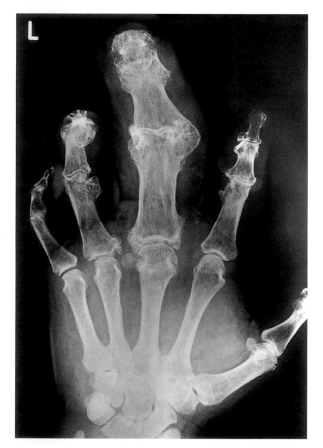

Fig. 2.**28**   Macrodactylia lipomatosa or fibrolipomatous hamartoma in a 73-year-old man without symptoms (incidental finding). (Courtesy of CA Priv. Doz. Dr. C.T. Muth, Cottbus.)

are unresponsive to parathyroid hormone (pseudohypoparathyroidism type 1–4, Freyschmidt 1997), Albright-type symptoms develop in association with proportional growth retardation and **disproportional brachymetacarpia** (e.g., of the first, fourth, and fifth rays).

The latter should be considered an associated anomaly rather than a result of the endocrine disorder.

A proportionately short hand skeleton with short, stubby fingers is also found in achondroplasia (Fig. 2.**31**).

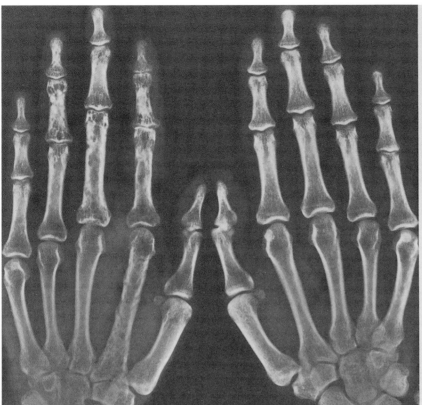
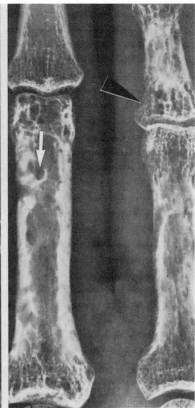

Fig. 2.**29 a–e**   Angiodysplasia of the Weber-type.
a The third finger is slightly elongated. The entire second ray and all of the third and fourth phalanges show marked structural changes.
b, c Magnification view of the phalanges and carpal bones shows a lacunar, honeycomb-like cancellous bone structure with an expanded nutrient canal (white arrow in **b**), incipient cortical striations and lacunar cortical defects (black arrow), cystlike lucencies in the carpal bones, and a cortical defect in the scaphoid (arrow in **c**).

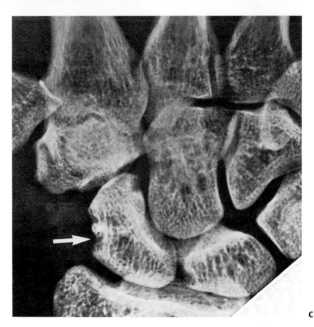

Fig. 2.**29 d** u. **e** ▷

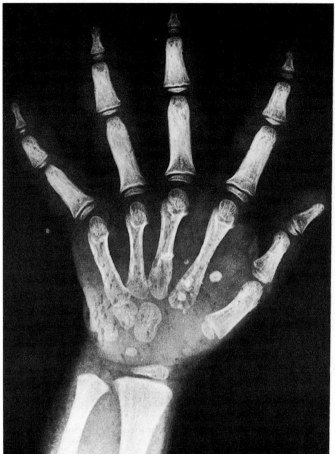

d

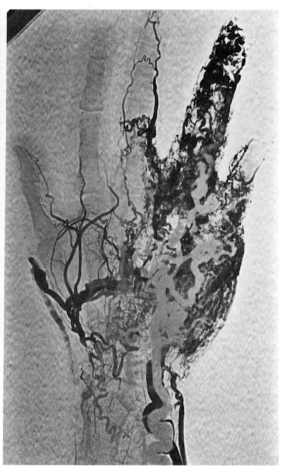

e

Fig. 2.**29 d, e** Angiodysplasia of the Servelle–Martorell type. **d** Film shows multiple cystlike lucencies, intracortical striations, and numerous phleboliths.

e Subtraction angiogram demonstrates severe arterial and venous vascular malformations in the first, second, and third rays and in the metacarpus.

A **disproportionately short hand skeleton**, usually confined to one side, occurs in **Servelle–Martorell-type angiodysplasia**. The length discrepancy can be as much as 2.5 cm (Langer and Langer 1982, 1985; Langer et al. 1981). This disease is based on a malformation of the arteries and veins (Fig. 2.**29 d,e**) leading to cystic, honeycomb-like cancellous bone destruction and intracortical linear striations. When the disease is periarticular, it can lead to very severe joint deformity. Plain radiographs may show multiple phleboliths within the hemangiomas (Fig. 2.**29 d**).

The radiographic features of various types of congenital angiodysplasia are compared in Table 2.**2**.

Dysplastic structural changes in the bones of the hand can occur not just in angiodysplasias but also in various **congenital anemias**. When marrow hyperplasia develops, it leads to widening of the medullary cavity with the resorption of cancellous and cortical bone. This usually results in coarse trabeculation or a reticular-honeycomb transformation of the cancellous bone. Marrow infarction can also occur, especially in sickle cell anemia, and is

Table 2.**2** Radiographic features of congenital angiodysplasias (from Langer and Langer 1982)

	Weber type	Klippel–Trenaunay type	Servelle–Martorell type
Gigantism	Proportionate	Disproportionate	–
Growth retardation	–	–	Disproportionate
Hemangiomas	–	Common	Common
Arteriovenous shunts	Consistently present	None (except for inactive microshunts)	None
Deep venous anomalies	–	Occasional	Common
Changes in cancellous and cortical bone	Lacunar cancellous bone structure, lacunar cortical defects	–	Foci of cancellous bone destruction, cortical destruction, intracortical striations, joint destruction
Prognosis	Uncertain	Favorable	Unfavorable

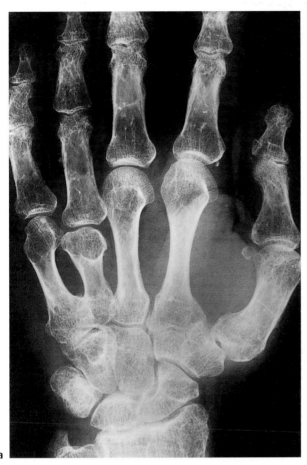
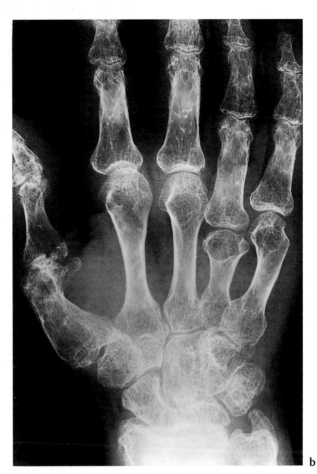

a

b

Fig. 2.**30a,b**   Short, thick metacarpals and phalanges in pseudohypoparathyroidism. The extremely short fourth metacarpals are virtually pathognomonic of the disease. Note the severe signs of osteopenia.

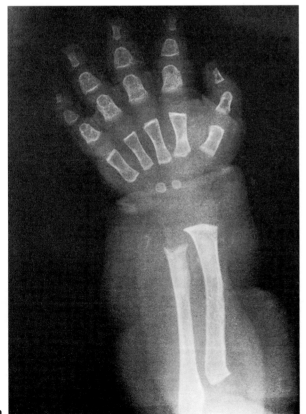
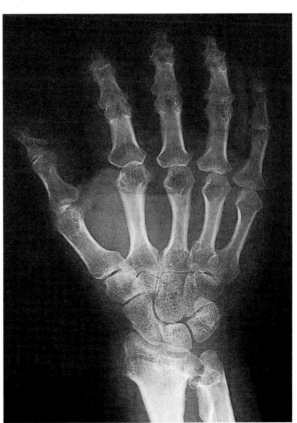

a

b

Fig. 2.**31a,b**   Typical short, thick phalanges and short metacarpals in achondroplasia. Note also the anomalous development of the distal radius and ulna.
a Child 4 months of age.

b Woman 53 years of age. Here the developmental anomalies of the distal radius and ulna have led to a kind of Madelung deformity.

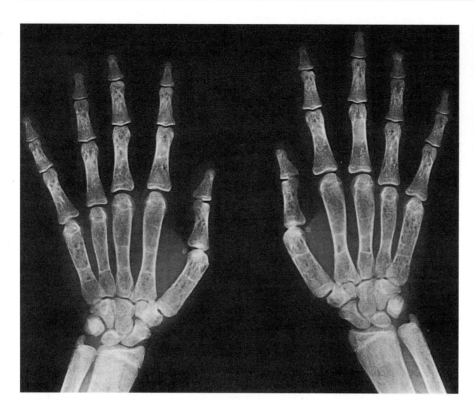

Fig. 2.**32** Typical skeletal changes in sickle cell anemia: marked widening of the medullary cavities and coarsening of the cancellous trabecular pattern. The patchy densities in the phalangeal shafts may represent dystrophic calcifications in circumscribed areas of marrow infarction.

manifested clinically by very painful swellings (hand-foot syndrome). **Infarctions** may be associated with **shortening of metacarpals, metatarsals, and phalanges** along with a general relative growth disturbance. The typical morphological and structural changes in thalassemia are illustrated in Fig. 2.**32**.

Oligoostotic and polyostotic **fibrous dysplasia** occasionally involve the bones of the hand. A combination of structural and morphological changes may be seen on radiographs (Fig. 2.**33**).

A generalized increase in bone density usually results from an increase in cortical thickness combined with an increase in the number and thickness of the cancellous trabeculae. A continuum exists between a **normal bone mass** and a **slight increase in bone mass**, which can be difficult to detect.

 Loss of the sharp cortical outline relative to the medullary cavity is indicative of disease (Fig. 2.**34a**).

In various Mediterranean ethnic groups and especially in black Africans, it can be normal for the bones of the hand to appear relatively dense on radiographic films.

One of the main causes of a uniform, generalized increase in bone density is **osteopetrosis** (Albers–Schönberg marble bone disease). A "bone-in-bone" appearance is characteristic of very severe cases. The less pronounced autosomal dominant forms present with a variable degree of cortical thickening and an increase in cancellous bone density (Fig. 2.**34a**).

In **pyknodysostosis**, the bones of the hand show a relatively uniform increase in density. The medullary cavity is preserved. The terminal phalanges become increasingly dysplastic during growth, resembling acro-osteolysis syndrome.

In **metaphyseal dysplasia** (Pyle disease), a slight increase in the density of the diaphyses, especially of the metacarpals, is accompanied by widening of the metaphyseal area due to deficient modeling (Erlenmeyer flask deformity). The cranial bones show increased sclerosis.

In **craniometaphyseal dysplasia**, cortical thickening and metaphyseal widening are observed in the bones of the hand. Cranial sclerosis is most pronounced in the base of the skull.

In **craniodiaphyseal dysplasia**, which produces coarse hyperostosis and sclerosis in the skull, the diaphyses of the tubular bones (especially the metacarpals in the hand) are expanded due to endosteal thickening of the cortical bone.

Endosteal hyperostosis (Worth type, van Buchem type, Fig. 2.**34c, d**) in the hand is marked by a generalized cortical hyperostosis with cortical thickening that progresses toward the medullary canal. The external shape of the tubular bone is usually preserved, but its total diameter may increase.

Besides these diseases, which are distinguishable by their genetic, clinical, and radiographic features, there are mixed presentations that do not fully conform to the entities listed above (**mixed sclerosing bone dysplasia**, Fig. 2.**38e, f**). In the hand, they can cause diverse skeletal changes with varying degrees of sclerosis and morphological changes.

An **acquired generalized increase in bone density** occurs rarely in advanced cases of **fluorosis**. **Osteomyelosclerosis** seldom causes an increase of bone density in the hand (Fig. 2.**34b**).

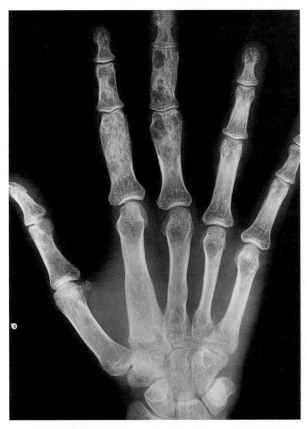

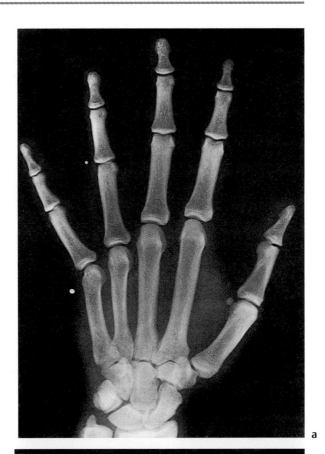

Fig. 2.**33** Polyostotic fibrous dysplasia (humerus and scapula are predominantly affected in this case). Note the coexistence of morphological and structural changes in the bones of the hand.

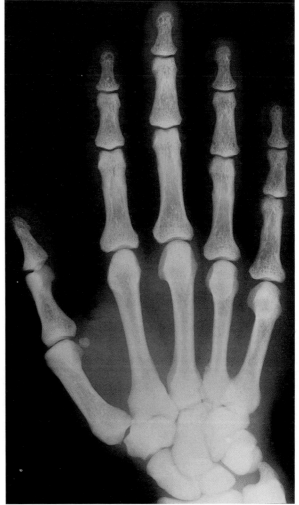

Fig. 2.**34 a–d** Various forms of hyperostosis. ▷
a Osteopetrosis, autosomal dominant form with a uniform, generalized increase in bone density. The ill-defined boundaries between the cortex and medullary cavity are typical. In extreme cases the uniform increase in density is accompanied by a "bone-in-bone" appearance.
b Osteomyelosclerosis.

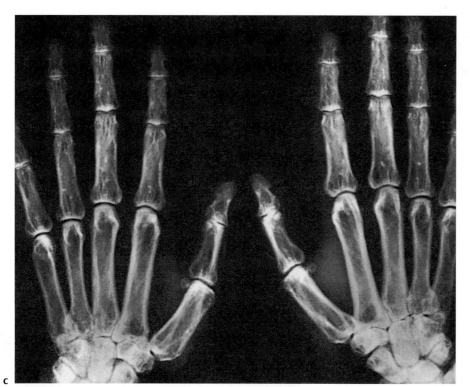

c

Fig. 2.**34 c, d**　Endosteal hyperostosis, van Buchem type. The 49-year-old father is in panel **c**, the 22-year-old daughter in panel **d**. An irregular increase in density is particularly evident in the daughter. In the father, the broadening of the tubular bones, especially the metacarpals, is a more conspicuous feature. The rest of the skeleton showed grotesque areas of bone expansion and zones of striated cancellous sclerosis. Clinically, both patients had diffuse, aching bone pain and hearing loss due to hyperostosis of the petrous bone with encasement of inner ear structures.

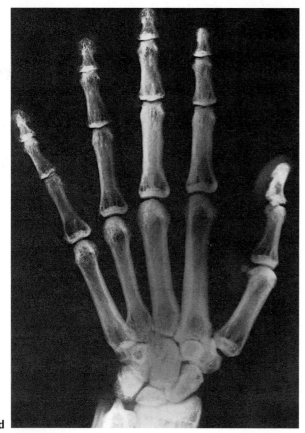

d

Fig. 2.**34 d**

Tuberous sclerosis is among the diseases that present with **irregular, patchy areas of increased density** and loss of corticomedullary differentiation, accompanied by irregular or cystlike lucencies and periosteal new bone formation (Fig. 2.**35**).

Sarcoidosis is characterized by **patchy sclerosis of the distal and middle phalanges** combined with cystlike lucencies in the metaphyses and destructive bone changes (Fig. 2.**36**). Less commonly, the dominant feature may be sclerosis with the expansion of one or more phalanges (Fig. 2.**37**). (See also p. 60, 76)

The hand is a site of predilection for skeletal sarcoidosis. The changes can be very diverse, and a detailed description would exceed our scope. Freyschmidt (1997) may be consulted for further details.

Multiple small foci of increased density are usually the result of **osteopoikilosis** (spotted bones). The round or oval areas of increased cancellous bone density measure 2–4 mm in size and generally occur near joints (Figs. 2.**38 a**, 2.**335 a, b**). More or less extensive changes are usually found in the carpal bones, the distal radius and ulna, and the periarticular portions of tubular bones. Generally this autosomal dominant condition is harmless and clinically asymptomatic, but cutaneous changes are occasionally described (dermatofibrosis lenticularis disseminata, keratoma hereditarium dissipatum palmare et plantare, proneness to keloid formation) (Freyschmidt and Freyschmidt 1996).

There are less pronounced, rudimentary forms of osteopoikilosis in which a few circumscribed areas of increased cancellous bone density occur in each hand, representing a true borderline condition between normal and pathological (Fig. 2.**38 b–d**).

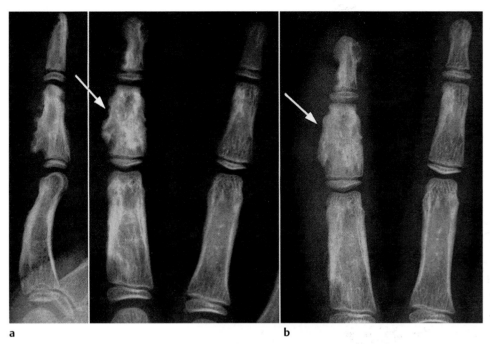

a   b

Fig. 2.**35 a, b** Serial radiographs of tuberous sclerosis with unusual changes in the bones of the hand. The boy presented at age 11 years with typical cutaneous lesions (angiofibromas, etc.) and neurological abnormalities (epilepsy, debility, etc.).
a Unusual periosteal new bone formation is seen along the proximal, middle, and distal phalanges of the index finger, with particularly heavy proliferation on the radial aspect of the middle phalanx. The diaphysis has lost its normal constriction or tubulation. Note the small cystic lucency on the ulnar side of the terminal tuft. When viewed in isolation, the changes in the middle phalanx resemble a florid reactive periostitis.
b Film three years later shows a slight increase and consolidation of the changes. Endosteal hyperostosis is also noted on the radial side of the adjacent middle phalanx of the third finger.

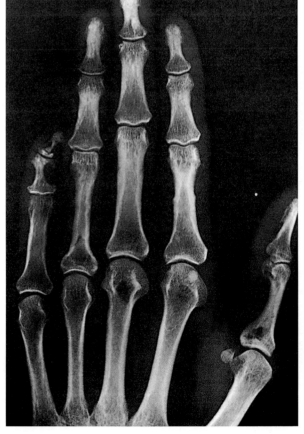

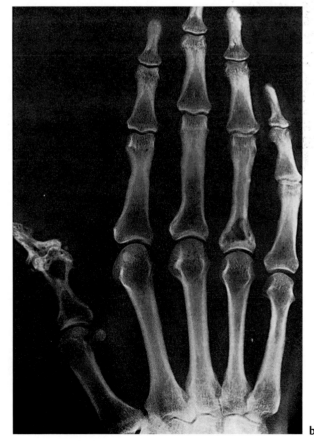

a   b

Fig. 2.**36 a, b** Typical manifestations of skeletal sarcoidosis in the bones of the hand: cancellous sclerosis in the distal phalanges, destructive changes in the fifth distal phalanx of the left hand, cystlike lucencies in the proximal phalanges of the thumb and fourth finger of both hands, and subperiosteal bone resorption with diaphyseal narrowing in the fourth proximal phalanx of both hands.

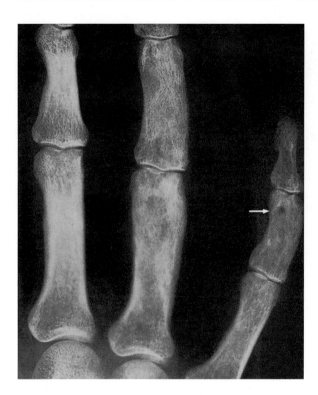

Fig. 2.**37** Sarcoidosis. All the phalanges of the third, fourth, and fifth fingers show ill-defined sclerosis. The fourth finger is expanded due to periosteal new bone formation. The small round lucency in the middle phalanx of the fifth finger (arrow) has been formed by confluent epitheloid cell granulomas.

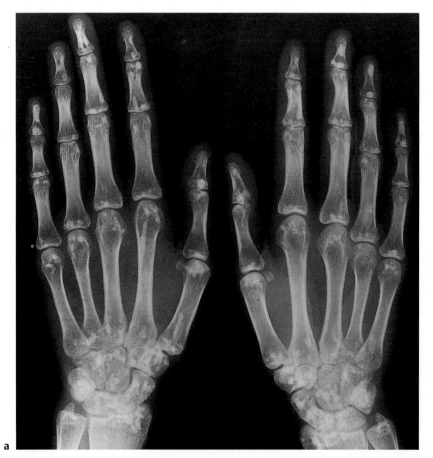

Fig. 2.**38 a–f** Osteopoikilosis and mixed sclerosing bone dysplasia.
a Fully developed form in an 18-year-old asymptomatic woman (incidental finding). Disseminated foci of increased density are seen in the cancellous bone near joints. There are also some linear areas of hyperostosis (e.g., in the second metacarpal and middle phalanx of the left hand) and coarse sclerotic foci in several terminal phalanges. The same patient had numerous foci of increased cancellous bone density scattered throughout the pelvis and the rest of the skeleton, especially near joints.

a

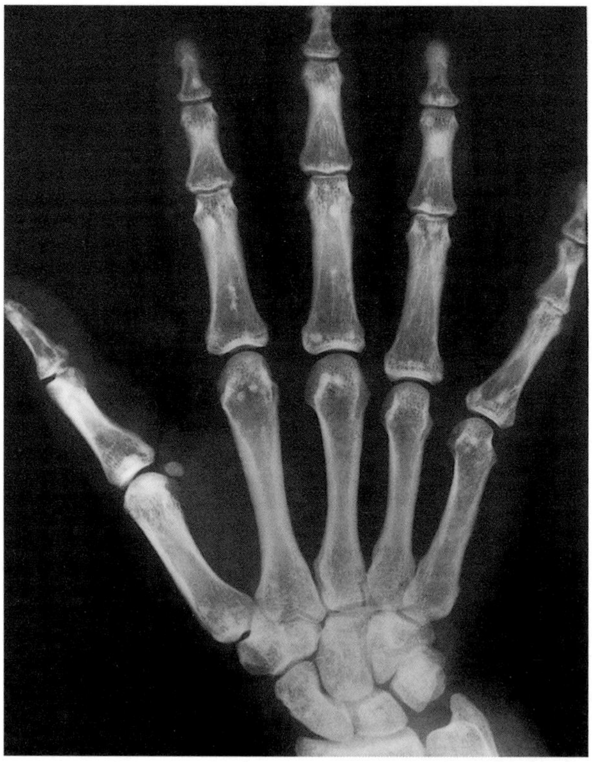
b

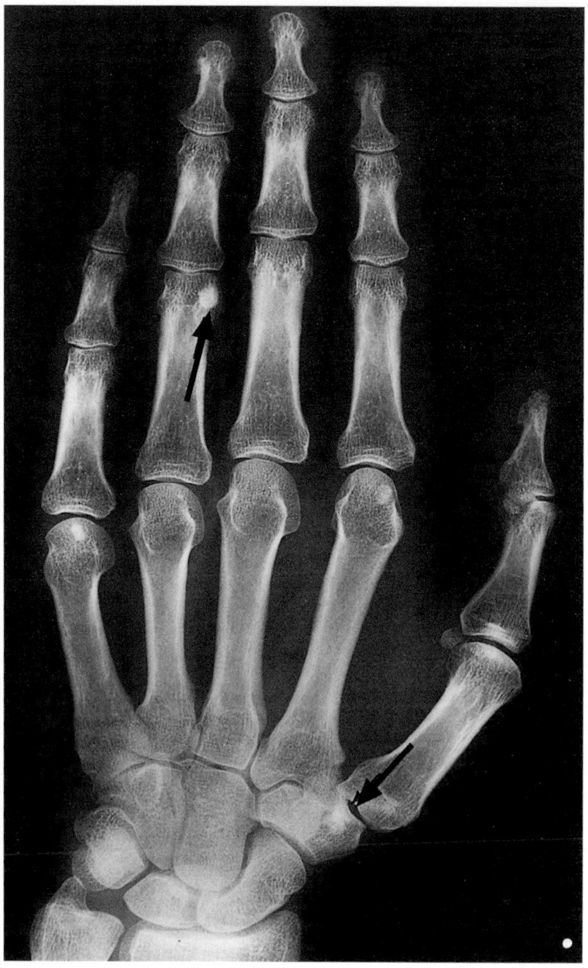
c

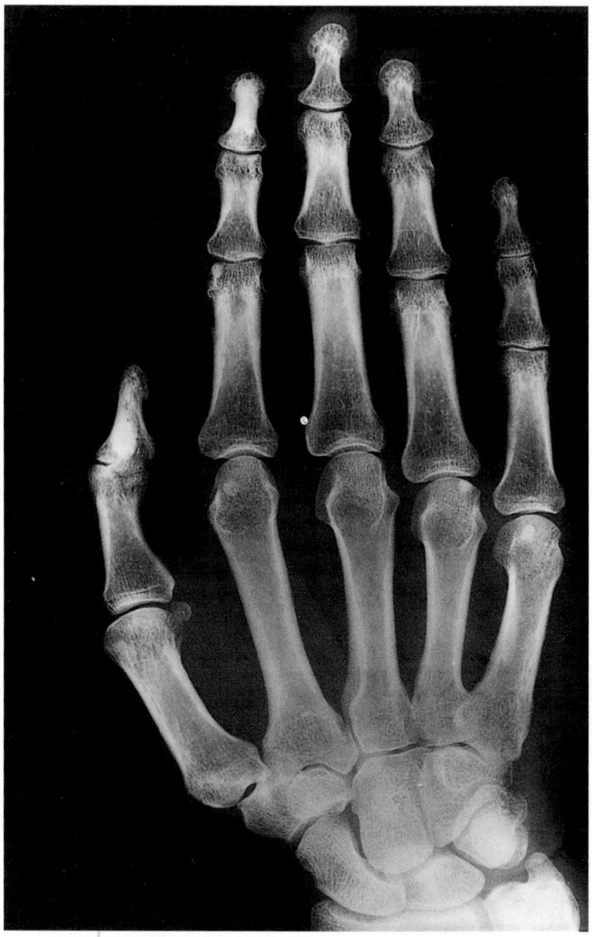
d

Fig. 2.**38 b–d** Panel **b** shows a less pronounced form of osteo-poikilosis; **c** and **d** show a rudimentary form with only isolated sclerotic foci. As in **a**, these patients had no skeletal symptoms.

Fig. 2.**38 e** and **f** ▷

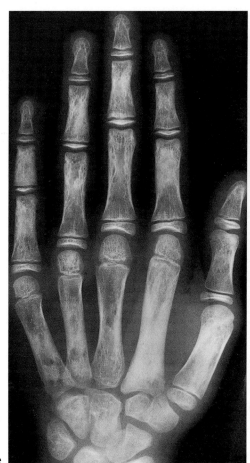
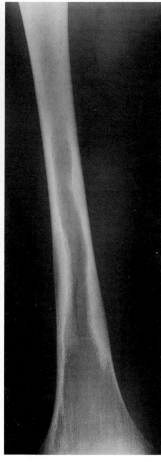

e   f

Fig. 2.**38 e, f**   Mixed sclerosing bone dysplasia, representing a mixed form of melorheostosis, osteopathia striata, and other hyperostoses.

Melorheostosis is characterized by sites of endosteal and periosteal new bone formation that resemble candle wax dripping down the bone (Fig. 2.**39**). Involvement of the hand is uncommon and is generally unilateral and confined to one or two rays, accompanied by manifestations in the rest of the arm. (Freyschmidt 2001)

The case of mixed sclerosing bone dysplasia shown in Fig. 2.**38 e, f** displays melorheostotic features.

Increased bone density in the hand can also result from purely **periosteal processes**, as in acquired **hypertrophic osteoarthropathy** (Fig. 2.**40**) or **EMO syndrome** (exophthalmos + myxedema pretibialis + osteopathy). It can also result from **congenital periostoses** such as **pachydermoperiostosis** (Fig. 2.**41**) or **hereditary palmoplantar keratosis** with clubbing of the fingers (watchglass nails) and bony hypertrophy (usually associated with acro-osteolysis, Fig. 2.**100**).

> Periosteal new bone formation in the hand is always a pathological sign. Not infrequently, the pathological process is not detectable on radiographs (despite clinical pain and swelling), but a radionuclide bone scan in these cases will usually show conspicuous, streaklike areas of increased tracer uptake (Fig. 2.**40 c**).

Fig. 2.**39**   Melorheostosis with extensive sites of endosteal ▷ and periosteal new bone formation in the fourth and fifth fingers. Radiographs showed additional changes in the right forearm and humerus of this 36-year-old man, who presented clinically with pain and subcutaneous changes.

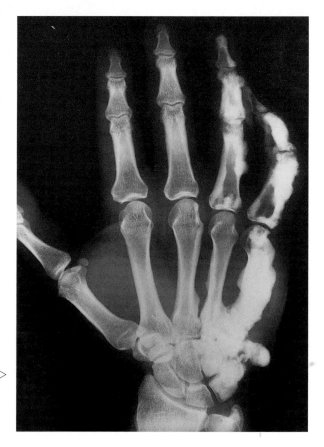

Fig. 2.**40a–c** Hypertrophic (pulmonary) osteoarthropathy and similar changes.
a Unusual manifestation of hypertrophic osteoarthropathy in a 6-year-old who presented clinically with neurodermatitis and severe asthma attacks. Note the solid periosteal new bone formations on the second and fourth metacarpals of the right hand. On several phalanges the periosteal new bone has already fused with the cortex, causing it to appear widened. Periosteal new bone was also visible on the right ulna. Extensive sites of periosteal bone formation were also found on the tibiae. The child presented clinically with variable pain and swellings on the hands and lower legs.

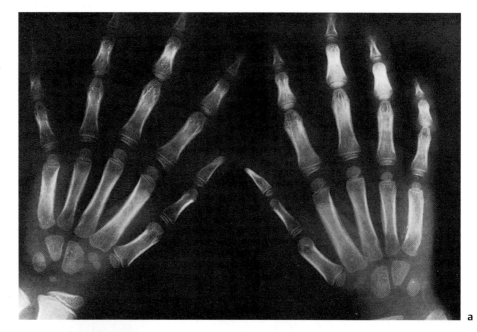

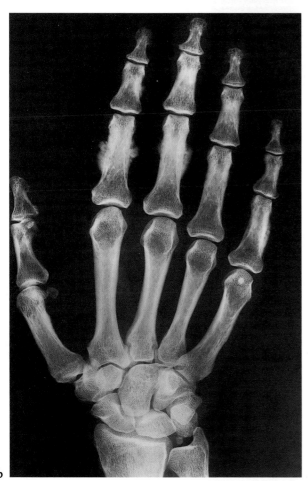

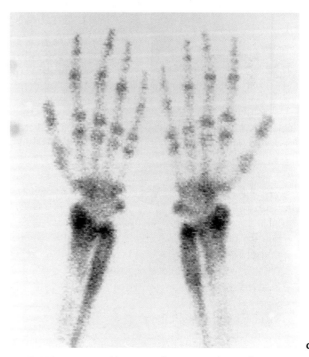

Fig. 2.**40b** Intestinal hypertrophic osteoarthropathy in a 73-year-old woman with Crohn disease. Extensive periosteal new bone formation is seen on the proximal phalanges of both hands and on the metatarsals (not shown).
c Bone scan of a generalized pathological periosteal process. Clinical findings included finger pain and swelling. Radiographs showed periosteal new bone on the radius and ulna. The bone scan shows a striated pattern of increased uptake with involvement of the metacarpals and phalanges. The underlying disease was identified as an hereditary palmoplantar keratosis with clubbing of the fingers and watchglass nails (see also Fig. 2.**100**).

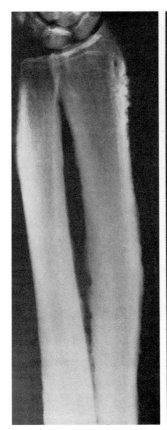
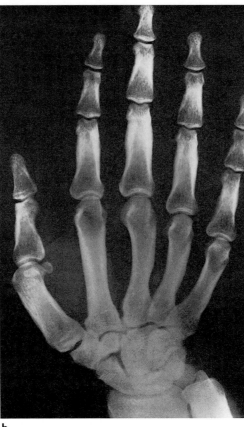

a   b

Fig. 2.**41 a, b** Pachydermoperiostosis with extensive periosteal new bone that has already fused with the cortex on the metacarpals, proximal phalanges, radius, and ulna, forming an irregular, undulating contour that is most conspicuous on the radius and ulna. The affected bone areas appear markedly broadened and thickened (undertubulation). Clinical findings included clubbing of the fingers, cutis verticis gyrata on the forehead and nuchal area, thickening of the upper eyelid, and thickened palmar skin.

Table 2.**3** Congenital or childhood-acquired diseases that are associated with oligo-ostotic or polyostotic periosteal new bone formation (from Freyschmidt 1997)

- Melorheostosis
- Camurati–Engelmann disease
- Pachydermoperiostosis
- Infantile cortical hyperostosis (Caffey disease)
- Rubella; infectious mononucleosis
- Congenital syphilis
- Chronic recurring multifocal periostotis
- Battered child syndrome
- Scurvy
- Vitamin A and D intoxication
- Inflammatory bowel diseases (e.g., ulcerative colitis)
- Leukemia
- Hemoglobinopathies
- Hemophilia
- Pulmonary hypertrophic osteoarthropathy (e.g., in honeycomb lung)
- Prostaglandin E-induced

Table 2.**5** Conditions associated with predominantly monostotic periosteal new bone formation (from Freyschmidt 1997)

- Inflammatory (osteomyelitis, osteitis, periostitis)
- Metaplastic/inflammatory (?): florid reactive periostitis
- Neoplastic (primary or secondary bone tumors)
- Impaired blood flow (e.g., unilateral varicose symptom complex, vascular malformations)
- Traumatic (mechanical, thermal, electrical)
- Pustulotic arthro-osteitis (SAPHO)
- Idiopathic

Table 2.**4** Adult diseases that are associated with oligo-ostotic or polyostotic periosteal new bone formation (usually solid, undulating, or straight-line pattern, rarely lamellar) (from Freyschmidt 1997)

- Pulmonary hypertrophic osteoarthropathy
- Gastrointestinal hypertrophic osteoarthropathy (ulcerative colitis, Crohn disease)
- Hypertrophic osteoarthropathy in cystic pancreatic fibrosis
- Pachydermoperiostosis
- EMO syndrome (exophthalmos, myxedema, osteopathy)
- Collagen diseases (especially polyarteritis, progressive scleroderma, lupus erythematosus)
- Rheumatoid arthritis
- Reiter disease, psoriasis (periarticular)
- Infectious mononucleosis
- Sarcoidosis (hands, feet)
- Multi-infarct processes (e.g., pancreatitis)
- Diabetes mellitus
- Acromegaly
- Disturbances of arterial and venous blood flow (e.g., varicose symptom complex)
- Lymphedema
- Retinoid induced
- Fluorosis
- Vitamin D hypervitaminosis in treatment of renal osteodystrophy
- Milk-alkali syndrome
- Hemoglobinopathies (especially with necrotic bone marrow changes)
- Coagulation disorders with subperiosteal bleeding
- Osteomyelosclerosis
- Syphilitic periostitis
- Periosteal new bone formation mimicked in hyperparathyroidism (by disruption of the outer cortex)

The etiologically diverse diseases that are associated with periosteal new bone formation are listed in Tables 2.**3**–2.**5**.

Generalized loss of bone density in the hand with cortical thinning and rarefaction of cancellous bone in the metaphyses is observed in osteopenia and osteoporosis. This loss of density is always very uniform and distinct. The value of the Barnett–Nordin index in differentiating borderline-normal from pathological findings was mentioned on p. 20. Congenital osteopenia is found in hypothyroidism, in various forms of pseudohypoparathyroidism (generally combined with shortening of the fourth and fifth metacarpals, Fig. 2.**30**), and in Klinefelter syndrome (Fig. 2.**42**).

In osteomalacia, the cancellous bone structures have a blurred or hazy appearance due to the presence of non-mineralized osteoid, as if rubbed with an eraser. They take on a ground-glass appearance. Intracortical striations may also be seen (Fig. 2.**43**).

In early forms of hyperparathyroidism (see also p. 88), the only radiographic findings are fraying of the cortex and ragged bone contours as a result of a "lacelike" subperiosteal resorption (Fig. 2.**44**).

Patchy periarticular demineralization occurs mainly in trophic disturbances (e.g., due to disuse, Figs. 2.**45**, 2.**46**), in Sudeck syndrome (Fig. 2.**47 a–c**), or with an exaggerated regional acceleratory phenomenon (RAP, Fig. 2.**47 d–f**). Karasik and Karasik (1982) described an unusual case of **"osteoporosis" confined to the fourth and fifth rays of both hands** in a woman with diabetes mellitus and peripheral ulnar neuropathy.

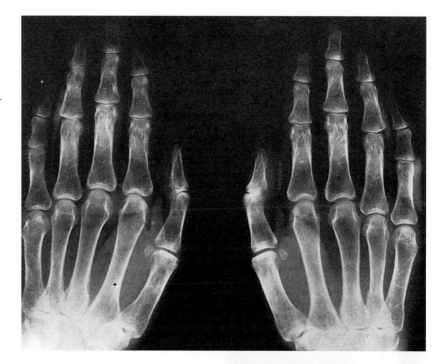

Fig. 2.**42** Pronounced osteoporosis in a 55-year-old man with Klinefelter syndrome. Radiograph shows severe thinning of the diaphyseal cortex, especially in the metacarpal region, with a peripheral Barnett–Nordin index less than 20% (index = ratio of cortical thickness to total midshaft diameter of the second or third metacarpal; 43–44% is normal; see text). The bony structures appear very distinct and sharp like "pencil tracings."

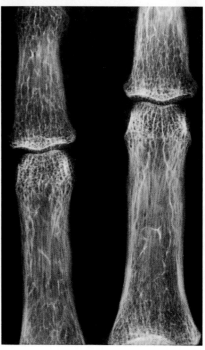

Fig. 2.**43** Hazy cancellous bone structures (ground-glass phenomenon) and cortical striations in incipient osteomalacia.

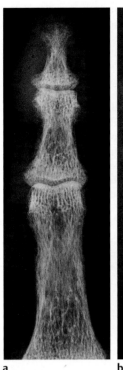
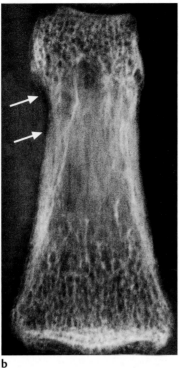

a   b

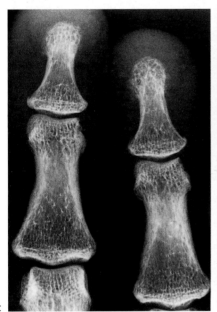
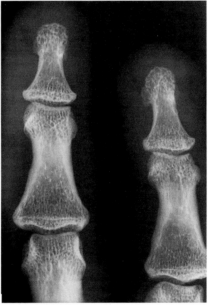

c

Fig. 2.44 a–c Secondary hyperparathyroidism with renal osteopathy.

a Subperiosteal bone resorption results in a fuzzy, spiculated outer cortical margin. Intracortical striations and cortical thinning are also present, along with severe acro-osteolysis.

b Close-up view of subperiosteal bone resorption at the metaphyseal-diaphyseal junction. Note the "roughening" of the cortical margin and the reticulostriate lucencies in the radial and ulnar aspects of the cortex. Direct magnification radiograph.

c Another case with 4-year follow-up. The subtle areas of cortical rarefaction in the film on the left, especially in the middle phalanges, are appreciated only when compared with the film on the right, which was taken four years later after parathyroidectomy. Note also the erosion of the phalangeal tufts in the left panel.

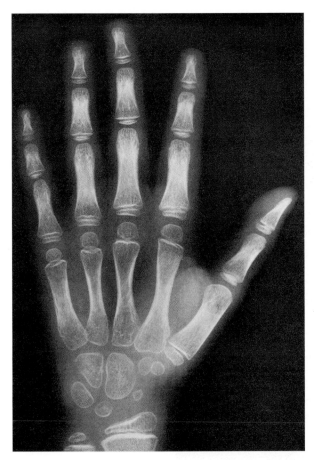

Fig. 2.**45**   Disuse osteoporosis in a 7-year-old child following prolonged cast immobilization after an injury.

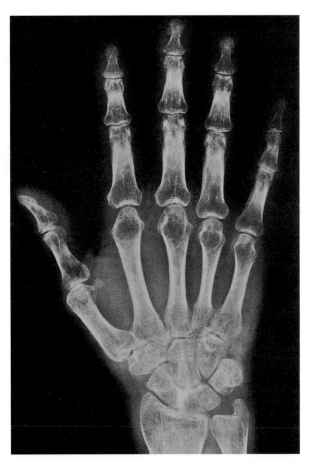

Fig. 2.**46**   Bandlike, periarticular disuse osteoporosis in a 36-year-old man after five weeks' immobilization for an elbow injury. The patient had no clinical symptoms of Sudeck atrophy.

Fig. 2.**47 a–f**   Trophic skeletal changes in the hand.
a Typical Sudeck changes with patchy demineralization affecting all periarticular segments. Remaining cancellous bone structures in the demineralized areas have a ground-glass appearance. Characteristic clinical symptoms were present.
Fig. 2.**47 b–f** ▷

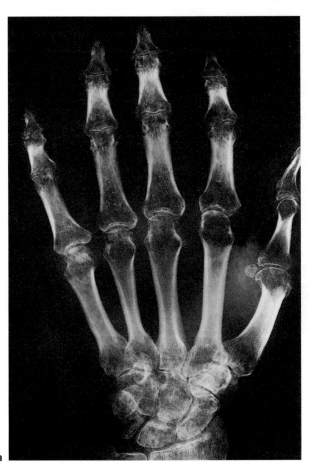

a

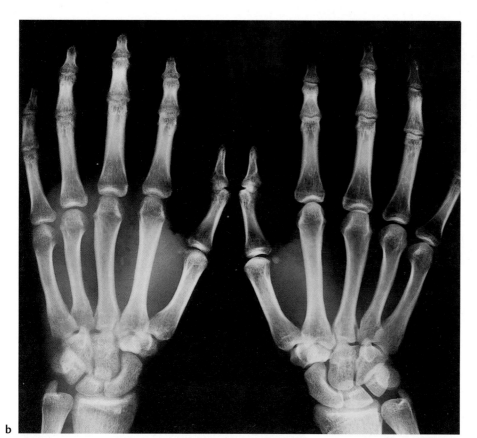

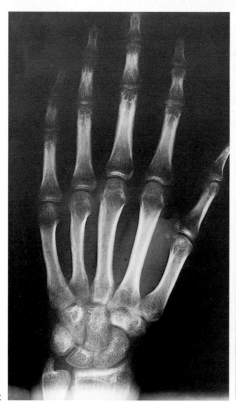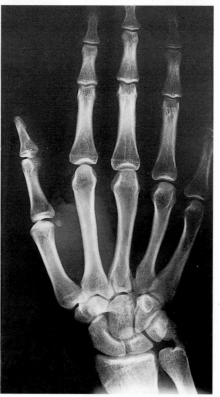

b

c

Fig. 2.**47 b, c** Development of Sudeck dystrophy in the left hand. Panel **b** shows initial "hazy" demineralization in the carpus and around the metacarpophalangeal and proximal interphalangeal joints. Soft-tissue swelling. All Sudeck criteria were present clinically. Panel **c** shows a massive increase in patchy periarticular demineralization three weeks later.

Fig. 2.**47 d–f**   Severe trophic changes but no Sudeck dystrophy following replantation of a traumatically amputated hand (**d** taken on 27 March 1997, **e** on 27 June 1997). Film two years later (**f**) shows almost completely normal bone structures in the left hand. The trophic demineralization reflects an exaggerated RAP. In contrast to the foot, where traumatic trophic changes tend to cause necrosis, the bones in the hand tend to undergo Sudeck-type changes with little if any necrosis. (Case courtesy of Dr. H. Vossmann, Bremen.)

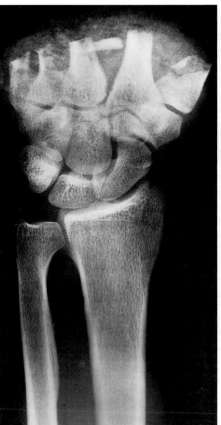

d

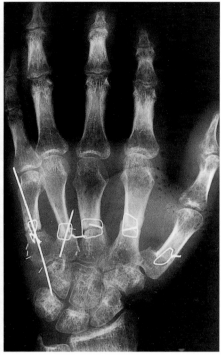

e

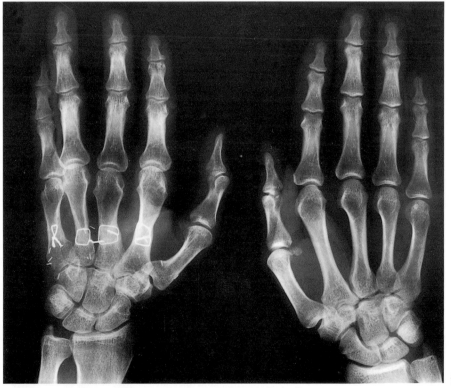

f

Fracture?

The nutrient canals and projection-related linear lucencies described above (Figs. 2.8, 2.9) should not be mistaken for fine fracture lines in patients with a prior history of trauma. A nutrient canal whose site of entry into the bone is projected clear on an oblique or lateral radiograph is particularly apt to be misinterpreted as a cortical fissure. Prominent bony tendon attachments should not be mistaken for fracture callus or periosteal pathology (see Figs. 2.3b, 2.9b, c, and 2.40b).

Metaplastic ossification, regardless of its cause, and small sesamoids can mimic bony ligament or capsule avulsions. A traumatic bone fragment should always be suspected if the geometry of the bony element is such that it could be fitted precisely into a defect in the adjacent bone.

The occasional duplication of a sesamoid (Fig. 2.48) can be misinterpreted as a fracture (Fig. 2.49). True sesamoid fractures are rare and are usually caused by extreme abduction of the thumb (e.g., in bracing or falling). This typically results in a flake fracture with a crescent-shaped fragment (Fig. 2.49), but comminuted fractures and simple avulsions (Fig. 2.50) can also occur.

Besides the rare sesamoid fractures of the thumb (q.v.), sesamoid fractures involving the index finger and small finger have also been described (Wood 1984). Mentally "fitting" the fragment back into the adjacent sesamoid, as described above, is a useful aid to diagnosis. If the bones are large enough, the fragment may display an irregular surface without a cortex and may be displaced by hematoma or posttraumatic soft-tissue swelling. Dislocations with interposition of the sesamoid into the metacarpophalangeal joint have been described (Sweterlitsch et al. 1959).

Contour defects, especially in the bases of the proximal phalanges, may signify an old injury (Figs. 2.51, 2.52). Very rarely, old healed erosions due to inflammatory joint processes may have the same appearance.

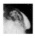

Necrosis?

During Growth

Dense **"ivory epiphyses"** (white epiphyses) may occur as a normal radiographic variant in children (Figs. 2.15, 2.54b). The distal phalanges are most commonly involved, followed by the proximal phalanges and fifth middle phalanx. The cause of these dense epiphyseal centers remains unclear (delayed differentiation of cancellous bone structures?). The reported prevalence of ivory epiphyses is 0.35% of 8536 children between 2.5 and 13 years of age. Ivory epiphyses may be inherited as an autosomal dominant trait (Poznanski 1984). They may also occur in skeletal growth retardation (hypothyroidism), trichorhinophalangeal syndrome, Cockayne syndrome, and also in renal osteodystrophy.

Some authors (e.g., v. d. Laan and Thijn 1986) have equated ivory epiphyses with **Thiemann disease** (Figs. 2.53, 2.54a), an autosomal dominant developmental disorder that occurs more in older children and adolescents. Characterized by increased density, widening, and fragmentation of the epiphyses, this disease may resolve

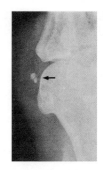
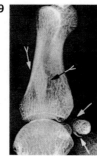
Fig. 2.48   Fig. 2.49

Fig. 2.48   Duplicated sesamoid.

Fig. 2.49   Flake fracture of a sesamoid (single arrows). The dense area in the proximal phalanx (double arrows) is a small bone island.

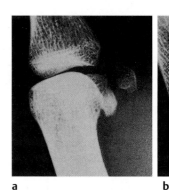
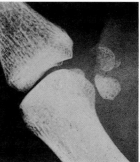

a   b

Fig. 2.50a, b   Sesamoid fracture.

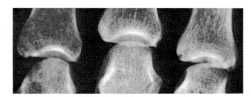

Fig. 2.51   Marked contour defects in the heads of the metacarpals (left) and in the ulnar base of the proximal phalanx (right). Very dense, slightly irregular subchondral plates are also visible along the proximal phalanges. The patient had engaged in heavy boxing workouts since childhood.

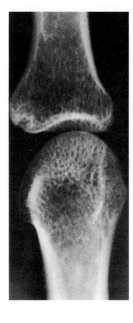

Fig. 2.52   Traumatic chip fracture from the medial base of a proximal phalanx, not to be confused with an arthritic erosion or a degenerative subchondral cyst.

completely but occasionally leaves permanent residual structural and morphological changes (Fig. 2.**55**).

Whereas ivory epiphyses are an incidental finding, Thiemann disease presents clinically with fusiform joint swelling that predominantly affects the interphalangeal joints. Gradually the swelling becomes painful and limits extension of the affected fingers. On radiographs the epiphyses show flattening, central fragmentation, and lateral displacement (Figs. 2.**53**, 2.**54a**). Occasionally the disease is associated with epiphyseal growth disturbances in other regions such as the hip. We feel that Thiemann disease merits the term "disease" because it is associated with clinical symptoms. Clinically and radiographically, it appears to involve a transient ischemic necrosis with a poten-

tial for full recovery, similar, for example, to the osteochondrosis of the knee joint that occurs in preadolescents.

When the radiographic changes of Thiemann disease occur in the metacarpal epiphyses, the condition is known as **Dieterich disease** (Fig. 2.**56**). It, too, is marked by pain, swelling, and limited motion.

Generally dense, fragmented epiphyses are characteristic of **stippled epiphyses** (Conradi–Hünermann disease, Fig. 2.**57**). Involvement of the hand is rare, however.

Generalized epiphyseal irregularities are also seen in **multiple epiphyseal dysplasia** (Fairbank disease), which may represent a tarda form of Conradi–Hünermann disease.

Fig. 2.**53** Juvenile epiphyseal abnormalities in the fingers and toes at age 16 years. (After Thiemann.)

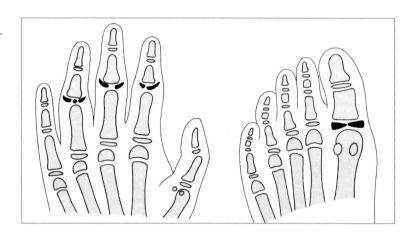

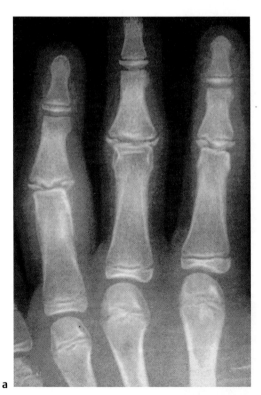

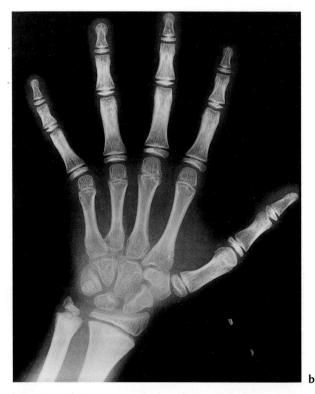

a   b

Fig. 2.**54a, b** Thiemann disease and ivory epiphyses.
a Thiemann disease presents with marked soft-tissue swelling, pain, and limited motion.

b Ivory epiphyses are usually detected incidentally in asymptomatic patients.

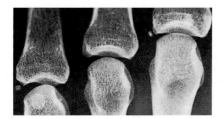

Fig. 2.**55**   Late findings after Thiemann disease.

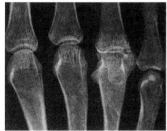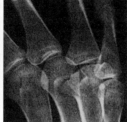

Fig. 2.**56**   Dieterich disease involving the head of the right fourth metacarpal in a 34-year-old woman.

Severe frostbite can lead to osteonecrosis of the hand bones, especially the distal phalanges, as a result of trophic disturbances (Wulle 1991). Figure 2.**58** shows a case in a growing child. The frostbite damaged the distal epiphyseal plates, stunting the growth of the distal phalanges.

Another disease marked by osteonecrosis of the growth cartilage is **Kashin–Beck disease** (Fig. 2.**59**). This disease is endemic mainly in Siberia, Russia, North Korea, and certain regions of China. It is a chronic, degenerative osteoarthropathy of unknown cause with a peak incidence between 5 and 13 years of age. Affecting the hyaline cartilage in bones formed by enchondral ossification, it can occur anywhere in the skeleton but has a predilection for the peripheral extremity bones. Atrophy and necrosis of the chondrocytes give way to reparative processes in the deeper zones of the growth cartilage (Wung et al. 1996), resulting in irregular epiphyseal contours, irregular calcification and contours of the metaphyses, premature closure of growth plates, etc. The epiphyses may appear cone-shaped in some cases. The features of Kashin–Beck disease in the wrist are discussed by Yu et al (2002). The presumed causes include malnutrition and extreme environmental conditions such as a short, wet summer or long, cold winter.

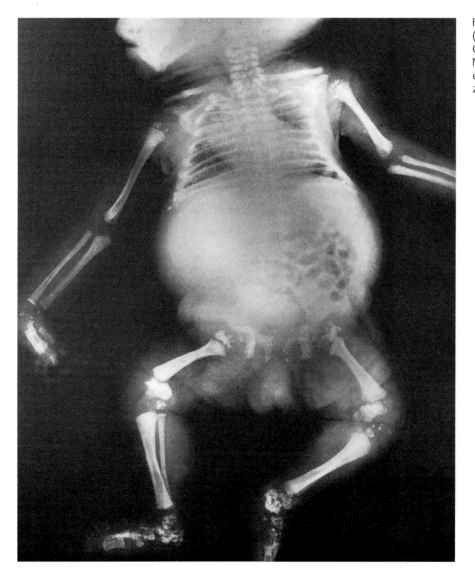

Fig. 2.**57**   Stippled epiphyses (chondrodysplasia punctata, Conradi–Hünermann disease). Note the small, fragmented epiphyseal centers in all growth zones.

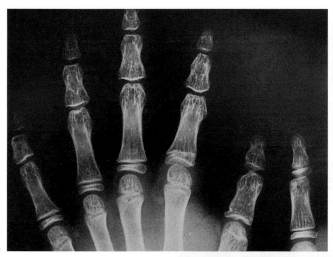
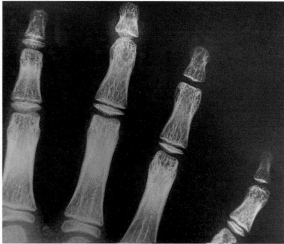
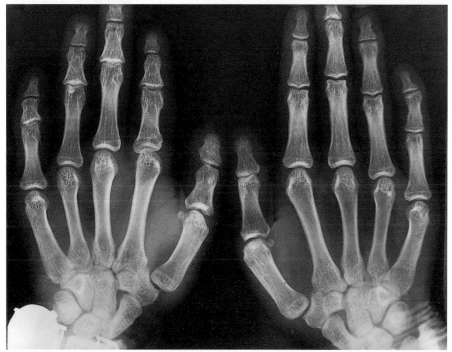

Fig. 2.**58 a–c**   Frostbite in a growing child.
a, b Radiographs taken three years after a severe frostbite injury (at age 7 years the boy lost his way in the snow) show closure of the epiphyseal plates of the third through fifth distal phalanges on the right side, along with radial deviation of the distal phalanx of the small finger due to uneven development of the head of the middle phalanx. On the left side, the head of the first metacarpal is deformed, and the epiphyseal plates of the first proximal phalanx, second through fifth middle pha-

langes, and all distal phalanges are closed. The terminal tufts are also deformed.
c Radiograph taken many years later shows marked deformity of almost all the fingers, especially in the left hand, where the distal phalanges and several other phalanges are short compared with the right hand. Note the similarities to Kashin–Beck disease. (With kind permission of Dr. C. Wulle, Nürnberg; see also Wulle 1991.)

The **phalangeal microgeodic syndrome** (see also p. 87) is another trophic disease in children that has been considered to be a transient disturbance of the peripheral circulation due to cold. The syndrome has been observed principally in Japan (Meller, et al. 1982). It frequently occurs in wintertime. The patients have frostbite-like symptoms (spindle-shaped swelling, redness, local heat and mild pain) in one or several fingers. Radiographically, the involved phalanges show sclerosis with multiple small areas of osteolysis ("microgeodes") and a widening of the bones. The middle or proximal phalanges of the second and third fingers are usually affected. Histological findings

reveal osteonecrosis and reparative processes in the cortex and bone marrow. The prognosis of the disease is excellent with regression of the clinical and radiological symptoms within several months. The differential diagnosis of the disease includes tuberculous osteitis and sarcoidosis.

Finally, **extreme mechanical stresses** on the epiphyses during growth can produce more or less circumscribed areas of osteonecrosis. Figure 2.**51** illustrates a case following years of boxing workouts.

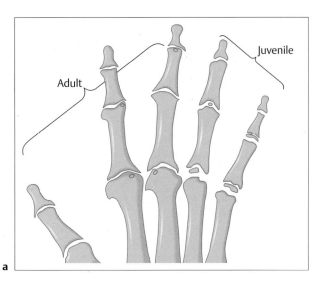

a

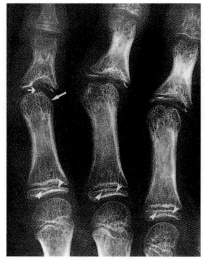

b

Fig. 2.**59 a, b**   Kashin–Beck disease.
a Schematic diagram (after Dihlmann). The features in adults are those of polyarticular degenerative arthritis.

b Kashin–Beck disease in a 10-year-old boy shows abnormal flattening of the metaphyses of the middle phalanges with fragmented residual epiphyses. Note the irregularities of the calcification lines around the epiphyses of the proximal phalanges. (From Wung et al. 1996.)

 ## In Adulthood

Osteonecrosis in specific bones of the hand and wrist, especially early forms, are discussed in the sections that deal with specific bones (e.g., metacarpus, lunate and scaphoid necrosis).

It should be noted that **sesamoids** can occasionally be affected by necrosis (Fig. 2.**60**). The early stage is characterized by demineralization and the late stage by increased density and fragmentation. If there are doubts as to the pathological significance of a somewhat dense or demineralized sesamoid, they can be resolved by radionuclide bone scanning with a pinhole collimator.

> If a dense sesamoid shows definite increased uptake on a bone scan, it is abnormal and should be surgically removed.

Another form of osteonecrosis is **acro-osteolysis**. Very early cases are manifested by loss of contour definition of the terminal tufts of one or more phalanges. These changes can be detected only on fine-detail radiographs (mammographic technique) that are viewed with a magnifying lens (e.g., Fig. 2.**44 c**). The most frequent causes of acro-osteolysis are listed in Table 2.**6**.

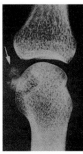

a

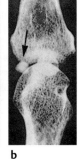

b

Fig. 2.**60 a, b**   Foci of osteonecrosis in the sesamoid of the thumb.
a Early form.
b Late "condensed" form.

Table 2.**6**   Principal causes of acro-osteolysis in the fingers and toes (from Freyschmidt 1997).

Trophic (vascular, neurogenic)
- Raynaud syndrome
- Scleroderma, Sharp syndrome
- Epidermolysis bullosa
- Ichthyosiform erythroderma
- Mutilating keratoderma
- Chronic acrodermatitis (Pick–Herxheimer)
- Neurosyphilis, syringomyelia, leprosy
- Hyperostosis with pachyderma (Uehlinger syndrome)
- Septic shock
- Hypertrophic osteoarthropathy

Traumatic
- Thermal burn or frostbite
- Electrical injury
- Chronic exposure to ionizing radiation
- Chronic excessive mechanical loads (e.g., in violinists or guitar players)

Hormonal
- Primary and secondary hyperparathyroidism
- Diabetes mellitus
- Pheochromocytoma

Toxic
- Occupational exposure to polyvinylchloride

Idiopathic (familial) (acro-)osteolysis

Gorham's disease (vanishing bone disease)

Other vascular malformations

Gorlin–Goltz syndrome

Ainhum syndrome

Pyknodysostosis

Sarcoidosis

Psoriasis

Gout

Tumors (metastases, squamous cell carcinoma, etc.)

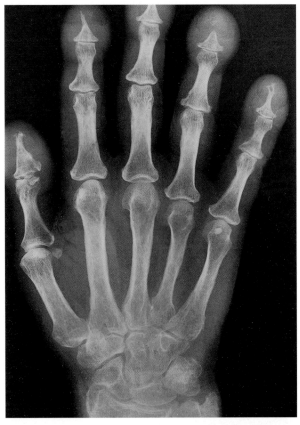

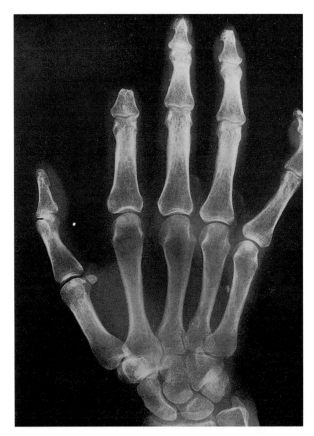

Fig. 2.**61**   Acro-osteolysis syndrome in pachydermoperiostosis.

Fig. 2.**62**   Acro-osteolysis in a collagen disease.

Figures 2.**61**, 2.**62**, and 2.**88** illustrate advanced stages of acro-osteolysis in patients with pachydermoperiostosis and a collagen disease.

 ## Inflammation?

Joints

Erosion is a definite radiographic sign of an inflammatory synovial process, regardless of whether the process is systemic or caused by bacterial infection (Figs. 2.**63**, 2.**132 a, b**, and 2.**133**).

Erosions require differentiation from older **traumatic contour defects** in periarticular bone (Figs. 2.**52**, 2.**64**). Traumatic bony avulsions and chip fractures generally have a solid sclerotic border, and no structural changes are found in the surrounding cancellous bone. Most of these lesions are solitary. Rarely they may involve multiple periarticular bone segments, especially in individuals who do very strenuous work with their hands. Inflammatory erosions usually are poorly demarcated from the exposed cancellous bone, and the surrounding bone shows patchy demineralization, as illustrated for rheumatoid arthritis in Fig. 2.63 **a** and for bacterial arthritis in Fig. 2.63 **b**. In inac-

tive cases of rheumatoid arthritis, reparative processes tend to resurface the erosive defects, simulating the appearance of a chip fracture (Fig. 2.**65**).

A detailed review of the diagnosis and differential diagnosis of inflammatory systemic joint changes in the hand is beyond our scope. It is important, however, to consider **polyarticular osteoarthritis** in the differential diagnosis of proximal and distal interphalangeal joint disease. Radiographs show more or less pronounced polyarticular degenerative changes in more than 60% of all adults over 50 years of age. Active phases are marked by pain and swelling (activated osteoarthritis) and can mimic a primary synovial inflammatory joint process.

Osteoarthritis of the distal interphalangeal joints (Heberden type) and proximal interphalangeal joints (Bouchard type) is characterized by varying degrees of symmetrical joint space narrowing, increased density of the subchondral bone plates, fine periarticular calcifications, and soft-tissue densities (Figs. 2.**66**, 2.**67**).

In more pronounced cases, productive bone changes lead to the formation of winglike osteophytes at the bases of the distal phalanges. These require differentiation from the "protuberances" seen in **psoriatic arthritis** (Figs. 2.**68**, 2.**133**).

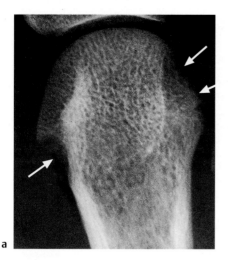

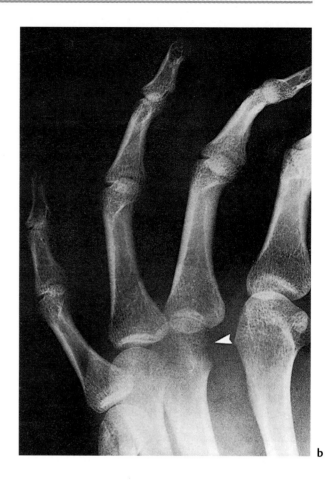

Fig. 2.**63 a, b** Joint erosions associated with inflammatory synovial processes.

a Rheumatoid arthritis.

b Articular panaritium. Note the erosion of the subchondral plate (arrow) and the narrowing of the associated joint space due to cartilage destruction.

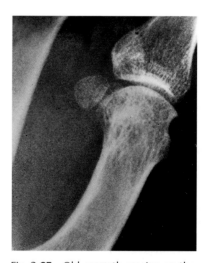

Fig. 2.**64** Marginal erosions in inactive rheumatoid arthritis. The erosions feature smooth edges and a reactive sclerotic rim, mimicking old avulsion fractures.

Fig. 2.**65** Old, smooth erosion on the radial side of the head of the first metacarpal.

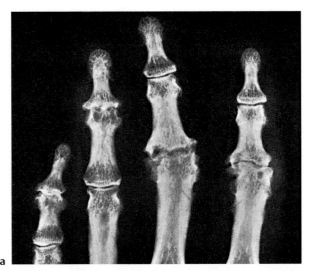

a

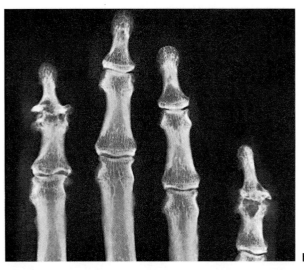

b

Fig. 2.**66 a, b** Polyarticular osteoarthritis. The winglike flaring of the bases of the distal phalanges at the affected joints is caused by bony proliferation, which is always accompanied by subchondral degenerative cysts in the same bone or in the ar-

ticulating bone. The affected distal interphalangeal joints show a mixed pattern of destruction, sclerosis, and small subchondral cysts.

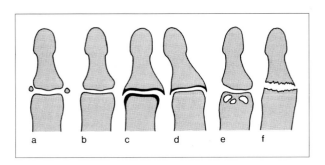

Fig. 2.**67 a–f** Radiographic signs of distal interphalangeal osteoarthritis, shown in the most common sequence of their development. (After Schacherl and Schilling.)
a Small periarticular ossicles.
b Joint space narrowing.
c Subchondral sclerosis and marginal spurs.
d Deviation of the distal phalanx.
e Subchondral cysts.
f Destructive joint changes.

The latter disease is also associated with productive bone changes involving, for example, the periosteum along the shafts of the small tubular bones. Figure 2.**69** shows the typical distribution patterns of early polyarticular changes in the hand that are observed in various diseases.

Chondrocalcinosis usually affects the metacarpophalangeal joints (Figs. 2.**70**, 2.**134**). If the cartilage does not calcify, the presence of beaklike or hanging-drop osteophytes on the radial aspect of the subchondral bone ("drooping osteophytes") can provide an important diagnostic clue. Similar productive bone changes can occur normally in hands that are subjected to heavy mechanical loads. Differentiation is aided by clinical symptomatology, since goutlike attacks can be a relatively specific sign of chondrocalcinosis. Also, chondrocalcinosis tends to involve different joints, especially in the carpus where scapholunate collapse is a typical finding.

Multicentric reticulohistiocytosis is associated with granulomatous changes in the skin and mucous membranes. The granulomatous synovial changes lead to predominantly central joint erosions that can progress rapidly to joint destruction (Freyschmidt and Freyschmidt 1996).

Bones

Inflammatory (osteomyelitic) changes in the bones of the hand are generally quite rare and mostly result from advanced inflammation due to bacterial arthritis. An early sign is conspicuous radiolucency of the affected bone, usually combined with fine periosteal new bone formation and adjacent intracortical bone resorption (cortical tunneling or striation). Reactive new bone formation does not occur until the reparative stage, when the bone shows a patchy, streaklike pattern of increased density.

A **bone felon** (osseous panaritium) most commonly occurs in the distal phalanx. Its early stage is generally marked by fine contour and structural irregularities (Fig. 2.**71**).

There is no danger of clinical confusion with acro-osteolysis syndrome, which generally is nonpainful. A bicompartment (bone and joint) inflammatory-destructive process following a bone and joint injury is shown in Fig. 2.**72**.

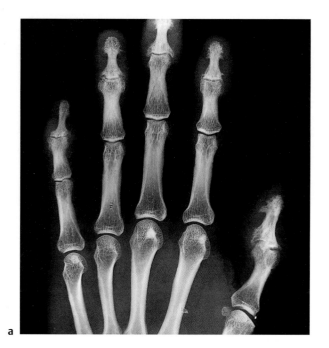

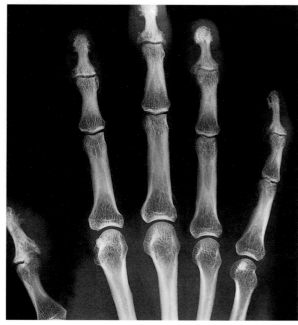

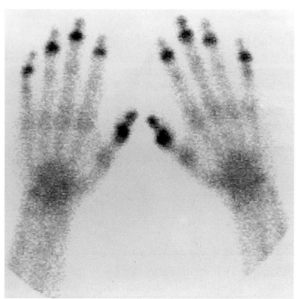

Fig. 2.**68 a–c** Psoriatic arthritis. Note the spiculated productive changes in the terminal tufts and the protuberances at the bases of the distal phalanges, most pronounced in the third and fourth fingers of the left hand and the second through fourth fingers of the right hand. The active proliferative changes are also vividly demonstrated in the bone scan shown in **c**.

Polyostotic **Paget disease** (very rarely monostotic) can present initially with rarefaction in one or more phalanges, followed by an increasing mixed pattern of coarsened trabecular structures, speckled or patchy densities and expansion, and culminating in conspicuous linear striations with bone expansion (Fig. 2.**73**).

Skeletal sarcoidosis (p. 40, 76) is the most important of the inflammatory-granulomatous processes that may be manifested in the bones of the hand. It usually shows a mixed radiographic pattern that may resemble dysplastic changes (Fig. 2.**36**). Sclerosis may be confined to the distal phalanges, as mentioned above, or additional sclerotic changes may occur in the bone or arise from the periosteum. Punched-out defects are seen in the cancellous bone of the phalanges, and radiographs occasionally show thinned areas due to bone erosion by subperiosteal granulomas or even frank destructive changes. At times, sarcoidosis can simulate the appearance of a chronic inflammatory (osteomyelitic) process (Fig. 2.**37**).

Cystic tuberculosis of bone can cause punched-out defects in the tubular bones of the hand and in the carpus but usually coexists with other skeletal lesions. The changes may resemble sarcoidosis due to the common underlying (pathoanatomic) granulomatous structure.

More or less extensive osteolytic changes in a phalanx, especially the distal phalanx in children, are usually a result of **spina ventosa**, a circumscribed expansile form of tuberculous dactylitis.

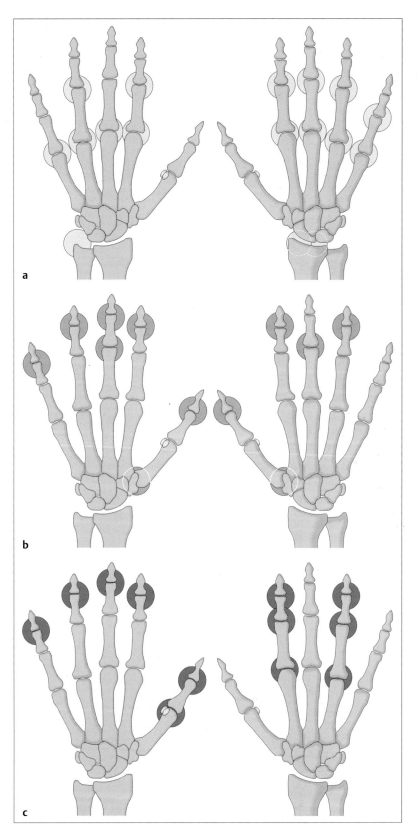

Fig. 2.**69 a–c**   Patterns of hand involvement by polyarticular joint changes in various diseases.
a In rheumatoid arthritis.
b In polyarticular osteoarthritis (Heberden and Bouchard type).
c In psoriatic arthritis.

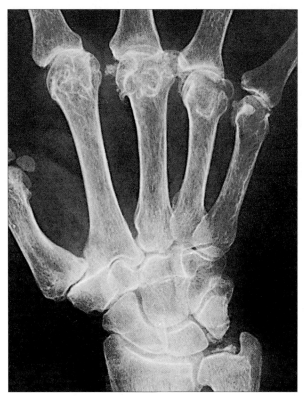

Fig. 2.**70**   Chondrocalcinosis with obliteration of the second through fifth metacarpophalangeal joint spaces, marked subchondral sclerosis, disruption of joint contours, and fine cyst-like lucencies, especially in the head of the second metacarpal. The head of the third metacarpal shows conspicuous productive bone changes. A drooping osteophyte is also seen. Note the calcifications in the triangular cartilage of the wrist and in the cartilage between the lunate and triquetrum. These findings are highly specific for chondrocalcinosis (see also Fig. 2.**283**). The "hard-working hand" may also show heavy sclerosis about the metacarpophalangeal joints with bone spurs and joint space narrowing. A case of secondary chondrocalcinosis in hemochromatosis is shown in Fig. 2.**134**.

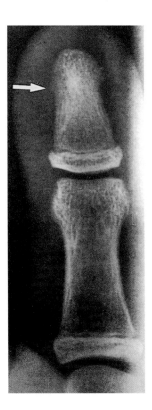

Fig. 2.**71**   Bone felon with lateral destruction of the terminal tuft and marginal sclerosis (arrow). The radiographic differential diagnosis should include osteoid osteoma.

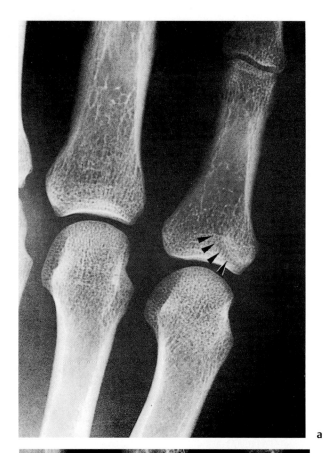

a

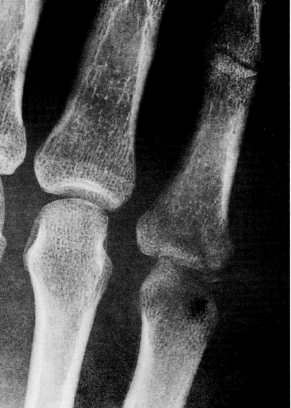

b

Fig. 2.**72 a, b**   Serial radiographs of an inflammatory bone and joint process following a blow to the ulnar border of the hand. Panel **a** shows an oblique subchondral fracture line at the base of the proximal phalanx. Film four weeks later shows extensive ostitis and arthritis, i.e., inflammatory-destructive changes in the bone ends accompanied by joint space narrowing due to destruction of the articular cartilage. Later, a complete ankylosis was seen.

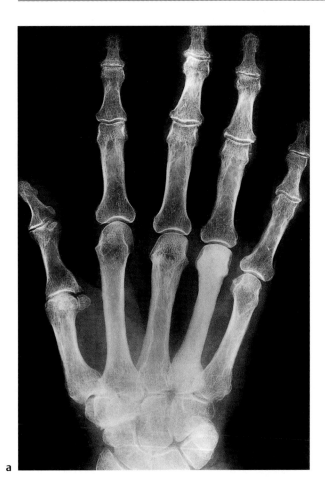

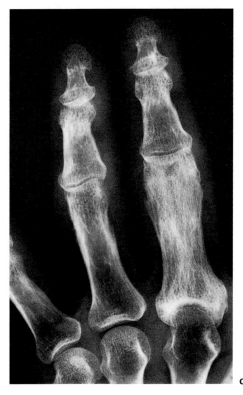

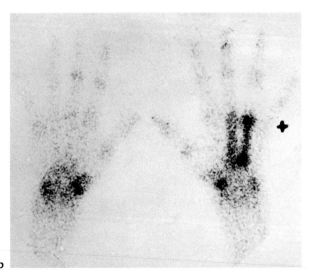

Fig. 2.**73a–c**   Paget disease in the hand.
a, b Involvement of the third and fourth metacarpals by poly-ostotic Paget disease.
c Unusual solitary manifestation of the disease in the proximal phalanx of the third finger.

Tumor?

Tumors and tumorlike lesions are not uncommon in the skeleton of the hand (Freyschmidt 1985).

In a series of 6464 primary bone tumors, we found that 7.8% of the lesions were located in the hand. The approximate percentages for specific types of primary tumor are listed below:

- Chondroma, 56%
- Osteoid osteoma, 9%
- Osteochondroma, 5%
- Osteoblatoma, 3%

Chondroblastoma, chondromyxoid fibroma, giant cell tumor, and hemangioendothelioma each accounted for less than 3% of bone tumors in the hand. We found that 14.5% of the 3271 benign tumors and 0.8% of the 3193 malignant tumors were located in the hand. The most common bone tumor in the hand is chondroma, followed by osteochondroma (only in cartilaginous exostotic disease) and osteoid osteoma. Chondromas occur most commonly in the phalanges, less often in the metacarpals, and very rarely in the carpus. Osteoid osteomas occur in the metacarpals and phalanges with about equal frequency. Osteochondroma predominantly affects the phalanges. In keeping with our theme, this section deals strictly with radiographic changes that may represent borderline situations with regard to productive or destructive tumors and tumorlike lesions.

Destructive Changes

Solitary or multiple **cystlike lucencies** 1–2 mm in diameter occur normally in the skeleton of the hand, especially in response to heavy mechanical loads. They show a predilection for the carpus but can also occur in the metacarpals and the bases of the proximal phalanges. These lucencies most likely represent small foci of osteonecrosis that undergo cystic transformation. We call these lesions **idiopathic hand cysts** (Fig. 2.**74**). Generally they have no pathological significance.

These idiopathic cysts should not be confused with cysts that accompany pathological conditions such as polyarticular osteoarthritis, the "sentinel" cysts of diseases such as rheumatoid arthritis, or with the brown tumors of hyperparathyroidism (Fig. 2.**75c**).

Whenever multiple cysts are found in the hand, the differential diagnosis should include **polycystic lipomembranous osteodysplasia** (Freyschmidt 1997).

Gout is commonly associated with subchondral intraosseous defects that may extend to the midshaft level (see below). They require differentiation from small enchondromas and, when multiple, from enchondromatosis (Fig. 2.**75b**). The differential diagnosis of cystlike bony lesions in the hand is reviewed in Table 2.**7**.

Large, solitary osteolytic processes with an epimetaphyseal location may represent the initial stage of a giant cell tumor, and osteolytic metastases should be

Table 2.**7**   Oligocystic and polycystic changes in the bones of the hand (from Freyschmidt 1997)

- Idiopathic hand cysts
- Sarcoidosis
- Polyarticular osteoarthritis
- Cystic form of rheumatoid arthritis
- Gout
- Certain forms of hemochromatosis
- Collagen diseases
- Amyloidosis
- Cystic tuberculosis
- Polycystic lipomembranous osteodysplasia
- Gorlin–Goltz syndrome
- Tuberous sclerosis
- Enchondromatosis

considered in adults. The latter can sometimes destroy entire phalanges, showing a predilection for the acral parts.

The following types of **pseudotumor** are observed in the hand with some regularity:

- Pseudotumorous forms of β_2-**microglobulin amyloid deposits** appear as cystlike lucencies in the skeleton of the hand, most commonly affecting the carpus (Fig. 2.**76**).

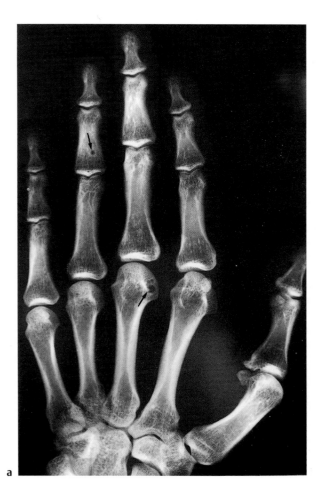

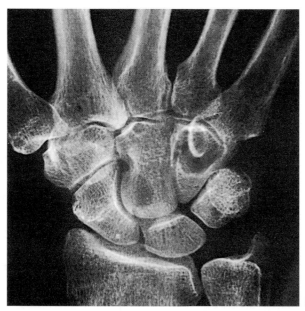

Fig. 2.**74a, b**   Idiopathic bone cysts in the hand. Usually without clinical significance, they can occasionally be an early sign of polycystic lipomembranous osteodysplasia or of β_2-microglobulin deposits in patients with a corresponding history. The latter have a predilection for the carpus and can fully mimic the appearance of idiopathic hand cysts (compare radiograph **b** with Fig. 2.**76**). The differential diagnosis of carpal cysts also includes enchondromas and, more rarely, large subchondral synovial cysts (intraosseous ganglia).

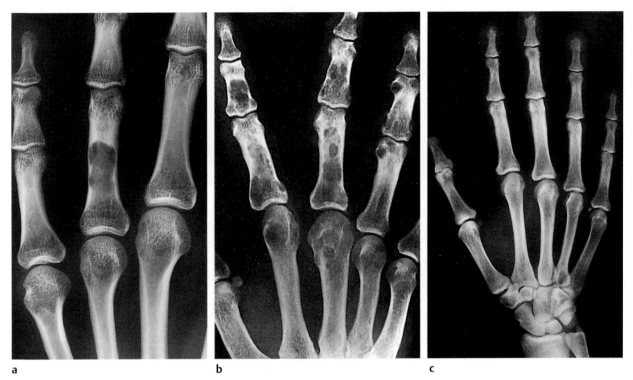

a   b   c

Fig. 2.**75a–c** Differential diagnosis of "cystic" lucencies in the tubular bones of the hand.
a Solitary enchondroma in the proximal phalanx of the fourth finger.
b Multiple enchondromas in Ollier disease.

c The osteolytic lesion in the base of the fourth metacarpal represents a brown tumor in hyperparathyroidism. Note the marked structural changes in the remaining bones, including acro-osteolytic lesions.

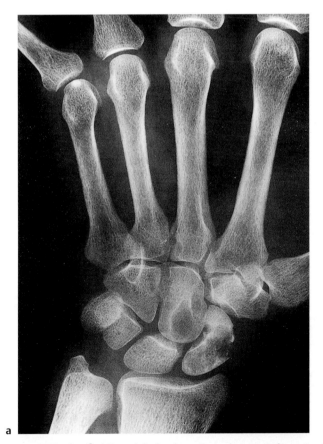

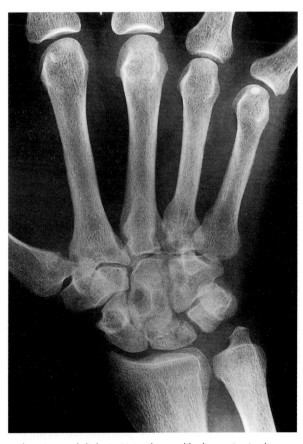

a   b

Fig. 2.**76a, b** β_2-Microglobulin deposits in the wrist of a patient on chronic renal dialysis. Note the cystlike lucencies in the scaphoid and hamate bones on both sides and in the lunate (with fracture line) and hamate bones of the right hand.

The majority of patients who have been on hemodialysis for approximately 10 years develop these pseudotumorous lucencies in the carpus.

- In the **pseudotumorous form of gout**, lucencies of varying size (medullary tophi) can appear in the shafts of the long bones of the hand (Fig. 2.77). These lesions may develop some distance from the joints.
- **Epidermoid cysts** (Fig. 2.78, 2.108) generally appear radiographically as sharply circumscribed osteolytic areas. Occasionally there is balloonlike expansion of the affected bone, which loses its internal architectural features. Many cases show a history of repetitive trauma to the soft tissues, periosteum, and bone (e.g., in seamstresses). It is assumed that epidermal elements, especially portions of the stratum germinativum with hyper-, para- or dyskeratosis, are introduced into the bone via a lymphoplasmocytic inflammation of the traumatized soft tissues, leading to bone erosion and cortical defects.

  Differentiation is mainly required from a purely intraosseous occurrence of glomus tumor, which is very rare. Glomus tumors in the soft tissues tend to erode the underlying bone (Fig. 2.79).
- **Inflammatory pseudotumors** can result from penetrating thorn injuries (e.g., rose-thorn induced pseudotumor, or punctures from other thorn-bearing plants).

Reparative giant cell granuloma is the most important example of **tumorlike lesions** that can involve the skeleton of the hand.

Subchondral synovial cyst or **intraosseous ganglion** is a relatively common tumorlike lesion that arises from the articular structures of the hand (Figs. 2.46b, 2.80). It occurs mainly in the carpus, where it requires differentiation from idiopathic hand cysts and amyloid deposits.

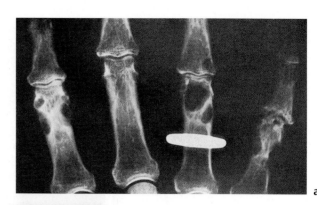

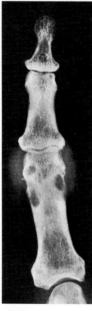

Fig. 2.**77 a, b**   "Cystic" lucencies in gout (confirmed by biopsy). Note the severe mutilation of the proximal phalanx of the small finger in panel **a**. Note also the marked soft-tissue swelling around the medullary tophi in the distal portion of the second proximal phalanx in panel **b**.

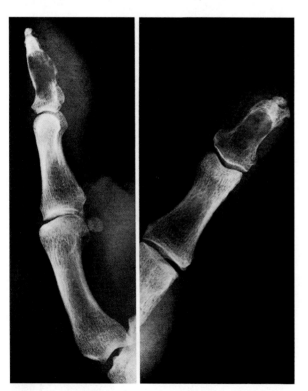

Fig. 2.**78**   Typical epidermoid cyst (epithelial cyst) in the distal phalanx of the thumb of a 48-year-old tailor.

Fig. 2.**79 a–c**   Glomus tumor of the dorsal subungual soft tissues with erosion of the underlying bone (star). Clinically, the site was extremely painful.

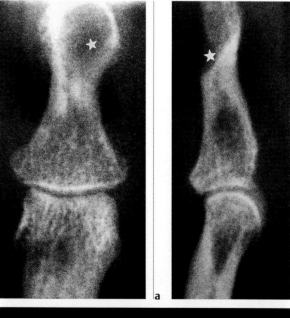

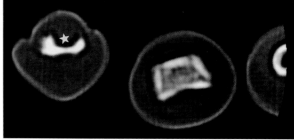

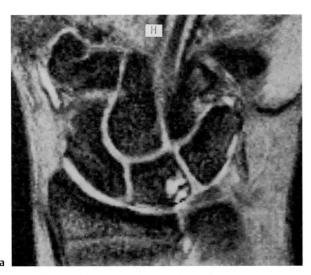

a

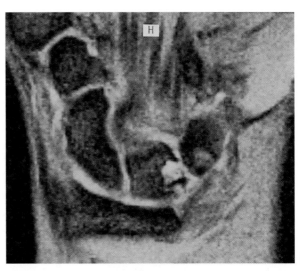

b

Fig. 2.**80 a, b**   Subchondral synovial cyst (intraosseous ganglion) in the lunate bone. Conventional radiographs showed a small lucency in the ulnar aspect of the lunate bone. The T2-weighted MR images demonstrate the ganglion as a mass of high (fluid-equivalent) signal intensity. The lesion has relatively broad contact with the lunotriquetral joint. See also Fig. 2.**165**.

Productive Tumorous and Tumorlike Lesions

Enostoses (medullary osteoma) or **bone islands** are the most frequent cause of circumscribed radiographic densities in the bones of the hand (Figs. 2.**38 c, d**, 2.**81**, 2.**82**).

This harmless lesion causes no clinical complaints, even when it occurs in the form of osteopoikilosis (Fig. 2.**38**). **Osteoid osteoma** can have a similar radiographic appearance (pure sclerosis), especially when the nidus is calcified and the sclerosis cannot be interpreted as response to an osteolytic tumor. Differentiation is aided in these cases by performing a three-phase bone scan (Fig. 2.**83 c**), which will generally show the double-density sign identifying the lesion as an osteoid osteoma. (In this sign the area of very heavy tracer uptake represents the nidus, and the surrounding area of less intense uptake represents reactive new bone formation.)

Florid reactive periostitis is a productive bone entity that has been diagnosed with increasing frequency in the hand (Spjut and Dorfman 1981). The reactive process most likely develops as a sequel to trauma (Fig. 2.**84**). Patients notice a progressive swelling as with a true inflammatory process, and a palpable thickening or lump soon develops over the affected bone (usually the proximal and middle phalanges). Radiographs initially show fine periosteal new bone formation, which later becomes solid and may increase over time before its deep layers finally may be incorporated into the underlying cortex. Differentiation from

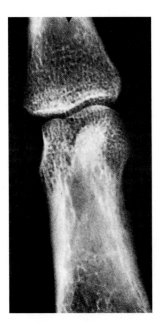

Fig. 2.**81**   Enostoma (bone island) in the distal middle phalanx of a finger.

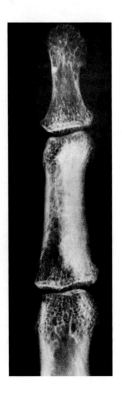

Fig. 2.**82**   Massive hyperostosis in the middle phalanx of the index finger detected incidentally in a 41-year-old woman. The hyperostosis, which has fused with the cortical bone, is most likely an unusually large example of an osteoma. The differential diagnosis in this case would include a rare digital manifestation of melorheostosis.

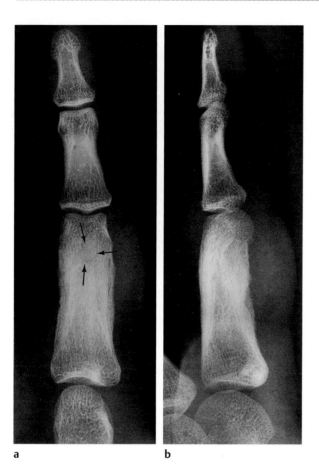

a

b

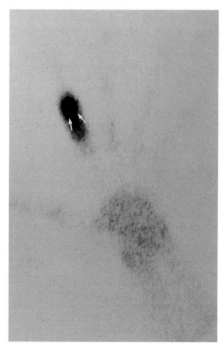

c

Fig. 2.**83 a–c**   Osteoid osteoma in the proximal phalanx of the index finger. The calcified nidus is faintly visible in the distal shaft (arrows) on conventional radiographs. Identification is aided by noting a relatively large nutrient canal that branches around the nidus. The bone scan (**c**) shows a typical double-density sign.

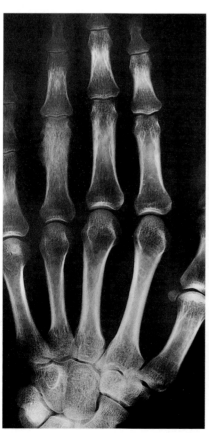

a

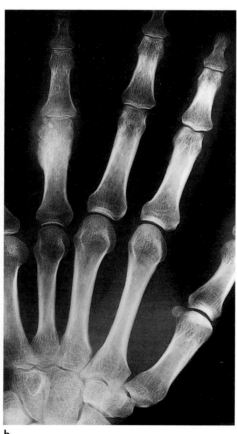

b

Fig. 2.**84 a, b**   Florid reactive periostitis. Film **a** was taken about 10 weeks earlier than film **b**.

osteoid osteoma can be difficult but is aided by bone scanning, which will not show a double-density sign if florid reactive periostitis is present. The histological features of florid reactive periostitis are sometimes confusing, as the proliferative, fibroblast-rich tissue may easily be mistaken for periosteal osteosarcoma, especially by an unexperienced pathologist. Similar productive bony processes in the hand have been described using various other terms (Nora et al. 1983, Nuovo et al. 1992, Schütte et al. 1990). A detailed description of proliferative processes in the hand and foot skeleton is given in our 1997 textbook on skeletal diseases, including the common etiological and pathogenetic features of the various disorders (Freyschmidt 1997). Finally, **osteochondromas** are a potential cause of productive tumorous changes in the bones of the hand (Fig. 2.**85**).

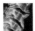
Degenerative Changes?

The differential diagnosis of polyarticular osteoarthritis was discussed previously, for didactic reasons, in the section on Inflammation. The present section expands the differential diagnosis by considering **productive bone changes in acromegaly**. The excessive production of somatotropic hormone by anterior pituitary adenomas in the mature skeleton leads to the additional growth and structural alteration of bone, cartilage, and soft tissues. The resulting enlargement is especially prominent in the acral parts of the skeleton. The overproduction of somatotropic hormone during skeletal growth leads to gigantism.

The somatotropin stimulates enchondral ossification at sites of tendon and ligament attachment to bone. It also stimulates the proliferation of articular cartilage, causing joint space widening on radiographs. As the subcutaneous fat is replaced by "water-equivalent" connective tissue, the soft tissues enlarge and the periarticular areas expand, accompanied by an overall thickening of the fingers. Radiographs (Fig. 2.**86**) show a broadening of the metacarpals and phalanges, and the muscle insertions become coarsened and irregular, especially in the subcapital area of the metacarpals.

The terminal tufts exhibit an anchorlike shape. Marginal osteophytes generally develop at the metacarpophalangeal and interphalangeal joints. Usually there is conspicuous widening of all joint spaces due to the thickened articular cartilage. This is an important differentiating criterion from osteoarthritis, which causes narrowing of the joint spaces.

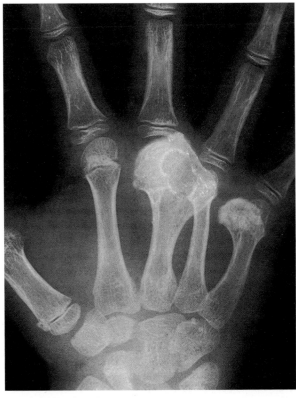

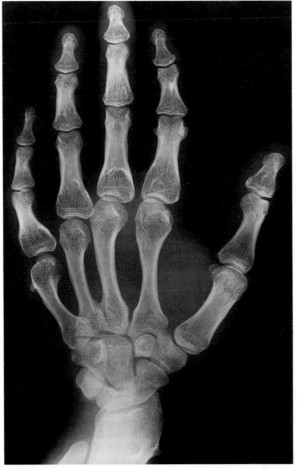

Fig. 2.**85 a, b**   Osteochondromas in the hand.
a Osteochondromas involving the distal metaphyses of the third and fifth metacarpals in a patient with multiple exostoses (osteochondromatosis). These lesions should not be mistaken for epiphyseal dysplasia. Note the narrowing of the fourth metacarpal.

b Numerous flat osteochondromas in a patient with multiple exostoses (osteochondromatosis). The ringlike densities at the bases of the second and third proximal phalanges represent the bases of the exostoses viewed end-on. The marked growth disturbance includes shortening of the fifth ray and a pseudo-Madelung deformity.

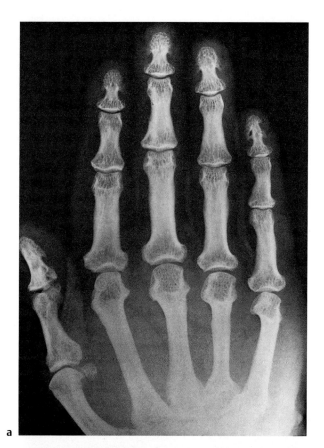

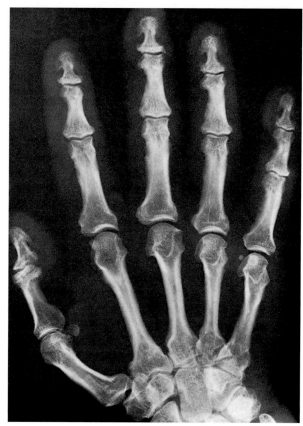

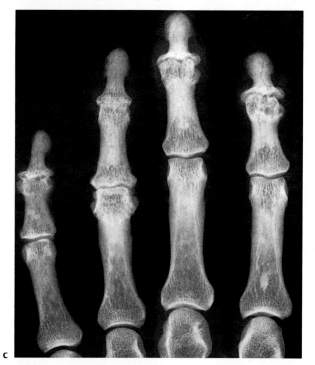

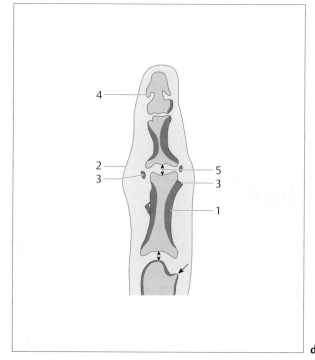

Fig. 2.**86 a–d**   Acromegaly and its differential diagnosis.
a, b Acromegaly (**a** 44-year-old woman, **b** 34-year-old man).
Note the anchorlike shape of the distal phalanges and the
prominent osteophytes, especially on the proximal interphalangeal and metacarpophalangeal joints. The joint spaces are
normal or widened, in contrast to osteoarthritis (**c**).

d Schematic diagram of typical acromegalic changes in the
phalanges.
1 Phalangeal shafts appear moderately thickened with prominent muscle attachments
2 Broadening of soft-tissue contours
3 Marginal osteophytes and periarticular calcifications
4 Anchorlike configuration of distal phalanges
5 Widening of joint spaces

Soft-Tissue Calcifications

There are three principal causes of soft-tissue calcifications in the hand:

- When the calcium phosphate product exceeds 70, calcium phosphate is precipitated in the soft tissues, especially around joints and vessels. This mechanism is found mainly in generalized osteopathies, particularly renal osteodystrophy, hypervitaminosis D, etc. Basically the same phenomenon occurs with calcium carbonate and calcium oxalate.
- Soft-tissue calcifications can result from local necrosis, since necrotic soft tissue is a potential "calcium catcher" due to its altered pH, etc. Necrotic soft-tissue changes in the subcutaneous tissue and muscles may be caused by trauma, impaired blood flow (e.g., due to vasculitis or a collagen disease), or may be the culmination of a destructive inflammatory process.
- Soft-tissue calcification can also result from mineralization of the matrix formed by a tumor or tumorlike process. This occurs mainly in association with cartilage- or bone-forming tumors and heterotopic bone formation. Mucus-forming metastases are also prone to ossification.

The radiographic morphology of soft-tissue calcifications can be fairly specific, and therefore the underlying mechanism can often be determined. For example, solid calcifications or, better, ossifications, with a definite shape and evidence of a cancellous trabecular structure most likely arose from a previously formed matrix due to heterotopic bone formation or a soft-tissue chondrosarcoma or osteosarcoma (etc.), whereas amorphous calcifications are more likely to have developed from a necrotic process. Further differentiation should rely on topographic data and clinical information.

Below we review several forms of soft-tissue calcification that are frequently encountered in the hand.

The most common is **interstitial calcinosis**, which is usually extra-articular. The classification of interstitial calcinoses is shown in Table 2.**8**.

In **calcinosis cicumscripta**, small amorphous calcifications are found **in the subcutaneous tissue**, especially on the palmar side of the distal phalanges (Fig. 2.**87 a, b**) and over the flexor tendon sheaths of the hands.

The condition is idiopathic in approximately 60% of cases, and only 40% are associated with scleroderma, dermatomyositis, or Raynaud disease (this combination is known as Thibiérge–Weissenbach syndrome). The calcifications may precede the onset of clinical symptoms. Older women appear to be at particularly high risk for **idiopathic calcinosis** cicumscripta, accounting for some 80–90% of cases.

Unlike the idiopathic circumscribed form in Fig. 2.**87 a, b**, circumscribed calcinosis involving the **tendon sheaths and bursae** of the hands are often associated with severe pain. These calcifications may regress spontaneously, especially after an inflammatory phase, similar to the course seen with calcifying periarthritis of the shoulder. The various radiographic manifestations of these tendon-sheath and bursal calcifications are illustrated in Fig. 2.**87 c–k**.

The **universal interstitial calcinoses** that most commonly affect the hand are those that are associated with collagen diseases (Thibiérge–Weissenbach syndrome, Fig. 2.**88**). They are particularly common in scleroderma,

dermatomyositis, Sharp syndrome, and Raynaud disease. External pressure on the subcutaneous calcium deposits may elicit a grayish-white discharge. When very prominent, the deposits can cause pressure erosion of the adjacent bone. More commonly, though, calcifications embedded in bony defects result from necrosis of the bone and adjacent soft tissue.

Interstitial calcinosis due to **calcium phosphate precipitation** occurs most frequently in the setting of renal osteodystrophy or long-term dialysis therapy. This interstitial calcinosis is sometimes associated with giant tumorlike calcifications in the periarticular soft tissue. In the case shown in Fig. 2.**89 a–c**, the changes in the hand are only the tip of the iceberg, for the patient also had large calcium phosphate deposits, some almost melon-size, about the shoulders, the greater trochanters, and other sites.

With well-circumscribed calcifications ranging down to the size of a pinhead, the differential diagnosis should include phleboliths, which occur almost exclusively in hemangiomatous lesions. These phleboliths, as well as mild regressive periarticular calcifications, should be differentiated from small traumatic bony avulsions whenever possible.

Intra-articular calcifications result from the **calcification of cartilage** in the great majority of cases. Cartilage calcification occurs normally in older individuals, especially in the triangular cartilage of the wrist but also at other sites (e.g., between the lunate and triquetrum). Rarely it affects the metacarpophalangeal joints (Fig. 2.**89 d–g**) and is often associated with polyarticular degenerative changes. The detection of cartilage calcification has pathological significance only in patients with **chondrocalcinosis** in the strict sense, known also as pseudogout (Fig. 2.**70**). Primary chondrocalcinosis (pseudogout, crystal synovitis, CPPD) is distinguished from a secondary or symptomatic form like that occurring in hemochromatosis or hemosiderosis, primary or secondary hyperparathyroidism, ochronosis, Wilson disease, etc.

Table 2.8   Classification of interstitial, mostly extra-articular soft-tissue calcifications

Primary interstitial calcinosis (idiopathic)
- Calcinosis cicumscripta (circumscribed calcinosis)
- Calcinosis universalis (universal calcinosis)
- Pseudotumorous interstitial calcinosis (Teutschlaender, tumoral calcinosis)
- Pseudotumorous form of pseudogout (chondrocalcinosis, CPPD[1])
Secondary interstitial calcinosis (symptomatic)
- Primary hyperparathyroidism (rare)
- Secondary hyperparathyroidism (in setting of renal osteodystrophy with dialysis therapy, featuring tumorlike calcifications in bursae, tendon sheaths, etc.)
- Hypervitaminosis D, especially in dialysis patients
- Milk drinker syndrome (Burnett syndrome)
- In collagen diseases
- Primary and secondary oxalosis

[1] CPPD Calcium pyrophosphate deposition disease

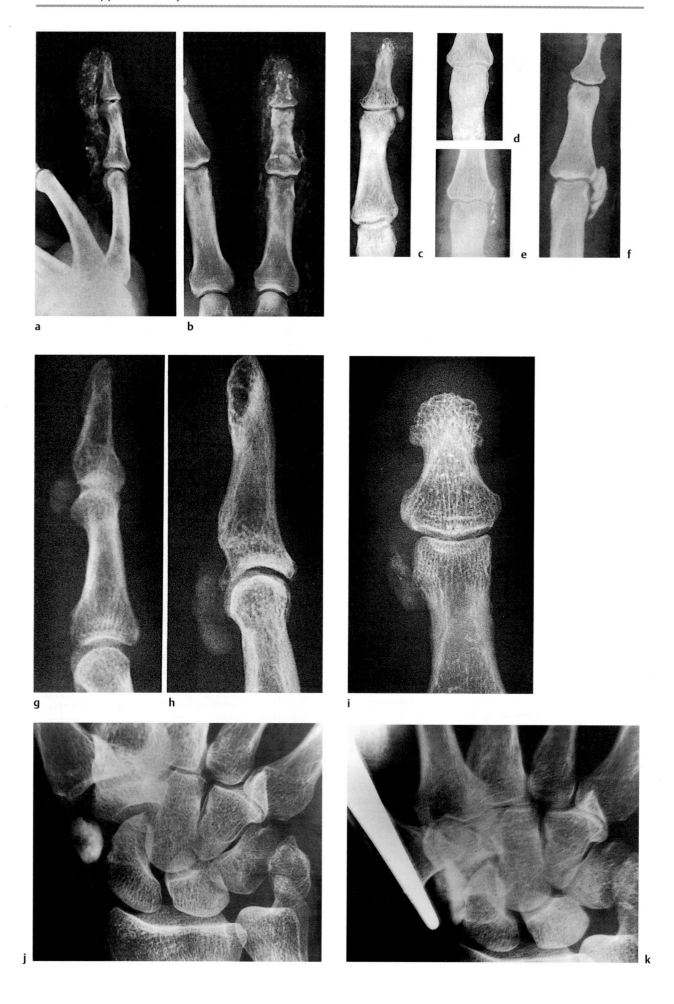

◁ Fig. 2.**87 a–k**   Calcinosis cicumscripta.

a, b Calcinosis cicumscripta in the left index finger of a 48-year-old woman who is otherwise healthy. The amorphous calcifications occur mainly on the palmar side. A pasty, grayish-white material can occasionally be expressed from the lesions. **c–i** Localized interstitial calcinosis predominantly affecting the periarticular bursae. Film **d**, taken eight years after **c**, documents spontaneous regression of the calcification. Film **f**, taken two years after **e**, shows a marked increase in the size and density of the calcifications. Film **g** shows calcifications on the palmar aspect of the distal interphalangeal joint of the index finger, which presented clinically with pain, redness, and swelling. Film **h** shows a periarticular bursal calcification on the palmar aspect of the distal interphalangeal joint of the small finger in an 80-year-old woman who was an artistic painter. Clinically the site was red, swollen, and tender. These symptoms and the radiographic calcifications regressed spontaneously in three weeks. Film **i** shows a periarticular bursal calcification next to the distal interphalangeal joint of the thumb (52-year-old woman), marked clinically by pain and swelling. A wasp sting to this site four weeks earlier may have incited the bursitis. Films **j** and **k** show an unusual "calcification" involving the abductor pollicus longus tendon sheath. The calcification appears very solid in the AP view (**j**) but can be pressed flat with a probe (**k**). This identifies the lesion as calcium-containing fluid in the tendon sheath or within a bursa. (Case courtesy of Dr. A. Nidecker, Basel.)

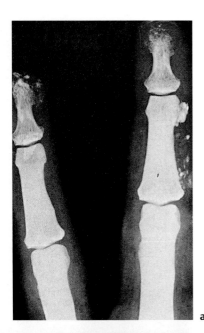

a

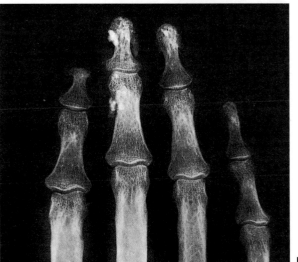

b

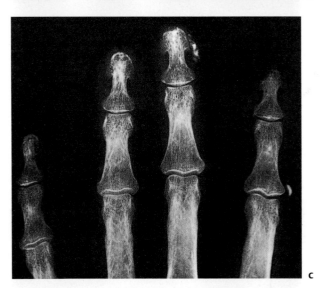

c

Fig. 2.**88 a–c**   Interstitial calcinosis in scleroderma. Note the acro-osteolytic lesions in the affected fingers.

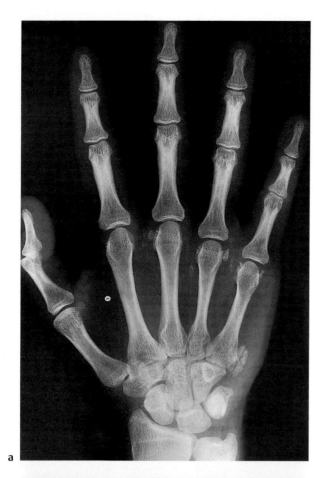

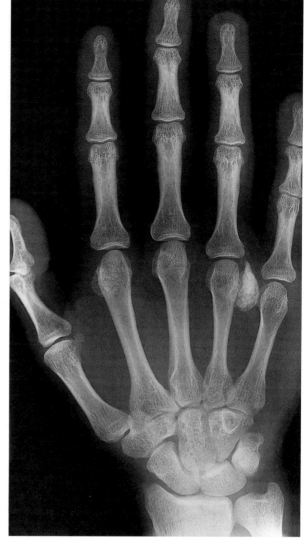

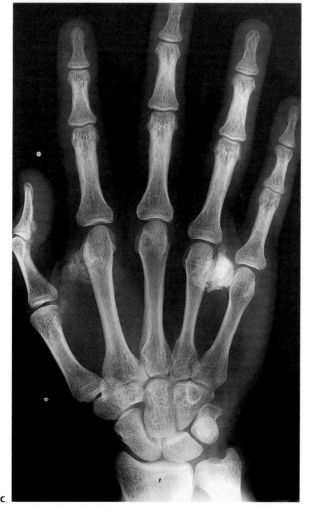

Fig. 2.**89 a–g**   Interstitial calcinosis and age-associated chondrocalcinosis.

a–c Interstitial calcinosis in a 27-year-old man with renal osteodystrophy. The patient was on long-term dialysis but received no treatment for hyperphosphatemia. Film **a** was taken about 18 months before **b**, and **b** was taken about one year before **c**. Besides an increase in calcification at some sites (e.g., lateral to the head of the fourth metacarpal), the serial films also show a decrease of calcification lateral to the base of the fifth metacarpal. This regression may occur spontaneously or in response to the spontaneous drainage of calcified material through small openings in the skin.

Fig. 2.**89 d–g** ▷

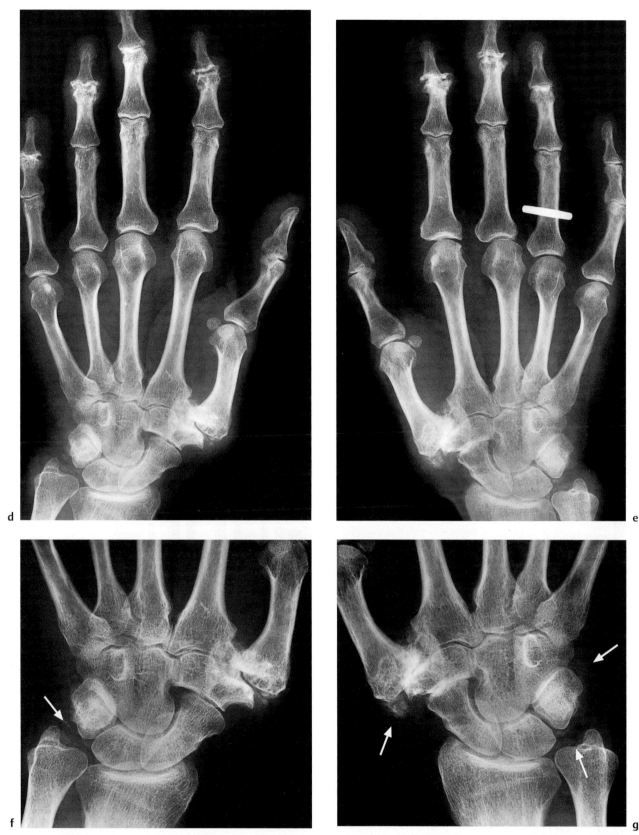

Fig. 2.**89d–g** Age-associated chondrocalcinosis in a moderately symptomatic patient with florid polyarticular osteoarthritis (affecting the distal interphalangeal joints). The close-up views of the carpi (**f, g**) show marked calcification of the triangular cartilage between the lunate and triquetrum, especially in the right hand, and calcifications adjacent to the carpometacarpal joint of the thumb in both hands. Note also the fine lateral bursal calcification in the niche between the hamate and triquetrum (arrows). The metacarpophalangeal joints, especially the second and third joints of the right hand, are slightly narrowed but show no calcifications and no subchondral structural changes. These features of age-associated chondrocalcinosis, especially in the metacarpophalangeal joints, differ markedly from the classic presentation of symptomatic chondrocalcinosis (pseudogout) shown in Fig. 2.**70**.

Specific Bones of the Hand

Distal Phalanges

▎ Normal Findings

The diaphysis of the distal phalanx is ossified at birth in full-term infants. The epiphyses become visible on radiographs between 5 months and 2 years of age and fuse with the shaft at age 17 years. When the epiphysis is fully developed, its width exceeds that of the bony shaft. The distal phalanges have an almost conical shape in children and adolescents (Fig. 2.**90**).

Very dense epiphyses ("ivory epiphyses," Figs. 2.**15**, 2.**54 b**, 2.**91**) are not necessarily pathological, especially in asymptomatic children (see p. 52).

 #### In Adulthood

The middle finger is normally longer than the index finger, and the distal phalanx of the ring finger is longer and thicker than that of the index finger.

As in all parts of the skeleton, the size (length and width) of the distal phalanges depends largely on constitutional factors (see p. 16 f). The shape of the phalanx and especially of the terminal tuft is also influenced by mechanical loads. With aging, the distal phalanx changes from the conical shape of adolescence to a more rounded, spadelike shape (Fig. 2.**90 c**). Spurlike excrescences of the tuft become more common with aging and are especially prominent on the palmar side (Fig. 2.**90 d, e**).

> ▎The terminal tuft of each finger normally has well-defined margins, and a definite line can be traced around its bony contour despite any lobulations and irregularities.

If this contour line is interrupted or if the margin of the tuft is ill-defined or disrupted by lucencies, it should be assumed that a pathological condition is present (e.g., primary or secondary hyperparathyroidism, necrosis due to a collagen disease, etc.; Figs. 2.**44 a, c**; 2.**61**; 2.**62**; p. 56).

Meanwhile, the terminal phalanges may exhibit a **marked osteosclerosis** in relation to the other phalanges, especially in their middle and distal portions, and this does not necessarily indicate pathology (Figs. 2.**3 c, d** and 2.**92**). Normally there is a smooth transition between the osteosclerotic area and the more proximal bone. A solitary osteosclerotic area with a very sharp transition probably represents enostoma (Figs. 2.**81**, 2.**82**). Osteosclerosis of the distal phalanges combined with cortical thickening of the metacarpals is a pattern occasionally seen in healthy individuals (Fig. 2.**3 c, d**). But dense osteosclerosis affecting all the terminal phalanges may also reflect an endocrine disorder, especially when combined with hyperostosis frontalis interna (Morgagni syndrome). Moreover, it is not uncommon to find distal phalangeal osteosclerosis in association with diseases such as sarcoidosis (Fig. 2.**36**). In some cases the patient's history may suggest that distal osteosclerosis is an exuberant reossification process following acro-osteolysis (Fig. 2.**93**).

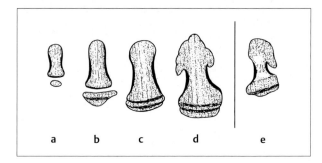

Fig. 2.**90 a–e** Development of the distal phalanges and terminal tufts.

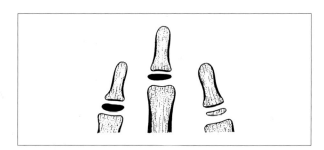

Fig. 2.**91** "Dense epiphyses." (After Brailsford.)

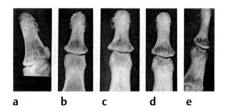

Fig. 2.**92 a–e** Examples of acro-osteosclerosis.

Sesamoid bones have been described as a normal finding at the distal interphalangeal joints of the second, fourth, and fifth fingers (see Fig. 2.**5**). One should be careful when interpreting a solid bony element projected over the third distal interphalangeal joint, because there have been no previous reports of a sesamoid occurring in that location. But 72.9% of the population have a sesamoid bone on the palmar aspect of the distal interphalangeal joint of the thumb (Fig. 2.**94**).

Fine central lucencies at the bases of the distal phalanges, usually surrounded by a sclerotic rim (when viewed with a magnifier), represent end-on projections of nutrient canals (Fig. 2.**8 b**).

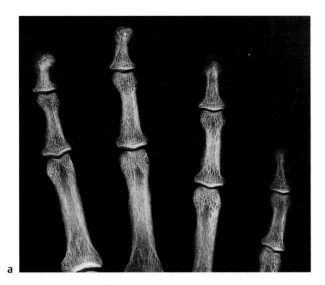

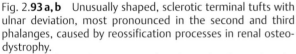

a

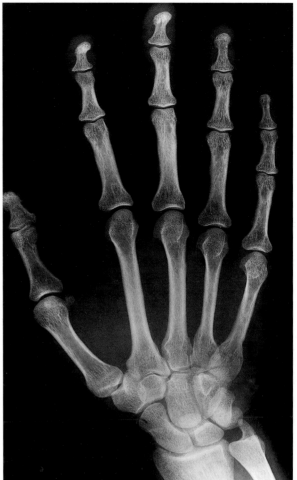

b

Fig. 2.**93 a, b**   Unusually shaped, sclerotic terminal tufts with ulnar deviation, most pronounced in the second and third phalanges, caused by reossification processes in renal osteo-dystrophy.
a Initial radiograph one year earlier shows distal osteolytic lesions (acro-osteolyses), but already there are signs of incipient reossification.
b The second radiograph cannot be interpreted without knowledge of the prior history. The cause of the deformity is indeterminate by radiography alone. This case illustrates how the bone matrix is basically preserved in acro-osteolysis due to hyperparathyroidism. Because the matrix is "soft," it is easily deformed.

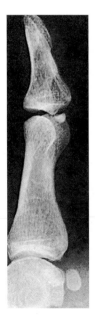

Fig. 2.**94**   Sesamoid bones adjacent to the interphalangeal joint and metacar-pophalangeal joint of the thumb.

▋ *Pathological Finding?*

Normal Variant or Anomaly?

As mentioned earlier, there is a large normal range of variation in the size and shape of the distal phalanges, and it is difficult to draw a sharp dividing line between normal and pathological. The phalangeal sign of Kosowicz (1965, Fig. 2.**4**) is occasionally helpful in making this distinction. The clinical presentation is also helpful in deciding whether remarkably long or short distal phalanges are pathological, and it is an important guide in making disability assessments. Table 2.**9** reviews the syndromic associations and other causes that are helpful in interpreting short, broad phalanges, narrow phalanges, and tuft erosions.

Bowing of the fingers is seen in clinodactyly and as one feature of Kirner deformity.

Clinodactyly is marked by radial or ulnar deviation of the distal phalanges. Often the cause is a trapezoid or delta configuration of the associated middle phalanx. Any finger may be involved, but radial deviation of the distal phalanx of the fifth digit is particularly common (Fig. 2.**26**). Clinodactyly of the small finger is a characteristic feature of trisomy 21 (Down syndrome).

Kirner deformity (dystelephalangia) is a special form of clinodactyly marked by dorsally convex bowing (clawlike deformity) of the distal phalanges of both small fingers. It can occur sporadically or may be inherited as an autosomal dominant trait (Figs. 2.**95**, 2.**96**). The distal phalanx may be very "white," and epiphyseal closure may be delayed.

In a book dealing with borderline findings and variants, it would go beyond our scope to discuss other less common deformities of the distal phalanges that occur in syndromes.

Figure 2.**93** shows an unusual case of tuft sclerosis with ulnar deviation, predominantly involving the second and third rays. The history and follow-up clearly identify the condition as reossifying acro-osteolysis in a setting of renal osteodystrophy. This case illustrates the fundamental importance of clinical findings in the interpretation of phalangeal deformities.

Conspicuous, acquired enlargement of the distal phalanges is a classic feature of acromegaly (p. 70). A typical finding is the anchor or spadelike configuration of the enlarged acral parts (Fig. 2.**97**).

Enlargement of the distal phalanges and terminal tufts has also been described as a feature of hyperthyroidism.

The hypertrophic changes at the bases of the distal phalanges in polyarticular osteoarthritis and psoriatic arthritis ("protuberances") were described in detail on p. 57 (Figs. 2.**66**, 2.**68**).

Fracture? Dislocation?

Tuft fractures of the distal phalanx usually result from crush injuries. The radiographic findings can be very subtle, consisting only of a tiny bone fragment distal to the tuft. The differential diagnosis should include a small, hyperdense particle of foreign material lodged beneath the nail (Fig. 2.**98**).

Trauma to the distal interphalangeal joints (e.g., jamming injury, forced flexion or extension) is often associated with the bony avulsion of flexor or extensor tendon attachments. These injuries are commonly observed in baseball players and in skiers who fall with their hand tangled in the skipole strap. **Mallet finger** refers to the deformity that results from an isolated extensor tendon rupture or a basal intra-articular fracture of the distal phalanx with avulsion of the extensor tendon (Fig. 2.**99**).

Even if there is no evidence of a bony avulsion, the extensor tendon injury can be recognized by noting the flexed position of the distal phalanx in relation to the other phalanges of the same finger. Occasionally it might be asked whether this deformity is a radiographic artifact. It should be noted, however, that most people can flex the distal interphalangeal joint only by simultaneously flexing the proximal interphalangeal joint. Isolated flexion of the distal phalanx without concomitant flexion of the proximal interphalangeal joint should be considered pathological until proven otherwise.

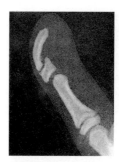

Fig. 2.**95** Clawlike curvature of the distal phalanx (Kirner deformity).

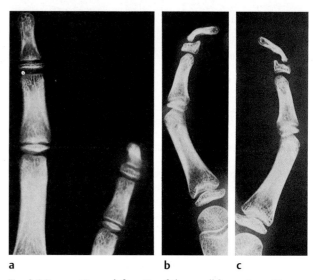

a   b   c

Fig. 2.**96 a–c** Kirner deformity of the small finger in an 11-year-old girl.

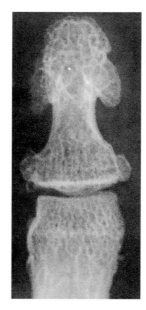

Fig. 2.**97** Anchorlike shape of the distal phalanx in acromegaly (see also Fig. 2.**86**).

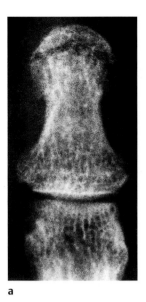 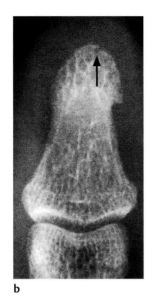

a   **b**

Fig. 2.**98 a, b**   Fractures?
a Dirt under the fingernail causes a Mach band phenomenon that mimics a tuft fracture.
b True avulsion fracture from the phalangeal tuft—a very subtle finding.

One should be careful in interpreting cases where there is accompanying hyperextension at the proximal interphalangeal joint. The resulting elongation of the extensor tendon permits isolated flexion of the distal interphalangeal joint (Fig. 2.**99 c**) as in a swan-neck deformity. Hyperextension of the proximal interphalangeal joint is not particularly unusual even in healthy individuals.

Hyperextension and hyperflexion trauma can also result in epiphyseal separation.

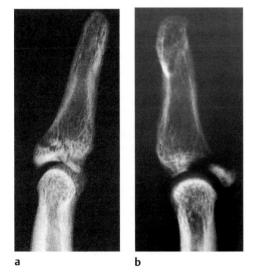

a   **b**

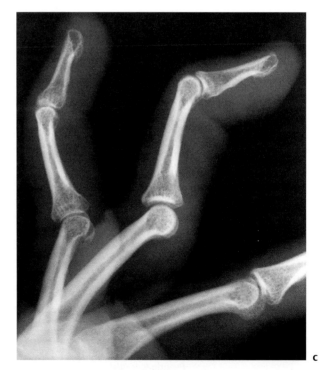

               c

Fig. 2.**99 a–c**   Basal intra-articular fracture, typical and simulated extensor tendon avulsion.
a Complete basal intra-articular fracture of a distal phalanx.
b Typical extensor tendon avulsion with slight flexion deformity of the distal interphalangeal joint.
c Simulated extensor tendon avulsion with deviation of the distal phalanx at the distal interphalangeal joint. Note, however, the hyperextension of the proximal interphalangeal joint,

causing a relative elongation of the extensor tendon that allows flexion at the distal interphalangeal joint ("swan-neck deformity"). This hyperextensibility of the proximal interphalangeal joint appears to be a normal variant, as the subject (an MRI technician at our center) was otherwise completely healthy.

Necrosis?

During Growth

We previously described the shortening and deformity of the distal phalanges (p. 54) that can result from frostbite or from Kashin–Beck disease with epiphyseal plate injury in the immature skeleton. An isolated "white" epiphysis, possibly combined with fragmentation, generally signifies some form of osteonecrosis. Radionuclide bone scanning can be used in doubtful cases to confirm or exclude pathology, since a pathological "white" epiphysis will generally show a circumscribed area of increased tracer uptake on bone scans. Developmental disturbances and deformities are listed in Table 2.**9**.

In Adulthood

Abnormal blood flow in the distal phalanx (hypoperfusion or hyperperfusion), regardless of its cause, can cause changes in the soft tissues of the fingertip and also in the underlying phalangeal tuft. The most typical change is osteolysis, marked by varying degrees of tuft destruction. This condition is known as **acro-osteolysis**. The principal causes of acro-osteolysis are listed in Table 2.**6**.

Acro-osteolysis can present clinically with **clubbing of the fingers** or thinning of the distal soft-tissue envelope. Clubbing results from an active or passive hyperemia of the fingertip and includes watchglass nails (Fig. 2.**100 a**).

Table 2.**9**   Developmental disorders and deformities of the distal phalanges, including tuft hypoplasia and erosions, and possible associated syndromes (after Poznanski)

Short, broad phalanges	
Limited to phalanges Primary involvement of the hands and feet	Bilginturan brachydactyly
Accompanying syndromes	Acrodysostosis Asphyxiating thoracic dysplasia Bilginturan Cheirolumbar dysostosis Cleidocranial dysplasia Coffin–Lowry[1] Diastrophic dysplasia DOOR (deafness, onychodystrophy, osteodystrophy, retardation) Fetal warfarin Hall Keutel Larsen Liebenberg Metaphyseal chondrodysplasia (Jansen) Pseudodermoperiostosis Pseudoachondroplasia Pseudohypoparathyroidism and pseudopseudohypoparathyroidism Rubinow Scalp defects Sensenbrenner
Acquired	Frostbite Trauma

Table 2.**9**   (Continue)

Thin, narrow phalanges	
Limited to phalanges Primary involvement of the hands and feet	With hypoplastic nails Symphalangism
Accompanying syndromes	Acrocephalosyndactyly (Carpenter) Asphyxiating thoracic dysplasia Chondroectodermal dysplasia Christian Coffin–Siris Fetal alcohol injury Fetal dilantin injury Fetal warfarin Hunter–Fraser Marshall Mucolipidosis II Osteodyplasia Pseudohypoparathyroidism Rüdiger Schinzel–Giedion Trisomy 9 p Trisomy 13 Trisomy 18 Zimmermann–Laband
Acquired	Frostbite

Tuft erosions or hypoplasia (see also Table 2.**6**)	
Limited to phalanges Primary involvement of the hands and feet	Brachydactyly B Osteolysis (phalangeal) (Hajdu–Cheney)
Accompanying syndromes	Cranioectodermal dysplasia Epidermolysis bullosa Lesch–Nyhan Mandibuloacral Mutilating palmoplantar keratoderma Pachydermoperiostosis Porphyria Progeria Pseudoxanthoma elasticum Pyknodysostosis Rothmund–Thomson Werner
Acquired	Chemical acro-osteolysis Endangiitis obliterans Gout Hyperparathyroidism Juvenile hyaline fibromatosis Collagen diseases Congenital insensitivity to pain Leprosy, sarcoidosis Neurotrophic disorders (e.g., hypertrophic osteoarthropathy) Psoriasis Irradiation Raynaud syndrome Burns, frostbite

[1] Broad tufts

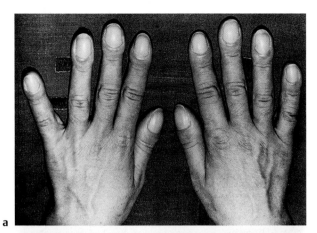

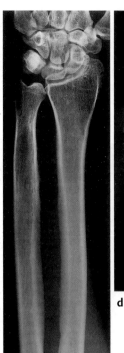

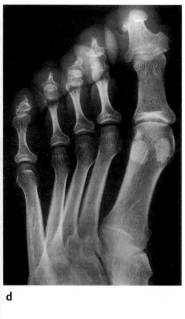

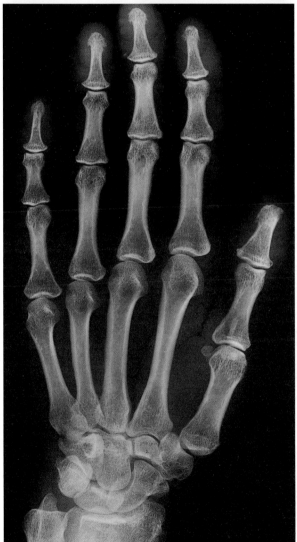

Digital clubbing is often seen in **hypertrophic osteoarthropathy** (pulmonary and intestinal type, Fig. 2.**40a**), pachydermoperiostosis (Fig. 2.**61**), angiodysplasias, and in a number of SKIBO diseases (Freyschmidt and Freyschmidt 1996).

The Yune soft tissue index can be used to quantitate narrowing of the distal soft-tissue envelope (Fig. 2.**101**). This occurs predominantly in collagen diseases (especially scleroderma and Sharp syndrome) and in certain SKIBO diseases such as **mutilating palmoplantar keratoderma** (Fig. 2.**100**) or epidermolysis bullosa dystrophica with acro-osteolysis (see *SKIBO Diseases* by Freyschmidt and Freyschmidt, 1996). The acro-osteolysis in hyperparathyroidism is clinically asymptomatic, resulting not from necrosis but from focal demineralization (with an intact matrix, Figs. 2.**112a**, 2.**44a**).

Fig. 2.**100a–d**   Clubbing of the fingers.
a Clinical appearance. Note the widening of the distal phalanges (probably caused by mucopolysaccharide deposits) and the watchglass deformity of the nails.
b Corresponding radiograph clearly shows the increased density of the distal soft tissues. There is only slight erosion of the terminal tufts, but the distal phalanges are remarkably slender.
c Note the periosteal new bone formation on the radius and ulna.
d The patient also had extensive acro-osteolysis in the foot. The patient was diagnosed with congenital **mutilating palmoplantar keratoderma**. A bone scan of the hands is shown in Fig. 2.**40c**.

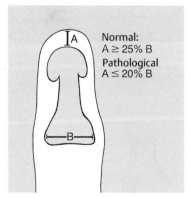

Fig. 2.**101**   Measurement of the Yune soft-tissue index.

A special form of acro-osteolysis that usually involves very severe trophic changes in the terminal tufts and surrounding soft tissues is **violin or guitar player's fingers**. The external hallmark is an atrophic fingertip with ulcerations and hyperkeratosis. Radiographs often show complete resorption of the terminal tufts. Destouet and Murphy (1981) described severe changes in an 18-year-old who had been a professional guitar player for eight years.

Radiographs showed bandlike areas of resorption across the distal phalanges of the second through fifth fingers, isolating the terminal tufts.

We cannot delve further into the specific clinical and radiographic features of the various forms of acro-osteolysis. Several cases are illustrated in Figs. 2.102–2.104 (see also Figs. 2.40a and 2.61).

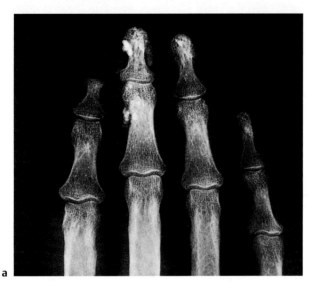 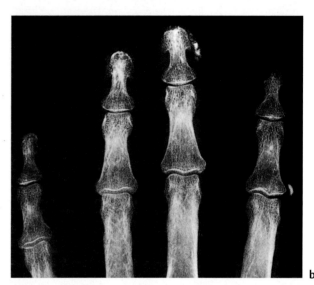

a   b

Fig. 2.**102 a, b**   Tuft defects and soft-tissue calcifications in scleroderma.

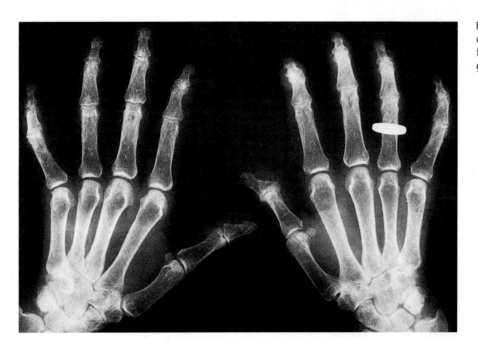

Fig. 2.**103**   Osteoporosis, cutaneous atrophy, and slight flexion deformity of the fingers in scleroderma.

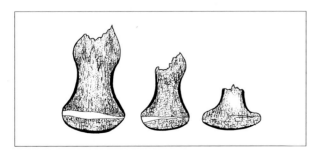

Fig. 2.**104 a–c**   Leprosy.

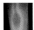 **Inflammation?**

Joints

The bases of the distal phalanges normally have smooth margins. Contour defects may result from trauma or from inflammatory processes (erosions, see p. 57). In generalized inflammatory joint diseases such as rheumatoid arthritis, erosive changes in the distal interphalangeal joints are usually seen only in advanced stages. By contrast, psoriatic arthritis affects these joints preferentially, and

erosive changes are generally accompanied by bone proliferation (Fig. 2.**105**).

The bony protuberances in psoriatic arthritis require differentiation from the marginal osteophytes of polyarticular osteoarthritis (Heberden arthrosis). In extreme cases these osteophytes are associated with subchondral degenerative cysts, which can become quite large in destructive (erosive) osteoarthritis. Advanced cases of destructive osteoarthritis (Fig. 2.**106**) are marked by ankylosis of the interphalangeal joints. Periarticular demineralization does not occur as it does in rheumatoid arthritis.

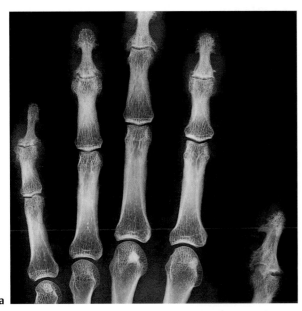

a

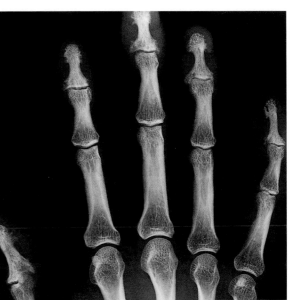

b

Fig. 2.**105 a, b** Typical appearance of psoriatic arthritis. Note how periarticular erosions are accompanied by bone proliferation in the form of protuberances and spiculated excrescences

on the terminal tufts. These changes differ markedly from those of polyarticular osteoarthritis shown in Figs. 2.**66** and 2.**106**.

Fig. 2.**106** Destructive osteoarthritis involving multiple interphalangeal joints. This case is unusual in that marked degenerative changes are also visible in the second metacarpophalangeal joint of each hand and, to a lesser degree, in the third through fifth metacarpophalangeal joints of the left hand. The proximal interphalangeal joint of the small finger of the right hand is ankylosed.

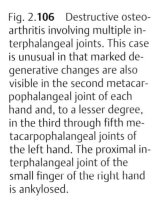

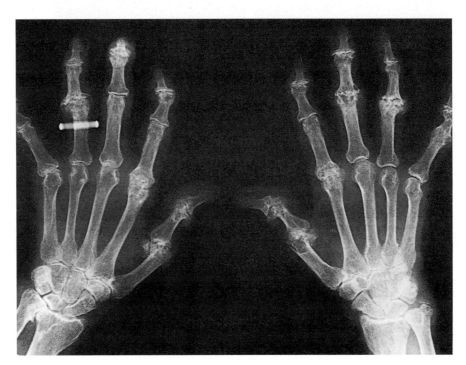

Bones

As mentioned earlier, a bone felon can have very subtle radiographic features in its early stage, which may consist only of circumscribed tuftal resorption.

> Clinically, however, these patients usually present with severe pain and swelling of the affected distal phalanx. This will direct the examiner's attention to possible subtle radiographic changes and may prompt the use of a magnifier (with mammographic technique) when the films are read.

Figure 2.**71** illustrates the early radiographic appearance of a bone felon. The lesion shown in Fig. 2.**107** has already caused significant bone destruction.

Fine osteolysis combined with marginal sclerosis, while always suspicious for an inflammatory process, is also observed with osteoid osteoma. This tumor rarely involves the distal phalanx, however.

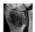 ## Tumor?

As in other body regions, tumors and tumorlike lesions of the distal phalanges are manifested by osteolysis, osteosclerosis, or a combination of both. Because the distal phalanges are very small bones, tumors tend to break out of them quickly, producing radiographic changes at an early stage. As a result, it is rare to encounter borderline findings between normal and pathological. The majority of malignant bone tumors in the distal phalanges are metastatic carcinomas, and most of these originate from the lung. All other tumor entities are very rare in the distal

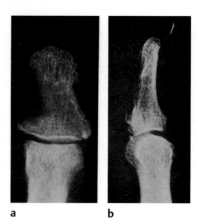

a   b

Fig. 2.**107 a, b**
Bone felon in the distal phalanx.

phalanges. This includes the extremely painful glomus tumor, which arises from the subcutaneous neuromyoarterial plexus and is located between the distal phalanx and the nail. This also characterizes its radiographic appearance, which consists of a dorsal defect below the nail (see Fig. 2.**79**). Purely intraosseous glomus tumors are very rare.

Subungual keratoacanthoma, like glomus tumors, can cause external erosion of the distal phalanx. Its radiographic features can be interpreted only within the context of the clinical presentation.

In the category of tumorlike lesions and pseudotumors, the dominant lesion is the epithelial cyst, described previously under General Aspects (Figs. 2.**78**, 2.**108**).

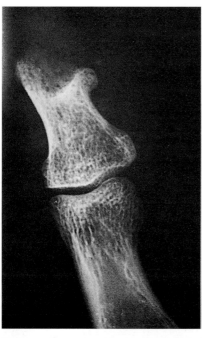 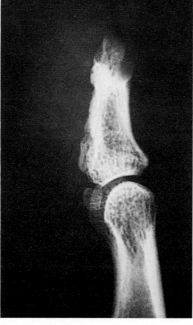

a   b

Fig. 2.**108 a, b**   Epithelial cyst with destruction of the terminal tuft. The differential diagnosis should include a metastasis from bronchial carcinoma.

Middle Phalanges

Normal Findings

 During Growth

The diaphysis of the middle phalanx is ossified at birth in full-term infants. The proximal epiphyses become radiographically visible later than in the distal phalanges and are not seen before the second to third year of life. They fuse with the shaft at age 17 to 18 years. The epiphyses of 13- to 15-year-old appear broader than the proximal shaft and have a denser structure.

 In Adulthood

The distal end of the middle phalanx, called the head, is formed by a trochlea with symmetrically shaped condyles. Just proximal to it is the narrowest portion of the shaft. As with all the bones of the hand, the size and shape of the middle phalanges show marked constitutional variations. This includes the prominence of the bony ridges to which the capsule and ligaments are attached (Fig. 2.**109**).

The middle phalanx also features a flat, Y-shaped ridge located at the center of the shaft on the palmar side (Fig. 2.**109a**), visible on lateral radiographs. The normal bony ridges and prominences should not be mistaken for pathological processes at fibro-osseous junctions (especially in acromegaly), for fracture callus, or periosteal pathology.

The nutrient canals in the distal half of the shaft run obliquely from the outer surface of the bone into the distal medullary cavity (Fig. 2.**8**). Nutrient canals that enter the bone on the palmar or dorsal side may be projected farther into the medullary region on radiographs (Fig. 2.**109c**).

Pathological Finding?

 Normal Variant or Anomaly?

Cone-shaped epiphyses are common in the middle phalanges, especially in the second and fifth digits (Fig. 2.**18**). It was noted on p. 24 that cone-shaped epiphyses are a normal variant and are rarely associated with clinical symptoms.

Brachymesophalangia is the most common hereditary anomaly of the middle phalanges. Short, occasionally stout middle phalanges (especially in the fifth finger) occur as a normal variant in approximately 20% of Japanese compared with 0.6–1% of the European population. There is a 62–67% incidence of brachymesophalangia in trisomy 21 (Down syndrome). The classification of brachymesophalangia is shown in Table 2.**10a**.

Table 2.**10b** lists the full spectrum of possible syndromic associations.

A wedged shape or trapezoidal configuration of the short middle phalanx inevitably results in **clinodactyly**, or angular deviation of the distal phalanx (Fig. 2.**110**).

Dubost et al. (1960) described aplasia of the middle phalanx combined with a short, hypoplastic distal phalanx and an extremely long proximal phalanx (perhaps as a compensatory mechanism).

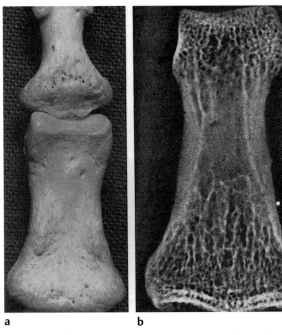
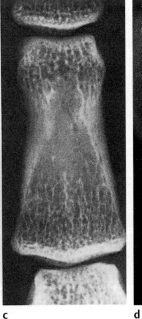
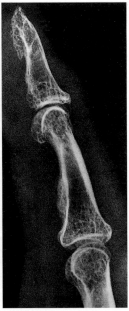

a　　　　　　　b　　　　　　　　　　　c　　　　　　　d

Fig. 2.**109a–d** Anatomic specimen and radiographs of middle phalanges. In panel **a**, note the many surface ridges and prominences and the nutrient canals. The lateral radiograph in **d** shows a superimposition view of the basal prominences that give attachment to the flexor digitorum profundus tendons.

Table 2.**10a** Classification of brachydactylies (after Bell)

Type	Description
A1	Brachymesophalangia II–IV and brachybasophalangia I Possible symphalangia of middle and distal phalanges or aplasia of middle phalanges
A2	Brachymesophalangia II Absence of epiphyses Delta phalanx with radial clinodactyly
A3	Brachymesophalangia V Radial clinodactyly
A4	Brachymesophalangia II–V Bifid distal phalanx of thumb Dystelephalangia V (Kirner deformity)
B	Brachymesophalangia and brachytelephalangia II–V (or absence of distal phalanges)
C	Brachymesophalangia II, III, and V Hyperphalangia of second and third proximal phalanges
D	Brachytelephalangia I with broadening
E	Brachymetacarpia III–V

Table 2.**10b** Spectrum of causes and syndromic associations in brachymesophalangia (after Poznanski)

Affecting the middle phalanx of the small finger	
Limited to the middle phalanges	Brachydactyly A3
Also involving other digits	Brachydactyly A1 Camptobrachydactyly Symphalangia Syndactyly type 3
Accompanying chromosomal syndromes	Trisomy 4 p Trisomy 9 p Trisomy 18 Trisomy 21 XXXXX XXXXY
Accompanying craniofacial syndromes	Ankyloglossia superior: Oculodentodigital Orofaciodigital I and II Otopalatodigital
Other accompanying syndromes	Aarskog Bloom Christian Coffin–Siris Progressive ossifying fibrodysplasia Goltz Hand–foot–genital syndrome Holt–Oram Laurence–Moon–Biedel Noonan Poland Popliteal pterygium Pseudothalidomide Seckel Shwachman Silver Thrombocytopenia with absent radius Williams
Acquired	Arthritis Neoplasms Trauma

Table 2.**10b** (Continue)

Affecting the index finger	
Limited to the middle phalanges	Brachydactyly A2
Also involving other digits	Brachydactyly A1
Accompanying chromosomal syndromes	
Accompanying craniofacial syndromes	
Other accompanying syndromes	Pseudohypoparathyroidism Pseudopseudohypoparathyroidism Sclerosteosis

Affecting other middle phalanges	
Limited to the middle phalanges	Brachydactyly A4
Also involving other digits	Brachydactyly A1 Brachydactyly B Brachydactyly C Symphalangia
Accompanying craniofacial syndromes	Acrocephalosyndactyly (Apert) Acrocephalosyndactyly (Carpenter)
Other accompanying syndromes	Aarskog Christian Frias Herrmann–Opitz Hollister–Hollister Hull Hunter–Frazer Cloverleaf skull Poland Saldino–Mainzer Symphalangia–brachydactyly Trichorhinophalangeal syndrome
Acquired	Arthritis Infection Neoplasms Sickle cell anemia Trauma

Delta phalanx can also affect the middle phalanges. Its features and syndromic associations were described on p. 26.

The original editor of this book, A. Köhler, observed unusual morphological changes involving the middle phalanges, and to a lesser degree the distal phalanges, in three generations of a family. There was no apparent syndromic association for these changes (Fig. 2.111), and Köhler noted that the family members were otherwise healthy. Broadening and deformity of the middle phalanges began between 7 and 10 years of age. The heads (trochleae) became rounded and oblique, causing angular deviation of the distal phalanges, and the heads of the proximal phalanges became squared-off. This condition affected the mother, five of her eight children, and five of eight grandchildren.

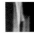 ## Fracture?

Several references have been made to the possibility of mistaking nutrient canals for fracture lines. Nutrient canals appear especially prominent when the cortical bone is very dense. Normal bony prominences and ridges may be mistaken for fracture callus.

Smoothly marginated defects at the corners of joints most commonly result from capsuloligamentous avulsions. A visible fragment is not always present, as it may have been spontaneously resorbed.

 ## Necrosis?

Very dense epiphysis (ivory epiphyses, white epiphyses) were discussed on p. 52. In patients with no clinical symptoms, dense epiphysis are considered a normal variant. They signify necrosis only if they are associated with clinical symptoms such as local swelling and pain, but even then the potential for recovery is excellent. **Thiemann disease** is characterized by dense, fragmented epiphysis occurring mainly in the middle phalanges (Figs. 2.53, 2.54). A single "white" epiphysis is always suspicious for necrosis.

Phalangeal microgeodic syndrome (of childhood) was first described by Maroteaux (1970) and Meller et al. (1982, see also p. 55). It is unclear whether the condition is a transient necrotic process or a true inflammatory disease. It is marked by sudden swelling, redness, heat, and pain occurring in the fingers of one or both hands and predominantly affecting the middle and proximal phalanges. The syndrome has been observed principally in Japan (Meller et al. 1982). Radiographs show sclerosis combined with small cystic lesions with honeycomb-like rarefaction of the cancellous and cortical bone. The authors state that the disorder occurs during the cold months of the year and resolves without treatment.

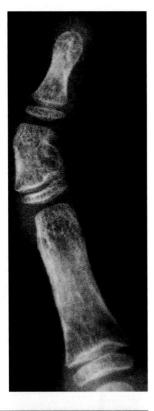

Fig. 2.**110** Brachymesophalangia of the small finger (A3, Table 2.**10**). The trapezoidal shape of the middle phalanx has caused radial deviation of the distal phalanx (clinodactyly). The lucent area on the radial side of the short middle phalanx could also be interpreted as a minimal variant of a delta phalanx (see p. 24).

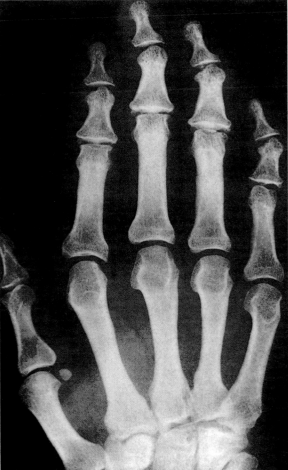

Fig. 2.**111** Deformities of the distal ends of the middle phalanges with consequent angulation of the distal phalanges. These unclassified changes were transmitted within the family as an autosomal dominant trait (observations by A. Köhler).

Inflammation, Tumor?

Inflammatory, neoplastic, and tumorlike changes in the skeleton of the hand were discussed earlier under General Aspects, with special emphasis placed on border-normal and borderline-pathological findings. Because these conditions can affect any of the phalanges and metacarpals, there is no need to review them here in detail. It is sufficient to note that proliferative processes of the phalanges, especially the subentity known as florid reactive periostitis, predominantly affect the middle phalanges (see p. ■).

Other Changes?

Resorptive changes on both the periosteal and endosteal sides in hyperparathyroidism mainly affect the middle phalanges and are most common on the radial side.

  Particularly the early features of hyperparathyroidism represent a true transition from the still-normal to the pathological.

In most cases, early resorptive changes can be seen only by obtaining microfocus magnification views or by using mammographic technique and then reading the films with a magnifier. Typical signs of primary and secondary hyperparathyroidism are loss of normal cortical definition along the radial margins, particularly on the middle phalanges of the second and third fingers, usually associated with rarefied and blurred cancellous trabeculae and intracortical bone resorption. In advanced cases the cortex is thinned from the outside, being replaced by spiculated bone remnants that create a shaggy contour. Sometimes the rarefied cortical bone can no longer be identified as such due to concomitant resorptive changes along the inner margin of the cortex. Figure 2.112 illustrates the processes in reverse order, proceeding from marked pathology in **a** to normal findings in **b** after the patient underwent a parathyroidectomy.

Figure 2.112 a also demonstrates acro-osteolytic lesions and a brown tumor in the head of the third metacarpal. The severe resorptive changes in renal osteodystrophy shown in Fig. 2.112 c can be seen and diagnosed only when proper radiographic technique is used. Radiographic examination of the hand is particularly important in renal osteodystrophy, because clinical and laboratory parameters (especially parathormone levels and alkaline phosphatase) are not always reliable depending on the duration of dialysis and coexisting disorders such as aluminum intoxication, adynamic bone disease, etc.

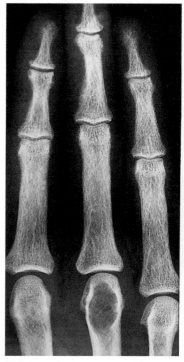
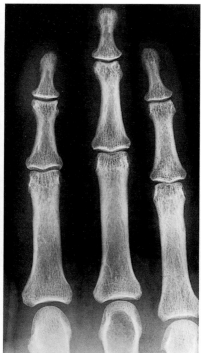
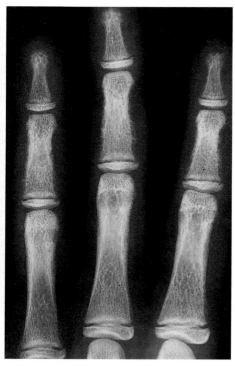

a   b   c

Fig. 2.112 a–c Secondary hyperparathyroidism in renal osteodystrophy.
a Florid stage with pronounced medial subperiosteal bone resorption of the middle phalanges and irregular, rarefied, blurred cancellous trabeculae. Tuft resorption is also present. Note the conspicuous brown tumor in the head of the third metacarpal. Marked changes are also visible in the proximal phalanges.

b Radiograph after parathyroidectomy shows an almost complete regression of changes except for the residual brown tumor in the third metacarpal and the somewhat dense, slightly ulnar-deviated reossified terminal tufts in the second and third digits.
c Florid form of renal osteopathy in a 4-year-old child with cortical resorption along the middle phalanges creating a shaggy, spiculated outer contour, especially on the middle finger.

Proximal Phalanges

Normal Findings

During Growth

The diaphysis of the proximal phalanx, like that of the distal and middle phalanges, is already ossified at birth. The diaphysis ossifies during the 11th week of intrauterine development. The epiphyses become radiographically visible between 27 and 30 months of age, or about the same time as in the middle phalanges. As in the other phalanges, the epiphyses of the proximal phalanges fuse with the shaft between 17 and 18 years of age.

The epiphyses of the proximal phalanges are slightly thicker on the palmar side than on the dorsal side, and they project slightly past the adjacent metaphysis and shaft (Fig. 2.**113**).

In Adulthood

The distal shaft of the proximal phalanges normally bears bony ridges that give attachment to tendons. The prominence of these ridges varies with the mechanical stresses on the hand (Figs. 2.**3 a, b**, 2.**114**). Normal bony prominences should not be mistaken for periosteal new bone formation, which usually occurs at the mid-shift level and always signifies a pathological process (e.g., Fig. 2.**40 b**).

The grooves located between these ridges and the adjacent cortex are occasionally projected as linear lucencies. These should not be mistaken for fracture lines (see Fig. 2.**9 a–c**).

The oblique **vascular (nutrient) canals** run proximally in the basal half of the phalanx and distally in the distal half. A nutrient canal projected end-on appears as a small round lucency. The lower third of the proximal phalanx is relatively bulky and contains abundant cancellous trabeculae. As a result, pathological changes are often first manifested in this region and may consist of an increase or decrease in the radiographic density of the spongiosa (e.g., periarticular demineralization due to metacarpophalangeal arthritis, osteopenia, osteomalacia, osteopetrosis, osteomyelosclerosis).

Pathological Finding?

Normal Variant or Anomaly?

Brachyphalangia, or shortening of the proximal phalanges, is usually accompanied by the shortening of other bones in the hand. Table 2.**11** lists the syndromes that may be associated with proximal brachyphalangia of the thumb and other fingers.

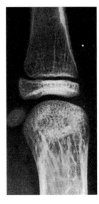

Fig. 2.**113**

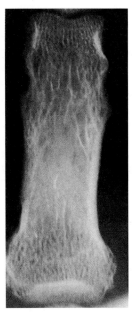

Fig. 2.**114**

Fig. 2.**113**   Shape of the basal epiphysis of the proximal phalanx.

Fig. 2.**114**   Magnification view of a proximal phalanx showing the physiological bony prominences on the distal, lateral aspects of the bone. These prominences should not be mistaken for abnormal periosteal new bone formation (extreme form shown in Fig. 2.**40 b**).

Table 2.**11**   Short proximal phalanges and possible syndromic associations (after Poznanski)

	Thumb alone	**Other or all fingers**
Involving other digits	Brachydactyly A1	Brachydactyly C[1] Brachydactyly A1 (sometimes) Brachydactyly A2 (sometimes)
Accompanying syndromes	Acrocephalopolysyndactyly (Carpenter) Acrocephalosyndactyly (Apert) Acrocephalosyndactyly (Pfeiffer) Diastrophic dwarfism Progressive myositis ossificans Nevoid basal cell carcinoma Rubinstein–Taybi (occasional) Trisomy 18	Diastrophic dwarfism
Acquired		Arthritis Infection Neoplasms Sickle cell anemia Trauma

[1] Proximal hyperphalangia of the second and third fingers

Fracture?

Reference was made earlier to the possibility of mistaking normal linear lucencies for fracture lines on oblique radiographs and mistaking normal bony ridges for callus.

True fractures in the form of bony capsuloligamentous avulsions occur predominantly in the basal portions of the proximal phalanges (Fig. 2.**115**). These small avulsions can be diagnosed on radiographic films by mentally fitting the fragment back into the defect in the adjacent bone. This also distinguishes an avulsed fragment from an accessory sesamoid bone. Occasionally, avulsed fragments may be spontaneously resorbed. Many avulsions never heal and remain isolated for the patient's lifetime, in which case the fracture surfaces become capped off (Fig. 2.**115 b**).

 Inflammation?

The basal articular portion of the proximal phalanges forms the distal side of each metacarpophalangeal joint. These joints are very commonly affected by rheumatoid arthritis and true chondrocalcinosis and provide a test region for radiographic confirmation of the clinical diagnosis.

 Marginal joint erosions are the basic radiological criteria for an inflammatory process.

In florid cases of rheumatoid arthritis, these defects are usually associated with erosions of the adjacent metacarpal heads (Figs. 2.**63**, 2.**116**), periarticular demineralization, and small sentinel cysts. Generally these changes involve both hands symmetrically and affect at least two or three metacarpophalangeal joints per side. Basically the following entities require differentiation from erosions and marginal joint defects (Figs. 2.**64**, 2.**117**):

- Traumatic avulsions with resorption of the avulsed fragment
- Residua of hand trauma sustained during skeletal growth (Fig. 2.**51**)
- Bone resorption and/or fractures in hyperparathyroidism, usually associated with similar changes in the opposing heads and structural changes in the other hand bones, especially the middle phalanges
- Healed erosions in which the cancellous bone exposed by the inflammation has been covered by a reparative "cap" (Fig. 2.**117**)

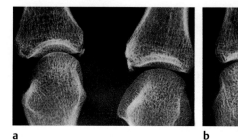

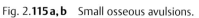
a   b

Fig. 2.**115 a, b**   Small osseous avulsions.

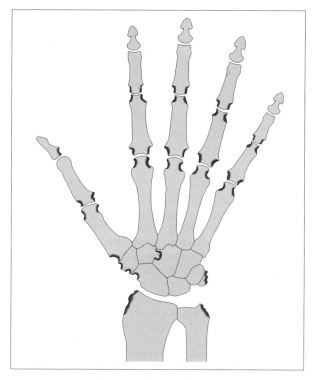

Fig. 2.**116**   Typical location of erosions in rheumatoid arthritis and multicentric reticulohistiocytosis. Both articular ends of the proximal phalanges are generally involved.

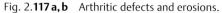

Fig. 2.**117 a, b**   Arthritic defects and erosions.   ▷
a Arthritic defect in the joint margin. There is no traumatic bone fragment.
b Older, smooth ("repaired") marginal erosion of the proximal phalanx in rheumatoid arthritis (right side of panel). The absence of periarticular osteoporosis shows that the acute component of the disease has resolved following treatment. Unrepaired erosions are still visible on the metacarpal head (arrows). Particularly the defect in the radial base of the proximal phalanx (right side of panel) may be mistaken for an old bony avulsion.

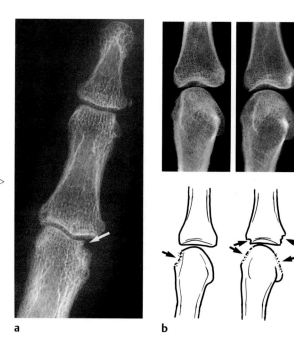

a   b

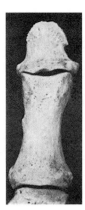

Fig. 2.**118** Clubbed thumb.

Erosions of the basal articular portions of the proximal phalanges occur not only in rheumatoid arthritis but also in chondrocalcinosis and multicentric reticulohistiocytosis. Whereas chondrocalcinosis predominantly affects the metacarpophalangeal joints, the other two diseases also involve the proximal interphalangeal joints and various joints in the wrist (Fig. 2.**116**). Unlike rheumatoid arthritis, multicentric reticulohistiocytosis does not cause significant periarticular demineralization (reflecting a trophic disturbance).

We conclude this brief discussion of rheumatological diagnosis with the following remarks on radiographic techniques, especially as they relate to issues of differential diagnosis.

- As a general rule, mammographic technique should be used for all radiographic examinations of the hands. If the differential diagnosis includes an inflammatory process, extra oblique views should be obtained in the "zither-player" position, i.e., a PA projection with the hand in 45° semisupination and the fingertips resting on the cassette. This gives an excellent view of dorsoulnar and radiopalmar erosions in the metacarpal heads and in the opposing ends of the proximal phalanges.
- In the Norgaard technique, erosions on the dorsoradial aspect of the second through fifth proximal phalanges (and of the joint between the pisiform and triquetrum) can be defined with an AP projection of both hands in 45° semisupination with the fingers spread wide apart ("catcher" position). Stelling et al. (1982) question the value of these extra views, however, noting that contour defects and loss of contour definition can occur physiologically at the sites of the Norgaard erosions.

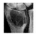 Tumor?

Since the proximal phalanges have a relatively large volume compared with the other phalanges, they are a relatively common site of involvement by tumors such as enchondromas (Fig. 2.**75a**). They are occasionally involved by giant cell tumors and by lesions that typically involve larger bones such as enostoma and osteoid osteoma (Fig. 2.**83**). The differential diagnosis should also include florid reactive periostitis (Fig. 2.**84**).

Thumb

Normal Findings

During Growth

The appearance and ossification of the diaphyseal and epiphyseal centers have the same timing as the corresponding processes in the middle and proximal phalanges (q.v.).

In Adulthood

In 73% of adults, a sesamoid bone is found adjacent to the interphalangeal joint of the thumb (see Figs. 2.**5** and 2.**6**). Figure 2.**7** shows a metacarpophalangeal thumb joint with two normal and two rudimentary sesamoid bones.

Aside from constitutional variants, the shape of the two phalanges of the thumb depends on manual stresses and levels of exertion at least as much as in the other fingers.

A short, broad thumb may be completely normal, but it is considered an anomaly when it occurs unilaterally or bilaterally in families. Then it is known as a **clubbed thumb** or "murderer's thumb" (Fig. 2.**118**). Clubbed thumb is a special form of **brachytelephalangia**, which is occasionally associated with partial duplication of the distal phalanx.

Pathological Finding?

Normal Variant or Anomaly?

The many possible congenital anomalies of the thumb are classified in Tables 2.**12**–2.**14**.

These tables are intended to provide a general overview without going into details. A thumb with a remarkably short distal phalanx may be a sign of a more complex dysplasia (Table 2.**14**). Syndromes associated with a short proximal phalanx are listed in Table 2.**11**. A short proximal phalanx often leads to deviation of the distal phalanx (pollex varus or valgus). In many of these cases the proximal phalanx shows a delta configuration (longitudinally bracketed diaphysis, Fig. 2.**119**), which can also be observed in the toes (q.v.). Shortening of the first digit is commonly seen in the Rubinstein–Taybi and acrocephalosyndactyly syndromes. The bony hypoplasia may be associated with absence of the thenar muscles, division of the flexor pollicis longus muscle including anomalous insertions, and lateral subluxation of the proximal phalanx of the thumb (Miura 1981, Rayan 1984, Martinez 1985). These anomalies may be inherited. The flexor pollicis longus may be completely absent (Miura 1977). A **triphalangeal** thumb has a prevalence of approximately 1 : 25 000 in the European population (Ferber 1953), and a familial incidence has been described. This condition may also be associated with duplication of the thumb, bilateral triphalangism, or aplasia of the contralateral thumb. Syndromes associated with triphalangism are listed in Table 2.**15**.

Table 2.**12**   Classification of anomalies of the thumb (after Swanson)

Grade	Anomaly
I	Failure of formation
A	Transverse deficiency

B	Longitudinal deficiency
	1. Radial ray defect: hypoplasia of the thumb
	2. Absence of musculature:
	  a. Extrinsic
	  b. Intrinsic

II	Failure of differentiation
A	Soft-tissue involvement: 1. Syndactyly 2. Congenital flexion contracture 3. Congenital trigger finger (snapping thumb or fixed flexion at the interphalangeal joint)
B	Skeletal involvement: 1. Angular deviation, delta phalanx (Fig. 2.**119**) 2. Symphalangia
III	Duplication: radial polydactyly (Fig. 2.**27 i, j**)
IV	Thumb too large: macrodactyly
V	Thumb too small: brachydactyly
VI	Ring constriction complex
VII	Miscellaneous anomalies and syndromes

Table 2.**13**   Classification of hypoplasia and aplasia of the thumb (after Blauth)

Grade	Anomaly
I	Minor hypoplasia of the thumb but all structures normal
II	Normal thumb skeleton, adduction contracture, MP joint instability, hypoplastic thenar muscles
III	Significant skeletal hypoplasia. CMCJ[1] may be present, or proximal portion of first metacarpal may be absent. Intrinsic tendons aplastic, extrinsic tendons rudimentary
IV	„Floating" thumb; rudimentary phalanx tethered on the second MP joint
V	Complete absence (aplasia) of the thumb

[1]MP joint   Metacarpophalangeal joint
CMCJ   Carpometacarpal joint

Table 2.**14**   Development disturbances with short distal phalanges primarily affecting the thumb (after Poznanski)

Short and broad	Narrow and thin
Acrocephalosyndactyly (Carpenter)	Cornelia de Lange syndrome
Acrocephalosyndactyly (Apert)	Cryptogenic brachymetacarpia
Acrocephalosyndactyly (Pfeifer)	Fanconi syndrome
Brachydactyly D[1]	Fibrodysplasia (myositis) ossificans congenita
Brachydactyly A4[1]	Holt–Oram syndrome
Cheirolumbar dysostosis	Radial hypoplasia
Christian brachydactyly	Trisomy 18
Cryptodontic metacarpalia	
Diastrophic dysplasia	
Fibrodysplasia (myositis) ossificans congenita	
Hand–foot–genital syndrome	
Osteodyplasitia (Melnick–Needles)	
Otopalatodigital syndrome	
Pseudohypoparathyroidism	
Pseudopseudohypoparathyroidism	
Robinow syndrome	
Rubinstein–Taybi syndrome	
Tabatznik syndrome	

[1] Possible longitudinal division

Table 2.**15**   Syndromes and other anomalies associated with a triphalangeal thumb (after Poznanski)

Syndromes
- Blackfan–Diamond anemia
- Cardiomelia (Holt–Oram)
- Duane
- Juberg–Hayward
- LADD (lacrima–auriculo–dento–digital syndrome)
- Thalidomide embryonopathy
- Goodman
- Trisomy 13–15 (occasionally)
- IVIC syndrome[1]
- Aase syndrome (congenitally deficient erythropoiesis)
- Nager acrofacial dysostosis
- Townes

Other accompanying anomalies
- Absence of the pectoralis muscle
- Absence of the tibia
- Duplication of the big toe
- Anal obliteration and deafness
- Congenital cleft foot (lobster claw)
- Preaxial polydactyly
- Polydactyly of the small toe
- Cleft hand

[1] IVIC Instituto Venezolano de Investigaciones Cientificas

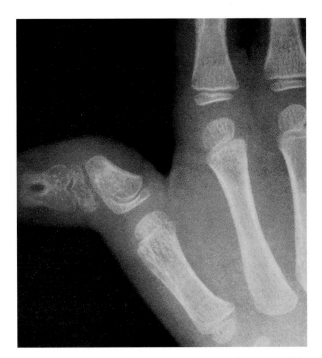

Fig. 2.**119**   Delta configuration of the proximal phalanx of the thumb with radial angulation of the distal phalanx in a 3-year-old girl. The findings were bilaterally symmetrical, and a proximal delta phalanx was also present in both big toes. Note the cleft deformity in the distal phalanx of the thumb, probably representing a minimal form of polydactyly ("distal phalanx type" described by Buck-Gramcko, p. 31).

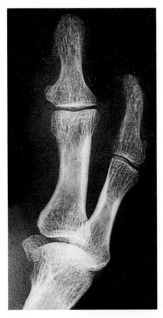

Fig. 2.**120**   Complete duplication of the thumb (MP-I type⁺ of Buck-Gramcko). A case of rudimentary polydactyly is shown in Fig. 2.**27**.

A case of radial polydactyly (duplication of the thumb) is shown in Fig. 2.**120**, which illustrates the MP-I-type⁺ of polydactyly described by Buck-Gramcko (1989). Other forms of radial polydactyly are shown in Fig. 2.**27**. The hand surgeon requires a precise morphological classification of the anomaly in order to plan corrective surgery (pp. 31, 32).

 ## Fracture?

One should be careful diagnosing a metacarpophalangeal subluxation of the thumb based on radiographs, since especially oblique projections may show an apparent offset of the joint contours (see also p. 132 f). Doubts can be resolved by comparing the films with contralateral views.

Gamekeeper's thumb is caused by a soft-tissue tear or bony avulsion of the ulnar ligament of the first metacarpophalangeal joint (Fig. 2.**122 b**). Similar injuries can be caused by the thumb getting tangled in the strap of a mechanical bull (Ginthner and Schabel 1981) or in the strap of a ski pole. The same injury has been observed in patients using a strapless ski pole (Primiano 1985). Wilhelm et al. (1982) described a similar "ski thumb" injury in children. Stress radiographs are needed to appreciate the extent of the ligamentous injury.

The rare **sesamoid fractures** were described under General Aspects and illustrated in Figs. 2.**49** and 2.**50**. Additional cases are shown in Figs. 2.**121** and 2.**122 a**.

 ## Necrosis?

Necrosis of the sesamoid bones was discussed under General Aspects (see Fig. 2.**60**).

Acro-osteolysis can affect the thumb as well as other digits and is also discussed fully under General Aspects (Table 2.**6**).

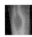 ## Inflammation?

The metacarpophalangeal joint of the thumb has a certain predisposition for gouty arthritis. Isolated inflammatory changes in the joint with signs of destruction, large medullary tophi, and especially fine paraosseous calcifications are always suspicious for gouty arthritis.

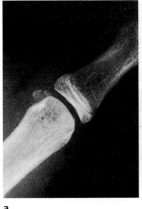 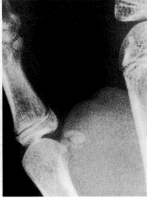

a   b

Fig. 2.**121 a, b**   Comminuted sesamoid fracture caused by a direct ski-pole injury in a 14-year-old girl.

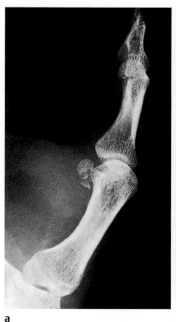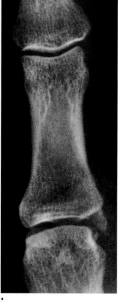

a   b

Fig. 2.**122 a, b**   Comminuted sesamoid fracture and bony avulsion of the ulnar ligament.
a Three-part fracture of the sesamoid in a 54-year-old woman.
b Bony avulsion of the ulnar ligament. If the bone fragment below the ulnar sesamoid were rotated 90° in a clockwise direction, it would fit precisely into the opposing edge defect.

 ## Other Changes?

Extreme occupational stresses on the interphalangeal joint of the thumb can lead to degenerative joint changes that are otherwise unusual at that location. Minuk et al. (1982) described this condition in laboratory technicians who repetitively flex and extend the interphalangeal joint of the thumb while using a pipette ("pipetter's thumb"). It presents radiographically with joint space narrowing, increased density of the subchondral bone plate, subchondral lucencies, and other osteoarthritic features. With the automation of laboratory procedures, it is unlikely that this type of joint degeneration is prevalent today.

Metacarpus

Normal Findings

 ### During Growth

The metacarpal ossification centers appear between 2 and 4 months of fetal development. The epiphyseal centers of the metacarpals become visible radiographically at 10 months to 2 years of age. The centers are located distally in the second through fifth rays and proximally in the first ray.

 ## In Adulthood

The first metacarpal is the shortest and thickest. The second metacarpal is the longest, and the fourth metacarpal is the most slender. A line drawn tangent to the radial margin of the first metacarpal should pass just radial to a line drawn tangent to the trapezium. This "step sign" can simulate the appearance of a subluxation on radiographs (Fig. 2.**123**).

The relatively broad, mortiselike or rooflike base of the second metacarpal articulates with the ridge of the trapezoid bone.

The cortex of the metacarpals is of variable thickness. The midshaft cortex in young, healthy individuals may be so thick that the marrow space is reduced to a slitlike space (Fig. 2.**3 c, d**). With aging, the metacarpal cortex decreases in thickness. This physiological thinning of the metacarpal cortex, as well as pathological cortical thinning, can be quantified with the Barnett–Nordin index (see p. 18 ff). Normally the cortex of the metacarpals is very solid, and intracortical striations are a sign of bone resorption, especially in hyperparathyroidism but also in osteomalacia (Figs. 2.**43**, 2.**44**, 2.**132 c**).

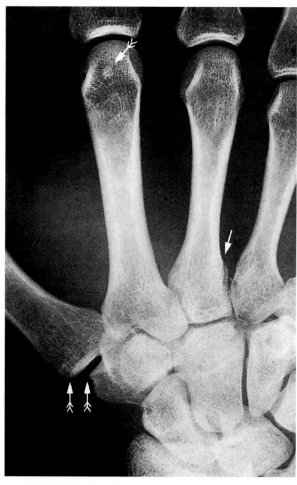

Fig. 2.**123**   Superficial fissure at the base of the third metacarpal (arrow). Sesamoid bone (double arrow) on the head of the second metacarpal. Note the simulated displacement of the adjacent "corners" of the first metacarpal and the trapezium (double arrows): the step sign.

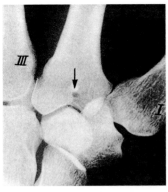

Fig. 2.**124**   Nutrient canal appears as a pinhole defect in the base of the second metacarpal.

The mechanical stresses at sites of capsular and tendon attachment can incite local proliferative changes. Exostosis-like prominences located at the head–shaft junction of the metacarpals are considered a normal finding (Fig. 2.**125**). Larger prominences should be considered pathological only when they are associated with narrowing of the joint spaces, especially in the second and third metacarpals. They can then be identified as the "drooping osteophytes" of chondrocalcinosis and are usually accompanied by small subchondral cystlike lucencies (p. 59, Fig. 2.**70**). The double head of the fifth metacarpal in Fig. 2.**125 c–e** is absolutely pathological and may be consistent with an osteochondroma or—more likely—with a rudimentary ulnar polydactylia (see also Fig. 2.**27 n**).

Pinhole defects located at the base of the second metacarpal and other metacarpals represent end-on projections of nutrient canals (Fig. 2.**124**). The nutrient canals in

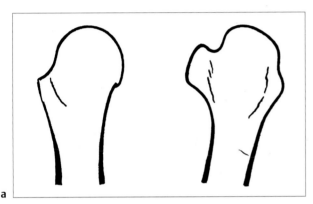

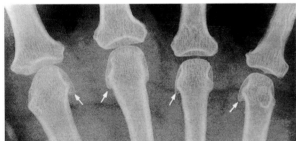

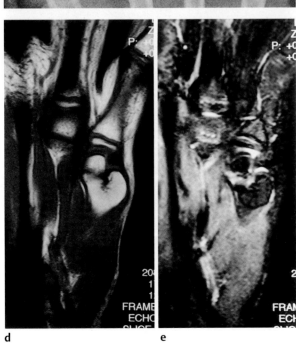

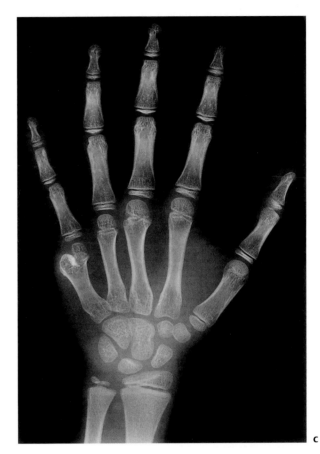

Fig. 2.**125 a–e**   Differential diagnosis of exostosis-like protuberances on the heads of the metacarpals.
a Typical exostosis-like prominence on the first metacarpal.
b Morphological variants of exostosis-like prominences on the metacarpal heads.
c–e "Double head" of the fifth metacarpal in a 9-year-old boy. We interpret it as a rudimentary ulnar polydactylia (see Fig. 2.**27 n**), but consider also an osteochondroma. (Case courtesy of Dr. Chr. Müller, Hamburg.)

the shafts of the metacarpals run obliquely from the cortex to the medullary cavity in a distal-to-proximal direction (see Fig. 2.**8b**).

> A rarefied, lucent area is frequently visible on the ulnar side of the base of the fifth metacarpal and is not an abnormal finding (Fig. 2.**10**).

In a recent publication Theumann et al (2002) discuss MR imaging of the metacarpophalangeal joints of the fingers.

Pathological Finding?

Normal Variant or Anomaly?

Accessory epiphyses, known also as pseudoepiphyses (p. 23 ff.), can occur as a normal variant, especially in the distal part of the first metacarpal and the proximal part of the second metacarpal (Figs. 2.**15**–2.**17**, 2.**126**). As mentioned under General Aspects, accessory epiphyses can also be a feature of hypothyroidism or Down syndrome. Accessory epiphyses are most commonly seen between 5 and 10 years of age and close years earlier than the normal epiphyseal plate in the same bone. They do not contribute to longitudinal bone growth, which is why they are called "pseudoepiphyses." Their development and maturation were discussed on p. 23 ff.

The shortening of one or more metacarpals usually has pathological significance. Table 2.**16** lists the syndromes that may be associated with a short first metacarpal (Table 2.**16a**) and other metacarpals (Table 2.**16 b**). The Kosowicz method for determining normal metacarpal length was explained earlier (see Fig. 2.**4**).

Shortening of the fourth metacarpal bone in adults is significant in the diagnosis of pseudohypoparathyroidism (Fig. 2.**30**). In these cases a tangent to the heads of the fourth and fifth metacarpals intersects the head of the third metacarpal.

Figure 2.**127** shows a case in which brachymetacarpia of the third metacarpal is combined with compensatory elongation of the proximal phalanx as an isolated anomaly.

Short, stout metacarpals that show proximal tapering are commonly seen in the various forms of mucopolysaccharidosis and mucolipidosis (Fig. 2.**128**).

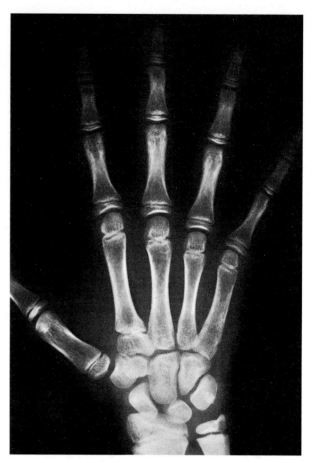

Fig. 2.**126** Large accessory epiphysis ("pseudoepiphysis") in the second metacarpal.

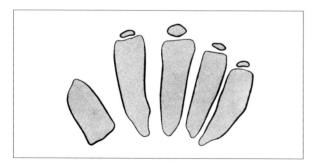

Fig. 2.**128** Metacarpal deformity in mucopolysaccharidosis.

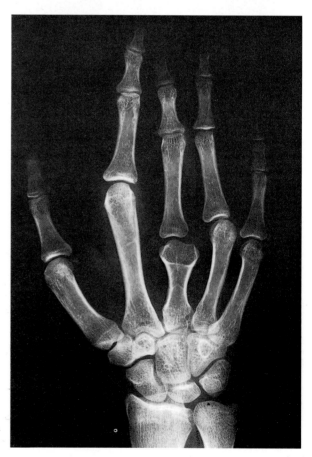

Fig. 2.**127** Short third metacarpal with compensatory elongation of the proximal phalanx. ▷

Table 2.**16 a, b**　Diseases and syndromes associated with short metacarpals (brachymetacarpia) (after Poznanski)

a　Short first metacarpal

	Thin	Normal width
Limited to the metacarpals	Isolated	
Also involving other bones in the hand	Radial hypoplasia syndromes	Brachydactyly C
Accompanying syndromes	Fanconi (pancytopenic dysmelia) Newberg–Hayward Radial hypoplasia Taybi–Lindner Trisomy 18q	André Christian brachydactyly Belange Diastrophic dysplasia Dyggve–Melchior–Clausen Dyssegmental dwarfism Fibrodysplasia (myositis) ossificans progressiva Hand–foot–genital syndrome Schinzel–Giedion Trisomy 9p Symphalangia–brachydactyly
Acquired		Arthritis Infection Neoplasms Sickle cell anemia Trauma

b　Other metacarpals

	Third, fourth, and fifth metacarpals	All or some metacarpals
Limited to the metacarpals	Brachydactyly E	
Also involving other bones in the hand	Brachydactyly A1 (sometimes) Brachydactyly C	
Accompanying syndromes	Beckwith–Wiedemann Biemond I Camptobrachydactyly Cheirolumbar Cryptodontic metacarpals Mseleni joint disease Multiple epiphyseal dysplasia Multiple exostoses Nevoid basal cell carcinoma Pseudo- and pseudopseudo-hypoparathyroidism Ruvalcaba Tabatznik Turner (XO) 5p (cri du chat)	Acrodysostosis Bilginturan brachydactyly Camptobrachydactyly Chondrodysplasia punctata Larsen Manzke (second metacarpal) Megaepiphyseal dwarfism Pseudo hypoparathyroidism and pseudopseudohypoparathyroidism Taybi–Lindner Trichorhinophalangeal I and II

Fracture?

Fractures of the metacarpal bones are classified as follows:

- Basal fractures of the first metacarpal
  - Bennett fracture (Fig. 2.**129 a–c**) (intra-articular)
  - Rolando fracture (intra-articular)
  - Winterstein fracture (extra-articular)
- Basal fractures of the second through fifth metacarpals (Fig. 2.**130**)
- Shaft fractures
- Subcapital fractures
- Head fractures

Fractures of the metacarpal heads themselves usually result from direct violence to the outstretched hand, whereas subcapital fractures are most often caused by a fall onto the closed fist. While displaced fractures generally present no problems of differential diagnosis, nondisplaced shaft fractures may occasionally be mistaken for nutrient canals.

Basal fractures of the first metacarpal are straightforward in terms of differential diagnosis, although an old nonunited fragment from a Bennett fracture-dislocation might be confused with an accessory bone element if the dislocation component of the fracture is no longer evident.

An important entity in the differential diagnosis of fractures and normal variants is the carpal boss, which is a bony protuberance on the dorsum of the wrist (discussed further on p. 138). Other accessory bone elements can also mimic fragments.

We close this section by recalling that complex injuries of the carpometacarpal region that involve multiple fracture lines and dislocations are extremely difficult to evaluate on conventional radiographic films. Most of these injuries will require CT evaluation in order to obtain sufficiently detailed information for appropriate treatment planning.

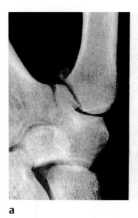 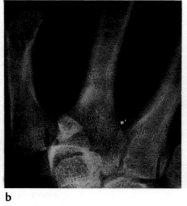 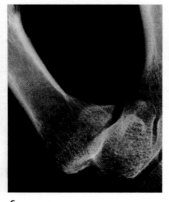 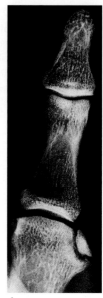

a   b   c

Fig. 2.**129 a–d** Traumatic changes in the thumb.
a–c Bennett fractures with fragments of varying size. Note particularly the radial dislocation of the base of the first metacarpal in panel **b** (see also text).
d Old avulsion fracture of the radial margin of the head of the first metacarpal. The geometric congruity of the bone fragment relative to the adjacent depression identifies it as an avulsed fragment rather than an accessory bone element.

d

 Necrosis?

Aseptic necrosis can occur in the metacarpal heads but is rare compared with the heads of the metatarsals. Best known is Dieterich disease, which is an epiphyseal necrosis of the metacarpals (p. 53, Fig. 2.**131 a**). Congenital anomalies of the epiphyses during skeletal growth (epiphyses too small or too large, "fragmented" epiphyses) require differentiation from necrotic changes. This is accomplished by noting that systemic epiphyseal growth disturbances (e.g., Conradi–Hünermann disease) generally affect all the epiphyses. By contrast, the involvement of individual epiphyses with increased density, fragmentation, etc. should always suggest aseptic necrosis. The potential for multiple epiphyseal necrotic changes in the setting of Kashin–Beck disease was noted on p. 54.

For completeness, Fig. 2.**131** illustrates an unusual case in which chronic recurring pancreatitis led to extensive infarctions not just in the large tubular bones but also in the hands and feet. Necrosis in the third and fourth metacarpals of the left hand resulted in extensive morphological and structural changes that simulate the appearance of fibrous dysplasia.

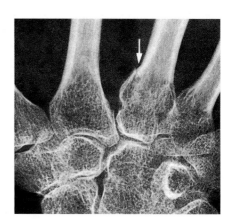

Fig. 2.**130** Traumatic fissure in the radial base of the third metacarpal (frequent site of injury).

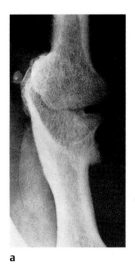

a

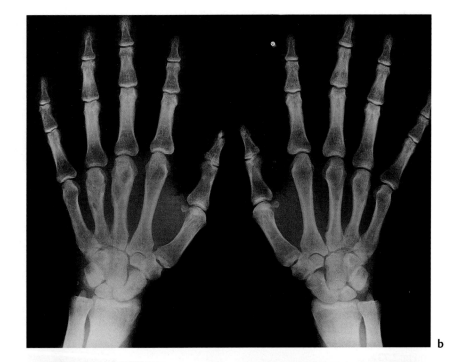

b

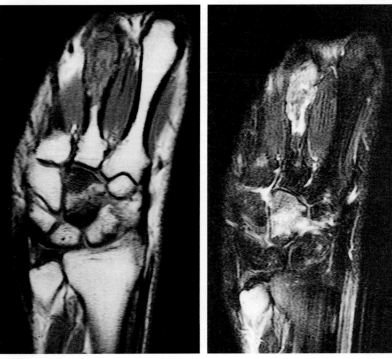

c

d

Fig. 2.**131 a–d**   Necrotic changes in the metacarpals.
a Late findings after aseptic necrosis of the metacarpal head (Dieterich epiphyseal necrosis). Note the severe head deformity and signs of secondary degenerative arthritis.
b–d Unusual morphological changes in the third and fourth metacarpals of the left hand, consisting of bone expansion and marked structural changes. These changes are based on extensive infarctions of the bone marrow and probably of the cortex as well, with later reparative processes in a patient with recurring bouts of pancreatitis. The MR images in **c** and **d** vividly demonstrate the florid soft-tissue changes within the third

metacarpal bone, which appear hyperintense (proton-rich) in the T2-weighted image. The streaklike areas of increased signal intensity in the T1-weighted image are probably due to intraosseous hemorrhage. Additional changes (also visible on conventional radiographs) are evident in the capitate and scaphoid bones, with the capitate showing conspicuous edema. Conventional radiographs also showed initial changes in the opposite hand and in numerous large tubular bones including the metaphyses and epiphyses. (Courtesy of Professor Dr. Terwey, Bremen.)

Inflammation?

As explained in the section on the proximal phalanges, the metacarpophalangeal joints are a site of predilection for systemic inflammatory changes, especially rheumatoid arthritis (Fig. 2.**132**) as well as cartilaginous disorders that lead to arthritis secondarily such as chondrocalcinosis and hemochromatosis (Fig. 2.**134**). The florid stage of rheumatoid arthritis is signaled by periarticular demineralization combined with sentinel cysts. Later stages, which are not detailed here, are marked by coarser destructive changes and osteolytic lesions leading to deformity. Chondrocalcinosis is almost always associated with joint space narrowing, since the disease originates in the cartilage. Increased density and erosion of the subchondral plates are accompanied by subchondral lucencies and frequent bone proliferation on the metacarpal heads (drooping osteophytes, Fig. 2.**70**). Psoriatic arthritis predominantly affects the distal and proximal interphalangeal joints, but advanced stages can also involve the metacarpophalangeal and carpal joints as shown in Fig. 2.**133**.

The potential for involvement of one or two metacarpal bones by Paget disease (osteitis deformans) was illustrated in Fig. 2.**73 a**.

Tumor?

There are no particular structures or variants in the metacarpal bones that can simulate a neoplastic process. True tumors and tumorlike lesions of the metacarpal region were discussed under General Aspects (p. 63 ff.). The differential diagnosis between an osteochondroma and an ulnar polydactylia is illustrated in Fig. 2.**125 c–e**.

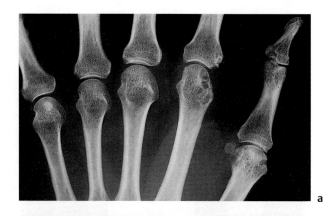

a

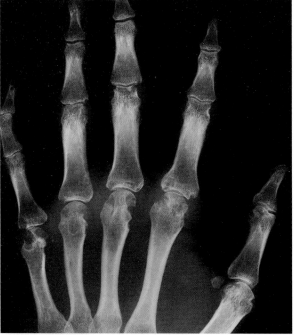

b

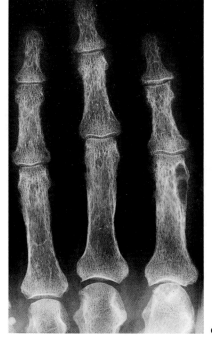

c

Fig. 2.**132 a–c** Differential diagnosis of rheumatoid arthritis. ▷
a, b Typical features of rheumatoid arthritis, with marginal erosions at the metacarpophalangeal joints and periarticular demineralization. Erosive changes are also visible around other joints in the hand.
c Coarse erosions of the metacarpal heads in a patient with florid hyperparathyroidism. The erosions or defects in the metacarpal heads result either from collapse of the "soft" bone or from crystal synovitis. Note the typical changes of hyperparathyroidism, especially in the middle phalanges. Note also the brown tumor in the second metacarpal and the acro-osteolytic lesions.

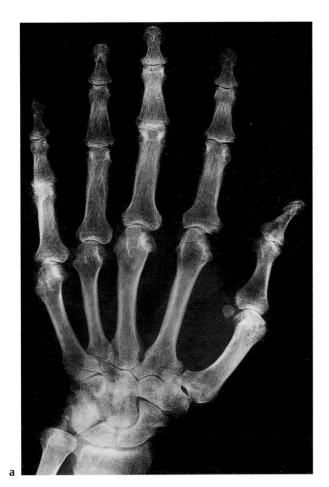

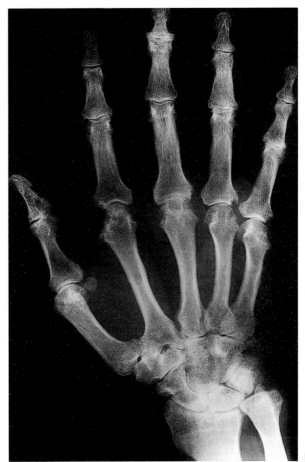

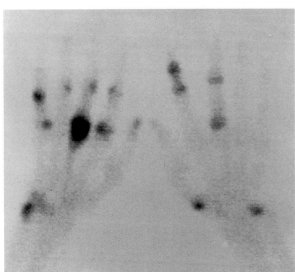

Fig. 2.**133 a–c** Psoriatic arthritis with a transverse pattern of metacarpophalangeal joint involvement. These joints show gross erosive and destructive changes, especially in the metacarpal heads, and small foci of periarticular demineralization. The fifth rays of both hands are involved, and ankylosis has developed across the proximal interphalangeal joints. Bilateral carpal involvement is also seen. Typical protuberances are visible on the distal phalanx of the third finger on each side, especially in the right hand. The pattern of involvement is defined very clearly by the bone scan in panel **c**.

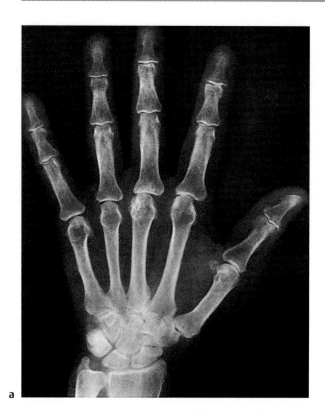

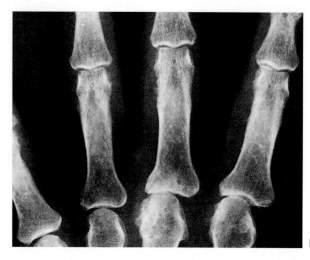

Fig. 2.**134a,b** Typical appearance of arthropathy in hemo-chromatosis with fine periarticular lucencies, especially in the head of the third metacarpal.
a Survey view.
b Enlarged view.

References

Ahn, J. M., D. J. Sartoris, H. S. Kang et al.: Gamekeeper thumb: Comparison of MR arthrography with conventional arthrography and MR imaging in cadavers. Radiology 206 (1998) 737

Albers, W., E. Schirner, H. Giedl: Das Plattenepithelkarzinom des Fingernagelbettes. Med. Welt 34 (1983) 1032

Austin, F. H.: Symphalangism and related fusions of tarsal bones. Radiology 56 (1951) 882

Bard, C., J. J. Sylvestre, R. G. Dussault: Hand osteomyelitis in pianists. J. Ass. Canad. Radiol. 35 (1984) 154

Brecht, G, H. U. Schweikert: Röntgenbefunde beim Pseudohypoparathyreoidismus. Fortschr.Röntgenstr. 136 (1982) 737

Buck-Gramcko,D., P. Behrens: Klassifikation der Polydaktylie für Hand und Fuß. Handchir. Mikrochir. plast. Chir.21 (1989) 195

Carrera, G. F.: Radiographic changes in the hand, following childhood frostbite injury. Skelet. Radiol. 6 (1981) 33

Clarke, P., E. Braunstein, Barbara N. et al.: Sesamoid fracture of the thumb. Case report. Brit. J. Radiol. 56 (1983) 485

Degen, S.: Über das Auftreten der Knochenkerne am Handskelett von der Geburt bis zur Reife. Med. Klin. 46 (1951) 1330

Destouet, J. M., W. A. Murphy: Guitar player acro-osteolysis. Skelet. Radiol. 6 (1981) 275

Dihlmann, W.: Gelenke, Wirbelverbindungen, 2.Aufl. Thieme, Stuttgart 1982

Dijkstra, R. F.: Analysis of metacarpophalangeal pattern profiles. Fortschr. Röntgenstr. 139 (1983) 158

Dreyfuss, U. Y., M. Singer: Human bites of the hand: a study of one hundred six patients. J. Hand Surg. 10-A (1985) 884

Dubost, E. et al.: Trois formes d'anomalies congènitales des membres. J. Radiol. Èlectrol 41 (1960) 579

Ferber, Ch.: Ein Beitrag zur Dreigliedrigkeit des Daumens. Z. Orthop. 83 (1953) 55

Fischer, E.: Akroosteosklerose der Finger, eine normale geschlechts- und altersabhängige endostale Reaktion. Fortschr. Röntgenstr. 137 (1982a) 384

Fischer, E.: Subunguale Verkalkungen. Fortschr. Röntgenstr. 137 (1982b) 580

Fischer, E.: Späte Knochen- und Weichteilveränderungen am Fingerendgelenk nach banalem Trauma. Fortschr. Röntgenstr. 138 (1983) 219

Fisher, M. R. et al.: Carpometacarpal dislocations. Crti. Rev. diagn. Imag. 22 (1984) 95

Freyschmidt, J.: Skeletterkrankungen – klinisch-radiologische Diagnose und Differentialdiagnose Springer, Berlin 1997

Freyschmidt, J.: Frèquence et diagnostic des tumeurs osseuses primitiveset des lésions pseudotumorales du squelette de la main. J. Radiol. CEPUR 5 (1985) 265

Freyschmidt, J., G. Freyschmidt: Haut-, Schleimhaut- und Skeletterkrankungen – SKIBO-DISEASES. Springer, Berlin 1996

Freyschmidt, J.: Melorheostosis: a review of 23 cases. Eur. Radiol. 11 (2001) 474

van Genechten, M.: Familial trigger thumb in children. Hand 14 (1982) 56

Giedion, A.: Zapfenepiphysen. Naturgeschichte und diagnostische Bedeutung einer Störung des enchondralen Wachstums. In Glauner, R., A. Rüttimann, P. Thurn, E. Vogler: Ergebnisse der medizinischen Radiologie. Thieme, Stuttgart 1968

Ginthner, T. P., S. I. Schabel: The "mechanical bull" thumb. Skelet. Radiol. 7 (1981) 131

Glass, T., S. E. Mills, R. E.Fechner et al.: Giant cell reparative granuloma of the hands and feet. Radiology 149 (1983) 65

Greulich, W. W., S. J. Pyle: Radiographic Atlas of Skeletal Developement of the Hand and Wrist, 2nd ed. Stanford University Press, Stanford 1959

Hertzog, K. P., S. M. Garn, S. F. Church: Cone-shaped epiphyses in the hand. Population frequences, anatomic distribution, and developmental stages. Invest. Radiol. 3 (1968) 433

Hoessly, M., R. Lagier: Anatomico-radiological study of intraossear epidermoid cysts. Fortschr. Röntgenstr. 137 (1982) 48

Kaibara, N., S. Masuda, I. Katsuki, T. Hotokebuchi, K. Shibata, H. Sada, M. Eguchi: Phalangeal microgeodic syndrome in childhood: report of seven cases and review of the literature. Eur. J. Pediatr. 136 (1981) 41

Karasick, S., D. Karasick: Case report 193. Skelet. Radiol. 8 (1982) 151

Khokhar, N., J. D. Lee: Phalangeal metastasis: first clinical sign of bronchogenic carcinoma. S. Med. J. 76 (1982) 927

Kosowicz,J.: The roentgen appearance of the hand and wrist in gonadal dysgenisis. Amer. J. Roentgenol.93 (1965) 354

v. d. Laan, J. G., C. J. P. Thijn: Ivory and dense epiphyses of the hand: Thiemann disease in three sisters. Skelet. Radiol. 15 (1986) 117

Lange, R. H., W.D. Engber.: Hyperextension Mallet Finger. Orthopedic 6 (1983) 1426

Langer, M., R. Langer: Radiologisch erfassbare Veränderungen der Angiodysplasie, Typ Klippel-Trénaunay und Typ Servelle-Martorell. Fortschr. Röntgenstr. 136 (1982) 577

Langer, M., R. Langer: Radiologic analysis of bone structure in congenital angiodysplasia. Europ. J. Radiol. 1 (1985) 195

Langer, M., R. Langer, H. Dewitz: Methodik des radiologischen Vorgehens bei klinischem Verdacht einer kongenitalen Angiodysplasie. Radiologe 21 (1981) 431

Lingg, G., A. Roessner, V. Fiedler et al.: Das reparative Riesenzellgranulom der Extremitäten. Fortschr. Röntgenstr. 142 (1985) 185

Lister, G.: The Hand, 3rd ed. Churchill Livingstone, Edinburgh 1993

Littlejohn, G. O., M. B. Urowitz, H. A. Smythe et al.: Radiographic features of the hand in diffuse idiopathic skeletal hyperostosis (DISH). Comparison with normal subjects and acromegalic patients. Radiology 140 (1981) 623

Lener,M., W. Judmaier, M. Galb et al.: Diagnostik des ulnokarpalen Komplexes im MR-Movie. Handchir. Mikrochir. plast. Chir. 26 (1994) 115

de Maeseneer, M., S. Jaovisidha,L.Lenchik et al.: Fibrolipomatous hamartoma: MR imaging findings. Skelet. Radiol. 26 (1997) 155

Maroteaux, P.: Cinq observation d'une affection microgèodic des phalanges du nourisson d'ètilogie inconnue. Ann. Radiol. 13 (1970) 229

Martinez, R., G. E. Ohmer: Bilateral subluxation of the base of the thumb secondary to an anusual abductor pollicis longus insertion: a case report. J. Hand Surg. 10-A (1985) 396

Meller, Y., J. Bar-Ziv, J. Goldstein, G. Torok: Phalangeal microgeodic syndrome in childhood. A case report. Acta Orthop. Scand. 53 (1982) 553

Minuk, G. Y. et al.: Pipetters thumb. New Engl. J. Med. 306 (1982) 751

Miura,T.: Congenital absence of the flexor pollicis longus—a case report. Hand 9 (1977) 272

Miura,T.: Congenital anomaly of the thumb—unusual bifurcation of the flexor pollicis longus and its unusual insertion. J. Hand Surg. 6 (1981) 613

Müller, K. T., A. Buchter, R. Gross et al.: Ergebnisse einer Studie an 17 Fällen von Langzeitexposition gegenüber Vinylchlorid. Med. Welt 27 (1976) 21

Nora, F. E., D. C. Dahlin, J. W. Beabout: Bizarre parosteal osteochondromatous proliferations of the hands and feet. Amer. J. surg. Pathol. 7 (1983) 245

Nòrgaard, G.: A follow-up study of the earliest radiological changes in rheumatoid polyarthritis. Brit.J.Radiol.53 (1983) 63

Nuovo, M. A., A. Norman, J. Chumas et al.: Myositis ossificans with atypical clinical, radiographic, or patholigc findings: a review of 23 cases. Skelet. Radiol 21 (1992) 87

Ogden, J. A., T. R. Light, G. J. Conlogue: Correlative roentgenography and morphology of the longitudinal epiphysial bracket. Skelet. Radiol. 6 (1981) 107

Ogden, J. A., T. M Ganey, T. R. Light et al.: Ossification and pseudo-epiphysis formation in the "nonepiphyseal" end of bones of the hands and feet. Skelet. Radiol. 23 (1994) 3

Poznanski, A. K., J. F. Holt: The carpals in congenital malformation syndromes. Amer. J. Roentgenol. 112 (1971) 443–459

Poznanski, A. K.: The Hand in Radiologic Diagnosis, 2nd ed. Saunders, Philadelphia 1984

Primiano, G. A.: Skeer's thumb injuries associated with flared skipole handles. Amer. J. Sports Med. 13 (1985) 425

Pritchett, J.W.: Bilateral symphalangism of the index fingers. J. Hand Surg. 10-A (1985) 619

Rahme, H.: Idiopathic avascular necrosis of the capitate bone—case report. Hand 15 (1983) 274

Rayan, G. M.: Congenital hypoplastic thumb with absent thenar muscles: anomalous digital neurovascular bundle. J. Hand Surg. 9-A (1984) 665

Ravelli, A.: Zur Ossifikation der Vieleckbeine. Fortschr. Röntgenstr. 83 (1955) 852

di Rocco, M., P. Thomà: L'acroosteolisi essenziale carpo-tarsale associata a nefropathia. Una rara affezione. Riv. ital. Pd. 9 (1983) 275

Rochels, R., F. Schmid: Morphologische und metrische Abweichungen der Handknochen beim Down-Syndrom – eine radiologische Studie. Fortschr. Roentgenstr. 133 (1980) 30

Sato, K., H. Sugiura, M. Aoki: Transient phalangeal osteolysis (microgeodic disease). Report of a case involving the foot. J. Bone Jt Surg. Am. 77 (1995 Dec.) 1888

Schäfer, H.: Zur röntgenologischen und klinischen Bedeutung der Pseudoepiphysenbildung am kindlichen Handskelett. Kinderärztl. Prax. 20 (1952) 77

Schmitt, R., U. Lanz: Bildgebende Diagnostik der Hand. Hippokrates, Stuttgart 1966

Schrader, M.: Polydaktylie der Hände. Vorschlag zu einer erweiterten Klassifikation. Handchir. Mirkrochir. plast. Chir. 23 (1991) 115

Schütte, H. E., R. O. van der Heul: Pseudomalignant, nonneoplastic osseous soft-tissue tumors of the hand and foot. Radiology 176 (1990) 149

Spjut, H. J., H. D. Dorfman: Floride reactive periostitis of the tubular bones of the hands and feet. Amer. J. surg. Pathol. 5 (1981) 423

Spranger, J. W., M. Langer, H. R. Wiedemann: Bone Dysplasias. Thieme, Stuttgart 1974 (p. 291)

Stecken, A.: Akroosteolysis bei einem Geiger. Fortschr. Röntgenstr. 80 (1954) 405

Steinberg, I: A simple screening test for the Marfan syndrome. J. Amer. med. Ass. 187 (1964) 118

Stelling, C. B., M. M. Keats et al.: Irregularities at the base of the proximal phalanges: false indicator of early rheumatoid arthritis. Amer. J. Roentgenol. 138 (1982) 695

Stotz, R., K. Kläy, J. Müller: Glomus-Tumoren der Hand. Helv. chir. Acta 50 (1983) 339

Sundaram, P. F. J., J. B. Shields, M. A. Riaz et al.: Terminal phalangeal tufts: earliest site of renal osteodystrophic finding in hemodialysis patients. Amer. J. Roentgenol. 133 (1979) 25

Swanson, A. B.: A classificaton for congenital thumb formations. J. Hand Surg. 1 (1976) 8

Sweterlitsch, P. R., J. S. Torg, H. Pollack: Entrapment of a sesamoid in the index metacarpophalangeal joint. J. Bone Jt Surg. 51-A (1959) 995

Tanner, J. M., R. H. Whitehouse, W. A. Marshall et al.: Assessment of Skeletal Maturity and Prediction of a Dult Hight (TW 2-Method). Academic Press, London 1975

Theander, G., N. Carstam: Longitudinally bracketed diaphyses. Ann. Radiol. 17 (1974) 355

Theander, G., N. Carstam, A. Rausing: Longitudinally bracketed diaphyses in young children. Acta radiol., Diagn. 23 (1982) 293

Theumann, N. H., W. A. Pfirrmann, J.-L. Drapé et al.: MR imaging of the metacarpophalangeal joints of the fingers. Radiology 222 (2002) 437

Trail, I.A.: Acute calcification in the fingers. J. Brit. Soc. Surg. Hand 10-B (1985) 263

Wilhelm, K., C. H. Feldmeier, W. Bracker: Der kindliche Skidaumen. Münch. med. Wschr. 124 (1982) 73

Wood, V. C.: The sesamoid bones of the hand and their pathology. J. Hand Surg. 9-B (1984) 261

Wulle, Chr.: Der Kälteschaden beim Kind. Handchir. Mikrochir. plast. Chir. 23 (1991) 144

Wung, Y., Z. Yang, L. A. Gilula et al.: Kashin-Beck disease: radiographic appearance in the hands and wrists. Radiology 201 (1996) 265

Yamamoto, T., M. Kurosaka, K. Mizuno, M. Fujii: Phalangeal microgeodic syndrome: MR appearance. Skeletal Radiol. 30(3) (2001 Mar.) 170

Yousefzadeh, D. K., J. H. Jackson: Organic foreign body reaction. Report of two cases of thorn induced "granuloma" and a review of the literature. Skelet. Radiol. 3 (1978) 167

Yu, W., Y. Wang, J. Jiang et al.: Kashin-Beck disease in children: radiographic findings in the wrist. Skletal Radiol 31 (2002) 222

Yune, H. Y., A. Vix, E. C. Klatte: Early fingertip changes in skleroderma. J. Amer. med. Ass. 215 (1971) 1113

Zguricas, J., P. Heutink, L. Heredeso et al.: Genetic aspects of polydactyly. Handchir. Mikrochir. plast. Chir. 28 (1996) 171

Carpus (wrist)

General Aspects

▌ Normal Findings

 During Growth

The sequence in which the carpal bones become radiographically visible is shown in Fig. 2.**1**. We refrain from discussing the problems of using the carpal ossification centers to determine skeletal age because any general discussion would necessarily involve some inaccuracies. We instead refer the reader to standard reference works that deal with skeletal age determination. Variants in the shape and size of the individual carpal bones during skeletal maturation are described under Specific Bones of the Carpus.

 In Adulthood

The carpus has been a subject of growing radiological interest during the past 10 years. There are two main causes, which are closely interrelated:

- The reliance of hand surgeons on diagnostic imaging procedures has increased with the expansion of surgical options in the hand.
- The evolution of diagnostic imaging in general, and its specific applications in the skeleton of the hand, especially the carpus, has made tremendous strides.

Diagnostic Methods

Today the following imaging modalities can be used as more specific adjuncts to plain-film radiography to answer the many clinical questions that may arise, especially in traumatology:

- CT
- MRI
- Arthrography
- CT and MR arthrography
- Ultrasonography
- Radionuclide bone scanning

Conventional tomography can be replaced by CT for all applications.

Valuable indications for **CT** in carpal imaging are listed below.

- The diagnosis of acute trauma–especially of fractures that are occult on conventional radiographs (Figs. 2.**255a-d**, 2.**270**)
- The monitoring of fracture healing
- The investigation of suspicious lucencies or densities (real or apparent) seen on conventional radiographs

CT is also very useful for investigating abnormalities detected by bone scan and MRI when conventional radiographic findings are equivocal.

MRI is an excellent modality for demonstrating soft-tissue structures (e.g., in the carpal tunnel, tendons and ligaments, cartilage, soft-tissue tumors), bone marrow changes, occult fractures with traumatic edema, avascular necrosis, and other types of pathology.

The **bone scan** can detect traumatic, radiographically occult changes in the carpus 3–4 days after the injury, thereby identifying a region that can be more selectively investigated by another modality such as CT. The bone scan can also be used in patients with unexplained pain to locate "vulnerable" points such as necrotic areas or accessory bone elements that interfere with normal patterns of movement.

A book whose subject is borderline-normal findings cannot delve too deeply into special techniques and image interpretation for the various modalities. For this the reader must consult the current specialized literature (see References for several selected works).

The following protocol is sufficient for a basic imaging workup, particularly in trauma cases:

- PA (dorsopalmar, DP) and lateral radiographs of the wrist.
- Stecher's projection of the scaphoid (fist closed and ulnarduction or ulnar deviation).
- Spiral CT if conventional findings are equivocal. It is sufficient to obtain uniplanar scans (e.g., axial) with a slice thickness of 1–1.5 mm. Additional planes can be reconstructed as required. If the scaphoid is of primary interest, it is better to use an oblique sagittal plane. Approximately 120 mAs, 120 kV.

MRI, CT arthrography, and MR arthrography are reserved for special investigations (ligament lesions, cartilage lesions, etc.).

There is no point discussing borderline findings based on simple static radiographs in two or more planes or in special projections (e.g., scaphoid quartet) unless attention is also given to the adjacent soft-tissue structures that form a functional unit with the bone.

For the first time, then, the current edition of *Borderlands* explores the anatomy and function of ligaments, joints, etc. in order to help the reader understand the normal and abnormal interrelationships of the individual bony elements in the wrist.

Morphometry of the Carpus

The determination of various angles in the carpus and the definition of various reference lines rely on **accurate radiographic projections**. All the angles indicated below are based on radiographs taken in the neutral position. Lateral radiographs are obtained with the elbow flexed and the upper arm adducted. PA (DP-dorsopalmar) radiographs are obtained with the upper arm abducted to shoulder height. Supination or pronation can significantly alter the projection, leading to inaccurate measurements. Various recent works may be consulted for details on radiographic positioning and projections, such as Schmitt and Lanz (1996) and Gilula and Yin (1996). Figure 2.**136 d** illustrates a typical diagnostic pitfall due to imprecise positioning.

The **angles of the distal radial articular surface** are shown in Fig. 2.**135**.

The radial articular surface normally slopes approximately 25° toward the ulna (normal range 15–35°, Fig. 2.**135 a**) and approximately 10° toward the palm (normal range 0–20°) relative to the long axis of the forearm (Fig. 2.**135 b**). This ulnar and palmar angulation would promote slippage of the carpus were it not for two opposing groups of ligaments:

- The palmar suspensory ligament This is composed of:
  - the radioscaphocapitate ligament (RSC)
  - the radiolunotriquetral ligament (RLT)
  - the ulnolunate ligament (UL)
  - the ulnotriquetral ligament (UT).
- The "carpal sling," which runs in a proximal-to-distal, radial-to-ulnar direction. It is composed of:
  - the radioscapholunate ligament (RSL)
  - the radiolunotriquetral ligament (RLT)
  - the radioscaphocapitate ligament (RSC)
  - the dorsal radiotriquetral ligament (RTD).

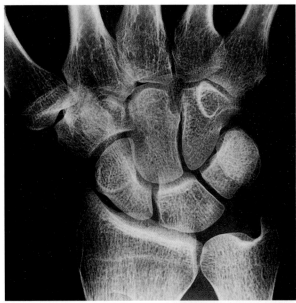

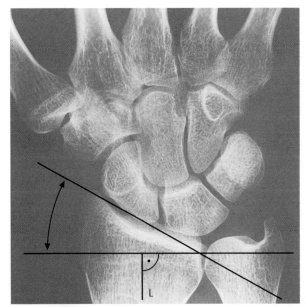

a

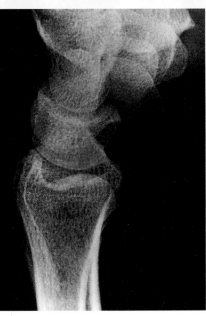

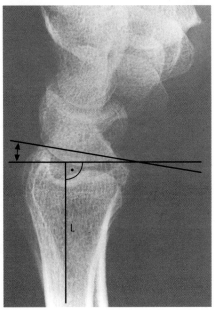

b

Fig. 2.**135 a, b** Normal angulation of the distal radial articular surface.
a The radial articular surface in the PA projection shows an average ulnar angulation of 25°.
b The average palmar angulation measured in the lateral projection is approximately 10° (Table 2.**17**).
L Longitudinal axis of the radius

When the carpal bones are normally positioned and aligned, smooth parallel arcs can be drawn through the proximal and distal rows of carpal bones on the PA radiograph (Fig. 2.**136a, b**) (Gilula and Yin 1996). **Arc 1** follows the proximal contours of the proximal carpal row, **arc 2** follows the distal contours of the proximal carpal row, and **arc 3** follows the proximal contours of the distal carpal row.

> Carpal instability should be strongly suspected if a radiograph in the neutral position shows stepoffs or discontinuities in the carpal arcs. Nonparallel arcs or a triangular configuration of the normally trapezoid-shaped lunate bone is also considered an abnormal finding.

Another useful reference line for radiographic evaluation is the **M-shaped carpometacarpal line** (Fig. 2.**136c**). This line follows the zigzag course of the carpometacarpal joint spaces across the hand. It should be noted that the base of the second metacarpal forms a concave arch and that the proximal joint of the fifth metacarpal shows about 30° of radial angulation. The first metacarpal articulates with the trapezium, the second metacarpal with the trapezoid, the third metacarpal with the capitate, the fourth metacarpal with the radial surface of the hamate, and the fifth metacarpal with the ulnar surface of the hamate.

The **carpal angles** are shown in Figs. 2.**137** and 2.**138**. They can be used to detect even mild degrees of carpal in-

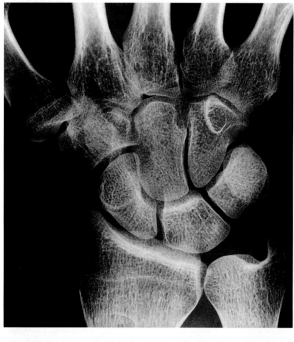

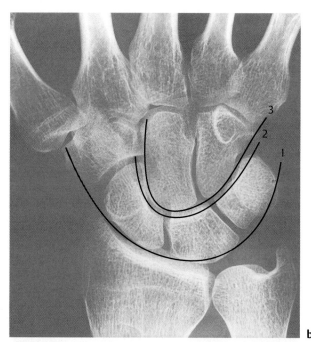

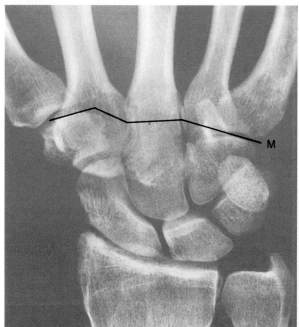

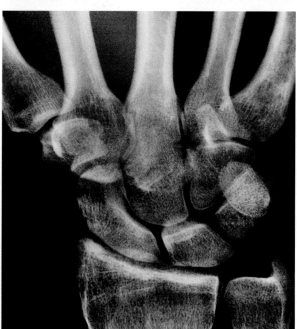

Fig. 2.**136a–d** Carpal lines.
a, b Carpal arcs (after Gilula). In the absence of carpal instability, smooth curvilinear lines can be drawn along the proximal row (1, 2) and distal row (3) of carpal bones. These lines are roughly parallel.

c M configuration of the carpometacarpal joints. **d** The wrist is held in a guarded position of hyperextension due to an extensor tendon injury. This alters the projection and simulates the appearance of a carpometacarpal dislocation.

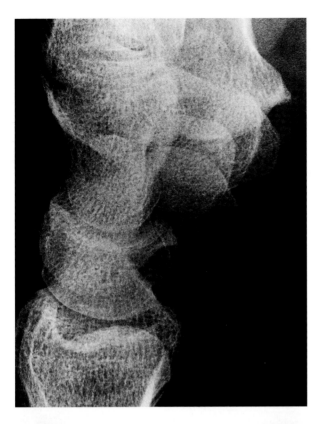
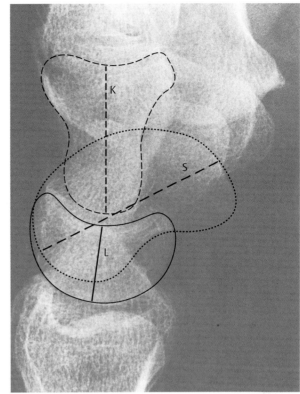

a

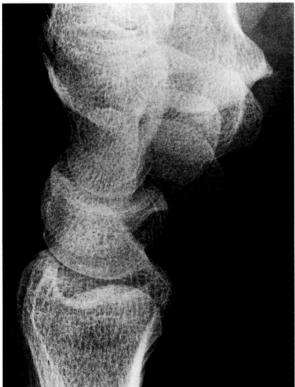
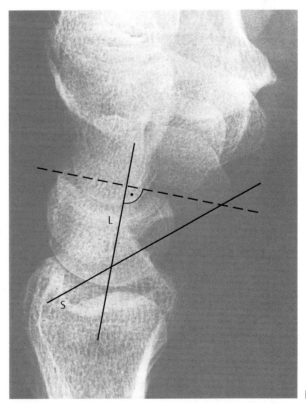

b

Fig. 2.**137 a, b**   Carpal angles.
a The lunate bone is outlined with a solid line, the scaphoid bone with a dotted line, and the capitate bone with a dashed line. The lines for measuring the carpal angles are drawn through the centers of the proximal and distal articular surfaces of the scaphoid and capitate bones ("axial method"). The normal values and their ranges are shown in Table 2.**17**.
K Capitate bone
L Lunate bone
S Scaphoid bone

b   Here the angles are determined by the "tangential method," in which one line is drawn tangent to the palmar surface of the scaphoid bone and another line is drawn tangent to the anterior and posterior horns of the lunate bone.

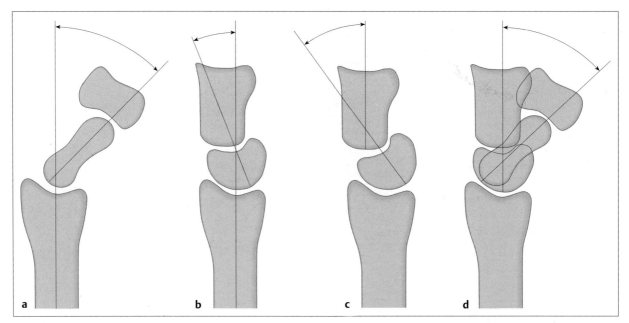

Fig. 2.**138a–d**   Practical application of carpal angle determination by the axial method.
a The radioscaphoid angle is 45°, which is normal. There is no evidence of carpal instability.

b The radiolunate angle is 22°. It is slightly increased due to a mild dorsiflexion carpal instability (DISI).
c The capitolunate angle, at 37°, is more than twice the upper limit of normal due to severe DISI.
d The scapholunate angle is 47°, which is within normal limits. (After Schmitt and Lanz.)

stability (see section on fractures and dislocations, p. 125 ff.). The following specific angles are defined (Table 2.**17**):

- Radiolunate angle
- Radioscaphoid angle
- Scapholunate angle
- Capitolunate angle

The **carpal height index**, which may be decreased in lunate necrosis, unstable scaphoid nonunions, and carpal instability, can be determined by either of two methods (Fig. 2.**139a**):

Table 2.**17**   Carpal angles (see Figs. 2.**137** and 2.**138**). In the DISI pattern, in which the lunate is tilted toward the back of the hand, the radiolunate angle is greater than 15° (e.g., in scapholunate dissociation; see also Fig. 2.**138c**). In the PISI pattern, in which the lunate is tilted toward the palm, the radiolunate angle is less than 15° (e.g., in mediocarpal and ulnar instabilities, especially lunotriquetral dissociation) (see text and Fig. 2.**138**).

Angle	Normal value	Range of variation
Radiolunate angle	0°	−15° to + 15°
Radioscaphoid angle	45°	30° to 60°
Scapholunate angle	47°	30° to 60°
Capitolunate angle	0°	−15° to + 15°

DISI Dorsal intercalated segmental instability
        (dorsiflexion carpal instability)
PISI Palmar intercalated segmental instability
        (palmar flexion carpal instability)

Determining the height index
➤ The carpal *height index of Youm* is defined as the ratio of carpal height (measured in line with the axis of the third metacarpal) to the length of the third metacarpal. The normal value is 0.54 ± 0.03.
➤ The modified *height index of Nattrass* allows for the fact that most carpal radiographs do not demonstrate the whole metacarpus. The Nattrass index is the ratio of carpal height (measured in line with the capitate axis) to the length of the capitate bone. The normal value is 1.57 ± 0.05 (Fig. 2.**139a**).

Two methods are also available for determining **carpal translation** in an ulnar direction, due for example to trauma or rheumatoid arthritis (Fig. 2.**139b**):

Determining the translation index
➤ The *translation index of Chamay* is based on the center of wrist rotation in the head of the capitate bone. It is measured on the radial side of the carpus. The distance from the center of rotation to a perpendicular line through the radial styloid process is divided by the length of the third metacarpal bone. Normal is 0.28 ± 0.03. Higher values are abnormal.
➤ The *translation index of McMurty* is measured on the ulnar side of the carpus. The distance from the center of rotation in the capitate bone to a perpendicular line through the center of the ulnar head is divided by the length of the third metacarpal bone. Normal is 0.30 ± 0.03. Lower values are abnormal.

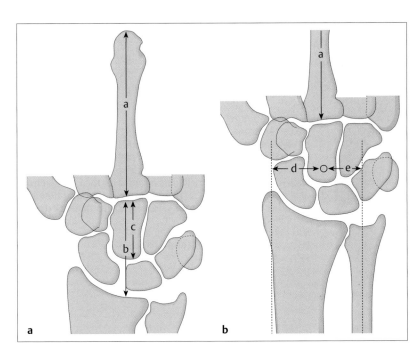

a
b

Fig. 2.**139 a, b** Indices for evaluating carpal height and carpal translation (after Schmitt and Lanz).

a In the diagram, *a* is the length of the third metacarpal, *b* is the overall height of the carpus, and *c* is the length of the capitate bone. The height index of Youm is the ratio *b/a* (normal = 0.54 ± 0.03), and the height index of Nattrass is the ratio *b/c* (normal = 1.57 ± 0.05).

b For evaluating translation, the circle in the capitate bone marks the center of rotation of the carpus. The dotted lines runs through the radial styloid process and through the center of the ulnar shaft. A perpendicular line is drawn through the center of rotation, and the distances from the center of rotation to the dotted lines (*d, e*) are measured. The Chamay translation index is the ratio *d/a* (normal = 0.28 ± 0.03), and the McMurty translation index is the ratio *e/a* (normal = 0.30 ± 0.03).

Three principal **joint compartments** can be identified in the carpus (Fig. 2.**140**):

- The midcarpal joint compartment, which is located between the proximal and distal rows of carpal bones and often communicates with the carpometacarpal and intermetacarpal joint spaces of the second through fourth fingers.

- The radiocarpal joint compartment, which is bounded proximally by the distal radial articular cartilage, ulnarly by the triangular fibrocartilage complex, and distally by the proximal carpal row with its associated bony elements and interosseous ligaments (scapholunate and lunotriquetral ligaments).

- The distal radioulnar joint compartment, which is bounded by the proximal surface of the triangular fibrocartilage complex and extends a variable distance proximally between the radius and ulna.

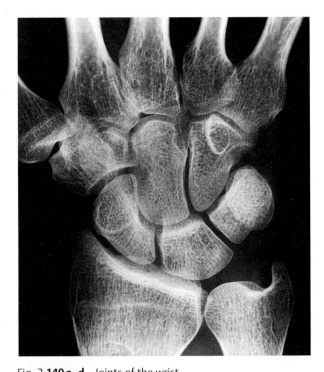

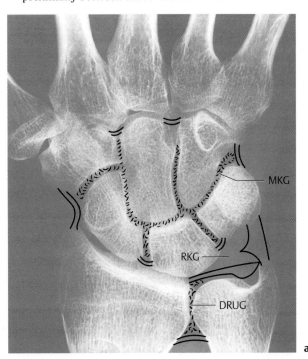

Fig. 2.**140 a–d** Joints of the wrist.

a Schematic view of the three major joint compartments in the wrist. The midcarpal joint (MKG) is located between the proximal and distal carpal rows. The radiocarpal joint compartment (RKG) is bounded proximally by the radial articular cartilage and triangular fibrocartilage complex and distally by the proximal carpal row with its articular cartilage and interosseous ligaments. The distal radioulnar joint compartment (DRUG) is bounded distally by the proximal surface of the triangular fibrocartilage complex and extends a variable distance proximally.

Fig. 2.**140 b–d** ▷

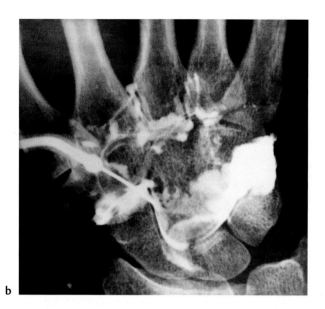

Fig. 2.**140 b–d** Arthrography of the hand. In **b** contrast medium has been injected into the midcarpal compartment. Very soon the medium defines physiological connections with the smaller carpometacarpal and intercarpal joint spaces. This is most clearly appreciated in the later radiograph (**c**), which shows better distribution of the contrast medium.

IMG   Intermetacarpal joint
KMG   Carpometacarpal joint
MKG   Midcarpal joint

d View after opacification of the radiocarpal joint compartment. Contrast medium has entered the distal radioulnar joint through a small perforation in the radial part of the radially displaced articular disc. Small tears account for the irregular margins of the articular disc. The resorptive tapering of the ulnar styloid process results from severe synovitis of the extensor carpi ulnaris tendon. For didactic reasons, the plain radiograph and MR images are shown in Fig. 2.**142**.

DT   Triangular discus (fibrocartilage)
RKG   Radiocarpal joint
DRUG   Distal radioulnar joint

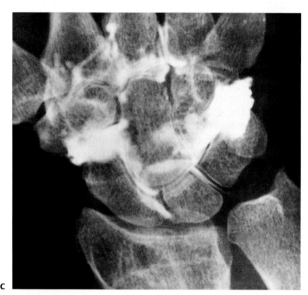

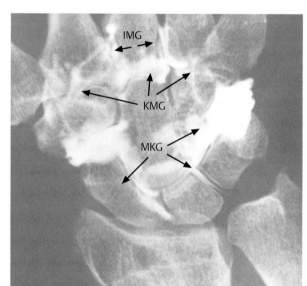

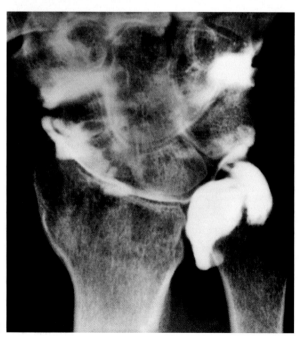

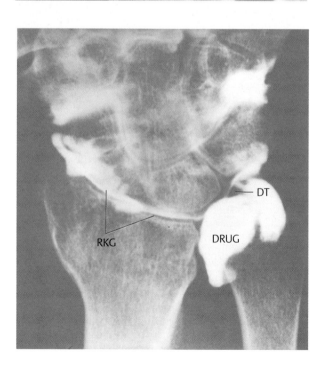

These three joint compartments are clearly visualized by **three-compartment arthrography** (Fig. 2.**140 b–d**). Normally the joint compartments do not communicate with one another, but they occasionally communicate with the following smaller joint spaces as a normal variant:

- Carpometacarpal compartment of the first ray
- Carpometacarpal compartments of the second through fifth rays
- Intermetacarpal compartments of the second through fifth rays
- Pisotriquetral compartment

It would exceed our scope to review normal arthrographic findings and their variants, age-related degenerative ligament changes, and especially the morphological diversity of the triangular fibrocartilage complex. The two large monographs by Schmitt and Lanz (1996) and Gilula and Yin (1969) are excellent references for this purpose.

The **triangular fibrocartilage complex** (TFCC) is composed of:

- The triangular fibrocartilage (articular disc)
- The ulnocarpalis muscle
- The ulnolunate and ulnotriquetral ligaments, the ulnar collateral ligament of the carpus, and the palmar and dorsal radioulnar ligaments
- The extensor carpi ulnaris tendon sheath

Thus, the TFCC is a very complex structure that is best examined today by MRI or, invasively, by CT-arthrography (multicompartment technique) or arthroscopy. The clinical questions that arise are based on mechanical instability in the distal radioulnar joint and unexplained ulnar-sided wrist pain (with negative skeletal radiographs). The TFCC forms a kind of buffer zone between the ulnar head and the ulnar portion of the proximal carpal row (the lunate and triquetrum). Much has been written in recent years on the diagnosis of traumatic and degenerative lesions of the TFCC. Anyone who uses MRI (Figs. 2.**141 e–g**, 2.**142**) should be familiar with the age-related normal variants and findings that can simulate pathology (e.g., Metz et al. 1992, Sugimoto et al. 1994, Totterman and Miller 1995, Timins et al. 1996). Recently Pfirrmann et al (2001) investigated the question "what happens to the triangular fibrocartilage complex during pronation and supination of the forearm", using MR arthrography.

The structural complexity of the TFCC accounts for the many possible injury patterns and degenerative changes (especially in the elasticity of the triangular fibrocartilage) that may be encountered in that region.

> As mentioned, a knowledge of the **carpal ligaments** is essential for understanding the normal and borderline-pathological radiographic anatomy of the radius, ulna, carpus, and metacarpal bones.

Besides the clinical examination, the diagnosis of ligament lesions (especially instabilities of the lunotriquetral and scapholunate ligaments) relies on stress radiographs, MRI, and/or CT-arthrography. A great many studies have been published on the comprehensive diagnosis of carpal ligament lesions (e.g., Smith 1994, Smith and Snearly 1994), including the monographs of Schmitt and Lanz (1996) and Gilula and Yin (1996).

The carpal ligaments can be classified as follows (Fig. 2.**141**):

- Anatomically, i.e., based on their relationship to the forearm and metacarpus
  - Extrinsic ligaments, which pass from the forearm to the carpus or from the metacarpal region to the carpus
  - Intrinsic ligaments, which stretch between the carpal bones (intercarpal ligaments)
- Functionally
  - Interosseous ligaments, which pass deeply between two bones
  - Proximal palmar V ligaments, which fan out from the radius and ulna to the lunate bone
  - Distal palmar V ligaments, which converge from the radius and triquetrum to the capitate
  - Dorsal V ligaments, which form a "transverse V" converging on the triquetrum from the radius and scaphoid.

It is important to note that most of the ligaments in the carpal region are intracapsular. The instability patterns that are associated with ligament ruptures are discussed under Fractures, Subluxations and Dislocations.

CT and MRI can provide **nonsuperimposed views of the carpus** in all dimensions. The indications for carpal CT were listed earlier in this chapter. As was the case in conventional tomography, the projection should be perpendicular to the bone surface of interest, and therefore the scan plane should be tailored to the specific clinical problem (Stewart and Gilula 1992).

Basically the following projections are available:

- Axial
- Coronal
- Sagittal
- Parallel to the long axis of the scaphoid bone
- Oblique scaphotrapezoidal projection (Stewart and Gilula 1992)

Each of these projections is optimal for visualizing certain bony structures in the wrist. It is not always easy to identify specific carpal bones by their location in the various image planes. Figure 2.**143** shows a series of axial scans and Fig. 2.**144** a series of sagittal scans with the various bones labeled. These figures are intended to demonstrate the complex spatial anatomy of the carpus.

> We have found it helpful in practice to refer to an actual hand skeleton when interpreting the various scan planes. Close scrutiny of the images will also show how the many spaces between the carpal bones, the various notches, etc. can mimic erosive or osteolytic lesions in a summation radiographic image (Figs. 2.**143**, 2.**147**).

Nakamura et al. (1996) described a modification of the radioulnar line method for diagnosing **subluxation of the distal radioulnar joint with CT**. Scanning is performed with the elbow extended and with maximum active pronation and supination of the forearm (Fig. 2.**145**).

With their modification of the radioulnar line method, the authors could drastically reduce the false-positive diagnosis of dorsal and palmar subluxations. They claim that their modified method makes it unnecessary to compare the symptomatic radioulnar joint with the opposite side.

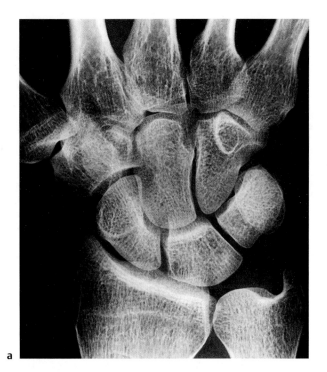

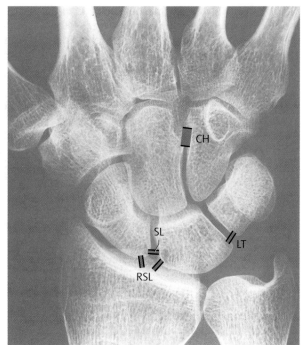

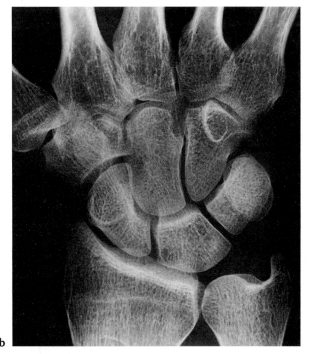

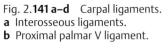

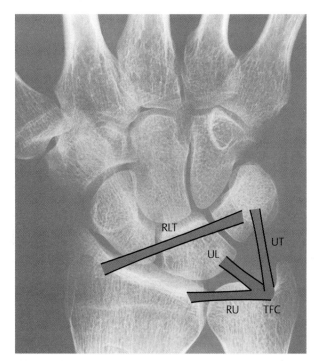

Fig. 2.**141 a–d**   Carpal ligaments.
a Interosseous ligaments.
b Proximal palmar V ligament.

CH	Capitohamate ligament
ICD	Dorsal intercarpal ligament
LT	Lunotriquetral ligament
pSTT	Palmar scaphotrapeziotrapezoidal ligament
RLT	Radiolunotriquetral ligament
RSC	Radioscaphocapitate ligament
RSL	Radioscapholunate ligament
RTD	Dorsal radiotriquetral ligament
RU	Radioulnar joint
SC	Scaphocapitate ligament
SL	Scapholunate ligament
TC	Triquetrocapitate ligament
TFC	Triangular fibrocartilage
UL	Ulnolunate ligament
UT	Ulnotriquetral ligament

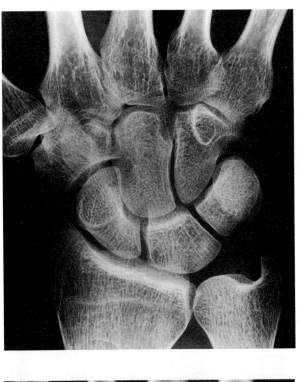
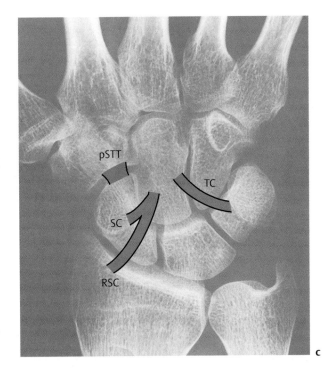
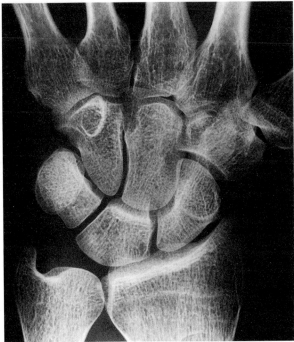
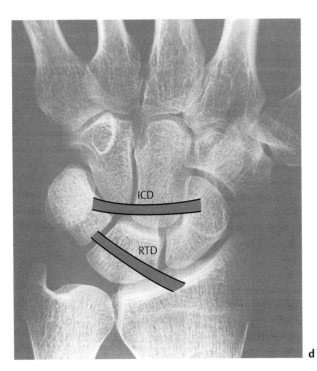

Fig. 2.**141 c, d**
c Distal palmar V ligament.
d Dorsal V ligament.

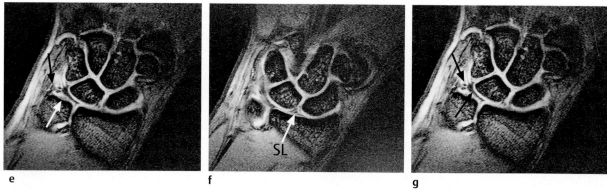

e   f   g

Fig. 2.**141 e–g** T2-weighted MR images of the intrinsic carpal ligaments. The arrows in images **e** and **g** indicate the triangular fibrocartilage complex. The arrow in **f** points to the scapholu- nate ligament. The lunotriquetral ligament is also visible in **e** and **g**.

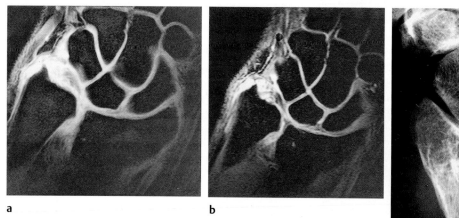

a   b

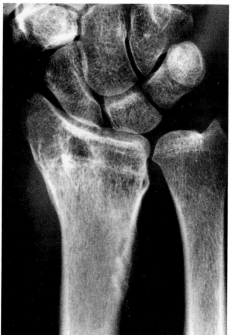

c

Fig. 2.**142 a–c** Disruption of the triangular fibrocartilage complex on MRI. The complex is avulsed and displaced radially. The ulnotriquetral ligament and ulnar collateral ligament are also torn. The tears are associated with massive effusion and edema. A radiograph taken at the same time (**c**) shows a pre- vious healed distal radial fracture (treated by internal fixation), slight distal protrusion (lengthening) of the ulna, and resorp- tive tapering of the ulnar styloid process. The ulnar portion of the wrist was painful with use. The correlative arthrograms for this case are shown in Fig. 2.**140 b–d**.

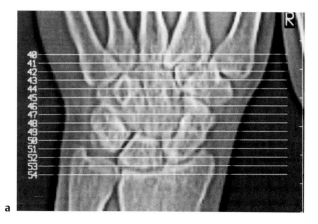

a

Fig. 2.**143 a–o** Axial CT survey of the carpus.

C	Capitate
H	Hamate
HH	Hook of the hamate
L	Lunate
MC	Metacarpal
PI	Pisiform
R	Radius
SC	Scaphoid
ST	Styloid process of the ulna
TO	Trapezoid
TR	Triquetrum
TZ	Trapezium
U	Ulna

Fig. 2.**143 b–o** ▷

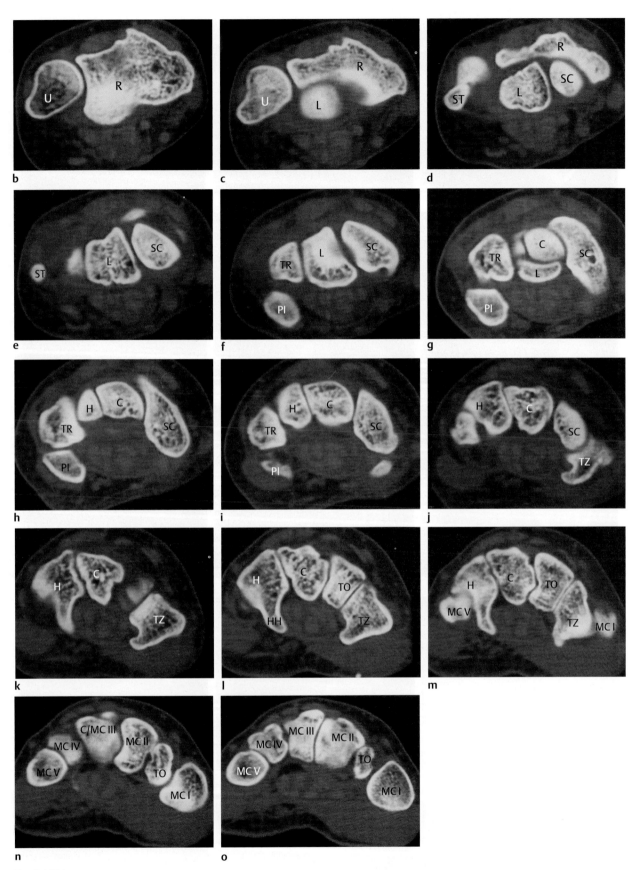

Fig. 2.**143 b–o**

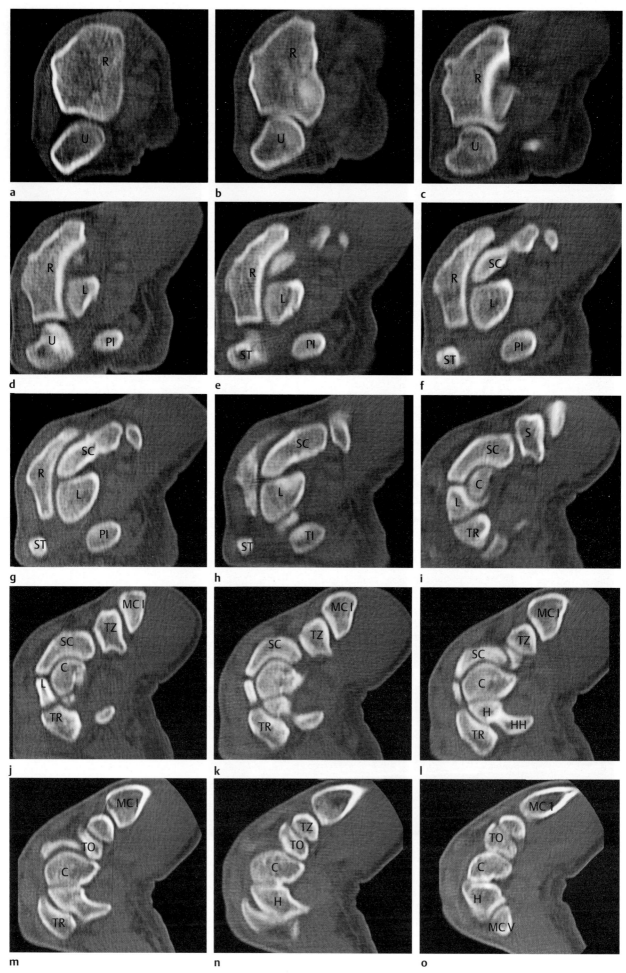

Fig. 2.**144 a–i**   Sagittal CT survey of the carpus. (See the label key in Fig. 2.**143**.)

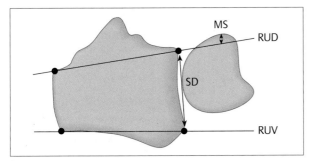

Fig. 2.**145** CT diagnosis of distal radioulnar joint subluxation by the method of Nakamura et al. (1996). In the standard radioulnar line method, the ulnar head should lie between RUD and RUV if the radioulnar joint is congruent. By that criterion, the drawing would indicate a dorsal subluxation. In the modified radioulnar line method, a subluxation is diagnosed only if MS equals more than one-fourth of SD. Thus, a subluxation should not be diagnosed in the case shown.

MS   Maximum width of the subluxated portion of the ulna
RUD   Radioulnar dorsal line
RUV   Radioulnar volar line
SD   Sigmoid notch diameter

Pathological Finding?

 ### Normal Variant or Anomaly?

Conventional radiographs of the carpus demonstrate a variety of **normal notches and recesses** (Fig. 1.**146**), as noted earlier in connection with the high spatial resolution of CT.

Especially when the radiographic parameters are less than ideal (focus too large, high speed screen, voltage too high), normal lucencies in the carpus may appear completely devoid of internal structure and can mimic the appearance of osteolytic lesions or erosions, depending on whether the projection is tangential or en face (Fig. 2.**147**).

Small round lucencies in individual carpal bones, usually surrounded by a sclerotic rim, are most likely nutrient canals (Fig. 2.**148**). These canals can also mimic fracture lines when viewed in tangential projection, as often occurs in the scaphoid bone.

Small circumscribed densities in individual carpal bones, especially the scaphoid and triquetrum, represent small bone islands and are considered a normal variant (Fig. 2.**148**). Of course, biplane views should always be obtained to check for superimposed soft-tissue calcifications.

Numerous **accessory bones** have been identified in the carpus (at least 24 to date, found in approximately 0.3–1.6% of the healthy population; O'Rahilly 1953), and these should not be mistaken for bone fragments. With a fresh avulsion fracture, both the fragment and the parent bone generally show an area of exposed cancellous bone that lacks a cortical boundary. Accessory bones, on the other hand, exhibit a complete and distinct cortical shell (on good-quality radiographs). Confusion can result, however, from an old avulsion fracture that has healed in a position of nonunion or from "mature" heterotopic new bone (Fig. 2.**235**). If doubt exists, radionuclide bone scans or MRI should be obtained. As a rule, bone scans are positive within 3–4 days after an avulsion fracture but are negative for ac-

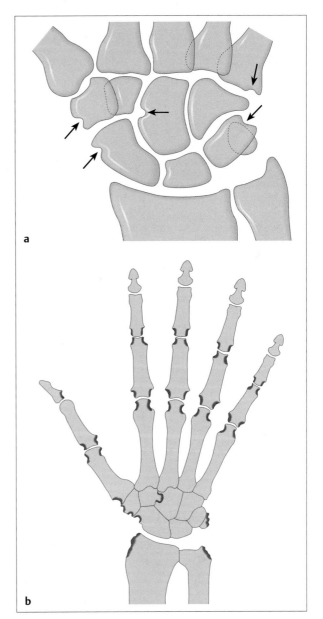

Fig. 2.**146 a, b** Differential diagnosis of physiological notches and concavities in the carpal bones.
a Drawing of physiological notches and concavities (after Dihlmann).
b Typical sites of occurrence of erosive lesions in rheumatoid arthritis. The scaphoid, trapezium, and capitate are particularly common sites of inflammatory erosions that match the location of normal concavities. Further information on differentiating erosions from normal features can be found in the text and Fig. 2.**147**.

cessory bones and old nonunions. The location of an isolated bone fragment is also an important consideration. *In an expert's report it would not go undiscussed if the examiner identified an accessory bone at a site where no such bone has previously been described (e.g., Fig. 2.**260**). At the same time, it is appropriate to question whether some of the "classic" accessory bones described by Pfitzner and some of the bones added by later authors (Figs. 2.**149**, 2.**150**) are indeed supernumerary bony elements as opposed to old avulsion fractures.*

Of course, the clinical findings are crucial in interpreting radiological images. Asymptomatic accessory bone el-

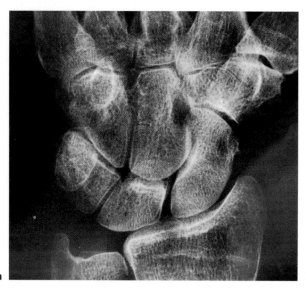

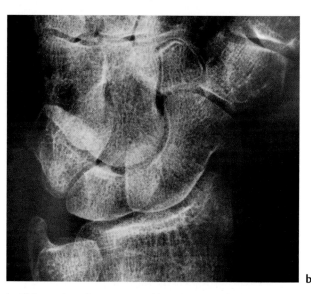

Fig. 2.**147 a, b** Emergency radiographs of the carpus using a 200-speed screen and a focal spot size of 1.2.
a In this film the physiological notch on the radial side of the capitate and the normal radiolucent area and notch in the distal radial portion of the scaphoid are very ill-defined and resemble osteolytic lesions.

b Oblique view shows a central lucent area in the hamate. Evidently the sulcus between the hamate and triquetrum has been projected into the hamate, creating an apparent lucency (see also Fig. 2.**143 b**, especially the ninth CT slice distal to the radius). Compare these technically poor films with the high-quality PA radiographs in Fig. 2.**140** and 2.**141**, which show fine trabecular details in the area of the notches, recesses, and radiolucent zones.

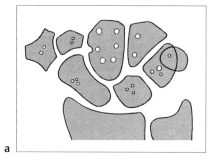

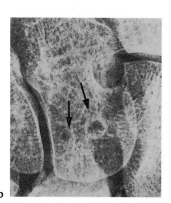

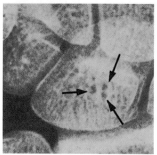

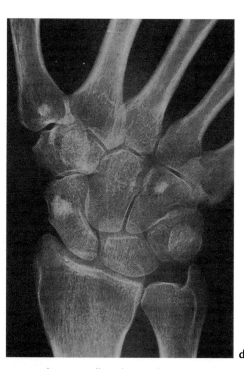

Fig. 2.**148 a–d** Normal structural variants in the carpal bones.
a–c Fine nutrient canals projected end-on. Schematic drawing in panel **a**, radiographs of the capitate and lunate bones in panels **b** and **c**.
d Small bone islands (enostomas) are visible in the capitate, scaphoid, and first metacarpal base. Close scrutiny reveals that the small bone islands have streaklike (anchorlike) attach-

ments to the surrounding cancellous bone. This sign is fairly definitive for small bone islands, which occur normally in these areas, but occasionally it may signify a rudimentary form of osteopoikilosis (see p. 40 and Fig. 2.**38**). The density in the scaphoid bone could also represent a palmar bursal calcification in principle, but its radiographic morphology does not support this interpretation. Any doubts are easily resolved by obtaining an oblique projection.

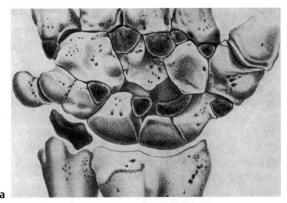

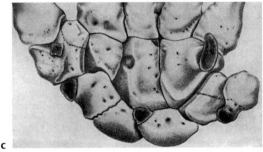

Fig. 2.**149 a–d** Dorsal and palmar aspects of the left hand, showing the accessory bones.
a, b Dorsal aspect (after Pfitzner).
c, d Palmar aspect (after Pfitzner).

C. sec.	Secondary capitate
Cap.	Capitate
Centr.	Os centrale carpi
Epl.	Os epilunatum
Epy.	Epipyramis
Ham.	Hamate
Hpl.	Os hypolunatum
Lun.	Lunate
Mst.	Metastyloid
Nav.	Navicular (scaphoid)
Os ham.	Hook of the hamate
Os. Gr.	Ossicle of Gruber
P.s.	Secondary pisiform
Pst.	Parastyloid
Ptp.	Pretrapezium
R.e.	Radiale externum
Styl.	Styloid
T.s.	Secondary trapezoid
Tp.	Trapezium
Tr. sec.	Secondary triquetral
Trq.	Triquetrum
Trzd.	Trapezoid
Ve.	Vesalian (Os vesalianum)
X	Secondary trapezium (?)

ements in the carpus have no significance and therefore do not require further imaging to establish the identity of the element.

The name of an accessory bone element has no bearing on the further treatment of a patient. It is important only that the accessory bone be identified as such. Following the practice in cerebral MRI of using the term "UBO" for an unknown bright object, one might refer to an unidentified accessory bone element as a "UBE" (unknown bony element) or more precisely as a "UABE" (unnamed accessory bone element).

One way to determine whether an accessory bone element is responsible for circumscribed pain is by the use of fluoroscopy.

Figure 2.**151** illustrates the problems that can arise when an unknown bony element is found. The radiographs are from a 28-year-old man who underwent the surgical removal of "supernumerary fingers" as a child. Nothing more was known about his history. The current radiographs, taken after an injury, show an isolated bony element located between the trapezium and the base of the right first metacarpal on the radiopalmar side. Almost as large as the trapezoid, the bony element might be a paratrapezium, a displaced external radial accessory bone, or a rudimentary duplication anomaly of the thumb. Because there were no local symptoms, the finding has no real sig-

nificance. But this case illustrates the familiar principle that accessory bones occur with greater frequency in syndromes than in normal individuals (Table 2.**18**).

Table 2.**18** Syndromes that are associated with accessory carpal bones (after Poznanski)

In the distal carpal row
• Arthro-ophthalmopathy
• Type A1 brachydactyly
• Diastrophic dysplasia
• Ellis–van Creveld syndrome
• Larsen syndrome
• Otopalatodigital syndrome
Os centrale—remnants of a central row
• Gorlin–Schlorf–Paperella
• Hand–foot–genital syndrome
• Hollister–Hollister
• Holt–Oram
• Larsen
• Otopalatodigital syndrome
Others
• Grebe
• Larsen
• Otospondylomegaepiphyseal syndrome

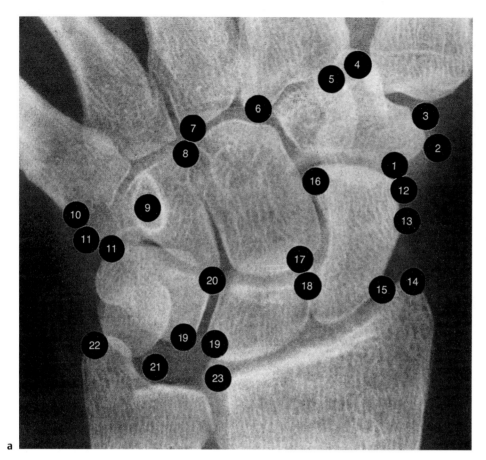

a

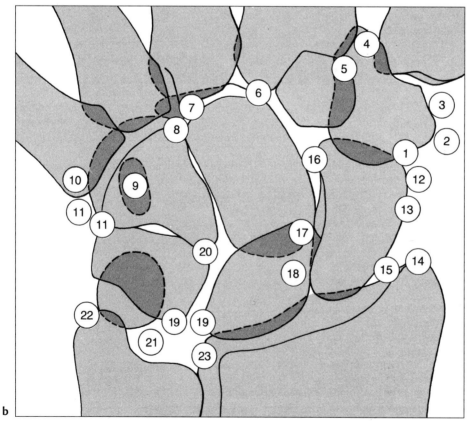

b

Fig. 2.**150 a–d** PA and lateral radiographs of the carpus.

a, b Locations of accessory bones that may be visible on PA radiographs of the wrist.

1 Epitrapezium
2 Calcification (bursa or tendon sheath of flexor carpi radialis)
3 Paratrapezium (pretrapezium?)
4 Secondary trapezium
5 Secondary trapezoid
6 Os styloideum
7 Gruber ossicle
8 Secondary capitate
9 Os hamuli proprium
10 Os vesalianum
11 Os ulnare externum (calcifications in bursa or tendon)
12 Os radiale externum
13 Traumatic avulsions
14 Persistent ossification center of radial styloid process
15 Wormian bone between the scaphoid and radius (paranavicular)
16 Os centrale carpi
17 Os hypolunatum
18 Os epilunatum
19 Accessory bone between lunate and triquetrum
20 Epipyramis
21 Os triangulare
22 Persistent ossification center of ulnar styloid process
23 Small bony element at the radioulnar joint

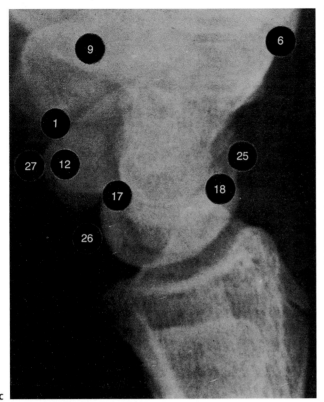

c

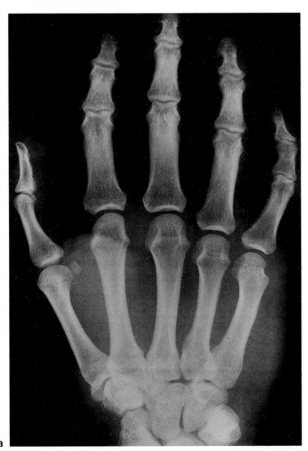

Fig. 2.**150c,d** Lateral radiograph.
  1 Epitrapezium
  6 Os styloideum
  9 Os hamuli proprium
  12 Os radiale externum

  17 Os hypolunatum
  18 Os epilunatum
  25 Triquetral avulsion (not an accessory bone)
  26 Tendon or bursal calcification
  27 Calcification on the pisiform

d

a

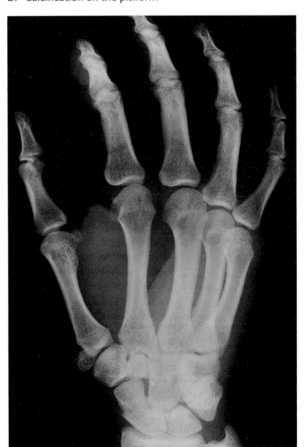

b

Fig. 2.**151 a,b** Unusual accessory bone element adjacent to the base of the first metacarpal, probably a rudimentary duplication anomaly of the thumb.

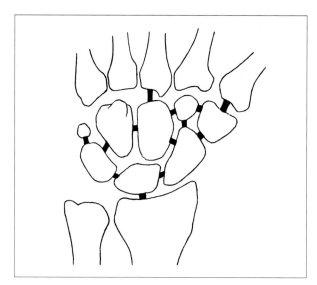

Fig. 2.**152**   Possible sites of carpal fusion (after Mestern).

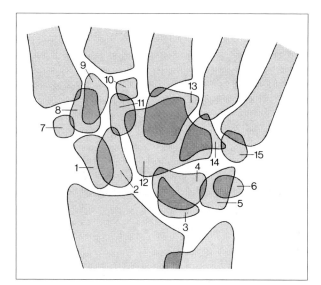

Fig. 2.**153**   Possible duplication anomalies of carpal bones. This drawing is from a radiograph of an 8-year-old child described by Ruckensteiner. The following interpretation has been modified:

1/2	Duplication of the scaphoid
3/4	Duplication of the lunate
5/6	Triquetrum and pisiform
7	Probably the epiphysis of the first metacarpal
8/9	Probably a duplication of the trapezium
10/11	Probably a duplication of the trapezoid
12/13	Duplication of the capitate
14	Epiphyseal center of the hamate
15	Probably a pseudoepiphysis

The various accessory carpal bones are discussed under Specific Carpal Bones in terms of their proximity to a particular major bone.

Carpal fusions (coalitions, synostoses) are classified along with accessory bone elements as normal variants of the carpal skeleton (Fig. 2.**152**). They occur in approximately 0.11 % of the white population, in 1.6 % of African-Americans, and in up to 8 % of Nigerians (Drewes and Günther 1966).

In a review of the literature on 127 cases of fusion between two carpal bones, 28 of the fusions were between the lunate and triquetrum (Fig. 2.**254**), 16 were between the capitate and hamate (Fig. 2.**194**), and all other combinations each accounted for 5 or fewer cases (Drewes and Günther 1966). Several types of **lunotriquetral fusion** have been identified:

- Complete fusion (type A)
- Fusion with a distal cleft (type B)
- Proximal fusion with a partial joint space (type C)
- Fusion with a ridge and distal cleft (type D)
- Incomplete fusion (type E) resembling a pseudarthrosis

Type E presents radiographically with narrowing of the lunotriquetral space and small subarticular lucencies (Resnick et al. 1986).

Stäbler et al. (1999) found marked edema of the affected bones on MRI in two symptomatic patients with an incomplete (fibrous) lunotriquetral fusion.

Lunotriquetral fusion may be associated with a widening of the distance between the scaphoid and lunate but no clinical symptoms of scapholunate dissociation. Metz et al. (1993) interpret this widening of the scapholunate space in lunotriquetral fusion as a normal variant.

Fusions involving three or more carpal bones are rare.

Combinations of carpal fusion with vertebral body fusions and vertebral dysplasia have been observed (Thakkar 1982). Perme et al. (1994) described a hereditary symphalangia with carpal and tarsal fusion and concomitant hearing loss. The latter may result from ankylosis of the stapes to the round window and fixation of the incus.

Bipartite carpal bones (or multipartite bones) can also occur as normal variants in the hand (Fig. 2.**153**).

> **Bipartite carpal bones, listed in descending frequency of occurrence (after Pfitzner)**
> ➤ Scaphoid
> ➤ Triquetrum
> ➤ Pisiform
> ➤ Trapezium
> ➤ Trapezoid
> ➤ Capitate

The following criteria should be met before an unusual bipartite scaphoid bone, for example, is diagnosed:

- No history of trauma.
- The cancellous bone architecture and density of the two bony elements should be identical (unequal densities signify a fracture with subsequent necrosis).
- Both elements should have a complete cortical shell and be separated by a jointlike interosseous space.
- There should be no evidence of osteoarthritis around the scaphoid bone, e.g., the radial styloid process and the joint between one part of the scaphoid and the trapezium and trapezoid.

Finding the same change in the contralateral wrist would support the diagnosis of an innocuous bipartite scaphoid bone.

Figure 2.**153** shows a tracing of a radiograph from an 8-year-old child who had multiple bipartite carpal bones in each hand (Ruckensteiner 1951). This case illustrates the diverse possibilities of this normal variant.

Figure 2.**215** demonstrates the problems with clarifying an anomaly of the scaphoid that may be a bipartite one.

Duplicated carpal bones have also been observed in a variety of **enchondral ossification disorders** (e.g., Schaaf and Wagner 1962). Of course, duplicated carpal bones can no longer be regarded as normal variants when discovered under these conditions (Fig. 2.**155 a**).

In **chondrodysplasia punctata** (Conradi–Hünermann disease), small punctate ossifications are seen in place of normal carpal ossification centers (Fig. 2.**57**). This condition should not be classified as a normal variant, but neither should it be mistaken for necrotic changes in the carpus.

Another differential diagnosis of duplication of carpal bones is **cretinism**, especially if the disturbance of the ossification center leads to fragmentation without coherence.

The correct diagnosis can be made based on the clinical symptoms and examination of radiographs of a radiological test region such as the hip.

Another epiphyseal enchondral ossification disorder may be associated with unusually pronounced foci of cartilage proliferation on the carpal bones, which later ossify. This is **dysplasia epiphysealis hemimelica** (Trevor disease), a special form of Fairbank disease (Fig. 2.**154**, 2.**244**). The tarsal bones and the tibial and femoral epiphyses are most commonly affected (Fig. 6.**147**). The disease is rare in the carpal bones, where it seems to have a proclivity for the scaphoid bone (Lamesch 1983). Pathogenetically, the unusual scaphoid deformity in Figs. 2.**154** and 2.**244** suggests that the growth cartilage has undergone an excessive proliferation and ossification at multiple centers, which later coalesced to produce a lobulated bony mass. Dysplasia

Fig. 2.**154 a, b**   Trevor disease of the scaphoid bone with exostosis-like proliferations in a 6-year-old boy (see also Fig. 2.**244**)

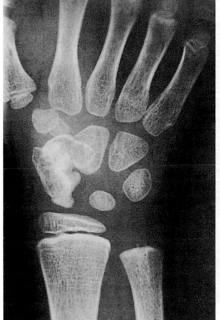
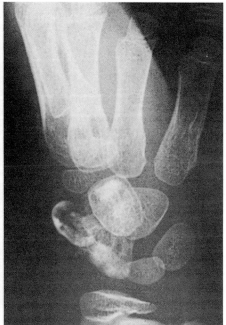

a

b

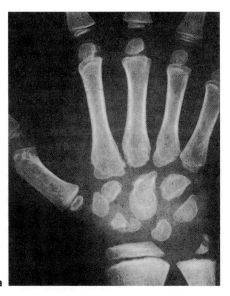
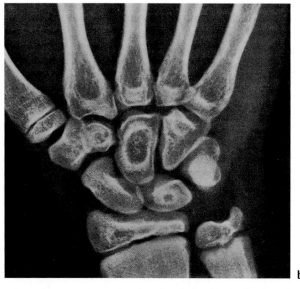

a

b

Fig. 2.**155 a, b**   Achondroplasia and marble bone disease (Albers–Schönberg, osteopetrosis).

a Irregular carpal bones in achondroplasia with duplication of the scaphoid.
b Bone-in-bone sign of marble bone disease.

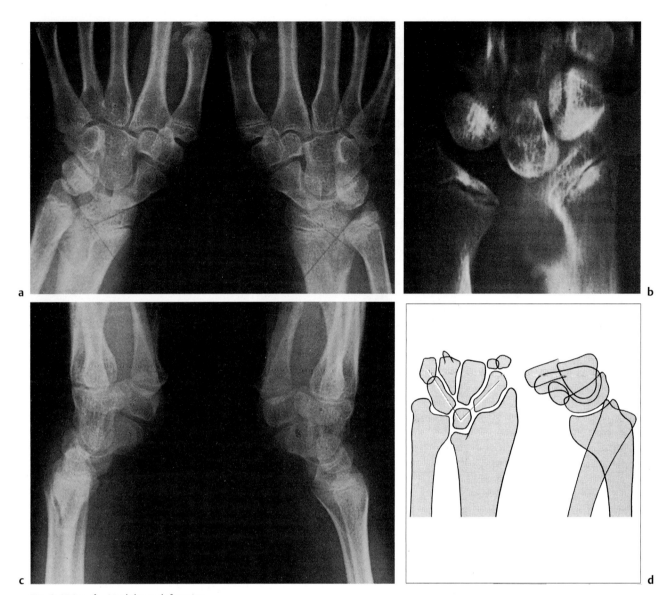

Fig. 2.**156a–d**   Madelung deformity.

epiphysealis hemimelica is easily mistaken for true osteo-chondromas.

The bone-in-bone sign occurs in **marble bone disease** (Fig. 2.**155b**) and should not be mistaken for osteonecrosis.

Reference is again made to **Madelung deformity**, a usually very severe dysostosis with significant carpal involvement (Figs. 2.**156**, 2.**157**). It is caused by an enchondral ossification disorder that probably involves premature closure of the ulnopalmar portions of the epiphyseal growth plate. This results in a bayonet-like deviation of the hand in relation to the forearm (palmar subluxation of the hand with dorsal protrusion of the ulna). Generally bilateral, the disease may be inherited as an autosomal dominant trait or may occur in the setting of enchondromatoses, Leri–Weill syndrome, Turner syndrome, and mucopolysaccharidoses. Females predominate. Clinical manifestations become evident between 8 and 14 years of age and consist more of visible deformity than actual complaints. However, extension, supination and radial abduction of the hand are limited due to faulty articulation in the radiocarpal and distal radioulnar joints. The bayonet-like deviation of the hand in the palmar direction (with simultaneous bowing in the radial or ulnar direction) is accompanied by dorsal protrusion of the ulnar head at the distal radioulnar joint. On lateral inspection, the dorsum of the hand and the flexor surface of the forearm appear to lie on the same plane.

Radiographically, the distal articular surfaces of the radius and ulna appear to "face" each other. The ulnar angulation of the distal radial surface is greater than the radial angulation of the ulnar surface. Additional features are palmar angulation of the distal radial articular surface and slight outward bowing of the distal radial shaft. The PA radiograph shows wedging of the carpus between the deformed articular surfaces of the radius and ulna. The lunate bone is at the apex of the wedge and may be interposed between the distal radial and ulnar epiphyses (Fig. 2.**156d**). Generally the ulna is too short, and the ulnar head is deformed and subluxated dorsally.

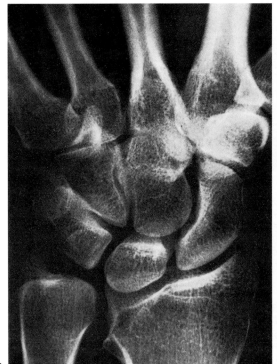

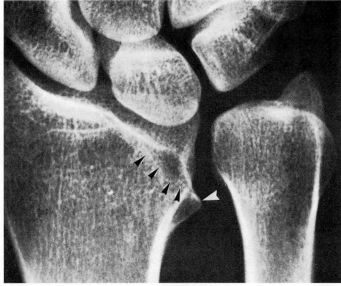

b

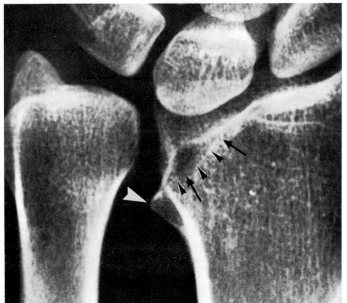

c

Fig. 2.**157 a–c** Madelung deformity in both hands.
a General view of the left carpus in the sagittal projection.
b, c Enlarged views of both sides in the same projection. The wedged carpus, with the lunate at the apex, glides into the corresponding ulnar-sided depressions on both radii.

The term **pseudo-Madelung deformity** is applied to cases in which the abnormal joint position has resulted from exostosis or a malunited forearm fracture (Figs. 2.**319**, 2.**320**).

 Fracture, Subluxation, or Dislocation?

A detailed discussion of fractures and dislocations in the distal forearm, carpus, and carpometacarpal joint region are beyond the scope of this monograph dealing with borderline findings. We again refer the reader to classic monographs on the subject (e.g., Schmitt and Lanz 1996, Gilula and Yin 1996). The special features of individual carpal fractures are described in the section on specific carpal bones. Of particular importance is the diagnostic differentiation of fractures and bony avulsions from accessory bone elements, and bipartite carpal bones (Fig. 2.**158**).

Some basic principles in the differential diagnosis of fractures and accessory bone elements are reviewed on p. 4.

> It should also be noted that trauma to the hand can cause the subluxation or dislocation of accessory bone elements, and these can produce complaints like those of a fracture.

This problem is extremely difficult to solve. CT can help sometimes, especially in the case of a fracture, by defining the defect in the fractured bone more clearly than on the projection radiographs (plane films).

Figure 2.**159** shows the **zones in which fractures, fracture-dislocations, and dislocations of the carpal bones most frequently occur**. The distal radial fracture, though common, is not shown in the diagram. When a distal radial fracture is evaluated, it should always be determined

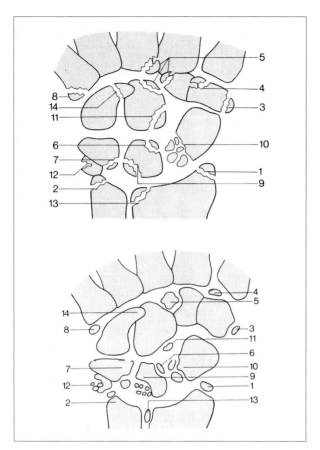

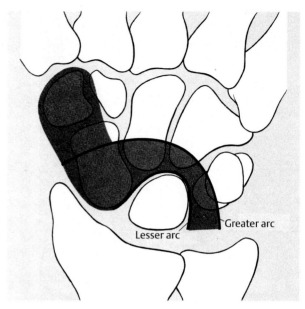

Fig. 2.**159** The shaded areas represent the "vulnerable zones" in which most fractures, fracture-dislocations, and dislocations of the carpal bones occur. Injuries along the lesser arc are mostly dislocations while those along the greater arc are fracture-dislocations.

Fig. 2.**158a,b** Common fractures of the carpal region and their differentiation from accessory bone elements (diagram from Zatzkin).

a Frequent carpal fractures

1	Radial styloid process
2	Ulnar styloid process
3, 4	Trapezium
5	Trapezoid, capitate, base of third metacarpal
6, 9	Lunate
7	Triquetrum
8	Base of fifth metacarpal
10	Scaphoid
11	Capitate
12	Pisiform
13	Radius
14	Hamate

b Differential diagnosis

1	Persistent ossification center: radial styloid process
2	Persistent ossification center: ulnar styloid process
3	Paratrapezium
4	Secondary trapezoid
5	Os styloideum
6	Os hypolunatum
7	Triquetrum, with an accessory bone radial to it
8	Os vesalianum
9	Osteonecrotic changes in the lunate
10	Multipartite scaphoid
11	Os centrale carpi
12	Multiple ossification centers in pisiform
13	Ossification centers at ulnar border of radius
14	Hook of the hamate

whether the fracture is extra-articular or intra-articular (involving the radiocarpal and/or radioulnar joint surface). The Frykman classification of distal radial fractures is based on the presence or absence of articular involvement. It is also important to determine the slope of the fractured radial articular surface, which normally is angled 15–35° toward the ulna in the coronal plane and 0–20° toward the palm. The difference between the radial length and ulnar length in the neutral position should be ± 2 mm, and the radioulnar joint space should measure 2 mm in the PA projection. The latter distance is important in diagnosing a Galeazzi fracture-dislocation. CT scanning should be used in all complicated fractures and potentially litigious situations, as it can accurately define the position of the fragments in specific planes while detecting any fractures or dislocations in the carpus. Radioulnar subluxation was discussed on p. 111 (Fig. 2.**145**). Subluxations and dislocations result from lesions of the dorsal and/or palmar radioulnar ligament caused by a rotational force acting on the pronated or supinated forearm while the hand is fixed or on the pronated or supinated hand while the forearm is fixed.

Very severe rotation can cause a complete avulsion of the triangular fibrocartilage complex. Injuries to this complex cannot be adequately evaluated with simple biplane radiographs. MRI has become the imaging procedure of first choice. If it is not available, CT-arthrography or arthroscopy makes an acceptable alternative.

The diagram in Fig. 2.**160** shows the **numerous dislocations and fracture-dislocations that can occur within the carpus**.

The most frequent combined injury is the transscaphoid–perilunate dislocation (of de Quervain), followed by the perilunate–transscaphoid–transcapitate fracture-dislocation. The Gilula lines in the PA radiograph (Fig. 2.**136**) are important in the diagnosis of carpal dislocations and fracture-dislocations. Any disruption of these lines signifies a dislocation or subluxation. Incongruities of joint contours and unusual overlaps of carpal bones are suspicious for a subluxation or dislocation. A typical sign in the PA projection is a triangular shape of the lunate bone, which overlaps the adjacent carpal bones.

Ligament ruptures are basically associated with the following patterns of instability (Schmitt and Lanz 1996):

- Isolated rupture of the scapholunate ligament with rotation of the lunate bone toward the dorsal side, creating a DISI pattern (dorsiflexed intercalated carpal instability, Fig. 2.**162**). Because of the dorsal tilt of the lunate bone, the radiolunate angle is greater than 15°. This pattern is most commonly seen in scapholunate dissociation (Fig. 2.**161 f**).
- Rupture of the lunotriquetral ligament causes the lunate bone to rotate toward the palm, creating a PISI pattern (palmar-flexed intercalated carpal instability, Fig. 2.**161 f**). The radiolunate angle is less than –15° due to the palmar tilt of the lunate bone.
- Rupture of the triquetrocarpal ligament results in midcarpal instability.
- Lesions of the proximal V ligaments generally lead to DISI, especially when complaints persist following a distal radial fracture.
- Rupture of the radioscaphocapitate ligament (the palmar suspensory ligament) leads to rotatory subluxation of the scaphoid.
- Rupture of the dorsal radiotriquetral ligament promotes ulnar translocation of the carpus in addition to a DISI configuration. Because the dorsal ligaments are attached to the triquetrum, triquetral avulsion fractures commonly occur.

Carpal instabilities due to any cause (traumatic with or without a fracture, with or without perilunar dislocation; chronic overload; chondrocalcinosis (Fig. 2.**283**); rheumatoid arthritis; congenital ligament weakness) may produce very subtle, borderline radiographic changes, which are outlined below.

A basic distinction is drawn between **dynamic and static forms** of carpal instability. Dynamic instability is apparent only when the wrist is moved, whereas static forms can be demonstrated even at rest. In a more recent approach, carpal instabilities are classified as dissociative or nondissociative. **Dissociative carpal instabilities** (CID) are based on a scapholunate or lunotriquetral dissociation in the proximal row of carpal bones. **Nondissociative carpal instabilities** (CIND) involve an abnormal position of the proximal row as a whole with no interosseous dissociations within the row (radiocarpal and midcarpal forms and ulnar translocation, Table 2.**19**).

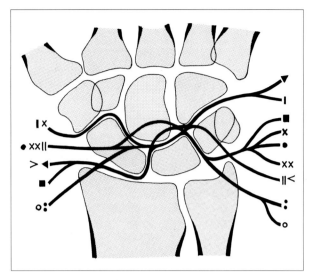

Fig. 2.**160**   Intercarpal dislocations and fracture-dislocations (from Dihlman 1987).
>–<   transtriquetral–perilunate
■–■   transcapitate–perilunate
◀–▶   peritriquetral–lunate
I–I   periscaphoid–triquetral–lunate
x–x   periscaphoid–lunate
•–•   transscaphoid–perilunate (de Quervain)
xx–xx   transscaphoid–capitate–perilunate
||–|| transscaphoid–capitate–triquetral–perilunate
:–:   transstyloid–perilunate
○–○   transstyloid–scaphoid–perilunate

Table 2.**19**   Classification of carpal instabilities (after Lanz and Schmitt)

Dissociative carpal instabilities (CID)
- Scapholunate dissociation
- Lunotriquetral dissociation

Nondissociative carpal instabilities (CIND)
- Radiocarpal instability
- Midcarpal instability
- Ulnar translocation (>50%)

Complex carpal instabilities (CIC)
- Perilunate dislocation (dorsal or palmar)
- Transscaphoid–perilunate fracture-dislocation

Axial carpal instabilities
- Ulnar (hamatocapitate) dissociation
- Radial dissociation
- Combined ulnar–radial dissociation

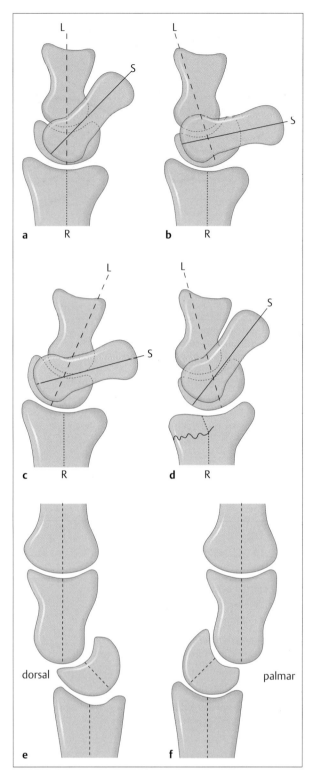

CID is characterized by a dissociation between the scaphoid and lunate or between the lunate and triquetrum, and CIND by a disruption of the articulation between the proximal and distal rows of carpal bones.

Whereas CID and CIND are chronic conditions, complex carpal instabilities (CIC) and axial instabilities are caused by acute dislocations or fracture-dislocations of the carpal bones. The descriptive acronyms DISI and PISI were explained previously (p. 127). They describe the abnormal position of the lunate bone within the proximal carpal row in the setting of a **zigzag deformity** (radial axis, lunate axis, capitate–third metacarpal axis, Fig. 2.**161 e, f**). The lunate is described as the interposed or "intercalated" bony element. The radiographic diagnosis of these instabilities demands a rigorous technique with biplane views of the wrist in the neutral position, PA stress radiographs in maximum radial and ulnar abduction, and lateral stress radiographs in maximum flexion and extension. The geometric relationships that exist in scapholunate dissociation, lunotriquetral dissociation, and radiocarpal instability are shown schematically from a lateral perspective in Fig. 2.**161**. The basic rule in the PA projection is that any discontinuity in the carpal arcs is suspicious for carpal instability. Other suspicious signs are a triangular lunate bone (see above) and nonparallel bony joint contours.

Conventional radiography of **scapholunate dissociation** is rewarding only in static forms of instability. Important radiographic signs are:

- Widening of the scapholunate space to more than 3 mm (2–3 mm is equivocal and should be compared with the opposite side). This is best demonstrated by the Moneim projection (palm resting on the cassette, small and ring fingers flexed to elevate the ulna slightly, beam perpendicular and centered on the radiocarpal joint).
- Palmar flexion of the scaphoid bone in the PA radiograph. The distal pole of the scaphoid is projected as a ringlike feature (the **ring sign**), and the scaphoid is foreshortened. The distance from the ring to the proximal pole of the scaphoid is less than 7 mm (Fig. 2.**162 b**). The radioscaphoid angle in the lateral radiograph is greater than 60° (Fig. 2.**162 d**).
- Dorsiflexion of the lunate bone (DISI). This is seen only in advanced stages. The PA radiograph shows a triangular-shaped lunate, the radioulnar angle in the lateral radiograph is greater than 15°, and the scapholunate angle is greater than 60°.

Fig. 2.161 a–f   Carpal instabilities.
a–d Longitudinal axes have been drawn through the radius, lunate, and scaphoid. Panel **a** shows a normal finding with a scapholunate angle of 45°. Panel **b** shows scapholunate dissociation. The scaphoid is rotated toward the palm, the lunate is rotated toward the dorsum of the hand, and the scapholunate angle is 96°. Panel **c** shows a typical case of lunotriquetral dissociation. The scaphoid and lunate are both tilted toward the palm. The scapholunate angle is normal, but the radiolunate angle is increased to 24° and the radioscaphoid angle to 78°. Panel **d** illustrates radiocarpal instability following a distal radial fracture. The dorsal inclination (deviation) has caused both

the scaphoid and lunate to rotate toward the back of the hand. The radiolunate angle is 22°, and the radioscaphoid angle is 37° (after Schmitt and Lanz).
e, f Schematic drawings of the DISI (**e**) and PISI (**f**) configurations. In DISI the lunate bone is flexed toward the back of the hand in an intercalated position. In PISI it is flexed toward the palm.

DISI   Dorsiflexed intercalated segmental instability
L   .   Lunate bone
PISI   Palmar-flexed intercalated segmental instability
R   Radius
S   Scaphoid bone

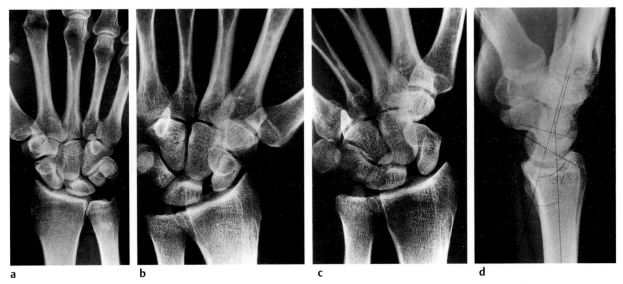

a   b   c   d

Fig. 2.**162 a–d**   Scapholunate dissociation with a DISI confi-guration. The radiolunate angle is 20°, the scapholunate angle is 74°, and the capitolunate angle is 0° (see Table 2.**17**). The
stress radiographs in **b** and **c** show marked displacement of the scaphoid. Note the "ring sign" in **a** and **b** (p. 128).

If projection radiographs (plane films) are unrewarding, the wrist should be evaluated by cineradiography, CT-arthrography, and/or MR imaging.

In **lunotriquetral dissociation**, the lunate bone is ro-tated toward the palm in a PISI configuration. This finding in itself, however, is insufficient to differentiate between lunotriquetral dissociation (CID-PISI) and hamato-triquetral instability (CIND-PISI). Lunotriquetral dissocia-tion is preceded by rupture of the lunotriquetral ligament, and adjacent extrinsic ligaments may also be affected when the instability is severe.

Lunotriquetral dissociation is associated with the fol-lowing radiographic findings (Fig. 2.**161 c**):

- The scaphoid and lunate bones are both flexed toward the palm (PISI). The PA view shows a triangular-shaped lunate. In the lateral view, the radiolunate angle is decreased to less than 15° while the radioscaphoid angle is increased to more than 60°.
- The triquetrum is flexed toward the dorsal side. The lunotriquetral angle in the lateral view is less than 15°, and the PA view shows the triquetrum displaced downward near the proximal pole of the hamate. In the advanced chronic stage of lunotriquetral dissociation, degenerative arthritic changes are found between the lunate and triquetrum and between the hamate and triquetrum.

In **radiocarpal instability**, disruption of the ligaments that stabilize the radiocarpal joint (RSL, RLT, RSC, TFCC, RTD, pp. 105 f and 111) leads to instability of the proximal carpal row, which may shift as a whole in the ulnar direction (due to the slope of the radial articular surface) or may rotated dorsalward. The instability is manifested clinically by a bayonet-like deformity of the wrist. Radiographs with an impacted, dorsally angulated radial fracture show dorsal rotation of the entire proximal carpal row and a flexion de-formity ("zigzag" deformity) of the midcarpal joint. The distal radioulnar joint shows axial subluxation with im-pingement of the distal ulna against the triquetrum. The DISI deformity affects the entire carpus (Fig. 2.**161 e**).

In **ulnar translocation**, the entire carpus drifts in an ulnar direction. The distance between the scaphoid bone and radial styloid process is increased to more than 2 mm (radioscaphoid diastasis), and the congruence between the articular surfaces of the radius and ulna is decreased. The degree of the shift can be measured using the methods of Chamay and McMurtry (Fig. 2.**139 b**). Occasionally the position of the scaphoid remains unchanged while the rest of the carpus shifts in an ulnar direction, creating a symp-tomatic scapholunate dissociation.

Midcarpal instability is a dynamic instability that oc-curs during abduction movements in the radiocarpal joint. It is characterized by a transient shifting of the articular surfaces of both rows of carpal bones. Only cineradiogra-phy can effectively document this finding.

We conclude this section on carpal injuries that often have subtle radiographic features ("borderline-pathologi-cal" findings) with a word about **carpometacarpal disloca-tions and fracture-dislocations**. These injuries may in-volve one or more joints, but the most common pattern is a dorsal dislocation affecting the fifth digit. Conventional radiographs may be relatively unrewarding, and therefore CT should be used as a primary study when this type of in-jury is suspected. The M-shaped carpometacarpal joint line shown in Fig. 2.**136 c** can be a helpful guide in conven-tional examinations. If the dislocation has reduced spon-taneously or if no dislocation has occurred, then the differ-ential diagnosis of isolated bony elements found in the mid-carpometacarpal region should include carpal boss-ing (p. 138) as well as accessory bones such as a secondary capitate.

Necrosis?

The carpus is a relatively common site of necrosis compared with the other bones in the hand. Most cases are posttraumatic, and the lunate bone is most commonly affected. The specific issue of lunate necrosis is discussed on p. 169 f. As a general rule, increased radiographic density and fragmentation of a carpal bone should raise suspicion of necrosis. These signs should be interpreted with caution in growing patients, however. As mentioned earlier, nonnecrotic stippled or fragmented carpal ossification centers may be found in diseases such as chondrodysplasia punctata (Conradi–Hünermann) and other complex disturbances of epiphyseal enchondral ossification.

The radiologic features of Kashin-Beck disease in the wrist of children were investigated by Yu et al (2002) (s. also p. 54).

 ## Inflammation?

The midcarpal joint compartment in particular has extensive connections with the carpometacarpal and intermetacarpal joint spaces (see Fig. 2.**140**), with the result that bacterial infections of a single joint can spread rapidly throughout the carpus. If untreated, the spreading infection can lead quickly to the destruction and eventual ankylosis of multiple joints (Fig. 2.**163**).

Sympathetic arthritis, precipitated, for example, by an osteoid osteoma in a carpal bone (Fig. 2.**164**), can also spread swiftly to involve all the neighboring joints.

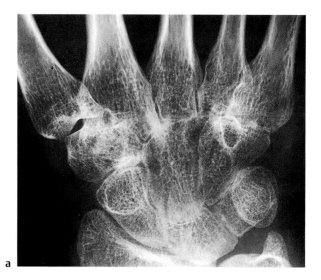

a

Fig. 2.**163 a–c** Typical features of carpal arthritis.
a PA radiograph shows extensive joint destruction and incipient ankyloses in a carpus previously affected by gonococcal arthritis. The changes involve the entire midcarpal joint space along with the carpometacarpal joints, which apparently communicate with it.
b Typical tuberculous carpal arthritis with cystlike bone defects, especially in the distal radius and scaphoid, and marked erosions of the joint contours, especially along the scaphoid. The ligaments between the radius and ulna and between the scaphoid and lunate have been destroyed, causing interosseous widening with carpal instability. The carpal arthritis, which may have arisen from the midcarpal joint compartment, has spread to involve the radiocarpal and ulnocarpal compartments and the neighboring carpometacarpal and intermetacarpal joints.
c Very severe tuberculous radiocarpal, intercarpal, and carpometacarpal arthritis with subtotal destruction of all affected bony structures and a significant reduction of carpal height. This case also demonstrates that joint infections in the carpus can spread rapidly to multiple compartments.

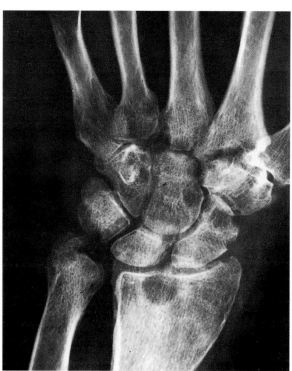

b

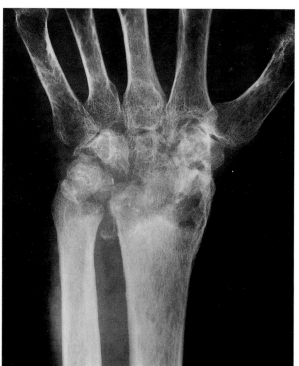

c

Finally, mention should be made of systemic disorders such as rheumatoid arthritis and psoriatic arthritis that may involve all or part of the carpus. Inflammatory erosions and destructive changes in the carpus require differentiation from physiological notches and depressions (Fig. 2.**146**). While erosions destroy the subchondral bone plate and portions of the adjacent cancellous bone with exposure of the rest of the spongiosa, notches have an intact cortical boundary. Inflammatory joint processes are generally accompanied by osteoporosis.

Inflammatory ankyloses require differentiation from congenital synostoses. They are difficult to distinguish from congenital lesions in cases where carpal arthritis in early childhood has led to hypoplastic carpal bone development and postinflammatory ankylosis.

 Tumor?

The differential diagnosis of cystic lesions in the hand and especially the carpus is reviewed in Table 2.**7**. Figure 2.**76** illustrates relatively large carpal "cysts" caused by β_2-microglobulin deposits following long-term hemodialysis. These cystic lesions are most commonly found in the carpal region, and "idiopathic" hand cysts (Fig. 2.**74**) also show a predilection for the wrist. Other lesions that frequently affect the carpus are simple chondromas (occasionally with calcified cartilage) and subchondral synovial cysts (Figs. 2.**80**, 2.**165**).

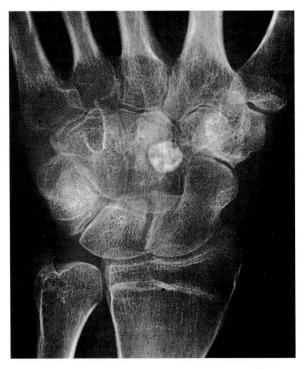

Fig. 2.**164**   Osteoid osteoma in the capitate bone. The nidus is almost completely ossified. There is considerable decalcification of all periarticular bone areas surrounding the carpus and of all the carpal bones, probably due to sympathetic arthritis. The patient presented clinically with carpal pain and swelling.

Fig. 2.**165 a–d**   Intraosseous ganglion with cortical erosion. The patient, a 36-year-old woman, presented with very severe pain. PA radiograph shows a lucent area in the central and proximal scaphoid, corresponding to the defects in the CT scans (**c, d**). The cortical perforation over the cyst has incited reparative bone formation, accounting for the intense tracer uptake in the bone scan (**b**).

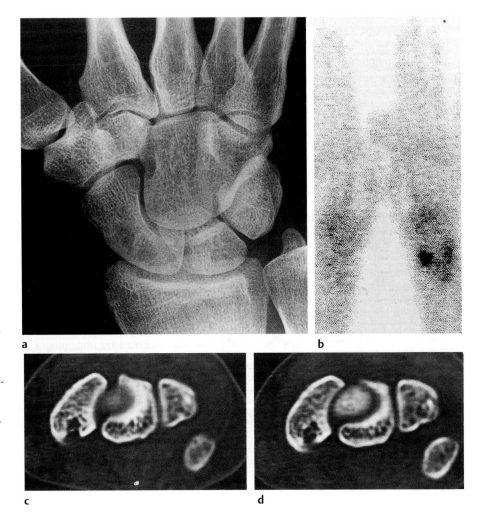

Osteoid osteomas (Figs. 2.**164**, 2.**248**) and osteoblastomas seldom affect the carpus, and malignant bone tumors such as osteosarcoma and chondrosarcoma are even rarer (Freyschmidt et al. 1998).

 It should be reemphasized that when radiographs of the carpus are technically poor, physiological notches and depressions, which are relatively radiolucent, may appear suspicious for pathology because their cancellous trabeculae are not defined. This can lead to further unnecessary and costly imaging studies (Fig. 2.**147**).

 ## Other Changes?

Calcifications of the triangular fibrocartilage (Fig. 2.**70**) do not necessarily have pathological significance in elderly patients but are almost always abnormal in patients under 50–60 years of age (e.g., posttraumatic with cartilage necrosis, chondrocalcinosis, etc.).

Specific Bones of the Carpus

Trapezium

Normal Findings

During Growth

The trapezium was formerly known as the os multangulum majus. Its first ossification center appears after 4 years of age, sometimes earlier, and may be duplicated. A transient increase in the density of the ossification center has no pathological significance in the absence of clinical symptoms (Fig. 2.**183**).

In Adulthood

The fully developed bone is shaped like a pentagon. Its distal articular surface is saddle-shaped and is "straddled" by the first metacarpal bone. Its most distal part projects like a gable between the bases of the first and second metacarpals. Its proximal part has surfaces that articulate with the scaphoid and trapezoid. The **tubercle** is located on the radial aspect of the palmar surface of the trapezium and is separated from the main body of the bone by a groove for the flexor carpi radialis tendon (Fig. 2.**166**, see also CT scans in Fig. 2.**143**).

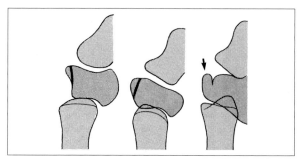

Fig. 2.**166**   Tubercle of the trapezium.

A special projection can be used to demonstrate the trapezium:

- The abducted thumb is placed on the cassette, and a wedge is placed beneath the metacarpus and fingers.
- The central ray is directed perpendicular to the cassette and centered on the radial third of the carpus.
- The two sesamoid bones of the first metacarpophalangeal joint must be superimposed.

This projection is recommended if there is suspicion of a trapezium fracture or a Bennett or Rolando fracture. A relatively good, clear projection of the trapezium can also be obtained by placing the dorsal side of the thumb on the cassette. In practice, however, primary use of CT is recommended.

Normal Variant or Anomaly?

There are morphological variants of the trapezium that have no significance as long as they do not cause carpal instability.

Synostoses (coalitions) with the first metacarpal, scaphoid, and trapezoid are known to occur as variants (Fig. 2.**167**).

A familial incidence of these synostoses has also been described. Delayed ossification of the scaphoid and trapezium after 4 or 5 years of age is believed to be a precursor of the synostosis. Projection-related effects can also simulate fusions and bony bridges between the trapezium, trapezoid, and capitate (Fig. 2.**167 c**). This can be appreciated by imagining a slightly oblique projection in the fourth row of CT images in Fig. 2.**143**.

Fracture or Dislocation?

The trapeziometacarpal joint (TMC), called also the first carpometacarpal joint or "basal joint," has a geometry that allows for maximum mobility of the thumb in flexion, extension, abduction, adduction, and axial rotation. This great freedom of motion naturally carries a risk of instabil-

Fig. 2.**167 a–c**
Synostosis.
a, b Synostosis between
the trapezium, trapezoid,
and scaphoid.
c Superimposition effect
mimicking a carpal syn-
ostosis.

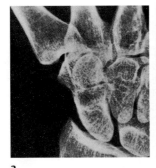
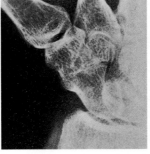
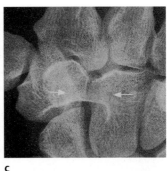

a b c

ity, especially in patients with lax ligaments (Fig. 2.**168**).
Subluxation is easily provoked in these individuals and can
be documented on stress radiographs. This phenomenon
does not necessarily have pathological significance and
may be a normal variant. However, if the first carpometacarpal joint is symptomatic, especially in menopausal or
postmenopausal women, and if subluxation can be demonstrated, it is reasonable to assume that the joint is affected by an early degenerative process that will eventually lead to joint space narrowing, loss of joint congruence,
subchondral sclerosis, and periarticular ossification (for
more on first carpometacarpal osteoarthritis see Cooke et
al. 1995; Figs. 2.**180** and 2.**181**).

Fractures of the trapezium are usually caused by a violent axial force on the thumb, as in a fall onto the outstretched hand. This kind of force can literally split the
trapezium in two. The impaction of the trapezium may be
transmitted across the scaphoid to the radius, resulting in
combined injuries with fractures of the scaphoid and
radial styloid process.

Several types of trapezium fracture may occur:

- Fractures of the body of the trapezium with vertical and
  horizontal fracture lines
- Fractures of the tubercle of the trapezium
- Avulsion fractures on the dorsoulnar or radial side of the
  bone

A burst fracture is shown in Fig. 2.**169**.

An important concern in the present monograph is the
differentiation of **avulsion fractures** from accessory bone
elements of a primary or secondary nature. The full spectrum of "accessory" bony elements (paratrapezium, secondary trapezium, secondary trapezoid), periarticular regressive ossifications, and capsular osteomas is illustrated
in Figs. 2.**170**–2.**181**.

Periarticular ossifications that accompany first carpometacarpal osteoarthritis (basal joint osteoarthritis) can
grow remarkably large. They are relatively easy to identify
as such by noting the degenerative process in the neighboring joint. The ossifications are sometimes palpable on
clinical examination. With many ossifications, especially
those located near the joint between the trapezium and
scaphoid bones, it may be impossible to distinguish an epitrapezium from a bursal calcification unless symptomatic
lesions are investigated further with CT for more accurate
localization. As mentioned earlier on p. 117 in connection
with a discussion of Fig. 2.**150**, bone scanning should additionally be used in potentially litigious situations and in
determining whether a radiographic finding correlates
with a particular clinical symptom. A negative bone scan
about 3–4 days after an injury always signifies a harmless
or inconsequential ossification. MRI can also be useful in
these situations (for detecting edema!).

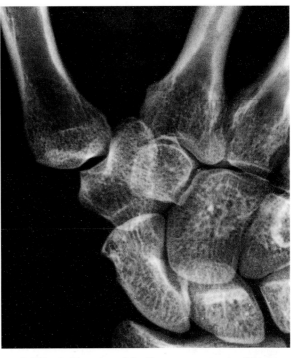

Fig. 2.**168** Subluxation of the first carpometacarpal joint in a
patient with lax ligaments. The proximal interphalangeal joints
were also hyperextensible in this otherwise healthy woman
(see Fig. 2.**99 c**).

Fig. 2.**169** Burst fracture of
the trapezium.

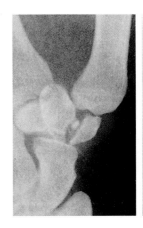

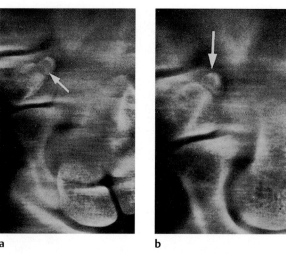
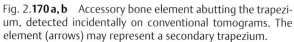

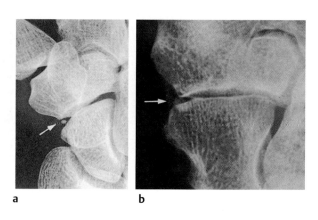

Fig. 2.**170 a, b**   Accessory bone element abutting the trapezium, detected incidentally on conventional tomograms. The element (arrows) may represent a secondary trapezium.

Fig. 2.**173 a, b**   Small, unidentified bony elements between the trapezium and scaphoid (arrows) (UBE = unknown bony element).

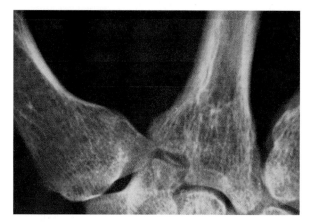

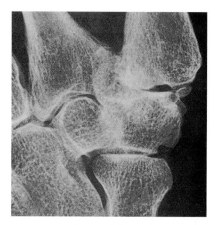

Fig. 2.**171**   Secondary trapezium. Incidental observation.

Fig. 2.**174**   The small bony element between the trapezium and first metacarpal may be either a paratrapezium or a remnant of an old avulsion fracture.

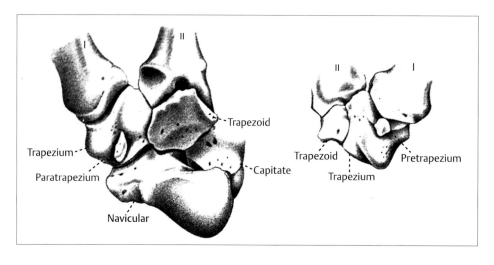

Fig. 2.**172**   Accessory trapezium bones in a diagram by Pfitzner.

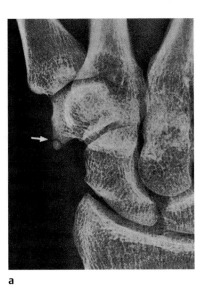
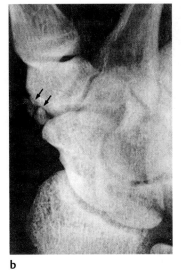
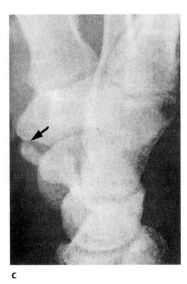

a b c

Fig. 2.**175 a–c** UBE in the area between the trapezium and scaphoid.
a The bony element could represent an old, small bony avulsion, since it fits well into an opposing crater in the trapezium (arrow).

b In this image the amorphous internal structure and multiplicity suggest heterotopic calcifications (arrows).
c Again, the somewhat amorphous mineralization could indicate a heterotopic process (arrow).

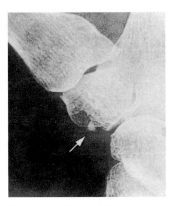

Fig. 2.**176** This relatively amorphous calcification probably represents a bursal calcification (arrow).

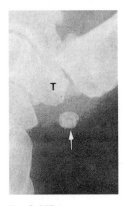
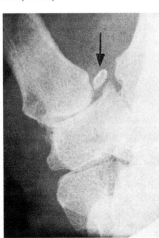

Fig. 2.**177**

Fig. 2.**178**

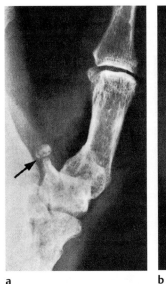
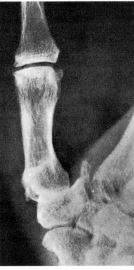

a b

Fig. 2.**179 a, b** Severe Heberden-type osteoarthritis with dystrophic calcifications in the periarticular tissue. The isolated elements could also be detached marginal osteophytes (arrow).

Fig. 2.**177** This accessory bone element shows a relatively good osseous structure and may be an osteoma in the joint capsule (arrow). The patient was clinically asymptomatic.

Fig. 2.**178** Marked first carpometacarpal osteoarthritis with an ossification in the periarticular tissue (arrow) (similar in appearance to a Heberden node, Fig. 2.**179**).

Fig. 2.**180** First carpometacarpal osteoarthritis. An osteophytic spur is visible on the radial margin (arrow). The feature on the ulnar side may be either a detached osteophyte or a structured ossification in the periarticular tissue (double arrow).

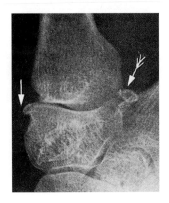

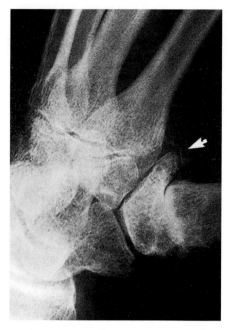

Fig. 2.**181**   Severe first carpometacarpal osteoarthritis with an isolated bony element directly adjacent to a large osteophyte—possibly a fragment broken from the osteophyte or a nonspecific ossification in the periarticular tissue (arrow). Note also the fine periarticular ossifications on the radial side.

 Necrosis?

A dense, irregularly calcified ossification center in the trapezium of a growing patient requires differentiation from necrosis. If the patient has no clinical complaints, findings like those shown in Fig. 2.**183** have no significance. Posttraumatic necrosis can occur in the trapezium as in any other carpal bone but has rarely been described. One such case is illustrated in Fig. 2.**182**.

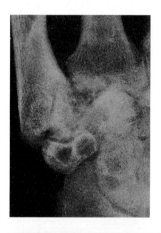

◁ Fig. 2.**182**   Posttraumatic necrosis of the distal trapezium fragment with severe regressive "cystic" transformation of the proximal fragment.

Fig. 2.**183 a, b**   The relatively dense ossification center of the trapezium (incidental finding) is a normal variant of the ossification process and does not signify necrosis.
▽

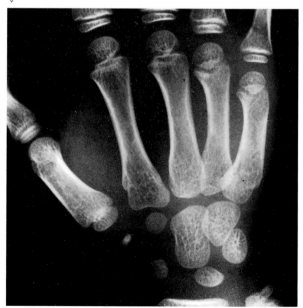

a   b

Tumor?

Coarse geodes can erode through the cortex in first carpometacarpal osteoarthritis (Fig. 2.**184**), mimicking destruction by a tumor.

True tumors are rare in the trapezium (Fig. 2.**184b**). Occasionally they may arise from tumors and tumorlike lesions in tendon sheaths (Fig. 2.**184c**).

Trapezoid

Normal Findings

The trapezoid was formerly termed the os multangulum minus.

 During Growth

The ossification center of the trapezoid, like that of the trapezium, is radiographically visible after 4 years of age.

 In Adulthood

The trapezoid is only slightly smaller than the trapezium. It is approximately wedge-shaped, its dorsal surface being broader than its palmar surface. It articulates with the trapezium, capitate, second metacarpal, and occasionally with the scaphoid.

Pathological Finding?

 Normal Variant or Anomaly?

Synostosis (coalition) between the trapezoid and capitate bones may occur as a normal variant (Neiss 1955, Buysch and Drewese 1971). But this coalition is as rare as trapezoid fusion with the second metacarpal (Leger 1955, Seibert-Daiker 1975). Coalitions involving the trapezoid are usually bilateral.

Another variant is a bipartite trapezoid divided into a palmar and a dorsal half, as described by Pfitzner (1885) and other authors.

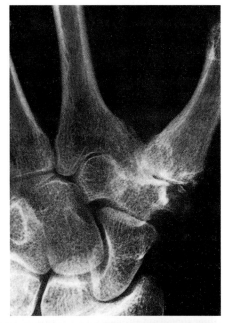

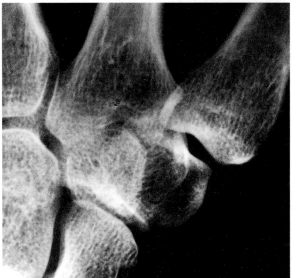

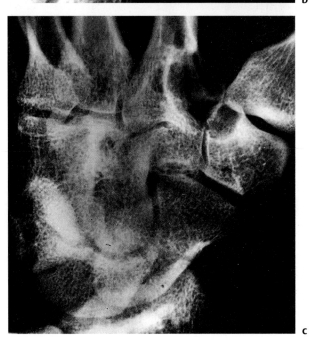

Fig. 2.**184a–c**   "Tumorous" lesions in the trapezium.   ▷
a A large geode in first carpometacarpal osteoarthritis has eroded through the trapezium cortex, mimicking a tumor.
b Lucent area in the trapezium with circumscribed perforation of the proximal cortex, caused by metastatic bronchial carcinoma.
c Nodular synovitis of the tendon sheath with erosion of the second metacarpal base on the radial side and of the opposing trapezium surface. The involvement of both bones marks the epicenter of tumorous destruction in the soft tissues. The site was extremely painful.

Fracture or Dislocation?

Fractures of the trapezoid are rare owing to the protected location of the bone. As in the case of the trapezium, most fractures are caused by an axial blow to the index finger.

Trapezoid fracture are classified into two main types:

- Vertical fractures
- Ligamentous avulsion fractures

Stress radiographs are excellent for trapezoid fractures as they can demonstrate both the fracture and associated capsuloligamentous injuries. If there is strong clinical suspicion of a trapezoid fracture but radiographs are negative, CT scans should be obtained.

Vertical fractures and avulsion fractures mainly require differentiation from accessory bone elements. The most familiar of these elements is the **os styloideum**, which is located between the trapezoid, capitate, and second and third metacarpals (Figs. 2.**185**, 2.**186**, 2.**198 e–h**).

Occasionally the os styloideum is fused with the second and third metacarpals. A radiograph in 30° supination and ulnar deviation provides a clear profile view of the bone (Fig. 2.**186**). The os styloideum can also be palpated as a dorsal bony protuberance at the base of the second and third metacarpals adjacent to the capitate and trapezoid bones. It is difficult to distinguish the os styloideum from **carpal bossing** (Foille 1931), a regressive process due to productive fibro-ostosis that arises from the second or third metacarpal and abuts the trapezoid, capitate and/or hamate bones on the dorsal side (Figs. 2.**187**, 2.**198 a–d**).

Carpal bossing is usually asymptomatic but may cause pain and limited motion, probably due to secondary inflammatory changes in the adjacent soft tissues. A carpal boss may coexist with an accessory ossification center, the os styloideum. If the term "carpal bossing" is viewed purely from a clinical perspective, however, it may be based entirely on the presence of an os styloideum.

Pfitzner described two other accessory bones that can occur close to the os styloideum: the metastyloid and parastyloid. These bones are radiographically indistinguishable from the os styloideum. Pfitzner also described a "**secondary trapezoid**" (Fig. 2.**188**). Nestled between the trapezoid, trapezium, and second metacarpal, this element is virtually indistinguishable from the trapezoid itself (see Fig. 2.**150**).

> We feel that it is unnecessary to assign a precise anatomic name to each of these bony elements. It is important only to differentiate them from a possible avulsion fragment.

Figures 2.**189**–2.**191** illustrate some of these small accessory bone elements, which may be classified as UBEs or UABEs on radiographs (p. 119).

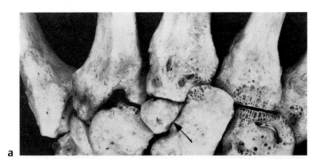
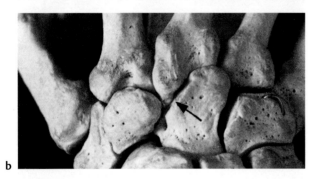

Fig. 2.**185 a, b**   Os styloideum.
a Relatively large os styloideum (arrow).
b Rudimentary os styloideum (arrow).

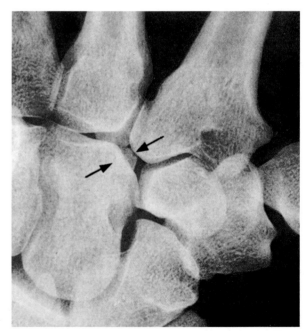

Fig. 2.**186**   Os styloideum (arrows).

Fig. 2.**187 a, b** Carpal bossing at the margins of the second and third carpometacarpal joints.

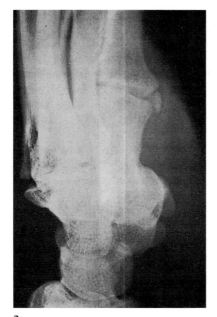
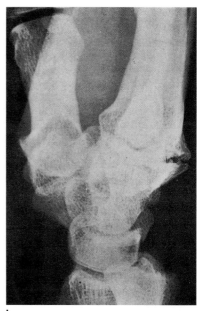

a

b

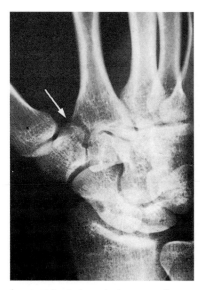

Fig. 2.**188** Secondary trapezoid as drawn by Pfitzner.

Fig. 2.**189** Secondary trapezoid (arrow)?

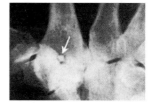

Fig. 2.**190** Relatively large, well-structured accessory bone element, probably a secondary trapezoid (arrow).

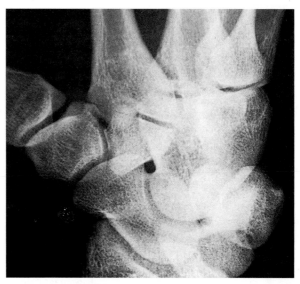

Fig. 2.**191** Secondary trapezoid or secondary trapezium.

Figure 2.**192** shows a small capsular osteoma or detached osteophyte in first carpometacarpal osteoarthritis, which might be confused with a secondary trapezoid or trapezium.

We again emphasize the importance of bone scans when clinical symptoms are present in association with an unidentified bony element. Accessory bones usually produce a negative scan, unless the element has been displaced due to trauma, or its anatomically unfavorable position has led to regressive changes. CT can also help localize and identify these elements.

Dislocations of the trapezoid bone are rare. They can occur after rupture of the dorsal ligaments, usually causing the trapezoid to displace dorsally. Palmar displacement has also been described (Goodman and Shankman 1983, Kopp 1985). Rarely, trapezoid displacement is associated with dislocation of the first metacarpal (Dunkerton and Singer 1985).

Standard criteria apply in the differential diagnosis of necrosis, inflammation, and tumors involving the trapezoid (see section on the Trapezium).

Capitate

Normal Findings

During Growth

The ossification center of the capitate bone becomes radiographically visible during the first months of life (on average, after three months). Irregular contours and slight densities that are detected incidentally on radiographs are not considered important in the absence of clinical symptoms.

In Adulthood

The proximal part of the capitate bone is somewhat rounded on its dorsal, radial aspect, and its more distal, palmar portion bears a kind of process (Fig. 2.**143**). On the PA radiograph, the radial surface of the capitate bears a notch at the level of the joint space between the scaphoid and trapezoid bones; this is explained by the spatial configuration shown in the CT scans in Fig. 2.**143** (images 9 and 10). This notch may be mistaken for an osteolytic lesion on a poor-quality film (Fig. 2.**147 a**). The ulnar side of the bone occasionally bears a small protuberance, corresponding to a small facet in the radial side of the hamate bone (Fig. 2.**193**).

Pathological Finding?

Normal Variant or Anomaly?

Fusion between the capitate and hamate bones is the second most frequent carpal coalition after lunotriquetral fusion (Fig. 2.**194**).

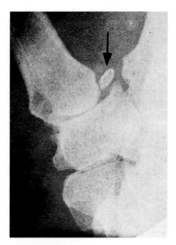

Fig. 2.**192**   First carpometacarpal osteoarthritis with a solid ossification in the capsule or periarticular tissue (not an accessory bone element).

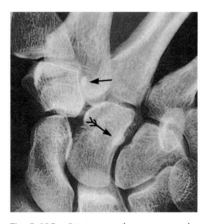

Fig. 2.**193**   Bony protuberance on the capitate (double arrow) as a normal variant. The single arrow points to an accessory bone element.

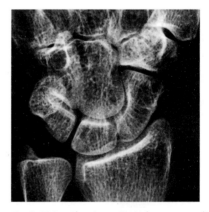

Fig. 2.**194**   Classic capitate-hamate coalition in an otherwise healthy and asymptomatic patient. The radioulnar dissociation was caused by trauma.

A slightly angled radiographic projection can simulate the appearance of a capitate–hamate fusion.

A bipartite capitate bone has been described by several authors (Ross 1954, Viehweger 1956).

As mentioned in the introductory section on the carpus, coalitions and bipartitions are generally asymptomatic and usually are not associated with any other skeletal abnormalities, allowing us to classify them as simple variants.

 ## Fracture or Dislocation?

Longitudinal and transverse fractures of the capitate (Fig. 2.**197b, c**) most commonly result from hyperextension trauma. They are very often combined with an avulsion fracture of the lunate horn and a lunate compression fracture and/or dorsal rim fracture of the radius. By contrast, the scaphoid-capitate fracture syndrome with 180° rotation of the capitate neck fragment is very rare (probably a variant of the de Quervain injury with a transcapital fracture and spontaneous resorption).

A bipartite capitate and its differentiation from a fracture were discussed under "Normal Variant or Anomaly?"

Fractures mainly require differentiation from a small accessory bone that may occur between the third and fourth metacarpals, hamate, and capitate. It is termed the **secondary capitate** (Fig. 2.**195**). It is mainly of academic interest that another accessory bone, the **Gruber ossicle**, can occur at a similar location as the secondary ossicle. It is believed to be considerably smaller, however (Fig. 2.**196**).

Carpal bossing, which arises from the second and/or third metacarpal and may occur dorsal to the capitate, was described in the section on the trapezoid (Fig. 2.**198**).

 ## Necrosis?

Idiopathic and posttraumatic necrosis of the capitate has been reported and may be bilateral (Rahme 1983, Bolton-Maggs et al. 1984, James and Burke 1984). Apparently there are critical perfusion zones in the capitate similar to those in the scaphoid and lunate. Necrosis most commonly occurs in the "head" segment of the capitate. Typical radiographic signs are irregular densities and lucencies with subsequent fragmentation, etc.

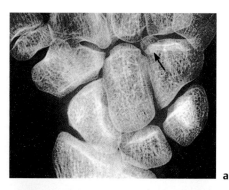

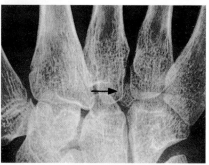

Fig. 2.**195a, b** Accessory bones located near the capitate. Each of the elements probably represents a "secondary capitate."

Small, cystlike lucencies in the capitate may be idiopathic bone cysts due to circumscribed osteonecrosis, especially in response to vibrational trauma (Fig. 2.**197**). Usually these cystic lucencies are considerably larger than end-on projections of nutrient canals. Larger, solitary circumscribed lucencies in the capitate usually represent subchondral synovial cysts or intraosseous ganglion cysts as described on p. 131 f. and 162.

Differentiation from inflammatory conditions and tumors is discussed under General Aspects. Particular note should be taken of the osteoid osteoma in Fig. 2.**164**.

Fig. 2.**196a, b** Gruber ossicle.
a Gruber ossicle as drawn by Pfitzner.
b Gruber ossicle (arrows)?

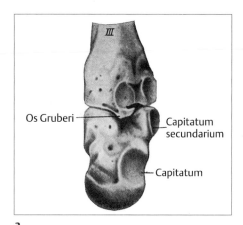

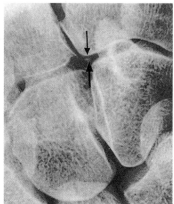

a

b

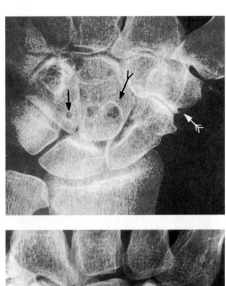

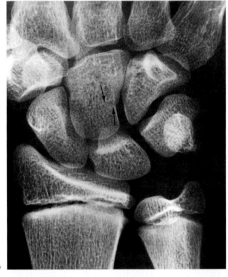

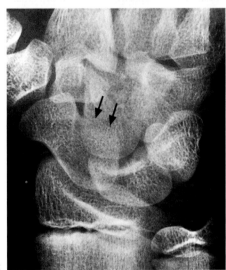

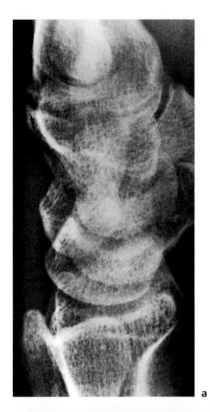

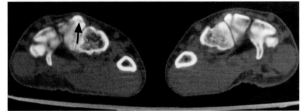

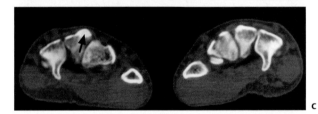

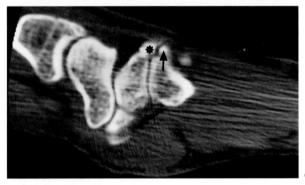

Fig. 2.**197 a–c**   Findings in the capitate bone.
a Marked structural irregularity and cystlike lucencies (end stage of osteonecrosis) are visible in the capitate and neighboring triquetrum, accompanied by significant osteoarthritis between the scaphoid and trapezium as a result of chronic vibrational trauma.
b, c Nondisplaced fracture of the capitate (arrows). This is not a nutrient canal or Mach band phenomenon.

Fig. 2.**198 a–h**   Differential diagnosis of fracture, carpal bossing, and os styloideum.
a–d Typical carpal bossing with productive bone changes on the opposing dorsal margins of the trapezoid and second and third metacarpals on the right side. The carpal bosses (star and arrows) should not be mistaken for avulsion fractures.

Fig. 2.**198 e–h** ▷

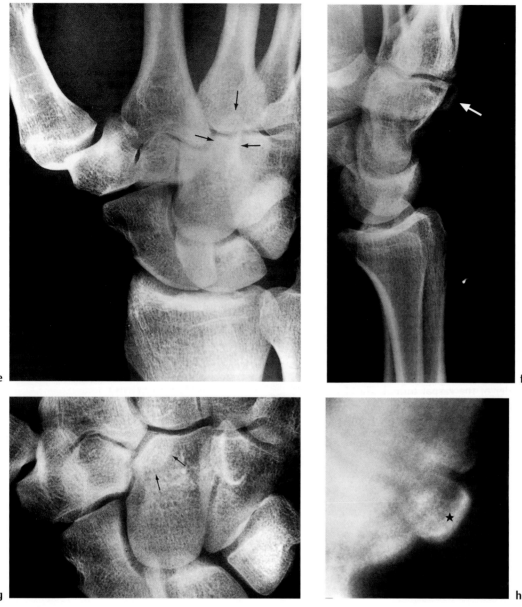

Fig. 2.**198 e–h** Well-developed os styloideum (arrows). In the overrotated lateral tomogram (**h**), the os is projected far dorsally (star) and is also palpable at that location. It is clinically indistinguishable from a carpal boss. Panel **f** also shows an old triquetral avulsion (white arrow).

Hamate

Normal Findings

During Growth

The hamate bone becomes radiographically visible after about three months of age.

In Adulthood

The small notch in the radial aspect of hamate, matching a small protuberance in the opposing capitate just distal to the center of both bones, was mentioned above (Fig. 2.**193**). The hooklike process of the hamate is called the hook of the hamate or the hamulus. The base of the hook appears as an elliptical or ringlike structure on PA radiographs (Fig. 2.**199**).

The carpal tunnel view is the only conventional radiographic view that gives a clear projection of the hook of the hamate. Axial CT scans (Fig. 2.**134**) are best for defining the topographic anatomy of the hamate and its hook, which forms the ulnar border of the **carpal tunnel**. The distal ulnar corner of the hamate bone may appear somewhat more radiolucent on technically poor radiographs and can mimic an erosion (Figs. 2.**147a**, 2.**200**).

Pathological Finding?

Normal Variant or Anomaly?

Coalition of the capitate and hamate bones, mentioned in the section on the capitate (Fig. 2.**194**), is the second most frequent carpal coalition after lunotriquetral fusion.

To our knowledge, a bipartite hamate has not yet been observed, although Greene and Hadied (1981) described a bipartite hamulus.

Two situations can cause atypical broadening of the hamate bone:

- Duplication of the fifth and sixth rays
- Broadening and bifurcation of the associated metacarpal bone, especially in Ellis–van Crefeld chondroectodermal dysplasia

Viehweger (1957) described bilateral hyperplasia of the hamate and pisiform.

A **separate joint facet to the lunate** (medial facet) occurs in 65% of individuals in cadaveric studies (Viegas et al. 1990, 1993) and can then be the cause of ulnar-sided wrist pain (Cerezal et al. 2001, see also p. 165).

Fracture or Dislocation?

Fractures of the body of the hamate are relatively rare. They most often occur in athletes in the hand that holds a club, racket, bat, or hockey stick (Blair et al. 1982, Schlosser and Murray 1984). Fractures of the hook of the hamate are more common. Bilateral hook fractures have also been reported. One case occurred in a golfer who struck the ground with a golf club held in both hands, the sudden deceleration trauma causing bilateral hook fractures (Bray et al. 1985). Axial violence to the fourth or fifth metacarpal can cause a dorsal avulsion fracture of the hamate. Fractures of the hamate present clinically with tenderness to pressure on the ulnar side.

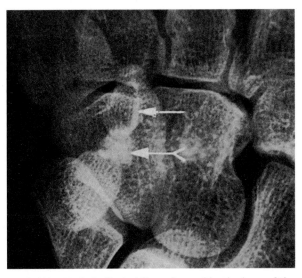

Fig. 2.**199**   Typical elliptical figure formed by the base of the hook of the hamate (arrow). In other cases it may appear as a more ringlike density, similar to the orthograde projection of an osteochondroma. The double arrow points to an innocuous bone island.

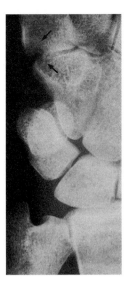

Fig. 2.**200**   Typical erosions at the base of the fifth metacarpal and opposing edge of the hamate in rheumatoid arthritis (compare with Fig. 2.**147b**).

Hamate fractures are classified as follows:

- Vertical fractures (medial or lateral to the hook, including tubercle fractures)
- Horizontal fractures

A distinction is also drawn between a dorsal avulsion fracture and a fracture of the hook of the hamate mentioned above.

The delayed union of a hook fracture is analogous to that of a scaphoid fracture (Schlosser and Murray 1984). For this reason, surgical excision of the hook fragment is recommended as a primary treatment for most cases (Schlosser and Murray 1984, Bray et al. 1985). Hook fractures as well as displaced fractures of the body of the hamate can lead to carpal tunnel syndrome (Schober and Bayard 1959, Tänzer 1959).

Fractures of the body of the hamate (Fig. 2.**209a**) are often missed on standard PA radiographs, especially when they are nondisplaced. Fractures through the proximal pole of the hamate should always raise suspicion of a more complex perilunate injury.

A **fracture of the hook of the hamate is relatively easy to diagnose** when the normally sharp, ringlike outline of the base of this process is not visible or is ill-defined. This signifies an angulated position of the hook, moving its base out of its normal end-on projection in the PA radiograph

(Norman et al. 1985, Fig. 2.**202**). Hook fractures are also relatively easy to identify on carpal tunnel views (Fig. 2.**202**). In doubtful cases, and especially if it is uncertain whether the finding is a fracture or an anomaly, CT scans should be obtained. This is particularly important given the fact that hamate and hook fractures tend to heal poorly and may produce a carpal tunnel syndrome.

Fractures of the body of the hamate mainly require differentiation from a congenital bipartite hamate, which is an obvious diagnosis but extremely rare. It is more difficult to distinguish avulsion fractures of the hook from accessory bones, particularly the **os hamuli proprium** (Figs. 2.**201**–2.**203**).

The hook of the hamate has its own ossification center, and the os hamuli proprium represents a hook that has failed to fuse with the body of the hamate. Bilateral occurrence supports a diagnosis of os hamuli proprium rather than fresh bilateral fractures (except in the golf injury mentioned above) (Fig. 2.**202**). Otherwise the differential diagnosis must rely on classic radiographic signs (see General Aspects). The value of bone scans is again emphasized in this regard.

Another accessory bone is the **os vesalianum**, located in the notch between the fifth metacarpal and the hamate (Figs. 2.**204**, 2.**205**). It requires differentiation from a fresh avulsion fracture or old nonunion.

Fig. 2.**201 a, b**   Os hamuli proprium: **a**, as drawn by Pfitzner; **b**, compared with a fresh avulsion of the tip of the hook (hamulus).

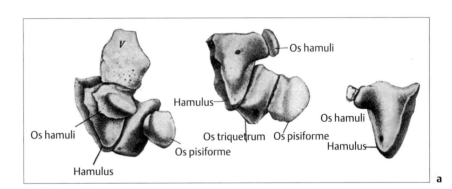

a

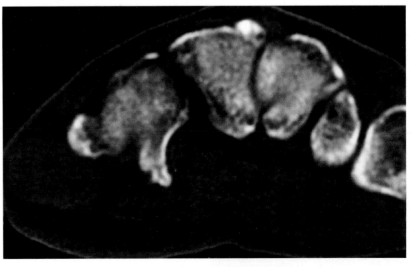

b

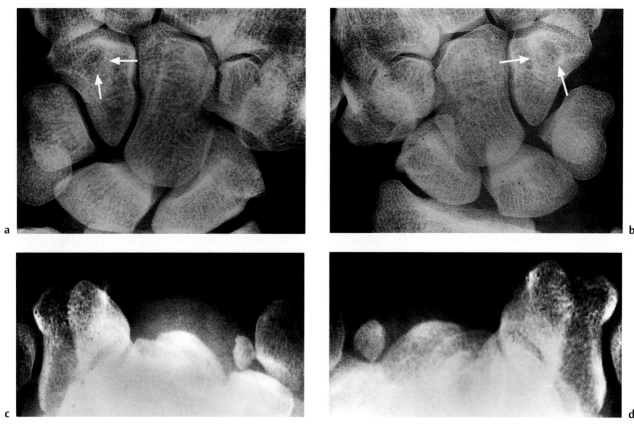

a

b

c

d

Fig. 2.**202 a–d** Unfused hook of the hamate (both sides), known also as the os hamuli proprium (Fig. 2.**203**). PA radiographs show an indistinct ringlike figure (arrows) in the area where the normally well-defined base of the hook should be. Fractures of the hook of the hamate can have a similar appearance when the fracture has occurred 1 or 2 mm distal to the actual base of the process. The case shown appears to be an os hamuli proprium, because on the tunnel views in **c** and **d**, the proximal margins of the small bony elements do not display typical fracture lines. Also, the patient had no prior history of a wrist fracture, although he presented clinically with an ulnar tunnel syndrome. (With kind permission of Dr. Helbig, Kiel.)

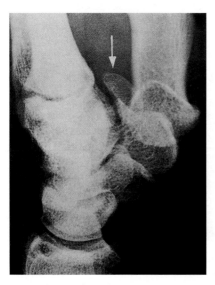

Fig. 2.**203**   Os hamuli proprium.

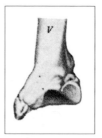

Fig. 2.**204**
Os vesalianum
(as drawn by
Pfitzner).

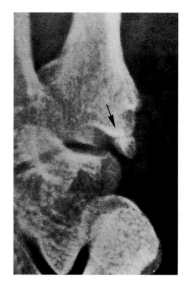

Fig. 2.**205**   Os vesalianum.

The os ulnare externum may also occupy a position similar to the os vesalianum. Ultimately, though, it is unimportant what we call an accessory ossicle as long as we can distinguish a harmless accessory bone or nonspecific bursal calcification from a finding that is definitely pathological. Figures 2.**206** through 2.**208** show examples of accessory bone elements that we have observed clinically over a period of years.

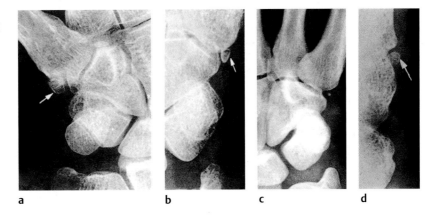

Fig. 2.**206 a–d**   Accessory bones adjacent to the base of the fifth metacarpal (arrows).

a   b   c   d

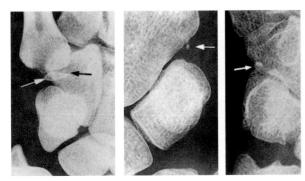

Fig. 2.**207**   Accessory bones adjacent to and projected over the hamate bone (arrows).

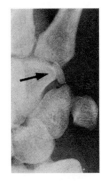

Fig. 2.**208**   Similar accessory bone detected on both sides (arrow).

Fig. 2.**209 a, b**   Fracture and necrosis of the hamate bone.
a Transverse fracture of the body of the hamate with an accompanying hook fracture and subsequent avascular necrosis, recognized by the irregular density of the distal fragment (arrow).
b Conspicuous necrosis of the hamate with marked fragmentation.

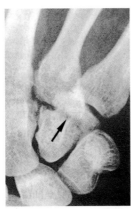

a

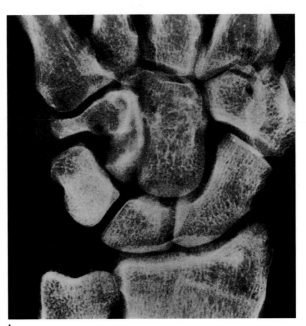

b

Fig. 2.**209 c, d** ▷

Necrosis?

Above we noted the similarities of the hamate bone to the scaphoid in terms of complicated fracture union, including ischemic necrosis. Irregular sclerotic structures projected over the hamate bone should always raise suspicion of a fractured, necrotic hamulus. Hamate necrosis is characterized radiographically by morphological changes, fragmentation, and irregular densities and lucencies ("motley pattern") (Fig. 2.**209**). Vogel (1963) described aseptic necrosis of the hamate.

 ### Inflammation? Tumor?

> There are no specific inflammatory or neoplastic changes in the hamate that would require the special differentiation of normal and borderline-pathological findings.

It is important to distinguish normal bony notches and concavities from inflammatory erosions, especially on the opposing ulnar margins of the fifth metacarpal and the hamate (Figs. 2.**146**, 2.**200**). Normal zones of relative lucency, especially on slightly oblique projections (Fig. 2.**147 b**), can mimic tumors and tumorlike lesions. This problem can be solved by obtaining technically optimum radiographs or, if these are equivocal, by proceeding with CT.

Intraosseous ganglia have not previously been described in the hamate bone, and other tumorlike and tumorous lesions such as osteoid osteoma, aneurysmal bone cyst (Lin et al. 1984, Fig. 2.**209 c, d**), and metastases (e.g., from bronchial carcinoma) are rare.

Scaphoid

Normal Findings

 ### During Growth

The scaphoid bone (formerly called the navicular) is not radiographically visible until after about five years of age (Fig. 2.**250**). Duplication of the ossification center is relatively common (Fig. 2.**210**).

As growth proceeds, the distal margin of the bone becomes oblique and irregular and may be associated with small, duplicated ossific nuclei (Figs. 2.**211**, 2.**213**).

The problem of differentiating duplicated ossification centers from necrosis and fractures is examined below in greater detail.

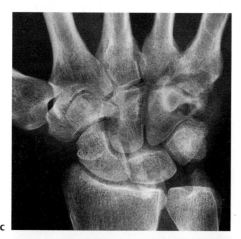

c

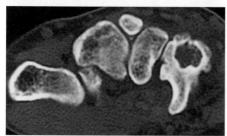

d

Fig. 2.**209 c, d**   Aneurysmal bone cyst in the hamate (original case). The histological diagnosis was surprising, as we had assumed that the lesion was an intraosseous ganglion.

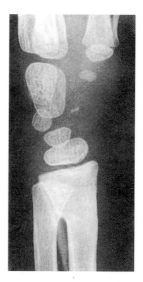

Fig. 2.**210**   Duplicate ossification centers in the scaphoid (radial fracture).

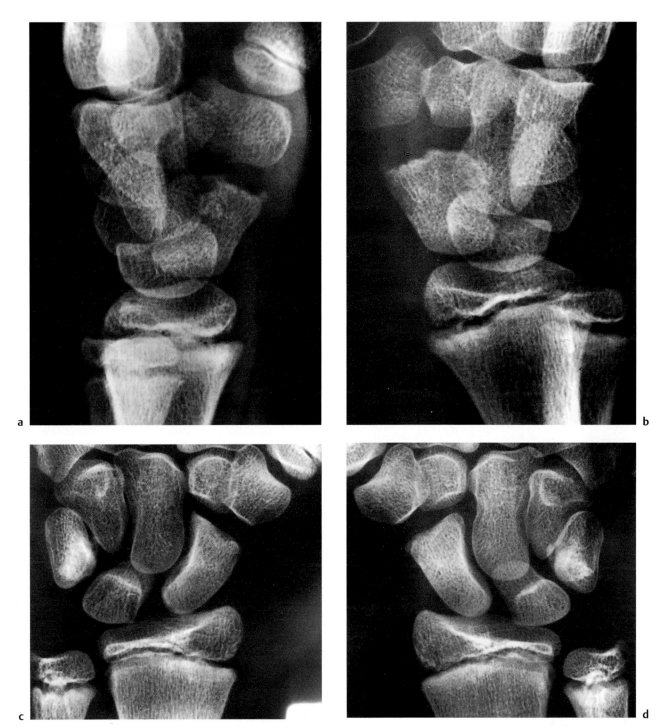

a b

c d

Fig. 2.**211 a–d** Physiological contour irregularities and small accessory centers in the distal scaphoid in a growing skeleton.

 In Adulthood

The scaphoid shows a considerable range of morphological variation in adults (Fig. 2.**212**).

If a separate ossification center for the tubercle fuses with the rest of the bone in a somewhat atypical manner, it can create a beaklike protuberance on that part of the bone (Fig. 2.**213 c–g**).

The spatial extent of the scaphoid is best appreciated on axial CT scans of the carpus (Fig. 2.**143**).

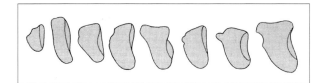

Fig. 2.**212** Morphological variants of the scaphoid bone.

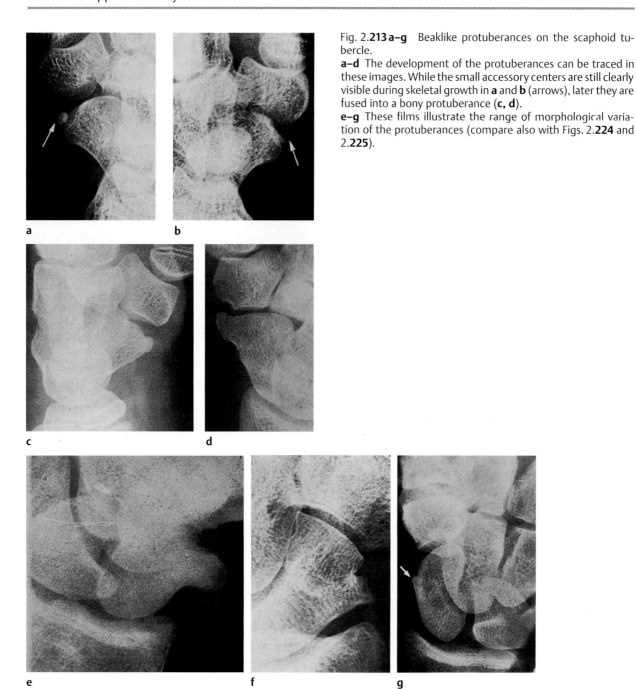

a   b

c   d

e   f   g

Fig. 2.**213 a–g** Beaklike protuberances on the scaphoid tubercle.
a–d The development of the protuberances can be traced in these images. While the small accessory centers are still clearly visible during skeletal growth in **a** and **b** (arrows), later they are fused into a bony protuberance (**c, d**).
e–g These films illustrate the range of morphological variation of the protuberances (compare also with Figs. 2.**224** and 2.**225**).

▌*Pathological Finding?*

 Normal Variant or Anomaly?

Bipartite and multipartite scaphoid bones have been described (Fig. 2.**153**). Even when bilateral, they constitute a normal variant. The same applies to coalitions of the scaphoid with one or more neighboring bones (Fig. 2.**152**). Figure 2.**215** shows an unusual case of scapholunate fusion with a nonunion at the junction of the middle and distal thirds of the composite bone (Krause 1949, Waugh 1950, Geyer 1962).

Hypoplasia of the scaphoid should also be considered an extreme morphological variant (Fig. 2.**214 a–e**), provided the patient has no associated syndromic signs or other manifestations of systemic disease.

It is difficult to classify scaphoid aplasias (Maier 1962, Knàkal and Chvojka 1970). Several authors have characterized them as "enchondral dysostoses." To date, the following patterns have been observed:

- Bilateral scaphoid and lunate aplasia
- Complete left-sided scaphoid aplasia, partial right-sided scaphoid aplasia with lateral displacement of the lunate bone and bilateral fusion of the lunate and capitate
- Bilateral scaphoid aplasia combined with an abnormal position of the proximal carpal row and atypical articulations
- Underdevelopment of the scaphoid with ulnar displacement of the lunate, combined with a wormian bone on the ulnar aspect of both radial epiphyses near the ulnar epiphysis

Fig. 2.**214 a–e**   Forms of scaphoid hypoplasia.
a The hypoplastic scaphoid ossification center is fused with
the radius.
b Bipartite scaphoid. The distal
portion, which developed from
the more distal of two ossification centers, is markedly hypoplastic. The trapezium is also hypoplastic, creating a large midcarpal gap on the radial side.
The findings were bilateral.

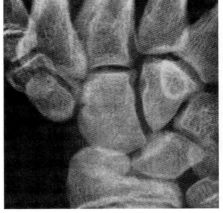

a

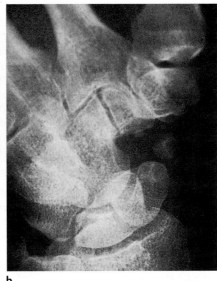

b

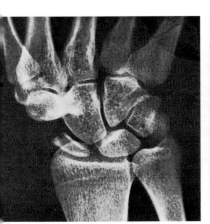

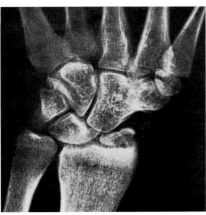

d

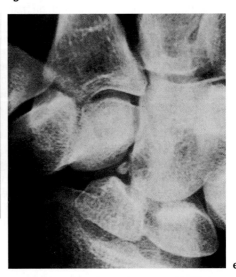

e

c, d Small hypoplastic scaphoid in each wrist. Bilateral hypoplastic scaphoids most likely occur in association with a more
complex anomaly or as an extreme variant. Additionally, the
trapezoids and capitates are fused, and the metacarpal bones
are markedly hypoplastic on both sides.
e Hypoplastic scaphoid with an adjacent os centrale.

Some authors use the term "partial aplasia" for a hypoplastic scaphoid in the belief that the bone developed from
dual centers. This may or may not be correct, and we feel
that it cannot be proved in any given case. It is conceivable
that hypoplastic scaphoids or their complete absence can
significantly alter the biomechanics of the carpus in some
cases. A **duplication** of the scaphoid is extremely rare (s.
also Fig. 2.**153**, p. 122). Trevor's disease should not be confused with the various forms of scaphoid bipartition and
other normal variants like duplication (see also p. 123).

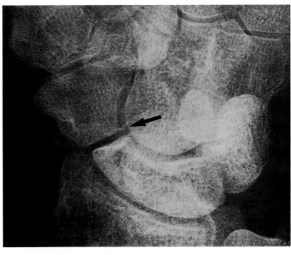

Fig. 2.**215**   Unusual fusion of the scaphoid and lunate with a ▷
posttraumatic nonunion (arrow) of the composite bone at the
junction of its middle and distal thirds.

Fracture or Dislocation?

Scaphoid fractures are among the most common carpal injuries. They are primarily an injury of young males. The ratio of scaphoid fractures to distal radial fractures is approximately 1 : 10.

Scaphoid fractures have two features that distinguish them from other carpal bone fractures (except the hamate):

- A high incidence of nonunion
- A high incidence of ischemic necrosis

This relates partly to the vascular supply of the scaphoid: the intraosseous blood supply diminishes toward the proximal end of the bone, whereas the distal and central portions of the bone each receive an adequate supply from one palmar and one dorsal branch of the radial artery. It is important to note that no anastomoses exist between the two vascular territories.

Scaphoid fractures are missed on radiographs with some frequency, especially when they are nondisplaced, impacted, or both. This is due in part to the physiological palmar tilt of the scaphoid, which means that the standard projection does not completely visualize the bone. Thus, whenever there is the slightest suspicion of a scaphoid fracture (tenderness in the anatomic snuffbox, pain on axial thumb compression, painful limitation of motion on radial deviation and extension of the wrist), an additional Stecher-view to the standard projection (PA, lateral radiographs) should be obtained to correct for the physiological palmar tilt and project the bone with its longitudinal axis parallel to the film plane. The so called "four view scaphoid" bears no advantages! If plain films are negative, we recommend the early use of CT, which can also demonstrate injury to other carpal bones (capitate, hamate, triquetrum, lunate, pisiform) and provide nonsuperimposed views showing any malalignment, dislocations, or subluxations of the bones. This particularly applies to the most frequent combined injury, the transscaphoid–perilunate fracture-dislocation of de Quervain. If the proper facilities are available, **bone scans** can also be obtained on the fourth day after the injury. The scans are usually positive if a fracture has occurred. A negative bone scan on the fourth day postinjury excludes a scaphoid fracture. **MRI** can also detect early scaphoid injuries, and spin-echo sequences are particularly useful for defining the fracture line (signal void) and associated soft-tissue injuries (Fig. 2.**223**).

It cannot be emphasized too strongly that the suspicion of a scaphoid fracture warrants an aggressive diagnosis due to the relatively high complication rates of undetected fractures (nonunion, necrosis). In litigations and disability assessments, it is common for attorneys to ask why an effective method was not used to diagnose the fracture promptly and institute appropriate treatment (reduction and immobilization) to protect the patient from serious sequelae.

We cannot explore all the problems that pertain to scaphoid fractures and refer the reader to the excellent monographs by Schmitt and Lanz (1996) and Gilula and Yin (1996). We limit our present discussion to the differentiation of scaphoid fractures from complete and incomplete bipartition, accessory bone elements, and other fracture-mimicking conditions.

A basic distinction is drawn among oblique, transverse, and vertical-oblique fractures of the scaphoid bone. The frequency distribution of fracture levels (distal, middle, and proximal third) is shown in Fig. 2.**216**.

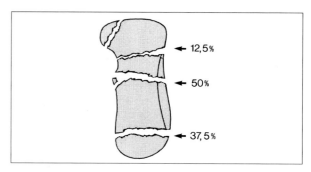

Fig. 2.**216**   Frequency distribution of typical scaphoid fractures.

Schmitt and Lanz (1996) report a similar distribution:

- Fracture of the scaphoid tubercle (extra-articular): 10% (Figs. 2.**222**, 2.**224**, 2.**225**)
- Fracture of the distal third of the scaphoid: 15%
- Fracture of the middle third of the scaphoid: 60% (Fig. 2.**221**)
- Fracture of the proximal third of the scaphoid: 15%

Evaluation of the **scaphoid (navicular) fat stripe** (Fig. 2.**217**) can be useful on conventional radiographs, especially for understanding later heterotopic bone formation in that area. The SFS (NFS) is a layer of fat approximately 1 mm thick, ulnarly convex, that runs between the radial collateral ligament of the wrist and the extensor pollicis brevis tendon. With fractures of the scaphoid (and of the radial styloid process, trapezium, and first metacarpal base; Lorenz and Fiedler 1982), a fracture-associated hematoma causes the fine lucent stripe to acquire a linear or radially convex shape. In Fig. 2.**235b**, which shows a basal fracture of the first metacarpal, the radial convexity of the SFS is apparently caused by the proximal extension of a hematoma from injured soft tissues. The solid cancellous bone in Fig. 2.**235a** results from heterotopic ossification that occurred later in the area of the hematoma.

Nutrient canals may be plainly visible in the scaphoid, especially on radiographs of high technical quality (Fig. 2.**218**). They require differentiation from fracture lines in trauma patients when corresponding clinical signs are present (Fig. 2.**221**).

Radionuclide bone scans obtained 4 days after the injury are excellent for making this differentiation. Partial bipartition of the scaphoid also requires differentiation from a fracture (Figs. 2.**219**, 2.**220**).

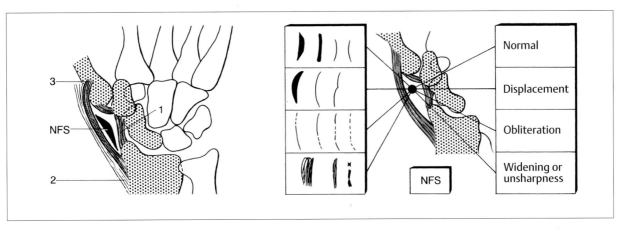

Fig. 2.**217 a, b**   Anatomy of the navicular (scaphoid) fat stripe (NFS).

a Anatomy of the NFS region.
1   Radial collateral ligament
2   Abductor pollicis longus tendon
3   Extensor pollicis brevis tendon

b Normal and pathological anatomy of the NFS (after Lorenz).

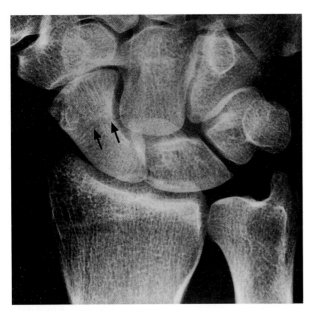

Fig. 2.**218**   Fracture-mimicking nutrient canal in the scaphoid (arrows) in the presence of a tubercle fracture.

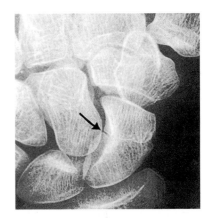

Fig. 2.**219**   Partially bipartite scaphoid (arrow).

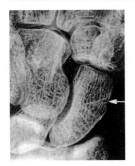

Fig. 2.**220**   Partially bipartite scaphoid (arrow).

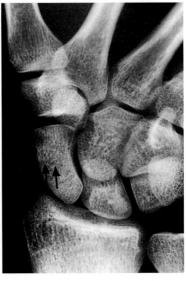

Fig. 2.**221**   Fresh scaphoid fracture (arrows) at a typical location (not a nutrient canal).

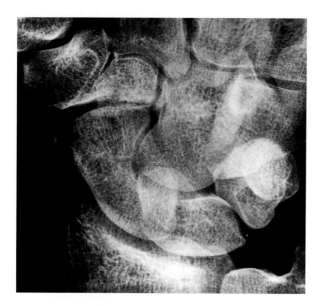

Fig. 2.**222**   Fresh fracture of the scaphoid tubercle.

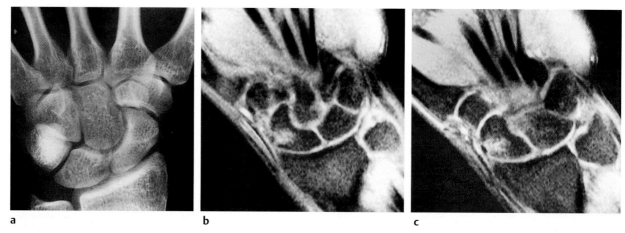

a   b   c

Fig. 2.**223 a–c**   Scaphoid contusion, marked clinically by severe pain in the anatomic snuffbox.
a Conventional radiograhshows no fracture or other apparent structural changes.

b, c T2-weighted MR images show an elliptical area of increased signal intensity at the center of the scaphoid, representing edema. A fracture is not visible.

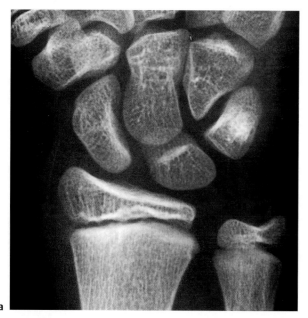

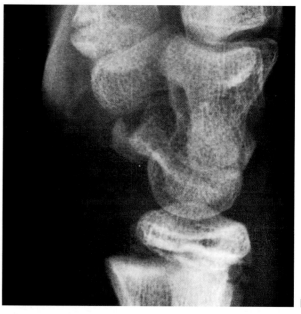

a   b

Fig. 2.**224 a, b**   Unusual avulsion fracture of the scaphoid tubercle combined with a traumatic fracture-separation of the distal radial epiphysis. A small accessory ossification center is

seen distal to the ulnar styloid process. Follow-up see Fig. 2.**225**. (Case from Dr. Schäfer, Oberhausen.)

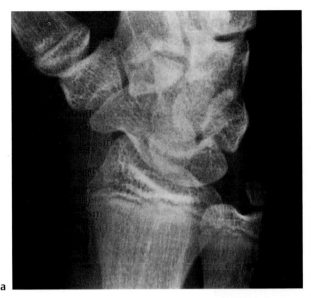

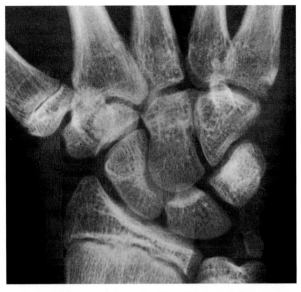

a

b

Fig. 2.**225 a, b**   Films of the case in Fig. 2.**224**, three years later. The prominent scaphoid tubercle in **a** results from a partially healed avulsion fracture. The accessory center of the ulnar styloid process shows marked and "harmonious" enlarge-

ment, suggesting that the earlier film (Fig. 2.**224**) did not portray an avulsed styloid tip (see also Fig. 2.**279**). (Case from Dr. Schäfer, Oberhausen.)

Unfused ossification centers (e.g., Fig. 2.**226**) and the os centrale should be differentiated from avulsion fractures of a bone in this region (gap between the scaphoid, trapezium, and capitate).

Pfitzner (1885) found an **os centrale carpi** in 1% of his autopsy material. This accessory ossicle is usually round, relatively dense, and lacks an internal trabecular structure (Figs. 2.**227**–2.**231**). It is located in the dorsal aspect of the space between scaphoid, capitate and trapezoidal bones.

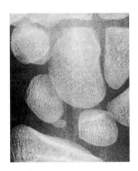

Fig. 2.**226**

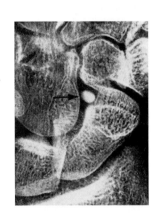

Fig. 2.**227**

Fig. 2.**226**   Ossification center at the proximal pole of the scaphoid (10-year-old boy).

Fig. 2.**227**   Os centrale (arrow).

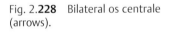

Fig. 2.**228**   Bilateral os centrale (arrows).

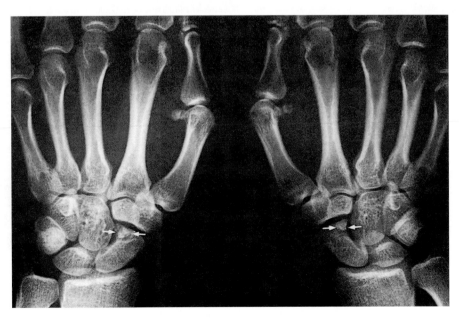

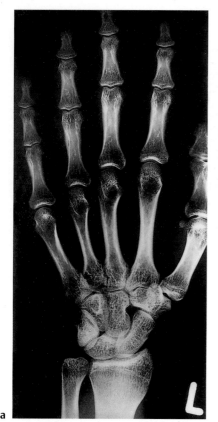

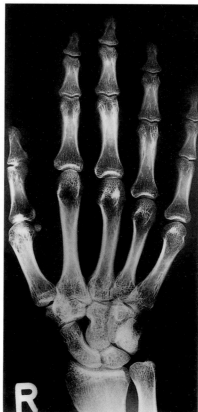

a

b

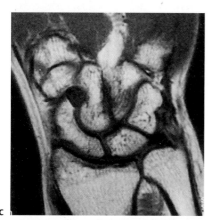

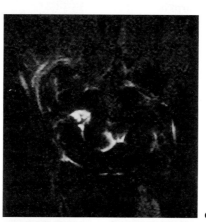

c

d

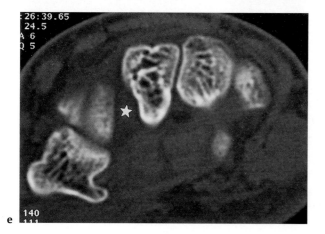

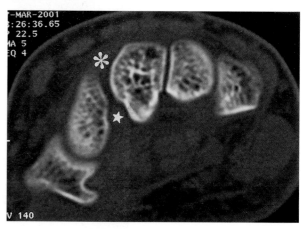

e

f

Fig. 2.**229** For the differential diagnosis of a radiographically occult carpal os centrale (see text). The unusually large gap between the distal scaphoid and a notch in the capitate contains only synovial structures and no cartilaginous anlage for an os centrale (see MR image in **d**). The gap is explained by the relative positions of the scaphoid and capitate, as the CT scans in **e** and **f** demonstrate (asterisks = gap between scaphoid and capitate; rosette in f = usual location of an os centrale). (Case courtesy of Dr. Marschall, Bremen.)

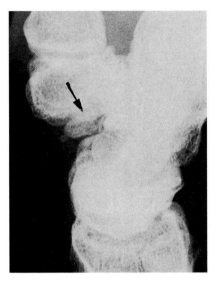

Fig. 2.**230**   Os centrale (arrow) shown in a lateral radiograph.

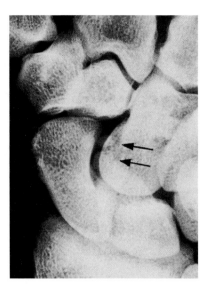

Fig. 2.**231**   Duplication of the os centrale (arrows).

A very dense os centrale may signify necrosis or a necrotic fragment, especially when clinical symptoms are present (bone scan, MRI [Abascal et al. 2001]). The os centrale may be overlapped by the capitate bone and therefore difficult to discern (Fig. 2.**231**). It may be present bilaterally (Fig. 2.**228**) and may be duplicated on one side (Fig. 2.**231**). According to Gerscovich et al. (1990) and Abascal et al. (2001), the os centrale carpi may also occur as an incompletely separated bony element with smooth contours or may be present as a radiographically empty space in the area of its usual appearance, if the cartilage anlage is not ossified. The latter situation may be simulated by an extreme "gap" between the distal scaphoid and a groove in the opposite capitatum (Fig. 2.**229**). According to Poznanski, the os centrale occurs with greater frequency in malformation syndromes. Bony fusion of the os centrale with

the scaphoid, capitate, or trapezium is occasionally observed. Poznanski found this pattern in 5 of 23 patients with Holt–Oram syndrome.

It is not important to differentiate an os centrale from an asymmetric bipartite scaphoid or from a scaphoid with an unfused accessory ossification center.

Fractures of the scaphoid tubercle (Fig. 2.**232**) mainly require differentiation from another accessory bone element, the **os radiale externum** (Figs. 2.**150**, 2.**233**, 2.**234**).

Another accessory bone that can mimic a tubercle avulsion fracture is the **epitrapezium** (Figs. 2.**150**, 2.**234**). Heterotopic bone formation as a sequel to trauma was noted above. The bony element seen in Fig. 2.**235**, though a product of heterotopic bone formation, could just as well represent a laterally displaced os radiale externum.

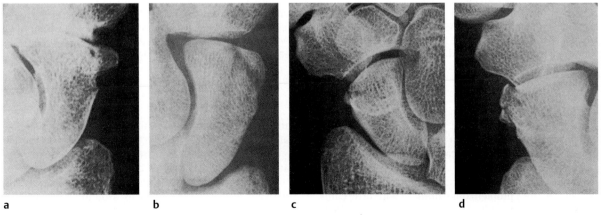

a   b   c   d

Fig. 2.**232 a–d**   Tubercle avulsion fractures (compare with Figs. 2.**222** and 2.**224**).

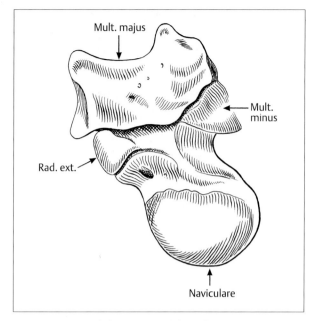

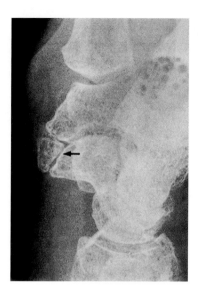

Fig. 2.**233**   Os radiale externum (after Pfitzner).

Fig. 2.**234**   Large epitrapezium or os radiale externum (arrow).

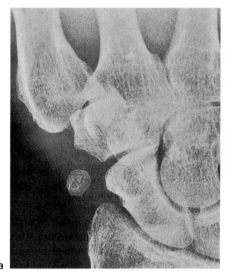

a

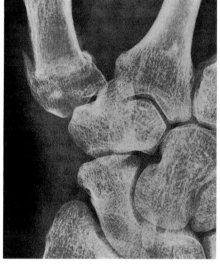

b

Fig. 2.**235 a, b**   Development of an "accessory" bony element, consisting of well-structured cancellous bone with a thin cortical shell located on the radial side adjacent to the space between the scaphoid and trapezium. The element could also represent an os radiale externum located in an unusual distance from the scaphoid. This bony element is not visible on a radiograph taken 17 years earlier (**b**), but we do see

a fracture at the base of the first metacarpal with displacement and unsharpness of the navicular fat stripe as a sign of concomitant hemorrhage and/or edema in that region. The bony element in **a** represents a focus of metaplastic (heterotopic) bone formation that developed gradually over a period of years (compare this case with Fig. 2.**87j, k**).

Finally there are dystrophic calcifications in tendon sheaths, which usually have an amorphous, stippled appearance on radiographs and can mimic small avulsions and accessory elements.

Differentiating a scaphoid nonunion from a bipartite scaphoid is really a problem only for those with little clinical or radiological experience. A **nonunion** always shows reactive changes in the cancellous bone under the bony cap, which appear as irregular structural densities along with tiny, usually cystic lucencies (resorption cysts, Figs. 2.**236**, 2.**237**). A partially consolidated scaphoid fracture (Fig. 2.**238**) may show similarities to a rudimentary bipartition.

Differentiation in these cases is generally aided by the patient's history. If a precise differential diagnosis is required for legal reasons, CT should be used to define the relatively fine structural changes around the nonunion. Scaphoid fractures in children are extremely difficult to diagnose. They are rarely detectable on conventional radiographs before 7 or 8 years of age (Gambel and Simmons 1982, Greene et al. 1984).

Necrosis?

We have mentioned the susceptibility of the injured scaphoid to osteonecrotic changes. Radiologically incipient necrosis is manifested by a slight increase in the density of the necrotic area. This occurs because the adjacent bone becomes demineralized due to inactivity or perifocal edema, but the necrotic area is not affected by this demineralization due to its lack of perfusion. In general, a necrotic area is not subject to physiological bone remodeling during the initial stage, resulting in a density contrast that occasionally involves a decrease of density within the necrotic area. Later stages are marked by the appearance of small, closely adjacent lucencies alternating with sclerosis, subchondral fracturing, and eventual fragmentation. Spontaneous repair is possible only before the fragmentation stage.

From the pathological-anatomic view, very early stages of scaphoid necrosis or partial necrosis are extremely difficult to detect on conventional radiographic films, and therefore MRI should be used when clinical suspicion exists. Both dynamic MRI and radionuclide scanning are useful for defining residual perfusion or reperfusion. Varying degrees of bone-fragment necrosis are shown in Figs. 2.**239**–2.**243**. Scaphoid nonunion in the fragmentation stage requires differentiation from fragmentary ossification in cretinism and other disturbances of enchondral ossification.

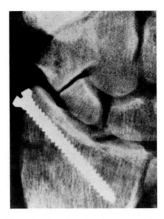

Fig. 2.**236** Bipartite scaphoid (not a fracture). The anomaly was detected incidentally on the radiograph of a distal radial fracture, which was stabilized with an internal fixation screw.

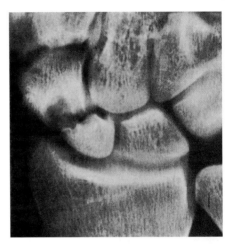

Fig. 2.**237** Typical scaphoid nonunion.

Fig. 2.**238 a, b** Incomplete union of a scaphoid fracture, leaving an unconsolidated gap filled with connective tissue. This condition is also termed a fibrous scaphoid nonunion.

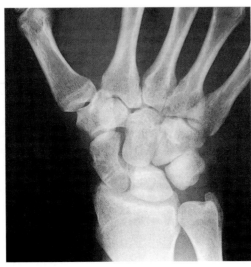

a

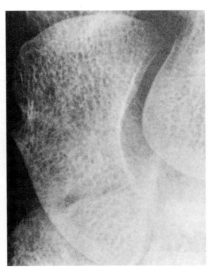

b

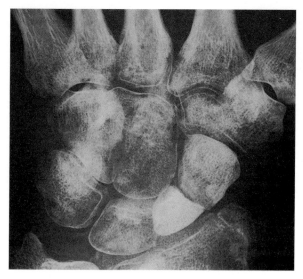

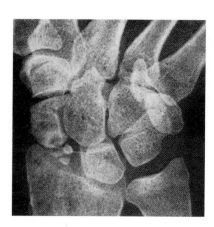

Fig. 2.**239 a, b**   Nonfragmented scaphoid necrosis. The proximal fragment in a scaphoid nonunion appears snowy white, contrasting sharply with the patchy demineralization in the surrounding bones. The patient had clinical manifestations of Sudeck dystrophy.

Fig. 2.**240**   Fragmentation of the proximal scaphoid fragment due to osteonecrosis.

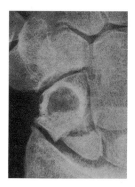

Fig. 2.**241**   Significant trophic disturbance in a distal scaphoid fragment (relatively white bone). The central cavity represents a large area of resorption.

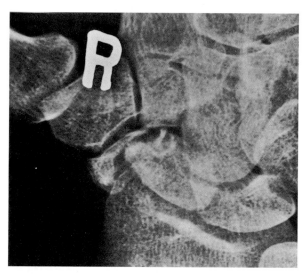

Fig. 2.**242**   Nonunion of a peripheral scaphoid fracture. Note the tilted peripheral fragment and the resorptive processes surrounding the nonunion.

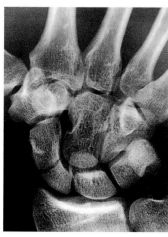

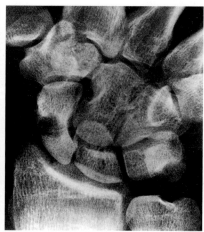

Fig. 2.**243 a, b**   Development of a scaphoid nonunion.
a Nondisplaced scaphoid fracture, seven days postinjury.
b Film seven months later shows massive resorptive processes with the development of a large cavity between the fragments. In most cases, continued mechanical stresses on the wrist will eventually displace the fragments as shown in Fig. 2.**237**.

a   b

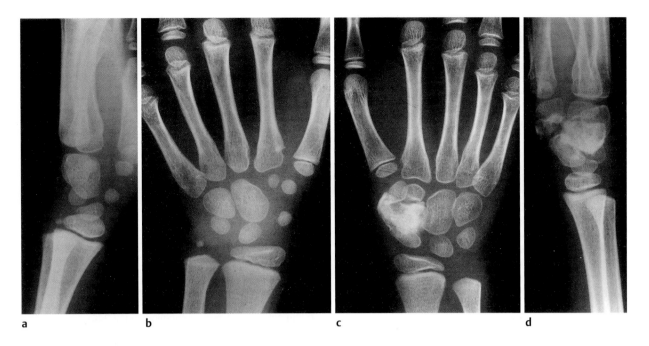

a   b   c   d

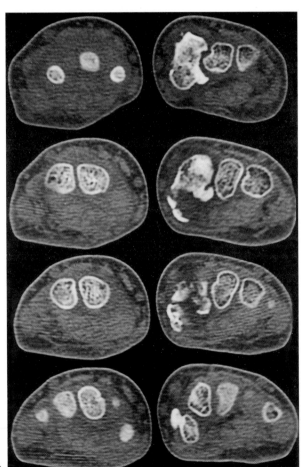

e

Fig. 2.**244 a–e**   Trevor's disease of the scaphoid in a 9-year-old girl, who suffered from pain while writing (see also Fig. 2.**154**). (Case courtesy of Dr. Plischewsky, Weserstede.)

Inflammation?

The differentiation of inflammatory erosions from physiological lucent zones in the scaphoid was mentioned above under Normal Findings. Scaphoid involvement is generally a feature of carpal inflammatory processes (bacterial carpal arthritis, rheumatoid arthritis, etc.).

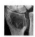 **Tumor?**

The most frequent causes of osteolytic changes in the scaphoid are cystic lesions, especially subchondral synovial cysts or intraosseous ganglions (Fig. 2.**246**). Idiopathic cysts are less common (Fig. 2.**245**).

Other causes of osteolytic changes are cystic lucencies resulting from β_2-microglobulin deposits (Fig. 2.**76**). The initial stages may present with very fine lucencies, which often can be seen only on magnification radiographs or by using mammographic technique and viewing the films with a magnifier. These lucencies are extremely difficult to

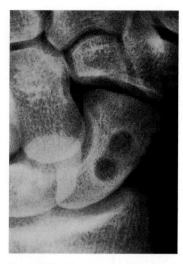

Fig. 2.**245** Two large, idiopathic cysts detected incidentally in the scaphoid of an otherwise healthy patient. CT or MRI should exclude a connection with surrounding structures, ruling out an intraosseous ganglion (Fig. 2.**246**).

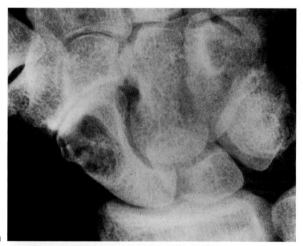

a

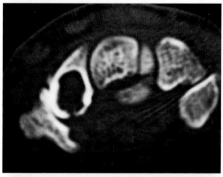

b

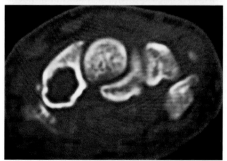

c

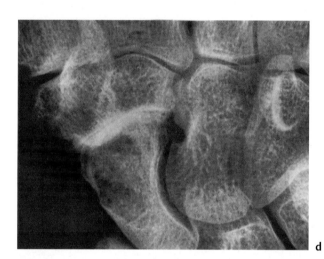

d

Fig. 2.**246 a–d** Large intraosseous ganglion in the scaphoid. The patient presented clinically with severe pain. Radiographs show significant osteoarthritis between the scaphoid, trapezium, and trapezoid bones. Apparently this osteoarthritis is unrelated to the development of the ganglion cyst, since the immediate subchondral portions of the scaphoid appear normal. Radiograph **d** was taken after cancellous bone grafting.

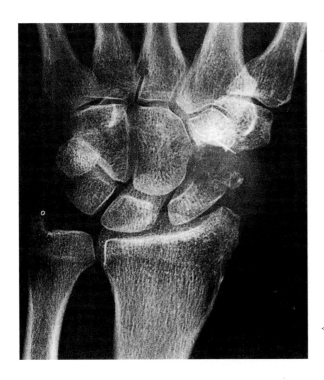

distinguish from idiopathic hand cysts, which probably are small circumscribed necrotic areas resulting from high mechanical stresses on the hand (Fig. 2.245).

In adults, osteolytic changes in the scaphoid may also result from acral metastases (e.g., due to bronchial carcinoma) (Fig. 2.247).

In adolescents, destructive changes in the scaphoid should raise immediate suspicion of osteoid osteoma. The case shown in Fig. 2.248 illustrates the spread of a "sympathetic" carpal arthritis.

Proliferative changes in the scaphoid are more often a result of Trevor's disease (Fig. 2.154, 2.244) than a true osteochondroma. The scaphoid is among the sites of predilection for involvement by Trevor disease in the upper extremity.

◁ Fig. 2.**247**   Gross destructive changes in the distal and central scaphoid caused by an acral metastasis from renal cell carcinoma.

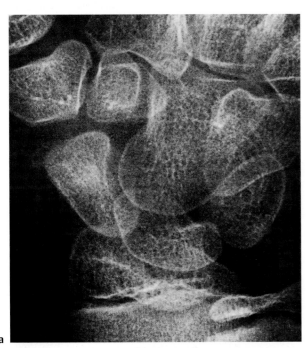

a

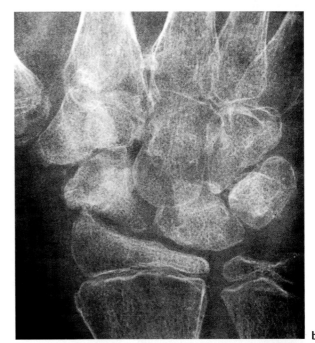

b

Fig. 2.**248 a–c**   Osteoid osteoma in the scaphoid of a 12-year-old child with a long history of complaints.

a The initial radiograph shows blurring of the trabecular pattern in the area of the scaphoid tubercle and fine calcification of the tumor matrix extending past the tubercle into the soft tissues.

b Radiograph eight months later shows dramatic progression of the changes. The distal portions of the scaphoid show patchy marginal sclerosis next to a large osteolytic process. All the carpal bones show subchondral plate irregularities due to a severe sympathetic carpal arthritis (compare with Figs. 2.**154** and 2.**244**).

c CT scans clearly demonstrate the extensive proliferative scaphoid changes. The heavily calcified nidus (arrows) forms a nodular mass projecting from the bone.

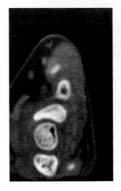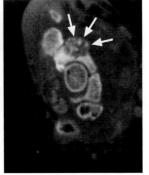

c

Lunate

Normal Findings

During Growth

The ossification center of the lunate bone is visible on radiographs after about 3–4 years of age. Double ossification centers may be observed (Fig. 2.**249**).

Duplication of the centers, known also as a bipartite lunate, may be unilateral or bilateral. Mordeja (1962) described the combination of a bipartite lunate bone with multicentric pisiform centers. The small ossification center palmar to the lunate in Fig. 2.**250** is not part of a double lunate center; it is the small ossification center of the scaphoid, which appears up to two years later than the lunate center and is therefore smaller.

> A central density in the lunate ossification center (Fig. 2.**251**) has no pathological significance. It is a normal finding and is not even considered a variant.

In children, small notches may be observed on the dorsal surface of the lunate (Fig. 2.**252**). They are a result of irregular ossification, much as in the scaphoid bone.

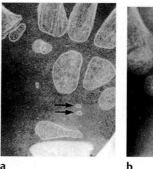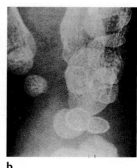

a   b

Fig. 2.**249a, b** Physiological duplication of the lunate ossification centers.

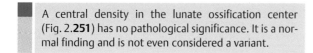

In Adulthood

Small "punched-out" lucencies in the lunate represent end-on projections of nutrient canals (Fig. 2.**253**).

The shape of the lunate is subject to little variation in adults. Its geometric configuration is best appreciated on CT scans (Fig. 2.**143**). A small distal process curves around the capitate on the palmar side, accounting for the overlap of these two bones in the PA radiograph.

When evaluating the lunate, especially in clinically symptomatic patients, the radiologist should particularly note its density in relation to the neighboring bones, since radiographically early osteonecrosis is manifested on plain films by a general or partial increase in the density of the bone compared with adjacent bones (see below).

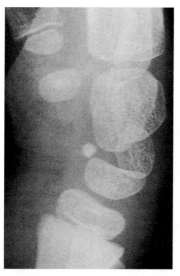 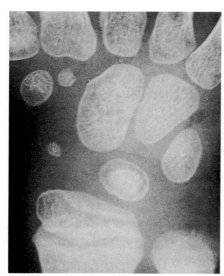 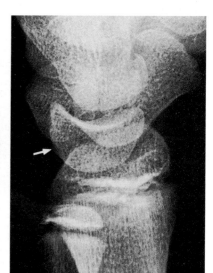

Fig. 2.**250**   Fig. 2.**251**   Fig. 2.**252**

Fig. 2.**250** What appears to be an accessory bone adjacent to the lunate is actually the ossification center of the scaphoid bone.

Fig. 2.**251** Physiological central density in the ossification center of the lunate. Occasionally this density is mimicked by a superimposed double ossification center on the palmar or dorsal side.

Fig. 2.**252** Small physiological notch in the dorsal surface of the lunate.

▌*Pathological Finding?*

Normal Variant or Anomaly?

It is relatively common to find the lunate fused with neighboring bones. The most frequent carpal coalition is lunotriquetral fusion (Fig. 2.**254a–c**).

Arens (1950) observed four cases of lunotriquetral fusion (coalition) in 5000 radiographs of the wrist. There are numerous variations, including distal and proximal fusions and complete and incomplete fusions (see also p. 122). An association with Madelung deformity is known (see also p. 124).

It is important to distinguish between an incomplete congenital fusion (coalition) and an acquired fusion (ankylosis) due for example to a previous inflammatory joint condition. Generally the history is helpful in making this differentiation. With a negative history, a confident radiographic differentiation cannot be made and is probably of no real consequence.

Becker (1935) and Girod (1964) described an unusual coalition between the lunate and radius with an underdeveloped scaphoid.

An anatomic variant consists of **an separate articulation between the hamate bone and the lunate bone** (socalled type II lunate bone, Viegas et al. 1990). This variant leads to a higher prevalence of chondromalacia of the proximal pole of the hamate bone than in wrists without

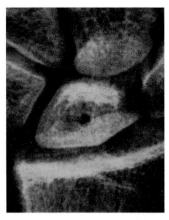

Fig. 2.**253**   Nutrient canal in the lunate.

this articulation (type I lunate bone) (Viegas et al. 1990, Sagerman et al. 1995). The suggested mechanism for the development of the chondromalacia is a repeated impingement and abrasion of the two bones, when the wrist is used in full ulnar deviation. (**hamatolunate impaction syndrome**) (Thurston et Stanley, 2000; Nakamura et al. 2000; Cerezal et al. 2002). Clinically patients suffer from ulnar-sided wrist pain, the imaging method of choice is MR (Fig. 2.**254d**). Early findings in plain film are subchondral lucencies within the proximal pole of the hamate, that faces the hamate facet of the lunate.

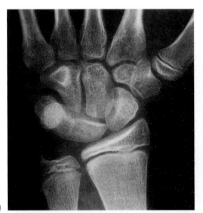

a

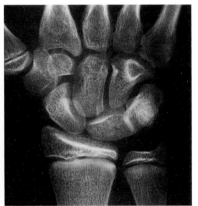

b

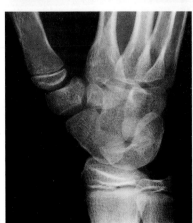

c

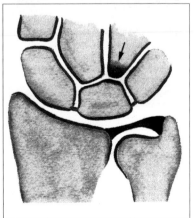

d

Fig. 2.**254a–c**   Bilateral lunotriquetral coalition. (Case courtesy of CA Dr. Schäfer, Obenhausen.)

Fig. 2.**254d**   Diagram of Viegas type II lunate with hamatolunate impaction syndrome (chondromalacia of the proximal pole of the hamate, subchondral sclerosis, and marrow edema) (After Cerezal et al. 2002)

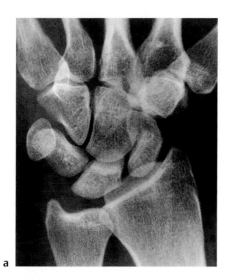

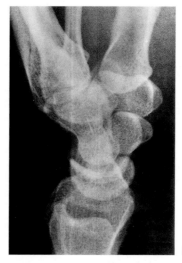

Fig. 2.**255 a–f** Fractures of the lunate.
a–d Complete vertical fractures of the lunate. **a,b** Invisible in the projection radiographs. Note the Mach-band in the scaphoid in **b**.
e, f Transverse lunate fracture several months old with incipient signs of nonunion (not an os hypolunatum). Note the widening of the space between the lunate and scaphoid as a result of scapholunate dissociation.

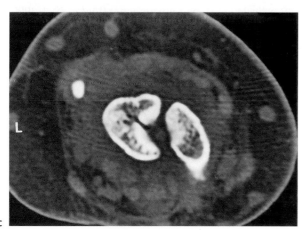

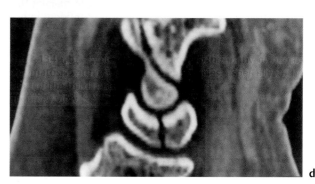

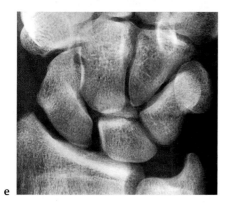

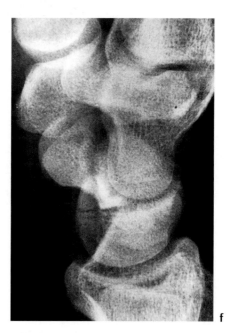

Fracture or Dislocation?

Severe axial trauma to the wrist can cause an isolated compression fracture of the lunate bone. Horizontal and vertical fracture patterns are less common, but avulsion fractures of the anterior or posterior horn combined with other carpal injuries are often caused by a fall onto the hyperextended or hyperflexed hand. Nondisplaced fractures are difficult to diagnose on conventional radiographs, and CT is superior for this purpose (Fig. 2.**255 a–d**). It can be difficult to distinguish the distal fragment of a transverse lunate fracture (Fig. 2.**255 e, f**) from an **os hypolunatum** (Fig. 2.**256**), especially in the case of a nonunion as shown in Fig. 2.**255 e, f**.

Radionuclide scanning can advance this differential diagnosis, since an accessory bone element like the os hypolunatum will yield a negative scan unless regressive changes have developed between the two elements. Morphological variants of the os hypolunatum are shown in

Figs. 2.**256** and 2.**257**. The case in Fig. 2.**257** is unusual in that the presence of a hypolunatum is combined with fusion of the scaphoid and trapezium.

Another accessory bone element requiring differentiation from an avulsion fracture (especially from a legal standpoint) is the **os epilunatum**, which usually appears as a rounded bony shadow at the dorsal horn of the lunate with flattening of the apposing bony margins (Fig. 2.**258**, 2.**259**).

Accessory bone elements should also be distinguished from necrotic fragments (Fig. 2.**267 c**) and from dystrophic calcifications in tendons, tendon sheaths, and bursae (Figs. 2.**261**, 2.**262**). No doubt there are even more accessory bone elements that have not yet been formally described (e.g., Figs. 2.**260** and 2.**263**) and that are probably clinically irrelevant. These elements have no importance when detected incidentally but should be distinguished from very small bony avulsions when found in trauma patients.

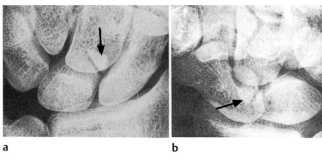

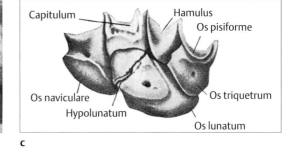

Capitulum
Hamulus
Os pisiforme
Os naviculare
Hypolunatum
Os triquetrum
Os lunatum

a b c

Fig. 2.**256 a–c**   Os hypolunatum as an accessory bone (arrows).

Fig. 2.**257 a, b**   Os hypolunatum in a carpus with a preexisting coalition between the scaphoid and trapezium. Without the coalition and bilateral findings, the accessory bone might well be interpreted as part of a nonunion owing to its precise "fit" with the lunate!

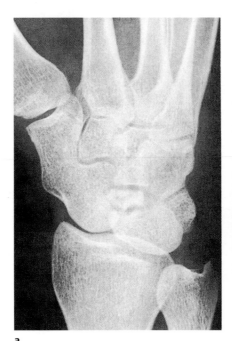

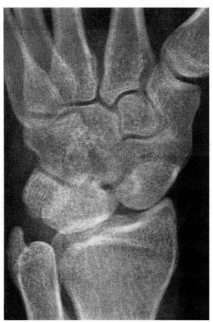

a b

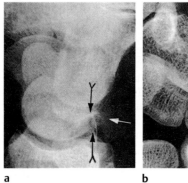
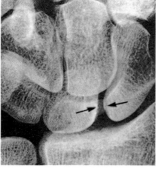

We cannot delve further into the complex subject of perilunar and lunar dislocations (Fig. 2.**264**). It may be noted, however, that this type of injury has been very accurately researched and defined and that excellent classifications can be found in the current literature (e.g., Schmitt and Lanz 1996).

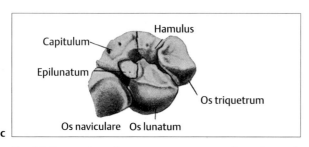

Fig. 2.**258 a–c**   Os epilunatum as an accessory bone (arrows).

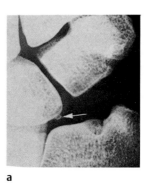
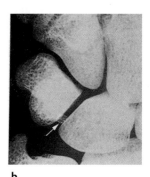

Fig. 2.**260 a, b**   Small, asymptomatic bony element of indeterminate origin (UBE, arrows).

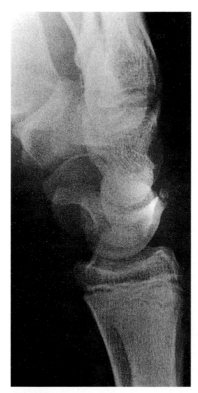

Fig. 2.**259**   Small accessory bone element in the area where the os epilunatum is normally projected. Differential diagnosis includes a still-unfused accessory ossification center of the lunate. The bony element was detected incidentally, so there was no follow-up.

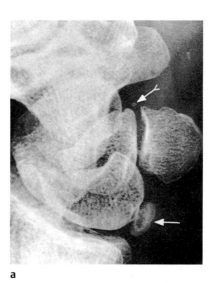
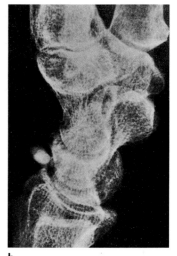

Fig. 2.**261 a, b**   Asymptomatic "accessory" bony elements palmar and dorsal to the lunate.
a Both bony elements may represent nonspecific regressive calcifications, capsular osteomas, etc. (arrows).
b The density and scant trabecular structure of the element in this film are more consistent with a dystrophic calcification or possibly a necrotic accessory bone. This is pure speculation, however, since in both cases the patients were free of clinical symptoms.

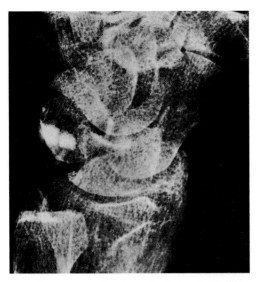

Fig. 2.**262** Dystrophic bursal calcifications dorsal to the lunate.

Fig. 2.**263** Unknown bony element (UBE) not associated with clinical symptoms (arrow).

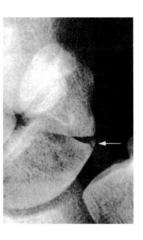

Fig. 2.**264a, b** Stage IV perilunar dislocation with palmar dislocation of the lunate bone. The other carpal bones have retained an essentially normal alignment.

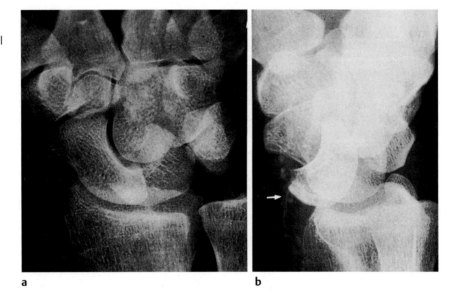

a   b

 Necrosis?

Necrosis of the lunate (formerly known as lunatomalacia or Kienböck disease) is one of the most common forms of osteonecrosis after avascular necrosis of the femoral head, osteochondritis dissecans, and bone-marrow infarction.

> Lunate necrosis in the borderline range between normal and pathological poses a great challenge to the diagnostician.

The predisposition of the lunate to avascular necrosis is based on the anatomic circumstance that, in 20% of the population, the bone has a palmar blood supply (from the ulnar and anterior interosseous arteries) but lacks a dorsal blood supply (from the radial artery). Thus the lunate has an end-arterial blood supply that cannot be replaced by collateral flow. If the wrist is subjected to chronic recurring microtrauma (e.g., pneumatic drilling) or even a single, more severe trauma, it is easy to see how vascular occlusions (primary occlusions due to a micro- or macrofracture, secondary occlusions due to intraosseous hemorrhage and edema) can interrupt the blood supply to the bone. Constitutional **negative ulnar variance** may be another predisposing factor, but this is controversial (Nakamura et al. 1991a, b). Negative ulnar variance means that the distal radius extends more than 2 mm beyond the distal ulnar surface, resulting in increased pressure on the lunate bone. It has been suggested that the less common positive ulnar variance can also contribute to lunate necrosis (probably due to ulnar impaction, see below). Other mechanisms such as Madelung deformity, a high radial ridge, and damage to the triangular fibrocartilage complex have also been suggested as having causal significance. "Idiopathic" lunate necrosis may relate to more or less latent endocrinological, metabolic, and neural disturbances.

Lunate necrosis occurs most commonly in males between 20 and 40 years of age. The initial symptoms are mild pain when using the wrist and limitation of motion. The dominant clinical sign is dorsal wrist tenderness. Since the onset of clinical symptoms is often quite delayed, very little is known about the early radiological manifestations of lunate necrosis. Conventional radiographs suggest the diagnosis only after initial subtle osteosclerotic changes appear, accompanied by a slight blurring of the trabecular pattern (Fig. 2.**265a**). MRI is of course positive at this stage, showing a signal void on T1-weighted images and increased signal intensity on T2-weighted images as a result of edema.

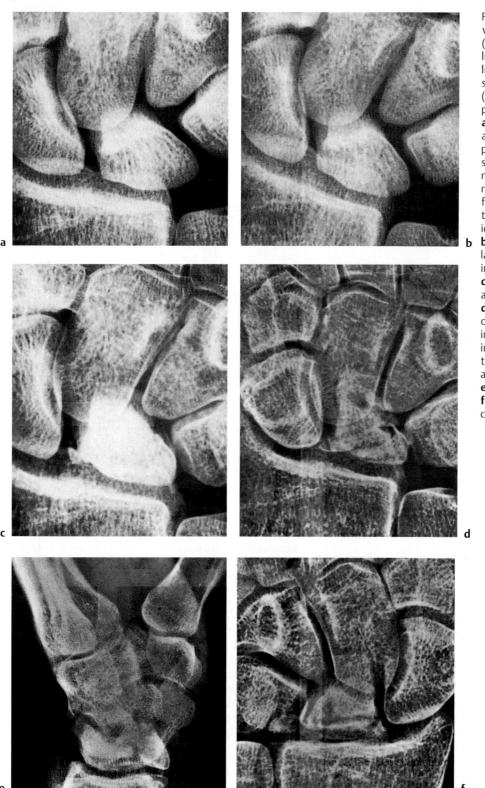

Fig. 2.**265a–f**   Serial observation of lunate necrosis (with concomitant scapholunate dissociation). Since lunate necrosis was also present on the opposite side (**f**), the necrosis may be idiopathic.

a This film, taken one hour after a minor injury, shows poorly defined trabecular structures of the lunate as a manifestation of reactive-reparative sclerosis. This finding is unrelated to the trauma and reflects previous idiopathic lunate necrosis.

b Radiograph one month later shows a slight increase in the osteosclerosis.

c Further density increase and incipient fragmentation.

d Complete fragmentation of the necrotic lunate. One indication of carpal shortening is the decreased distance between the capitate and radius.

e Lateral aspect of **d**

f Lunate necrosis in the contralateral wrist.

Radiographic stages of lunate necrosis described by Decoulx et al. (1957) and Lichtman et al. (1977)	
Stage I	Diffuse osteosclerosis with loss of normal trabecular markings and no alteration of bone shape
Stage II	Cystic lucencies along with patchy sclerosis and no alteration of bone shape
Stage IIIa	Proximal fragmentation with some deformation of the bone
Stage IIIb	Proximal fragmentation with increasing deformation and increased tilting of the scaphoid (Fig. 2.**265 d**)
Stage IV	Greatly increased density of the collapsed lunate bone with degenerative changes in the adjacent joints

The individual stages in the progression of lunate necrosis are illustrated in Fig. 2.**265**.

Figure 2.**266 a–d** shows that the process can be reversible, with a regression from stage IIIa to stage I or even to normal.

Dynamic MRI with gadolinium enhancement yields excellent information on the stage of disease progression. Thus, homogeneous signal enhancement indicates the presence of an edematous stage, patchy nonhomogeneous enhancement indicates partial necrosis, and the absence of enhancement signifies complete necrosis. A three-phase radionuclide bone scan also provides information on perfusion status. With very early necrosis, perfusion is reduced and tracer uptake on delayed scans is less than in the other carpal bones. This stage is very rarely encountered, however. In the majority of cases, lunate uptake is in-

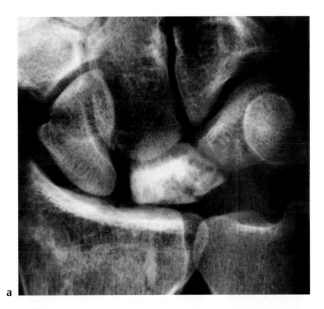

a

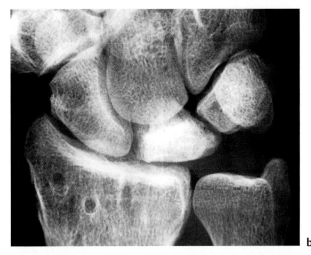

b

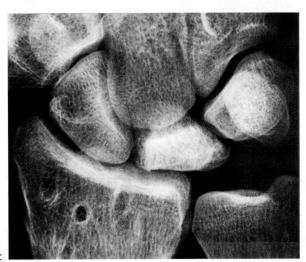

c

d

Fig. 2.**266 a–f**   Regression or repair of lunate necrosis.
a Film showing incipient fragmentation of the necrotic lunate was taken to evaluate a radial fracture. The patient (a manual laborer) had apparently been asymptomatic prior to that time. The radial fracture was treated by internal fixation, with shortening of the ulna.

b Film three years later shows increasing, uniform sclerosis of the osseous structures, which are more sharply defined. No further fragmentation is evident.
c After another three years, the lunate appears almost normal aside from a slight increase in density and straightening of the proximal margin.
d Four years later, the lunate displays an almost normal trabecular structure.

Fig. 2.**266 e, f** ▷

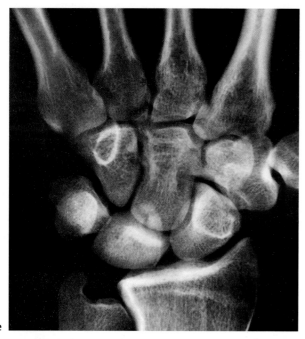

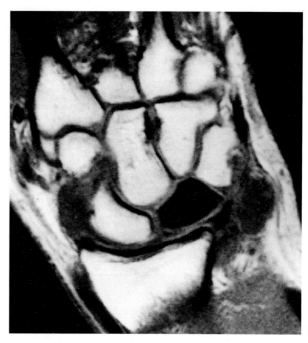

e

f

Fig. 2.**266 e, f**   Lunate necrosis with distal fragmentation in a 34-year-old physician. The main body of the lunate shows slight but definite sclerosis. MRI (**f**) shows a complete fat signal void in the lunate. Note chronic synovitis with associated edema around the scaphoid bone and distal to the ulnar head.

creased due to reactive reparative processes. Figure 2.**267 a–e** illustrates other cases of lunate necrosis in various stages that have varying radiographic appearances.

Circumscribed subchondral sclerosis affecting ulnar portions of the lunate generally signifies an **ulnar impac-tion syndrome** rather than incipient lunate necrosis (Figs. 2.**268**, 2.**314**, 2.**316**–2.**318**, 2.**386 d**). The sclerosis in these cases is a reactive subchondral sclerosis that develops in response to increased pressure loads. Ulnar impaction syndrome (also called ulnar abutment syn-

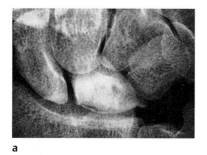

a

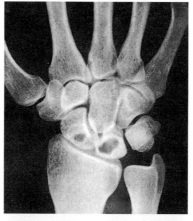

b

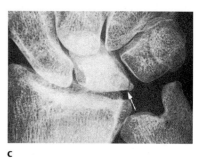

c

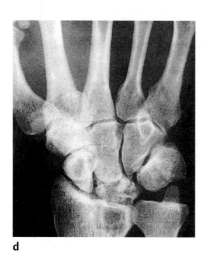

d

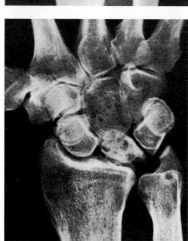

e

Fig. 2.**267 a–e**   Radiographs illustrating various stages and appearances of lunate necrosis.

drome) has diverse causes that include a congenital or acquired (e.g., radial fracture) positive ulnar variance, decreased elasticity of the triangular fibrocartilage, lesions of the suspensory apparatus of the triangular fibrocartilage, and many more. All cases involve some degree of damage to the triangular fibrocartilage complex (p. 111). The subchondral ulnar portion of the triquetrum is involved as frequently as the lunate. Lener et al. (1994) used MRI to document the entrapment and compression of the triangular fibrocartilage in various functional positions of the hand, showing how the fibrocartilage is caught between the ulnar head and triquetrum during ulnar deviation of the hand and between the ulnar head and lunate during radial deviation. They described a third group in which the fibrocartilage was caught between the ulnar notch of the radius and the triquetrum during ulnar deviation. This appears to be a more common pattern in patients with negative ulnar variance.

We see, then, that a positive length discrepancy of the ulna or damage to the triangular fibrocartilage complex increases the pressure load that is transmitted to the lunate and/or the triquetrum, eventually leading to chondromalacia and reactive subchondral changes. These changes are manifested clinically by ulnar-sided wrist pain. Palmer (1989) described the following stages in the progression of the impaction syndrome resulting from chronic repetitive ulnar loads:

Stages in the progression of ulnar impaction syndrome (after Palmer)
(see series of images in Figs. 2.**316**–2.**318**)
Stage I — Degenerative changes in the horizontal part of the triangular fibrocartilage complex, initially without perforation
Stage II — Further degeneration and chondromalacia of the ulnar head and proximal aspect of the lunate
Stage III — Perforation of the triangular fibrocartilage complex, progressive degeneration of the articular surfaces of the ulnar head and lunate, and destruction of the lunotriquetral ligament.
Final stage — Osteoarthritis of the distal radioulnar joint.

Imaeda et al. (1996) and Escobedo et al. (1995) have described the MR imaging findings of ulnar impaction syndrome (see p. 190 ff., Figs. 2.**316**–2.**318**).

Ulnolunate or Ulnocarpal Impaction versus Ulnoradial Impingement

In the literature, the terms ulnar impaction and ulnar impingement are used interchangeably, although they are mutually exclusive phenomena (Gilula and Yin 1996). We cite the same authors: "Whereas **ulnar impaction** is primarily due to ulnar positive variance with abnormalities between the adjacent articulating surfaces of the ulna and radius, lunate and/or triquetrum, **ulnar impingement** is characterized by a shortened distal ulna that articulates with the distal radius proximal to the sigmoid notch. Perhaps the initial confusion has resulted from the similar clinical presentation of these two groups of patients. As in ulnar impaction, patients with painful ulnar impingement present with ulnar-sided wrist pain and there may be wrist clicking. However, in contrast to ulnar impaction patients, the latter group has been noted to have a narrow wrist on physical examination.

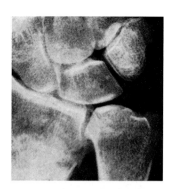

Fig. 2.**268** Ulnar impaction syndrome with sclerosis of the distal subchondral portions of the ulna and opposing subchondral portions of the lunate (see also Figs. 2.**314**, 2.**316**–2.**318**). The "positive ulnar variance" (posttraumatic "lengthening") results from a distal radial fracture that healed with bone shortening.

 Inflammation?

We know of no cases of isolated osteitis or osteomyelitis involving the lunate bone. Inflammatory changes in the lunate generally occur as an accompanying feature of purulent forms of carpal arthritis. Initial radiographic changes were described under General Aspects in the chapter on the carpus. Erosive destruction of the lunate occurs in conditions such as rheumatoid arthritis and psoriatic arthritis.

 Tumor?

The lunate is not predisposed to involvement by tumors or tumorlike lesions. Cystlike lucencies are seen in association with intraosseous ganglions (Fig. 2.**269**), β_2-microglobulin deposits, chondromas, etc.

Small round lucencies, especially when sharply marginated, are usually end-on projections of nutrient canals rather than early tumor-associated destructive changes (Fig. 2.**253**).

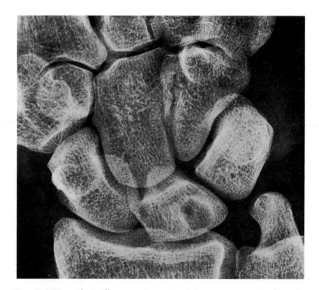

Fig. 2.**269** Clinically symptomatic intraosseous ganglion in the lunate.

Triquetrum

Normal Findings

During Growth

The ossification center of the triquetrum can be seen on radiographs after one year of age, and thus later than the centers of the capitate and hamate. Two ossification centers have been observed.

In Adulthood

The geometry and relative location of the triquetrum are best appreciated on axial CT scans (Fig. 2.**143**). Sometimes the bone is difficult to identify on lateral radiographs.

Pathological Finding?

Normal Variant or Anomaly?

Several references have been made to fusion between the lunate and triquetrum (Fig. 2.**254**, pp. 122 and 165). Anderson and Bowers (1985) described a case of congenital absence of the triquetrum accompanied by scapholunate dissociation and triquetral hypoplasia on the contralateral side.

Fracture or Dislocation?

Fractures of the triquetrum are caused by direct ulnar-sided trauma or by axial trauma due to a fall onto the outstretched hand. Two main types of triquetral fracture are distinguished:

● Fracture of the body of the triquetrum (longitudinal or transverse, Figs. 2.**271**, 2.**272**)
● Dorsal avulsion fracture or chip fracture (Fig. 2.**273**)

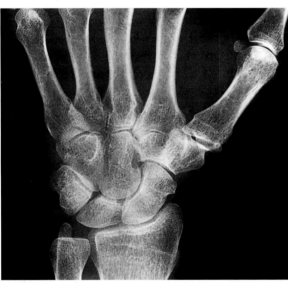

a

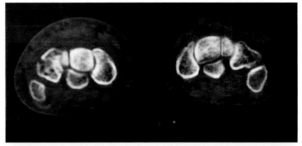
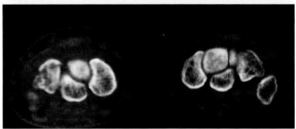

b

Fig. 2.**270 a, b**   Comminuted fracture of the triquetrum. The PA radiograph, though of high technical quality, shows only a slight structural irregularity that could almost be interpreted as a normal variant. But because the patient had diffuse swelling of the wrist and point tenderness over the triquetrum, a

CT examination was performed. CT clearly demonstrates a comminuted fracture or at least a multipart fracture of the triquetrum. The healthy opposite side is also shown for comparison.

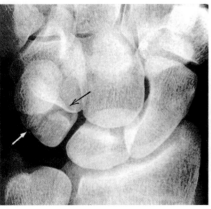

a

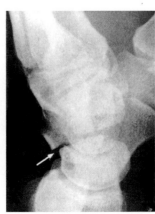

b

Fig. 2.**271 a, b**   Transverse fracture of the triquetrum. Displacement is evident in the lateral view.

The latter account for approximately 90% of all triquetral fractures. They involve a bony avulsion of the radio-triquetral ligament or dorsal intercarpal ligament (Figs. 2.**273**, 2.**275**).

Comminuted fractures of the triquetrum, usually impacted, may be undetectable on standard PA radiographs or may present only with structural irregularities (Fig. 2.**270a**). In the lateral projection, multiple superimposed carpal bones usually make it impossible to evaluate the position of the fragments, and therefore early CT examination is advised (Fig. 2.**270b**). Triquetral avulsion fractures are easier to diagnose on lateral radiographs

(Fig. 2.**273**). Figure 2.**274a** shows a somewhat unusual, superficial avulsion fracture of the proximal lunate surface of the triquetrum. It is easy to imagine the strange groovelike feature in Fig. 2.**274b** and **c** as a healed, superficial triquetral avulsion.

That feature was identified as a normal variant in the previous edition of *Borderlands*, but today this interpretation appears incorrect when we consider the radiographic features of the case as a whole.

With the triquetrum as with other carpal bones, it is important to distinguish congenital **accessory bones** from fragments. The only accessory bones that can be classified

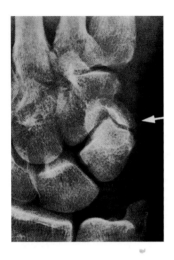

Fig. 2.**272** Peripheral transverse fracture of the triquetrum (arrow). The distal fragment projects past the contour of the pisiform. The hook of the hamate is also fractured.

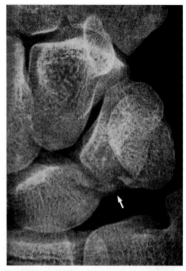

a

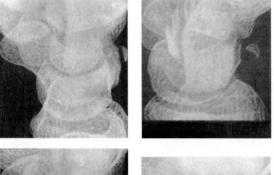

a

b

c

d

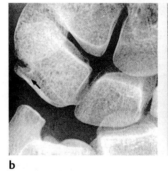

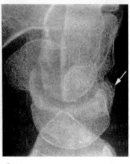

b

c

Fig. 2.**274a–c** Superficial avulsion fracture of the proximal triquetrum (arrow in **a** and **c**). The curious groovelike lucency along the proximal margin in panel **b**, ending in a kind of distal process, most likely represents the osseous union of an old avulsion. It is easy to imagine this developing from the fresh shell-like avulsion in panel **a**.

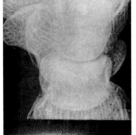
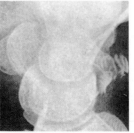

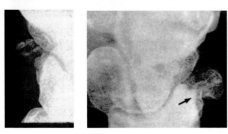

e

f

Fig. 2.**273a–f** Recent (**a–c**) and older (**d–f**) avulsion fractures of the triquetrum. The irregularity and "multiplicity" of the triquetral avulsions shown in **d–f** apparently result from additional heterotopic ossifications.

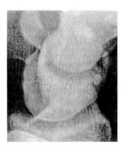

Fig. 2.**275** Triquetral avulsion (distal bony element) with an adjacent os epilunatum (proximal rounded element).

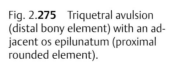

as such with some confidence are the **epipyramis** and the **os epitriquetrum** (Figs. 2.**150**, 2.**284**). Reports on these two bony elements can be found in de Cuveland (1962b) and O'Rahilly (1953). A curious accessory bone is the **os daubentonii** (Fig. 2.**285**), which is extremely rare in humans and actually represents an atavistic bone that occurs normally in the gibbon and other ape species.

The **os triangulare** (Fig. 2.**278**) definitely exists as such (Riva 1949, Ravelli 1956). The problem is that it may occur between the ulnar styloid process and the triquetrum, an area that is commonly "inhabited" by fractured bone elements (e.g., from the ulnar styloid process, Figs. 2.**276**, 2.**279**, 2.**280**) and various ossifications. The latter include dystrophic and heterotopic calcifications (Figs. 2.**277**, 2.**281**, 2.**286a**, 2.**287**), chondrocalcinosis (Fig. 2.**283**) as well as osteomas and chondromas that show varying degrees of lamination (Figs. 2.**282**, 2.**286b,c**).

As long as the bony element is detected incidentally, there is no need to identify it precisely. The unknown bony elements (UBEs) mentioned in previous sections can generally be distinguished from fresh avulsions either by a lack of internal trabecular structure (high-quality radiographs viewed with a magnifying lens) and/or by lamination, especially in slow-growing chondromas or capsular osteomas. If a UBE is not associated with trauma but does show local tenderness, a bone scan should be obtained to check for pathology (e.g., necrosis of an accessory bone, mechanical irritation). If necessary, the symptomatic UBE can be surgically removed without a detailed diagnostic workup, since further preoperative differentiation is of little value and probably could not be accomplished even by CT or MRI.

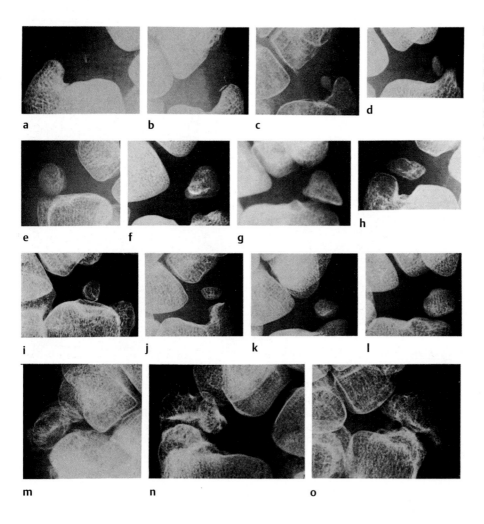

Fig. 2.**276a–o** Isolated bony elements of varying size and shape following injuries of the ulnar styloid process. The hypertrophic nonunions in **m** and **o** show pronounced regressive changes with an increase in the volume of the distal fragments (compare with Figs. 2.**225** and 2.**311**).

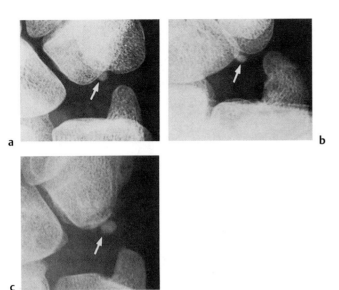

a

b

c

Fig. 2.**277 a–c** Unstructured heterotopic ossifications abutting the proximal margin of the triquetrum (arrows). They were detected incidentally and thus have no clinical significance.

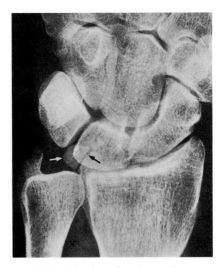

Fig. 2.**278** Os triangulare (arrows).

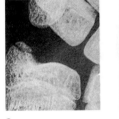 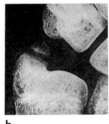

a b

Fig. 2.**279 a, b** Radiographic follow-up of an avulsion fracture of the tip of the ulnar styloid process.
a Postinjury radiograph.
b Radiograph one year later shows marked enlargement of the fragment. This enlargement cannot be explained entirely by possible increased angulation of the fragment. (But compare with Fig. 2.**225**, in which the element has an almost spherical shape, suggesting an accessory bone.)

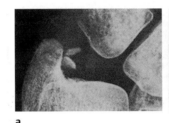 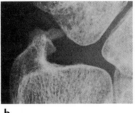

a b

Fig. 2.**280 a, b** Radiographic follow-up of two isolated bone fragments from the ulnar styloid process.
a Postinjury radiograph.
b Radiograph one year later shows irregular healing and enlargement of the original fragments.

Fig. 2.**281 a–f** Examples of various bony elements that may be found in the angle between the ulnar styloid process and the triquetrum (compare these images with Fig. 2.**276**).
a–c The larger elements in these films definitely represent "hypertrophic" avulsions with smaller avulsions nearby. All of the larger avulsions are nonunions.
d–f The rounded, less structured bony elements in these films are undoubtedly heterotopic ossifications. The bony elements adjacent to the styloid process in panel **f** are difficult to interpret. They probably represent two-stage or fragmented styloid avulsions.

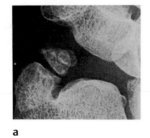 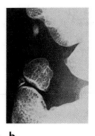

a b

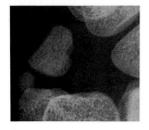 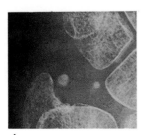 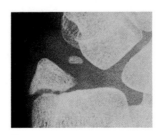 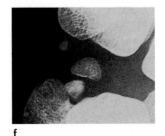

c d e f

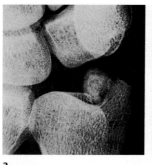 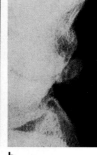 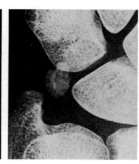

a   b   c

Fig. 2.**282 a–c** Targetoid ossifications in the area between the ulnar styloid process and triquetrum, probably representing capsular osteomas or chondromas.

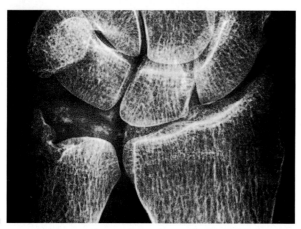

a

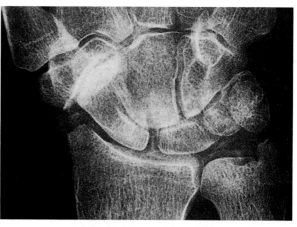

b

Fig. 2.**283 a, b** Typical appearance of chondrocalcinosis with calcifications in both the hyaline cartilage and triangular fibrocartilage. Scapholunate dissociation has developed in panel **b**, where, interestingly, the articular cartilage of both op- posing bones has become calcified. Marked degenerative changes are evident in the joint between the scaphoid, trapezium, and trapezoid. This joint is frequently involved by chondrocalcinosis.

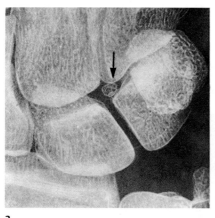

a

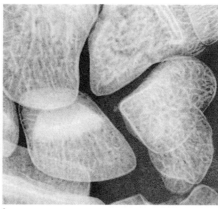

b

Fig. 2.**284 a, b** The small accessory bone elements most likely represent an os epipyramis.

Fig. 2.**285** Os daubentonii. The elongated bony element lat- ▷
eral to the triquetrum shows a peripheral transverse fracture.

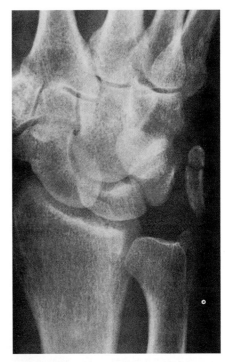

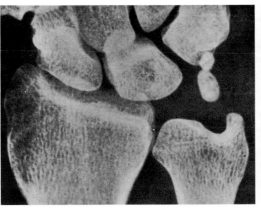
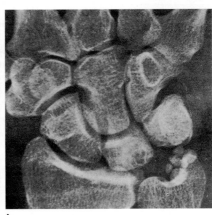
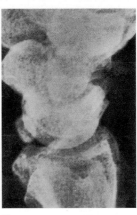

a   b   c

Fig. 2.**286 a–c** Symptomatic bony elements between the ulna and triquetrum.
a Here the two isolated bony elements proximal to the triquetrum are relatively amorphous and represent heterotopic ossifications, probably secondary to a hematoma. The surrounding soft tissues show increased density due to synovitis.

b, c The numerous small ossifications most likely represent
secondary capsular osteomas that developed from the fragmentation of a partially necrotic lunate bone.

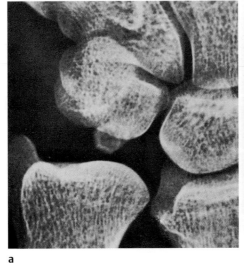
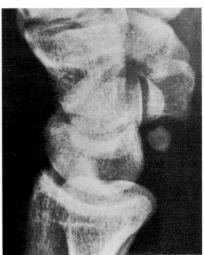

Fig. 2.**287 a, b** Bursal calcification located distal to the ulnar
head on the palmar side.

a   b

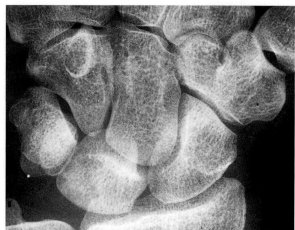

a

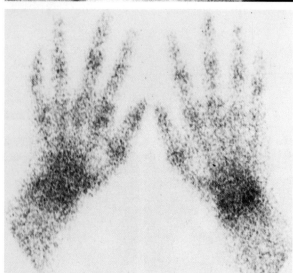

b

Fig. 2.**288 a, b** Irregular lucencies at the center of the trique-trum in a bus driver with a duplicated pisiform. The region was severely painful, and the patient said that she had frequently struck the steering wheel with her left hand during her many years as a driver. We interpret the triquetral lucencies as partial necrosis caused by repetitive microtrauma and apparently re-lating to the duplication of the pisiform in that hand.

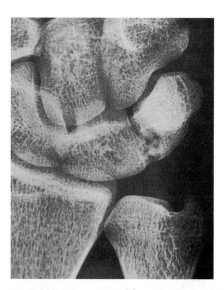

Fig. 2.**289** Necrosis and fragmentation of the proximal por-tion of the triquetrum.

 Necrosis?

Complete necrosis of the triquetrum is rare (Fig. 2.**289**). Circumscribed necrosis associated with fine lucencies and no fragmentation can occur as a repetitive stress injury, as shown in Fig. 2.**288**.

Pisiform

Normal Findings

 During Growth

The ossification center of the pisiform appears relatively late, after 8 or 9 years of age. Generally the bone has multi-ple ossification centers, and it is normal for the pisiform to have a "crumbly" appearance on radiographs (Figs. 2.**290**, 2.**291**).

On PA radiographs the ossification center is projected adjoining or partially overlapping the triquetrum (Fig. 2.**290 a**). Oblique films can provide a clear projection of the pisiform in the soft tissues or may project it in the space between the hamate, lunate, and triquetrum (Fig. 2.**290 c**). Lateral films may show a primary ossification center on the palmar side with a number of additional crumbly or eggshell-like ossification centers toward the carpus (Figs. 2.**291**, 2.**292**).

The pisiform gives attachment to the flexor carpi ulnaris and abductor digiti minimi tendons. The transverse carpal ligament is also attached to the pisiform.

 In Adulthood

The adult pisiform is elliptical in shape and usually has smooth margins. It is best seen in a slightly oblique projec-tion with the dorsum of the hand positioned on a 60° wedge in slight dorsiflexion. The beam is perpendicular to the cassette and centered on the lower third of the wrist. The pisotriquetral joint should be projected clear.

Pathological Finding?

 Normal Variant or Anomaly??

The ossification of the pisiform was described above (Figs. 2.**290**–2.**292**). Fusion with the triquetrum or hamate is rare but may occur. While we have no reports of aplasia or extreme hypoplasia, Viehweger (1957) described bi-lateral hyperplasia of the pisiform combined with hyper-plasia of the hook of the hamate.

Keats (1979) noted the possibility of a bipartite pisiform and also described an unusual exostosis-like process pro-jecting distally from the distal end of the bone and termi-nating at the level of the fourth metacarpal. We have per-sonally observed one such case, in which this process was fractured on the left side (Fig. 2.**293**).

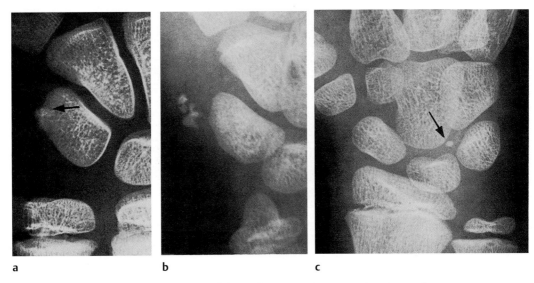

a   b   c

Fig. 2.**290 a–c**   Stages in the ossification of the pisiform in various projections (arrows).

Fig. 2.**291 a, b**   Stage in the ossification of the pisiform.

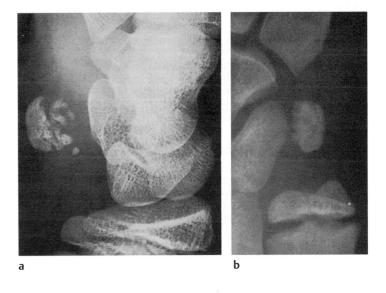

a   b

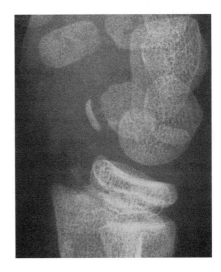

Fig. 2.**292**   Shell-like additional pisiform ossification center ▷ palmar to the main body of the pisiform. The gap between these two structures contains two additional small ossification nucleoli. The radiograph was taken to investigate an Aitken type 1 distal radial fracture.

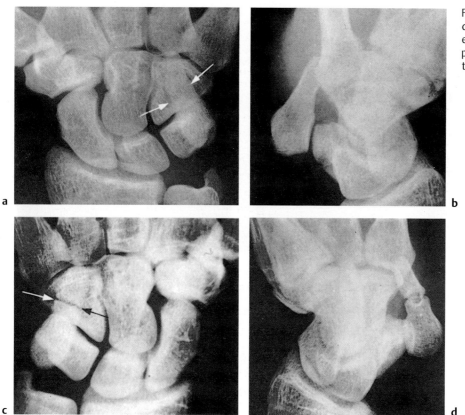

Fig. 2.**293 a–d**   Pisiform with a distal exostosis-like process in each hand. On the left side the process is fractured and shows the features of a nonunion.

 Fracture or Dislocation?

Pisiform fractures are caused by direct trauma to the ulnar aspect of the wrist. They may also accompany fractures of the radius, triquetrum, and hamate. Ligamentous injuries can lead to loss of congruity of the pisotriquetral joint. Three main types of pisiform fracture have been identified:

- Linear fractures (longitudinal and transverse, Fig. 2.**294**)
- Comminuted fractures
- Depressed articular fractures

The finding shown in Fig. 2.**295** may represent an old superficial avulsion fracture or nonspecific metaplastic bone formation, similar to that in Fig. 2.**298**. In comminuted fractures with one or two isolated fragments, the differen-

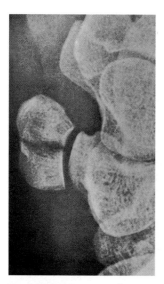

Fig. 2.**294**   Transverse fracture of the pisiform.

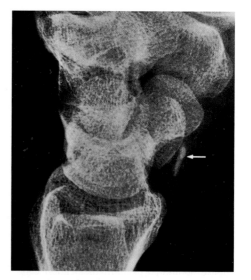

Fig. 2.**295**   Old superficial avulsion fracture of the palmar surface of the pisiform (arrow). The differential diagnosis should include heterotopic ossification. The bony element was detected incidentally and caused no clinical symptoms.

tial diagnosis would naturally include an accessory bone, although no specific accessory bones are known to occur in that area (besides the unassimilated double pisiform centers mentioned earlier). Since nothing has yet been published on accessory bones in the pisiform region despite years of enthusiasm in seeking and describing these bones, it is reasonable to assume that accessory bones do not occur in that area with any regularity. The finding in Fig. 2.296 is probably an old avulsion fracture owing to the congruity of the fragment with the opposing pisiform defect. The morphological and contour changes shown in Fig. 2.297 are consistent with old avulsion fractures or chip fractures that have gone on to bony union.

 ## Necrosis?

Reference was made earlier to the possibility of mistaking "crumbly" ossification centers in the pisiform during skeletal growth for necrotic changes (Figs. 2.290, 2.291).

Otherwise, idiopathic necrosis of the pisiform is not known to occur. Posttraumatic avascular necrosis is always a possibility, however.

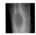 ## Inflammation?

Any inflammatory carpal processes may involve the pisiform. Guly and Azam (1983) described an isolated case of pisotriquetral arthritis as an unusual finding.

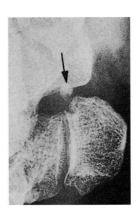

Fig. 2.**296** Avulsion fracture of the distal articular margin of the pisiform. The small, rounded bony element fits precisely into an opposing defect in the pisiform.

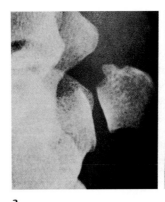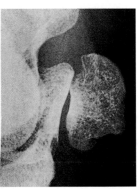

a   **b**

Fig. 2.**297 a, b**   Sequelae of pisiform injuries.
a Old bony avulsion that has healed in an exostosis-like form.
b The marked shape distortion of this pisiform has resulted either from an old longitudinal fracture or from the malunion of distal and proximal avulsions.

Fig. 2.**298** Metaplastic ossifications in the palmar soft tissues over the pisiform. The irregular, crumbly configuration justifies this diagnosis.

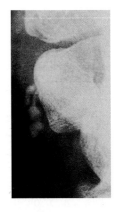

References

Abascal, F., L. Cerezal, F. del Pinal, et al.: Unilateral osteonecrosis in a patient with bilateral os centrale carpi: imaging findings. Skeletal Radiol. 30 (2001) 643

Anderson, W. J., W. H. Bowers: Congenital absence of the triquetrum: a case report. J. Hand Surg. 10 A (1985) 620

Arens, W.: Über die angeborene Synostose zwischen dem Os lunatum und dem Os triquetrum. Fortschr. Röntgenstr. 73 (1950) 772

Balague, F., I. Radi: Unusual erosive osteoarthopathy of a single midcarpal joint. Clin. exp. Rheumatol. 3 (1985) 89

Becker, A.: Über eine ungewöhnliche Handgelenksverbindung (angeborene Radius-Lunatum-Synostose). Fortschr. Röntgenstr. 52 (1935) 245

Blair, W. F., W. C. Kilpatrick, G. E. Omer: Open fracture of the hook of the hamate. Clin. Orthop. 163 (1982) 180

Bolton-Maggs, B. G., B. H. Helal, P. A. Revell: Bilateral avascular necrosis of the capitate. J. Bone Jt Surg. 66-B (1984) 557

Bray, T., A. R. Swafford, R. L. Brown: Bilateral fracture of the hook of the hamate. J. Trauma 25 (1985) 174

Buysch, K. H., J. Drewes et al.: Synostosen zwischen Multangulum minus und Capitatum. Fortschr. Röntgenstr. 115 (1971) 267

Carlson, D. H.: Coalition of the carpal bones. Skelet. Radiol. 7 (1981) 125

Cerezal, L., F. del Piñal, F. Abascal et al.: Imaging findings in ulnar-sided wrist impaction syndromes. Radiographics 22 (2002) 105

Cooke, K. S. et al.: Degenerative changes of the trapeziometacarpal joint: radiologic assessment Skelet. Radiol 24 (1995) 523

de Cuveland, E.: Os radiale externum. Forschr. Röntgenstr. 97 (1962 a) 392

de Cuveland, E.: Als Epipyramis bzw. Epitriquetrum bezeichnete Skelettstücke und -abschnitte im und um den medialen (ulnaren) Interkarpalraum. Fortschr. Röntgenstr. 97 (1962 b) 507

Decoulx, R., M. Marchand, P. Minet et al.: La maladie de Kienböck chez le mineur. Lille chir. 12 (1957) 65

Drewes, J., D. Günther: Über angeborene Synostosen im Handwurzelbereich. Radiologe 6 (1966) 64

Dunkerton, M., M. Singer: Dislocation of the index metacarpal and trapezoid bones. J. Hand. Surg. 10-B (1985) 377

Escobedo, E. M., A. G. Bergmann, J. C. Hunter: MR imaging of ulnar impaction. Skelet. Radiol. 24 (1995) 85

Fischer, E.: Neues Skelettelement dorsal am Radio-Carpalgelenk. Fortschr. Röntgenstr. 91 (1959) 530

Foille, J.: Le carpe bossu. Bull. Mem. Soc. Nat. Chir.57 (1931) 1687

Fowler, C., B. Sullivan, L. A. Williams: A comparison of bone scintigraphy and MRI in the early diagnosis of the occult scaphoid waist fracture. Skelet. Radiol 27 (1998) 683

Freeland, A. E., J. S. Finley: Displaced vertical fracture of the trapezium treated with a small cancellous lag screw. J. Hand Surg. 9-A (1984) 843

Freyschmidt, J., H. Ostertag, G. Jundt: Knochentumoren, 2. Aufl. Springer, Berlin 1998

Gainor, B. Simultaneous dislocation of the hamate and pisiforme: a case report: J. Hand Surg. 10-A (1985) 88

Gambel, J. G., S. C. Simmons III.: Bilateral scaphoid fracture in a child. Clin. Orthop. 125 (1982) 125

Gerscovich, E. O., A. Greenspan: Case report 598: Os centrale carpi. Skeletal Radiol. 19(2) (1990) 143

Geyer, E.: Kritische Betrachtung zur Differentialdiagnose Naviculare bipartitum—Naviculare-Pseudarthrose. Mschr. Unfallheilk. 65 (1962) 149

Gibson, P. H.: Scaphoid-trapezium-trapezoid dislocation. J. Hand. 15 (1983) 267

Gilula, L. A., Y. Yin: Imaging of the Wrist and Hand. Saunders, Philadelphia 1996

Girod, E.: Beitrag zur Radius-Lunatum-Synostose. Fortschr. Röntgenstr. 100 (1964) 282

Gombert, H. J.: Rechtsseitige kongenitale Verschmelzung des Os naviculare und lunatum mit der Radiusepiphyse. Fortschr. Röntgenstr. 91 (1959) 527

Goodman, M. L., G. B. Shankman: Palmar dislocation of the trapezoid. A case report. J. Hand. Surg. 8 (1983) 606

Gottlieb, Ph. D., Sh. J. Parikh, J. K. Singh: Metastatic disease of the carpus (primary site: bronchogenic carcinoma). Skelet. Radiol. 13 (1985) 154

Greene, M. H., A. M Hadied: Bipartite hamulus with ulnar tunnel syndrome—case report and literature review. J. Hand Surg. 6 (1981) 605

Greene, M. H., A. M. Hadied, R. L. Lamont: Scaphoid fractures in children. J. Hand Surg. 9-A (1984) 536

Guly, H. R., M. A. Azam: Pisotriquetral arthritis:a case report. Hand 15 (1983) 294

Gunn, R. S.: Dislocation of the hamate bone. J. Hand Surg. 10-B (1985) 107

Hastings, H., B. P.Simmons: Hand fractures in children. Clin. Orthop. 188 (1984) 120

Heimsöth, G.: Os radiale externum. Fortschr. Röntgenstr. 96 (1962) 306

Hodgkinson, J. P., W. Parkinson, D. R. A. Davies: Simultaneous fracture of the carpal scaphoid and trapezium—a very unusual combination of fractures. J. Hand Surg. 10-B (1985) 393

Imaeda,T., R. Nakamura, K. Shinonoya et al.: Ulnar impaction syndrome: MR imaging findings. Radiology 201 (1996) 495

James, E. T. R., F. D. Burke: Vibration disease of the capitate. J. Hand Surg. 9-B (1984) 169

Jones, W. A., M. S. Ghorbal: Fractures of the trapezium. A report of three cases. J. Hand Surg. 10-B (1985) 227

Keats, Th. E.: An Atlas of Normal Roentgen Variants that May Simulate Disease, 3rd ed.Year Book, Chicago 1979

Knàkal, St., J. Chvojka: Doppelseitige Kahnbeinaplasie. Fortschr. Röntgenstr. 112 (1970) 837

Kopp, J. R.: Isolated palmar dislocation of the trapezoid bone. J. Hand. Surg. 10-A (1985) 91

Krause,G. P.: Os naviculare bipartitum beider Hände. Fortschr. Röntgenstr. 71 (1949) 359

Lamesch, A. J.: Dysplasia epihphysealis hemimelica of the carpal bones. J.Bone Jt Surg. 65-A (1983) 398

Leger, Z.: Beobachtung einer angeborenen Synostose zwischen Multangulum minus und Metakarpale 2. Z. Orthop. 87 (1955) 70

Lichtman, D. M., G. R. Mack, R. J. McDonald et al.: Kienböck's disease: the role of silicone-replacement arthroplasty. Amer. J. Bone Jt Surg. 59 (1977) 899

Lin, E., J. Engel, J. J. Bubis et al.: Aneurysmal bone-cyst of the hamate bone. J. Hand Surg. 9-A (1984) 847

Lener, M., W. Judmaier, M. Galb et al.: Diagnostik des ulnokarpalen Komplexes im MR-Movie. Handchir. Mikrochir. plast. Chir. 26 (1994) 115

Lorenz, R., V. Fiedler: Der Navikularefettstreifen (NFS). Fortschr. Röntgenstr. 137 (1982) 286

Magee, T. H., A. M. Rowedder, G. G. Degnan: Intraosseus ganglia of the wrist. Radiology 195 (1995) 517

Maier, K.: Gibt es eine Navikulare-Aplasie an der Hand? Fortschr. Röntgenstr. 97 (1962) 52

Mann, F. A., A. J. Wilson, L. A. Gilula: Radiographic evaluation of the wrist: What does the hand surgeon want to know? Radiology 184 (1992) 15

Marsh, A. P., P. J. Lampros: The naviculo-capitate fracture-syndrome. Amer. J. Roentgenol. 82 (1959) 255

Metz, V. M., M. Schratter, W. I. Dock et al.: Age-associated changes of the triangular fibrocartilage of the wrist: evaluation of the diagnostic performance of MR Imaging. Radiology 184 (1992) 217

Metz, V. M., S. M. Schimmerl, L. A. Gilula et al.: Wide scapholunate joint space in lunotriquetral coalition: A normal variant? Radiology 188 (1993) 557

Mordeja, J.: Das Lunatum bipartitum und die multizentrische Kernanlage des Os pisiforme. Z. Orthop. 95 (1962) 492

Murken, J. D.: Fehlen von Handwurzel-Knochenkernen, Ringknorpeldysplasie und Veränderungen von Femurepiphyse und Becken – ein eigenes Krankheitsbild? Radiologe 9 (1969) 227

Nakamura, K., M. Beppu, R.M. Patterson et al.: Motion analysis in two dimensions of ulnar-sided deviation of type I versus type II lunates. J. Hand Surg [Am] 25 (2000) 877

Nakamura, R., Y. Tanaka, T. Imaeda et al.: The influence of age and sex on ulnar variance. J. Hand. Surg. 16-B (1991 a) 84

Nakamura, R., T. Imaeda, K. Suzuki et al.: Sports-related Kienböck's disease. Amer. J. Sports Med. 19 (1991 b) 88

Nakamura, R., E. Horii, T. Imaeda et al.: Criteria for diagnosing distal radioulnar joint subluxation by computed tomography. Skelet. Radiol. 25 (1996) 649

Neiss, A.: Doppelseitige Synostose zwischen dem Os multangulum minus und dem Os capitatum. Fortschr. Röntgenstr. 82 (1955) 925

Norman, A., J. Nelseon. St. Green: Fractures of the hook of hamate: radiographic signs. Radiology 154 (1985) 49

North, E. R., W. M. Rutledge: The trapzeium-thumb metacarpal joint: the relationship of joint-shape and degenerative joint disease. J. Hand. 15 (1983) 201

O'Rahilly, R. J.: Survey of carpal and tarsal anomalies. J. Bone Jt Surg. 35-A (1953) 626

O'Rahilly, R.: Epitriquetrum, hypotriquetrum and lunato-triquetrum. Acta radiol. 39 (1953) 401

Palmer, A.: Tiangular fibrocartilage lesions: a classification. J. Hand Surg. 14-A (1989) 594

Pennes, D. R.,E. M. Braunstein, K. K. Shirazi: Carpal ligamentous laxity with bilateral perilunate dislocation in Marfan syndrome. Skelet. Radiol. 13 (1985) 62

Perme, Ch. M., St. P. Johnson, A. S. Weinstein: Hereditary symphalangism with carpal and tarsal fusions and deafness. Skelet. Radiol. 23 (1994) 468

Pfirrmann, C. W. A., N. H. Theumann, C. B. Chung et al.: What happens to the triangular fibrocartilage complex during pronation and supination of the forearm? Analysis of its morphology and diagnostic assessment with MR arthrography. Skeletal Radiol 30 (2001) 677

Pfitzner, W.: Beiträge zur Kenntnis des menschlichen Extremitätenskeletts. VIII. Die morphologischen Elemente des menschlichen Handskeletts. Abschnitt I: Allgemeiner Teil. Z. Morphol. Anthropol. 2 (1900) 77

Pfitzner, W.: Beiträge zur Kenntnis des menschlichen Extremitätenskeletts. VIII. Die morphologischen Elemente des menschlichen Handskeletts. Abschnitt II: Spezieller Teil. Z. Morphol. Anthropol. 2 (1900) 365

Pfitzner, W.: Beiträge zur Kenntnis des menschlichen Extremitätenskeletts. Dritte Abteilung: Die Varietäten. VI. Die Variationen im Aufbau des Handskeletts. Morphol. Arb. IV (1885) 347

Poznanski, A. K., J. F. Holt: The carpals in congenital malformation syndroms. Amer. J. Roentgenol. 112 (1971) 443

Poznanski, A., K.: The Hand in Radiologic Diagnosis, 2nd ed. Saunders, Philadelphia 1984 (p. 198)

Ravelli, A.: Zur Ossifikation der Vieleckbeine. Fortschr. Röntgenstr. 83 (1955) 852

Rahme, H.: Idiopathic avascular necrosis of the capitate bone—case report. Hand 15 (1983) 274

Ravelli, A.: Zur Deutung und Bedeutung überzähliger Karpalelemente. Fortschr. Röntgenstr. 84 (1956) 630

Riva, G.: Ein Fall von doppelseitigem Os tiangulare carpi. Radiol. clin. 18 (1949) 78

Resnick, Ch. S., R. H.Gelberman, D. Resnick: Transscaphoid, transcapitate, perilunate fracture dislocation (scaphocapitate syndrome). Skelet. Radiol. 9 (1983) 192

Resnick, Ch. S., J. D. Grizzard, B. P. Simmons et al.: Incomplete carpal coalition. Amer. J. Roentgenol. 147 (1986) 301

Ross, E.: Os capitatum bipartitum. Fortschr. Röntgenstr. 81 (1954) 224

Ruckensteiner, E.: Über multiple Handwurzelknochen. Röntgen-Bl. 4 (1951) 236

Sagerman, S. D., R. M. Hauck, A. K. Palmer: Lunate morphology: can it be predicted with routine x-ray films? J. Hand Surg [Am] 20 (1995) 38

Schaaf, J., A. Wagner: Multiplizität von Handwurzelknochen bei drei Geschwistern mit polytoper enchondraler Dysostose. Fortschr. Röntgenstr. 97 (1962) 497

Schiltenwolf, M, A. K. Martini: Der Spontanverlauf der Lunatumnekrose. Orthopädie 23 (1994) 243

Schmitt, R., U. Lanz : Bildgebende Diagnostik der Hand. Hippokrates, Stuttgart 1996

Schlosser, H., J. F. Murray: Fracture of the hook of the hamate. Canad. J. Surg. 27 (1984) 587

Schober, R., C.A. Bayard: Hamulusfrakturen und Karpaltunnelsyndrom. Fortschr. Röntgenstr. 90 (1959) 266

Seibert-Daiker, F. M.: Anlage eines Os hypolunatum beiderseits bei kongenitaler Konkreszenz des Scapoideum und Trapezium. Fortschr. Röntgenstr. 122 (1975) 463

Shirazi, Kh. K., F. P. Agha, M. A. Amendola: Isolated fracture of greater multangular. Brit. J. Radiol. 35 (1982) 923

Smith-Hoefer, E.: Isolated carpal synchondrosis of the scaphoid and trapezium. J. Bone Jt Surg. 67-A (1985) 317

Smith, D. K., W. N. Snearly: Lunotriquetral interosseous ligament of the wrist: MR appearances in asymptomatic volunteers and arthrographically normal wrists. Radiology 191 (1994) 199

Smith, D. K.: Scapholunate interosseous ligament of the wrist: MR appearances in asymptomatic volunteers and arthrographically normal wrists. Radiology 192 (1994) 217

Stäbler, A.: Der pathologische Entstehungsmechanismus der destruierenden Handgelenksarthropathie bei Gicht. Fortschr. Roentgenstr. 156 (1992) 73

Stäbler, A., C. Glaser, M. Reiser et al.: Symptomatic fibrous lunato-triquetral coalition. Europ. Radiol. 9 (1999) 1643

Stewart, N. R., L. A. Gilula: CT of the wrist: a tailored approach. Radiology 183 (1992) 13

Sugimoto, H., T.Shinozaki, T. Ohsawa: Triangular fibrocartilage in asymptomatic. subjects: Investigation of abnormal MR signal intensity. Radiology 191 (1994) 193

Tänzer, A.: Hamulusfraktur und Karpaltunnelsyndrom. Fortschr. Röntgenstr. 91 (1959) 283

Thakkar, D. H.: Lunato-triquetral fusion and associated spinal abnormality. Hand 1 (1982) 89

Thurston, A. J., J. K. Stanley: Hamatolunate impingement: an uncommon cause of ulnar-sided wrist pain. Arthroscopy 16 (2000) 540

Timins, M. E., St. E. O'Connell, S. J. Erickson et al.: MR imaging of the wrist: Normal findings that may simulate disease. Radio Graphics 16 (1996) 987

Totterman, S. M. S, R. J. Miller: Triangular fibrocartilage complex: Normal appearance on coronal three-dimensional gradient-re-called-echo MR images. Radiology 195 (1995) 521

Viegas, S. F., K. Wagner, R. M. Patterson et al.: Medial (hamate) facet of the lunate. J. Hand Surg [Am] 15 (1990) 564

Viegas, S. F., R. M. Patterson, J. A. Hokanson et al.: Wrist anatomy: incidence, distribution, and correlation of anatomic variation, tears, and arthrosis. J. Hand Surg [Am] 18 (1993) 463

Viehweger, G.: Beitrag zur Spaltbildung an den Handwurzelknochen. Fortschr. Röntgenstr. (1956) 376

Viehweger, G.: Doppelseitige Hyperplasie des Os pisiforme und des Hamulus ossis hamati. Fortschr. Röntgenstr. 86 (1957) 407

Vogel, K. H.: Aseptische Nekrose am Os hamatum. Fortschr. Röntgenstr. 99 (1963) 112

Waugh, R. L., R. F. Sullivan: Anomalies of the carpus with particular reference to the bipartite scaphoid (navicular). J. Bone Jt Surg. 32-A (1950) 682

White, S. J., D. S. Louis, E. M. Braunstein et al.: Capitate-lunate instability. Amer. J. Roentgenol. 143 (1984) 361

Yu, W., Y. Wang, Y. Jiang et al.: Kashin-Beck disease in children: radiographic findings in the wrist. Skeletal Radiol 31 (2002) 222

Forearm

Distal Radius and Ulna

▌ Normal Findings

 During Growth

The ossification centers of the radial and ulnar shafts appear in the 6th to 8th week of fetal development. The ossification center of the distal radial epiphysis appears from 8 to 18 months after birth, and that of the distal ulnar epiphysis appears between 5 and 7 years of age. There is a relatively large range of variation in the times of appearance of these centers.

The distal epiphyseal center of the radius and ulna fuses with the metaphysis at about 17 years of age. The epiphyseal plate ossifies more rapidly in its ulnar portion.

At 5 years of age the distal epiphyseal center of the radius is extremely small in relation to the adjacent metaphysis. The epiphyseal growth plate is normally of variable thickness, and a wide epiphyseal (cartilage) plate (physis) should not be mistaken for an epiphyseal separation (see under Fracture, Subluxation or Dislocation). In the lateral projection, the metaphysis forms a slightly cup-shaped expansion below the epiphysis (Fig. 2.**299**).

At 14 years of age the distal radial epiphysis is almost as wide as the metaphysis. By 18 years of age, the radial epiphysis has reached its definitive size. It is broader than the metaphysis and bears a typical spur on its radial surface just prior to fusion (Figs. 2.**299 b**, 2.**300**).

The epiphyseal plate (growth plate) of the ulna usually appears wider than that of the radius on radiographic films (Fig. 2.**301**). Small, fine bony structures are found with some consistency at the center of the ulnar epiphyseal plate (Fig. 2.**302 a**). Sometimes they appear to form a columnlike structure that spans the physis like a bridge (Fig. 2.**302 b**).

Similar structures are found less frequently in the radial epiphyseal plate (Fig. 2.**302 c**).

Ghantus (1951) published relatively precise data on the size and length of the shaft of the radius and ulna during the first two years of life. Hafner et al. (1989) calculated the range of variation of ulnar length from 1.5 to 15.5 years of age based on 535 radiographs of the hand. The values found by the authors (distance from the most proximal point of the distal radial metaphysis to the most proximal point of the distal ulnar metaphysis, and distance from the most distal point of the distal radius to the ulnar metaphysis) have proven helpful in objectifying and following ulnar

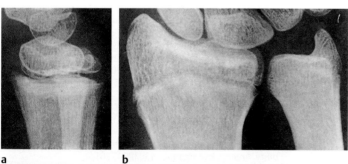

a   b

Fig. 2.**299 a, b**   Typical radiographic appearance of the epiphyses and metaphyses of the distal radius and ulna in a 17-year-old boy. Note the cup-shaped configuration of the radial metaphysis in the lateral view (**a**) and the normal metaphyseal bone spur on the lateral aspect of the radius (**b**).

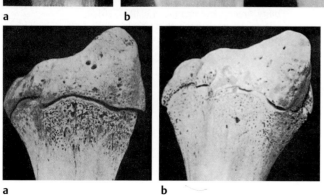

a   b

Fig. 2.**300 a, b**   The distal radial growth zone in anatomic specimens. Note particularly the spur on the radial side of the metaphysis in panel **b**.

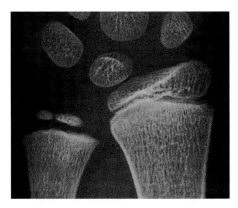

Fig. 2.**301**   Physiologically very broad epiphyseal plate in the distal ulna with two ossification centers.

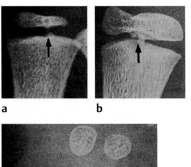

Fig. 2.**302 a–c**
Normal variants in the distal, ulnar and radial epiphyseal plates. **a, b** Fine ossifications in the distal epiphyseal plate of the ulna. **c** Normal fine ossification forming a "bony column" in the epiphyseal line of the distal radius.

shortening in conditions such as rheumatoid arthritis or exostosis disease (Fig. 2.**303**).

The portions of the radial and ulnar metaphysis that directly border the epiphyseal plate often appear very dense before 2 years of age. This **metaphyseal ring** represents a kind of amorphously calcified cuff of perichondral structures, also termed the "virole" (Fig. 2.**304**).

The metaphyseal ring is seen most clearly when the central ray is parallel to the end plane of the radial metaphysis. This is accomplished by angling the central ray about 5° distally. An off-angle projection can create the appearance of a "cushion epiphysis" (Fig. 2.**305**) like that seen in various developmental disorders (Buttenberg 1967). Nonorthograde projections can also create the erroneous impression of rickets or intracancellous callus formation.

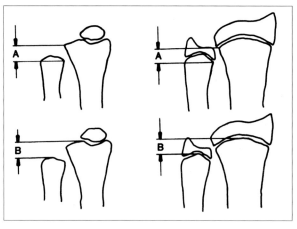

Fig. 2.**303**   Method used to measure the ulnar variance. *A* is the distance from the most proximal point of the ulnar metaphysis to the most proximal point of the radial metaphysis. *B* is the distance from the most distal point of the ulnar metyphysis to the most distal point of the radial metaphysis. (From Hafner et al. 1989.)

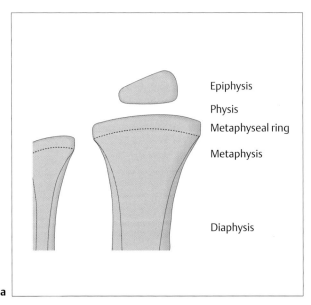

Epiphysis

Physis

Metaphyseal ring

Metaphysis

Diaphysis

Fig. 2.**304 a, b**   The metaphyseal ring.
a Diagram of the radiographic appearance of the distal forearm of a 2-year-old child. The "metaphyseal ring" forms a cylindrical, full-width base for the more proximal metaphysis.

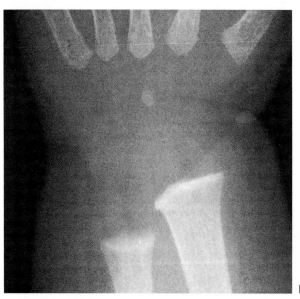

b Wrist radiograph of a 10-month-old child. A dense metaphyseal ring is visible in the radius and ulna. (From Laval-Jeantet et al. Ann. Radiol. 11 [1968] 327.)

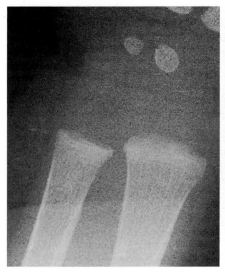
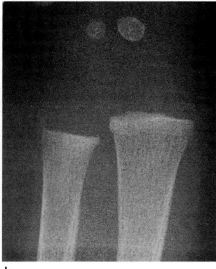

a   b

Fig. 2.**305 a, b** So-called "cushion epiphyses" in the wrist radiograph of a 2-month-old infant.
a In this film the central ray strikes the distal metaphyses of the radius and ulna at a 90° angle, causing dense, bandlike structures to appear on the ends of the bones. This is a projection-related phenomenon with no pathological significance (as proved by panel **b**).
b When the x-ray tube is angled 5° cephalad, the projection-related changes disappear.

 ## In Adulthood

We referred earlier to the spurlike prominence on the radial side of the radial epiphysis, seen around the time the epiphysis fuses with the metaphysis (Fig. 2.**299 b**). This spur is more prominent in adults and may form a knoblike protuberance (Fig. 2.**306**).

A narrow "ridge" is often visible along the ulnar surface of the radial metaphysis and appears to merge distally with the radioulnar joint contour. This is a projection-related effect that should not be mistaken for a zone of subperiosteal resorption like that associated with a subperiosteal ganglion (Fig. 2.**307**).

The normal degrees of palmar and ulnar angulation of the distal radial articular surface were reviewed in the chapter on the carpus (p. 105). It should be recalled that the range of variation of these angles is extremely large (0–20° for palmar angulation, 15–35° for ulnar angulation).

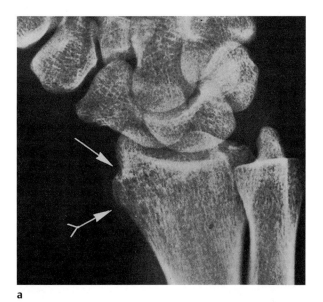
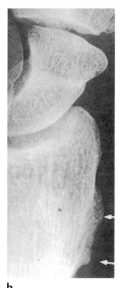

a   b

Fig. 2.**306 a, b** Bone spur and bony prominence.
a Physiological bone spur on the radial side of the radial metaphysis (arrows) (compare with Fig. 2.**300 b**).
b Normal ridgelike bony prominence at the level of the former epiphyseal growth plate (arrows). This ridgelike protuberance is actually a variant of the bone spur in radiograph **a**.

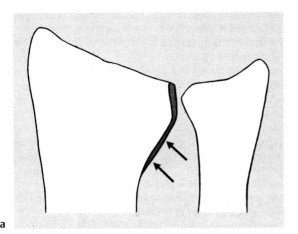

a

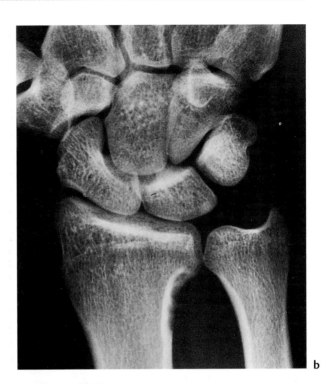

b

Fig. 2.**307 a–d**   Normal and pathological contours of the distal ulnar side of the radius.

a An apparent ridge along the ulnar contour of the distal radius (arrows) is a typical projection-related phenomenon that occurs when the plateaulike ulnar surface of the radial epiphysis and metaphysis is imaged in a nonorthograde projection.

b Subperiosteal ganglion on the ulnar side of the radius in a young physiotherapist. This pathological finding should not be mistaken for a projection phenomenon as in **a** because the ganglion caused an unequivocal erosion in the radial cortex.

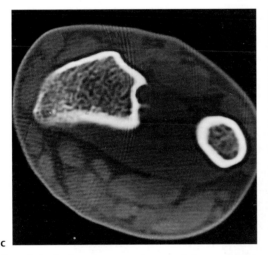

c

d

Fig. 2.**307 c**   Note the relatively deep bony erosion or pit in the CT scan.

d The associated soft-tissue lesion shows high, fluid-equivalent signal intensity on T2-weighted MRI (25-year-old masseuse).

Pathological Finding?

 ### Normal Variant or Anomaly?

The distal radial and ulnar epiphyses may have two ossification centers that do not fuse but persist as separate centers (Figs. 2.**301**, 2.**308**–2.**311**). These persistent centers are known as the ossa styloides radii or ulnae. They are distinguished from tip avulsions of the styloid process by the prior history, palpable findings, and possibly by associated injuries (Fig. 2.**312**).

Information on accessory bone elements around the radial and ulnar styloid processes can be found on p. 175 f. and in Figs. 2.**224**, 2.**225**, and 2.**279**–2.**282**. Congenitally small styloid processes (Fig. 2.**235 c, d**) as well as large, stout processes are considered a normal variant. If the

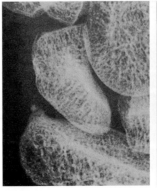
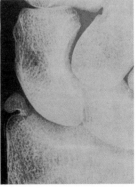

a   **b**

Fig. 2.**308 a, b**   Isolated ossification centers at the tip of the radial styloid process.

patient in Fig. 2.**335 a, b** did not have a suggestive prior history, the pathological changes in the ulnar styloid processes would have been classified as a normal variant.

An excessively long styloid process can lead to an **ulnar styloid impaction syndrome** with ulnar-sided wrist pain because of an impaction between the excessively long ulnar styloid process and the triquetrum (Topper et al). This entity is distinctly different from the more well known form of **ulnar impaction syndrome** (p. 173 and below) in

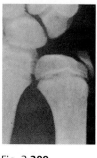 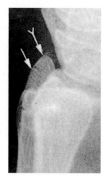

Fig. 2.**309**

Fig. 2.**310**

Fig. 2.**309**   Ossification center of the ulnar styloid process.

Fig. 2.**310**   Persistence of ossification centers on the ulna (arrows).

that the radiographic evidence of chondromalacia does not involve the proximal pole of the lunate bone and ulnar head, but rather the proximal pole of the triquetrum bone and ulnar styloid process (Cerezal et al. 2002). A typical radiographic sign of ulnar styloid impaction syndrome is subcortical sclerosis of the styloid process. The normal length of the ulnar styloid process varies between 2–6 mm. Garcia–Elias (1987) has developed a method of assessing the relative size of the process (USPI = Ulnar Styloid Process Index). An exessively long ulnar styloid process has an USPI greater than 0.21 ± 0.07 or an overall length greater than 6 mm.

Small, isolated ossification centers in asymptomatic patients with no trauma history are occasionally found on the ulnar articular margin of the distal radius (Fig. 2.**313**).

A positive congenital (nontraumatic) length discrepancy of the ulna relative to the radius is called **positive ulnar variance**, and a negative length discrepancy is called **negative ulnar variance** (Fig. 2.**315**; p. 169). An extreme negative ulnar variance is transitional with Madelung deformity (p. 124 f.). Strictly speaking, positive and negative ulnar variance should be distinguished from **posttraumatic ulnar lengthening** due to shortening of the radius (Fig. 2.**314**) and from posttraumatic ulnar shortening.

Positive ulnar variance and posttraumatic ulnar advancement show a striking association with **ulnar impaction syndrome**, known also as ulnar abutment syndrome (Definition, see p. 173). Normally, the ulna transmits ap-

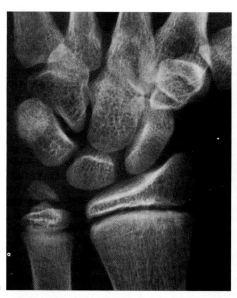 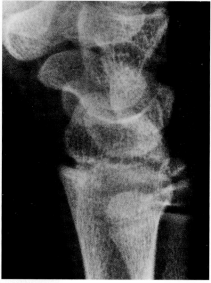

Fig. 2.**311 a, b**   Two persistent ossification centers of the ulnar styloid process, simulating the appearance of a styloid process avulsion (compare with Figs. 2.**224**, 2.**225**, 2.**279**–2.**282**).

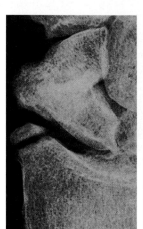 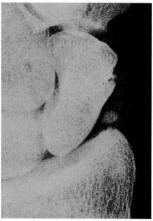

Fig. 2.**312 a, b**   Differential diagnosis of persistent epiphyseal centers in the radial styloid process.
a This isolated bony element is easily interpreted as a rim fragment owing to its congruence with the adjacent radial surface. The film also shows an old scaphoid fracture as an associated injury (or vice versa).
b This film shows no associated injury and no change in the tip of the radial styloid process. Hence, the very small bony element should be interpreted as an accessory bone (compare with Fig. 2.**235**).

proximately 20 % of axial forces from the wrist to the forearm (Palmer 1984). Even a slight lengthening of the ulna relative to the radius will dramatically increase the forces that are transmitted along the ulna, placing unphysiologically high loads on structures that are distal to the ulna. These structures include:

- The triangular fibrocartilage complex (TFCC, p. 111)
- The lunate and triquetrum and their attached ligaments

Palmer (1989) described the ulnar impaction syndrome as a spectrum of changes in the ulnar aspect of the wrist that progress in definable stages (p. 173). The changes are the

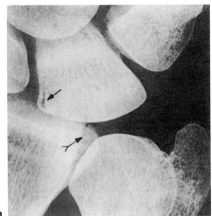
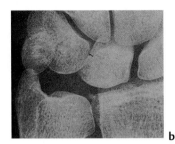

Fig. 2.**313 a, b**
Small ossification centers at the ulnar border of the radius (double arrow).
a The single arrow points to a subchondral "fissure" in the lunate, apparently caused by a circumscribed rarefaction of the cancellous bone and fatty replacement in the clinically asymptomatic patient.
b This radiograph shows another obvious small accessory ossification center at the ulnar border of the radius.

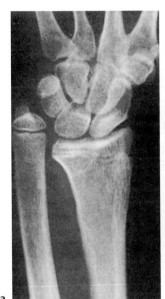
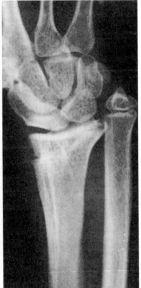
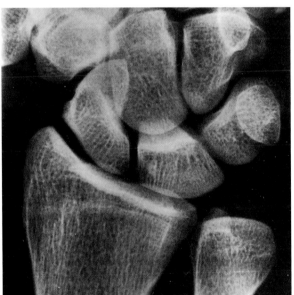
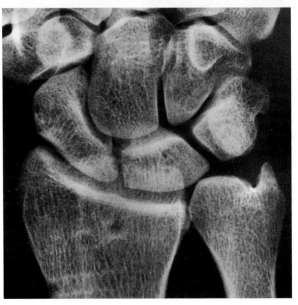

Fig. 2.**314 a–c** Posttraumatic "positive ulnar variance" or, more accurately, posttraumatic ulnar lengthening.
a Marked posttraumatic "positive ulnar variance" in a clinically asymptomatic patient. The short radius is probably a result of previous growth plate injuries.
b, c Development of "positive ulnar variance" in a 28-year-old man. Image **b** is a postinjury radiograph taken on 5 February 1998. The distal radial shaft fracture is not shown. Radiograph taken six months later after internal fixation, fracture healing, and removal of the fixation material (**c**) shows definite ulnar lengthening (the radial fracture healed with bone shortening) and incipient ulnar impaction. Note the fine subchondral sclerosis and blurred cancellous trabeculae in the lunate, which is abutted by the ulnar head.

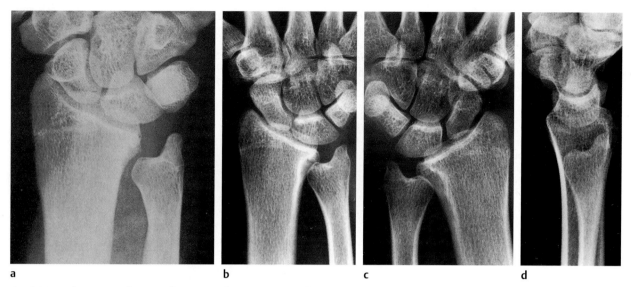

a   b   c   d

Fig. 2.**315 a–d**   Various degrees of negative ulnar variance. Radiographs **b–d** are from a 17-year-old asymptomatic patient. In **b**, signs of radioulnar impingement on the radius (bone resorption, sclerosis).

end result of chronic, repetitive, excessive ulnar loads. The initial stage is marked by degenerative changes in the horizontal portion of the TFCC without perforation. In the next stage these degenerative changes increase, accompanied by the development of chondromalacic changes in the ulnar head and in the proximal ulnar portion of the lunate. With passage of time, a TFCC perforation occurs. Progressive degenerative changes develop in the lunate bone and in the articular surface of the ulnar head, and the lunotriquetral ligament is destroyed. Ultimately, degenerative changes may also develop in the distal radioulnar joint. Positive ulnar variance has much greater causal significance in ulnar impaction syndrome than acquired distal radial shortening (e.g., due to a Colles fracture). Patients with an ulnar impaction syndrome present clinically with ulnar-sided wrist pain, especially on pronation, supination, or ulnar deviation. Focal swelling may be evident between the ulnar head and the lunate and triquetral bones. Patients often feel a click or crepitus when rotating the wrist. Palmer classified the degenerative

changes in the TFCC into five subcategories of increasing severity (class 2 A through 2 E) (Palmer 1989, 1990).

The radiographic signs of ulnar impaction syndrome are as follows:

- Positive ulnar variance or "posttraumatic ulnar lengthening"
- Cortical and subchondral sclerosis
- Subchondral cystlike lucencies in the ulnar head and beneath the opposing articular surfaces of the lunate and triquetrum (Figs. 2.**316 a**, 2.**318 a**, 2.**386 d**)

These pathological changes generally represent an advanced stage of ulnar impaction syndrome.

> Very early radiographic changes can be seen only in radiographs of excellent technical quality that are viewed with a magnifying lens, and sometimes they are indistinguishable from normal findings (Figs. 2.**316 a**, 2.**317 a**).

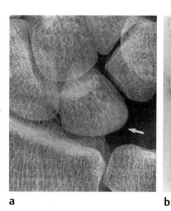
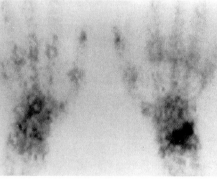
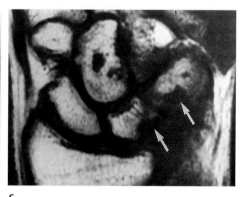

a   b   c

Fig. 2.**316 a–c**   Ulnar impaction syndrome.
a This radiograph shows subtle sclerotic changes in the subchondral ulnar portions of the lunate. The sclerosis obscures the normal trabecular pattern (arrow).
b ^{99m}Tc diphosphonate bone scan shows asymmetrical increased uptake in the area of the left lunate and triquetrum with a normal-appearing opposite side (AP projection).

c Coronal T1-weighted MRI shows foci of low signal intensity in the lunate and triquetrum (arrows). The hypointense foci in the capitate are normal variations due to focal increased cancellous bone density. (From Escobedo et al. 1995.)

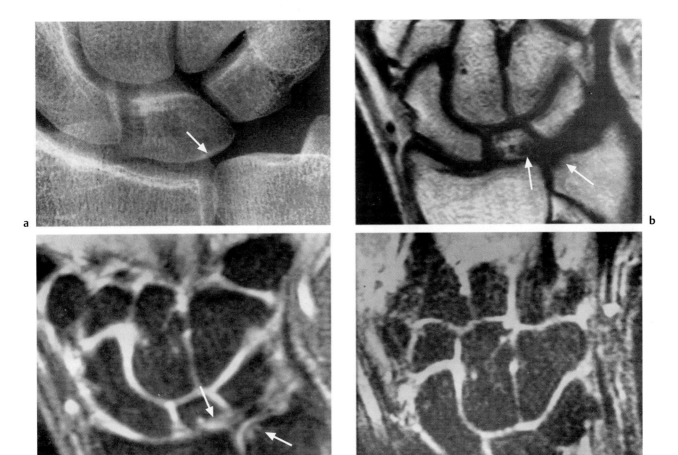

Fig. 2.**317 a–d**   Ulnar impaction syndrome.
a Positive ulnar variance with mild subchondral sclerosis in the ulnar aspect of the lunate (arrow).
b Coronal T1-weighted MRI shows a circumscribed zone of low signal intensity in the ulnar aspect of the lunate and opposing ulna (arrows).
c Coronal fat-suppressed image shows increased signal intensity in the proximal lunate and distal ulna (straight arrows). A

synovial fluid communication exists between the radiocarpal and distal radioulnar joints (proximal arrow) caused by a rupture of the TFCC.
d Coronal STIR sequence nine months after an ulnar shortening osteotomy shows regression of signal changes in the lunate and ulna and decreased effusion in the carpus. The destruction of the TFCC is more clearly visualized. (From Escobedo et al. 1995.)

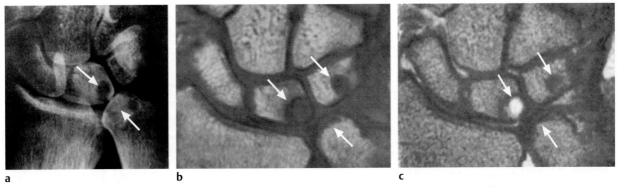

Fig. 2.**318 a–c** Ulnar impaction syndrome.
a Marked positive ulnar variance with a large subchondral (degenerative) cyst in the lunate, surrounded by sclerosis. Sclerosis is also visible in the opposing ulnar head (arrows).
b Coronal T1-weighted image demonstrates low signal intensities in the lunate, triquetrum, and ulna (arrows).

c On the corresponding T2-weighted image, the lunate cyst appears hyperintense as expected, while the zones of low signal intensity previously seen in the triquetrum and ulnar head remain hypointense, apparently a result of circumscribed sclerosis. (From Imaeda et al. 1996.)

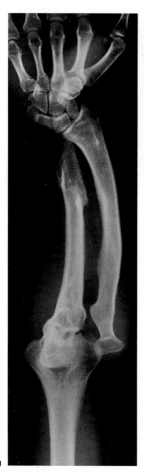
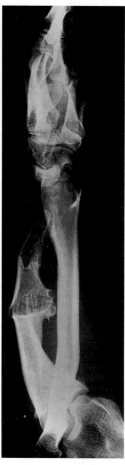

a   b

Fig. 2.**319 a, b** Cartilaginous exostoses (different patients with hereditary osteochondromatosis) with pseudo-Madelung deformity caused by distal ulnar exostosis leading to inhibition of ulnar growth. Dislocation of the radial head is also present. A broad cartilaginous cap over the radial-sided exostosis in **a** is responsible for the marked bowing of the radius. The cartilage cap of this larges exostosis is not visible, because it is not calcified.

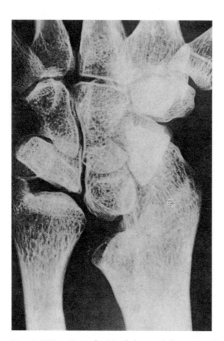

Fig. 2.**320** Pseudo-Madelung deformity after an epiphyseal plate fracture.

Bone scans show increased tracer uptake in the involved bones, although this is a nonspecific finding (Fig. 2.**316 b**). MRI can help in this situation by accurately defining the TFCC and also by detecting early changes in the affected bones (Escobedo et al. 1995, Imaeda et al. 1996). T1-weighted images usually show low signal intensities in the subchondral portions of the ulnar head, lunate, and triquetrum. T2-weighted MRI may show low signal intensities representing sclerosis or fibrosis in the corresponding subchondral bone areas, or it may show high signal intensities representing edema, subchondral cysts, or a combination of both (Figs. 2.**316**–2.**318**).

The differential diagnosis of the above radiological signs mainly includes age-related changes (Uchiyama and Terayama 1991, Viegas et al. 1993). The clinical presentation must be considered in order to interpret the signs correctly. The differential diagnosis also includes incipient lunate necrosis (p. 169), but generally this is associated with negative rather than positive ulnar variance and affects the entire bone (especially on MRI).

Madelung deformity was discussed previously in the chapter on the carpus. It should not be confused with **pseudo-Madelung deformity**. Whereas the growth disturbance in Madelung deformity involves the medial, palmar portion of the distal radial epiphysis, which shows increased ulnar and palmar angulation (with bayonet-like palmar deviation of the hand relative to the forearm and subluxation of the ulnar head), pseudo-Madelung deformity can result from cartilaginous exostoses on the radial side of the ulnar metaphysis, for example (Fig. 2.**319**), or from a cessation of growth on the ulnar side following a radial epiphyseal plate fracture (Fig. 2.**320**).

A **short ulna** is most commonly encountered in the more complex skeletal dysplasias (e.g., achondroplasia, Morquio type IV mucopolysaccharidosis).

Fracture, Subluxation, or Dislocation?

Traumatic epiphyseal separations are often very difficult to diagnose radiographically. They are usually seen better in the lateral view than in the PA projection (Fig. 2.**321**).

Subtle displacement of the epiphysis relative to the metaphysis or an asymmetric width of the physis (gaping) can often be appreciated only by comparison with the opposite side (Fig. 2.**322**).

Epiphyseal slip and separation should be distinguished from **stress-induced widening of the physis** (Fig. 2.**323**).

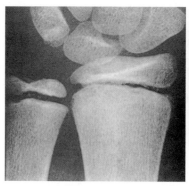
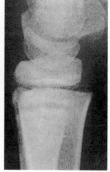

a   b

Fig. 2.**321 a, b** Epiphyseolysis, appreciated only in the lateral radiograph (**b**) which shows dorsal displacement.

During growth, the epiphyseal growth plate is particularly susceptible to acute and chronic stresses because the articular capsule and ligaments are two to five times stronger than the growth cartilage (Harsha 1957). Stress-induced widening of the physis is generally associated with stress fractures of the growth cartilage or with metaphyseal fractures (Fliegel 1986, Carter et al. 1988, Mandelbaum et al. 1989, Caine et al. 1992).

In Europe, **chronic stress-induced changes in the radial physis** are particularly common in patients who engage in strenuous gymnastic floor exercises, apparatus exercises, or breakdancing. Besides physeal widening, radiographs show irregular marginal fraying of the metaphysis. The ulnar physis may also be involved. Shih et al. (1995) described the MR imaging appearance of chronically stressed radial and ulnar physes in adolescent gymnasts at a Chinese opera school. The children did two hours of floor exercises daily for six days during ten months of the year, including up to 45 minutes of handstands. In addition to the conventional radiographic signs noted above, MRI showed horizontal metaphyseal fractures and physeal cartilage extension into the metaphysis. In another study in

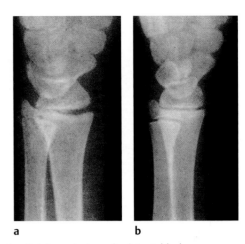

Fig. 2.**322 a, b** Epiphyseolysis, only detectable by an asymmetric widening of the palmar part of the epiphyseal space in **a**. Diagnosis is aided by comparison with the opposite side.

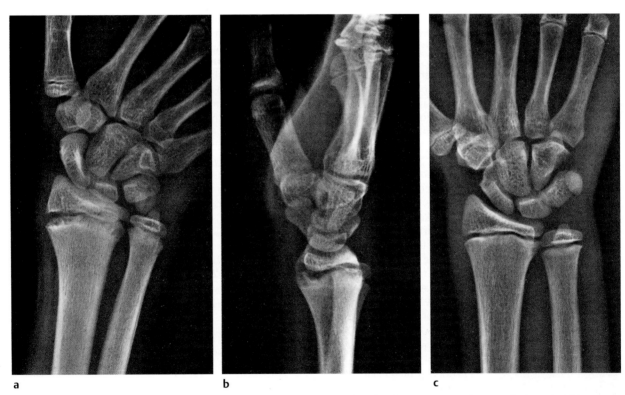

Fig. 2.**323 a–c** Effects of chronic stress on the physis.
a, b Biplane views.

c When the chronic stress is eliminated, physeal width returns to normal.

Fig. 2.**324 a, b** Fresh impacted radial fracture.
a The radial fracture cannot be positively identified, especially with the slight projection error.
b Three weeks later, initial callus appears in the form of a dense transverse band.

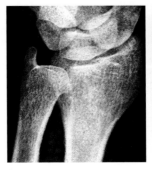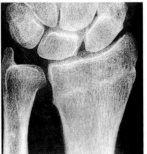

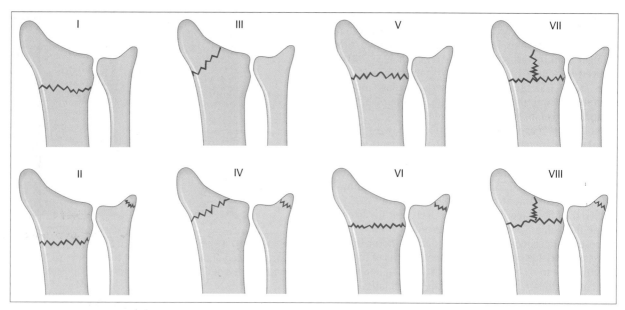

Fig. 2.**325**   Frykman classification of distal radial fractures.

the same population, Chang et al. (1995) found additional radiological changes that included metaphyseal sclerosis, gaps in the metaphysis, and small fragments within the physis.

Subluxation of the distal radioulnar joint can be difficult to detect on conventional radiographs despite marked clinical symptoms. It is essential to obtain an accurate projection and avoid supination or pronation of the wrist. The lateral radiograph should be taken without shoulder abduction, with the elbow flexed 90°, and with the forearm in neutral rotation (Mino et al. 1983, Mino et al. 1985, Nakamura et al. 1995). In many cases, however, it is technically impossible to obtain a neutral lateral radiograph, and CT should be used to detect subluxation by the modified radioulnar line method (Fig. 2.**145**; Nakamura et al. 1996). Staron et al. (1994) reported on the normal and abnormal geometry of the distal radioulnar joint based on MRI findings in symptomatic and asymptomatic patients.

The Frykman classification is one of several systems that have been devised for the classification of distal radial fractures (Fig. 2.**325** and Table 2.**20**). A **Barton fracture** is an intra-articular dorsal rim fracture of the radius caused by **hyperextension trauma** (Figs. 2.**327**, 2.**328**). If there is dorsal angulation of the articular fragment, the injury is called a **Colles fracture**. A palmar rim fracture caused by **hyperflexion trauma** is termed a **reverse Barton fracture**, and palmar angulation of the distal fragment is termed a **Smith fracture**. Further details on distal radial fractures would exceed our scope, especially since there are generally no problems of distinguishing them from normal variants (except for small marginal avulsion fractures). Nondisplaced compression fractures of the distal radius can be extremely difficult to diagnose on conventional radiographic films (Fig. 2.**324**). This underscores the value of early CT, especially for confirming or excluding articular involvement. Subperiosteal fractures (greenstick fractures) (Fig. 2.**326**) may be missed on an improper lateral projection in which the buckled cortex is rotated out of view.

Avulsion fractures of the ulnar and radial styloid processes (Fig. 2.**276**, 2.**279**–2.**282**) should be differentiated from **persistent accessory ossification centers** (Fig. 2.**225**, 2.**309**–2.**312**; see also p. 175 and 189).

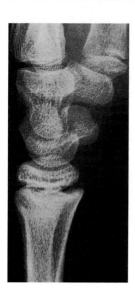

Fig. 2.**326**   Typical subperiosteal fracture with the presence of a step or bulge on the dorsal metaphyseal border (Aitken type 1 or Salter–Harris type II fracture).

> Whenever an isolated bone fragment is not completely enclosed by an intact cortical boundary, it should be assumed that a fracture is present.

Table 2.**20**   Frykman classification of distal radial fractures

Fracture line	Fracture type	Articular involvement	Ulnar styloid process
Extra-articular	I, II	–	Not fractured (= odd number)
Intra-articular	III, IV	Radiocarpal	
	V, VI	Distal radioulnar joint (DRUJ)	Fractured (= even number)
	VII, VIII	Radiocarpal + distal radioulnar joint (DRUJ)	

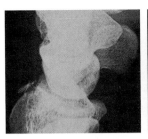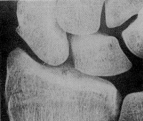

Fig. 2.**327**   Small Barton fracture.

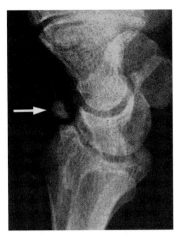

Fig. 2.**328**   Small Barton fracture (arrow). Complex radiocarpal disruption with a DISI configuration.

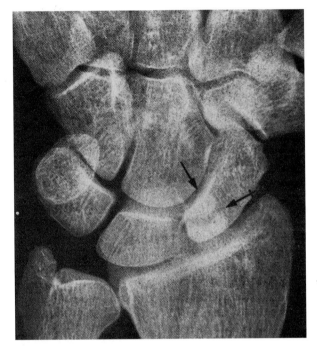

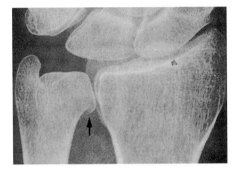

Fig. 2.**330**   Interruption of the proximal ulnar head contour by a fracture.

◁ Fig. 2.**329**   Accessory bone element (arrows) projected over the medial end of the scaphoid. The history was negative, making an old Barton fracture unlikely. Unfortunately we do not have a lateral radiograph, but it is reasonable to assume that the element is dorsal to the scaphoid.

Dorsal rim fractures of the distal radius caused by hyperextension trauma (Barton fracture, see above and Figs. 2.**327** and 2.**328**) require differentiation from rare accessory bone elements such as the os epilunatum (history, Fig. 2.**329**).

Isolated fractures of the ulnar head are rare and can be difficult to diagnose (e.g., Fig. 2.**330**).

 Necrosis?

Necrosis of the distal radial and ulnar epiphyses and especially of the styloid processes is an occupational hazard in workers exposed to significant repetitive stresses (e.g., jack-hammer operators). The necrotic area consists radiographically of very dense, crumbly bone fragments accompanied by irregular lucencies in the adjacent bone (Figs. 2.**331**–2.**333**).

Hypertrophic or duplicated processes and unfused ossification centers appear to be especially susceptible to necrosis (Figs. 2.**332**, 2.**333**). Necrotic bony elements are distinguished from persistent accessory epiphyseal centers of the radius and ulna by their increased density or

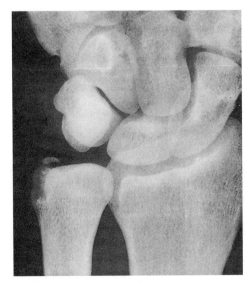

Fig. 2.**331**   Necrosis of the ulnar styloid process.

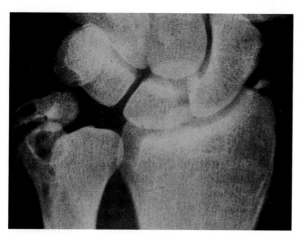

Fig. 2.**332** Osteonecrosis of an apparently congenitally hypertrophic ulnar styloid process and its persistent apophysis. The radial styloid process is also necrotic. (Figure 2.**333** shows the opposite wrist in the same patient.)

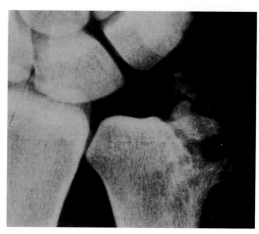

Fig. 2.**333** Osteonecrosis of the right ulnar styloid process. (Same patient as in Fig. 2.**332**.)

their nonhomogeneous density. The complicated term "aseptic necrotic ulnar styloidosis" was used in some earlier studies to describe aseptic necrosis of the ulnar styloid process (Müller 1941, Wuensch 1957). Of course, the isolated necrosis of a bony element located distal to the ulnar styloid process must be differentiated from a necrotic portion of the styloid process that has broken away from the parent bone.

Osteochondritis dissecans of the ulnar head was described by Schöneich (1952).

 ## Inflammation?

Along with the tibia and femur, the distal radial metaphysis is among the most common sites of involvement by inflammatory bone changes, including chronic lesions such as Brodie's abscess. These changes should not be difficult to distinguish from normal, as there are no normal structural variants in the distal radial metaphysis and epiphysis that resemble inflammatory changes.

The situation is different with the **styloid processes**, in which **erosions** can occur due to inflammatory changes in the adjacent bursa. This particularly applies to the ulnar styloid process. The extensor carpi ulnaris tendon sheath, located adjacent to this process, is frequently involved by inflammatory processes, especially rheumatoid arthritis. The earliest radiographic change is a loss of sharp cortical outlines, followed later by destructive changes in the form of marginal erosions of the ulnar styloid process (Fig. 2.**334**).

In advanced cases the styloid processes may completely disappear. If the inflammatory process subsides, bone regeneration can occur, marked radiographically by hypertrophic, fungiform new bone formation (Fig. 2.**335 a, b**).

> The differentiation of very early erosions, marked by irregular, ill-defined bony margins, from a borderline-normal styloid process requires extremely high-quality radiographs viewed with a magnifying lens.

The destructive cartilage changes in **chondrocalcinosis** (pseudogout) are accompanied in late stages by "reactive" or consecutive arthritis. This leads to an involvement of the distal radial joint contours, which show increasingly severe erosive and destructive changes. Typically the scaphoid bone subluxates into the groovelike excavated articular surface of the radius. The detection of cartilage calcifications, especially in the triangular fibrocartilage, is among the findings that support this diagnosis (see also Fig. 2.**70**).

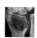 ## Tumor?

Neither the distal radius nor the distal ulna has physiological concavities or intraosseous rarefied areas that could mimic a tumor. But the distal radial metaphysis is not an infrequent site of involvement by bone tumors, apparently because it is an active growth region that contributes approximately 80% to the longitudinal growth of the radius. This makes the distal radial metaphysis, like the metaphyses about the knee joint, a site of predilection for osteosarcomas, chondrosarcomas, giant cell tumors, and a number of tumorlike lesions. Figure 2.**307 b** shows a subperiosteal ganglion, which should not be mistaken for the physiological ridge at that location (Fig. 2.**307 a**).

We referred earlier to the bony prominence that normally occurs on the radial side of the former epiphyseal growth plate. Again, this feature should not be confused with a flat exostosis, for example, or with abnormal periosteal processes.

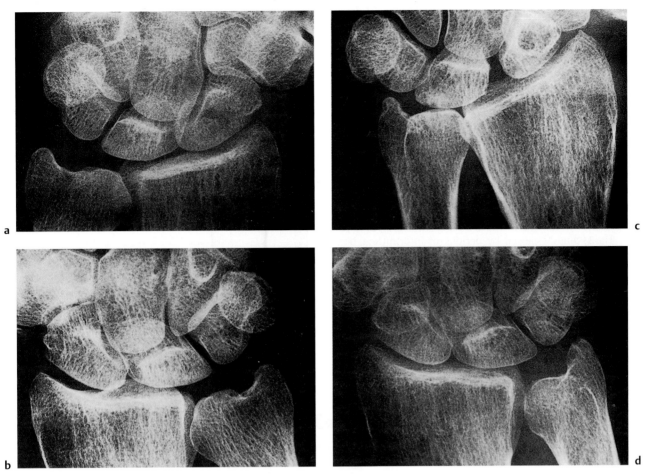

a

b

c

d

Fig. 2.**334a–d** Rheumatoid arthritis.
a, b Normal-appearing ulnar styloid process on each side. Soft-tissue swelling was present on the left side.

c, d Radiographs one year later show erosions of both ulnar styloid processes.

Fig. 2.**335a–d** Variable morphology of the ulnar styloid process.
a, b Reactive hypertrophic ulnar styloid processes in a woman with a history of severe, bilateral stress-related extensor carpi ulnaris tendinitis 10 years before. Earlier radiographs showed subtotal destruction of the ulnar styloid process on both sides. The patient is now free of complaints. New films show pronounced, bilateral, clinically palpable hypertrophy of the ulnar styloid processes. If the history were negative, it would have been reasonable to interpret the large, stout processes as normal variants. Osteopoikilosis is noted as an incidental finding.
c, d The small, short ulnar styloid processes in this patient are a normal variant.

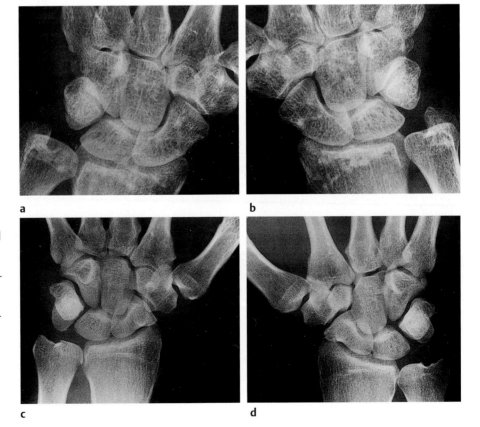

a

b

c

d

Other Changes?

The distal ends of the radius and ulna are of special diagnostic importance in various metabolic disorders and inflammatory diseases in the pediatric age group. For example, the early stage of **rickets**, before there is visible cupping of the distal radial metaphysis, presents radiographically with intracortical striations and a gradual disappearance of the metaphyseal ring (p. 187).

The features that distinguish rickets from scurvy and syphilis are described in Table 2.**21** and shown schematically in Fig. 2.**336**. Radiographs illustrating different stages of rickets are shown in Figs. 2.**337** and 2.**338**.

Transverse striations in the cancellous bone, especially in the distal radius, represent "growth lines" ("Harris lines") caused by periods of intermittent bone growth. They may be an entirely normal phenomenon, or they may reflect transient growth disturbances in various diseases.

Osteoarthritic changes in the distal radioulnar joint are relatively rare, especially when there is no predisposing condition such as a posttraumatic deformity of the articulating bone ends. Osteoarthritic changes have been described in occupations that involve repetitive twisting movements of the radioulnar joint (Fig. 2.**339**).

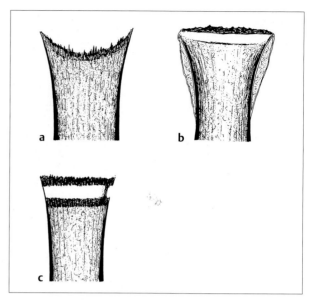

Fig. 2.**336a–c**   Differential diagnosis of rickets (see also Figs. 2.**348c** and 2.**350**).
a Rickets.
b Scurvy.
c Congenital syphilis.

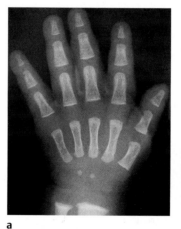

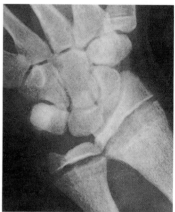

Fig. 2.**337a,b**   Classic appearance of rickets in relatively early radiological stages. In **a**, a 5-month-old girl; in **b**, a 12-year-old girl.   ▷

a   **b**

Table 2.**21**   Differentiation of rickets, scurvy, and syphilis (after Holthausen)

Rickets	Scurvy	Syphilis (congenital)
Rare in the first 3 months (except in premature and growth-retarded infants)	Rare before 5 months (except in premature infants)	Pronounced during the first 3 months
Epiphyseal centers poorly calcified, „delayed" maturation	Isolated decalcification of the epiphyseal centers	No involvement of epiphyses
Cupping, blurring, and fraying of the metaphysis with absence of the metaphyseal ring	Dense, irregular metaphyseal ring accompanied by a broad lucent zone on the diaphyseal side ("scurvy line", Trummerfeld zone)	Metaphyseal ring is dense, irregular, and sometimes spiculated; lucent zone with contour defects toward the diaphysis (Wimberger's sign)
Generalized decalcification		
Bowing of bones		
Frequent fractures (without subperiosteal hemorrhage)	Frequent metaphyseal fractures and epiphysiolysis	Fractures are rare
Cortical striations, periosteal reaction only in the healing stage	Extensive subperiosteal hemorrhage with calcification of hematomas	Always inflammatory periosteal reaction along the shaft

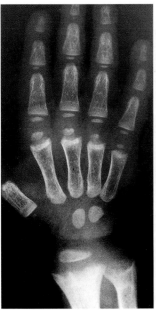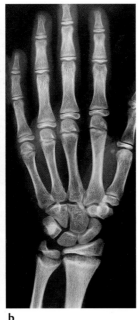

a   b

Fig. 2.**338 a, b** Examples of advanced rickets.
a Metaphyseal cupping not only of the distal radial and ulnar metaphyses but also of the metacarpals in a 4-year-old child.
b "Immigrant rickets" with secondary, regulative hyperparathyroidism in an 11-year-old girl who always wore a veil outdoors.

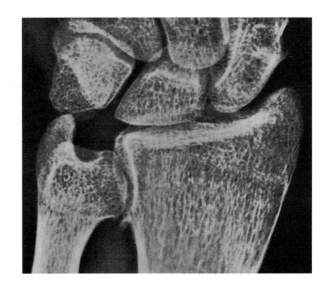

Fig. 2.**339** Radioulnar osteoarthritis caused by repetitive occupational pronation-supination of the left hand. The diagnosis of this case is not based entirely on the proximal osteophytes but also on signs such as increased density of the subchondral bone plate of the radius and fine subchondral lucencies in the ulna.

It should be added that **synovial chondromatosis** can apparently involve the distal radioulnar joint (Ballet et al. 1984). The calcified cartilage spheres that initially appear in this tumorlike joint process should not be mistaken for accessory bone elements.

References

Ballet, F. L., H. K. Watson, J. Ryu: Synovial chondromatosis of the distal radioulnar joint. J. Hand Surg. 9-A (1984) 590

Bugyi, B.: Atypische Veränderungen der Handgelenkknochen bei Preßluftwerkzeugarbeitern. Fortschr. Röntgenstr. 117 (1972) 346

Buttenberg, H.: Zur Bedeutung von Polsterepiphysen bei entwicklungsgestörten Kindern. Fortschr. Röntgenstr. 107 (1967) 786

Caine, D., S. Roy, K. M. Singer et al.: Stress changes of the distal radial growth plate: a radiographic survey and review of the literature. Amer. J. Sports Med. 20 (1992) 290

Carter, S. R., M. J. Aldridge, R. Fitzgerald et al.: Stress changes of the wrist in adolescent gymnasts. Brit. J. Radiol. 61 (1988) 109

Chang, Ch.-Y., Ch. Shih, I.-W. Penn et al.: Wrist injuries in adolescent gymnasts of a chinese opera school: radiographic survey. Radiology 195 (1995) 861

Chunhsi, Sh., Ch.-Y. Chang, I. W. Penn: Chronically stressed wrists in adolescent gymnasts: MR imaging appearance. Radiology 195 (1995) 855

de Cuveland, E.: Epiphysènnekrose des Radius. Z. Orthop. 83 (1953) 279

Dihlmann, W.: Der Processus styloides ulnae – ein röntgenologischer Indikator für chronische rheumatische Polyarthritiden. Fortschr. Röntgenstr. 109 (1968) 199

Escobedo, E. M., A. G.Bergmann, J. C. Hunter: MR imaging of ulnar impaction. Skelet. Radiol. 24 (1995) 85

Fischer, E.: Neues Skelettelement dorsal am Radio-Carpalgelenk. Fortschr. Röntgenstr. 91 (1959) 530

Fliegel, C. P.: Stress related widening of the radial growth plate in adolescents. Ann. Radiol. 29 (1986) 374

Frahm, R., M. Schwarz, M. Geishauser: Seltene Hypersupinationsluxation im distalen radioulnaren Gelenk. Fortschr. Röntgenstr. 150 (1989) 746

Gerber, S. D., P. P. Griffin, B. P. Simmons: Break dancer's wrist. Case report. J. pediat. Orthop. 6 (1986) 98

Ghantus, M. K.: Growth of the shaft of the human radius and ulna during the first two years of life. Amer. J. Roentgenol. 65 (1951) 784

Gollasch, W.: Osteochondritis dissecans des Handgelenkes. Röntgenpraxis 14 (1942) 468

Gumbs, V. L., D. Segal, J. B. Halligan et al.: Bilateral distal radius and ulnar fractures in adolescent weight lifters. Amer. J. Sports Med. 10 (1982) 375

Hafner, R., A. K. Poznanski, J. M. Donovan: Ulnar variance in children—standard measurements for evaluation of ulnar shortening in juvenile rheumatoid arthritis, hereditary multiple exostosis and other bone or joint disorders in childhood. Skelet. Radiol. 18 (1989) 513

Harsha, W. N.: Effects of trauma upon epihyses. Clin. Orthop. 10 (1957) 140

Horvàth, F., T. Kàkosy: Arthrose des distalen radioulnaren Gelenkes bei Motorsägenbetreibern. Fortschr. Röntgenstr. 131 (1979) 54

Imaeda, T., R. Nakamura, K. Shionoya et al.: Ulnar impaction syndrome: MR imaging findings. Radiology 201 (1996) 495

Le Veau, B.F., D. B. Bernhardt: Developmental biomechanics: effects of forces on the growth, development, and maintenance of the human body. Phys. Ther. 64 (1984) 1874

Mandelbaum, B. R., A. R. Bartolozzi, C. A. Davis et al.: Wrist pain syndrome in the gymnast: pathogenetic, diagnostic, and therapeutic considerations. Amer. J. Sports Med. 17 (1989) 305

Magee, Th. H., A. M. Rowedder, G. G. Degnan: Intraosseus ganglia of the wrist. Radiology 195 (1995) 517

Mino, D. E., A. K. Palmer, E. M. Levinsohn: The role of radiography and computed tomography in the diagnosis of subluxation and dislocation of the distal radioulnar joint. J. Hand Surg. 8 (1983) 23

Mino, D. E., A. K. Palmer, E.M. Levinsohn: Radiography and computerized tomography in diagnosis of incongruity of the distal radio-ulnar joint. J. Bone Jt Surg. 57-A (1985) 247

Müller, J. H.: Die Styloidosis ulnae aseptica necroticans. Röntgenpraxis 13 (1941) 419

Nakamura, R., E. Horii, T. Imaeda et al.: Criteria for diagnosing distal radioulnar joint subluxation by computed tomography. Skelet. Radiol. 25 (1996) 649

Nakamura, R., E. Horii, T. Imeada et al.: Distal radioulnar joint subluxation and dislocation diagnosed by standard roentgenography. Skelet. Radiol 24 (1995) 91

Palmer, A. K., F. Werner: Biomechanics of the distal radioulnar joint. Clin. Orthop. 187 (1984) 26

Palmer, A. K.: Triangular fibrocartilage lesions: a classification. J. Hand Surg. 14-A (1989) 594

Palmer, A. K.: Triangular fibrocartilage disorders: injury patterns and treatment. Arthroscopy 6 (1990) 125

Pitt, M. J.: Rachitic and osteomalacic syndromes. Radiol. Clin. N. Amer. 19 (1981) 581

Roy, St. R., D. Caine, K. M. Singer: Stress changes of the distal radial epiphysis in young gymnasts. Amer. J. Sports Med. 13 (1985) 301

Schöneich, R.: Osteochondritis dissecans am Ulnaköpfchen. Fortschr. Röntgenstr. 76 (1952) 268

Shih, Ch., Ch.-Y.Chang, I.-W. Penn et al.: Chronically stressed wrists in adolescent gymnasts: MR imaging appearance. Radiology 195 (1995) 855

Staron, R. B., F. Feldmann, N. Haramati et al.: Abnormal geometry of the distal radioulnar joint: MR findings. Skelet. Radiol. 23 (1994) 369

Uchiyama S., K. Terayama: Radiographic changes in wrists with ulnar plus variance observed over a ten-year period. J. Hand Surg. 16-A (1991) 45

Viegas, S. F., R. M. Patterson, J. A. Hokanson et al.: Wrist anatomy: incidence, distribution, and correlation of anatomic variations, tears, and arthrosis. J. Hand Surg. 18-A (1993) 463

Diaphysis of the Forearm

▌ *Normal Findings*

Linear or punched-out lucencies in the radial and ulnar shaft usually represent nutrient canals when detected incidentally. They may be seen in an end-on or tangential projection (Figs. 2.**340**, 2.**341**).

On closer inspection, a nutrient canal in the tangential projection passes through the entire cortex and is then lost in the medullary cavity (Fig. 2.**341**). Fissures, on the other hand, usually run a longer distance through the cortex and are also projected into the medullary cavity. Nutrient canals are most clearly demonstrated in a macerated specimen by bending open a paperclip, inserting the wire into the canal, and then rotating the specimen during fluoroscopic imaging (Fig. 2.**414**). The radial shaft generally shows a gentle curve with the convexity directed radially and toward the flexor side. The ulnar shaft is gently curved toward the ulnar side in its middle and distal thirds, and its proximal third is curved toward the extensor side. The **interosseous crest** arises from the medial cortex of the radial shaft. The greater the curvature of the bone, the more prominent the crest (Fig. 2.**343**). A similar crest is present on the ulnar shaft. The extent of the interosseous crest is clearly demonstrated on CT scans (Fig. 2.**342**).

▌ In the lateral projection, the overlap of the radius and ulna may create a linear lucency (Mach band phenomenon). This should not be misinterpreted as a fracture.

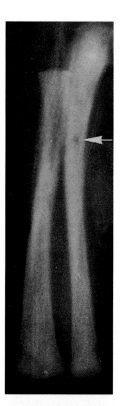

Fig. 2.**340** End-on projection of a nutrient canal in the ulna of a 6-day-old infant (arrow).

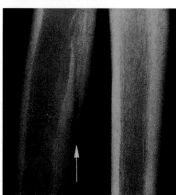

Fig. 2.**341** Tangential projection of a nutrient canal at the center of the radial-shaft (arrow).

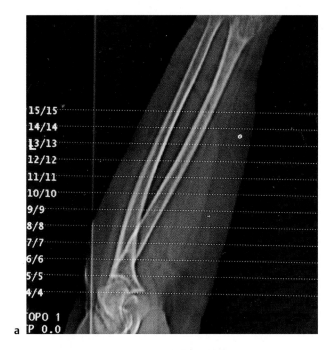

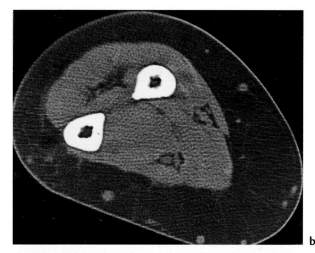

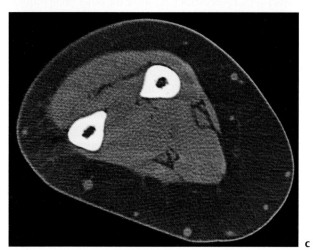

Fig. 2.**342 a–c** CT scans through the middle third of the radis and ulna, showing the location and extent of the interosseous crests (**b, c**). The flexor side is downward. The corresponding scout view is shown in panel **a**.

Fig. 2.**343 a, b** Radiographic appearance of the interosseous ▷ crest.

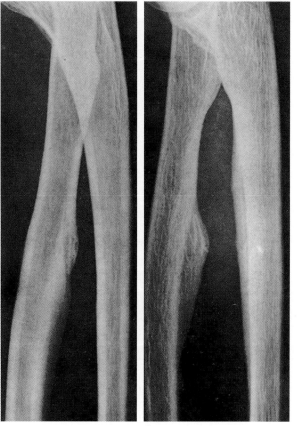

Pathological Finding?

Normal Variant or Anomaly?

The normal, gentle curvatures of the radius and ulna were described above.

> This physiological "bowing" should not be confused with **acute plastic bowing** of the forearm, which is definitely pathological and is caused by multiple traumatic microfractures whose summation effect is a more or less generalized bowing (Fig. 2.**346a**).

Not infrequently, the bowing of one forearm bone is combined with a greenstick fracture of the other bone (Borden 1975, Crowe and Swischuk 1977, Braune 1985). If doubt exists, the diagnosis can be confirmed by investigating the opposite side or obtaining a bone scan (Miller and Osterkamp 1982). A positive bone scan will show greatly increased tracer uptake throughout the diaphysis.

The forearm is subject to numerous dysplasias and deformities, the most important of which are listed in Table 2.**22**. Figure 2.**344** illustrates Holt–Oram syndrome, and Fig. 2.**345** shows the typical features of Nievergelt syndrome.

Radial clubhand is a congenital deformity characterized by hypoplasia or aplasia of the radius. The deficiency may involve the thumb. The wrist deviates markedly toward the radial side due to the absence of a normal buttress on that side. The mode of inheritance is unknown. The deformity is bilateral in 50–70% of cases. The thumb may be hypoplastic in unilateral cases. The condition has various clinical and functional sequelae that need not be discussed here.

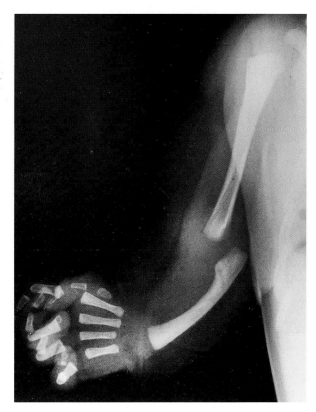

Fig. 2.**344**   Radial aplasia (reduction deformity) in a 5-day-old child with Holt–Oram syndrome.

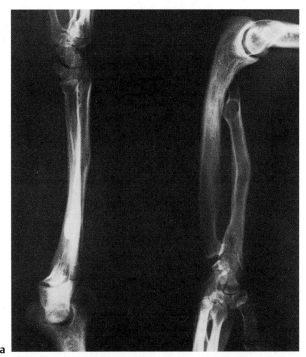

a

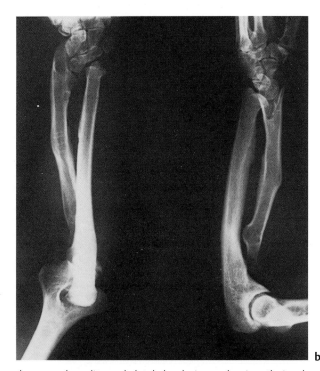

b

Fig. 2.**345a, b**   Nievergelt yndrome (mesomelic dysplasia). Note the proximal shortening of the radius, the bowing of the radius and ulna, and the anomalies and malalignments in the wrist. Radioulnar synstosis is also common in Nievergelt syn-drome, a hereditary skeletal dysplasia predominantly involving the midportions of the extremities and associated with synostoses.

Table 2.**22** Dysplasias and deformities of the forearm and important syndromic associations or other causes

Hypoplasia or aplasia of the radius and/or thumb
- Cornelia de Lange syndrome
- Fanconi syndrome (pancytopenia–dysmelia syndrome, Fig. 2.**388**)
- Holt–Oram syndrome (Fig. 2.**344**)
- Isolated anomaly (may be associated with ulnar hypoplasia)
- Phocomelia (e.g., thalidomide embryopathy)
- Thrombocytopenia-absent radius syndrome

Radioulnar synostosis (p. 225)
- Ehlers–Danlos syndrome
- Holt–Oram syndrome
- Idiopathic, isolated anomaly
- Multiple cartilaginous exostoses
- Trauma (ossification of interosseous membrane)

Forearm deformities
- Traumatic
- Enchondromatosis, exostoses
- Madelung deformity
- Osteogenesis imperfecta
- Over- and underconstriction (over- and undertubulation)[1] in numerous congenital and acquired diseases (see Kozlowski and Beighton 1984).

[1] Overconstriction (overtubulation) refers to a long, thin bone; underconstriction (undertubulation) has the opposite meaning.

The radiographic signs of radial clubhand are listed below (after Schmitt and Lanz 1996).

- Radial anomaly
  - Type I: absence of the distal radial epiphysis
  - Type II: radius present but shortened (hypoplastic)
  - Type III: only the proximal radius is present (partial aplasia)
  - Type IV: complete radial aplasia
- Ulna bowed toward the radial side, thickened, and approximately 60% of normal length
- Thumb absent or hypoplastic
- Carpal bones fused or partially absent (scaphoid, trapezium)
- Humerus shortened and distally deformed

Ulnar clubhand is a sporadically occurring congenital anomaly affecting the ulnar portions of the hand and forearm. It is relatively rare. Because the humeroulnar joint is absent or deficient, the function of the elbow joint is usually seriously impaired while the wrist is stable.

The radiographic signs of ulnar clubhand are as follows (after Schmitt and Lanz 1996):

- Ulnar anomaly
  - Type I: ulna present but shortened (hypoplastic)
  - Type II: only the proximal ulna is present (partial aplasia)
  - Type III: complete ulnar aplasia
  - Type IV: radiohumeral synostosis
- Ulnar bowing of the radius in types II and IV
- Radius subluxated at the elbow in types I and III
- Aplasia or syndactyly of the ulnar fingers and wrist (hamate, capitate, triquetrum, pisiform)

 Fracture, Subluxation, or Dislocation?

We cannot explore all the aspects of radial and ulnar fractures within the scope of this monograph. It is sufficient to point out that transverse fractures of the ulna alone as well as combined, nondisplaced midshaft fractures of the radius and ulna are usually parry fractures. A radial shaft fracture at the junction of the distal and middle thirds combined with a distal radioulnar joint dislocation and with possible avulsion of the ulnar styloid process is called a **Galeazzi fracture**.

The features of a complete avulsion of the interosseous crest of the ulna can be found in specialized publications (e.g., Kácl and Kolàr 1958).

Congenital pseudarthrosis of the ulna occurs typically in neurofibromatosis (Ostrowski et al. 1985).

Stress fractures are not limited to the lower extremity and are seen with increasing frequency in the upper extremity as well, especially in high-performance athletes. The ulna is most commonly affected (Mutoh et al. 1982). This type of fracture is particularly common in female volleyball players and male body builders (Hamilton 1981).

At sites where stress fractures occur, so-called Looser zones (pseudo-fractures) may also be found due to pathological structural changes in the bone (e.g., rickets, osteomalacia, renal osteodystrophy) (Fig. 2.**346**). They usually appear on radiographs as an indistinct, transverse lucent area surrounded by fluffy, usually hypertrophic callus.

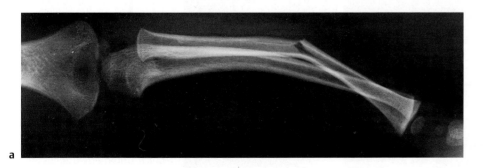

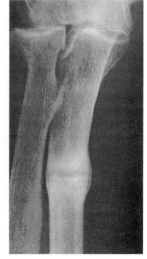

Fig. 2.**346 a, b** Acute plastic bowing in a radial shaft fracture and a so-called Looser zone.
a Acute plastic bowing of the ulna associated with a radial shaft fracture in a 2.5-year-old child. The bowed ulna does not appear to be fractured.
b Looser zone (pseudofracture or chronic insufficiency fracture) at a typical location in the proximal third of the ulnar shaft.

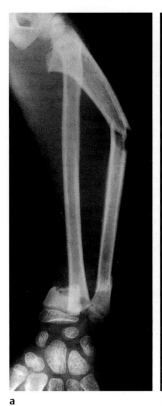
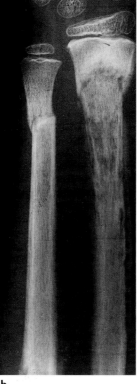

a   b

Fig. 2.**347 a, b**   Regional acceleratory phenomenon (RAP) mimicking ostenecrosis of he distal radial shaft following a complex forearm fracture in a 7-year-old boy. The radiograph **b** was taken about three weeks after the radiograph in **a** to monitor progress. Eight weeks later the radius was completely healed.

 Necrosis?

Necrosis of the radial and ulnar diaphysis is extremely unusual and occurs almost exclusively as a result of trauma. Its radiographic features pose no problems of differentiating normal findings from borderline-pathological findings and need not be discussed here. An exception is the **regional acceleratory phenomenon** (RAP) in the healing of pediatric fractures. The marked transient bone resorption that occurs in this phenomenon can simulate the appearance of osteonecrosis (Fig. 2.**347**).

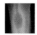 **Inflammation?**

Inflammatory bone processes involving the shafts of the radius and ulna are rare and occur almost entirely in adults. These changes do not play a role in the differential diagnosis of borderline findings in skeletal radiology.

In infants, periosteal new bone formation in conditions such as **Caffey syndrome** (infantile cortical hyperostosis, Fig. 2.**348 a, b**), **battered child syndrome** (Fig. 2.**349**), **syphilis** (Fig. 2.**350**), and **subperiosteal hemorrhage** (e.g., due to vitamin C deficiency, Fig. 2.**348 c**) can easily mimic an inflammatory process.

Most of these children present at a stage when the changes are already advanced and the radiographic findings are no longer borderline. We illustrate these findings with representative images, thereby continuing the *Borderlands* tradition of covering the rare and unusual.

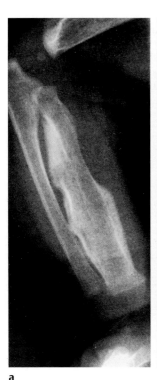
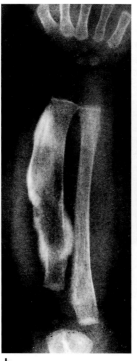
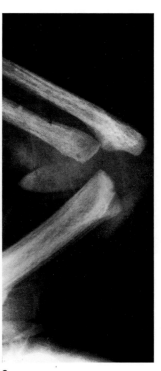

a   b   c

Fig. 2.**348 a–c**   Perioseal new bone formation on a pediatric forearm.
a, b Caffey syndrome (infantile cortical hyperostosis). Note the conspicuous periosteal bone formation on the radius, typically sparing the metaphyses and epiphyses.
c Extensive new periosteal bone formation on the humerus and forearm bones in scurvy (the same child also had extensive new periosteal bone formations on the lower extremities). Note that the periosteal new bone formation includes the metaphyses, in which Trummerfeld zones are also visible.

Fig. 2.**349 a, b** Battered child syndrome. Radiographs show considerable periosteal ossification on the humerus and subtle, smooth periosteal reactions on the radius and ulna.

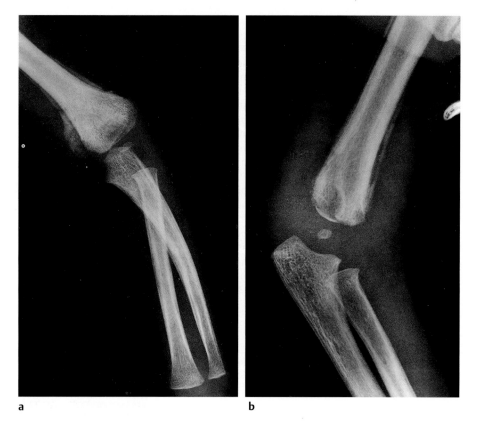

a   b

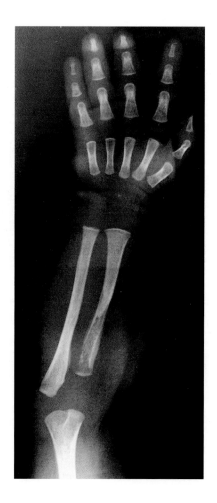

Fig. 2.**350** Osteolytic changes in the proximal radial shaft of ▷ a child with congenital syphilis (syphilitic osteitis). Note the accompanying periosteal reactions.

Tumor?

The radius and ulna are susceptible to marked trophic changes that are characterized by patchy demineralization on radiographs (Fig. 2.**351**) and may mimic tumorous destruction. They may involve a **regional osteoporosis** or osteodystrophy and are especially common in patients with obstructed lymphatic drainage (e.g., following mastectomy and radiotherapy in breast cancer patients). Also, Sudeck (reflex sympathetic) dystrophy may affect the radius and ulna without involving the hand. These changes are also seen in advanced hyperparathyroidism, whose manifestations include multiple foci of bone resorption that may show a patchy configuration (Fig. 2.**352**).

Among the resorptive processes that are caused either by primary osteoclastic hyperactivity and/or by excessive perfusion is **Paget disease** (osteitis deformans). Involvement of the forearm bones is unusual with this disease and usually occurs in polyostotic cases (Fig. 2.**353**).

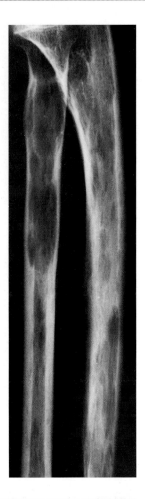

Fig. 2.**351**   Pseudomalignant osteoporosis of the forearm bones. The osteolytic lesions are a result of severe regional resorption, caused in turn by extensive trophic disturbances. This case presented clinically with severe lymphedema following a previous mastectomy and postoperative radiation.

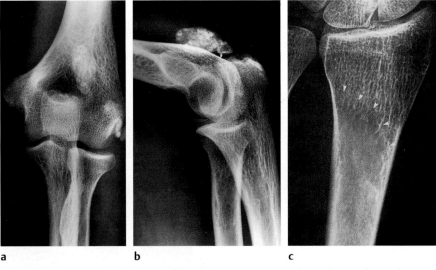

a   b   c

Fig. 2.**352a–c**   Secondary hyperparathyroidism in a patient with renal osteodystrophy.
a, b The ulna shows fine intracortical striations and a raryfied, lacy metaphyseal trabecular pattern, note the bursal calcifications.
c Marked rarefication of the cancellous bone (arrowheads).

Fig. 2.**353**   Paget's disease (osteitis deformans) of the ulna in a patient with polyostotic involvement. Note the generalized bone expansion and coarsened trabecular pattern throughout the ulnar shaft and proximal metaphysis. There is marked concomitant bowing of the ulna.   ▷

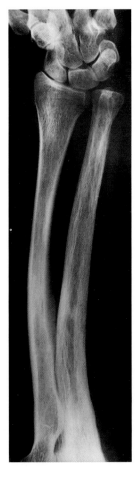

References

Borden, S.: Roentgen recognition of acute plastic bowing of the forearm in children. Amer. J. Roentgenol. 125 (1975) 524

Braune, M.: Maskierte Frakturen im Säuglings- und Kindesalter. Radiologe 25 (1985) 97

Cerezal, L., F. del Piñal, F. Abascal et al.: Imaging findings in ulnar-sided wrist impaction syndrome. Radiographics 22 (2002) 105

Crowe, J. E., L. E. Swischuk: Acute bowing fractures of the forearm in children. A frequently missed injury. Amer. J. Roentgenol. 128 (1977) 981

Garcia–Elias, M.: Dorsal fractures of the triquetrum: Avulsion or compression fractures? J. Hand Surg [Am] 12 (1987) 266

Hamilton, H. K.: Stress fracture of the diaphysis of the ulna in a body builder. Amer. J. Sports Med. 12 (1984) 405

Kácl, J., J. Kolàr: Eine ungewöhnliche Form der Ulnafraktur. Fortschr. Röntgenstr. 88 (1958) 244

Kemperdick, H., F. Majewski: Mesomeler Zwergwuchs vom Typ Langer als homozygote Form der Dyschondrosteose. Fortschr. Röntgenstr. 136 (1982) 583

Kozlowski, K., P. Beighton: Gamut Index of Skeletal Dysplasia. Springer, Berlin 1984

Miller, J. H., J. A. Osterkamp: Scintigraphy in acute plastic bowing of the forearm. Radiology 142 (1982) 742

Mutoh, Y., T. Mori, Y. Suzuki et al.: Stress fractures of the ulna in athletes. Amer. J. Sports Med. 10 (1982) 365

Ostrowski, D. M., R. E. Eilert, G. Waldstein: Congenital pseudarthrosis of the ulna: a report of two cases and a review of the literature. J. pediat. Orthop. 5 (1985) 463

Perry, C. R., H. M. Perry III, R. E. Burdge: Stress fracture of the radius following a fracture of the ulna diaphysis. Clin. Orthop. 187 (1984) 193

Topper, S. M., M. B. Wood, L. K. Ruby: Ulnar styloid impaction syndrome. J. Hand Surg [Am] 22 (1997) 699

Schmitt, R., U. Lanz: Bildgebende Diagnostik der Hand. Hippokrates, Stuttgart 1996

Tredwell, S. J., K. van Peteghem, M. Clough: Pattern of forearm fractures in children. J. pediat. Orthop. 4 (1984) 604

Elbow Region

Normal Findings

During Growth

A notch typically appears in the proximal end of the radius at 2–4 years of age and disappears by about 9–10 years of age (Fig. 2.**355**). The epiphyseal center of the radial head appears at about 4–5 years of age. Its morphology is highly variable, and multiple centers can occur (Fig. 2.**355**).

The proximal end of the ulna is blunt and stubby until about age 9 or 10, at which time a small ossification center for the olecranon becomes radiographically visible. It is best seen in the lateral projection (Fig. 2.**356**). Multiple centers may be present (Fig. 2.**357**) and located up to 5 mm from the main bone. When the centers fuse, fine bony trabeculae initially form cordlike structures that bridge the space to the proximal metaphysis (Figs. 2.**358**, 2.**359**). The fusion starts on the anterior (flexor) side, initially leaving a deep gap or groove posteriorly (Fig. 2.**360**). At 16–20 years of age, the ossification centers of the olecranon fuse completely with the shaft. There may be a small ossifica-

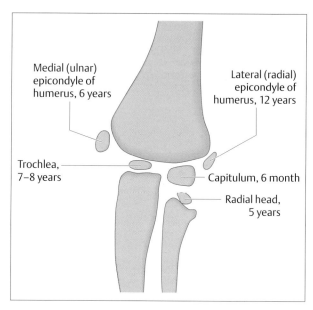

Fig. 2.**354** Ages at which ossification centers appear about the elbow joint in boys.

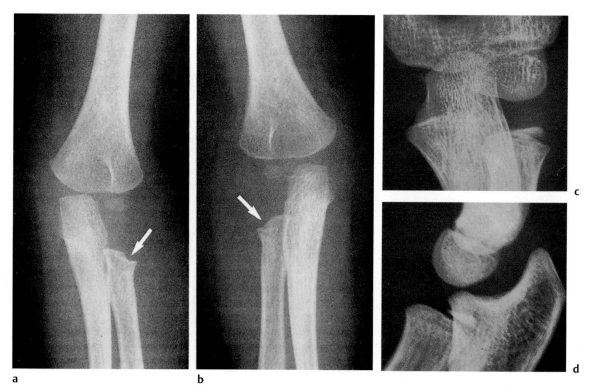

a b

Fig. 2.**355 a–d** Osseous development of the proximal radius. **a, b** Temporary, physiological notch in the radial head (arrows) of a 2-year-old girl.

c, d Atypical epiphyseal center of the radial head in a 10-year-old boy.

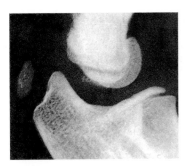

Fig. 2.**356** Ossification center of the olecranon.

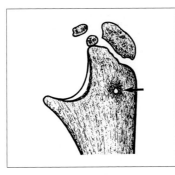

Fig. 2.**357** Multiple ossification centers of the olecranon tip. Nutrient canal (arrow).

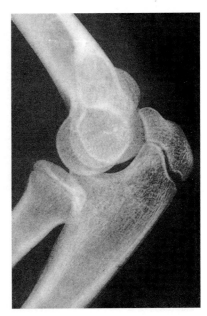

Fig. 2.**358** Fusion of the olecranon tip, here commencing on the flexor side of the growth plate.

tion center in the coronoid process that fuses earlier (at about 9–10 years of age?), but this is uncertain (see p. 218).

The epiphyseal and apophyseal centers about the elbow joint appear with some consistency in the following sequence in boys (Fig. 2.**354**):

- Capitulum of humerus: 6th month (1–12 months)
- Trochlea of humerus (usually multicentric): 8th year (6–10)
- Medial (ulnar) epicondyle of humerus: 6th year (4–8)
- Lateral (radial) epicondyle of humerus: 12th year (11–14)
- Olecranon: 10th year (8–12)

Radiographically visible ossification occurs up to two years earlier in girls.

The ossification center of the trochlea may occasionally appear before the ossification center of the medial (ulnar) epicondyle.

The ossification centers of the pediatric elbow and their variants are reviewed by Resnik and Hartenberg (1986). The radiographs in Fig. 2.**361** illustrate the development of the ossification centers about the elbow joint from 5 to 11 years of age.

A knowledge of the times of appearance of the various ossification centers is of major importance in the radiological diagnosis of pediatric trauma (see below).

The ossification center of the capitulum (known also as the capitellum) in small children occupies a relatively anterior position between the end of the humerus and the coronoid process (Fig. 2.**362a**). Posterior gaping of the epiphyseal cleft is a normal finding when the center is fully developed (Fig. 2.**362b**). The trochlea of the humerus often arises from multiple centers (Fig. 2.**362c, d**).

A small process extending from the ossification center of the medial (ulnar) epicondyle toward the trochlea is considered a normal finding (Bánki 1967, Fig. 2.**363**).

The ossification center of the lateral (radial) epicondyle is normally located relatively far from the end of the humerus.

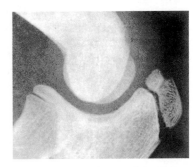

Fig. 2.**359** A small ossification center at the tip of the olecranon has fused with a larger center, and both centers have started to fuse with the rest of the olecranon. Note the fine ossifications within the growth plate.

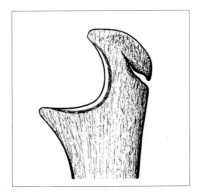

Fig. 2.**360** The olecranon center has already fused on the anterior side, leaving a deep gap on the posterior side (see also Fig. 2.**358**).

 The growth centers about the elbow joint contribute only about 10–20% to the longitudinal growth of the corresponding bones (humerus, radius, and ulna).

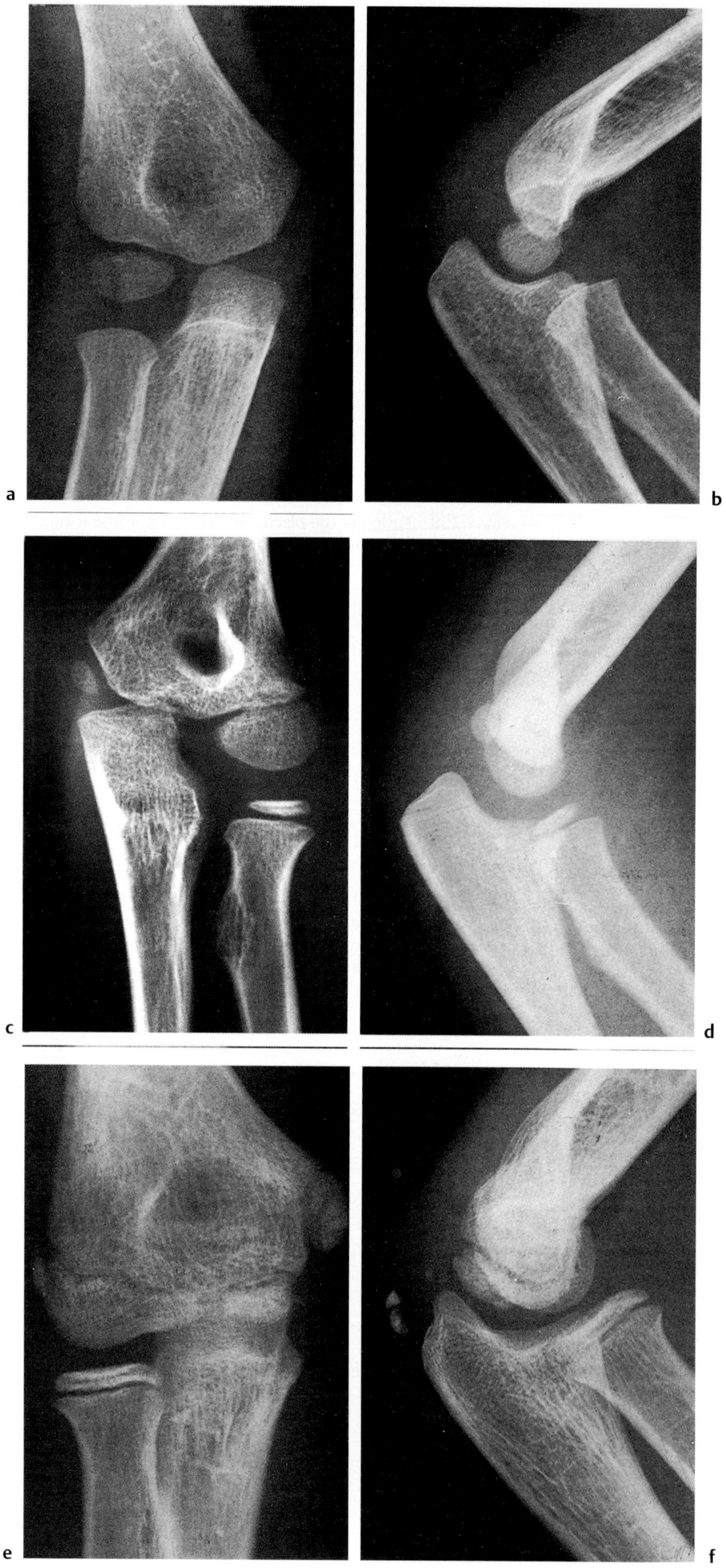

Fig. 2.**361 a–f**   Elbow ossification at different ages.
a, b Boy 5 years of age.
c, d Boy 7 years of age.
e, f Girl 11 years of age.

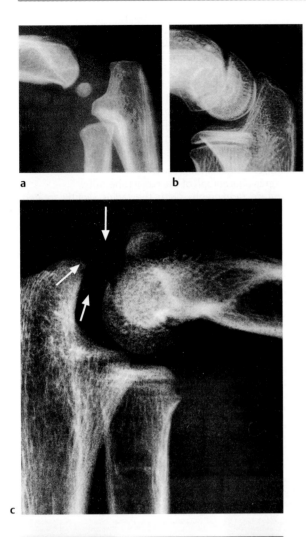

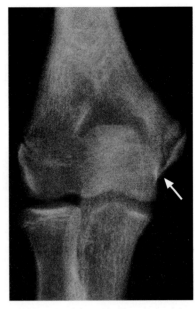

Fig. 2.**363** Distal processlike extension of the epicondylar epiphysis (arrow).

◁ Fig. 2.**362a–d** Development of the ossification centers of the capitulum and trochlea.
a At 3 years of age.
b At 8 years of age.
c, d Multiple ossification centers of the trochlea. In the lateral radiograph, three centers are projected into the humeroulnar joint space (arrows).

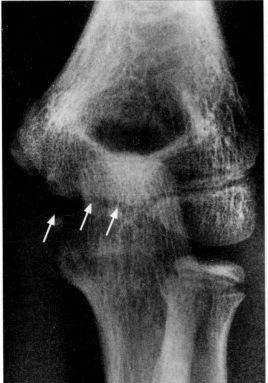

In Adulthood

The **radial tuberosity** appears on tangential projections as a broad-based, sharply defined prominence on the flexor surface of the radius. It is directed somewhat medially (ulnarly) in the sagittal projection. Physiologically, cancellous bone structures are relatively sparse below the radial tuberosity, typically causing the tuberosity to appear as a lucent area in the en-face projection (Fig. 2.364).

Anterolateral to the radial tuberosity is a bony fossa that also appears as a lucent area when projected en face (Fig. 2.364 g, h). This hollow usually receives the bicipito-radial bursa, which is located between the bone and the biceps tendon, which "wraps" around it during pronation. The more prominent the radial tuberosity, the deeper the fossa appears (Fig. 2.365 a–c).

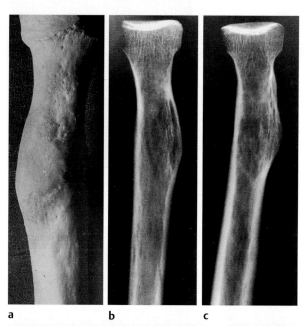

a   b   c

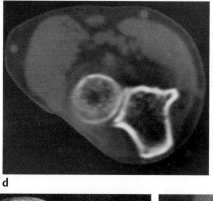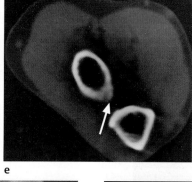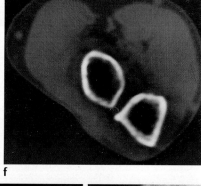

d   e   f

Fig. 2.**364 a–j**   Radial tuberosity.
a Anatomic photograph of the radial tuberosity.
b, c En-face radiographs (with the radius slightly rotated) show a lucent zone in the area of the tuberosity caused by the relatively scant trabeculae in this bony prominence.
d–f Axial CT scans of the proximal radius and ulna. Scan **d** is at the level of the radioulnar joint, scan **e** at the level of the radial tuberosity. Note the relative lucency of the tuberosity caused by the sparse cancellous trabeculae in that area (arrow). Scan **f** is at a somewhat more distal level, showing the prominent radial ridge on the ulna.
g, h Specimen photograph and radiograph in the same position show a small fossa in the radial cortex anteroradial to the tuberosity (arrow), probably caused by the bicipitoradial bursa.
i, j Unusual sclerosis of a nutrient canal, possibly a result of vascular thrombosis. Radiograph **j** shows an end-on projection of the "white" line in **i** (arrow). (Case courtesy of Professor Dr. S. Feuerbach, Regensburg.)

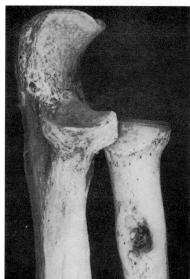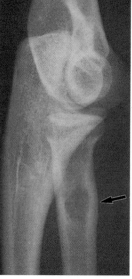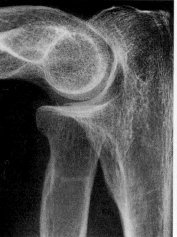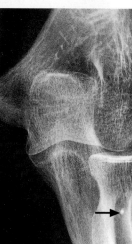

g   h   i   j

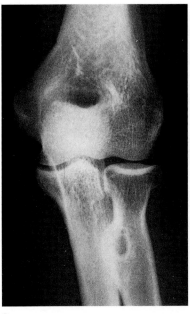
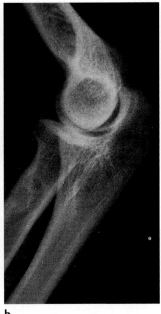
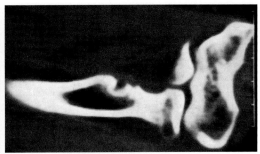

a

b

Fig. 2.**365 a–c** Very prominent radial tuberosity flanked by a bony fossa that appears as a conspicuous lucency when projected en face (**a**). The CT scan (**c**) shows how a more prominent tuberosity causes the fossa to appear deeper.

Level with the proximal end of the tuberosity is a physiological nutrient canal that runs in a sagittal direction, appearing as a bandlike lucency in the lateral projection and as a small hole in the PA projection. Sclerosis of the nutrient canal is unusual (Fig. 2.**364 i, j**).

Radiographs normally show a well-circumscribed elliptical lucency below the "confluence" of the olecranon and coronoid process (Fig. 2.**366**). It is not unusual to find nutrient canals in this area that appear as punched-out defects in the lateral projection.

It is also normal to find a small notch or incisure at the center of the ulnar articular margin (radiographic contour of the trochlear notch of the ulna, see below) (Figs. 2.**367**, 2.**401 b**).

A small transverse ridge is normally visible between the articular portion of the ulna formed by the olecranon and that formed by the coronoid process (which together form the trochlear notch or incisura semilunaris) when this area is viewed in the lateral projection (Figs. 2.**367 d**, 2.**368**).

A circumscribed, rounded lucency distal to the radial notch of the ulna (the articular facet for the radial head) marks the site of attachment of the radial annular ligament. This site may be fossa-shaped and seems most pronounced in patients who have an exceptionally large range of forearm supination.

The **shape of the distal humerus** is asymmetrical. The medial epicondyle forms a salient projection while the lateral epicondyle has a flattened, truncated shape. The projection of the lateral border of the capitulum over the medial epicondyle creates a double outline in the lateral radiograph.

The articular surface of the medial (ulnar) condyle (the trochlea) in the humeroulnar joint is somewhat broader than the articular surface of the lateral condyle (the capitulum) in the humeroradial joint. A cartilage-covered eminence separates the articular surfaces of the two humeral condyles. It may be flattened or spike-shaped, in the latter case appearing as a small intra-articular process when viewed in a tangential projection (Fig. 2.**368 b**).

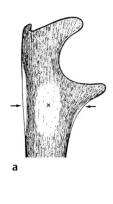

a

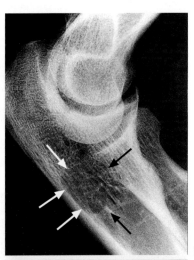

b

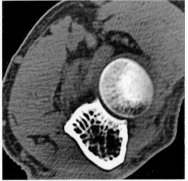

c

Fig. 2.**366** Physiological lucency in the proximal ulna.

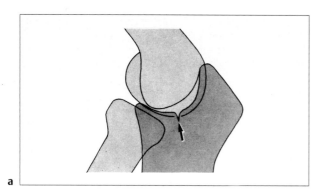

a

Fig. 2.**367 a–d**   Notch or groove in the articular margin of the ulna.

a A small notch or groove is visible in the articular margin of the ulna in the lateral projection (arrow).

b–d The photographs show that this notch is formed by a medial prominence of the articular margin at the junction of the olecranon and coronoid portions of the trochlear notch of the ulna (incisura semiluminaris ulnae), at the base of the coronoid process. A typical radiograph of the small notch is shown in Fig. 2.**401 b**.

Asterisk	Coronoid process of ulna
Arrow	Radiographic notch at junction of olecranon and coronoid process
Two arrows	Ridge lateral (radial) to the notch (see also Fig. 2.**368 a**).

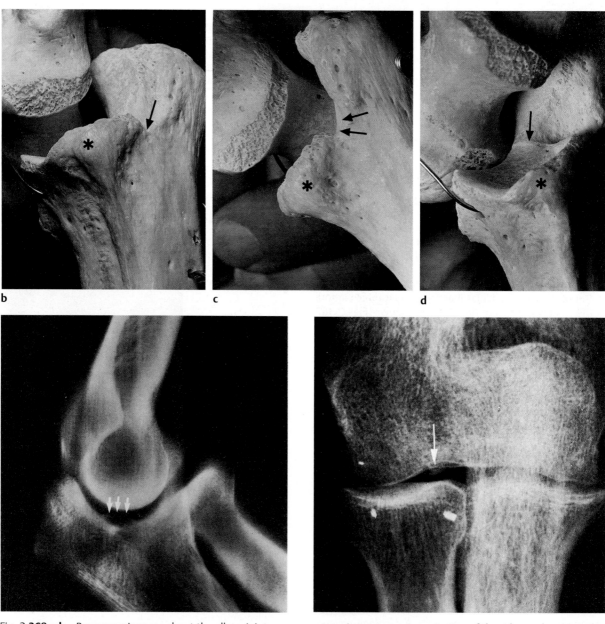

b

c

d

a

b

Fig. 2.**368 a, b**   Bony prominences about the elbow joint.

a Small pysiological ridge in the middle of the ulnar joint margin, occasionally visible in the lateral projection. It is located somewhat more anterior and superior on radiographs than the notch described above (Fig. 2.**67**). Anatomically, it corresponds to a ridgelike prominence in the trochlear notch that fits into the groove of the humeral trochlea (arrows). This tomo-

gram givs an accurate projection of the ridge and consequently does not show the notch in the articular rim (Fig. 2.**367**), which is located almost 1 cm medially (ulnar).

b Small prominence (arrow) represents a tangential projection of the intercondylar eminence in the articular surface of the humerus. This eminence is clearly visible on the anatomic specimen in Fig. 2.**370**.

In the lateral projection, the medial margin of the humeral trochlea may be superimposed over the medial peripheral ridge of the ulnar coronoid process (described in the legend to Fig. 2.**367 b–d**), simulating the appearance of a crescent-shaped density (Fig. 2.**369**).

The **ridgelike lateral border of the distal humerus** presents a very sharp edge from the lateral epicondyle to the humeral shaft (see anatomic specimen and CT scans in Fig. 2.**370 a**), with a correspondingly thin cortex. This feature should not be mistaken for periosteal new bone formation.

A **small notch** is normally seen **proximal to the medial epicondyle**, occasionally accompanied by thinning of the metaphyseal cortex. This notch corresponds to the gap between the attachments of the pronator teres and brachialis muscles. The greater the loads on these muscles (i.e., the more prominent their attachments), the more conspicuous is the notch or depression (Fig. 2.**370 b, c**).

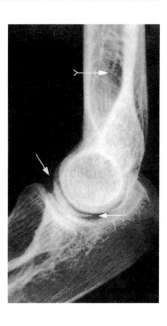

Fig. 2.**369** Apparent crescent-shaped "density" in the humeroradial joint (arrows). Normal structural lucency (double arrow).

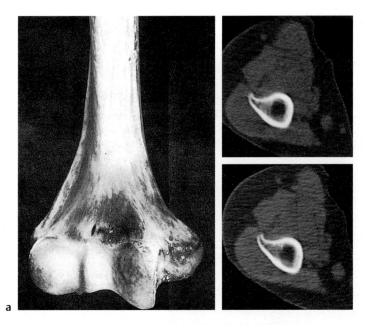

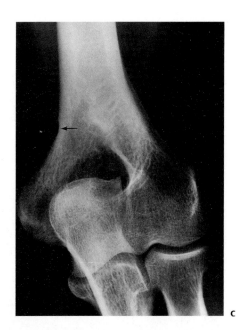

a

c

b

Fig. 2.**370 a–c** Radial intermuscular septum and notched contour of the medial epicondyle of the humerus.

a The lateral border of the distal humeral metaphysis is sharp and ridgelike toward the anterior side, forming the radial intermuscular septum. The brachioradialis ad extensor carpi radialis longus muscles are among the structures hat are attached to the septum. Because of its lucent, "fibrous" appearance on rdiographs, this rige is eaily mistaken for periosteal pathology (sealso panel **c**).

b, c Physioloical notch in the humeral border proximal to the medial (ulnar) epicondyle (arrow; also see text). (Radiograph **c** with kind permission of Dr. G. F. Jacobs, Düsseldorf.)

▌ *Pathological Finding?*

 Normal Variant or Anomaly?

Persistent ossification centers of the olecranon can occur as a variant, especially when there is a stress-related delay in the fusion of the olecranon center (similar to other apophyses and epiphyses, Fig. 2.**372**). Another variant is the **enlargement of a persistent olecranon ossification center**. This bony element was formerly called the "patella cubiti" in analogy to the patella of the knee. It is distinguished from a nonunited olecranon fracture by the history and clinical findings.

Occasionally the **ossification center of the olecranon tip** (p. 211) persists as an isolated bony element (Figs. 2.**371**, 2.**378**).

The olecranon spur is a result of productive fibro-ostosis and should be classified as a normal variant (Fig. 2.**373 a**). Like a spur on the calcaneal tuberosity, it is usually asymptomatic and is seen in almost 20–30% of all radiographs in adults over 45–50 years of age.

Olecranon spurs also occur in pathological conditions such as DISH syndrome and metabolic disorders (e.g., gout, diabetes mellitus) that are associated with metaplastic ossification at sites of tendon attachment. Occasionally, olecranon spurs break off spontaneously or in response to minor trauma (Fig. 2.**373 b**).

Persistence of the ossification center of the coronoid process could also be classified as a variant if there were

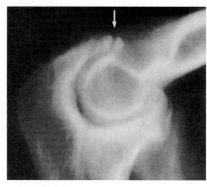

Fig. 2.**371**   Persistent ossification center for the tip of the olecranon (arrow) (lateral tomogram).

definite proof that this ossification center exists (p. 211) (Rumpold 1964). This finding was formerly called the "os cubiti anterius."

Persistent ossification centers also occur in the **epicondyles** as a normal variant (Günsel 1952, de Cuveland 1955, Hillger and Hamm 1956, Schröder 1956, Sieckel 1956; Figs. 2.**374**, 2.**375**).

By contrast, the unusually large bony element in the area of the medial epicondyle in Fig. 2.**376** most likely represents an old nonunion of a medial epicondyle fracture. One reason for this interpretation is the small ossicle that is projected into the bony element. Apparently it represents a persistent apophyseal center, similar to that on the lateral side.

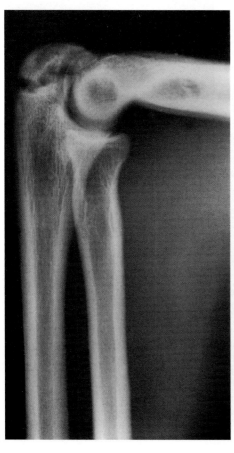

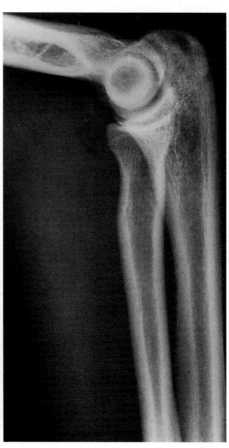

a   b

Fig. 2.**372 a, b**   Asymmetrical delay of olecranon ossification in a 17-year-old wrestler on the German olympic team. Note the widely gaping apophyseal cleft in this right-handed adolescent. Because the finding was painful and the ossification center shows some irregularities, the differential diagnosis included incipient necrosis of the ossification center. Radiograph taken six months after the suspension of training shows complete regression of the structural changes and fusion of the ossification center.

Fig. 2.**373 a, b**   Olecranon spur.
a Typical olecranon spur, actually considered a normal finding in adults.
b This very prominent spur has been broken from the olecranon due to trauma.

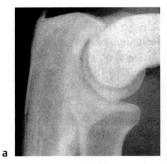

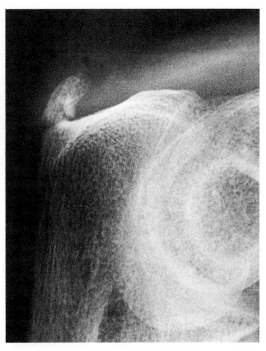

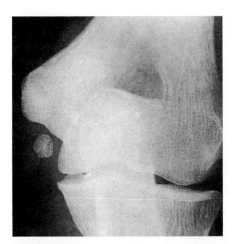

Fig. 2**374**   Ossicle locted at a tpical sitedistal tohe medial (ulnar) epicondyle.

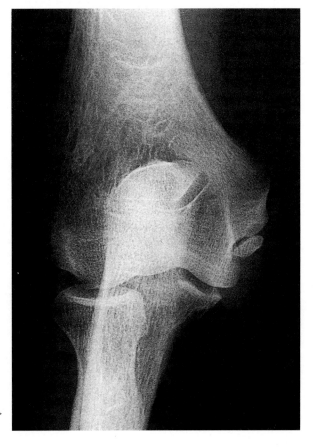

Fig. 2.**375**   Ossicle located at a typical site distal to the medial ▷ (ulnar) epicondyle.

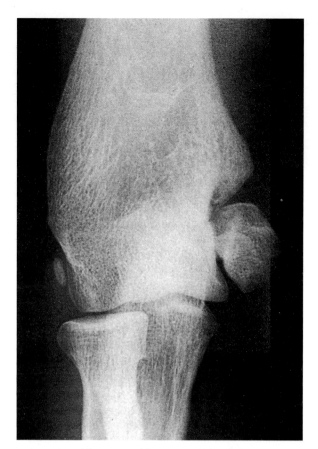

Fig. 2.**376** Old nonunited fragment of the ulnar epicondyle, onto which a small ossicle is projected. Another ossicle is visible adjacent to the radial epicondyle.

The epicondyles occasionally contain lucent areas that can mimic osteolytic lesions, especially in older patients (Fig. 2.**377**). These are areas in which the fine cancellous trabeculae have been replaced by fatty tissue.

The coronoid fossa and olecranon fossa may be separated by a bony layer only a few millimeters thick or in some cases by a paper-thin membrane that forms an apparent orifice on radiographs called the **supratrochlear foramen** (Figs. 2.**378**–2.**379**). The CT scans in Fig. 2.**380** clearly demonstrate the anatomic correlate of this feature.

When the membrane is absent, the arm can be hyperextended at the elbow joint. A familial tendency has been reported for this phenomenon.

The olecranon fossa and coronoid fossa may contain accessory bone elements that are called **ossa supratrochleare** (Fig. 2.**381**).

The small bony elements located within the olecranon fossa and anterior to the proximal olecranon in Fig. 2.**380** may represent accessory and persistent ossification centers of the olecranon. Later these centers may migrate proximally and develop into an os supratrochleare like that shown in Fig. 2.**381**. The os supratrochleare mainly requires differentiation from an articular chondroma (Fig. 2.**382c–h**) or an osteochondral fragment that has mi-

Fig. 2.**377 a–d** Focal lucent area in the lateral epicondyle of ▷
the humerus in a 68-year old woman with clinical signs of humeral epicondylitis. The lucent area that mimics osteolysis is actually caused by cancellous bone loss and fatty replacement; hence it is an incidental finding.

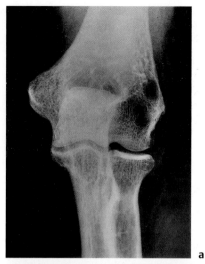

a

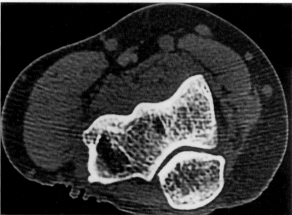

b

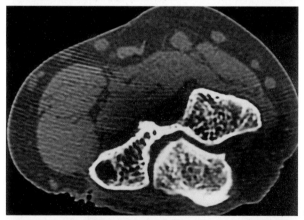

c

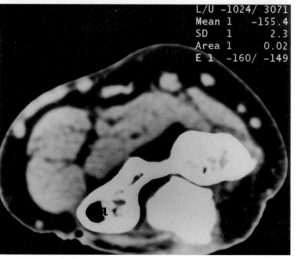

d

Fig. 2.**378 a–c**   Supratrochlear foramen. **a** Anatomic specimen. **b, c** Supratrochlear foramen in a 10-year-old boy. Note also the ossification center at the olecranon tip.

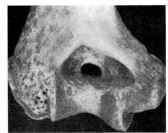

a

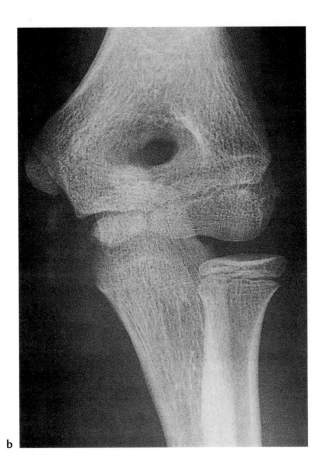

b

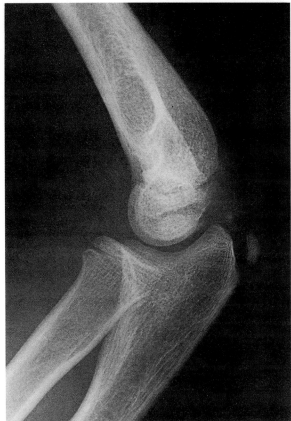

c

grated to that site from an area affected by osteochondritis dissecans (Fig. 2.**401 a, b**).

A typical normal variant is the **supracondylar process** (or trochlear process), a hook-shaped, exostosis-like bony structure located in the area of the diaphyseal-metaphyseal junction (Figs. 2.**383**, 2.**384**). It is probably an atavistic structure, as it occurs in monkeys and various other mammals. It is connected to the medial epicondyle of the humerus by a ligament (Struthers ligament), which is turn gives origin to a supernumerary portion of the pronator teres muscle. The presence of a supracondylar process is more common in individuals with upper extremity dysmelias (Fig. 2.**385**) than in the general population (approximately 1–2%).

The supracondylar process differs from a cartilaginous exostosis in that it is based directly on the cortex. With an osteochondroma, the spongiosa of the tumor-bearing bone is continuous with the spongiosa of the exostosis. Trauma to the region of the supracondylar process can lead to neurological complications due to the proximity of the median nerve (Fig. 2.**383**; Gantert and Alzheimer 1956). Traumatic avulsion of the process can also occur (Fig. 2.**384 b**).

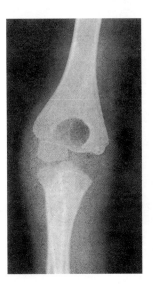

Fig. 2.**379**   Large supratrochlear foramen in a child.

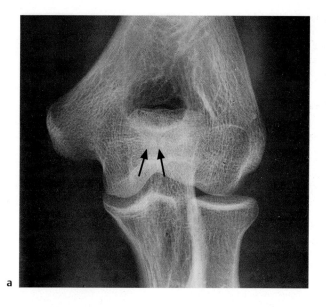

a

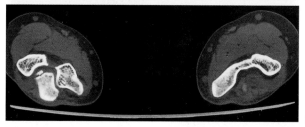

b

c

d

e

Fig. 2.**380 a–e**   CT sections through the region of the supra-trochlear foramen. The anatomic scan levels differ slightly between the sides due to unequal arm lengths. Scans **b** and **c** in the left arm and scans **d** and **e** in the right arm clearly demonstrate a bone defect spanned by a thin, ossified membrane. Associated findings include very small ossification centers anterior to the proximal part of the both olecranons within the olecranon fossa. We believe they represent unusual, unfused accessory centers in this 18-year-old male rather than fragments from osteochondritis dissecans. The small ossification centers are also visible in the plain film (arrows).

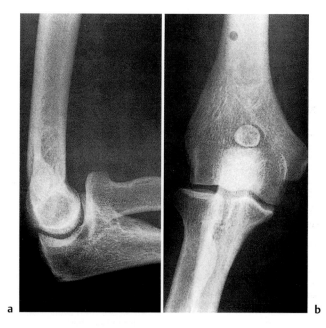

a   b

Fig. 2.**381 a, b**   Os supratrochleare in the olecranon fossa.

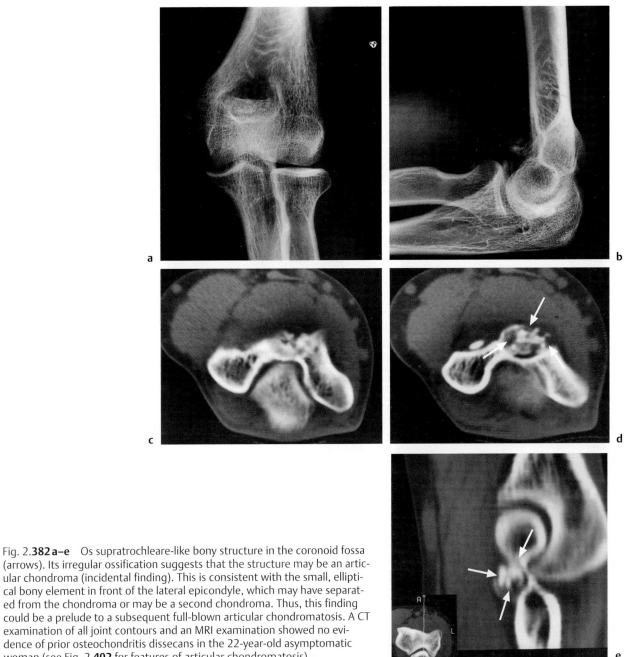

Fig. 2.**382 a–e**   Os supratrochleare-like bony structure in the coronoid fossa (arrows). Its irregular ossification suggests that the structure may be an articular chondroma (incidental finding). This is consistent with the small, elliptical bony element in front of the lateral epicondyle, which may have separated from the chondroma or may be a second chondroma. Thus, this finding could be a prelude to a subsequent full-blown articular chondromatosis. A CT examination of all joint contours and an MRI examination showed no evidence of prior osteochondritis dissecans in the 22-year-old asymptomatic woman (see Fig. 2.**402** for features of articular chondromatosis).

Fig. 2.**383**   Supracondylar process with blood vessel and nerve.   ▷

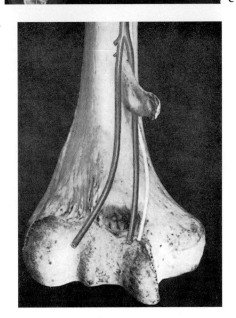

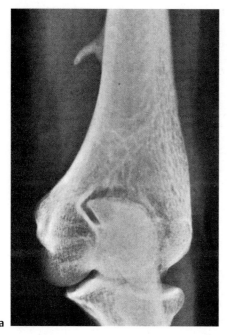

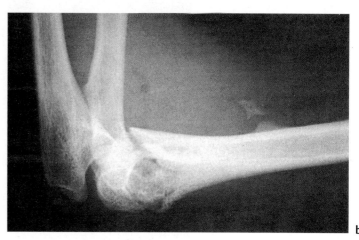

Fig. 2.**384a,b**   Supracondylar process.
a Supracondylar process in a 29-year-old man.

b Avulsion of the supracondylar process in a transcondylar fracture (9-year-old girl).

◁ Fig. 2.**385**   Supracondylar process in dysmelia.

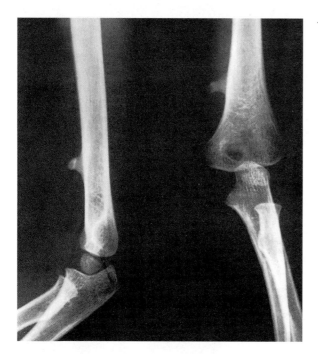

Congenital **dislocation of the radial head** can no longer be classified as a normal variant, especially when one considers its frequent association with certain complex dysplasias. It is usually bilateral, and the radial head may be dislocated in the anterior or posterior direction (see diagram in Fig. 2.**386a**).

Dislocation of the radial head is particularly well known in **nail–patella syndrome** (Fig. 2.**386b–d**) and also in otopalatodigital syndrome, Cornelia de Lange syndrome, and others. **Radioulnar synostosis** is a congenital anomaly involving an osseous fusion of the **proximal radius and ulna** (Figs. 2.**387**, 2.**388**; Miura et al. 1984).

Radioulnar synostoses are commonly associated with carpal and tarsal coalitions. Cleary and Omer (1985) published an informative review of the radiographic patterns and clinical manifestations of proximal radioulnar synostoses (Table 2.**22**).

To date, **hypoplasia of the humeral trochlea** has been described as a definite anomaly only in Japanese patients (27 cases) (Tanabu et al. 1985). This hypoplasia may be associated with ulnar nerve palsy. Deformities of the periarticular epiphyses due to **hemophilia** (bleeders' joint) should not be confused with epiphyseal dysplasia (Fig. 2.**389**).

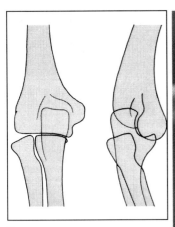

a

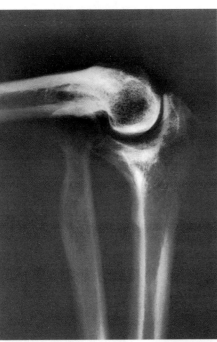

b

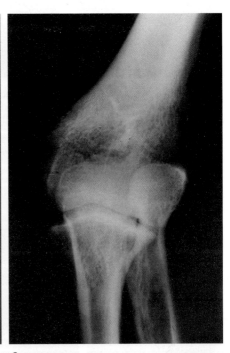

c

Fig. 2.**386a–d** Dislocation of the radial head.
a Schematic diagram.
b–d Proximal radial dislocation in nail-patella syndrome (bilateral). Note the extreme positive ulnar variance on both sides (**d**) with marked signs of ulnar impaction syndrome (pp. 173 and 190). Bilateral patellar dysplasia was also present.

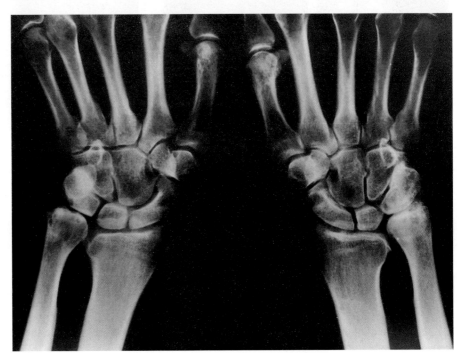

d

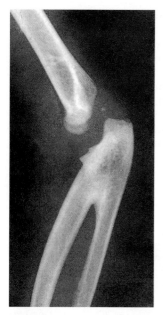

Fig. 2.**387**   Radioulnar synostosis, showing very pronounced osseous fusion of the proximal segments of the radius and ulna.

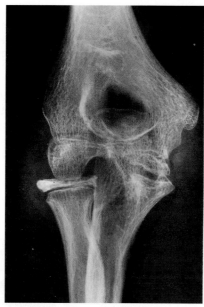
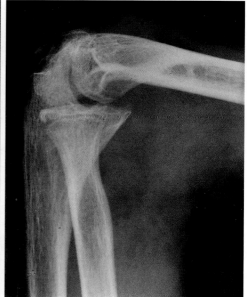

Fig. 2.**389a, b**   Unusual deformities of the distal humeral epiphysis and radial head, expansion of the olecranon fossa, and periarticular osteoporosis. These changes are a result of type A hemophilia (13-year-old boy) rather than epiphyseal dysplasia.

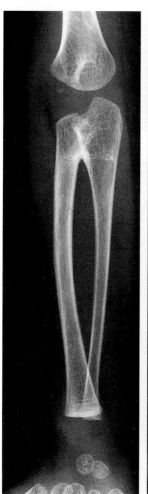
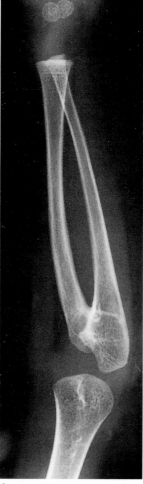

a

b

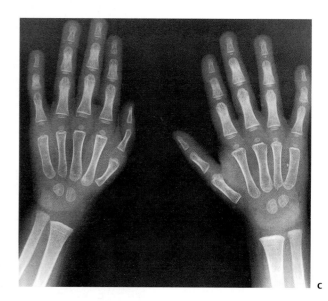

c

Fig. 2.**388a–c**   Proximal radioulnar synostosis (less pronounced than in Fig. 2.**387**) in a 3-year-old boy with Fanconi anemia. Note the typical associated skeletal deformities in the hands: hypoplasia of the thumb (especially on the left side) and short fifth metacarpals on both sides.

Fracture, Subluxation, or Dislocation?

A knowledge of the **times of appearance of the various apophyseal and epiphyseal centers** is of fundamental importance in diagnosing bony injuries of the pediatric elbow.

For example, a bony element found adjacent to the lateral (radial) epicondyle of the humerus in a 9-year-old child cannot be an ossification center (which is not yet present at this age) and should definitely be interpreted as an avulsion fracture, with corresponding therapeutic implications. On the other hand, a bony element adjacent to the humeral trochlea in a 9-year-old child might well represent a displaced ossification center of the medial (ulnar) epicondyle, which is already present at this age (Fig. 2.**390 a**).

The presence of **multiple ossification centers** in various apophyses and epiphyses is also of practical importance in interpreting radiographs of the pediatric elbow (e.g., Figs. 2.**357**, 2.**359**, 2.**361**, 2.**362**).

In another example from daily practice, a bony element found distal to the medial portion of the humeral metaphysis (in the area of the future trochlea) in a 7-year-old boy does not represent the trochlea itself but a displaced apophyseal center of the medial epicondyle, since the ossification center for the trochlea does not appear on radiographs until 8 to 10 years of age (Fig. 2.**390 b**).

A **linear lucency between the tip of the olecranon and the adjacent bone** should always be interpreted as a fracture, rather than an apophyseal line, if the patient is less than 10–13 years old, because normally the apophyseal center does not become radiographically visible until the teen years (Fig. 2.**391**).

Pure **metaphyseal fractures of the distal humerus** are also extremely difficult to diagnose in children (Fig. 2.**392**), especially since the normal metaphyseal contours often have an "unsettled" appearance in 7- to 12-year-olds.

The **cubital fat pad sign** can be helpful in diagnosing trauma to the pediatric elbow joint. The anterior and posterior cubital fat pad sign, visible on the lateral radioulnar elbow radiograph in 90° flexion, is produced by fatty layers (pads) located between the synovial membrane and fibrous capsule, making the fat pads intracapsular and extrasynovial in location (Goswami, 2002). The anterior fat pad in a healthy joint appears as a bandlike or teardrop-shaped dark feature about 5 mm wide that is level with and just anterior to the coronoid process (Fig. 2.**393 a**).

The posterior fat pad is projected into the olecranon fossa, so normally it is not visible (Fig. 2.**393 a**). Any expansion of the joint cavity, whether due to hemarthrosis or an inflammatory effusion, pushes the fat pad anteriorly, and the posterior fat pad becomes visible behind the articular margin of the humerus (Figs. 2.**392 b**, 2.**393 b**, 2.**394 a**). If the capsule is torn in the presence of an effusion, the fat pad sign remains negative.

Another soft-tissue sign in the elbow joint is the supinator fat line (Fig. 2.**392 b**), which runs over the supinator muscle to the proximal radius. In both traumatic and inflammatory joint effusions, the supinator fat line is displaced anteriorly, distorted, broadened, or ill-defined.

The relative weakness of the annular ligament in small children predisposes to subluxation of the radial head. **Anterior subluxation of the radial head** is a particularly well-known injury that occurs when an adult yanks upward on the hand of a stumbling child. This can even cause a painful paralysis of the arm. In evaluating the position of the radial head, it should be noted that the axis of the radius should run precisely through the center of the humeral trochlea (Schmidt 1952, Dahm 1953).

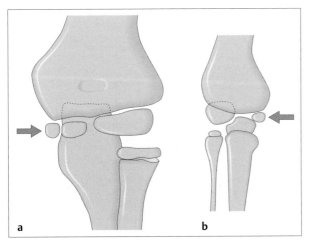

Fig. 2.**390 a, b**   Traumatic displacements of the ossification center of the ulnar epicondyle are easily missed, because the radiographs appear "normal" with no evidence of fracture lnes.

a Posttraumatic displacement in a 9-year-old child. At this age the ossification center of the ulnar epicondyle should already be distinctly visible. Because it is absent in a normally developed child, it is wrong to interpret the bony element next to the trochlear center as a duplication of the trochlea. Actually it is an inferiorly displaced apophyseal center of the ulnar epicondyle.

b Normally developed 7-year-old boy who fell while playing at school (the exact mechanism of the injury could not be determined). The bony element shown by the arrow is not the humeral trochlea, which is not yet ossified at this age, but an inferiorly displaced ossification center of the medial epicondyle.

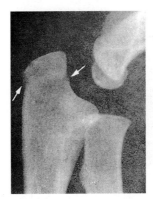

Fig. 2.**391**   Postinjury radiograph of a 6-year-old boy. The faint linear lucency (arrow) below the tip of the olecranon is not the apophyseal growth plate center of the olecranon (which does not appear before 10–11 years of age) but a metahyseal fracture.

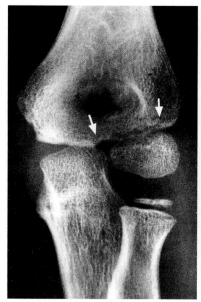
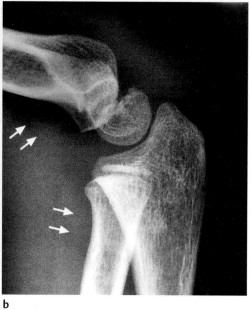

a   b

Fig. 2.**392 a, b**   Typical fracture of the distal humeral metaphysis. This injury is easily missed because the metaphysis often has irregular contours, especially in relation to the trochlea. Note the displaced fat pad signs in radiograph **b**.
Proximal arrows: anterior cubital fat sign
Distal arrows: supinator fat line

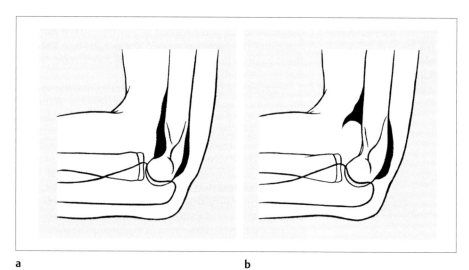

a   b

Fig. 2.**393 a, b**   Diagram of the soft-tissue signs about the elbow.
a Normal.
b Posttraumatic elevation of the anterior cubital fat pad.

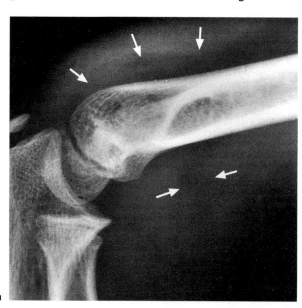
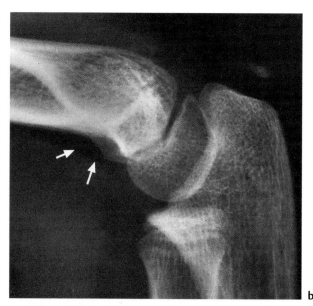

a   b

Fig. 2.**394 a, b**   Elbow injury and the cubital fat pad sign.
a Injury of the right elbow joint. The cubital fat pad has been markedly displaced anteriorly and posteriorly (arrows).

b The arrows indicate the normal position of the cubital fat pad sign.

Anterior or posterior dislocations of the capitulum are often very difficult to diagnose. The following reference lines are helpful:

- An extension of the anterior (palmar) contour of the humerus passes through the posterior third of the ossification center of the capitulum.
- The capitulum should be anterior to a line drawn along the humeral axis and through the apposing outlines of the coronoid and olecranon fossae.

Fractures of the radial head can be very difficult to diagnose in children as well as adults, because the head and neck of the radius are generally superimposed by the ulna in the lateral projection (Fig. 2.**394**). Generally a radial head-capitulum lateral projection with the x-ray tube angled 45° proximally (forearm flexed 90° at the elbow) will provide a clear projection of the radial head. This projection also gives a clear view of the capitulum and the coronoid process of the ulna. If the clinical signs strongly suggest a bony injury of the elbow joint but conventional radiographs (including special views) do not show a definite fracture, CT scans should be obtained. Figure 2.**395** illustrates how the superimposed structures of the elbow joint can obscure a fracture on conventional radiographs. Only a precise orthograde projection of the ulnar fracture line caused by avulsion of the radial annular ligament would permit a diagnosis to be made. A mere 2–3° of rotation about the longitudinal axis would be enough to obscure the fracture line on a conventional radiograph.

 Necrosis?

The **apophyseal and epiphyseal ossification centers** about the elbow joint can be extremely **variable** both in their anatomy (one or multiple centers) and in their density. Increased density of the ossification centers combined with fragmentation ("crumbling") should raise suspicion of osteonecrosis, especially if the finding is asymmetrical.

> Because the normal range is so broad, however, such findings can be interpreted only by taking the clinical presentation into account. Generally they have no significance when detected incidentally (Figs. 2.**396**–2.**398**).

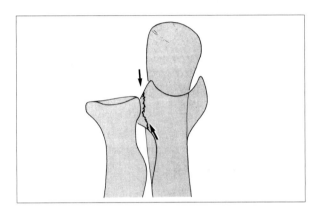

Fig. 2.**395** Easily missed fracture line separating the radial notch (the ulnar portion of the proximal radioulnar joint) from the ulna (avulsion-type fracture; arrows).

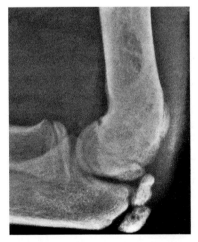

Fig. 2.**396** What appears to be necrotic ossification centers of the olecranon apophysis is actually an asymptomatic normal variant.

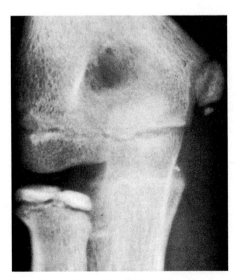

Fig. 2.**397** The "white" bipartite radial head epiphysis is a normal variant and does not signify necrosis.

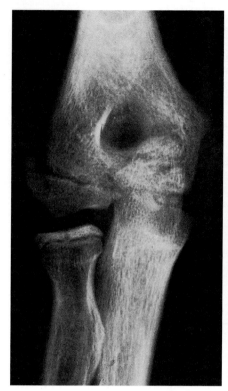
a

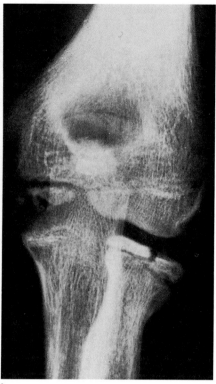
b

Fig. 2.**398**   The relatively "white" double epiphyses of the radial head on each side are normal variants and do not signify necrosis. Note also the "crumbly" ossification centers of the trochlea.

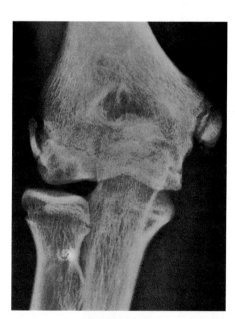

Fig. 2.**399**   Advanced idiopathic necrosis of the capitulum humeri (Panner disease), still without fragmentation. In many cases this disease resolves spontaneously without fragmentation. Clinically the elbow was painful with use. Ultrasound showed a small effusion.

Lucent areas in the subchondral bone combined with irregular surrounding sclerosis, with or without fragmentation, generally signify **osteonecrosis** in symptomatic patients. The most common form about the elbow is osteonecrosis of the capitulum, known also as Panner disease (Figs. 2.**399**, 2.**400**).

As a rule, only late stages can be detected on conventional radiographs. Early stages can be detected more accurately by MRI. Although necrosis of the small ossification centers in the growing elbow skeleton has no active therapeutic implications (e.g., drilling to relieve pressure), MRI can at least furnish a diagnosis in patients with unexplained pain.

If an osteochondral fragment develops from a necrotic lesion, the condition is described as **osteochondritis dissecans**, which also occurs in adults (e.g., air-hammer operators). The capitulum and trochlea are most commonly involved; the radial head is rarely affected. If the fragment separates from its bony bed, it can migrate and become an intra-articular loose body (Figs. 2.**401**, 2.**402a, b**).

Occasionally these cases are difficult to distinguish from primary articular chondromatosis (Figs. 2.**402c–h**), which is a tumorlike lesion of the joint membrane. These typically rounded, laminar, ossified bodies do not originate from the bone. They may separate from the synovial membrane and migrate within the joint.

Fig. 2.**400 a, b** Progression of an initial osteonecrosis of the capitulum humeri in a 13-year-old boy. When radiograph **a** was taken, the elbow joint was markedly painful with use. When the film is viewed with a magnifying lens, slight haziness can be seen in the area that appears four months later (**b**) as a subchondral lucency.

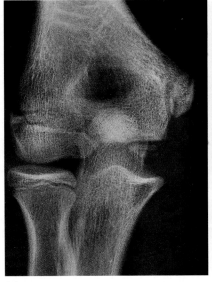
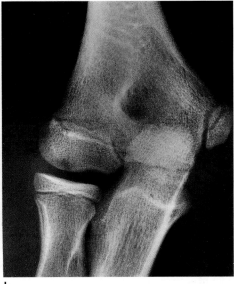

a b

Fig. 2.**401 a, b** Osteochondritis dissecans (arrow). A normal notch is visible in the articular surface of the ulna (double arrow).

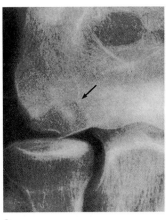
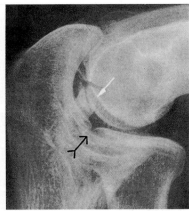

a b

Fig. 2.**402 a–h** Synovial chondromatosis.
a, b This case of synovial chondromatosis developed from an osteonecrotic lesion of the medial condyle (trochlea) of the humerus. Osteochondral fragments in the anterior joint recess migrated upward into the coronoid fossa, where they enlarged to produce a secondary chondromatosis.

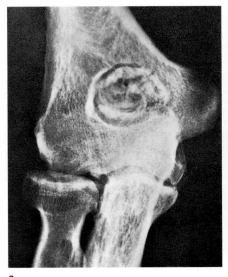
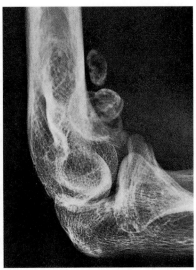

a b

Fig. 2.**402 c–h** ▷

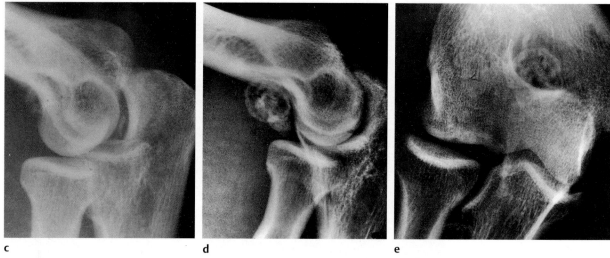

c   d   e

Fig. 2.**402 c–e** Primary synovial chondromatosis without any signs of necrotic changes in the bones that form the joint. Be- tween fig. c and fig. d/e there are 1.5 years, in which the chon- dromas at the flexion side have rapidly grown.

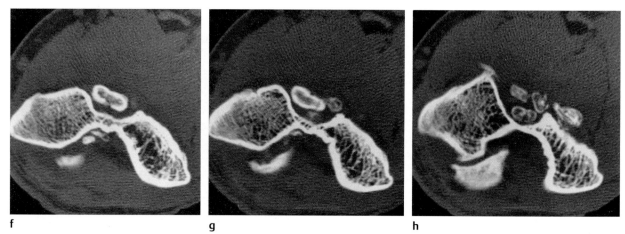

f   g   h

Fig. 2.**402 f–h** CT scans of synovial chondromatosis show intra-articular "loose bodies" in the coronoid fossa and in the olecranon fossa, although the latter may represent persistent ossification centers of the olecranon (see also Fig. 2.**380**).

Note the differentiated structural features of the osteochon- dromatous bodies. The patient, a 25-year-old man, presented clinically with intermittent arrest of the elbow joint.

 Tumor?

We referred earlier to the physiological lucencies in the area of the radial tuberosity (Figs. 2.**364**, 2.**365**), the small notch in the medial surface of the humeral metaphysis (Fig. 2.**370 b, c**), the variable depth of the supratrochlear foramen (Figs. 2.**377**–2.**379**), and the normally rarefied trabecular structure of the proximal ulnar metaphysis (Fig. 2.**366**) as well as in the epicondyles of the humerus (Fig. 2.**377**). These normal findings should not be mistaken for tumor-associated bone destruction. Conversely, a phys- iological prominence such as the supracondylar process (Figs. 2.**383**–2.**385**) should not be interpreted as a car- tilaginous exostosis (osteochondroma).

Otherwise there are no structures about the elbow joint that might be confused with tumors. Occasionally an osteoid osteoma may be missed on conventional radio- graphic films (Fig. 2.**403**).

Sharply circumscribed "white specks" up to 5 mm in di- ameter in the metaphyseal portions of the bones compris- ing the elbow generally represent **osteopoikilotic foci** rather than osteosclerotic metastases (Fig. 2.**404**).

A radiograph of the opposite site or of the hand can quickly establish the presence of osteopoikilosis by show- ing additional lesions at typical locations.

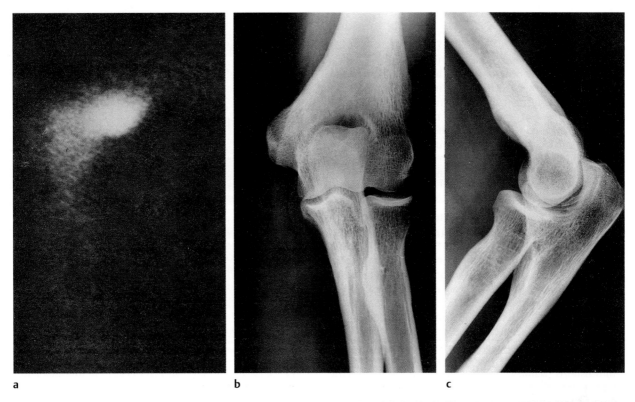

a   b   c

Fig. 2.**403 a–d**   Osteoid osteoma of the anterior side of the left distal humeral metaphysis, virtually undetectable on conventional radiographs. The patient, a 60-year-old man, had more than a one-year history of pain in the left elbow joint, had seen various doctors, and had received several intra-articular injections, which were of no benefit. The patient claimed that the pain was dramatically relieved by aspirin. These signs indicate an osteoid osteoma.

a Bone scan shows greatly increased tracer uptake in the anterior part of the distal humerus. Note the double-density sign that is of high specificity for an osteoid osteoma.

b, c Conventional radiographs. The lateral view (**c**) shows circumscribed hyperostosis in the distal humeral metaphysis.

d CT clearly demonstrates the calcified nidus (between the arrows). The tumor was surgically removed, immediately relieving the patient's complaints.

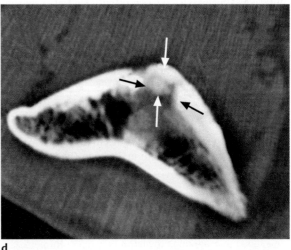

d

Fig. 2.**404 a, b**   Foci of osteopoikilosis appear as "white specks" in the cancellous bone near the elbow joint of an asymptomatic adult woman. The lesion are not osteoblastic metastases.

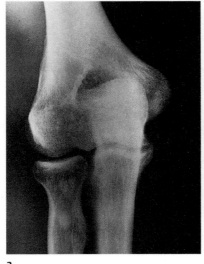

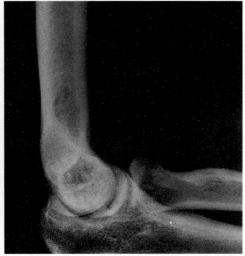

a   b

Inflammation?

In the section on tumors, we described the physiological lucencies that may be confused with lesions. These lucencies may also be mistaken for foci of inflammatory destruction. Additionally, the ridgelike cortical extensions on the lateral aspect of the distal humeral metaphysis (Fig. 2.**370a**) should not be confused with the periosteal bone deposition that may accompany an inflammatory or neoplastic process.

The importance of the fat pad sign was discussed earlier (Fig. 2.**392**–2.**394**).

Soft-Tissue Calcifications and Ossifications, Changes at the Fibro-osseous Junction

Punctate and streaklike calcifications that run parallel to the joint contours in the articular cartilage of the humerus and especially of the radius are a sign of **chondrocalcinosis** (Fig. 2.**405**). When it involves the elbow joint, it is usually only one feature of a generalized disease (with sites of predilection in the joints of the hand, knee, etc.).

Productive bone changes in the epicondyles showing a pencil- or flame-shaped configuration are an expression of fibro-osteitis (clinical epicondylitis). In asymptomatic patients who do not recall elbow pain, these changes can almost be considered a normal variant. They are especially common in tennis players, and they are an expression of enthesopathy in patients with seronegative spondylarthritis (Fig. 2.**406**).

Marked productive bone changes involving the medial epicondyle with ossifications in the surrounding soft tissues are particularly common in javelin throwers (Fig. 2.**407**).

Shell-like ossifications near the epicondyles are attributed to metaplastic bone formation in response to soft-tissue trauma (Fig. 2.**408**), analogous to the Köhler–Stieda–Pellegrini shadows that occur in the knee. **Osteophytes** ap-

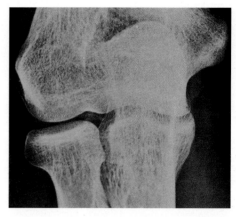

Fig. 2.**405**   Chondrocalcinosis with subtle calcification above the ulnar side of the radial head. The pattern suggests a circumscribed calcification of the articular cartilage in the area of the lateral epicondyle opposite the radial head.

pear as sharp excrescences at joint margins, as shown schematically in Fig. 2.**409**. When intracapsular, they reflect an incipient osteoarthritis; when extra-articular (involving the metaphysis away from the joint margins), they are interpreted as traction phenomena.

Shell-like ossifications as well as streaklike or punctate ossifications on the palmar aspect of the radial head represent **heterotopic bone formation in the ruptured annular ligament or anterior joint capsule** (Earwaker 1992; Fig. 2.**410**). The causative dislocation of the radial head is not always obvious on radiographs. A cuff of calcification around the radial neck signifies a rupture of the oblique cord (Earwaker 1992).

These calcifications or ossifications do not appear until 2–3 weeks after an injury. They can be important in compensation evaluations, especially in cases where a radial head dislocation has been missed.

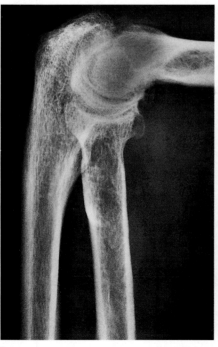

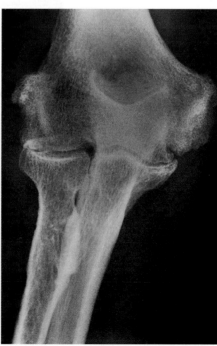

Fig. 2.**406a, b**   Pronounced enthesopathy in psoriatic arthritis with marked productive ossifications on the epicondyles, olecranon, and capsular attachment (see also Fig. 2.**409**).

a

b

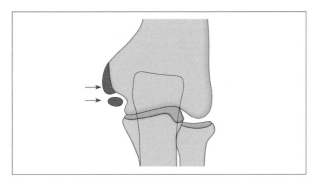

Fig. 2.**407**   Javelin-thrower's elbow, marked by periostosis on the ulnar side of the joint and heterotopic bone formation (shaded, arrows).

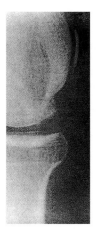

Fig. 2.**408**   Plaquelike calcification on the lateral epicondyle.

More solid ankylosing ossifications, often a sequel to trauma, are a manifestation of myositis ossificans (Fig. 2.**411**).

Rounded multicentric calcifications as well as homogeneous calcifications adjacent to the epicondyles and proximal to the olecranon generally represent calcified bursitis or calcium phosphate or carbonate deposits in hyperparathyroidism (Fig. 2.**412**).

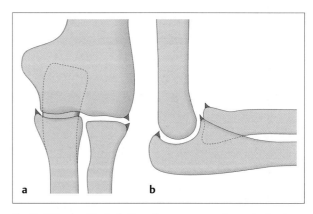

Fig. 2.**409 a, b**   Typical sites of occurrence of marginal osteophytes about the elbow joint.

Fig. 2.**410 a–d**   Heterotopic posttraumatic ossification of the radial annular ligament. **a, b** Missed anterior dislocation of the radius. Three weeks later a shell-like ossification is visible anterior to the proximal radius, representing heterotopic bone formation in the torn annular ligament or anterior joint capsule. The main factors precipitating the heterotopic ossification are probably local hemorrhage and edematous changes in the injured area. **c, d** Cuff of calcification around the radial neck, caused by a rupture of the oblique cord. (From Earwaker 1992.)

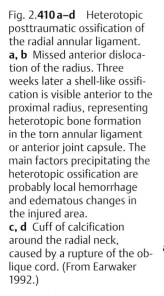

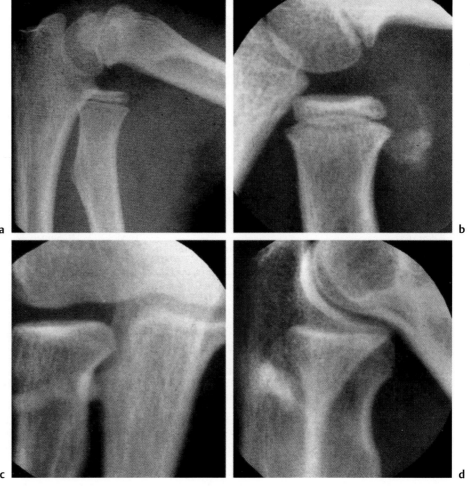

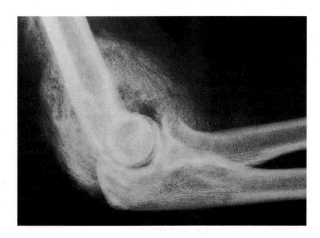

Fig. 2.**411**   Typical myositis ossificans or ankylosing heterotopic ossification in a multiple-injury patient. Since a severe head injury was present, the condition is classified as a neuropathic myositis ossificans. The radiograph was taken 19 days after the trauma.

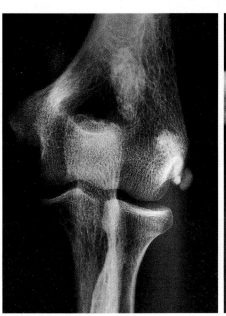 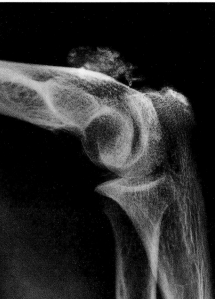

Fig. 2.**412 a, b**   Bursal calcifications in severe renal osteodystrophy with excessive vitamin D replacement.

a   b

References

Bánki, Z.: Die Apophyse mit Fortsatzbildung des Epicondylus medialis humeri. Fortschr. Röntgenstr. 107 (1967) 815

Bassett, L. W., J. M. Mirra, M. Forrester et al.: Posttraumatic osteochondral "loose body" of the olecranon fossa. Radiology 141 (1981) 635

Bohrer, St. P.: The fat pad sign following elbow trauma. Its usefulness and reliability in suspecting "invisible" fractures. Clin. Radiol. 21 (1970) 90

Buse, H.: Beitrag zur Persistenz der Olekranonapophyse. Fortschr. Röntgenstr. 104 (1966) 867

Canigiani, G., J. Wickenhauser, W. Czesch: Beitrag zur Osteochondrosis dissecans im Foramen supratrochleare. Fortschr. Röntgenstr. 117 (1972) 66

Cleary, J. E., G. E. Omer: Congenital proximal radioulnar synostosis. J. Bone Jt Surg. 67-A (1985) 539

de Cuveland, E.: Persistierende Knochenkerne des Epicondylus ulnaris und radialis. Fortschr. Röntgenstr. 82 (1955) 125

Dahm, M.: Das Röntgenbild bei Luxation des Radius im Kindesalter. Fortschr. Röntgenstr. 79 (1953) 224

D'Ambrosia, R., W. Zink: Fractures of the elbow in children. Pediat. Ann. 11 (1982) 541

Earwaker, J.: Posttraumatic calcification of the annular ligament of the radius. Skelet. Radiol. 21 (1992) 149

Eitel, F., L.Schweiberer: Olekranonfrakturen. Unfallheilkunde 86 (1983) 143

Foster, D. E., J. A. Sullivan, R. H.Gross: Lateral humeral condylar fractures in children. J. pediat. Orthop. 5 (1985) 16

Fowles, J. V., N. Sliman, M. T. Kassab: The Monteggia-lesion in children. J. Bone Jt Surg. 65-A (1983) 1276

Gantert, F., Ch. Alzheimer: Der Processus supracondylaris humeri und Foramen supracondyloideum. Nervenarzt 27 (1956) 349

Gaston, S. R., F. M. Smith, O. D. Baab: Epiphyseal injuries of the radial head and neck. Amer. J. Surg. 85 (1953) 266

Giustra, P. E., J. Killoran, R. S. Furmann et al.: The missed Monteggia-fracture. Radiology 110 (1974) 45

Goswami, G. K.: The fat pad sign. Radiology 222 (2002) 419

Greenspan, A., A. Norman, H. Rosen: Radial head-capitellum view in elbow trauma. J. Roentgenol. 143 (1984) 355

Grundy, A., G. Murrphy, A. Barker et al.: The value of the radial-head-capitellum view in radial head trauma. Brit. J. Radiol. 58 (1985) 965

Günsel, E.: Persistierende Apophyse des Epicondylus medialis humeri. Fortschr. Röntgenstr. 76 (1952) 660

Hillger, H., H. Hamm: Persistierende Knochenkerne des Epicondylus ulnaris und radialis. Fortschr. Röntgenstr. 84 (1956) 650

Höffken, W.: Eine Varität der Ulna und ihre Täuschungsmöglich-keit. Fortschr. Röntgenstr. 76 (1952) 259

Kattan, K. R., D. S. Babcock: Bilateral patella cubiti. Case report 105. Skelet. Radiol. 4 (1979) 249

Lawson, J. P.: Symptomatic radiographic variants in extremities. Radiology 157 (1985) 613

Letts, M., R. Locht, J. Wiens: Monteggia fracture dislocation in children. J. Bone Jt Surg. 67-B (1985) 724

Miura, T., R. Nakamura, M. Suzuki et al.: Congenital radio-ulnar synostosis. J. Hand Surg. 9-B (1984) 153

Neiss, A.: Abrißfraktur eines Processus supracondylicus humeri. Fortschr. Röntgenstr. 83 (1955) 120

Obermann, R. W., H. W. C. Loose: The os supratrochleare dorsale: a normal variant that may cause symptoms. Amer. J. Roentgenol. 141 (1983) 123

Papavasiliou, V. A.: Fracture-separation of the medial epicondylar epiphysis of the elbow joint. Clin. Orthop. 171 (1982) 172

Papavasiliou, V. A., Th. A. Beslikas: Fractures of the lateral humeral condyle in children—an analysis of 39 cases. Injury 16 (1985) 364

Piroth, P., M. Gharib: Die traumatische Subluxation des Radius-köpfchens. Dtsch. med. Wschr. 101 (1976) 1520

Resnik, C. S., M. A. Hartenberg: Ossification centres of the pediatric elbow: a rare normal variant. Pediat. Radiol 16 (1986) 254

Rosenberg, Z. S., J. Beltran, Y. Y. Cheung: Pseudodefect of the capitellum: potential MR imaging pitfall. Radiology 191 (1994) 821

Rumpold, H.-J.: Die Persistenz des Verknöcherungszentrums im proximalen Gelenkabschnitt der Ulna. Fortschr. Röntgenstr. 100 (1964) 651

Rutherford, A.: Fractures of the lateral humeral condyle in children. J. Bone Jt Surg. 67-A (1985) 851

Schiele, H. P., R. B. Hubbard, H. M.Bruck: Radiographic changes in burns of the upper extremity. Radiology 104 (1972) 13

Schmitt, H. G.: Persistierende Apophyse des Olecranons. Fortschr. Röntgenstr. 74 (1951) 241

Schmitt, H.: Über die durch Zug bedingte schmerzhafte Armläh-mung bei Kleinkindern. Med. Klin.47 (1952) 867

Schröder, G.: Persistierende Apophyse des Epicondylus medialis humeri. Fortschr. Röntgenstr. 84 (1956) 262

Schröder, G.: Zum Problem der persistierenden Knochenkerne des Epicondylus humeri ulnaris et radialis. Fortschr. Röntgenstr. 85 (1956) 716

Schwarz, G. S.: Bilateral antecubital ossicles (fabellae cubiti) and other rare accessory bones of the elbow. With a case report. Radiology 69 (1957) 730

Sieckel, L.: Über die persistierenden Knochenkerne am Ellenbo-gengelenk. Fortschr. Röntgenstr. 85 (1956) 709

Simmons, B. P., W. W. Southmaid, E. J. Riseborough: Congenital radioulnar synostosis. J. Hand Surg. 8 (1983) 829

Skaf, A. Y., R. D. Boutin, R. W. M. Dantas et al.: Bicipitoradial bursitis: MR imaging findings in eight patients and anatomic data from contrast material opacification of bursae followed by routine ra-diography and MR imaging in cadavers. Radiology 212 (1999) 111

Swischuk, L. E.: Emergency radiology of the acutely ill of injured child. Williams & Wilkins, Baltimore 1979 (p. 288)

Tanabu, F., Y. Yamanuchi, M. Tukushima: Hypoplasia of the trochlea of the humerus as a cause of ulnar nerve palsy. J. Bone Jt Surg. 67-A (1985) 151

Wieser, R., H. Scheier, R. P. Meyer: Knochennekrosen am Ellenbo-gen. Orthopädie 10 (1981) 68

Wiley, J. J., J. P. Galey: Monteggia injuries in children. J. Bone Jt Surg. 67-B (1985) 728

Zimmers, T. E.: Fat plane radiological signs in wrist and elbow trauma. Amer. J. Emerg. Med. 2 (1984) 526

Upper Arm

Diaphysis

▌ Normal Findings

During Growth

It is normal for radiographs of the upper arm in children and adolescents to show double outlines along the lateral or medial aspect of the proximal diaphyseal–metaphyseal junction of the humerus (Fig. 2.**413**). Apparently these double lines relate to the crests of the greater and lesser tuberosities, whose contours blend with the surrounding cortex with passage of time.

Depending on the projection, these crests appear as distal extensions of the greater and lesser tuberosities and are a product of muscular traction (from the pectoralis major and deltoid).

A shallow notch in the medial aspect of the proximal humeral metaphysis with an irregular, frayed, or absent cortex is a normal finding in children 10 to 16 years of age. Variously described as the "upper humeral notch" or "metaphyseal cortical irregularities," these features should not be mistaken for destructive lesions (Ozonoff and Ziter 1974, Keats and Joyce 1984, p. 258 and Fig. 2.**443**).

Nutrient canals as a source of diagnostic error are discussed below (Fig. 2.**414b**).

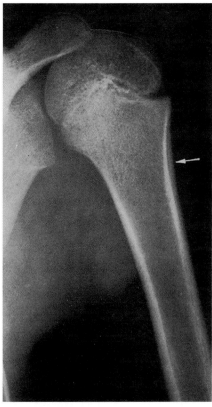

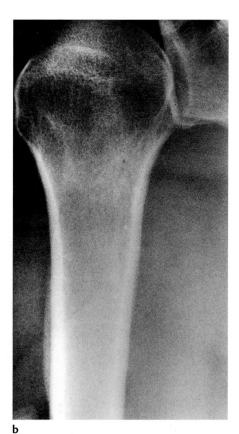

a   b

Fig. 2.**413a, b**   Abnormal periosteal processes?
a Normal double outline of the humerus during skeletal growth (compare with Fig. 2.**421b**).
b Superimposed soft tissues resemble an abnormal periosteal reaction along the lateral cortex of the proximal humeral shaft. A repeat radiograph was normal, and CT scans were negative.

In Adulthood

A nutrient canal is consistently found in the middle third of the humeral diaphysis, starting at the medial circumference of the bone and running distally (Fig. 2.**414**). Generally it is visible on radiographs taken of the humeral shaft in 45° of external rotation.

Very often a radiolucent area can be seen in the proximal portion of the middle third of the diaphysis. This lucency may be caused by overlying muscle groups, super-

imposed soft tissues of the lateral chest wall, or voluminous breasts (Fig. 2.**415 a**). Changing the projection will eliminate the lucency (e.g., slight abduction or axial image, etc.). Superimposed soft tissues can also mimic periosteal densities (Fig. 2.**413 b**).

The deltoid tuberosity is a frequent source of confusion for inexperienced examiners. Giving attachment to the deltoid muscle, the tuberosity is an extension of a ridge (crest) that runs distally from the greater tuberosity. The stronger the muscle groups that attach to the bony ridges, the more prominent the ridges appear (Figs. 2.**416**–2.**418**).

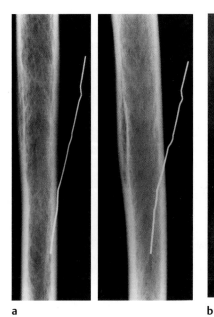
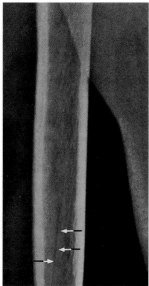
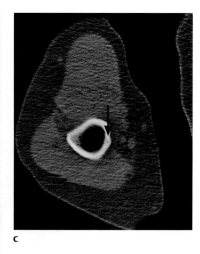

a   **b**   **c**

Fig. 2.**414 a–c**   Nutrient canal in the middle third of the humeral diaphysis.
a A paperclip has been bent open and inserted into the nutrient canal to define its path. The nutrient canal runs obliquely through the cortex for a considerable distance and continues as a fine linear lucency along the endosteal cortical surface. In

the image on the right, the base of the more proximally and laterally situaed deltod tuberosty appears as acent line (see also Fig. 2.**419 a, b**).
b Appearance of the nutrient canal in an 11-year-old girl.
c The intracortical nutrient canal appears on CT as a tiny round lucency (arrow).

Fig. 2.**415 a–d**   Lucencies in the humeral shaft.
a Triangular lucency caused by superimposed soft tissues.
b–d CT shows an unusual endosteal notch in the cortex of the humeral shaft, completely filled with intramedullary fat. Incidental finding, possibly a normal variant. (Case courtesy of Dr. H. Ch. Wulke, Frechen.)

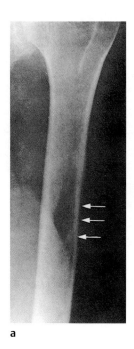
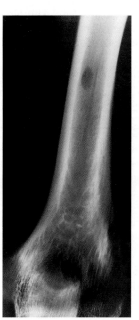
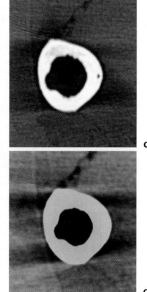

a   **b**   **c**   **d**

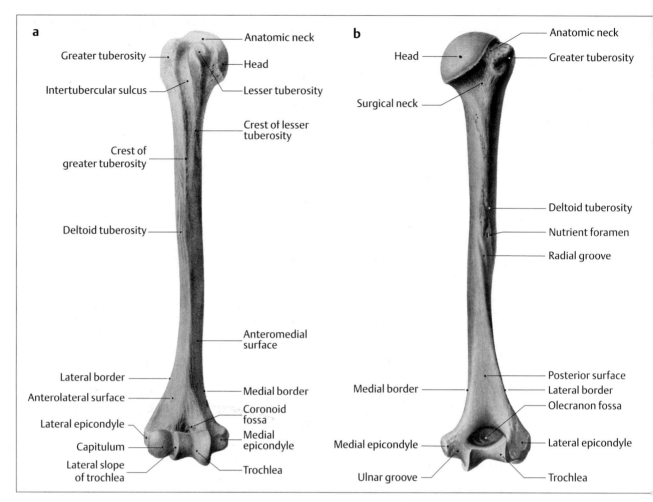

a

Greater tuberosity

Intertubercular sulcus

Crest of greater tuberosity

Deltoid tuberosity

Lateral border

Anterolateral surface

Lateral epicondyle

Capitulum

Lateral slope of trochlea

Anatomic neck

Head

Lesser tuberosity

Crest of lesser tuberosity

Anteromedial surface

Medial border

Coronoid fossa

Medial epicondyle

Trochlea

b

Head

Surgical neck

Medial border

Medial epicondyle

Ulnar groove

Anatomic neck

Greater tuberosity

Deltoid tuberosity

Nutrient foramen

Radial groove

Posterior surface

Lateral border

Olecranon fossa

Lateral epicondyle

Trochlea

Fig. 2.**416 a, b**   Surface anatomy of the humerus. Note the ridgelike prominences formed by the crests of the greater and lesser tuberosities and the "roughness" of the deltoid tuberosity.

The structure of the bone below the prominent contour of the tuberosity can appear irregular and mottled, especially in a tangential projection (see especially Fig. 2.**417 a, b**). These structural irregularities are explained by axial sections showing the relative porosity of the bony structures that underlie the tuberosity (Fig. 2.**419**). Similar irregularities are seen below the crests of the greater and lesser tuberosities (Figs. 2.**419**, 2.**420**, 3.**15**).

A tremendous range of variation is found in the distribution of MRI signal intensities, especially in the proximal humeral diaphyses, and the radiologist must know these patterns to avoid diagnostic errors (Fig. 2.**441 d, e**). In equivocal cases, it is always helpful to image the opposite side for comparison. Of course, clinical criteria should also be considered in interpreting the radiological findings.

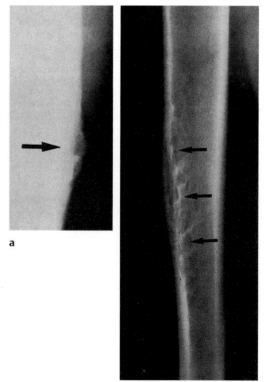

a

b

Fig. 2.**417 a, b**   Structural and contour irregularities at the attachment of the deltoid muscle.
a Circumscribed.
b More extensive.

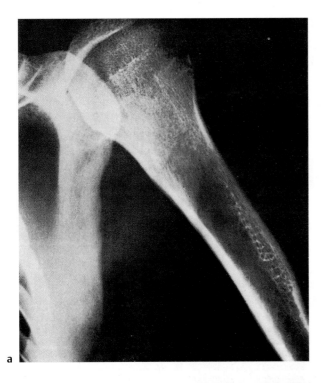

a

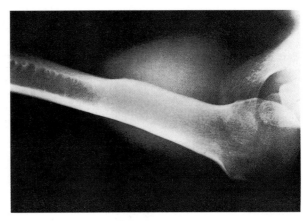

b

Fig. 2.**418 a, b**   Very prominent deltoid tuberosity.

Fig. 2.**419 a, b**   Axial CT scans of the proximal humeral diaphysis show the deltoid tuberosity posteriorly and the crest of the greater tuberosity anteriorly. The endostal part of the cortex below the tuberosity and crest appears markedly thin and porous; this accounts for the imaging phenomena seen in Figs. 2.**417** and 2.**420**.

a

b

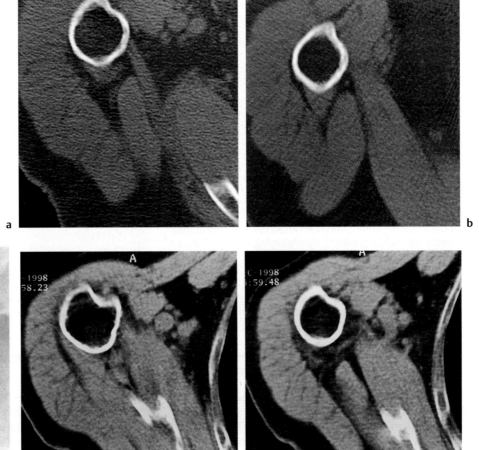

a

b

c

Fig. 2.**420 a–g**   Normal and stressed attachments of the pectoralis and deltoid muscles.
a Lucency at the attachment of the pectoralis muscle to the crest of the greater tuberosity or at the deltoid attachment as normal variant or as a stress-related phenomenon that mimics circumscribed bone destruction.

b The crest of the lesser tuberosity appears on axial CT as an anteromedial prominence. CT also shows the physiological porosity and irregularity of the bony structures in this region.
c On a CT scan 5 mm distal to the plane in **b**, the crest of the greater tuberosity is still very prominent while that of the lesser tuberosity appears flatter.

Fig. 2.**420 d–g** ▷

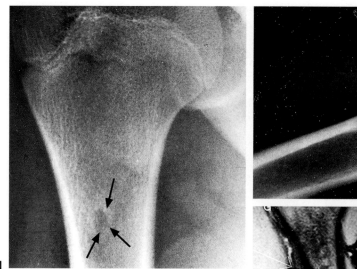
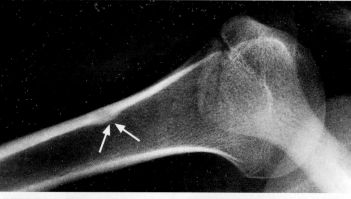
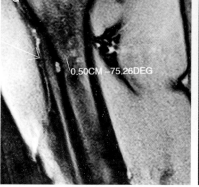
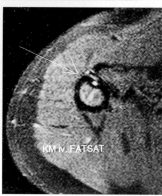

d

e

Fig. 2.**420 d–g**   Chronic traction trauma at the attachment of the pectoralis or deltoid muscle (arrows) in a 13-year-old girl. Not a bone tumor.

f

g

Pathological Finding?

Fracture

Nutrient canals can sometimes resemble fracture lines. The differential diagnosis relies chiefly on a possible trauma history and the clinical findings. Generally it may be said that fracture lines are very unusual in the segment of the humerus where nutrient canals typically occur. Any doubts are easily resolved by obtaining a few CT scans (Fig. 2.**414 c**).

Inflammation, Tumor?

The double outline of the proximal humeral shaft and proximal metaphysis seen in children and adolescents (see Fig. 2.**413**) may be mistaken for smooth periosteal new bone formation like that observed in osteomyelitis (Fig. 2.**421**).

Variants of the deltoid tuberosity and of the crests of the greater and lesser tuberosities can lead to similar confusion in adults (see above, Figs. 2.**417**, 2.**418**). The differential diagnosis in children and adolescents can be resolved by ultrasound examination of the soft tissues surrounding the "periosteal change." If necessary, MRI can be added to check for intra- and extraosseous edema and a possible abscess. It is essential that the differential diagnosis be completed within 1–2 days. This also applies to early small-cell and round-cell tumors in the medullary cavity, such as Ewing sarcoma, which does not radiologically af-

fect the cortex in its early stages but can easily incite a periosteal reaction by penetrating the various vascular canals of the cortex.

Rarely, a **shallow notch** may be seen in the endosteal surface of the cortex as an incidental finding. The explanation for this feature is unclear (partially healed eosinophilic granuloma? obliterated intraosseous varix?) (see Fig. 2.**415 b–d**).

> The fact that an endosteal cortical notch is completely filled with medullary fat proves that the finding is harmless.

Chronic traction trauma at the site of attachment of tendinous fibers can lead to cortical bone resorption resembling a tumor (Fig. 2.**420 a, d–g**).

Soft-Tissue Calcifications

Regressive paraosseous calcifications can occur at sites of tendon attachment, especially that of the deltoid muscle to the deltoid tuberosity, as the result of a calcifying tendinitis (similar to that occurring on the linea aspera of the femur, q.v., Fig. 2.**422**). Usually the adjacent cortex shows circumscribed structural irregularities caused by focal reactive hyperperfusion (Neumann et al. 1996). The necrotic calcifications should not be mistaken for myositis ossificans or for areas of heterotopic bone formation. Heterotopic ossification affects the upper extremity with some frequency, especially in the neuropathic form.

Fig. 2.**421 a–c** Periosteal and cortical changes in hematogenous osteomyelitis. The 15-year-old boy presented clinically with severe shoulder pain.
a Expansion of the haversian canals appears as faint striated lucencies, most pronounced along the lateral cortex.
b Spot film shows a thin, lamellar periosteal reaction (compare with Fig. 2.**413**).
c Tomogram taken 14 days later already shows gross cortical bone resorption, especially on the lateral side. By this tme a soft-tssue abscess had developed in the upper arm, marked by skin redness and fluctuation. Cultures from the abscess yielded *Staphylococcus aureus*.

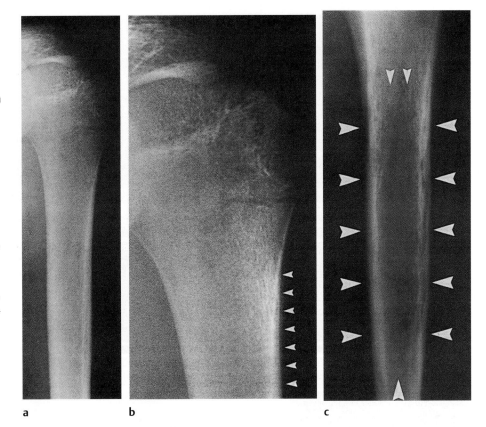

a   b   c

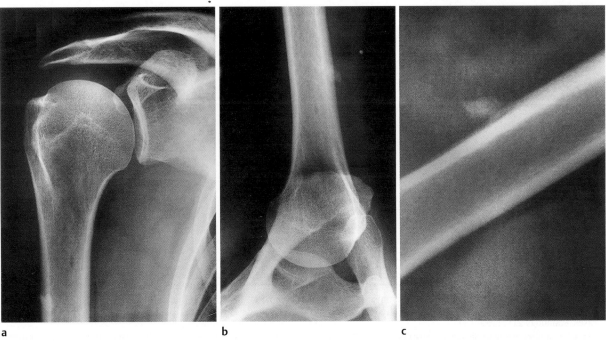

a   b   c

Fig. 2.**422 a–i** Typical cases of calcifying tendinitis in the deltoid insertion.
a–c 43-year-old patient with pain in his right upper arm.
d–i 47-year-old female with severe pain and tenderness in the left upper arm. Note the circumscribed destruction of the cortex under the soft tissue calcification, mimicking a tumorous lesion. MRI pictures demonstrate the relationship between the extraosseous inflammatory process and the intraosseus part of the lesion.

Fig. 2.**422 d–i** ▷

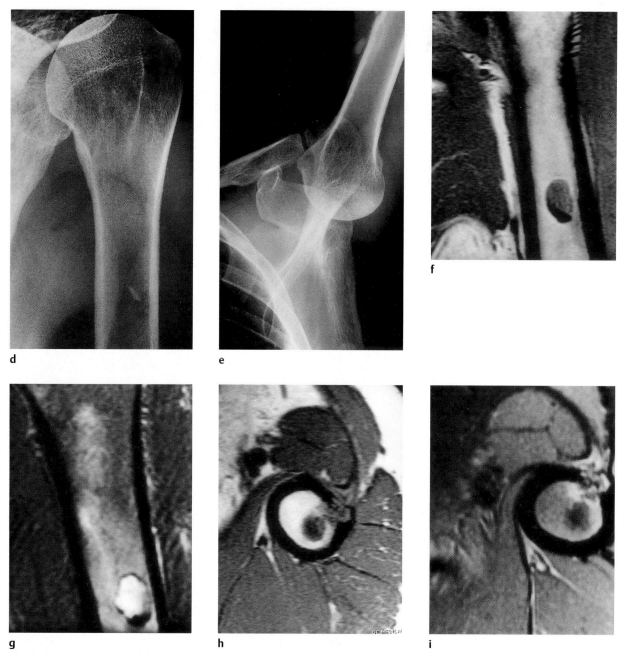

d

e

f

g

h

i

Fig. 2.**422 d–i**

References

Donnelly, L. F., C. A. Helms, G. S. Bisset III: Chronic avulsive injury of the deltoid insertion in adolescents: imaging findings in three cases. Radiology 211 (1999) 233

Keats, Th. E.: Metaphyseal cortical irregularities in children: a new perspective on a multifocal growth variant. Skelet. Radiol. 12 (1984) 112

Neumann, St., J. Freyschmidt, B. R. Holland: Die kalzifizierende Tendinits am Femur – Diagnose und Differentialdiagnose am Beispiel von 5 Fällen. Z. Rheumatol 55 (1996) 114

Ozonoff, M. B., F. M. H. Ziter jr.: The upper humeral notch: a normal variant in children. Radiology 113 (1974) 699

Rettig, A. C., H. F. Beltz: Stress fracture in the humerus in an adolescent tennis-tournament player. Amer. J. Sports Med. 13 (1985) 55

Proximal Humerus

Normal Findings

During Growth

The main ossification center of the humeral head generally becomes visible on radiographs between 4 and 8 months of age. It is located on the medial side of the upper humerus, adjacent to the glenoid fossa (Fig. 2.**423a**). Very rarely, this center is radiographically visible in newborns. The lateral ossification center for the greater tuberosity appears between birth and 2 years of age (Fig. 2.**423b**), and another center for the lesser tuberosity appears between 2 and 4 years of age. Only a very favorable projection can demonstrate the ossification center for the lesser tuberosity, as it is usually superimposed on the center for the greater tuberosity (Cocchi 1950).

The ossification centers for the tuberosities fuse with each other between 4 and 8 years of age and with the capital humeral epiphysis at 12–14 years of age, forming one large epiphysis that fuses with the proximal humeral metaphysis in about the 20th year.

The epiphyseal growth plate does not run perpendicular to the shaft. Due to the location of the tuberosity ossification centers, the lateral portion of the growth plate has the shape of an inverted V with the point up, giving the metaphysis the shape of a gabled roof (Fig. 2.**423d**).

The **geometry of the growth plate** is a frequent source of **annoyance in CT imaging**, because any given scan plane will show only a portion of the plate and adjacent solid bony structures. This results in a juxtaposition of low and high densities that should not be misinterpreted as a pathological process. If the epiphyseal plate is already closed (calcified), a pathological osteosclerotic process can be simulated (Fig. 2.**424**).

Multiplanar reformations can be helpful in doubtful cases. The shallow humeral notch or metaphyseal cortical irregularities were described on p. 238. Further details can be found on p. 258 and in Fig. 2.**443**.

In Adulthood

The radiographic morphology of the proximal humerus depends on the various positions and techniques that are used in different radiology departments.

In the standard AP projection with the central beam perpendicular to the cassette, the greater tuberosity should always appear on the lateral side (Fig. 2.**425a**).

In the lateral projection, the lesser tuberosity (on the front of the bone) appears as a prominence on the flexion surface of the humerus (Fig. 2.**426**).

With strong internal rotation of the humerus, the crest of the lesser tuberosity (giving attachment to the teres major and latissimus dorsi muscles) appears as a medial protuberance (Fig. 2.**427**). This anatomic feature should not be mistaken for exostosis.

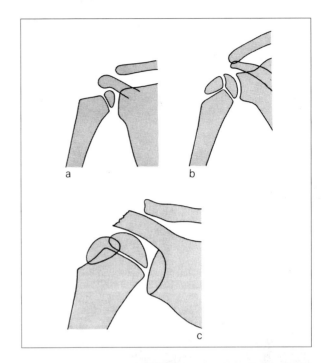

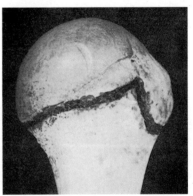

Fig. 2.**423a–d**   Normal epiphyseal ossification of the humerus. **a–c** See text.
d Anatomic specimen showing the inverted V shape of the proximal humeral epiphyseal plate.

Figure 4.**428** shows how the **radiographic morphology of the humeral head varies** (from club-shaped to elliptical) as the head is **rotated about the axis of the shaft**.

Other morphological variants are produced by angling the central beam 30° caudally, for example, to better evaluate the anterior inferior surface of the acromion (e.g., in the diagnosis of impingement syndrome) or by elevating the contralateral shoulder to correct for the natural obliquity of the glenoid fossa in the AP projection and obtain a tangential view of the glenoid.

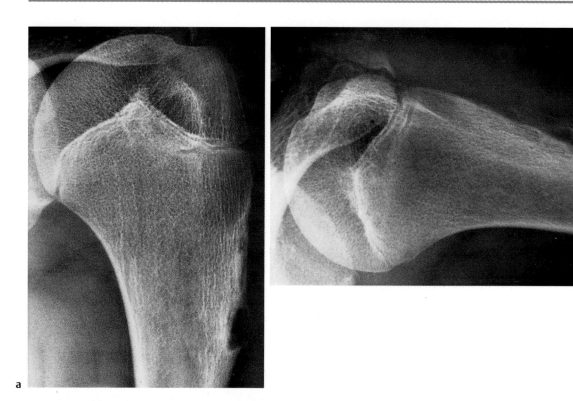

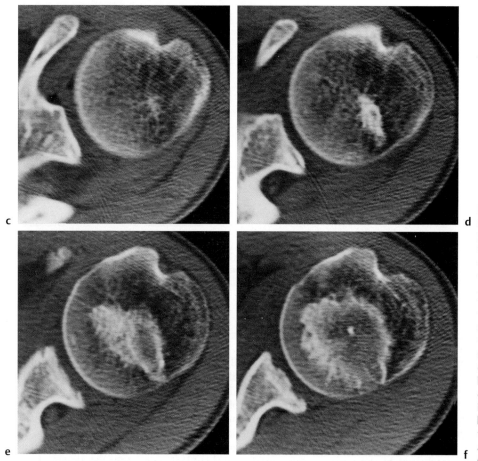

Fig. 2.**424a–p**   Variable appearance of the unfused epiphyseal growth plate and adjacent bone of the upper humerus in various CT planes. The male patient is 16 years old in panels **a–h** and 20 years old in panels **i–p**. The CT scans were obtained for a periosteal chondroma of the lateral proximal humeral shaft and metaphysis. Radiographs **a** and **b** demonstrate the tumor as a shallow excentric craterlike defect with an overhanging distal edge. The ridge or peak of the growth plate at the center of the humeral head appears in planes **c** and **d** as an irregular, circumscribed central density. As the scan plane moves distally, the bony boundaries of the growth plate acquire a more rosettelike appearance with a central lucency and irregular peripheral density (**f, g**). Thereafter, the central lucency disappears as the growth plate ossifies, appearing on CT as a more or less homogeneous central density with "cribriform extensions" at the center of the humerus (**j–p**).

Fig. 2.**424g–p** ▷

Fig. 2.**424 g–p**

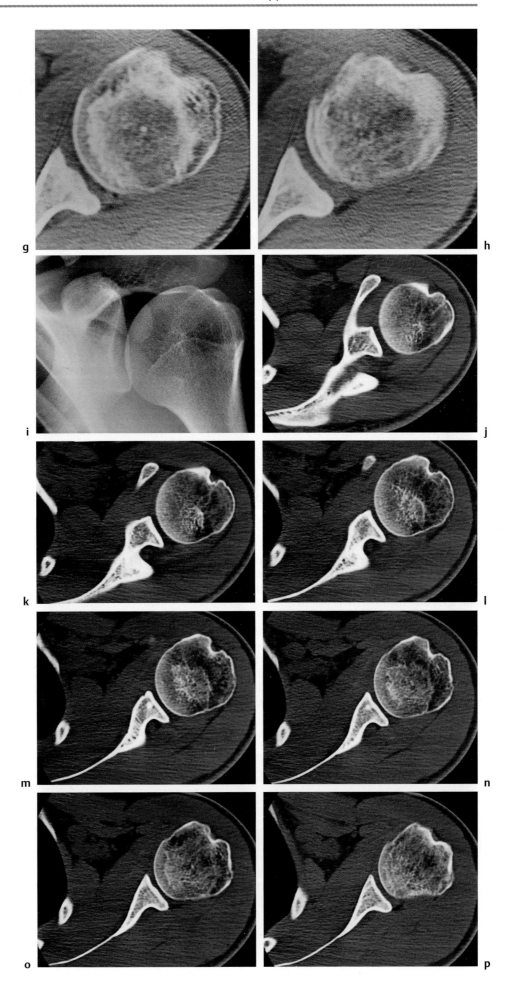

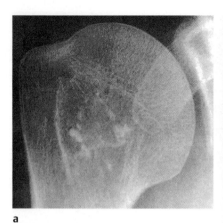

a

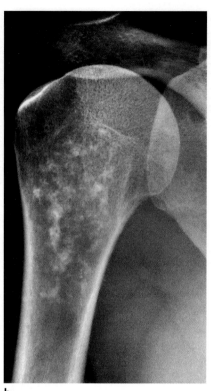

b

Fig. 2.**425 a, b**   Typical AP projection of the humeral head, illustrating the differential diagnosis of metaphyseal "calcifications."

a Lateral position of the greater tuberosity. Note the fine irregular densities in the proximal humeral metaphysis below the anatomic neck. Once known as "normal stippling," these densities most likely represent small bone marrow infarction. In several cases that we examined by MRI, the stippled areas appeared as signal voids on T1- and T2-weighted images. This is inconsistent with calcified cartilaginous matrix, where T2-weighted MRI would usually show hyperintense areas between the calcifications.

b This radiograph shows a calcifying enchondroma in the proximal humeral shaft and metaphysis. The calcifications of the tumorous cartilaginous matrix clearly extend into the shaft, which is not observed in radiograph **a**.

Since both patients were asymptomatic, the differentiation of "stippling" from a calcified enchondroma is of purely academic interest, especially since the maximum extent of the affected areas is no more than 2–3 cm.

The diagram in Fig. 2.**429** shows the radiographic anatomy of the axial projection. This is a caudocranial projection in which the central beam is coaxial to the long axis of the body and the cassette is placed on the shoulder perpendicular to the central beam.

A radiograph with the arm slightly elevated and internally rotated can provide a tangential view of the bicipital groove, which is flanked by the superior cartilage-bearing portion of the humeral head on one side and the greater tuberosity on the other (Fig. 2.**430a**). This feature should not be mistaken for an erosion (Fig. 2.**430b, c**), especially when the contour of the groove is solid.

The **relationship of the humeral head to the glenoid is particularly variable in elderly patients** and can sometimes mimic a shoulder subluxation. Carpenter and Millard (1982) observed both superior and inferior excursion of the humeral head in geriatric patients. Inferior subluxation in particular is probably a result of lax musculature, a phenomenon that is also seen in the initial weeks following trauma to the shoulder joint (e.g., subcapital humeral fracture). Inferior subluxation in these cases, then, is not entirely the result of intra-articular effusion.

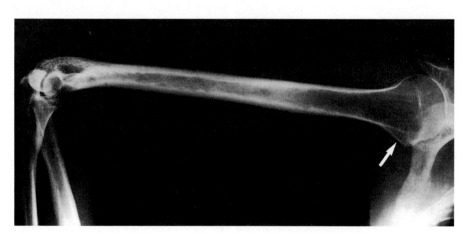

Fig. 2.**426**   Lesser tuberosity on the flexor aspect of the upper humerus.

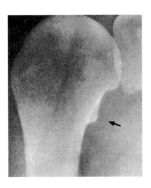

Fig. 2.**427** With the humerus internally rotated, the crest of the lesser tuberosity (giving attachment to the teres major and latissimus dorsi muscles) appears as a prominence on the medial side of the bone (arrow).

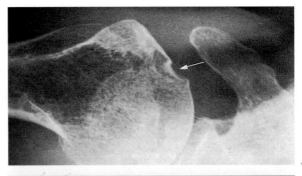

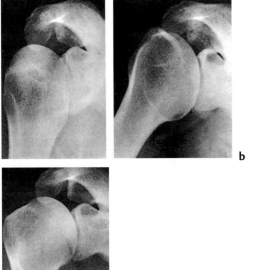

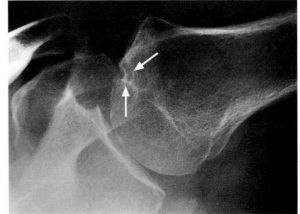

Fig. 2.**428 a–c** Variation of shape of the humeral head in different projections.
a Internal rotation.
b External rotation.
c Neutral position.

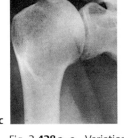

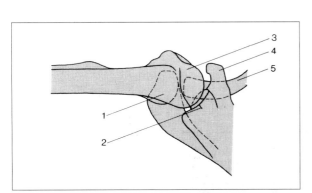

Fig. 2.**429** Radiographic anatomy in an axial projection of the shoulder joint.
1 Acromion
2 Glenoid fossa
3 Humeral head
4 Coracoid process
5 Clavicle

Fig. 2.**430 a–c** Normal and eroded intertubercular sulcus.
a Tangential view of the intertubercular sulcus in an asymptomatic patient. Note the solid contours of the sulcus.
b, c In these radiographs the sulcus has indistinct margins due to inflammatory erosion resulting from long biceps tenosynovitis. Film **b** is from a man with rheumatoid arthritis, and film **c** is from a woman with multicentric reticulohistiocytosis. Neither of these standard projections shows whether the poorly marginated depression is actually the intertubercular sulcus or a marginal erosion in the bare area of the upper humerus.

The **trabecular architecture of the humeral head** is normally uniform, but the cancellous trabeculae are relatively sparse in the region of the tuberosities, forming a rounded lucent area that can mimic an osteolytic lesion (Fig. 2.**431**).

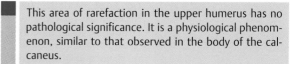

This area of rarefaction in the upper humerus has no pathological significance. It is a physiological phenomenon, similar to that observed in the body of the calcaneus.

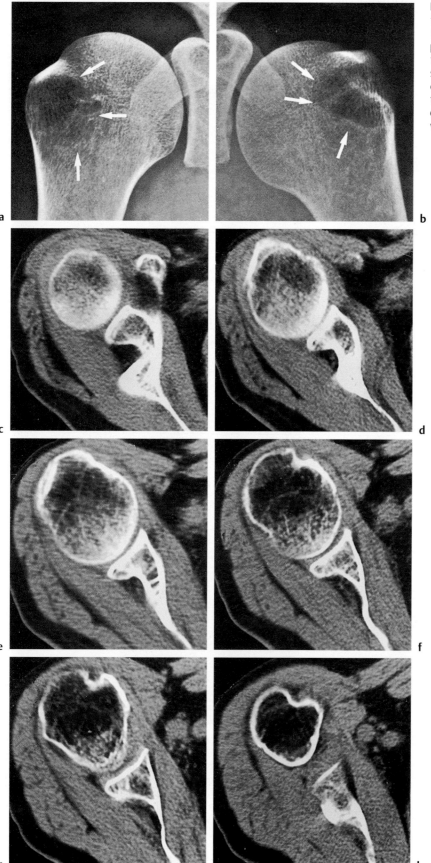

Fig. 2.**431 a–h**   Normal area of rarefaction in the region of the tuberosities (arrows), not to be confused with pathological osteolysis. The lucent effect is explained by the series of CT scans in **c–h**, which clearly show the diminution of cancellous trabeculae in this region and the relative abundance of fatty tissue (compare films **a** and **b** with the series in Fig. 2.**432 a–e**).

Formerly, these areas of rarefaction in the humerus and calcaneus were called pseudocysts—a term that is misleading since the rarefied area is not a fluid-filled space but an area with a relative abundance of fat and relatively sparse trabeculae per unit volume. This is illustrated by the series of CT scans in Fig. 2.**431**. True osteolytic lesions caused by tumors have a different radiographic appearance (Fig. 2.**432**).

The area below the **anatomic neck** of the humerus occasionally contains amorphous, patchy densities that are usually located in the medial portion of the lucent area described above and most likely represent small fat-marrow infarcts (Fig. 2.**425**). They have no pathological significance and generally are detected incidentally.

Fig. 2.**432 a–j** Differentiating the normal lucency in the proximal humerus from osteolytic processes.
a–c Grade I chondrosarcoma, easily distinguished from normal lucency by its destruction of the lateral metaphyseal cortex and the sclerotic margin separating it from surrounding bone (seen most clearly in **b**). The CT appearance is shown in **c**.
d Epiphyseal chondroma appears as a multicentric lucency in the humeral head (i.e., closer to the joint) combined with a calcified cartilage matrix.
e Giant cell tumor shows relatively gross destruction of the entire proximal humeral metaphysis with osteolytic lesions extending into the shaft. The "lucency" is not confined to the intertubercular region (arrows).

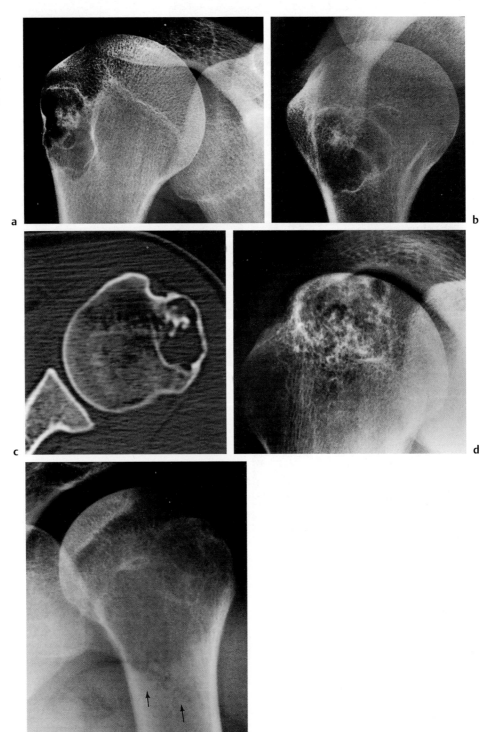

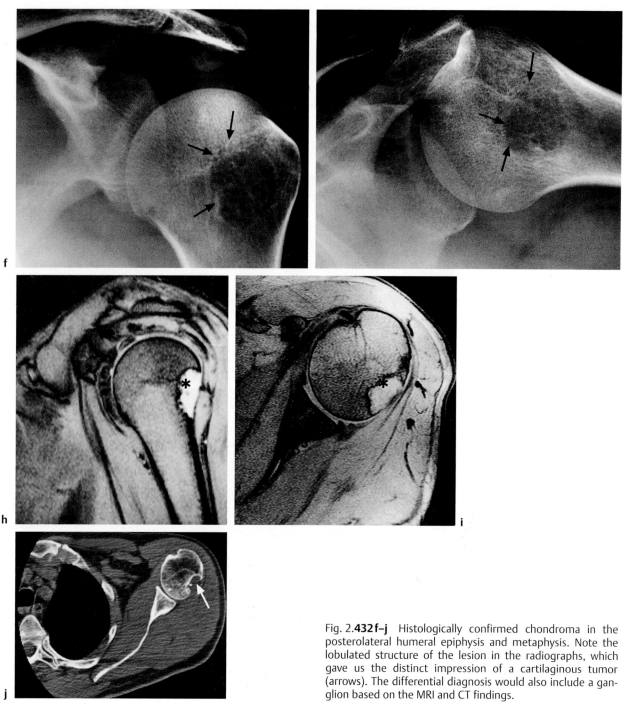

Fig. 2.**432f–j** Histologically confirmed chondroma in the posterolateral humeral epiphysis and metaphysis. Note the lobulated structure of the lesion in the radiographs, which gave us the distinct impression of a cartilaginous tumor (arrows). The differential diagnosis would also include a ganglion based on the MRI and CT findings.

Pathological Finding?

Normal Variant or Anomaly?

The angle formed by the axis of the humeral shaft and that of the humeral head (line through the anatomic neck, after Keats 1966) is normally 60–62°. A smaller angle is defined as **humerus varus**, one of the most common deformities of the proximal humerus (Fig. 2.**433**).

This deformity may be one feature of a congenital syndrome (e.g., achondroplasia), or it may be acquired as a result of arthritis, avascular necrosis, or trauma during the skeletal growth period (Fig. 2.**434**).

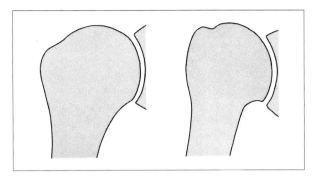

Fig. 2.**433 a, b**   Humerus varus.
a Normal humerus.
b Humerus varus.

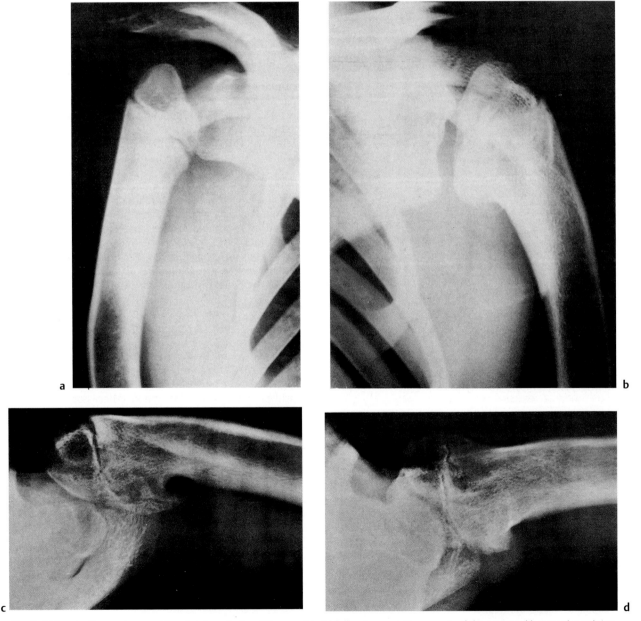

Fig. 2.**434 a–d**   Severe humeral head deformity in a 15-year-old girl following aseptic necrosis of the proximal humeral epiphysis. The deformity closely resembles the late stage of aseptic necrosis of the femoral head (Perthes disease).

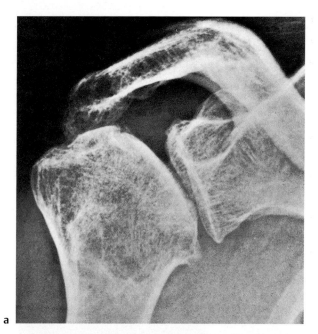

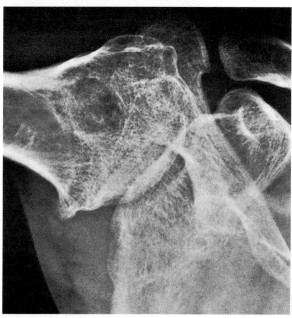

Fig. 2.**435 a, b**   Flattened, necrotic humeral head following an injury, with signs of secondary osteoarthritis of the glenohumeral joint (compare with Fig. 2.**428**).

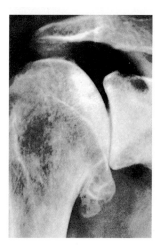

Fig. 2.**436**   Humeral head deformity in syringomyelia.

Congenital varus deformity may be combined with a shallow or aplastic glenoid or with a spade-shaped glenoid. While isolated humerus varus is not necessarily symptomatic, its combination with a glenoid anomaly invariably predisposes to recurrent dislocation of the shoulder.

Humeral head fractures and necrosis due to trauma or other causes in adults can lead to acquired deformities as shown in Figs. 2.**435** and 2.**436**.

Increased **retroversion** of the humeral head decreases contact between the head and the scapular articular surface and correlates with recurrent anterior dislocation of the humeral head (Cyprien et al. 1983). In the section on normal findings in adults, it was noted that the **shape of the proximal humerus depends strongly on the radiographic projection**. Oblique projections and rotation of the humeral head can easily create a false impression of dysplasia. Thus, an accurate standard projection as described above is one of the prerequisites for evaluating the anatomic shape of the proximal humeral epiphysis and metaphysis.

 Fracture, Subluxation, or Dislocation?

We cannot fully explore the complex issues relating to **shoulder dislocations** in the context of normal variants. The various types of dislocation and associated bony injuries of the humerus and glenoid are reviewed in the section on the Shoulder Joint as a Whole. Here we shall briefly describe the **Hill–Sachs lesion**, which is easily missed on standard AP radiographs of the shoulder joint. It occurs when the humeral head dislocates anteriorly and becomes impacted against the inferior glenoid rim, creating an impression defect in the posterolateral aspect of the head. Radiographically, the Hill–Sachs lesion is best demonstrated on internally rotated spot films of the humeral head (Fig. 2.**437**).

The Hill–Sachs lesion is found in approximately 95% of patients with recurrent shoulder dislocations. Three radiographic types are distinguished:

- Notch type
- Groove type
- Flat type

The first two are easily differentiated from normal variants, but the flat type can present difficulties. It should be diagnosed only by correlating the radiographic findings with the clinical presentation and, if necessary, by obtaining confirmatory CT scans.

Specific details on the various **fracture patterns in the proximal humerus** are beyond our scope, but it is helpful to review the **Neer classification**, which is the most widely used system for classifying proximal humeral fractures. This classification subdivides the proximal humerus into four major segments (Fig. 2.**438 a**).

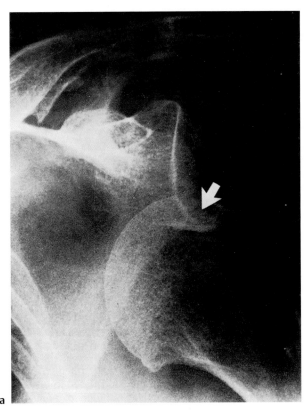

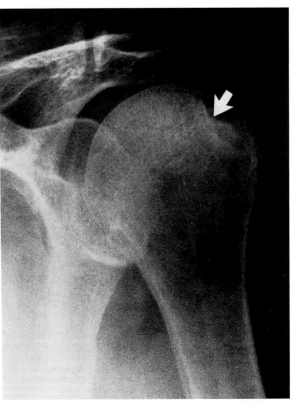

a

b

Fig. 2.**437 a, b**   Hill–Sachs lesion following an anterior subglenoid shoulder dislocation with impaction of the humeral head against the inferior glenoid rim (arrow). The postreduction film (**b**) shows the posterolateral impression defect in the humeral head.

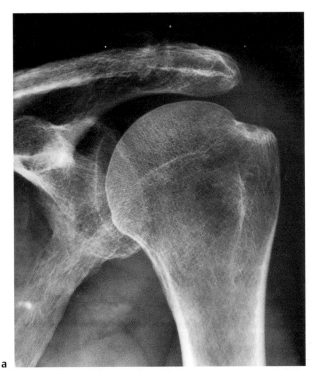

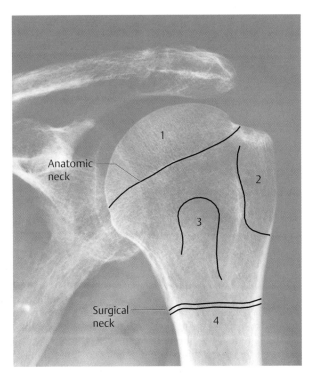

a

Fig. 2.**438 a, b**   Segments of the proximal humerus used in the classification of fractures.
a The four segments are shown schematically in the image on the right.

1 Articular segment (anatomic neck)
2 Greater tuberosity
3 Lesser tuberosity
4 Shaft segment (surgical neck)

Fig. 2.**438 b** ▷

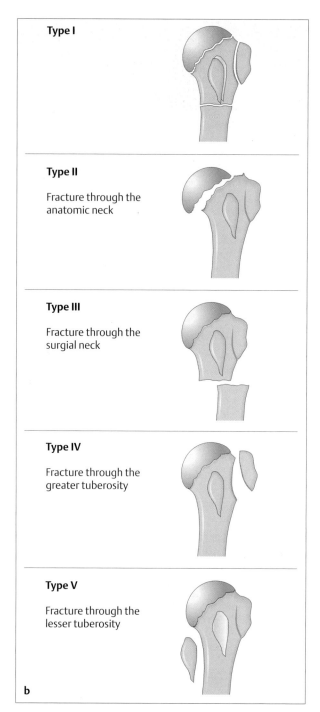

Type I

Type II

Fracture through the
anatomic neck

Type III

Fracture through the
surgial neck

Type IV

Fracture through the
greater tuberosity

Type V

Fracture through the
lesser tuberosity

b

Fig. 2.**438b** Neer classification of proximal humeral fractures. Type VI is a fracture-dislocation.

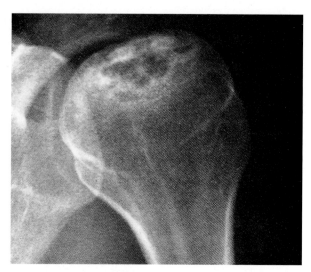

Fig. 2.**439** Fully developed osteonecrosis of the humeral
head, marked by a combination of lucencies, sclerotic changes, and fragmentation of the subchondral bone.

These segments have practical importance only if one or
more segments are displaced more than 1 cm or angulated
more than 45°. Six fracture types are distinguished
(Fig. 2.**438b**). A type I fracture is one in which there is no
significant displacement. This fracture is classified by stat-
ing the type and the number of parts, i.e., the number of
fractured segments. If just one segment is displaced in relation to the three remaining segments, the fracture is assigned to type II–V, depending on the displaced segment.
The number of fractured segments that are not displaced
or angulated is also stated. If two or more segments are displaced or angulated, the numerically higher fracture type

determines the type assignment, and the fracture is described as three-part (two segments displaced in relation
to the remaining two) or four-part (all four segments are
displaced). For example, a displaced fracture through the
surgical neck combined with a displaced fracture of the
lesser tuberosity would be classified as a three-part type V
fracture. Fracture-dislocations of the proximal humerus
are always classified as type VI.

Only avulsion fractures of the tuberosities have real importance in the differential diagnosis of borderline-pathological findings. Fractures through the anatomic neck or
surgical neck should be easy to identify. Tuberosity avulsions require differentiation from intra-articular loose
bodies at unusual locations and from very solid bursal calcifications (see Figs. 3.**65** and 3.**66**).

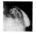 **Necrosis?**

The **humeral head** is a relatively common site of
osteonecrosis, especially following the systemic use of
steroids. In the latter case the humeral head is the third
most common site of involvement after the femoral head
and the knee. The humeral head also seems particularly
sensitive to barotrauma, developing more or less pronounced signs of necrosis and eventual deformity. Fully
developed osteonecrosis of the humeral head presents
radiographically with lucencies, sclerotic changes, one or
more subchondral fractures, and fragmentation
(Fig. 2.**439**). Generally these changes present no difficulties
in terms of differential diagnosis.

It is critical to detect **early osteonecrosis**, which typically appears in the humeral head as a relatively homogeneous subchondral density ("snowcap" sign, Fig. 2.**440**).
Although the radiographic change is subtle, the density in
fact represents an advanced necrotic process. True early
forms can be detected only by MRI or radionuclide scanning (Fig. 2.**441**).

Idiopathic avascular necrosis of the humeral head appears to be extremely rare. The eventual deformity closely
resembles Perthes disease of the femoral head (Fig. 2.**434**).

Fig. 2.**440 a, b**   Osteonecrosis of the humeral head.

a   This humeral head is necrotic but not yet fractured. Note the "white" trabecular structures in the subchondral bone (snowcap sign).

b   Radiograph several weeks later demonstrates a subchondral fracture. The necrotic area is demarcated by a heavy, reactive sclerotic border.

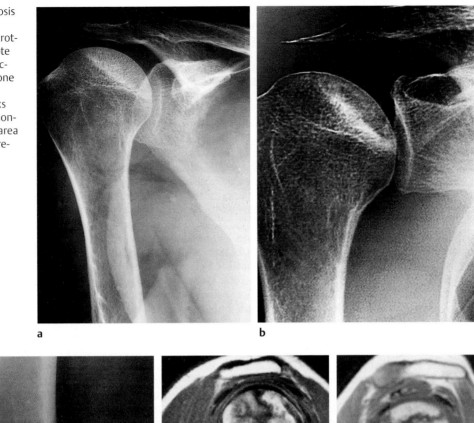

a

b

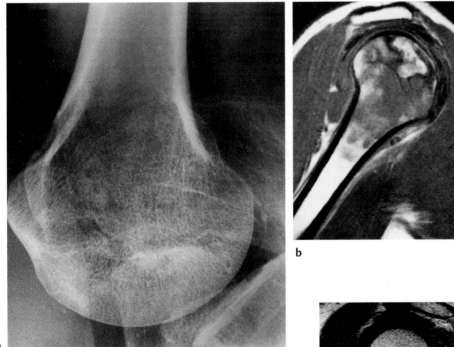

a

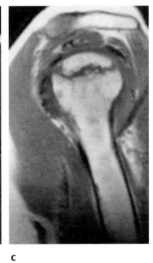

b

c

Fig. 2.**441 a–e**   Differential diagnosis of osteonecrotic changes in the proximal humerus.

a–c   Early osteonecrosis in a patient treated with steroids for a collagen disease. Radiograph with the arm elevated shows no obvious subchondral changes (**a**), but on MRI the subchondral necrotic area is already demarcated from healthy bone (**b, c**). Note the signal void caused by extensive edema about the proximal humeral epiphysis and metaphysis in image **b**. Marked enhancement is observed after contrast administration (**c**).

d, e   These images show an extreme normal variant of bone marrow reconversion (fat > red marrow) in an asymptomatic 58-year-old woman (not marrow necrosis or tumor infiltration of the medullary cavity). Note the patchy pattern of low signal intensity in the T1-weighted image (**d**) and the hyperintensity of the same areas in the T2-weighted image (**e**).

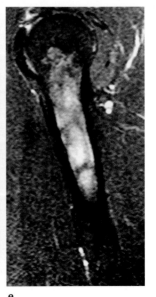

d

e

Osteochondritis dissecans (subarticular avascular necrosis) of the humeral head is rarely diagnosed, and involvement of the opposing glenoid fossa is much more common. It is unclear if osteochondritis dissecans of the humeral head is indeed rare or if traditional diagnostic methods have been inadequate. Current MRI studies in young patients with unexplained shoulder pain should help to clarify this issue.

An osteonecrotic component plays a significant role in the pathogenesis of **neurogenic arthropathy**. The humeral head is a site of predilection for neurogenic arthropathy, especially in patients with syringomyelia (Fig. 2.**436**). Both a neurogenic component (based on the "neurovascular theory") and an osteonecrotic cofactor contribute to the pathogenesis of the **Milwaukee shoulder**. This syndrome, known also as "rapidly destructive osteoarthritis" (omarthrosis), occurs predominantly in older women. Within a matter of months, the disease leads to joint space narrowing followed by superior migration of the humeral head, massive joint effusion, and eventual osteonecrosis of the humeral head (Fig. 2.**442**). There are no typical osteoarthritis-related phenomena such as geodes or osteophytes.

Another subtype of osteonecrosis occurs in the form of **bone marrow necrosis** with small dystrophic calcifications in the proximal humeral metaphysis, as shown in Fig. 2.**425**. Most of these cases involve a necrosis of the marrow fat as the consequence of abundant fat accumulation but no real clinical significance. Differentiation is required from ossified cartilaginous matrix in enchondromatosis and from an enchondroma (see below).

 Tumor?

Cortical irregularities are a frequent source of diagnostic error. Described as "metaphyseal cortical irregularities" by Keats and Joyce (1984) or as the "upper humeral notch" by Ozonoff and Ziter (1974), they are found in the proximal medial humeral metaphyseal cortex of adolescents. Although cortical irregularities occur mainly in the distal femoral metaphysis, they have also been observed in the distal humeral metaphysis of children 10–16 years of age. Other sites of occurrence are the distal radial and ulnar metaphysis and the proximal and distal metaphysis of the tibia and fibula. They can also occur in younger children. It is reasonable to speculate that cortical irregularities occur in response to heavy stresses, but this has not yet been proved. Keats and Joyce (1984) observed irregularities of the underlying cancellous bone with absence or marked reduction of the overlying cortex, so that the cancellous bone bordered almost directly on the periosteum. In a histological study, Brower et al. (1971) found only connective tissue in the area of the irregular or deficient cortex. Cortical irregularities in the distal femur and proximal humerus are usually bilateral and self-limiting, persisting for a period of several weeks to a few years. The outer medial contour of the proximal humerus has a frayed and irregular appearance and sometimes bears a shallow indentation (humeral notch) (Fig. 2.**443**). Cortical irregularities do not cause clinical symptoms.

These findings should not be mistaken for a neoplastic process (e.g., arising from the periosteum). They are negative on radionuclide bone scans.

As the series of images in Fig. 2.**431** illustrates, the **physiological lucent area** in the tuberosity region is to be distinguished from **true osteolytic lesions**. A comparison of Fig. 2.**431 a, b** with Fig. 2.**432 a, b** shows that the differential diagnosis is straightforward, provided of course that the clinical presentation is also considered. While the lucencies in Fig. 2.**431** blend smoothly with the proximal lateral aspect of the metaphysis with no cortical violation or peri-

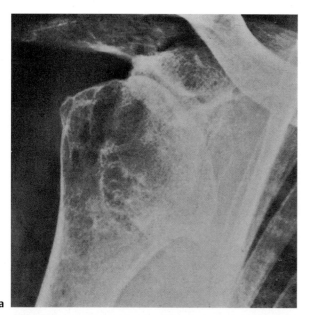

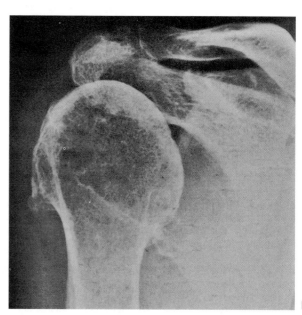

a   b

Fig. 2.**442 a, b**   Milwaukee shoulder in a 68-year-old woman with a marked necrotic component and deformity of the humeral head.

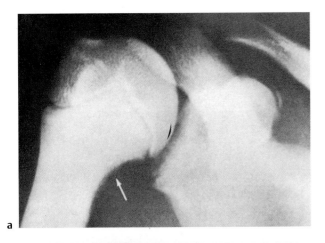
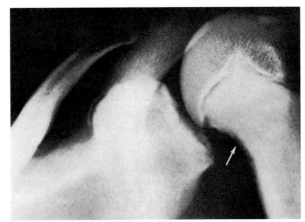
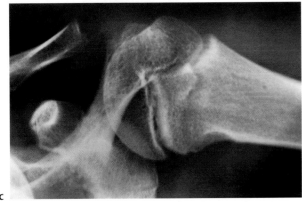
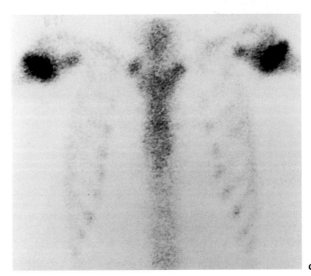

Fig. 2.**443 a–d**   Metaphyseal cortical irregularities and defects as physiological phenomena.
a, b Cortical irregularities in the medial humeral metaphysis of a 14-year-old girl. This feature should not be misinterpreted as destructive changes. (From Keats and Joyce 1984.)

c, d Picture **c** shows a "notch" or "pit" in the anterior cortex of an 11-year-old girl. Although this was detected incidentally on a posttraumatic radiograph, it was interpreted as a destructive process. But when the finding was checked by bone scanning (**d**), it proved to be a normal variant.

osteal reaction, a grade I chondrosarcoma is distinguished by cortical erosion and central ossification of the cartilaginous matrix, similar to the appearance of an epiphyseal chondroma (Fig. 2.**432 d**). Also, the chondroma in Figure 2.**432** involves the epiphysis rather than the metaphysis. With a giant cell tumor of the proximal humeral metaphysis (about 10% of cases), a detectable tumor margin is generally present on radiographs (Fig. 2.**432 e**), whereas physiological lucencies blend smoothly with the surrounding, denser trabecular network. The chondroma in Fig. 2.**432 f–j**, which was confirmed by CT-guided percutaneous biopsy, has a very distinct, lobulated sclerotic margin and a "honeycomb" internal structure (peripheral ossified septa between cartilaginous lobules en face).

Juvenile bone cysts in the proximal humerus are tumor-like lesions that normally involve the shaft-metaphyseal region and generally appear as a very lucent area that "expands" the bone (by new cortical bone formation).

A classic calcifying enchondroma of the proximal humeral shaft and metaphysis is shown in Figs. 2.**425 b** and 2.**444**.

 Inflammation?

Omarthritis, regardless of its cause, is usually associated with demineralization of portions of the humeral head, especially in the subchondral area. This process begins within a matter of days (in children) to weeks (in adults). Omarthritis is generally distinguished from a normal variant by a slight blurring of the demineralized areas; this can be detected by scrutinizing the radiograph with a magnifying lens. The problem of differentiating inflammatory erosions from a normal intertubercular sulcus was discussed on p. 248 and in Fig. 2.**430 a–c**.

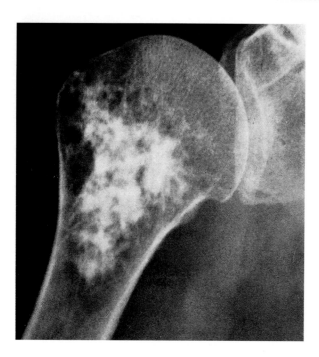

Fig. 2.**444** Typical calcifying enchondroma in the proximal humeral shaft and metaphysis (compare this finding with Fig. 2.**425 a, b**).

References

Anderson, W. J., W. Bonner-Guilford: Osteochondritis dissecans of the humeral head. Clin. Orthop. 173 (1983) 166

Bricout, P. B., M. Simanovsky, M. I. Feldmann et al.: Necrosis of the humeral head following postoperative supervoltage irradiation and chemotherapy in carcinoma of the breast. Brit. J. Radiol. 58 (1985) 562

Brower, A. C., J. E. Culver, T. E. Keats: Histological nature of the cortical irregularity of the medial posterior distal femoral metaphysis in children. Radiology 99 (1971) 389

Brown, W. H., J. M. Dennis, C. N. Davidson et al.: Posterior dislocation of the shoulder. Radiology 69 (1957) 815

Carpenter,G. I., P. H. Millard: Shoulder subluxation in elderly inpatients. J. Amer. Geriat. Soc. 30 (1982) 441

Cocchi, U.: Zur Frage der Epiphysenossifikation des Humeruskopfes. Das Tuberculum minus. Radiol. clin. (Basel) 19 (1950) 18

Cone, R. O., L. Danzig, D. Resnick et al.: The bicipital groove. Amer. J. Roentgenol. 141 (1983) 781

Cruess, R. L.: Corticosteroid-induced osteonecrosis of the humeral head. Orthoped. Clin. N. Amer. 16 (1985) 789

Cyprien, J. M., H. M. Vasey, A. Burdet et al.: Humeral retrotorsion and glenohumeral relationship in the normal shoulder and in recurrent anterior dislocation (scapulometry). Clin. Orthop. 175 (1983) 8

Garth, W. P., C. E. Slappy, Ch. W. Ochs: Roentgenographic demonstration of instability of the shoulder: the apical oblique projection. J. Bone Jt Surg. 66-A (1984) 1450

Gould, R., A. T. Rosenfield, G. E.Friedlaender: Loose body within the glenohumeral joint in recurrent anterior dislocation: CT-demonstration. Case report. J. Comput. assist. Tomogr. 9 (1985) 404

Halverson, P. B., D. M. McCarty, H. S. Chung et al.: Milwaukee shoulder syndrome: eleven additional cases with involvement of the knee in seven (basic calcium phosphate crystal deposition disease). Semin. Arthr. Rheum. 14 (1984) 36

Hansen jr., N. M.: Epiphyseal changes in the proximal humerus of an adolescent baseball pitcher. Amer. J. Sports Med. 10 (1982) 380

Heyser, K., E. Günther, B. Rumpf: Progrediente Nekrose am Humeruskopf bei Syringomyelie. Fortschr. Röntgenstr. 123 (1975) 280

Jobe, F. W., Ch. M. Job: Painful athletic injuries of the shoulder. Clin. Orthop. 173 (1983) 117

Keats, Th. E., M. Joyce: Metaphyseal cortical irregularities in children: a new perspective on a multifocal growth variant. Skelet. Radiol. 12 (1984) 112

Kerr, R., D. Resnick, C. Pineda et al.: Osteoarthritis of the glenohumeral joint: a radiologic-pathologic study. Amer. J. Roentgenol. 144 (1985) 967

McCarthy, D. J., P. B. Halveson, G. F. Carrera et al.: "Milwaukee shoulder": association of microspheroids containing hydroxyapatite crystals, active collagenase, and neutral protease with rotator cuff defects. Arthr. and Rheum. 24 (1981) 464

Ozonoff, M. B., F. M. H. Ziter jr.: The upper humeral notch. Radiology 113 (1974) 699

Podesva, K., H. Ritter: Seltene Beobachtung einer Humeruskopfnekrose. Unfallheilkunde 85 (1982) 120

Poser, H., P. Gabriel-Jürgens: Knochen- und Gelenkveränderungen durch Druckluft bei Tauchern und Caissonarbeitern. Fortschr. Röntgenstr. 126 (177) 156

Resnick, D., R. O. Cone: The nature of humeral pseudocysts. Radiology 150 (1984) 27

3

Shoulder Girdle and Thorax

J. Freyschmidt

Scapula

Normal Findings

During Growth

The first ossification center of the scapula appears in the area of the scapular neck during the seventh or eighth week of fetal development. At birth, the central portion of the scapula is ossified along with part of the acromion. Significant portions of the glenoid, the medial border of the scapula, the scapular angle, the coracoid process, and the acromion are still cartilaginous at that stage. Details on the

postnatal development of the scapula are reviewed in Odgen and Phillips (1983).

The **glenoid cavity** (glenoid, glenoid fossa) is poorly differentiated in infants and slightly convex or shallow (Fig. 3.**1**).

By 8 to 13 years of age, the subchondral bony contour of the glenoid fossa appears heavily rippled (Fig. 3.**2**), similar to the acetabulum of the hip joint.

The epiphysis is ring-shaped, similar to the marginal ridges or rings of the vertebral bodies. The radiographically visible ossification phase lasts only a short time and then can be seen only in certain projections (Figs. 3.**3**, 3.**4**), for soon the epiphyseal ring fuses with the body of the scapula.

Ziegler (1957) described the ossification of the cartilaginous glenoid labrum, which is completed by 18 years of age.

The **scapular angles** (see Fig. 3.**14**) have **apophyseal centers** that appear between 16 and 18 years of age. If the apophyseal center of the inferior angle persists, it is termed the **os infrascapulare** (Fig. 3.**5**).

Occasionally an ossification center also occurs at the superior medial angle (Fig. 3.**6**).

The medial border of the scapula frequently appears undulated in the growing skeleton and occasionally presents double contours. Fine apophyseal ridges have also been described.

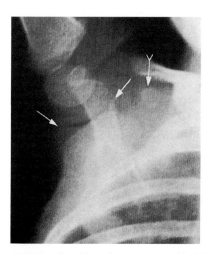

Fig. 3.**1** Shoulder of a 3-month-old child. True joint space (arrows), coracoid center (double arrow).

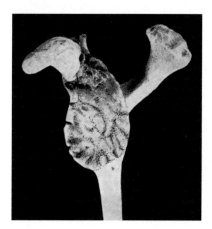

Fig. 3.**2** Glenoid fossa in an anatomic specimen from an adolescent.

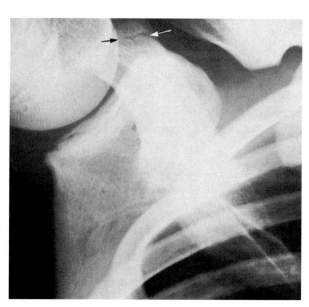

Fig. 3.**3** Irregular, undulant contour of the glenoid. Apical ossification center of the coracoid process (arrows).

The **coracoid process** develops from a center that appears before one year of age and remains unfused until 15 to 20 years of age (Fig. 3.**7**).

The zigzag apophyseal plate remains visible for a relatively long time (Fig. 3.**8**).

Another isolated center, called the os infracoracoideum, is occasionally visible in continuity with the apophyseal plate toward the glenoid cavity between 10 and 14 years of age (Fig. 3.**9**). Two years after its appearance, this center disappears by fusing with the scapula or coracoid (Lossen and Wegner 1936). An **apical coracoid center** has also been described (Fig. 3.**10**).

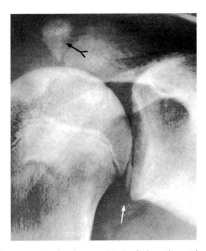

Fig. 3.**4** Epiphyseal center in the lower third of the glenoid cavity (arrow) and an isolated center at the tip of the acromion (double arrow).

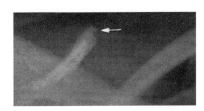

Fig. 3.**6** Ossification center at the superior medial angle of the scapula (arrow) (compare with Fig. 3.**22**).

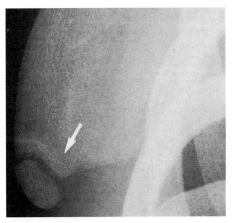

Fig. 3.**5** Os infrascapulare (arrow).

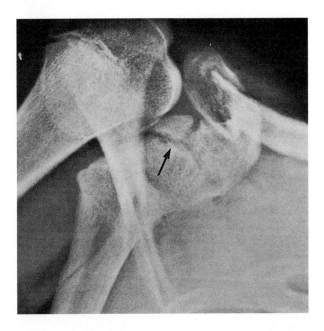

Fig. 3.**7** Triangular apophyseal center of the coracoid in a 14-year-old boy. A traumatic fracture is visible at the acromial end of the clavicle (arrow).

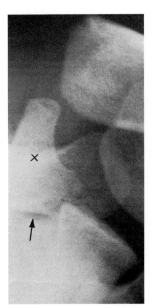

Fig. 3.**9**

Fig. 3.**8**

Fig. 3.**8** Synchondrosis (arrow) at the base of the coracoid process (×).

Fig. 3.**9** Isolated ossification center in the apophyseal cartilage of the coracoid process.

Two or three ossification centers, and sometimes more, appear at the lateral end of the **acromion** in the 15th to 18th years of life (Fig. 3.**11**). They fuse with one another at 20–25 years of age (Fig. 3.**12a**) and later with the scapular spine. As a result, the articular end of the acromion may be capped by a large ossification zone that is separated from it by a gap of variable width (Figs. 3.**12b**, 3.**13**). This apophyseal plate gapes considerably in children.

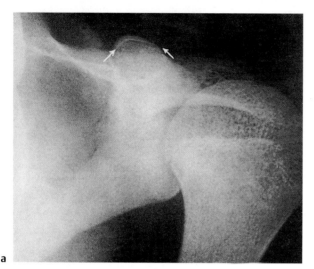

a

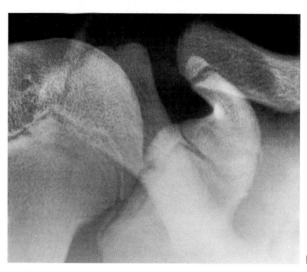

b

Fig. 3.**10a, b**   Apophyseal and epiphyseal growth centers.
a Apical ossification center of the coracoid process (arrows).

b All growth centers of the shoulder region in a 15-year-old boy.

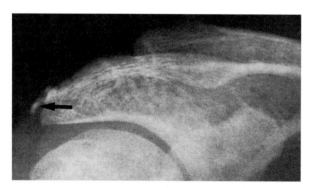

Fig. 3.**11**   Ossification centers of the acromion (arrow).

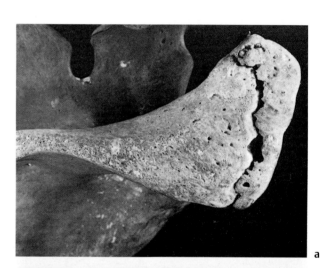

a

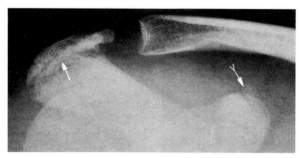

Fig. 3.**13**   Apophyseal centers of the acromion (arrow) and coracoid process (double arrow).

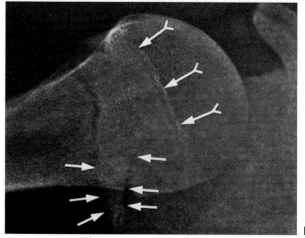

b

Fig. 3.**12a, b**   Development of the acromion (arrows).
a Platelike configuration of the acromial apophysis.
b Acromial apophysis or epiphysis in axial projection.

In Adulthood

The specimen photographs in Fig. 3.**14** illustrate the complex anatomy of the scapula. CT is the only imaging modality that can provide views of comparable detail (Fig. 3.**15**).

Conventional radiographs can define only certain portions of the scapula in nonsuperimposed views. In the **AP projection**, the scapula is correctly visualized if the glenoid cavity appears as a line or narrow ellipse. The **axial scapular view** (horizontal projection between the scapula and ribs, central ray perpendicular to the center of the medial scapular border and center of the cassette) is best for demonstrating the scapular spine, acromion, and the scapula itself. The **cephaloscapular projection**, obtained with the upper body bent 45° forward and the cassette fixed in a holder perpendicular to the projection, gives a nonsuperimposed view of all portions of the scapula (Oppenheim et al. 1985). The neck and body should be turned slightly toward the contralateral side, and the injured shoulder should be slightly elevated.

With injuries of the coracoid process, the affected shoulder should be rotated 20° posteriorly and obliquely while the central ray is angled 20° cephalad (Goldberg and Vicks 1983). The **transscapular Y view**, which Neer (1972) modified and called the supraspinatus outlet view, is useful for evaluating the curvature of the inferior surface of the acromion (p. 272 f. and Fig. 3.**16**).

The radiographic technique for a suspected Bankert lesion (the Bernageau view) is described on p. 299 f.

Scrutiny of the photographs in Fig. 3.**14** and the CT scans in Fig. 3.**15** reveals several notable features:

- The scapula itself is highly variable in its thickness.
- The muscular lines appear as ridgelike prominences between thinner areas of the bone.
- The scapula normally contains vascular foramina of varying size (Figs. 3.**17**, 3.**18**), especially in the junctional area between the neck and body of the scapula and the base of the coracoid process.

When nutrient canals are viewed in a tangential projection, they can appear as paired lucent lines. Some double lines may be a projection-related effect caused by the superimposed inferior border of the coracoid process (Fig. 3.**19**).

A physiological lucency in the upper portion of the scapular neck (Fig. 3.**20**) is often mistaken for an osteolytic lesion. It is explained by the series of CT scans in Fig. 3.**15** (e_1 through e_3), which show a fossa placed between the upper part of the scapular neck and the coracoid process.

A similar "defect" based on a superimposition effect is seen near the scapular neck on an axial projection of the shoulder joint (Fig. 3.**21**).

The **axillary or lateral border** between the glenoid cavity and inferior angle has a distinctly undulated contour. The **infraglenoid tubercle** is an exostosis-like prominence located 0.5–1 cm below the glenoid cavity. It gives attachment to the long head of the biceps brachii muscle (Fig. 3.**14**).

The **superior angle** of the scapula is often somewhat blunt and frequently asymmetrical. It sometimes presents a bifid tip (Fig. 3.**22**).

The base of the coracoid process appears round or elliptical in the orthograde projection (Fig. 3.**23**), similar to an orthograde projection of the base of an osteochondroma.

The **acromion** is among the skeletal structures that show the greatest morphological variety. Its lateral border may form a smooth convex arch; it may be scalloped, zigzag, or irregular; or it may even present a large, shallow indentation. These variants have no functional importance, unlike the morphological variations of the anterior third (flat, curved, hook-shaped), which significantly affect the underlying space for the rotator cuff (for details, see Normal Variant or Anomaly and Fig. 3.**28**).

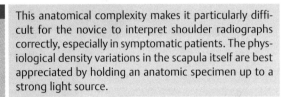

This anatomical complexity makes it particularly difficult for the novice to interpret shoulder radiographs correctly, especially in symptomatic patients. The physiological density variations in the scapula itself are best appreciated by holding an anatomic specimen up to a strong light source.

The acromioclavicular joint is discussed on p. 287 ff.

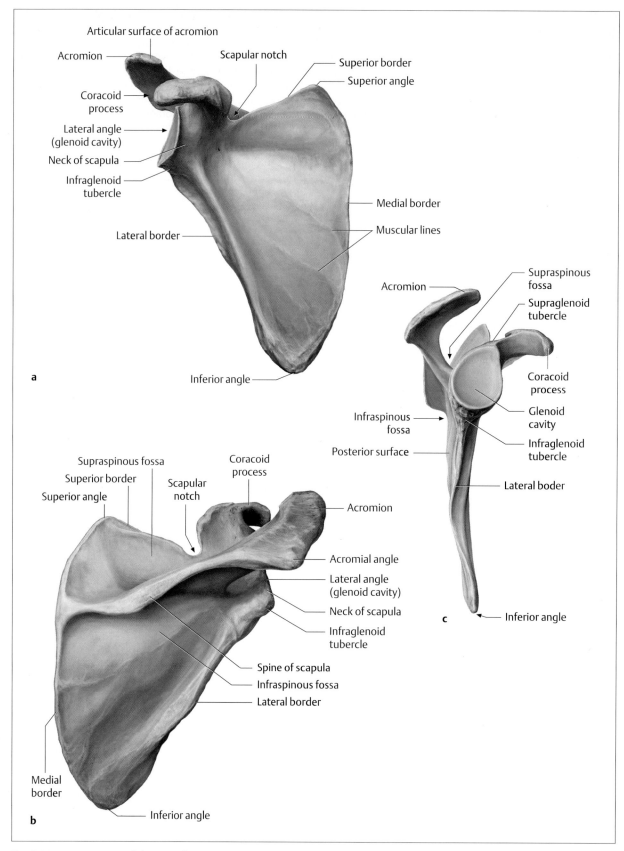

Fig. 3.**14 a–c**   Anatomy of the scapula.
a   Anterior aspect.
b   Posterior aspect.
c   Lateral aspect.

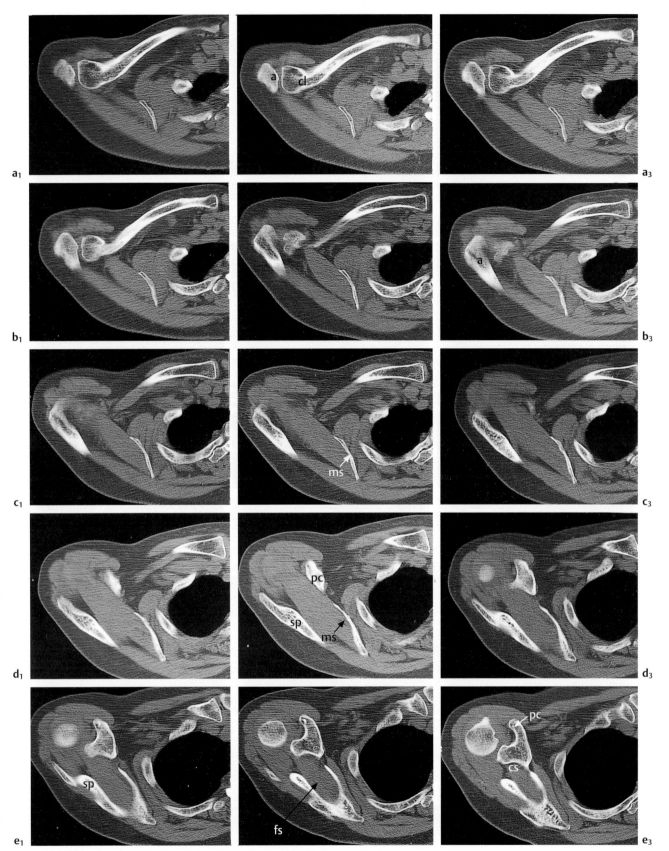

Fig. 3.**15 a–k** Series of CT scans through the scapula. The arm of the patient (an adult woman) is adducted and internally rotated. The scans are spaced at intervals of 1–2 mm from a_1 to g_2 and 3–4 mm from g_3 to h_3. Images **i–k** are coronal reformatted images.

a   Acromion
cl Clavicle

cs Neck of scapula
fs Suprascapular (supraspinous) fossa
gl Glenoid
ms Superior border of scapula
pc Coracoid process
sp Scapular spine

Fig. 3.**15 f–k** ▷

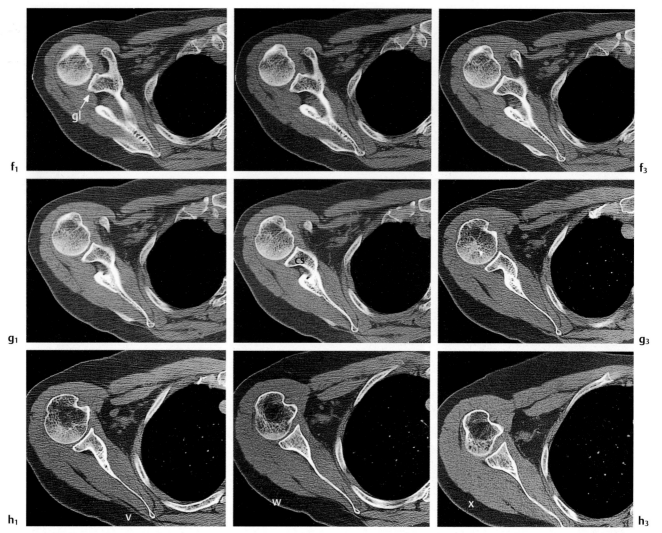

Fig. 3.**15 f–h**

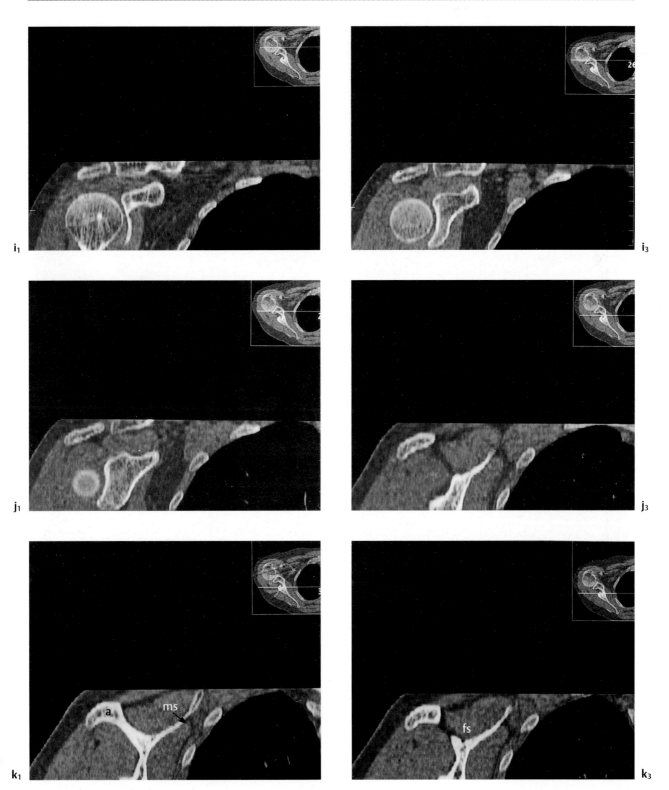

Fig. 3.**15 i**–**k**   Coronal reformatted images.

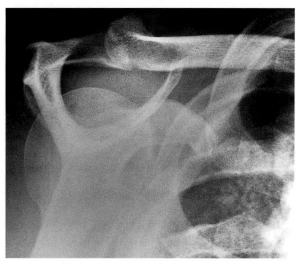

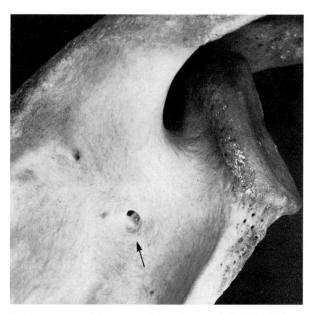

Fig. 3.**16** Transscapular Y view of the shoulder. Note the good, clear projection of the anterior portions of the acromion in this somewhat cranially centered view. In contrast to the "classic" Y view, the scapular spine rather than the coracoid process forms one limb of the Y. The acromion forms the other. The glenoid cavity is located at the intersection of the two short limbs with the long limb of the Y. A "vacant glenoid" signifies a luxation. To the soft tissue signs of the supraspinatus muscle (superior contour and homogeneity) see p. 296.

Fig. 3.**17** Typical location of nutrient canals (entry sites) in the scapula.

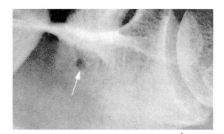

Fig. 3.**18** Radiographic appearance of the entry site for a nutrient canal in the scapular neck and coracoid base (arrow).

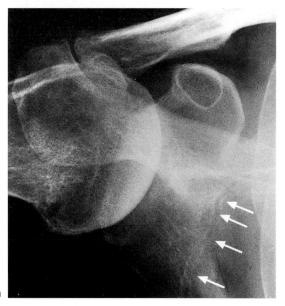

a

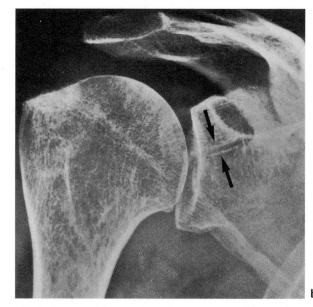

b

Fig. 3.**19a, b** Differential diagnosis of nutrient canals viewed in a tangential projection.

a Typical tangential projection of a nutrient canal (arrows).
b Not a nutrient canal in the scapular neck, but a projection effect caused by the coracoid process (arrows).

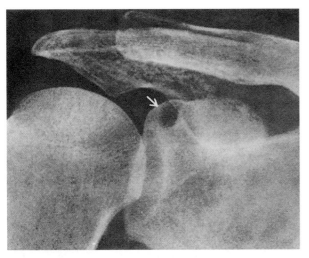

Fig. 3.**20**   Normal lucency (arrow) (see also Fig. 3.**38**).

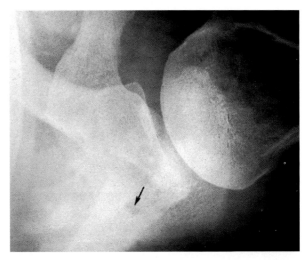

Fig. 3.**21**   Normal lucency (arrow).

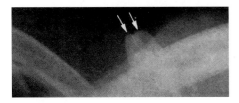

Fig. 3.**22**   Bifid tip (arrows) of the superior angle of the scapula (compare with Fig. 3.**6**).

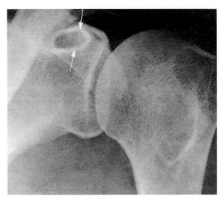

Fig. 3.**23**   Orthograde projection through the base of the coracoid process (arrows).

Pathological Finding?

 ### Normal Variant or Anomaly?

Variants

The following are considered true **variants of the scapula**:

A **scaphoid scapula** is one that has a concave medial border between the scapular spine and inferior angle.

With **ossification of the superior transverse scapular ligament**, the underlying scapular notch (between the superior border and coracoid process) assumes a foramen-like appearance (Fig. 3.**24**). A familial incidence of this ligamentous ossification has been reported (Giordano 1962). Figure 3.**25** shows a similar variant involving the superior border of the scapula.

Ossification of the coracoclavicular ligament is a relatively common variant (Fig. 3.**26**). This ligament is composed of a lateral part (trapezoid ligament) and a medial part (conoid ligament). Both ligaments may become partly or completely ossified (Villanyi 1970). Congenital ossification of the ligament should always be assumed if there is no history of trauma. But if there has been trauma to the shoulder girdle, subsequent ossification of the ligaments is not unusual. It may occur 3–5 weeks after an injury or may

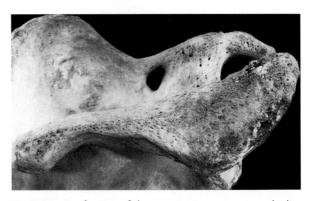

Fig. 3.**24**   Ossification of the superior transverse scapular ligament in an anatomic specimen.

result from repetitive microtrauma to the shoulder girdle. The partial ossification shown in Fig. 3.**26b** has a traumatic etiology. Schulte (1960) described **a jointlike connection between the coracoid process and the clavicle** (coracoclavicular joint, Fig. 3.**27**). This feature probably has both a congenital and an acquired form, the latter most likely consisting of a pseudarthrosis (e.g., associated with an ossified ligament).

Pratesi (1963) described an **ossification along the lateral border of the scapula** as a variant.

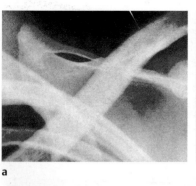
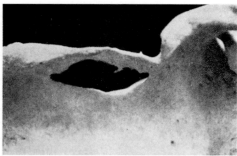

a   b

Fig. 3.**25 a, b**   Bridgelike superior scapular border: radiograph and anatomic specimen.

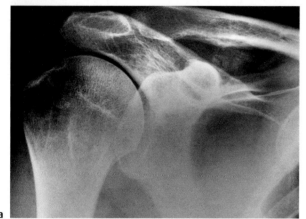
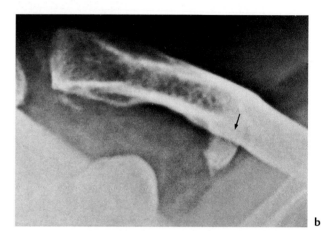

a   b

c   d

Fig. 3.**26 a–d**   Ossification of the coracoclavicular ligament.
a Since the patient gave no history of trauma, either the ossification is a congenital variant or the history is wrong. It is common for patients to forget shoulder trauma that occurred more than five years before.
b Ossification in the conoid (medial) portion of the coracoclavicular ligament. The film shows an acromioclavicular disrup-

tion with a bony avulsion from the inferior surface of the clavicle (arrow).
c, d Posttraumatic Y-shaped ossification of the coronoid (medially) as well the trapezoid (laterally) part of the coracoclavicular ligament. The radiograph in **c** was performed just after the trauma (14 months before the radiograph in **d**) and shows a separation of the AC joint.

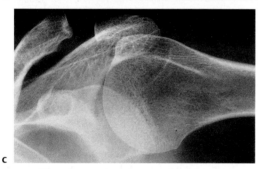

Fig. 3.**27**   Coracoclavicular joint.

Since the publication by Neer (1972) on anterior acromioplasty, the variable **arched shape of the acromion** (the acromial arch) is known to have causal significance in

chronic impingement syndrome of the rotator cuff. The variability of the bony acromial arch, plus the ability of MRI to define the underlying soft tissue structures in excellent detail, has sparked considerable interest in diagnostic imaging of the acromion. Of course, the acromial arch is only one component of the space traversed by the rotator cuff, since the arch (known technically as the **coracoacromial arch**) is completed by the acromioclavicular joint, the coracoid process, and the coracoacromial ligament.

Bigliani et al. (1991) classified the acromion into three morphological types:

Morphological types of the acromion described by Bigliani et al. (Fig. 3.**28 a–c**):
➤ *Type I* Flat
➤ *Type II* Curved
➤ *Type III* Hook-shaped

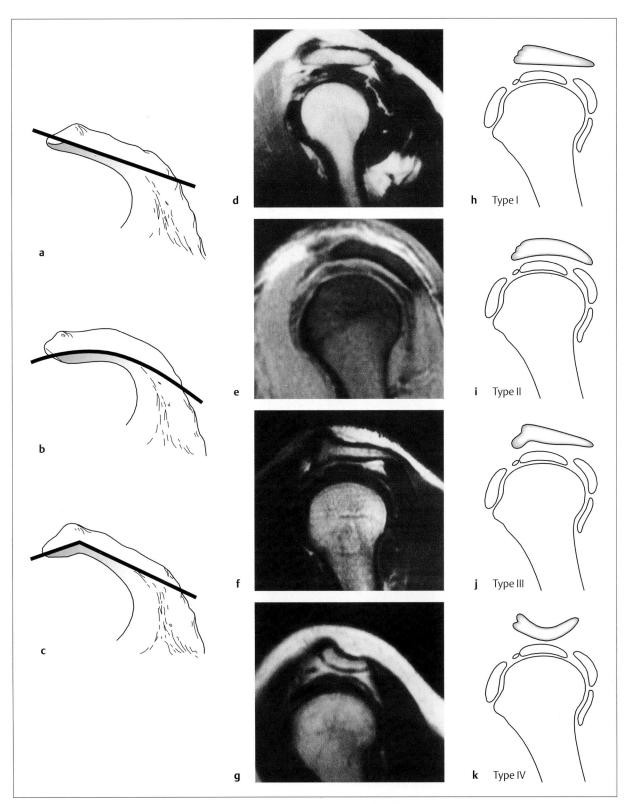

Fig. 3.**28 a–k** Morphology of the acromial arch.

a–c Schematic diagram of the classification of Bigliani (1986):

a Type I = flat.

b Type II = curved.

c Type III = hook-shaped.

d–k MR images of the various types of acromion:

d, h Type I (flat configuration) on T1-weighted oblique sagittal MRI.

e, i Type II (gently curved with a concave undersurface) on T2-weighted oblique sagittal MRI.

f, j Type III (hook-shaped anterior configuration) on T1-weighted oblique sagittal MRI scan through the acromion. Impingement was present clinically.

g, k Type IV (convex undersurface) on T1-weighted oblique sagittal MRI scan through the acromion (after Farley et al.).

In examinations of 140 cadaveric shoulders, Bigliani et al. (1986) found type I in 18.6%, type II in 42.0%, and type III in 38.6%. In cadaveric studies as well as clinical examinations, these authors found a strong correlation between the type III acromion and tears of the rotator cuff. This confirms the hypothesis of Neer (1972, 1983) that a hook-shaped acromion can narrow the subacromial space, allowing the rotator cuff to become entrapped between the acromion and humeral head. Neer stated that this repetitive or chronic impingement would also promote secondary osteophytic lipping on the undersurface of the anterior third of the acromion (p. 296 and Fig. 3.**60**). Later studies could not fully substantiate these findings. For example, Getz et al. (1996) found the following distribution of acromial types: type I = 22.8%, type II = 68.5%, type III = 8.6%.

Getz et al. (1996) examined 394 cadaveric scapulas. Type III was more prevalent in males, occurring in 10.2% of specimens versus 6.9% in females. Type I had a respective prevalence of 18.5% and 27.5% in males and females. Osteophytes were seen in 59% of type III cases, versus 42.6% in type II and 24% in type I. Acromial morphology was symmetrical in 70.7% of the specimens studied. Farley et al. (1994) found the following distribution of acromial types in MRI examinations of 45 patients with a partial or complete rotator cuff tear: type I 38%, type II 40%, and type III 18%.

These authors also identified a type IV acromion with a convex undersurface (Fig. 3.**28g, k**), which they noted in 4% of patients. In a comparative examination of 57 asymptomatic volunteers, they found type I in 44%, type II in 35%, type III in 12%, and type IV in 9%.

Peh et al. (1995), in a study comparing supraspinatus outlet radiographic views (a modified Y view) of the shoulder with parasagittal MR images, noted minor changes in the shape of the acromion caused by slight variations in the radiographic and MR imaging techniques.

> This means that the significance of acromion shape should not be overemphasized, especially in patients with clinical signs of impingement syndrome.

Peh et al. (1995) also point out that the detection of a type II or III acromion on radiographs is not sufficient for predicting the risk of rotator cuff problems or referring the patient for an MRI examination.

Persistent apophyses and accessory bone elements are discussed below (Fracture, Subluxation, or Dislocation?).

Deformities

Sprengel deformity refers not just to unilateral or bilateral elevation of the scapula but also to an abnormally broad, short scapula whose superior angle is curved like a hook (Fig. 3.**29**).

The deformity results from a failure of normal descent of the scapula, which remains in its original embryological position (Ogden et al. 1979, Laumann and Cire 1985). Sprengel deformity rarely occurs in isolation and is usually associated with muscular anomalies and with malformations of the cervical vertebrae and ribs. Ogden et al. (1979) published a very informative review of the radiological and pathoanatomic features of Sprengel deformity.

Congenital shoulder dysplasias may be characterized by a concave humeral head articulating with a convex glenoid, or there may be a flattened inferior glenoid rim with humerus varus (Owen 1953; Fig. 3.**30a**). Possible associated deformities include a hypoplastic scapular neck (Resnick et al. 1982; Fig. 3.**30b**) and occasional malformations of the clavicle and coracoid (Wörth 1959, Moser 1962; Fig. 3.**31**).

An excellent review of glenoid dysplasias can be found in Kozlowski et al. (1985).

Common and rare congenital syndromes that are associated with scapular abnormalities, generally hypoplasia, are listed in Table 3.**1**.

A less spectacular deformity is **circumscribed hypoplasia of the posterior glenoid rim**, which predisposes to recurrent (atraumatic) posterior shoulder instability (Edelson 1995, Weishaupt et al. 2000). Weishaupt et al. (2000) discovered that hypoplasia of the posterior rim with a craniocaudal length more than 12 mm and increased retroversion at the midglenoid level are important in the pathogenesis of recurrent (atraumatic) posterior instability (Fig. 3.**30d–f**).

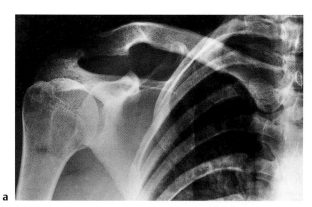
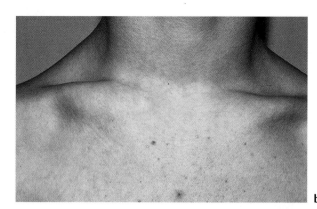

a   b

Fig. 3.29 a–e Sprengel deformity in the setting of Klippel–Feil syndrome with disproportionate elevation of the scapulae. Note the abnormal prominence of the superior angle and the abnormal projection of the clavicles, which appear to be rotated and displaced upward. The clinical photographs in **b–d** (different case from in panel **a**, with less pronounced radiographic signs) show the superiorly "rotated" clavicles (**b**), the sharply projecting superior angle (**c**), and the prominent medial border (**d**), signs that are very typical of Sprengel deformity. **e** Correlative MRI for panel **c** shows the prominent, exostosis-like superior angle of the scapula. Figure 5.**171** shows possible associated spinal deformities and omovertebral ossifications.

Fig. 3.**29 c–e**

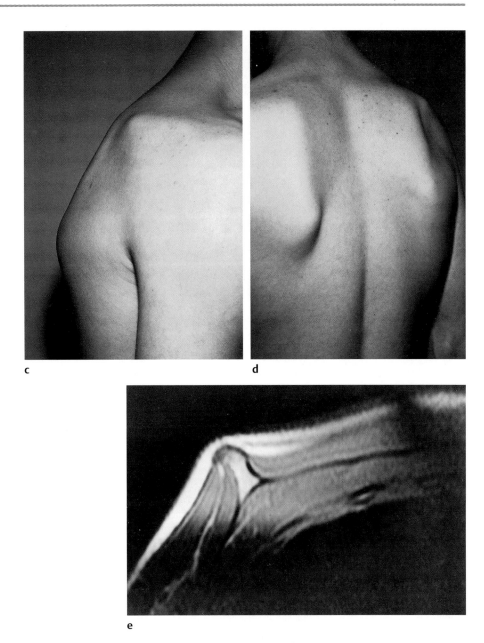

c

d

e

Fig. 3.**30 a–f** Deformities of the shoulder joint.
a Convex glenoid and concave humeral head.
b Shallow glenoid due to short or absent scapular neck.
c Humerus varus combined with aplasia of the scapular neck.
d–f The spectrum of the different anatomic forms of the posterior glenoid rim at the base of the glenoid (after Weishaupt et al. 2000). Schematic drawings from CT-arthrograms.
d Pointed form without bony deficiency.
(**e, f**) Hypoplasia of the dorsal glenoid rim: rounded glenoid deficiency ("lazy J" form), and triangular bony deficiency ("delta" form).

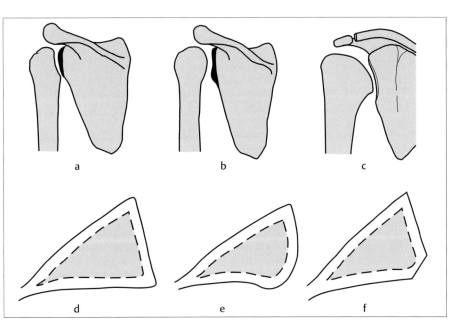

a

b

c

d

e

f

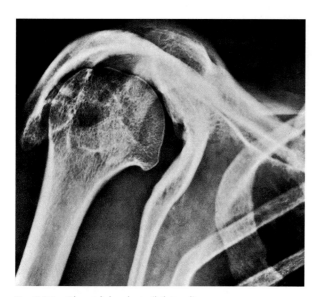

Fig. 3.**31** Glenoid dysplasia (bilateral).

Table 3.**1** Common and rare congenital syndromes that are associated with scapular abnormalities

Common congenital syndromes	Rare congenital syndromes
• Cleidocranial dysplasia • Mucopolysaccharidoses • Nail–patella syndrome • Sprengel deformity • Klippel–Feil syndrome	• Achondrogenesis • Achondroplasia (flat inferior angle) • Basal cell nevus syndrome (Gorlins syndrome) • Camptomelic dysplasia • CHILD[1] syndrome • Dyggve–Melchior–Clausen syndrome • Dysegmental dysplasia • Fetal varicella syndrome • Hallermann–Streiff syndrome • Holt–Oram syndrome • Kinky hair syndrome (Menkes syndrome) • LEOPARD[2] syndrome • Mucolipidosis II, fucosidosis • Poland syndrome • Proteus syndrome • Scapuloiliac dysostosis • Short rib–polydactyly syndrome • Thanatophoric dysplasia

[1] CHILD Congenital hemidysplasia, ichthyosiform nevi, limb defect
[2] LEOPARD Lentiginosis, electrocardiographic disorders, ocular disorders, pulmonary stenosis, abnormalities in formation of the genitalia, retardation of growth, deafness

 Fracture, Subluxation, or Dislocation?

Given the complex three-dimensional anatomy of the scapula and the tendency for the humerus and adjacent ribs to overlap other structures on radiographs, Mach band effects are difficult to avoid (e.g., Figs. 3.**19** and 3.**32**).

Structures that can mimic fractures on radiographs include apophyseal growth plates and lines in children and adults (Figs. 3.**3**, 3.**4**, 3.**6**–3.**13**), persistent apophyses in adults (Figs. 3.**5**, 3.**33**, 3.**34**), and accessory bone elements (Figs. 3.**35**, 3.**36**).

> It should be assumed that a persistent apophysis is present if the adjacent bony elements are separated by solid cortical contours and if the bony element in question (e.g., a persistent coracoid center) is not appreciably larger or smaller than normal (e.g., compared with the opposite side).

The latter is a typical feature of an **accessory bone element**: the surrounding anatomic structures are normal and the accessory bone actually represents a supernumerary element. Occasionally the basal element is hypoplastic, however, as illustrated in Fig. 3.**36**.

Persistent Apophysis (Fig. 3.**34a–d**)

Persistence of the ossification center at the **free end of the acromion** is observed in 7% to 15% of all radiographs of the region. A persistent ossification center or apophysis of the acromion is also termed an **os acromiale**. According to studies by Park et al. (1994), this variant can be a **significant cause of rotator cuff impingement**. In MRI studies of 10 patients over age 25 with an os acromiale, the authors detected a lesion of the supraspinatus tendon in every case (tendinitis in four patients, tendon tear in six patients). The os acromiale is most clearly demonstrated on oblique sagittal or oblique coronal MR images.

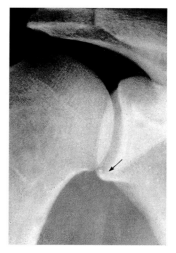

Fig. 3.**32** Not an isolated accessory bone but an apparent separation caused by a Mach effect.

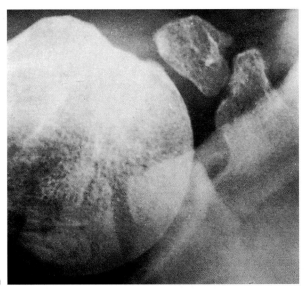

a

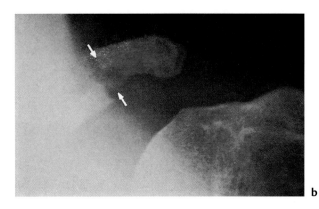

b

Fig. 3.**33a,b**   Differentiating a variant from a fracture of the coracoid process.

a Persistent coracoid center.
b Fracture (arrows).
The patient in **a** gave no history of trauma, and the irregular margins of the center and base are more consistent with a variant than a fracture. Of course, the clinical presentation should always be considered when the images are interpreted.

Fig. 3.**34a–h**   Persistent apophyses distinguished from stress fractures and pathological fractures of the scapula.

a The ossification centers of the acromion and the various ossification patterns that may be encountered (after Park et al.). Assuming that the acromion is ossified from three centers, a preacromion can be distinguished from a mesoacromion and a meta-acromion. A failure of fusion at one or more levels can result in seven possible configurations (labeled I–VII in the diagram).
BA   Basiacromion
MSA   Mesoacromion
MTS   Meta-acromion
PA   Preacromion

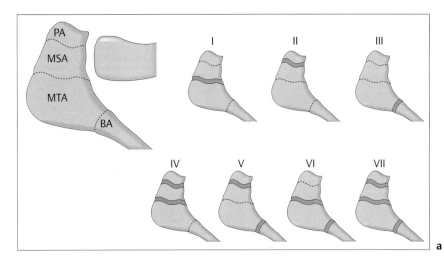

a

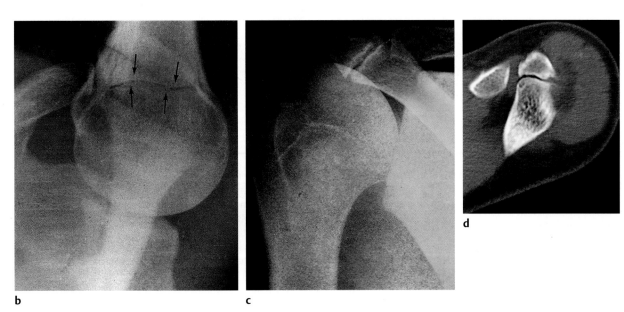

b   c

d

b Typical os acromiale corresponding to the type II pattern (arrows).
c–d Type II os acromiale in an asymptomatic adult woman. Not a fracture.

Fig. 3.**34e–h** ▷

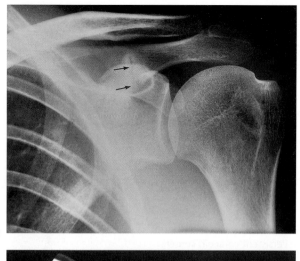

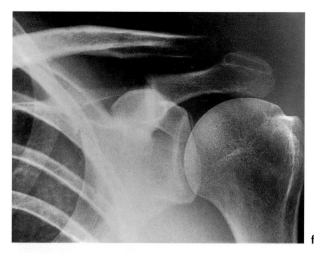

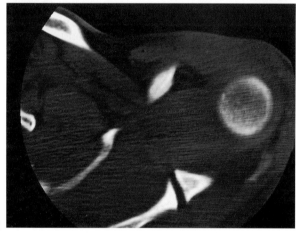

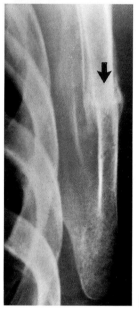

Fig. 3.**34 e–h**   Unusual stress fracture at the base of the acromion in a 47-year-old man who had done heavy "body building" for six months. Radiograph **e** shows the typical appearance of a stress fracture (arrows). In the follow-up X-ray in **f**, the acromion is completely separated and displaced. CT (**g**) was performed on the same day that film **e** was obtained. **h** Looser zone (pseudofracture) in the scapula of a patient with osteomalacia.

Three ossification centers can be distinguished in the acromion:

- Preacromion
- Mesoacromion
- Metaacromion

Park et al. (1994) identified seven types of os acromiale based on the location of the fusion defect (Fig. 3.**34 a**). The os acromiale may be connected to the rest of the acromion by connective tissue, cartilage, periosteum, or by a synovial joint. Conventional radiographs demonstrate the os acromiale most clearly in axial projections. Osteophytic lipping at the margins of the gap between the os acromiale and the acromion signifies instability of the os acromiale, which in turn can lead to a **supraspinatus impingement syndrom**e (Mudge et al. 1984, Edelson et al. 1993, Park et al. 1994). Instability of the os acromiale can incite regressive changes in the acromioclavicular joint (Grass 1992). Contractions of the deltoid muscle can pull downward on the acromial end, causing rotator cuff impingement. Osteophytes at the margins of the acromial gap can also cause erosive lesions of the rotator cuff.

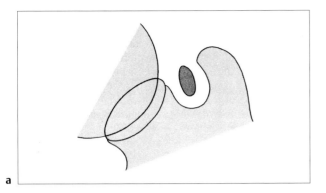

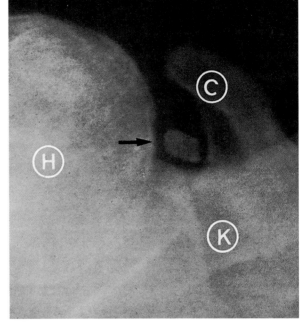

Fig. 3.**35 a, b**   Accessory bones.
a Accessory bone located between the coracoid process and glenoid rim (drawing from an axial shoulder radiograph).

b Accessory bone located anterior to the clavicle between the humeral head and coracoid process (arrow) in a 70-year-old woman.
C   Coracoid process
H   Humeral head
K   Clavicle

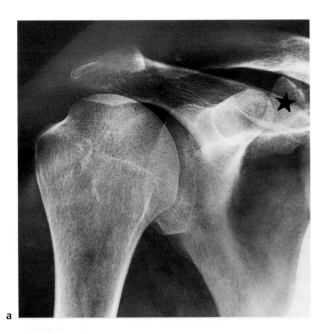

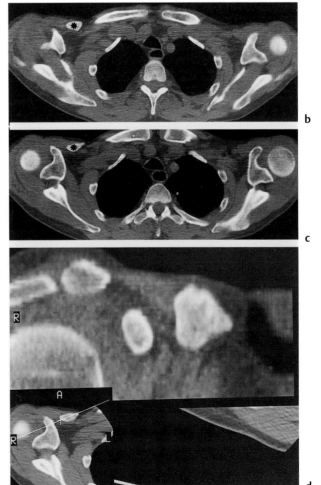

Fig. 3.**36 a–d**   This accessory bone element, located anterior to the coracoid process, was detected incidentally in a patient with no trauma history. The bony element labeled with a star displays well-rounded contours and is located anteromedial to the coracoid process, which looks hypoplastic compared with the opposite side. The small proliferation at the tip of the coracoid process is probably an enthesiopathy at the attachment of the pectoralis minor, secondary to the functional effects of the coracoid hypoplasia. The academic question of whether the isolated bony element might also be a displaced persistent apophysis is pointless, since neither entity can be proved and the patient is asymptomatic.

Accessory Bone Elements (Figs. 3.**35**–3.**38**)

Accessory bone elements about the superior and inferior glenoid rim can be very difficult to distinguish from bony avulsions of the capsule (Figs. 3.**37**, 3.**38**).

> It should be assumed that an **accessory bone element** is present if the element is located near the glenoid rim but bears no geometric relationship to the shape of the bony glenoid, as illustrated in Figs. 3.**37** and 3.**38**.

It should be added, however, that when such bony elements are detected in adults, they may well result from heterotopic bone formation following an intracapsular hemorrhage caused by a forgotten shoulder injury. They could also represent avulsed, extracapsular bony excrescences or osteophytes that are unrelated to osteoarthritis. Bankart lesions are discussed more fully in the section on the shoulder joint as a whole.

Fractures

Fractures of the scapula **most commonly involve the scapular neck** and sometimes can be confirmed only by obtaining special views or CT scans. Fractures of the acromion can result from birth trauma and child abuse (Swischuk 1980). The radiological findings are almost identical to those of irregular bone development or unfused ossification centers.

Figure 3.**34e–g** illustrates an unusual stress fracture of the acromion.

Bezold (1956) and Viehweger (1957) described displaced fractures of the superior border of the scapula, producing a ridgelike fragment.

Fractures of the coracoid process are distinguished radiographically from a persistent coracoid center by the irregular, often jagged boundaries of the fractured bone ends. A persistent coracoid center has intact cortical margins (Fig. 3.**33**). Of course, the clinical presentation should also be taken into account.

Epiphyseal or apophyseal separation of the coracoid process without acromioclavicular dislocation is described by Holst and Christiansen (1998).

Fractures of the coracoid process are generally rare and have been the subject of sporadic reports (e.g., Froimson 1978). Coracoid fractures may occur in isolation or may be associated with acromioclavicular dislocation (Bernard et al. 1983) or with anterior dislocation of the shoulder (Benchetrit and Friedman 1979). Most fractures of the coracoid process occur through the base and show little displacement due to the stabilizing action of the coracoclavicular ligament.

Fractures and dislocations involving the acromioclavicular joint are discussed on p. 288.

In patients with osteomalacia, the scapula is a site of predilection for the development of **Looser zones** (pseudo- or insufficiency fractures) (Fig. 3.**34h**).

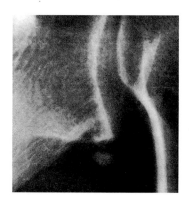

Fig. 3.**37**   Accessory bone at the inferior rim of the glenoid cavity.

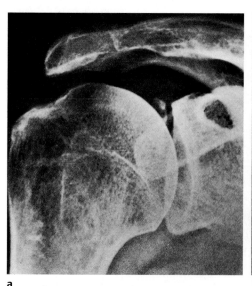
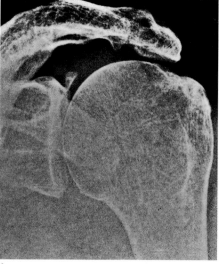
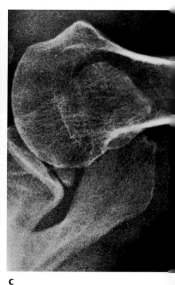

a   b   c

Fig. 3.**38a–c**   Accessory bone at the superior and anterior glenoid rim.

Necrosis?

The irregular contours of the glenoid cavity in childhood should not be mistaken for osteonecrosis or osteochondritis dissecans (focal subchondral osteonecrosis) (Figs. 3.**3**, 3.**4**, 3.**39**).

Similarly, slight irregularities of the epiphyseal centers (e.g., of the coracoid process, Fig. 3.**7**) should not be misinterpreted as necrosis. In questionable cases where clinical symptoms are present, a diagnosis can be established by MRI or radionuclide scanning.

It is not uncommon for radiotherapy in breast cancer patients to cause dystrophic changes in the bony structures about the shoulder (osteoradiodystrophy), which may or may not be accompanied by necrosis (Fig. 3.**40**).

Acro-osteolysis due to a variety of causes (see Table 2.**6**) can completely obliterate the bony structures of the acromion.

 Inflammation?

The scapula is a relatively rare site of involvement by primary hematogenous osteomyelitis. On the other hand, bacterial arthritic processes in the acromioclavicular or glenohumeral joint can easily spread to the adjacent bone, in which case the radiographic changes depend on the acuteness of the process.

We have personally observed five cases of nonspecific, aseptic chronic osteitis of the scapula in the setting of **pustulotic arthro-osteitis** (PAO, also called SAPHO, see

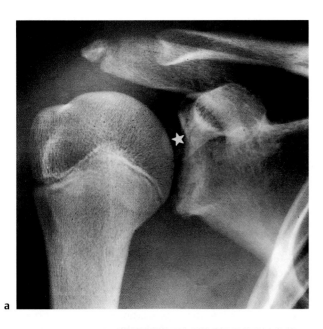

a

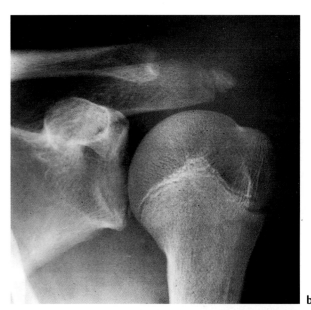

b

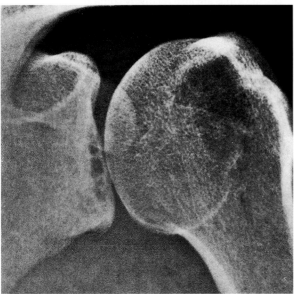

c

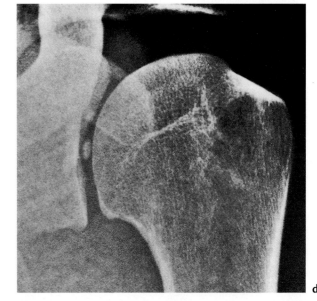

d

Fig. 3.**39 a–d**   Differential diagnosis of osteochondritis dissecans (focal subarticular or subchondral avascular osteonecrosis).
a, b Normal irregular contour of the glenoid. The bony structure labeled with a star on the right side (**a**) is caused by

an "elongated" view of the peripheral portions of the coracoid process in an atypical projection. Postinjury radiographs in a patient with an otherwise negative history.
c, d Osteochondritis dissecans of the glenoid, with "mouse bed" (**c**) and detached fragment (**d**).

p. 315). In a series that totaled more than 80 cases, this was a relatively high prevalence. The diagnosis was based on clinical manifestations (presence of pustulosis palmoplantaris and/or psoriasis) and on radionuclide scans, which consistently showed associated sternocostoclavicular hyperostosis or other nonspecific inflammatory bone changes along with spondylarthritis.

Conventional radiographs in the initial stage of **Paget disease** (without significant deformity) show few if any changes. The disease should be suspected if radionuclide scanning shows intense, continuous, homogeneous uptake (as an incidental finding). The case shown in Fig. 3.**41** should not be difficult to diagnose.

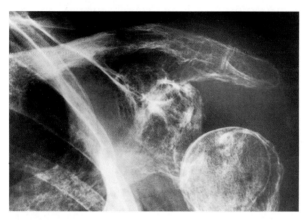

Fig. 3.**40**   Severe osteoradiodystrophy involving the entire scapula, the humeral head, clavicle, and ribs following postoperative radiotherapy for breast carcinoma. Laxness of the capsule and ligaments has led to subluxation of the humeral head. Without knowing the prior history, one could also interpret the changes as the lytic stage of Paget disease, although the lack of bony enlargement would be unusual.

Tumor?

Reference was made earlier to the physiologically thin portions of the scapula and projection-related lucencies (e.g., Figs. 3.**20**,3.**21**, 3.**23**) and how they might be confused with areas of bone destruction. Incipient destructive changes in the scapula are extremely difficult to detect on plain films. If clinical suspicion exists (e.g., a tumor patient with scapular pain), sectional imaging studies should be performed without delay.

> In **elderly patients**, the acromion may be so atrophic (osteoporotic) that it cannot be identified on standard radiographs, even when a halogen iris diaphragm is used. In tumor patients, the signs and symptoms should dictate the further course of action.

Three special circumstances should be noted:

● **Subchondral synovial cyst** (intraosseous ganglion cyst) is a potential cause of osteolytic changes near the glenoid. This lesion shows a certain predilection for the scapula and is mentioned here because it is often detected as an incidental finding, placing it in the category of borderline-normal variants. The cysts appear as subchondral osteolytic lesions up to 1–2 cm in diameter, usually located near the joint margin and surrounded by a sclerotic rim. CT or MRI can often confirm the proximity of the lesion to the joint space. The subchondral lucencies often contain air bubbles, since "vacuum air" in the glenohumeral joint (from blood gases out of solution by reduced pressure) can enter the cyst through fine fissures in the articular cartilage (Figs. 3.**42**–3.**44**).

● **Osteochondromas** and **cartilaginous exostoses** are not uncommon in the scapula (where approximately 5% of all osteochondromas occur, Fig. 3.**45**). It has been suggested that these lesions represent a local "growth disturbance" rather than autochthonous tumors. Chondrosarcomas are also relatively common in the scapula, with 5% occurring in this flat bone. They are almost al-

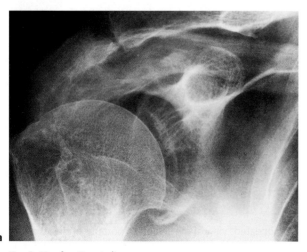

a

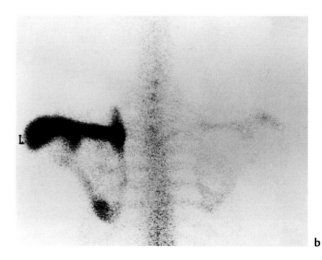

b

Fig. 3.**41 a, b**   Paget disease.
a Enlargement of the acromion and scapular spine with a coarsened trabecular pattern.

b Typical bone scan showing an extended area of intense, homogeneous uptake.

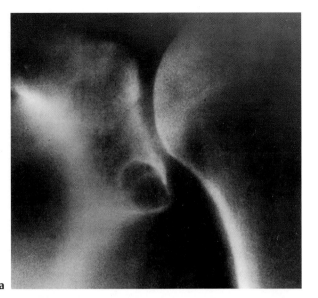 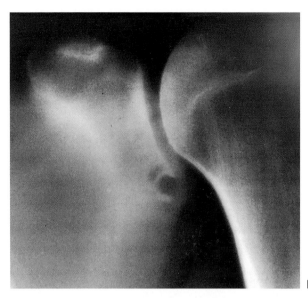

a   b

Fig. 3.**42 a, b**   Subchondral synovial cyst (intraosseous ganglion cyst) below the inferior part of the glenoid cavity. Incidental finding on conventional tomograms.

ways symptomatic. Ossification centers and projection-related effects (e.g., an orthograde projection through the coracoid process) should not be mistaken for osteochondromas (Figs. 3.**6**, 3.**7**, 3.**10**, 3.**23**).

- **Posttraumatic defects (clefts or gaps)** in the scapula are found with some frequency in disability examinations of young adults (Fig. 3.**46**). They can result from incomplete fracture healing or interposed tissues (organized hematoma, muscle, etc.). They should not be confused with bone destruction by eosinophilic granuloma (focus of Langerhans cell histiocytosis) or another tumor.

Fig. 3.**43 a–d**   Painful ganglion cyst at the posterior attachment of the joint capsule (arrow, star). This ganglion was not visible on conventional radiographs. The pain is caused by irritation of the suprascapular nerve, which runs directly over this region. Differentiation is mainly required from an unusual bursa (p. 294 f.), but the visible defect in the scapula is more consistent with an intraosseous ganglion cyst.

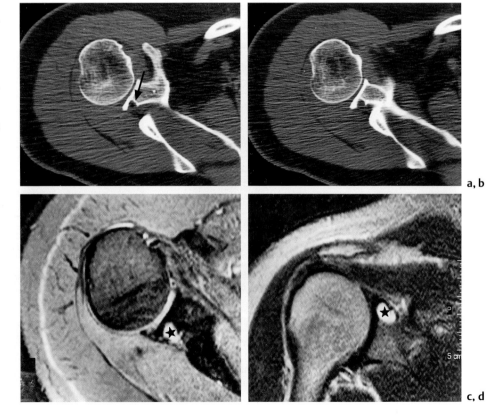

a, b

c, d

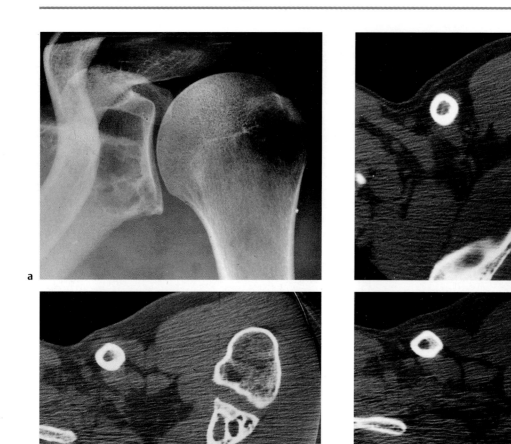

Fig. 3.**44 a–d**   Intraosseous ganglion cyst below the inferior glenoid in the scapular neck. Stabbing joint pain occurred with certain shoulder movements. The CT scan in **d** shows de-struction of the anterior bony labrum; that is probably where the cyst communicates with the joint.

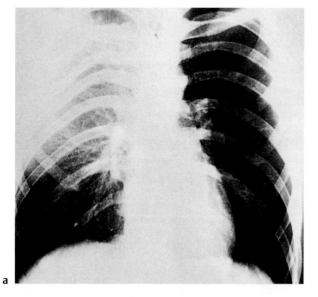

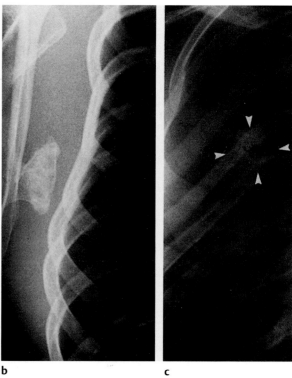

Fig. 3.**45 a–d**   Osteochondromas of the lower scapula (arrowheads).
a   This patient has severe bursitis emanating from a bursa located over the head of the exostosis.
b, c   Spot views of **a**.

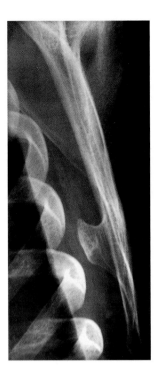

Fig. 3.**45 d** Another asymptomatic case of an osteochondroma.

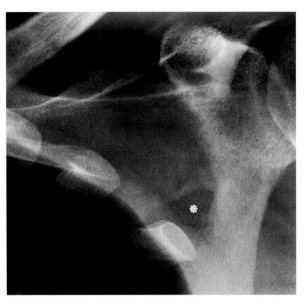

Fig. 3.**46**   Posttraumatic defect in the scapula (not a tumor).

References

Andrews, J. R., Th. J. W. Byrd, S. P. Kupfferman et al.: The profile view of the acromion. Clin. Orthop. 263 (1991) 142

Benchetrit, E., B. Friedman: Fracture of the coracoid process associated with subglenoid dislocation of the shoulder: a case report. J. Bone Jt Surg. 61-A (1979) 295

Bernard, T. N., M. E. Brunet, R. J. Haddad: Fractured coracoid process in acromioclavicular dislocations: report of four cases and review of the literature. Clin. Orthop. 175 (1983) 227

Bezold, K.: Die Abrißfraktur der Margo cranialis scapulae. Fortschr. Röntgenstr. 85 (1956) 423

Bigliani, L. U., D. S. Morrison, E. W. April: The morphology of the acromion and rotator cuff impingement. Orthop. Trans. 10 (1986) 228 (abstract)

Bigliani, L. U., J. B. Ticker, E.L. Flatlow et al.: The relationship of acromial architecture to rotator cuff disease. Clin. Sports Med 10 (1991) 823

Edelson, J. G.: Localized glenoid hypoplasia. Clin. Orthop. 321 (1995) 189

Edelson, J. G., J. Zukerman, I. Hershkovitz: Os acromiale: anatomy and surgical implication. J. Bone Jt. Surg. 75-B (1993) 551

Farley, T. E., C. H. Neumann, L. S. Steinbach et al.: The coracoacromial arch: MR evaluation and correlation with rotator cuff pathology. Skelet. Radiol. 23 (1994) 641

Fazekas, P., M. Ferjentsik: Lochförmiger Defekt des Schulterblattes mit einer schwalbenschwanzähnlichen Deformität des unteren Abschnitts. Fortschr. Röntgenstr. 121 (1974) 657

Fischer, E.: Lochförmiger Defekt im Schulterblatt. Fortschr. Röntgenstr. 86 (1957) 530

Froimson, A. I.: Fracture of the coracoid process of the scapula. J. Bone Jt Surg. 60-A (1978) 710

Getz, J. D., M. P.Recht, D. W. Piraino et al.: Acromial morphology: Relation of sex, age, symmetry and subacromial enthesophytes. Radiology 199 (1996) 737

Giordano, A.: Zwei familiäre Fälle von Ossifikation des „Ligamentum transversum scapulae superius". Fortschr. Röntgenstr. 96 (1962) 834

Goldberg, R. P., B. Vicks: Oblique angled view for coracoid fractures. Skelet. Radiol. 9 (1983) 195

Grass, A.: The incidence and role of the os acromiale in the acromiohumeral impingement syndrome. Radiol. med. 84 (1992) 567

Hall, R. J., P. T. Calvert: Stress fracture of the acromion: an unusual mechanism and review of the literature. J. Bone Jt Surg. 77-B (1994) 153

Hirschfeld, P., G. Dimanski: Die Schulter: funktionelle Diagnostik und kausale Therapie in der ärztlichen Praxis. PERIMED, spitta, Balingen 1994

Holst, A. K., J. V. Christiansen: Epiphyseal separation of the coracoid process without acromioclavicular dislocation. Skelet. Radiol. 27 (1998) 461

Hutchinson, M. R., M. A. Veenstra: Arthroscopic decompression of shoulder impingement secondary to os acromiale. Arthroscopy 9 (1993) 28

Keats, Th. E., L. Thomas, Jr. Pope: The acromioclavicular joint: normal variation and the diagnosis of dislocation. Skelet. Radiol. 17 (1988) 159

Klever, H.: Apophysenpersistenz im Bereich beider Schultergelenkspfannen. Fortschr. Röntgenstr. 95 (1961) 419

Koch-Holst, A., J. V. Christiansen: Epiphyseal separation of the coracoid process without acromioclavicular dislocation. Skelet. Radiol. 27 (1998) 461

Kozlowski, K., N. Colavita, L. Morris et al.: Bilateral glenoid dysplasia. Aust. Radiol. 29 (1985) 174

Laumann, U., B. Ciré: Der angeborene Schulterblatthochstand. Z. Orthop. 123 (1985) 380

Lossen, H., R. N. Wegner: Die Knochenkerne der Skapula, röntgenologisch und vergleichend-anatomisch betrachtet. Fortschr. Röntgenstr. 53 (1936) 443

Moser, F.: Beitrag zur kongenitalen Schulterdysplasie. Fortschr. Röntgenstr. 97 (1962) 661

Mudge, M. K., V. E. Wood, G. K. Frykmann: Rotator cuff tears associated with os acromiale. J. Bone Jt Surg. 66-A (1984) 427

Neer, C.S.: Anterior acromioplasty for the chronic impingement syndrome in the shoulder. J. Bone Jt Surg. 54-A (1972) 41

Neer, C.S.: Impingement lesions. Clin. Orthop. 173 (1983) 70

Ogden, J. A., G. J. Conlogue, St. B. Phillips et al.: Sprengel's deformity. Radiology of the pathologic deformation. Skelet. Radiol. 4 (1979) 204

Ogden, J. A., St. B. Phillips: Radiology of postnatal development. VII. The scapula. Skelet. Radiol. 9 (1983) 157

Oppenheim, W. L., E. G. Dawson, Ch. Quirlain et al.: The cephaloscapular projection. Clin. Orthop. 195 (1985) 191

Owen, R.: Bilateral glenoid hypoplasia. J. Bone Jt Surg. 35-B (1953) 262

Park, J. G., J. K. Lee, C. T. Phelps: Os acromiale associated with rotator cuff impingement: MR imaging of the shoulder. Radiology 193 (1994) 255

Pate, D., S. Kursunoglu, D. Resnick et al.: Scapular foramina. Skelet. Radiol. 14 (1985) 270

Peh, W. C. G., T. H. R. Farmer, W. G. Totty: Acromial arch shape: assessment with MR imaging. Radiology 195 (1995) 501

Pratesi, A. C.: Ein Fall von bilateraler Dysmorphie der Scapula. Fortschr. Röntgenstr. 99 (1963) 571

Rask, M. R., L. H. Steinberg: Fracture of the acromion caused by muscle forces. J. Bone Jt Surg. 60-A (1978) 1146

Resnick, D., R. D. Walter, A. S. Crudale: Bilateral dysplasia of the scapula neck. Amer. J. Roentgenol. 139 (1982) 387

Schulte, E.: Beitrag zum Korakoklavikulargelenk. Fortschr. Röntgenstr. 92 (1960) 463

Swischuk, L. E.: Radiology of the Newborn and Young Infant, 2nd ed. Williams & Wilkins, Baltimore 1980

Taga, I., M. Yoneda, K. Ono: Epiphyseal separation of the coracoid process associated with acromioclavicular sprain: a case report and review of the literature. Clin. Orthop. 207 (1986) 138

Teichert, G.: Persistierende Apophyse der Schultergelenkspfanne oder Pfannenrandbruch? Fortschr. Röntgenstr. 85 (1956) 357

Viehweger, G.: Röntgenologische Beobachtungen und Untersuchungen bei Scapulaverletzungen im Bereich des Margo cranialis. Fortschr. Röntgenstr. 86 (1957) 226

Villanyi, G.: Seltener Fall der Verkalkung des Ligamentum coracoclaviculare. Fortschr. Röntgenstr. 112 (1970) 695

Weisshaupt, D., M. Zanetti, R. W. Nyffeler, et al: Posterior glenoid rim deficiency in recurrent (atraumatic) posterior shoulder instability. Skeletal Radiol. 29 (2000) 204

Wörth, D.: Über seltene Schultergelenksdysplasien. Bericht über drei Beobachtungen von Fehlbildungen des Schultergelenkes. Z. Orthop. 92 (1959) 224–233

Ziegler, G.: Ossifikation im Bereich der knorpeligen Gelenklippe der Schultergelenkpfanne. Fortschr. Röntgenstr. 86 (1957) 270

Acromioclavicular Joint

In contrast to the treatment in previous editions of this book, the peripheral bony portions of the acromion and clavicle that make up the acromioclavicular joint are not included in the chapters on the scapula and clavicle but are discussed separately as the components of a functionally important joint. The acromioclavicular joint with its capsule and ligaments is also an integral part of the anatomic tunnel or arch that covers such delicate structures as the rotator cuff, bursae, and tendon sheaths. The radiological detection of bony abnormalities is of little value unless they are considered in relation to potential injuries of the underlying soft-tissue structures.

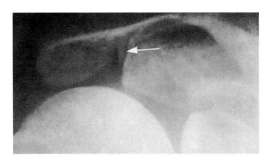

Fig. 3.**47**   Calcification of the articular disk in the acromioclavicular joint (arrow).

▌ Normal Findings

During Growth

The ossification of the acromion (apophyseal centers appear at 15–18 years of age and fuse at 20–25 years) was described on p. 264. The lateral end of the clavicle normally has an isolated ossification center that contributes very little to the longitudinal growth of the clavicle and generally is not visible on radiographs (p. 305).

In Adulthood

The acromial end of the clavicle is slightly convex, forming the acromial articular surface of that bone. This convex, cartilage-covered surface articulates with the reciprocally concave articular surface of the acromion. The fibrous joint capsule is attached to both bones and is lined by synovial membrane. The articulation is therefore classified as a synovial joint, which can be important in patients with rheumatoid disorders. Sometimes a disk is interposed between the articular surfaces (Fig. 3.**47**).

The joint is reinforced by the acromioclavicular ligament and stabilized by the coracoclavicular ligament (consisting of the lateral trapezoid ligament and medial conoid ligament, Fig. 3.**56a**).

The clearest radiographic projection of the acromioclavicular joint is obtained by angling the central ray about 10–15° caudocranially so that the scapula is not superimposed on the clavicle. Functional stress testing of the joint is described below.

▌ Pathological Finding?

Normal Variant or Anomaly?

According to studies by Pettrone and Nirschl (1978), the inferior borders of the apposing ends of the clavicle and acromion are at exactly the same level (forming a straight line) in approximately 80% of the population (Fig. 3.**48**).

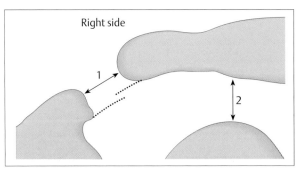

Fig. 3.**48**   Instability of the acromioclavicular joint. Schematic diagram of possible measurements.
1   Width of the acromioclavicular joint space (normally 1–3 mm, with an extreme range of 0.5–7 mm).
2   Distance between the inferior border of the clavicle and the superior border of the coracoid process. With a Tossy type II separation, the distance is increased by a maximum of 50%; with a type III separation, it is increased by more than 50 % (compared with the opposite side).
Dotted lines: tangents to the inferior borders of the clavicle and acromion. Failure of the tangents to meet (as in the diagram) has no significance unless compared with the opposite side or, if necessary, evaluated by stress views.

The authors observed a high clavicle in 7% of a normal population (140 people), a low clavicle in another 7%, and overriding of the acromion by the clavicle in 5% of cases. Of course, this makes it extremely problematic to diagnose an acromioclavicular joint injury based on the relative position of the articulating bone ends.

 Fracture, Subluxation, or Dislocation?

As mentioned above, the relationship of the acromion to the clavicle is extremely variable, and even an overriding clavicle may be seen in normal individuals (Keats and Pope 1988). This underscores the necessity of comparing radiographic findings with the opposite side and, in some circumstances, obtaining stress radiographs (weight of 5–10 kg in both hands, arms slightly externally rotated, 10–15° caudocranial projection; Fig. 3.**49**).

> If stress radiographs show displacement of the acromion relative to the clavicle when compared with the opposite side and a history of trauma is present, it is reasonable to assume that the capsule and ligaments have been injured. It should be noted that the radiographic joint space is 1–3 mm wide in most individuals, but that extreme values ranging from 0.5 to 6–7 mm may be observed.

Harrison et al. (1980) found that muscle spasms can mask an acromioclavicular dislocation. The authors therefore suggest relaxing the acromioclavicular joint by local anesthesia before obtaining stress radiographs.

Acromioclavicular dislocations (in which the lateral end of the clavicle is dislocated superiorly or sometimes posteriorly by direct or indirect forces) are classified into three types based on the Tossy classification.

> **Tossy classification of acromioclavicular dislocations (separations)**
> ➤ *Type I* Rupture of the joint capsule with no significant ligamentous injury.
> ➤ *Type II* Additional disruption of the acromioclavicular ligament. The coracoclavicular ligament may be sprained, but its continuity is preserved.
> ➤ *Type III* Additional disruption of the coracoclavicular ligament.

Rockwood et al. (1996) added several more types of injury to the Tossey classification: type IV (posterior displacement of the clavicle into or through the trapezius muscle), type V (extreme vertical displacement of the clavicle), and type VI (inferior displacement of the clavicle to a subacromial or subcoracoid position).

> **Radiology of the Tossy classification:**
> ➤ *Type I* Normal findings on nonstress and stress radiographs.
> ➤ *Type II* Normal position of the acromioclavicular joint on nonstress radiographs. When stress is applied, the clavicle is displaced upward by no more than one-half the height of the joint space. Its distance from the coracoid process is increased by a maximum of 50% compared with the opposite side.
> ➤ *Type III* Elevation of the shoulder. When stress is applied, the dehiscence is greater than in type II, and the distance from the coracoid process is increased by more than 50% (Figs. 3.**49**, 3.**50**).

A rare injury of the acromioclavicular joint in children with **pseudodislocation** can occur when the clavicle subluxates upward through a superior tear in the periosteal sleeve (Neu and Krämer 1981; Fig. 3.**51**). The cartilaginous articular end of the clavicle remains apposed to the acromial apophysis, and the capsule and ligaments are intact.

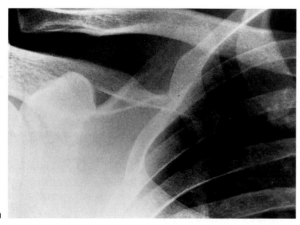

a

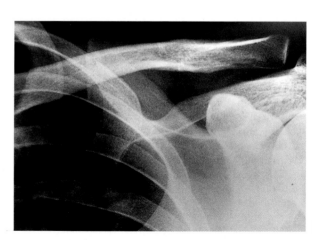

b

Fig. 3.**49a, b**   Tossy type III dislocation of the right acromioclavicular joint. Findings on nonstress radiographs were equivocal. Radiographs were then taken of both sides with a 10-kg weight in each hand. The right acromioclavicular joint space widens markedly from 4 to 8 mm. The clavicle is displaced upward by 8 mm, and the coracoclavicular distance is increased by more than 50%.

Necrosis?

The outer end of the clavicle is very prone to necrotic changes, especially in the form of acro-osteolysis. This may occur in the setting of a familial acro-osteolysis syndrome, collagen diseases, or various other disorders (Table 2.**6**). The most common form, however, is **spontaneous post-traumatic osteolysis of the peripheral end of the clavicle** (Hermanns et al. 1981, Puente et al. 1999; Fig. 3.**52**). But repeated stress or microtrauma to the shoulder are also a potential pathomechanism (Sopov et al. 2001).

The initial radiographic change is a circumscribed resorption of the clavicular subchondral plate, occurring approximately two months after the injury (Fig. 3.**52b**). This

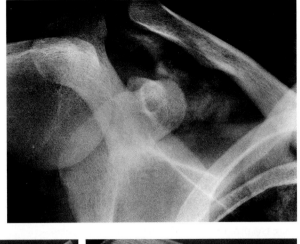

a

Fig. 3.**50 a–e**   Posttraumatic ossification, consisting of heterotopic bone formation secondary to acromioclavicular separation. The width of the acromioclavicular joint space is increased to at least 1 cm in both the radiograph and CT scan (**b**). The heterotopic ossifications extend into the joint and below the clavicle, terminating in front of the coracoid process. Apparently there is also a full-thickness tear of the coracoclavicular ligament.

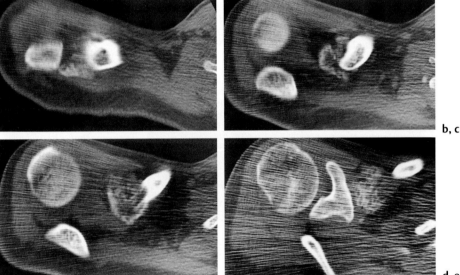

b, c

d, e

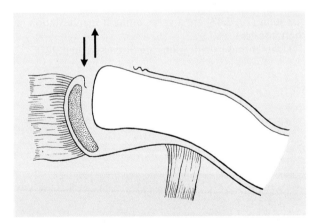

Fig. 3.**51**   "Pseudodislocation" of the clavicle through a periosteal tear in a 10-year-old child.

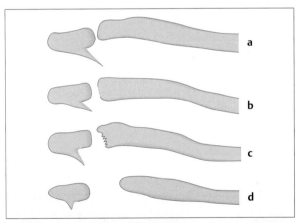

a

b

c

d

Fig. 3.**52 a–e**   Acro-osteolysis of the clavicle.   ▷
a–d Evolution of posttraumatic acro-osteolysis of the clavicle.
e Posttraumatic osteolysis at the acromial end of the clavicle with necrotic bone debris in the joint space.

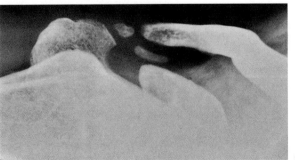

e

is followed by a progressive erosion over the next four weeks (Fig. 3.**52c**) until finally about 1–2 cm of bony substance has disappeared or vanished from the distal end of the clavicle (Fig. 3.**52d**). The margin of the lesion is tapered or looks conelike or pencil-like.

 ## Inflammation?

Bacterial arthritis of the acromioclavicular joint is not uncommon, particularly in immunocompromised patients (Fig. 3.**53**).

Early diagnosis is based on signs and symptoms, most notably a painful swelling of the acromioclavicular joint. Radiographs show an increasing loss of subchondral bone. The articulating bone ends acquire jagged contours, and there is a progressive widening of the joint space.

Because the acromioclavicular joint is synovial, it is also involved by **rheumatic disorders**. This process takes a slower course than bacterial arthritis and starts with marginal erosions. The end stage is marked by joint space

widening with destruction of the capsule and ligaments (Fig. 3.**69**).

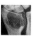 ## Tumor?

Various causes of radiographic bone loss about the acromioclavicular joint, especially at the end of the clavicle, were mentioned above. But the "loss of joint contours" can also have a purely technical cause, as in slightly overexposed radiographs of atrophic peripheral bone in older patients.

The principal causes of vanishing bony contours and structures about the acromioclavicular joint are listed below:

- Inflammation
- Tumor
- Necrosis, especially posttraumatic
- Hyperparathyroidism (Fig. 3.**54**)
- Age-related atrophy
- Gout, psoriasis

 ## Other Changes?

The acromioclavicular joint is among the articular structures that show early, frequent signs of **degenerative change** in nonarthritic patients. This probably relates to the fact that this rudimentary spheroidal joint is subject to exceptionally heavy loads, especially from shear forces. It is unclear why this process is not associated with concomitant synovitis, which would mark the transition from degenerative to (an unspecific) inflammatory arthritis.

Given the frequency with which degenerative changes in the acromioclavicular joint are seen on radiographs, it is appropriate to ask whether this finding should still be considered a normal variant in asymptomatic elder patients (Fig. 3.**55**).

Calcifications of the articular disk of the acromioclavicular joint (Fig. 3.**47**) are a very common manifestation of chondrocalcinosis.

Ligamentous calcifications are discussed on p. 271f.

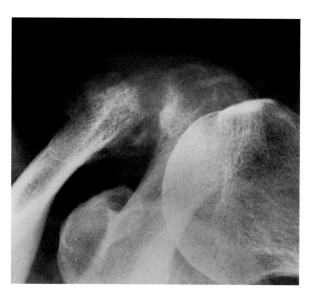

Fig. 3.**53** Typical acromioclavicular arthritis with widening of the joint space and destruction of the bone ends. Metaplastic ossifications have formed in the capsule. Painful swelling was present clinically, and needle aspiration yielded pus with *Staphylococcus aureus*.

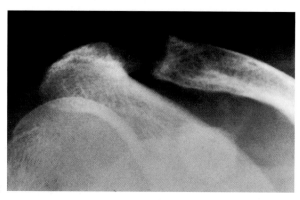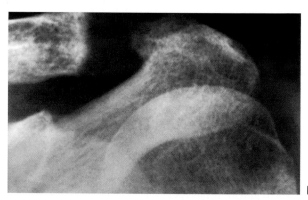

Fig. 3.**54a, b**   Apparent widening of the acromioclavicular joint space caused by subchondral resorption due to secondary hyperparathyroidism in a patient with renal osteodystrophy.

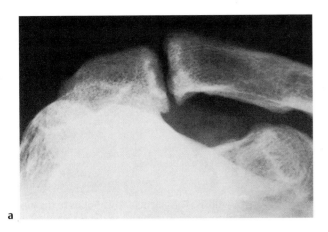
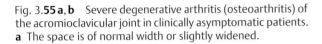

a

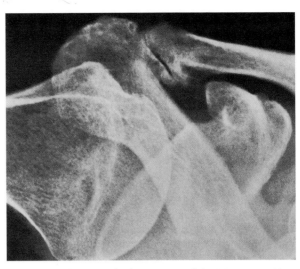

b

Fig. 3.**55a, b**   Severe degenerative arthritis (osteoarthritis) of the acromioclavicular joint in clinically asymptomatic patients. **a** The space is of normal width or slightly widened.

b This case shows marked narrowing of the joint space. Note the subchondral lucencies, sclerotic areas, marginal osteophytes, and other features of osteoarthritis.

References

Deutsch, A. L., D. Resnick, J. H. Mink: Computed tomography of the glenohumeral and sternoclavicular joints. Orthop. Clin. N. Amer. 16 (1985) 497

Falstie-Jensen, S., P. Mikkelsen: Pseudodislocation of the acromioclavicular joint. J. Bone Jt. Surg. 64-B (1982) 368

Harrison, R. B., H. O. Riddervold, E. D. Willett et al.: Acromioclavicular separation masked by muscle spasms. Virginia med. Mth. 107 (1980) 337

Hermanns, P. H., R. Beeger, D. Kötter: Posttraumatische Osteolyse des distalen Klavikulaendes. Röntgenblätter 34 (1981) 399

Keats, T. E., T. L. Pope: The acromioclavicular joint: normal variation and the diagnosis of dislocation. Skelet. Radiol. 17 (1988) 159

Neu, K., H. Krämer: Die Pseudoluxation des Akromioklavikulargelenkes – eine Sonderform der Epiphyseolysis. Z. Kinderchir. 34 (1981) 80

Oláh, J.: Das Röntgenbild des akromioklavikulären Gelenkes im Alter. Fortschr. Röntgenstr. 127 (1977) 334

Petersson, C. J., I. Redlund-Johnell: Radiographic joint space in normal acromioclavicular joints. Acta orthop. scand. 54 (1983) 431

Pettrone, F. A., R. P. Nirschl: Acromioclavicular dislocation. Amer. J. Sports Med. 6 (1978) 160

Post, M.: Current concepts in the diagnosis and management of acromioclavicular dislocations. Clin. Orthop. 200 (1985) 234

Puente, R., R. D. Boutin, D. J. Theodorou et al.: Post-traumatic and stress-induced osteolysis of the distal clavicle: MR imaging findings in 17 patients. Skelet. Radiol. 28 (1999) 202

Rockwood, C. A., G. R. Williams, D. C. Joung et al.: Injuries to the acromioclavicular joint. In Rockwood, C. A. et al.: Fractures in Adults, 4th ed. Lippincott-Raven, Philadelphia 1996

Sopov, V., D. Fuchs, E. Bar-Meir, et al.: Stress induced osteolysis of distal calvicle: imaging patterns and treatment using CT-guided injection. Eur. Radiol. 11 (2001) 270

Tossy, J. D., N. C. Mead, H. M. Sigmond: Acromioclavicular separations: Useful and practical classification for treatment. Clin. Orthop. 28 (1963) 111

The Shoulder Joint as a Whole

The chapters on the proximal humerus, scapula, and acromioclavicular joint reviewed the bony structures of the shoulder with regard to normal anatomy, normal variants, and significant (mainly borderline) findings. The radiographic evaluation of these structures is of little value, however, unless we view the findings against the background of the associated soft-tissue structures. In other words, an abnormal skeletal finding is generally only the tip of the iceberg; the changes in adjacent soft tissues are equally important and may have a greater impact on the patient's prognosis. This particularly applies to the glenoid labrum and rotator cuff, which are the primary focus of this chapter along with bursitic and other soft-tissue calcifications.

This chapter is not intended to give a comprehensive review of impingement syndrome, acute shoulder dislocations, chronic instability, etc. Its purpose, rather, is to offer a supplemental description that will enhance our understanding of the bony structures covered in the preceding chapters.

Soft-Tissue Anatomy of the Shoulder Joint

With Doppler ultrasound and especially MRI, we can define in considerable detail the soft-tissue structures that stabilize the shoulder joint. This fact, plus advances in orthopedic surgery and arthroscopy, have revolutionized our understanding of the complex traumatic and degenerative changes that can affect the shoulder joint.

The glenohumeral joint is inherently unstable due largely to the shallowness of the glenoid cavity. Ultimately the joint is stabilized by the articular capsule, the glenohumeral ligaments, the glenoid labrum, and the rotator cuff. While the glenoid labrum was once considered to have a major role in stabilizing the joint, today it is believed that this function is accomplished more by the anterior portion of the capsule.

The Anterior Capsular Complex

The stabilizing **anterior capsular complex** consists of the following structures:

- Biceps tendon
- Coracohumeral ligament
- Glenohumeral ligaments
- Subscapularis tendon (Fig. 3.**56**)

The biceps tendon is but one example of the extreme variability of the soft-tissue anatomy of the glenohumeral joint. The tendon may insert on the posterior labrum alone, on the anterior and posterior labrum, or on the anterior labrum alone. The glenohumeral ligament is composed of the superior, middle, and inferior ligaments (Fig. 3.**56a**). The inferior glenohumeral ligament appears to contribute most to the stability of the glenohumeral joint.

Glenoid Labrum

The glenoid labrum is a fibrous condensation of the joint capsule that deepens the glenoid cavity and augments the coverage of the humeral head (Fig. 3.**56b, c**).

The following two normal anatomic structures may be misidentified as an anterior labrum tear on MR images:

- The hyaline articular cartilage below the labrum. Normally the articular cartilage covers the surface of the glenoid and extends somewhat past its outer edges. The anterior labrum lies on the surface of the cartilage, and the underlying hyaline cartilage appears as a small zone of high signal intensity that can mimic a tear or avulsion of the labrum (Fig. 3.**59d, e**).
- The middle glenohumeral ligament anterior to the labrum (Fig. 3.**59d**). A thickening of the anterior capsule, this ligament is located directly in front of the anterior labrum and is separated from it by a thin layer of fluid that appears hyperintense on MRI.

It would exceed our scope to go into the specific imaging features that are used to avoid these pitfalls. An actual review article about the normal anatomy, variants and pathology of the middle glenohumeral ligament was presented by Beltran et al. (2002).

The glenoid labrum is highly variable in its shape (Fig. 3.**57**). A table on the morphological variants of the labral ligamentous complex can be found in Shankman et al. (1999).

Attachment of the Anterior Capsule

The anterior capsule (Fig. 3.**56b, c**) may be attached just medial to the glenoid labrum (type I attachment), up to 1 cm farther medially (type II), or at a site farther down the scapular neck (type III). The type III attachment may predispose to glenohumeral instability and dislocation. The posterior capsule, however, is almost always attached to the labrum or just medial to it.

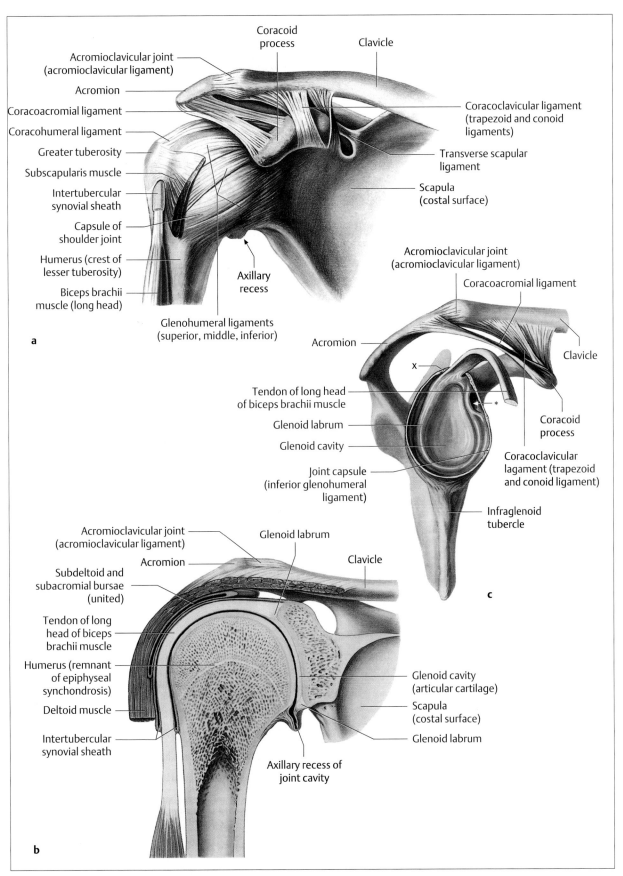

Fig. 3.**56a–c**   Anatomy of the shoulder joint (after Wolf-Heidegger).

a Anterior aspect.
b Coronal view.
c Lateral view of the glenoid.

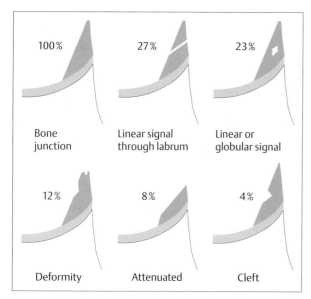

Fig. 3.**57** Morphological and signal variability of the labrum (after McCauley et al.).

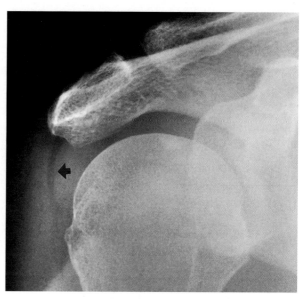

Fig. 3.**58** Physiological fat stripe on the subdeltoid bursa (arrow).

Rotator Cuff

The rotator cuff is formed by four muscles that arise from the anterior and posterior surfaces of the scapula and insert on the humeral head (Figs. 3.**56**, 3.**59**):

● Subscapularis (inserts on the lesser tuberosity)
● Supraspinatus (inserts on the proximal greater tuberosity)
● Infraspinatus and teres minor (insert on the middle and distal greater tuberosity)

The subscapularis is responsible for internal rotation and adduction, the supraspinatus and infraspinatus/teres minor for external rotation. The supraspinatus also assists the deltoid muscle in abduction and external rotation.

Bursae About the Shoulder Joint

The bursae about the shoulder joint consist of small sacs lined by a synovial membrane that secretes a fluid film (Figs. 3.**56**, 3.**59**). Interposed between adjacent anatomic structures, the bursae keep the structures from rubbing against each other and help tendons, for example, to glide smoothly past adjacent ligaments.

Bursae are not always present at birth. They can develop in response, say, to a cartilaginous exostosis that is impinging on adjacent bony structures or a nearby muscle (Fig. 3.**45**).

The bursae located about the shoulder joint are the following.

Subacromial–Subdeltoid Bursa

This bursa is actually composed of two bursae: the subacromial bursa and the subdeltoid bursa. The two bursae communicate with each other in approximately 95% of the population.

The subacromial–subdeltoid bursa has a relatively large surface area and facilitates movement between the rotator cuff tendons and coracoacromial arch on the one hand and between the rotator cuff tendons and deltoid muscle on the other. The bursa extends medially toward the coracoid process. Its lateral and inferior portions near the deltoid muscle are variable and may extend up to 3 cm below the greater tuberosity. Anteriorly, the bursa covers the groove of the biceps brachii muscle. Normally the subacromial–subdeltoid bursa is not visible on conventional radiographs. But since a fatty layer 1–2 mm wide is normally present between the outer fibrous layers of the bursa and the rotator cuff tendons and deltoid muscle, the bursa can be identified indirectly as a structure located medial to the fat stripe (Fig. 3.**58**).

The fat stripe is best demonstrated on internally rotated views of the shoulder. Partial or complete obliteration of the fat stripe is not a specific criterion for a soft-tissue abnormality of the shoulder. Coronal MR images usually provide an excellent view of the fat stripe (Fig. 3.**59 b**).

If the bursa is free of abnormal fluid collections, generally it can be identified only indirectly (below the fat stripe) with MRI.

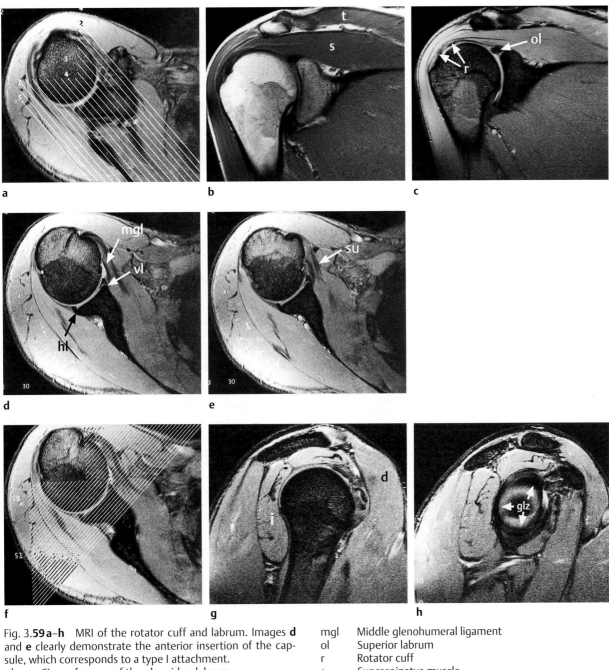

Fig. 3.**59 a–h**   MRI of the rotator cuff and labrum. Images **d** and **e** clearly demonstrate the anterior insertion of the capsule, which corresponds to a type I attachment.

glz	Circumference of the glenoid or labrum (direct view in **h**)
hl	Posterior labrum
i	Infraspinatus muscle
mgl	Middle glenohumeral ligament
ol	Superior labrum
r	Rotator cuff
s	Supraspinatus muscle
su	Subscapularis tendon
t	Trapezius muscle
vl	Anterior labrum

Subcoracoid Bursa

The subcoracoid bursa is located above the subscapularis tendon and below the coracoid process and the common tendon of the short biceps head and coracobrachialis. The bursa extends posteriorly below the coracoid process. It facilitates motion between the subscapularis tendon and the tendons of the short biceps head and coracobrachialis during rotation of the humeral head.

Coracoclavicular Bursa

The coracoid process and clavicle are interconnected by the coracoclavicular ligament, which, as mentioned earlier, consists of two parts (the conoid and trapezoid ligaments). The coracoclavicular bursa, sometimes called the supracoracoid bursa, is located in the angle between the two ligaments, embedded in fibrofatty tissue. It forms a cushion between the clavicle above and the posterior coracoid surface below.

Supra-acromial Bursa

The supra-acromial bursa is located on the upper surface of the acromion and normally does not communicate with the glenohumeral joint.

Other Bursae

There are usually two and occasionally three openings (foramina) in the glenohumeral joint capsule:

- One opening communicates with the subscapular bursa (through the foramen described by Weitbrecht between the superior and middle glenohumeral ligaments, Fig. 3.56 c).

- A second opening is located between the humeral tuberosities at the level of the bicipital groove. It gives passage to the long biceps tendon and its sheath.
- A third, inconstant opening is posterior and connects the glenohumeral joint with a bursa separating the infraspinatus tendon and joint capsule.

When bursal disease is present (bursitis with or without calcium deposits), the anatomy of the bursae is clearly delineated on radiographs, CT scans, and MR images (Figs. 3.**65**, 3.**68**–3.**71**).

Shoulder Impingement and Rotator Cuff Tears

In shoulder impingement syndrome, the rotator cuff (especially the supraspinatus muscle) impinges against the anterior acromion or coracoacromial ligament, and less commonly against the acromioclavicular joint, during forward flexion of the arm. The chronic, repetitive trauma leads to degeneration and eventual tearing of the rotator cuff. In other cases the rotator cuff may be ruptured by a single traumatic episode.

Neer stages of shoulder impingement syndrome
➤ *Stage I* Supraspinatus intramuscular hemorrhage and edema. Most patients are under 25 years of age.
➤ *Stage II* Rotator cuff tendinopathy and fibrosis plus thickening of the subacromial bursa. Patients are between 25 and 40 years of age.
➤ *Stage III* Tendon rupture, occurring mainly in patients over 40 years of age.

In another type of impingement called **subcoracoid shoulder impingement**, the distance between the humeral head and coracoid is diminished (congenital, posttraumatic, etc.).

Finally, a **posterosuperior impingement** has been described that occurs mainly in throwing athletes. Each time the arm is raised to the throwing position (humerus externally rotated and abducted 90°), the supra- and infraspinatus tendon insertions are compressed against the posterior superior rim of the glenoid. The pathoanatomic effects of this recurrent impingement are partial tearing of the rotator cuff, subchondral resorption of the greater tuberosity, and regressive changes in the posterior glenoid rim and labrum.

It should be reemphasized that the term "impingement syndrome" refers entirely to clinical manifestations. The radiologist examines the rotator cuff and its surroundings with ultrasound, MRI, or both in order to identify the pathoanatomic changes that underlie the clinical manifestations.

The cardinal symptom of impingement syndrome is a stabbing pain when the arm is abducted (more than 70–20°) and externally rotated (more than 20–30°) or elevated (more than 70–120°) and internally rotated (more than 30°). Crepitus is occasionally noted over the convexity of the shoulder, caused by impingement of the greater tuberosity against the acromioclavicular arch.

Conventional radiographs contribute relatively little information because they tend to show the effects rather than the cause of the constriction of the subacromial space (Fig. 3.**60**).

The Neer modification of the Y shoulder view is useful for defining the curvature of the acromion (p. 272 ff. and Fig. 3.**16**, 3.**28**). Angling the x-ray tube 30° caudad gives a clear view of the lower portions of the acromion and will reveal osteophytes located on the anterior undersurface of the acromion ("subacromial spurs," Figs. 3.**16**, 3.**60**). Stallenberg et al. (2001) found significant concordances between the assessments of the superior contour and the heterogeneity of the muscle radiodensity, respectively, on the outlet view radiograph (Fig. 3.16) and MR images: A flattened or ill-defined contour and a heterogenous density of the supraspinatus muscle may be signs of a rotator cuff tear. On the other hand, a bulging muscle contour and homogeneity appear to be the most suitable features for excluding atrophy and fatty infiltration of the muscle, caused by a full-thickness tear.

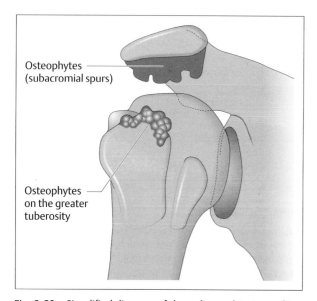

Osteophytes (subacromial spurs)

Osteophytes on the greater tuberosity

Fig. 3.**60**   Simplified diagram of the radiographic signs of impingement syndrome: subacromial osteophytes accompanied by sclerosis and irregular excrescences on the greater tuberosity. The diagram corresponds to a radiograph with the tube angled 30° downward.

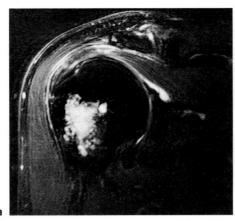
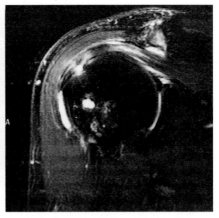

a

b

Fig. 3.**61 a, b** Man 61 years of age presented with right shoulder pain that gave the clinical impression of an impingement syndrome. Coronal T2-weighted fat-suppressed MR images show conspicuous, streaklike areas of increased signal intensity in the rotator cuff and fluid in the subdeltoid and subacromial bursae. The increased signal intensities in the rotator cuff represent tears. The hyperintense area in the humeral head with racemose extensions is a benign cartilaginous tumor (enchondroma).

Fluoroscopy during abduction of the externally rotated arm will occasionally reveal a painful impingement of the greater tuberosity against the osteophytes. These roentgen signs are at best suggestive, however. The proof of a rotator cuff lesion must rely on **ultrasonography** (not discussed here) or on **MRI** and **MR arthrography** (Figs. 3.**61**, 3.**62**). The most suitable imaging planes are listed below.

- Axial images (to demonstrate the subscapularis muscle, the intertubercular portion of the biceps tendon, the labrum, and the joint capsule)
- Oblique coronal images (perpendicular to the glenoid and parallel to the supraspinatus muscle)
- Oblique sagittal images (parallel to the glenoid)

The standard protocol consists of T1- and T2-weighted spin-echo sequences. MR arthrography can be performed directly or indirectly (after the intravenous injection of gadolinium).

Fresh partial or complete rotator cuff tears appear on T2-weighted images as sharply defined areas of high signal intensity (Fig. 3.**62**). Older tears in which edema has cleared are not hyperintense on T2-weighted images, but they can be recognized in T1-weighted sequences by the increased signal intensity of the muscle due to fatty atrophy. These changes in signal intensity require differentia-

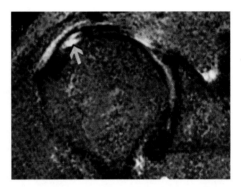

Fig. 3.**62** Fresh partial rotator cuff tear. Oblique coronal MRI shows a partial, hyperintense disruption in the part of the supraspinatus tendon that faces the joint (arrow).

tion from high tendon signals caused by partial volume averaging or the "magic angle" effect (angle of tendon relative to the magnetic field). MR arthrography permits a more confident differentiation between degenerative changes and a partial or complete tear. As in conventional shoulder arthrography, a complete tear is associated with contrast extravasation into the adjacent bursa.

Shoulder Dislocation and Shoulder Instability

Eighty-five percent of all shoulder dislocations involve the glenohumeral joint, 12% the acromioclavicular joint, and only 3% the sternoclavicular joint. Ninety-five percent of all glenohumeral dislocations are anterior, 2–4% are posterior, 1–2% are inferior, and fewer than 1% are superior.

Anterior glenohumeral dislocations are further classified as follows:

- Subcoracoid dislocations
- Subglenoid dislocations
- Subclavicular dislocations
- Intrathoracic dislocations

Subcoracoid and subglenoid dislocations may be associated with injuries to the posterolateral aspect of the humerus (Hill–Sachs lesion) and the anterior rim of the glenoid (Bankert lesion). The **Hill–Sachs lesion** is actually the result of a violent initial dislocation of the humeral head to a subglenoid position (Figs. 2.**437**, 3.**63**).

Once this lesion has occurred, it can predispose to the development of recurrent anterior glenohumeral dislocations.

> The Hill–Sachs lesion should not be confused with a fossa that is normally present in the posterolateral aspect of the humerus. Typically this feature appears below the axial scan plane of the coracoid process on CT and MR images. A typical Hill–Sachs lesion is located at or above the level of the coracoid process (Fig. 3.**15 g, h**, versus 3.**63**).

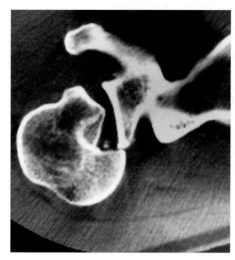

Fig. 3.**63**   Typical Hill–Sachs indentation caused by impaction of the humeral head against the inferior rim of the glenoid.

The term "**Bankert lesion**" (Fig. 3.**64**) originally referred to a **purely cartilaginous lesion** at the attachment of the anterior part of the inferior glenohumeral ligament. Adjacent osseous lesions are called **bony Bankert lesions** (Fig. 3.**64 c**).

Posterior glenohumeral dislocations are classified as follows:

- Subacromial dislocations
- Subglenoid dislocations
- Subspinous dislocations

Chronic recurrent (atraumatic) posterior shoulder instability may be caused by a bony deficiency (hypoplasia) of the posterior glenoid rim (see p. 274).

Inferior dislocations of the glenohumeral joint are also known as "luxatio erecta" because the arm is held above the patient's head with the elbow flexed.

Superior dislocations occur when the humeral head is driven upward through the rotator cuff. Associated injuries of the humerus, clavicle, and acromion are observed.

With any shoulder dislocation and chronic instability, the lesions described above are generally accompanied by injuries to the joint capsule and glenohumeral ligaments, which can be clearly demonstrated by MRI.

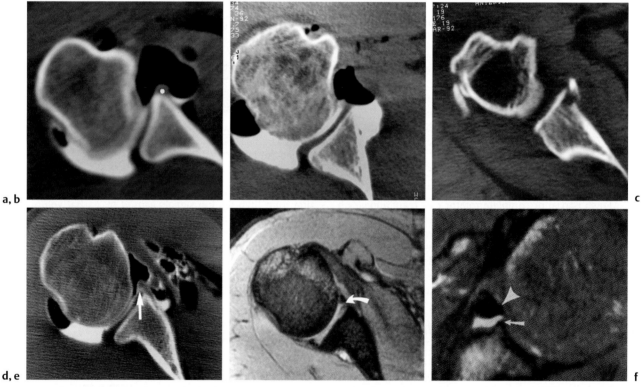

Fig. 3.**64 a–f**   Bankert lesion and its differential diagnosis.
a CT arthrogram shows anteromedial displacement of the anterior labrum (asterisk).
b Here the anterior air bubble is in direct contact with the articular cartilage, and the contrast pool behind the air bubble directly abuts the glenoid bone. This confirms the absence of the labrum, which apparently has been completely avulsed from the glenoid.
c Typical bony Bankert lesion.
(Panels **a–c** with kind permission of Professor Dr. Erlemann, Duisburg-Hamborn)

d, e An arrow in the CT arthrogram (**d**) marks the labral tear, which MRI (**e**, fat-suppressed T2-weighted sequence) demonstrates as a hyperintense line (arrow). Not a morphological variant.
f MRI in another patient with a "sublabral foramen" reveals articular fluid between the detached anterosuperior labrum (arrowhead) and the glenoid rim (arrow). The middle glenohumeral ligament is indistinguishable from the detached labrum. This type of labral variant is found in approximately 10% of the population. (From Tuite and Orwin, 1996.)

Clinically, the differential diagnosis of shoulder disloca-tion, particularly recurrent dislocations, should include impingement syndrome, intra-articular loose bodies, glenohumeral osteoarthritis, and especially a rotator cuff tear. It is the task of the radiologist to "untangle" this broad spectrum of differential diagnoses.

Radiological Examination Technique

The radiological examination in shoulder dislocation and instability consists of the following:

- **AP radiograph** (with the patient turned toward the af-fected shoulder). **Neer modification of the Y view** (p. 265). The **Bernageau view** is best for demonstrating a bony Bankert lesion (avulsion fracture of the anterior inferior glenoid rim). A Hill–Sachs lesion can be demon-strated on tangential views of the posterior superior humeral head or **fluoroscopically guided views** in in-ternal rotation.

- **CT** can be used to define a bony Bankert lesion, Hill–Sachs lesion, or other injuries of osseous structures. **CT arthrography** (with the injection of air or air plus con-trast medium) can define all relevant soft-tissue struc-tures such as the labrum, joint capsule, and gleno-humeral ligaments (Bachman et al. 1998; Fig. 3.**64 a, b**). The region should be meticulously scanned at 2-mm in-tervals from the superior border of the humeral head to the axillary recess.

- We cannot offer specific details on techniques of **MRI** examination, particularly since certain techniques are highly controversial. It is clear, however, that transaxial images have the greatest value. Typical protocols in-clude a conventional spin-echo sequence, a fast spin-echo sequence, a two-dimensional gradient-echo sequence, and three-dimensional gradient-echo sequences. **MR arthrography** can be a necessary study, especially for imaging the glenohumeral ligaments. As a general rule, MRI is inferior to CT for demonstrating small bony Bankert lesions.

Calcifications and Ossifications in the Soft Tissues of the Shoulder

The causal spectrum of soft-tissue calcifications in the shoulder region is extremely broad and ranges from harm-less bursal calcifications, which generally are detected in-cidentally, to neoplastic processes (e.g., synovial chondro-matosis).

The principal regressive changes and ossifications about the shoulder are shown schematically in Fig. 3.**65**.

The precise differentiation between calcifications in the supraspinatus, infraspinatus and teres minor tendons is ultimately of no clinical importance, even in patients with symptoms of "humeroscapular periarthritis" (pain and palpable induration of tendons and bursae, or even perifo-cal edema). "Humeroscapular periarthritis" occasionally may take the form of an acute bursitis or tenosynovitis that is not associated with calcifications. Tendon and bursal cal-cifications are usually detected incidentally in older patients (Fig. 3.**66**).

In other cases tendon calcifications may be resorbed, especially if they have entered the subacromial–subdel-toid bursa, and are no longer visible on radiographs (Fig. 3.**67**).

If the findings are detected incidentally, they should probably be classified as **periarthropathia calcificans**. Not infrequently, these changes coexist with sites of bone pro-liferation on the anterior undersurface of the acromion and on the greater tuberosity (productive fibro-ostosis; Fig. 3.**65**). The acuteness of these changes can be quickly evaluated by performing an ultrasound scan of the rotator cuff (to check for fluid in the bursa, rotator cuff tears, etc.). The diagram in Fig. 3.**65** shows additional bursal calcifica-tions, generally in the form of hydroxyapatite. If these cal-cifications are very dense, they may be mistaken for foci of ligamentous ossification or even bony avulsions.

Fig. 3.**65 a, b**   Diagram of various calcifications and ossifications that can occur about the shoulder.
a Standard AP projection.
1   Bony proliferation below the an-terior border of the acromion
2   Bony proliferation on the greater tuberosity
3   Calcification in the supraspinatus tendon
4   Fine, diffuse calcifications or cal-cium deposits due to massive in-flammation of the subdeltoid bursa
5   Calcifications in the subcoracoid bursa
6   Calcifications in the coracoclavic-ular bursa

b Internal rotation view.
1   Calcifications in the supraspinatus tendon
2   Calcifications in the infraspinatus tendon
3   Calcifications in the teres minor tendon

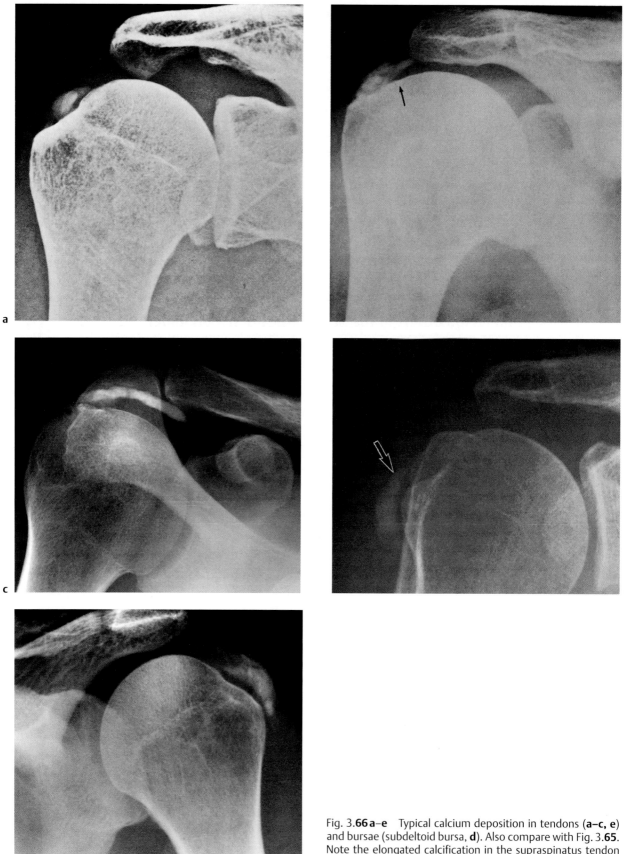

Fig. 3.**66 a–e** Typical calcium deposition in tendons (**a–c, e**) and bursae (subdeltoid bursa, **d**). Also compare with Fig. 3.**65**. Note the elongated calcification in the supraspinatus tendon in radiograph **c**.

Fig. 3.**67 a–d**   Calcifications and ossifications about the shoulder.
a, b Radiographs taken at three-month intervals show the partial spontaneous regression of calcifications in the supraspinatus tendon.
c, d Unusual metaplastic bone formation in the inferior joint capsule.

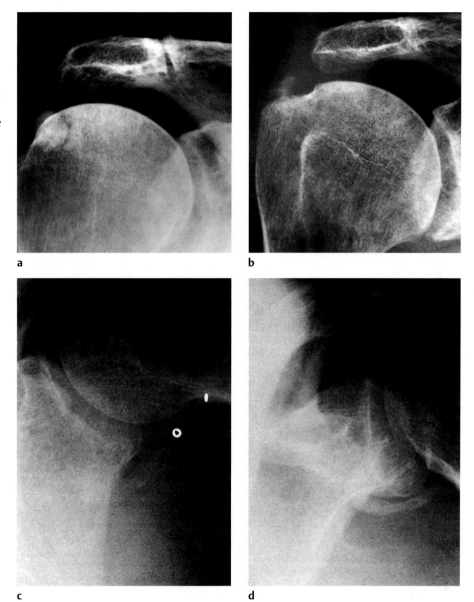

a

b

c

d

Calcium deposits in the bursae of the shoulder girdle also occur in the setting of **interstitial calcinosis** in patients with **renal osteodystrophy** (Fig. 3.**68**) and also in **primary chondrocalcinosis**.

Interstitial calcinosis in the setting of Thibierge–Weissenbach syndrome does not occur in the bursae but between the deep muscles and periarticular region.

Rice bodies that form in chronically inflamed joints and bursae (e.g., in patients with rheumatoid arthritis) are usually not visible on radiographs. Rice bodies consist of fibrin clumps whose pathogenesis is not fully understood. Figure 3.**69** illustrates a case of rice body synovitis that also vividly defines the anatomy of the bursae.

Ossifications in ligaments (e.g., the coracoclavicular ligament, see p. 271 and Fig. 3.**26**) may be purely regressive in nature, may result from trauma, and may occur in diseases that are associated with productive fibro-ostitic changes, such as seronegative spondylarthritis.

Ligamentous ossifications require differentiation from heterotopic bone formation (myositis ossificans, Fig. 3.**50**).

More solid "calcifications" in the shoulder soft tissues may represent **intra-articular loose bodies** due to osteochondritis dissecans (Fig. 3.**39**) or may result from extensive necrosis of the humeral head (Fig. 3.**70**). Another potential cause is primary synovial chondromatosis (Fig. 3.**71**).

While these disorders are significant from the standpoint of differential diagnosis, we cannot explore them more fully in a monograph that deals primarily with borderline findings.

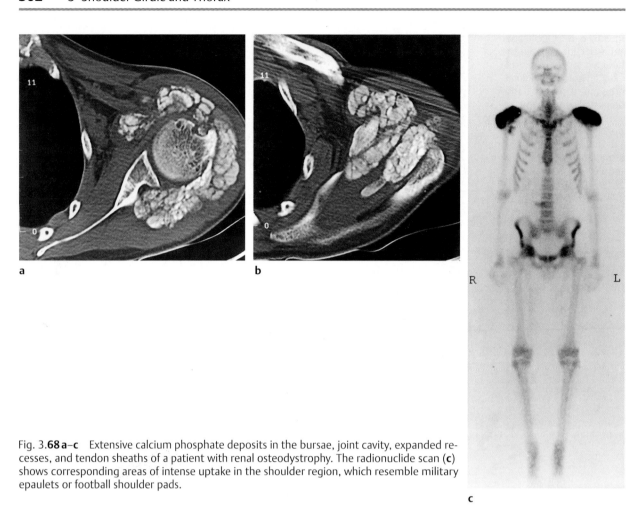

Fig. 3.**68 a–c**   Extensive calcium phosphate deposits in the bursae, joint cavity, expanded recesses, and tendon sheaths of a patient with renal osteodystrophy. The radionuclide scan (**c**) shows corresponding areas of intense uptake in the shoulder region, which resemble military epaulets or football shoulder pads.

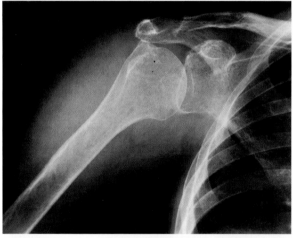

Fig. 3.**69 a–d**   Unusually conspicuous rice bodies in an elderly woman with rheumatoid arthritis. Note the destruction of the acromioclavicular joint in panel **a**. The joint space and its recess are markedly expanded and filled with small rice bodies. Note the communication between the subacromial–subdeltoid bursa and the coracoclavicular bursa in image **c**.

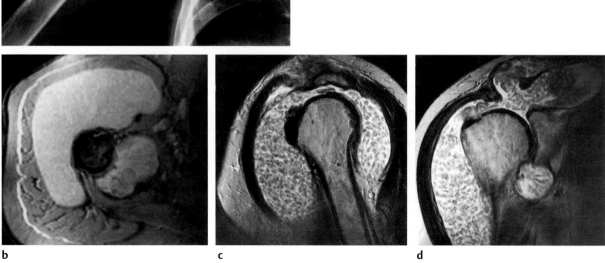

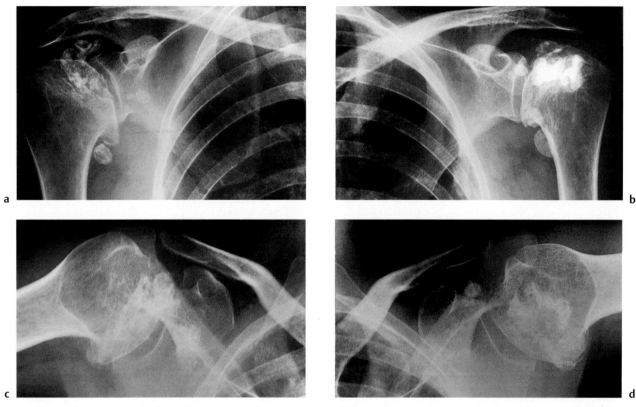

Fig. 3.**70 a–d** Intra-articular loose bodies secondary to severe humeral head necrosis (in the setting of a collagen disease). The numerous loose bodies, some displaying well-defined bony structures, bear a marked resemblance to the bodies in articular chondromatosis (Fig. 3.**71**).

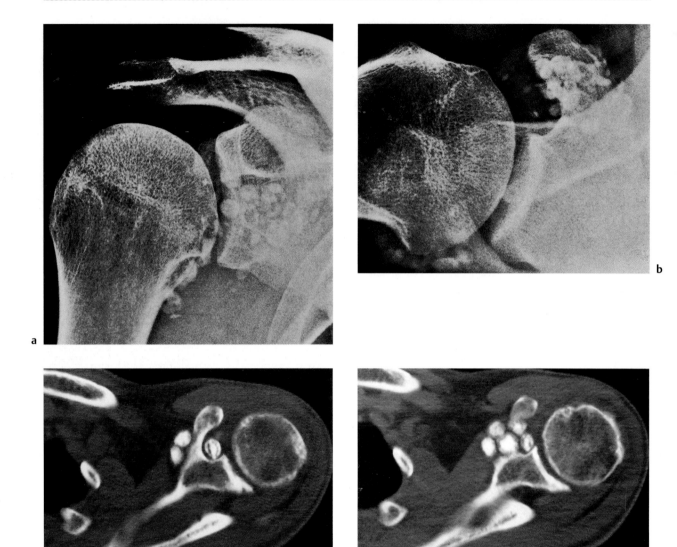

Fig. 3.**71 a–d**   Typical articular chondromatosis. The CT scans in **c** and **d** are from a different patient. Some of the intra-articular loose bodies in these images are located in the axillary recess and perhaps in the expanded subcoracoid bursa.

References

Bachmann, G., T. Bauer, I. Jürgensen et al.: Diagnostische Sicherheit und therapeutische Relevanz von CT-Arthrographie und MR-Arthrographie der Schulter. Fortschr. Röntgenstr. 168 (1998) 149

Beltran, J., Z. S. Rosenberg, V. P. Chandnani et al.: Glenohumeral instability: evaluation with MR arthrography. Radiographics 17 (1997) 657

Beltran, J., J. Bencardino, M. Padron et al.: The middle glenohumeral ligament: normal anatomy, variants and pathology. Skeletal Radiol. 31 (2002) 253

Gusmer, P. B., H. G. Potter, J. A. Schatz et al.: Labral injuries: accuracy of detection with unenhanced MR imaging of the shoulder. Radiology 200 (1996) 519

Hirschfeld, P., G. Dimanski: Die Schulter. Funktionelle Diagnostik und kausale Therapie in der Praxis. Perimed-spitta, Balingen 1994

Kaplan, P. A., K. C. Bryans, J. P.Davick et al.: MR imaging of the normal shoulder: variants and pitfalls. Radiology 184 (1992) 519

McCauley, T. R., C. F. Pope, P. Jokl: Normal and abnormal glenoid labrum:assessment with multiplanar gradient-echo MR imaging. Radiology 183 (1992) 35

Neumann, C. H., R. G. Holt, L. S. Steinbach et al.: MR imaging of the shoulder: appearance of the supraspinatus tendon in asymptomatic volunteers. Amer. J. Roentgenol. 158 (1992) 1281

Shankman, St., J. Bencardino, J. Beltran: Glenohumeral instability: evaluation using MR arthrography of the shoulder. Skelet. Radiol. 28 (1999) 365

Stallenberg, B., J. Rommens, C. Legrand, et al.: Radiographic diagnosis of rotator cuff tear based on the supraspinatus muscle density. Skeletal Radiol. 30 (2001) 31

Stiles, R. G., M. T. Otte: Imaging of the shoulder. Radiology 188 (1993) 603

Stoller, D. W.: MR-Arthrography of the glenohumeral joint. Radiol. Clin. N. Amer. 1 (1997) 97

Tuite, M. J., J. F. Orwin: Arterosuperior labral variants of the shoulder. Radiology 199 (1996) 537

Vahlensieck, M.: Indirekte MR-Arthrographie der Schulter. Radiologe 36 (1996) 960

Wolf-Heidegger, G.: Atlas der systematischen Anatomie des Menschen, Bd. I, 2. Aufl. Karger, Basel 1961

Clavicle and Sternoclavicular Joint

Normal Findings

During Growth

The clavicle is a long bone that is preformed in connective tissue and contains a medullary canal. It starts to ossify before any other bone in the body. It is ossified from two primary centers, one medial and the other lateral, which appear in the fifth and sixth weeks of intrauterine life and fuse during fetal development. Enchondral (epiphyseal) ossification takes place at both the acromial and sternal ends of the bone. In the clavicle, then, we have the unusual situation of membranous diaphyseal and metaphyseal ossification coexisting with enchondral longitudinal growth in the same bone. Membranous ossification of the diaphysis contributes most to longitudinal growth during both the intrauterine and postnatal periods. Longitudinal growth at the acromial end of the clavicle is insignificant by comparison.

Sonographic measurements by Yarkoni et al. (1985) showed a linear correlation between the length of the fetal clavicle and gestational age.

> These studies indicate that, as a general rule of thumb, the gestational age of a fetus in weeks is approximately equal to the length of the clavicle in millimeters.

The **secondary epiphyseal ossification center** at the medial end of the clavicle can be useful for **age determination**, especially between late adolescence and the third decade of life.

In their retrospective CT study of 380 subjects under 30 years of age, Kreitner et al. (1998) discovered that the medial ossification center of the clavicle appears between 11 and 22 years of age. They observed partial fusion between 16 and 24 years of age (Fig. 3.**74**) and complete fusion no earlier than 20 years of age; fusion occurred in 100% of cases by age 27. On comparing their data with the previous literature, the authors found no ethnic differences in the onset of ossification, the duration of partial fusion, or the timing of complete fusion. Despite the relatively long time needed for bony maturation of the medial epiphysis, the authors claim that the ossification pattern of the clavicle can be used forensically to determine whether an individual is in his or her late teens or early twenties (e.g., for referral to a penal institution for juveniles or adults). The same criteria can also be used for the age determination of human torsos.

As in adults, the juvenile clavicle is anteriorly convex in its medial two-thirds and posteriorly convex in its lateral third. The individual segments of the clavicle can show varying radiographic densities, depending on the projection (Fig. 3. **72**).

The sternal end of the clavicle undergoes distinct morphological changes with aging:

- In the first decade of life, the sternal end is shaped somewhat like a mushroom with smooth or irregular contours (Fig. 3.**73 a**).
- In the second decade of life, it becomes more cup-shaped and often has irregular borders (Fig. 3.**73 b**).

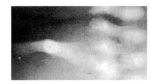
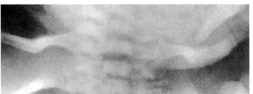

Fig. 3.**72 a, b**   The pediatric clavicle.
a The increased density at the center of the clavicle in an infant is a projection-related effect.
b Normal curvature of the pediatric clavicle.

In Adulthood

After about 25 years of age, the medial end of the clavicle is radiologically shaped somewhat like a pestle, often bearing a central notch or groove in its articular surface (Figs. 3.**75 b**, 3.**76**).

In adults as in children, the three-dimensional curvature of the clavicle should be considered when the bone is evaluated. This is necessary to avoid the misinterpretation of deformities, especially in atypical projections (e.g., an elevated scapula in the AP projection, etc.).

An approximately 4-mm-wide band of soft-tissue density is normally seen parallel to the superior border of the clavicle. It represents an orthograde projection of the skin that overlies the clavicle.

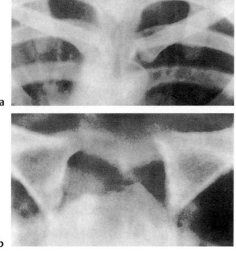

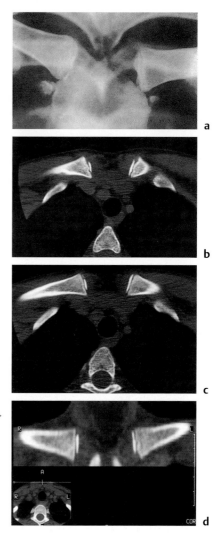

Fig. 3.**73a,b**   Morphological changes in the medial clavicle during growth.
a The medial end of the clavicle is mushroom-shaped during the first decade of life (9-year-old boy).
b The medial end of the clavicle is cup-shaped in the second decade of life (12-year-old girl).

Fig. 3.**74a–d**   Ossification of the medial clavicular epiphysis.   ▷
a Radiograph in a 21-year-old man shows partial ossification of the medial epiphyseal center of the clavicle.
b–d CT scans from a convicted criminal of unknown age. The scans were taken to determine whether the individual should be placed in a juvenile or adult penal facility. The partially fused medial clavicular epiphysis proves that the patient must be between 16 and 26 years of age. If the epiphysis were completely fused, he would have to be over 20 years of age.

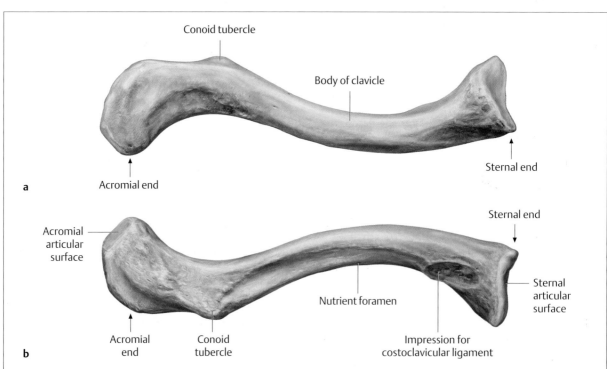

Fig. 3.**75a,b**   Anatomy of the clavicle.
a Superior aspect.
b Inferior aspect.

Note the pronounced S-shaped curvature of the clavicle and the configuration of the medial articular end.

On atypical projections, superimposed portions of the scapula can lead to strange or confusing findings (Fig. 3.**77**).

A small defect is occasionally seen in the superior border of the middle third of the clavicle. It represents the foramen of a canal that transmits the medial fascicle of the supraclavicular nerve (Fig. 3.**78**). According to anatomists, this nerve canal is present in 2–6% of the population. Duplication of the canal was described by Pahl (1955) (Fig. 3.**79**).

Besides neural foramina, nutrient canals also occur in the clavicle and are most conspicuous at the junction of its middle and lateral thirds (Figs. 3.**75 b**, 3.**89 a, b**).

The site where the coracoclavicular ligament attaches to the clavicle may exhibit pits, cortical irregularities, or a normal conoid tubercle (called also the coracoid tubercle; Fig. 3.**75**).

The site where the costoclavicular ligament attaches to the inferior medial border of the clavicle (Fig. 3.**81**) normally bears a notch (Fig. 3.**75 b**) that can be quite conspicuous in some individuals, especially those who subject the shoulder to heavy loads (Fig. 3.**80 a, b**).

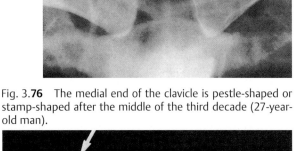

Fig. 3.**76**   The medial end of the clavicle is pestle-shaped or stamp-shaped after the middle of the third decade (27-year-old man).

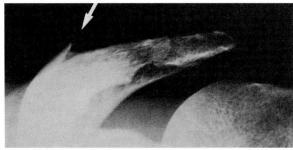

Fig. 3.**77**   Apparent "exostosis" at the superior border of the clavicle: a projection-related artifact.

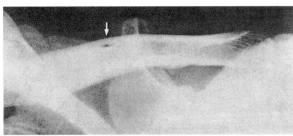

a

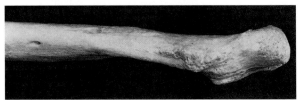

b

Fig. 3.**78 a, b**   Canal for the medial fascicle of the supraclavicular nerve (arrow).

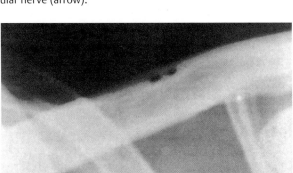

Fig. 3.**79**   Duplication of the neural foramen for the supraclavicular nerve fascicle (observation by Pahl).

Fig. 3.**80 a–c**   Ligament attachments.   ▷
a Relatively deep notch at the attachment the costoclavicular ligament (arrow).
b Appearance in an anatomic specimen.
c "Roughness" at the attachment of the sternohyoid and sternocleidomastoid muscles.

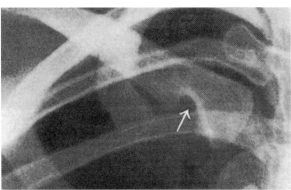

a

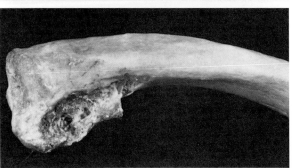

b

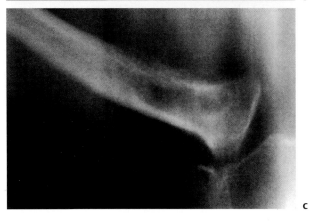

c

The differential diagnosis of this feature should always include a rarefying fibro-ostosis or fibro-ostitis (i.e., an enthesiopathy). The cortex also appears rough or spongy in the superomedial portion of the clavicle that gives attachment to the sternohyoid and sternocleidomastoid muscles (Fig. 3.**80c**).

The medial or sternal end of the clavicle cannot be considered without noting its importance as a component of the **sternoclavicular joint** (Fig. 3.**81**). This joint is the only true articulation that exists between the trunk and the shoulder girdle. The sternal side bears an extremely shallow joint cavity that is only partially congruent with the slightly convex but sometimes concave sternal end of the clavicle. As a result, the joint is inherently unstable. An interposed **articular disk** compensates for the lack of stable congruence. It also serves as a shock absorber for forces that are transmitted through the clavicle to the sternum. The articular disk undergoes regressive changes as early as 20–30 years of age, and after age 50 these "normal"

changes can be extremely pronounced without causing clinical symptoms. The possible clinical significance of the articular disk is discussed on p. 310.

The capsule of the sternoclavicular joint is relatively broad and is lined by a synovial membrane. The joint is stabilized chiefly by the anterior and posterior sternoclavicular ligament, which is basically a thickening of the fibrous capsule. Other known thickenings of the capsule anchor the medial end of the clavicle to the sternum, and the extra-articular costoclavicular ligament helps stabilize the joint by binding the medial clavicular metaphysis to the first rib.

Normal CT-measured values for the width of the sternoclavicular joint space are listed in Table 3.**2**.

An intra-articular vacuum phenomenon (Fig. 3.**95**) can be observed as early as 20 years of age but usually is not seen until age 40 (in approximately 8% of healthy subjects) (Hatfield et al. 1984).

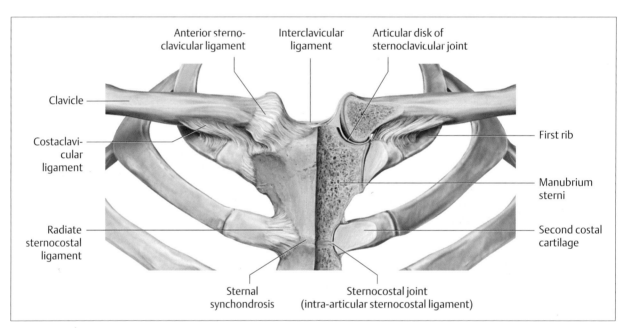

Fig. 3.**81**   Anatomy of the sternocostoclavicular region. Note the many ligament attachments, the composition of the sternoclavicular joint with its articular disk, and the sternal synchondrosis (after Wolf-Heidegger).

Table 3.**2**   Normal CT dimensions of the sternal region in millimeters (soft-tissue window, level 30 HU, window 500 HU, after Hatfield et al.). The values are approximately 10% higher than measurements using a bone window

	N	Overall mean	Male mean[1]	Female mean[1]	Minimum	Maximum
Sternal size:						
• AP	354	21.0	21.8	19.8	5	38
• Transverse	354	59.0	62.0	55.1	8	120
• Craniocaudal	354	159.0	166.0	149.0	40	230
Cortical thickness:						
• Manubrium sterni	311	9.5	9.7	9.1	4	21
• Body of sternum	306	6.1	6.6	5.6	2	13
Sternoclavicular joint distance	335	6.4	6.9	5.8	1	14

[1] Average age of subjects: males 45.1 years, females 44.7 years. Youngest subject 9 days, oldest subject 94 years

Pathological Finding?

Normal Variant or Anomaly?

The **medial epiphysis of the clavicle**, like most epiphyses in the shoulder girdle region, is subject to pronounced morphological variations, ranging in appearance from small nuclei in fossa-like depressions (Fig. 3.**82a**) to disk-shaped structures. The persistence of these centers has also been observed (Fig. 3.**82b**).

In extreme cases the medial end of the clavicle may show a forklike or fish-mouth configuration, even if there is no persistent epiphyseal center (Ravelli 1955).

Another variant is the **costoclavicular joint**, which may occur in place of the normal ligamentous attachments between the clavicle and first rib (Redlund-Johnell 1986).

Complete absence of the clavicle is classified as a true dysplasia. A large defect in the acromial end of the clavicle, combined with malformations of the skull and hands, can occur as part of a cleidocranial dysplasia. Congenital **unilateral hypoplasia** of the clavicle with pseudarthrosis formation between the hypoplastic segments is another type of dysplasia that probably has an autosomal dominant mode of inheritance (March 1968, Höcht et al. 1979).

Another anomaly, the **lateral clavicle hook**, consists of a hooklike accentuation of the lateral curvature of the bone. This type of anomaly may be associated with Holt–Oram syndrome, osteodysplastia, or trisomy 18 (Igual and Giedion 1979). These conditions cannot be covered here in detail, but the principal anomalies are summarized in Tables 3.**3** and 3.**4** (after Reeder 1993).

A final possible normal variant is **duplication of the clavicle** (Golthamer 1957, Twigg 1981).

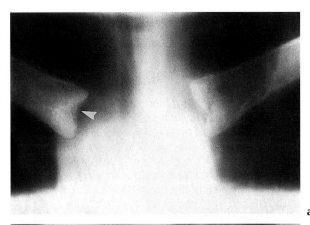

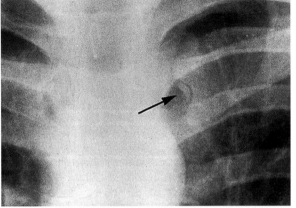

Fig. 3.**82a,b** Isolated and persistent ossification centers in the medial end of the clavicle.
a Isolated center in a 16-year-old boy (arrowhead).
b Persistent center in an adult (arrow).

Table 3.**3** Etiological spectrum of thin or hypoplastic clavicle

Common	Rare
• Cleidocranial dysplasia • Holt–Oram syndrome • Osteodysplastia (Melnick–Needles syndrome) • Pyknodysostosis • Progeria (thin clavicle)	• Brachial plexus paralysis (unilateral) caused by birth trauma • CHILD[1] syndrome • Cockayne syndrome (thin clavicle) • Congenital clavicular pseudarthrosis • Coffin–Siris syndrome • Goltz–Gorlin syndrome (focal dermal hypoplasia) • Fucosidosis • Larsen syndrome (thin clavicle) • Scapuloiliac dysostosis • Spondyloepiphyseal dysplasia (delayed ossification) • Trisomy 13 syndrome (thin clavicle) • Trisomy 18 syndrome (thin clavicle) • Turner syndrome (thin lateral clavicle)

[1] CHILD Congenital hemidysplasia, ichthyosiform nevi, limb defect

Table 3.**4** Hypoplastic stocky ("handlebar-like") clavicle

- Diastrophic dysplasia
- Holt–Oram syndrome
- Thrombocytopenia-absent radius syndrome
- Trisomy 18 syndrome
- Normal variant

Fracture, Subluxation, or Dislocation?

Fractures?

Clavicular fractures can occur as a result of **birth trauma** (Enzler 1950, Köster 1957). Initial callus becomes visible on radiographs in just 8–9 days. Clavicular fractures are not uncommon in children, especially before age 10, and comprise perhaps 50% of all injuries in the shoulder girdle region. The middle of the clavicle is a site of predilection for fractures. Often these pediatric fractures are very difficult to detect radiographically, especially since the majority are of the greenstick type.

As explained on p. 288, a superior tear in the periosteal sleeve of the lateral clavicle can allow the end of the clavicle to displace upward, leaving the cartilaginous portions in the acromioclavicular joint. The ligaments and capsule of the acromioclavicular joint are not disrupted. Basically this injury involves an epiphyseal separation corresponding to a Salter–Harris type I epiphyseal injury. A **sternoclavicular epiphyseal separation (epiphysiolysis)** can occur at the medial end of the clavicle (Lemire and Rosmann 1984).

In **adults**, 80% of all **clavicular fractures** involve the middle third of the clavicle. Fifteen percent involve the lateral third and may or may not be associated with a tear of the coracoclavicular ligament. The fracture line may extend into the acromioclavicular joint.

Only about 5% of clavicular fractures involve the sternal end, where they are very difficult to detect radiographically. Clavicular fractures mainly require **differentiation** from unusually prominent **nutrient canals**, **nerve canals**, and simple **projection-related effects** (Fig. 3.**83**).

Stress fractures of the clavicle most commonly occur after a radical neck dissection.

Subluxations and Dislocations

Traumatic dislocations of the sternoclavicular joint account for approximately 1% of all dislocations (Nettles and Linscheid 1968). The joint typically dislocates anteriorly and superiorly. **Posterior dislocations** are very rare (Fig. 3.**84**). They may be associated with severe clinical complications caused by pressure from the dislocated clavicle on the major vessels, trachea, esophagus, etc. (Cope and Riddervold 1988). Sternoclavicular dislocations are difficult to document with plain films, and we feel that a CT examination should be performed routinely whenever this injury is suspected.

Anterior and superior subluxation of the medial end of the clavicle due to regressive changes is a difficult diagnostic problem. Most patients are women 50 years of age or older who suddenly notice a "lump" over the medial end of the clavicle. The subluxation may indeed develop suddenly, or it may actually be present for some time before the patient becomes aware of it.

The clinical hallmark of these cases is a marked prominence of the clavicular head (Fig. 3.**85a**), which often feels somewhat springy to the touch. It may or may not be painful. Conventional radiographs are usually unrewarding due to the difficulty of obtaining a clear projection. A bone scan may show slightly increased tracer uptake in the region of the manubrium-clavicular joint. The most conclusive study is CT, which can document the anterior and superior displacement of the clavicular head (Fig. 3.**85b–d**). In many cases CT will also show definite regressive changes at the ends of the joint with subchondral sclerosis, small subchondral cysts, and marginal osteophytes. Etiologically, we feel that a painless subluxation is based on an age-related regressive process similar to the marginal osteophytes that develop along the acromioclavicular joint (see p. 290). The underlying cause may well be a constitutional laxity of the capsule and ligaments. We often confront this problem in cases that have been referred to us for consultation. The situation is different in patients who present clinically with pain and swelling. This implies a true pathological process in the sense of an active osteoarthritis with subluxation, similar to the changes that can affect joints elsewhere in the body.

Aumann and Brüning (1980) shed new light on this problem with their operative findings in six patients. They noted significant morphological disk changes (flattening and thinning, fragmentation, swelling) with otherwise normal-appearing bone and cartilage in the sternoclavicular joint. Clinically, the authors described transient joint swelling, severe pain, and crepitus during joint movements. In some cases the pain radiated throughout the shoulder girdle and to the back of the neck. The authors attributed the symptoms to the severe disk changes and believed that edema of the capsule and ligaments was responsible for the swelling that is seen in cases of degenerative subluxation.

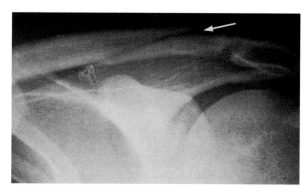

Fig. 3.**83** Mach effect produced by the superimposed clavicle and acromion.

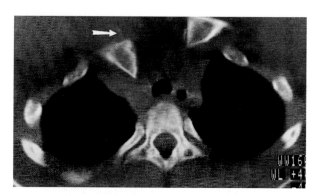

Fig. 3.**84** Posterior dislocation of the clavicle at the sternoclavicular joint. The arrow indicates the detached medial epiphysis (from Cope and Riddervold 1988).

Generally, **regressive subluxation with prominence of the clavicular head** as well as the **disk abnormalities** described by Aumann and Brüning (1980) require differentiation from **aseptic necrosis** (Friedrich disease) and from an early stage of unilateral sternocostoclavicular hyperostosis. If there is demonstrable swelling of the sternoclavicular joint but no redness, it is unlikely that arthritis is present.

 ## Necrosis?

Densities at the inferior medial end of the clavicle may be purely regressive in nature, but in symptomatic patients they may signify **aseptic necrosis** at that location (Friedrich disease). This condition presents clinically with a soft to firm swelling over the sternoclavicular joint. The earliest radiographic change is sclerosis involving the inferior medial end of the clavicle (stage I, Fig. 3.**86a**). With further progression, radiographs demonstrate fragmentation or demarcation of the necrotic end (stage II, Fig. 3.**86b**).

The necrotic process culminates in stage III, which displays the features of manubrioclavicular osteoarthritis (Heinemeier et al. 1979, Lingg and Heinemeier 1981).

Differentiation is mainly required from the condition known as osteitis condensans of the clavicle (Brower et al. 1974) and from early sternoclavicular hyperostosis (see below). Some cases of "aseptic necrosis" (Friedrich disease) that we have observed appeared to represent an initial stage of sternocostoclavicular hyperostosis, which became more obvious as the years progressed (see below). These patients developed dermatological changes such as pustulosis palmoplantaris or classic psoriasis, or the changes were already present when the patients were first seen.

Interestingly, Friedrich disease is observed predominantly in females.

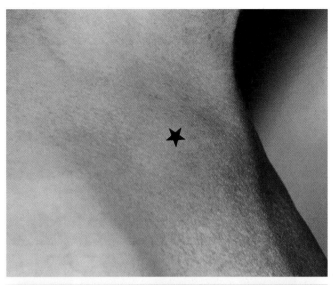

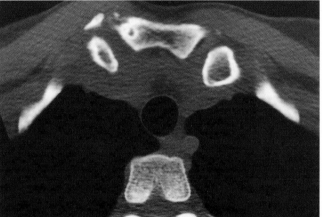

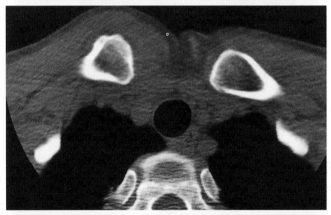

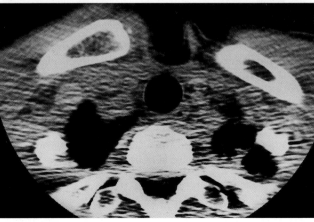

Fig. 3.**85a–d** Nonpainful subluxation of the right sternoclavicular joint. While dressing, the patient suddenly noticed a prominence of the medial end of the right clavicle (star). CT shows an obvious anterior-superior subluxation of the clavicular head (**b**). New bone formation is apparent in the area where the capsule and ligaments attach to the clavicular head on the right side. Compare this finding with Fig. 3.**94**, and contrast with the features of aseptic necrosis in Fig. 3.**86**.

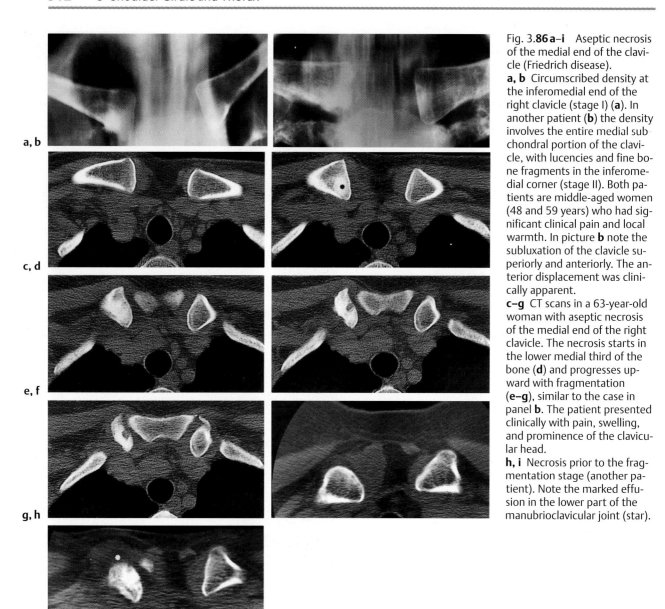

a, b

c, d

e, f

g, h

i

Fig. 3.**86 a–i**   Aseptic necrosis of the medial end of the clavicle (Friedrich disease).

a, b Circumscribed density at the inferomedial end of the right clavicle (stage I) (**a**). In another patient (**b**) the density involves the entire medial subchondral portion of the clavicle, with lucencies and fine bone fragments in the inferomedial corner (stage II). Both patients are middle-aged women (48 and 59 years) who had significant clinical pain and local warmth. In picture **b** note the subluxation of the clavicle superiorly and anteriorly. The anterior displacement was clinically apparent.

c–g CT scans in a 63-year-old woman with aseptic necrosis of the medial end of the right clavicle. The necrosis starts in the lower medial third of the bone (**d**) and progresses upward with fragmentation (**e–g**), similar to the case in panel **b**. The patient presented clinically with pain, swelling, and prominence of the clavicular head.

h, i Necrosis prior to the fragmentation stage (another patient). Note the marked effusion in the lower part of the manubrioclavicular joint (star).

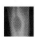 **Inflammation?**

Generally there should be little difficulty in distinguishing inflammatory diseases of the clavicle from normal variants. We include a section on inflammatory conditions because, at most, there may be some confusion with initial findings.

Infantile Cortical Hyperostosis

After the mandible, the clavicle is the second most frequent site of involvement by infantile cortical hyperostosis (Caffey disease). Most cases are bilateral.

Chronic Recurring Multifocal Osteomyelitis

Another inflammatory disorder with a predilection for the clavicle is chronic recurrent multifocal osteomyelitis. Initially, this disease usually presents radiographically as a subacute to chronic osteomyelitis without sequestrum formation (Figs. 3.**87**, 3.**88**).

Generally the diagnosis is established by the radionuclide detection of additional sites of involvement, especially in the metaphyses of the long bones of the lower extremity. Not infrequently, the condition is associated with pustulosis palmoplantaris (Freyschmidt and Freyschmidt 1996).

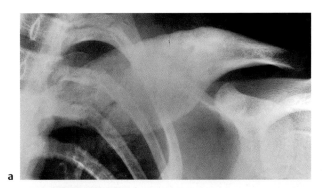

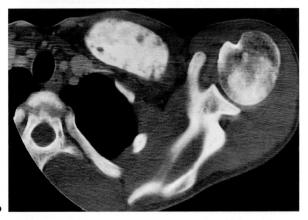

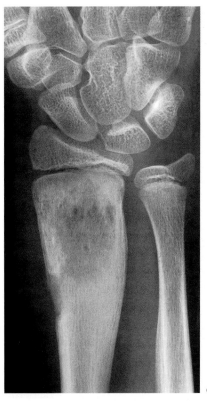

Fig. 3.**87 a–c**   Chronic recurrent multifocal osteomyelitis. The patient, a 13-year-old boy, presented clinically with massive prominence of the left clavicle but no inflammatory redness of the skin. Note the grotesque enlargement and increased den- sity of the left clavicle and the concomitant involvement of the distal radius (**c**). The lucency on the radial side of the metaphy- seal-diaphyseal junction is a postsurgical defect.

Osteitis condensans of the Clavicle

Osteitis condensans of the clavicle is a nonbacterial inflam- matory disease (Brower et al. 1974, Franquet et al. 1985). Usually there is isolated involvement of the clavicular head, which has a homogeneous roentgen appearance with no destructive changes or obvious periosteal reac- tions (Fig. 3.**89 a**). We doubt whether this entity actually exists as such and suggest that it may represent aseptic necrosis without fragmentation or incipient sternocosto- clavicular hyperostosis.

Paget Disease

In polyostotic cases of Paget disease (osteitis deformans), the clavicle may be involved in addition to other bones. The classic features are bony enlargement and a coarsened trabecular pattern with loss of clear delineation between the cortex and medullary canal (Fig. 3.**89 c, d**).

Bacterial Diseases

Bacterial osteomyelitis of the clavicle (usually caused by *Staphylococcus aureus*) is rare but occurs with some frequency in immunocompromised patients (diabetes mellitus, chronic hemodialysis, drug abuse, etc.). Hunter et al. (1983) described the development of clavicular osteo- myelitis following the insertion of a Swan–Ganz catheter.

In **congenital syphilis**, the clavicle is a site of predilec- tion for osseous involvement (Fig. 3.**90**).

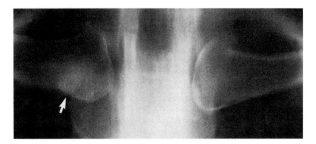

Fig. 3.**88**   Chronic recurrent multifocal osteomyelitis. The process started in the right clavicle. There is a relative paucity of destructive changes and new bone formation (arrow). Me- tachronous changes in other skeletal regions appeared during subsequent years. Differentiation is required from aseptic ne- crosis of the medial end of the clavicle (Fig. 3.**86**).

Bacterial arthritis of the manubrioclavicular joint is also relatively common in immunocompromised patients. The pattern of involvement with destruction of the bone ends, accompanying periosteal reaction, etc. is the same as in other forms of bacterial arthritis.

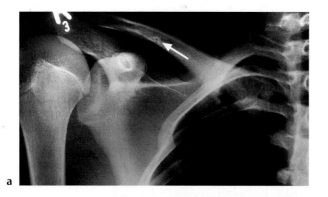

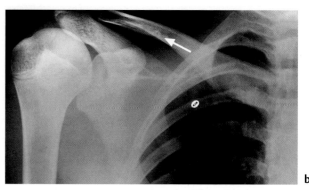

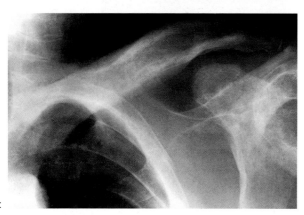

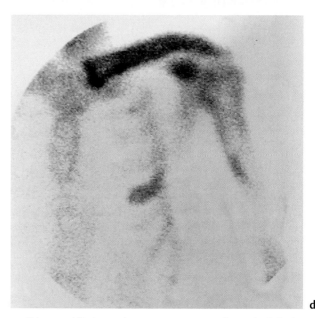

Fig. 3.**89 a–d** So-called osteitis condensans of the clavicle and Paget disease.
a, b So-called osteitis condensans of the clavicle in a 17-year-old male. Follow-up (**b**) for one year showed increasing sclerosis of the medial end of the clavicle.

The case presented clinically with swelling and little pain. The absence of other skeletal manifestations, even years later, distinguishes this condition from chronic recurrent multifocal osteomyelitis (CRMO). Note the nutrient canal in the lower mid-clavicle (arrow).

c, d Involvement of the clavicle by polyostotic Paget disease in a 61-year-old man. Note the coarsened trabecular pattern throughout the left clavicle and in the coracoid process (**c**). The humeral head also exhibits structural change. The radio-

nuclide scan (**d**) shows the most intense uptake in the left clavicle and coracoid process, apparently because the disease is still in a florid stage at those locations. Additionally, giant-cell tumorlike lesions were found in the humeral head and proximal diaphyseal-metaphyseal junction of the left humerus. This case is fully documented in Freyschmidt (1997, Fig. 14.42 c–n).

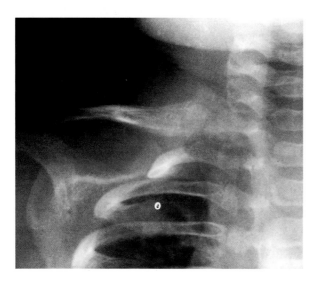

Fig. 3.**90** Stage III syphilitic osteitis of the right clavicle in a 2-month-old infant with congenital syphilis. The large tubular bones were also involved. Note how destructive lesions in the medial third of the clavicle are combined with extensive periosteal new bone formation, which apparently preceded the destructive changes (stage II).

Sternocostoclavicular Hypertostosis

Sternocostoclavicular hypertostosis is an inflammatory disease that we and other authors have observed with increasing frequency in the sternoclavicular region during recent years (Sonozaki et al. 1981, Kasperczyk and Freyschmidt 1993, Dihlmann 1993, Freyschmidt and Freyschmidt 1996, Freyschmidt and Sternberg 1998, Schilling and Kessler 1998). The swelling and redness are based on an inflammatory destructive process that involves the sternum, the medial ends of the clavicles, and the ligament and tendon attachments, especially between the ribs and clavicles (Figs. 3.**91**, 3.**123**).

This abacterial process is always associated with concomitant reactive-reparative and ankylosing bone formation in the affected region, leading to a progressive limita-

tion of motion in the joints between the manubrium and clavicles. Eventually the sclerotic changes spread to the clavicles and anterior ribs, the interosseous ligaments (e.g., the costoclavicular ligaments) ossify, and finally a plaque-like ossification affects the entire region (Fig. 3.**91 a**).

Sternocostoclavicular hypertostosis may occur by itself with no other disease manifestations, but most cases are associated with **pustulosis palmoplantaris** and/or **psoriasis**, which may coincide with or follow the clinical and radiological changes in the sternoclavicular region.

From a clinical standpoint, we describe the entire process as a **pustulotic arthro-osteitis** (PAO) while other authors prefer the term **SAPHO syndrome** (synovitis, acne, pustulosis, hyperostosis, osteitis).

We interpret pustulotic arthro-osteitis as a subtype of **seronegative spondylarthritis** owing to the frequency of

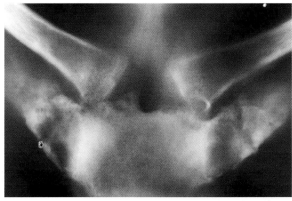
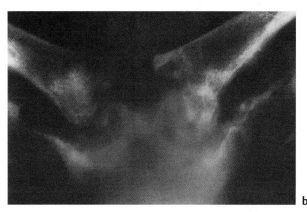

a   b

Fig. 3.**91 a–h**   Sternocostoclavicular hypertostosis.
a Advanced changes with staghorn-like ossification, especially of the manubriocostal attachments. Note the destructive changes in the manubrioclavicular joints. There was also inflammatory widening of the manubriosternal synchondrosis (not demonstrated here: see Fig. 3.**123 e, h**).

b Predominantly destructive form of sternocostoclavicular hypertostosis with complete destruction of the sternoclavicular joints accompanied by bone proliferation.

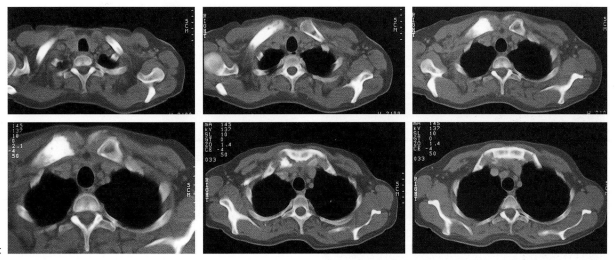

c

Fig. 3.**91 c**   Series of CT scans in sternocostoclavicular hyperostosis (**c**). The right clavicle and manubrioclavicular joint are predominantly affected in this patient. The whole-body radionuclide scan (**f**) shows predominant involvement of the right medial clavicle and manubrium. It also demonstrates foci in both lower thoracic vertebrae, in both lower lumbar vertebrae,

and in the sacrum consistent with a nonspecific spondylitis/spondylodiscitis (**g**). Note the typical sites of syndesmophyte formation on the affected vertebral bodies, indicating that this disease should be classified as a seronegative spondylarthritis.

Fig. 3.**91 d–h** ▷

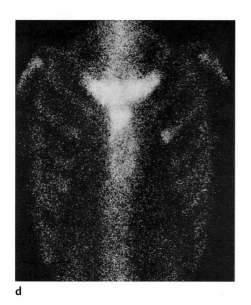

d

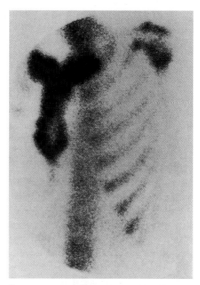

e

Fig. 3.**91 d, e**   These scans show the typical bull's head pattern of radionuclide uptake in the sternocostoclavicular region. Scan **d** goes with the radiograph in **a**, and scan **e** goes with the radiograph in **b**.
h Clinical appearance of sternocostoclavicular hypertostosis in the patient imaged in **a** and **d**: marked redness and swelling in the sternocostoclavicular region, accompanied by a conspicuous inflammatory prominence over the manubriosternal synchondrosis.

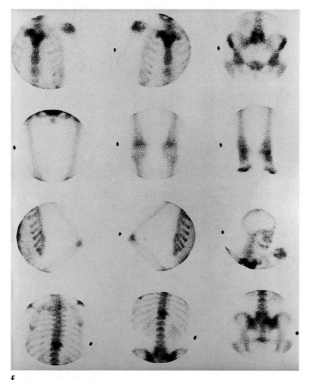

f

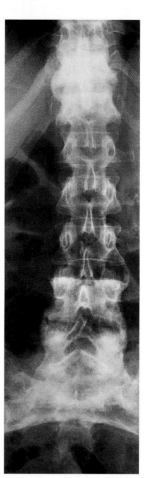

g

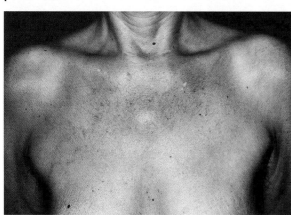

h

associated spondylarthritic changes, which may even progress to the classic picture of ankylosing spondylitis. In contrast to classic forms of spondylarthritis, this form involves the shoulder girdle more than the sacroiliac region, and the shoulder girdle is the primary site of involvement by inflammatory destructive and proliferative changes. Unusual tumorlike lesions occur in the tubular bones (Kasperczyk and Freyschmidt 1993). A detailed description of the features of pustulotic arthro-osteitis can be found in Freyschmidt and Freyschmidt (1996, 1998) and other sources. Most patients present at a relatively late stage, because usually the diagnosis is not routinely considered. Only CT and radionuclide scans can reliably detect the disease in its early stages. Whenever initial destructive and proliferative changes are found in the sternocostoclavicular region on clinical and radiological examination, a radionuclide scan should be obtained to check for the typical "bull-head" pattern of intense uptake in the sternocostoclavicular region (Freyschmidt and Sternberg 1998). The advantage of the radionuclide scan is that it also permits the early detection of other inflammatory skeletal changes.

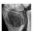

Tumor?

Basically all types of primary and secondary bone tumors may involve the clavicle. Early osteosclerotic and even osteolytic changes are often very difficult to detect on plain films. The following figures show typical examples of neoplastic changes in the clavicle:

- Figure 3.92: Langerhans-cell histiocytosis in a small child
- Figure 3.93a: Fibrous dysplasia
- Figure 3.93b: Bone metastasis

Pseudotumors of the clavicle can develop as a sequel to radical neck dissection (Fini-Storchi et al. 1985). Ultimately they are the result of a stress fracture with hemorrhagic areas and reactive changes.

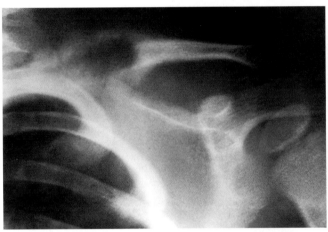

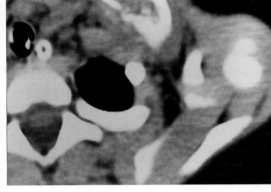

Fig. 3.**92a,b** Medial destruction of the left clavicle in a 3-year-old child with Langerhans-cell histiocytosis (eosinophilic granuloma). The cufflike periosteal reaction bridging the gap caused by bone destruction is a typical feature of Langerhans-cell histiocytosis. The CT scan (**b**) shows bony debris (sequestrum) within the periosteal cuff. The changes resolved spontaneously during the following year.

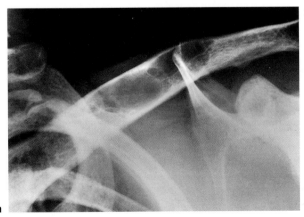

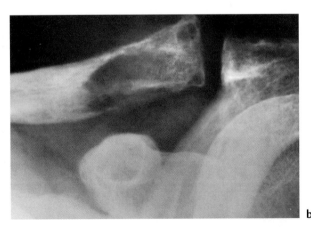

Fig. 3.**93a,b** Fibrous dysplasia and metastatic bone destruction.
a Fibrous dysplasia appears as a lucent (cystlike) area in the middle third of the clavicle with slight expansion of the bone. The lesion is sharply marginated. The medial portion shows a typical ground-glass appearance, distinguishing it from a true bone cyst.
b Metastatic destruction of the acromial segment of the clavicle in a patient with renal cell carcinoma.

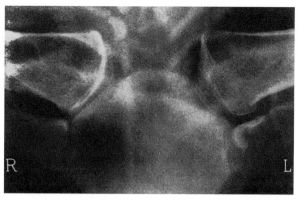

Fig. 3.**94** Painful degenerative arthritis with joint space narrowing and sclerosis of the articular surface in a 63-year-old man.

 Other Changes?

Degenerative arthritis of the sternoclavicular joint is not an unusual finding in radiographic examinations (Figs. 3.**94**, 3.**95**). Lately we have seen it quite often on digital thoracic images (owing to the large dynamic range). The patients denied having symptoms referable to the degenerative changes, so we interpreted the condition as an incidental finding or **age-associated variant**. Painful degenerative changes are uncommon (Fig. 3.**94**).

The problem of regressive disk changes in the sternoclavicular joint and the features of subluxation combined with osteoarthritis are covered under Fractures, Subluxations and Dislocations.

Calcifications and ossifications of the ligaments attached to the clavicle are illustrated in Figs. 3.**26** and 3.**50**.

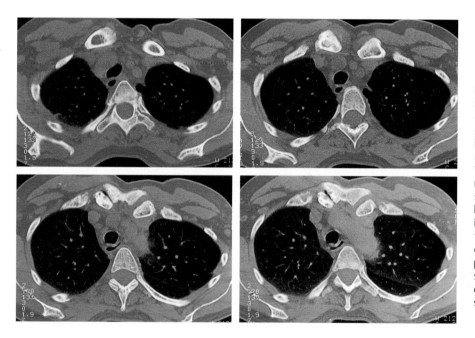

Fig. 3.**95 a–d** Classic sternoclavicular osteoarthritis in a 61-year-old woman who had done heavy physical labor all her life. She presented clinically with prominence of the right medial clavicle. She had occasional pain and crackling on joint motion but no swelling. The manubrium may be congenitally asymmetrical or "tilted," as its transverse axis is not horizontal. The CT scans show marked productive new bone formation on the superiorly subluxated medial end of the clavicle. The joint space (**c, d**) shows a definite vacuum phenomenon along with small subchondral degenerative cysts that confirm the presence of osteoarthritis.

References

Appell, R. G., H. C. Oppermann, W. Becker et al.: Condensing osteitis of the clavicle in childhood: a rare sclerotic bone lesion. Pediat. Radiol. 13 (1983) 301

Aumann, U., W. Brüning: Die Discopathie des Sternoclaviculargelenkes. Chirurg 51 (1980) 722

Brower, A. C., D. E. Sweet, T. E. Keats: Condensing osteitis of the clavicle: a new entity. Amer. J. Roentgenol. 121 (1974) 17

Clavo, E., D. Fernandez-Yruegas, L. Alvarez et al.: Bilateral stress fracture of the clavicle. Skelet. Radiol. 24 (1995) 613

Cone, R. O., D. Resnick, Th. G. Goergen et al.: Condensing osteitis of the clavicle. Amer. J. Roentgenol. 141 (1983) 387

Cope, R., H. O. Riddervold: Posterior dislocation of the sternoclavicular joint: report of two cases, with emphasis on radiologic management and early diagnosis. Skelet. Radiol. 17 (1988) 247

Dihlmann, W.: Akquiriertes Hyperostose-Syndrom (sogenannte pustulöse Arthroosteitis). Literaturübersicht einschließlich 73 eigener Beobachtungen. Wien. klin. Wschr. 105 (1993) 127

Enzler, A.: Die Claviculafraktur als Geburtsverletzung des Neugeborenen. Schweiz. med. Wschr. 80 (1950) 1280

Fini-Storchi, O., D. Lo Rùsso, V. Agostini: „Pseudotumors" of the clavicle subsequent to radical neck dissection. J. Laryngol. Otol. 99 (1985) 73

Fischer, E.: Persistierende Klavikulaapophyse. Fortschr. Röntgenstr. 86 (1957) 532

Fischer, E.: Tubercula für Muskel- und Bandansätze am Schlüsselbein. Fortschr. Röntgenstr. 88 (1958) 71

Franquet, T., F. Lecumberry, A. Rivas et al.: Condensing osteitis of the clavicle. Report of two new cases. Skelet. Radiol. 14 (1985) 184

Fràter, L., Z. Czipott, L. Fodor: Hämangiom des Schlüsselbeines. Fortschr. Röntgenstr. 115 (1971) 686

Freyschmidt, J.: Skeletterkrankungen – klinisch-radiologische Diagnostik und Differentialdiagnose. Springer, Berlin 1997

Freyschmidt, J., G. Freyschmidt: Haut-, Schleimhaut- und Skelett-erkrankungen – SKIBO-Diseases –, Springer, Heidelberg 1996

Freyschmidt, J., G. Freyschmidt: SKIBO-Diseases. Disorders affecting the skin and bones. Springer, Berlin 1998

Freyschmidt, J., A. Sternberg: The bullhead sign—scintigraphic pattern of sternocostoclavicular hyperostosis and pustulotic arthro-osteitis. Europ. Radiol. 8 (1998) 807

Golthamer, C. R.: Duplication of the clavicle ("Os subclaviculare"). Radiology 68 (1957) 576

Hatfield, M. K., B. H. Gross, G. H. Glazer, et al.: Computed tomography of the sternum and its articulations. Skeletal Radiol. 11 (1984) 197

Heinemeier, G., G. Delling, D. v. Torklus: Osteonekrose des sternalen Klavikulaendes – Morbus Friedrich. Orthop. Prax. 15 (1979) 278

Hermanutz, K. D., P. Ehlenz, B. Verburg: Morphometrie und Bestimmung kortikodiaphysärer Indices der Klavikula im konventionellen Thoraxröntgenbild bei Gesunden und Knochenerkrankungen. Fortschr. Röntgenstr. 137 (1982) 281

Höcht, B., B. Gay, R. Arbogast: Die Behandlung der kongenitalen Claviculapseudarthrose durch Plattenosteosynthese. Z. Kinderchir. 28 (1979) 158

Horváth, F.: Über die auf dem sternalen Drittel und kaudal befindlichen „Usuration" der Klavikula. Fortschr. Röntgenstr. (1972) 836

Hunter, D., J. F. Moran, F. R. Venezio: Osteomyelitis of the clavicle after Swan-Ganz-Catherization. Arch. intern. Med. 143 (1983) 154

Igual, M., A. Giedion: The lateral clavicle hook. Ann. Radiol. 22 (1979) 136

Jurik, A. G., H. Graudahl, A. de Carvalho: Monarticular involvement of the manubriosternal joint. Skelet. Radiol. 14 (1985 a) 99

Jurik, A. G., A. de Carvalho, H. Graudahl: Sclerotic changes of the sternal end of the clavicle. Clin. Radiol. 36 (1985 b) 23

Kaplan, Ph. A., D. Resnick: Stress-induced osteolysis of the clavicle. Case report. Radiology 158 (1986) 139

Kasperczyk, A., J. Freyschmidt: Pustulotic arthro-osteitis: Spectrum of bone lesions with palmoplantar pustulosis. Radiology 191 (1993) 207

Kaye J. J., P. E. Nance jr, N. E. Green: Fatigue fracture of the medial aspect of the clavicle: an academic rather than athletic injury. Radiology 144 (1982) 89

Köster, H. J.: Die Claviculafraktur des Neugeborenen. Röntgen-Bl. 10 (1957) 117

Kreitner, K.-F., F. J. Schweden, T. Riepert et al.: Bone age determination based on the study of the medial extremity of the clavicle. Europ. Radiol. 8 (1998) 1116

Lemire, L., M. Rosmann: Sternoclavicular epiphyseal separation with adjacent clavicular fracture. J. pediat. Orthoped. 4 (1984) 118

Lingg, G., G. Heinemeier: Morbus Friedrich – Aseptische Knochennekrose des sternalen Klavikulaendes. Beobachtung von 6 Fällen. Fortschr. Röntgenstr. 134 (1981) 74

March, H. C.: Congenital pseudarthrosis of the clavicle. J. Canad. Ass. Radiol. 19 (1968) 167

Nettles, J. L., R. L. Linscheid: Sternoclavicular dislocations. J. Trauma. 8 (1968) 158

Pahl, R.: Doppelter Nervenkanal der Klavikula als diagnostische Fehlerquelle. Fortschr. Röntgenstr. 82 (1955) 487

Pritchett, J. W.: Ossification of the coracoclavicular ligaments in ankylosing spondylitis. J. Bone Jt Surg. 65-A (1983) 1017

Ravelli, A.: Über die eigenartige Form des sternalen Schlüsselbeines („Fischmaulform"). Fortschr. Röntgenstr. 82 (1955) 827

Redlund-Johnell, I: The costoclavicular joint. Skelet. Radiol. 15 (1986) 25

Reeder, M. M.: Reeder and Felson's Gamuts in Bone, Joint and Spine Radiology. Springer, Berlin 1993

Rockwood, C. A., D. P. Green: Fractures in Adults, Vol.1, 2nd ed. Lippincott, Philadelphia 1984 (p. 920)

Schilling, F., H. G. Fassbender: Sterno-kosto-klavikuläre Hyperostose – pustulotische Arthro-Osteitis – Pustulosis palmaris et plantaris: eine enthesiopatische Extremform der psoriatischen Spondarthritis? Z. Rheumatol. 44 (1985) 483

Schilling, F., S. Kessler: Die Spondarthritis hyperostotica pustulo-psoriatica. Nosologische Studie mit klinischer und radiologischer Darstellung innerhalb des SAPHO-Syndroms. Fortschr. Roentgenstr. 169 (1998) 576

Solovay, J., C. Gardner: Involvement of the manubriosternal joint in Marie-Strümpel disease. Amer. J. Roentgenol. 65 (1951) 749

Sonozaki, H., H. Mitsui, Y. Miyanaga et al.: Clinical features of 53 cases with pustulotic arthroosteitis. Ann. rheum. Dis. 40 (1981) 547

Twigg, H. L.: Duplication of the clavicle. Skelet. Radiol. 6 (1981) 281

Vándor, F.: Aseptische Nekrose der Clavicula nach Dissektionsoperationen des Halses. Fortschr. Röntgenstr. 94 (1961) 656

Yarkoni, Sh., W. Schmidt, Ph. Jeanty et al.: Clavicular measurement: a new biometric parameter for fetal evaluation. J. Ultrasound Med. 4 (1985) 467

Sternum

Normal Findings

During Growth

To understand the anatomy and radiographic appearance of the sternum and its numerous variants, it is necessary to review its embryological development:

The ventral ends of the first through seventh ribs, which are still composed of mesenchyma, bend slightly to form bilateral sternal plates (Ruge 1980, Odita et al. 1985). The manubrium develops from the upper portions of both sternal plates and also from an interclavicular blastema, which forms a funnel-shaped interface between the two plates. The interclavicular blastema gives rise to the cranial and central portions of the manubrium, both sternoclavicular joints and their disks, the cartilage covering the medial part of the clavicular head, and the suprasternal structures (Fig. 3.96).

Segmentation of the sternum occurs during the cartilaginous stage. The first ossification centers appear during the fetal period, and some do not appear until after birth. Their appearance follows a chronological progression from above downward (left half of Fig. 3.97). By contrast, fusion of the ossification centers starts inferiorly and progresses upward (right half of Fig. 3.97).

The segments of the body of the sternum start to undergo bony fusion at the center, which usually appears as a cone-shaped area. In adults this cone-shaped central ossification can often be identified on radiographs as a particularly dense sclerotic zone.

Ossification of the xiphoid is independent of age and the ossification of the other sternal segments, and it shows certain parallels with the ossification of the rib cartilage.

Dual ossification centers are reportedly more common in boys than in girls and usually ossify first on the right side. Paired ossification centers apparently occur only below unpaired centers, never above them (Fig. 3.98).

In newborns, multiple ossification centers are found in the manubrium in 21% of cases, in the first and second body segments in 50%, and in the third body segment in 74%. It is very unusual to find multiple centers in the xiphoid process. The paired centers mentioned above are usually located at the same level.

The shape and number of the ossification centers and their times of fusion are highly variable, as indicated by the numerical data in Fig. 3.97.

It is apparent, then, that the sternum of the growing child is extremely pleomorphic in its radiographic appearance, containing bony elements of highly variable size and configuration except for the manubrium, which has only one ossification center in most cases (approximately 80%). A "missing" sternal ossification center may be a potential

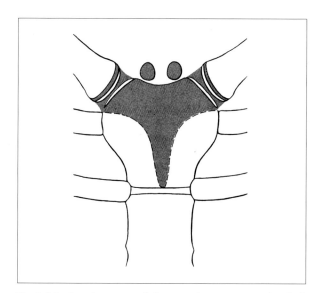

Fig. 3.96 Development of the manubrium sterni. The dark area represents the interclavicular blastema.

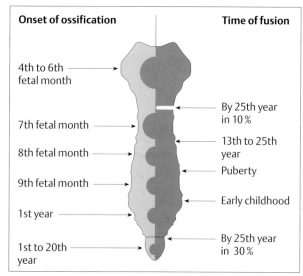

Fig. 3.97 Diagram showing the ossification and fusion of the individual sternal segments (after Fischer).

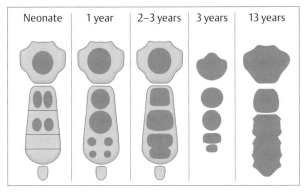

Fig. 3.**98** Schematic diagram of the normal ossification of the sternum (after Herdner).

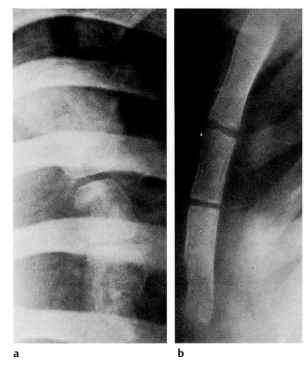

a　　　　　　　　　　　　b

Fig. 3.**99 a, b** Typical appearance of the sternum in a child.

mimicker of disease in young children (Rush et al. 2002). Such a missing sternal ossification center most commonly occurs at the segments 2 (1,5%) and 4 (1,5%) (Rush et al. 2002). The typical radiographic appearance of the pediatric sternum is shown in Fig. 3.**99**.

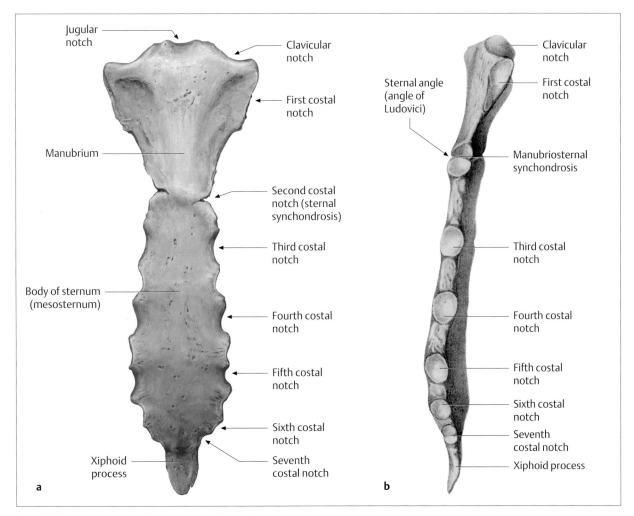

Fig. 3.**100 a, b**　Anatomy of the sternum. (From Wolf-Heidegger 1961.)

a Anterior aspect.
b Lateral aspect.

In Adulthood

The manubrium is the broadest and thickest part of the sternum (Fig. 3.**100**). Its superior border has a central depression, the jugular notch, and two lateral depressions, the clavicular notches. The superior contour of the manubrium, defined by the jugular and clavicular notches, is extremely variable in shape. Each lateral border of the manubrium bears a costal notch for the first rib. Until middle age, a fibrocartilage-filled space called the sternal symphysis or sternal synchondrosis separates the manubrium from the body of the sternum. The manubrium and body form an angle at the synchondrosis, called the sternal angle. It is at this level that the manubrium and the body of the sternum each bears a facet that helps form the notch for the second rib. The **sternal angle (angle of Ludovici)** is clinically important in that it forms a ridge that is easily palpated and can be used to locate the anterior second rib. The first rib is too deep to be palpated through the skin. The opposing borders of the manubrium and sternal body show a relatively diverse morphology in the coronal plane (conventional tomograms or images reformatted from axial CT; top row in Fig. 3.**101**). Lateral views of this junction (bottom row in Fig. 3.**101**) also show normal morphological variants including increased density of subchondral bone structures and bone spurs.

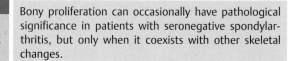

Bony proliferation can occasionally have pathological significance in patients with seronegative spondylarthritis, but only when it coexists with other skeletal changes.

The body of the sternum is narrower and thinner than the manubrium. Each of its lateral borders bears 5.5 notches for the second through seventh ribs. It is broadest in its lower half. The craniocaudal length of the body determines the sites of attachment of the sixth and seventh ribs. In a long sternum, both ribs attach to the lateral borders. If the sternum is short, they attach to its lower end. Lateral rib attachments with a solitary ("free") xiphoid process have been found in 65% of cases (male:female ratio of 3 : 1) and low rib attachments in 35% (male:female ratio of 4 : 7) (Versé 1910). **Replacement of the costal notches by bony prominences** (costal processes) is normal and is not even considered a variant. The **xiphoid process** varies greatly in its shape. The distal pole may have clefts, or may be bifid, there may be central perforations and the distal part may be broad and teardrop-shaped (Fig. 3.**102**).

The xiphosternal synchondrosis is as variable as the process itself. In 50% of cases it is completely fused to the lower end of the sternal body. Also the position of the xiphoid in relation to the sternum has a broad spectrum of variation (Fig. 3.**113**).

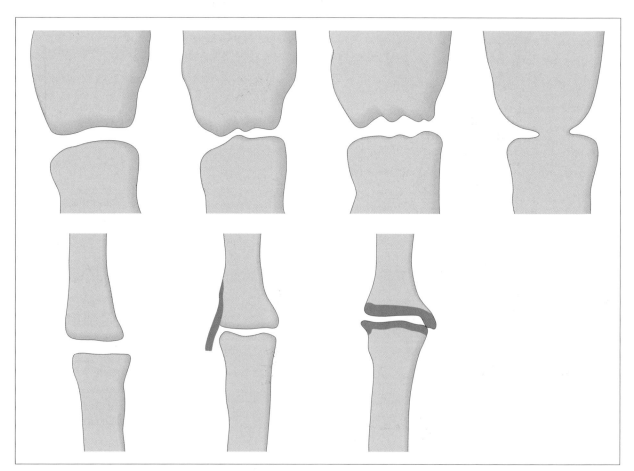

Fig. 3.**101**   Normal morphological variations of the opposing surfaces of the sternal manubrium and body that form the manubriosternal synchondrosis: anteroposterior or coronal view (top), lateral or sagittal view (bottom).

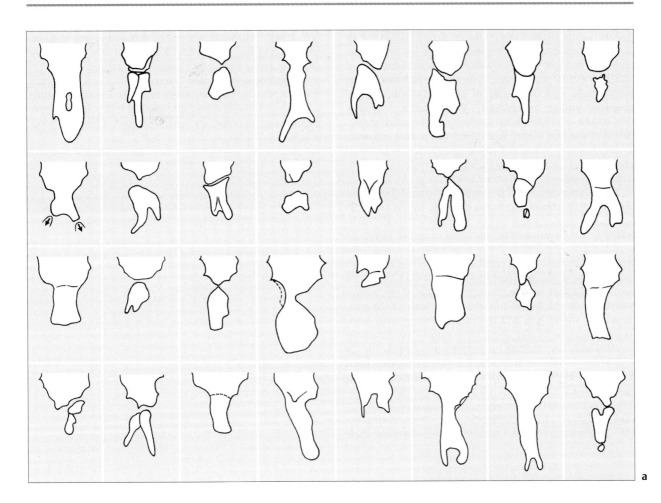

a

Examination Techniques

Conventional radiographic examination of the sternum poses considerable difficulties due to multiple overlaps with the spinal column, ribs, and lungs. The lateral sternal radiograph can provide information on the gross anatomy of the bone (size, position, shape). But since most patients, especially the elderly, have mild deformities of the chest wall and because the rib cartilage increasingly calcifies with aging, often the lateral radiograph will not provide a nonsuperimposed view. Foci of circumscribed bone destruction and other abnormalities can easily escape conventional detection. The current method of choice for optimally defining the bony structures of the sternum is **CT**. The radiologist must be familiar with CT imaging of the sternum, however, to avoid mistaking normal anatomy for pathology. The **normal dimensions** of the sternum are listed in Table 3.**2**. The size of the sternum increases linearly until age 25 and undergoes no further changes thereafter. The cortical thickness of the sternum correlates with the height and body weight of the patient (Hatfield et al. 1984). The cortical thickness increases until age 24 and thereafter remains constant. In approximately 70% of cases, the medullary cavity of the manubrium cannot be adequately visualized with a soft-tissue window setting in children under 5 years of age, but this situation improves as the child grows older. By 20 years of age the medullary cavity can be successfully evaluated with CT in approximately 90% of all patients. The manubrium and body of the sternum are clearly distinguishable on CT scans by their

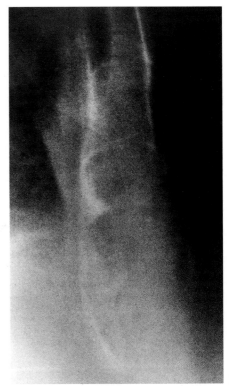

b

Fig. 3.**102 a, b** Morphological variations of the xiphoid process.
a The process at upper left has a central perforation.
b Lateral radiograph of the xiphoid process, which appears to have a solid bony attachment to the lowest sternal segment.

size and shape. In the study by Hatfield et al. (1984), the xi-phoid process could be identified in just 9% of patients under 15 years of age, as opposed to more than 80% of patients over 30 years of age. Typically the **junction of the manubrium and body and of the body and xiphoid process shows increased radiographic density** (Fig. 3.**103a–e**). This is because the normal manubriosternal synchondrosis may contain subchondral sclerotic areas, especially in adults, and because the fusion of the xiphoid process to the body creates relatively dense, unstructured areas of ossification.

The relative density of the structures about the manubriosternal synchondrosis is also based on the fact that the medullary cavity in this region is relatively small. Additionally, the sternum itself contains zones of increased density that represent vestigial sites of bony fusion. The sternum presents a sharp contour in more than 80% of all patients examined. **Cortical unsharpness** on CT scans is occasionally seen on the posterior surface of the manubrium and on the lateral surfaces of the body of the sternum (Figs. 3.**103f, g, h**, 3.**125b**). Lateral unsharpness is apparently caused by the slight indentations of the costal notches and their oblique projection on CT scans. The CT studies by Hatfield et al. (1984) indicate that **costochondral calcifications are much more pronounced in men than women** and, as we know from conventional radiography, tend to increase with aging. The **parasternal soft tissues**, consisting mainly of the costal cartilages, often present a relatively broad, spindle-shaped configuration

(Fig. 3.**103**), which should not be mistaken for a mass lesion. Generally these broadenings of the soft-tissue shadows show a bilateral symmetrical arrangement.

On **radionuclide scans**, the manubriosternal synchondrosis normally shows a slight increase in tracer uptake, apparently because the slight mobility at this junction promotes an increase in cartilage and bone turnover (Fig. 3.**103**).

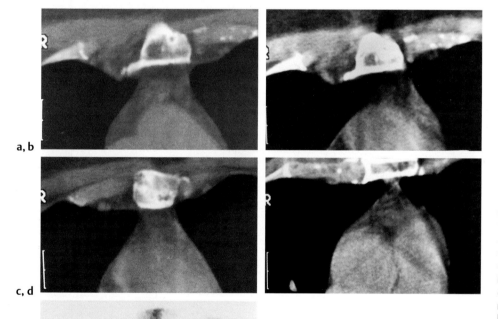

a, b

c, d

e

Fig. 3.**103a–h** Typical CT images of the manubrium and body of the sternum.
a–e Bony sclerosis at the transitions from manubrium to body. Scan **c** passes through the synchondrosis, and scan **d** cuts the top of the sternal body. The patient is a 46-year-old woman with non-Hodgkin lymphoma. The radionuclide scan in **e** raised suspicion of bone involvement. The region of the manubriosternal synchondrosis shows increased uptake on the oblique projection, but this is still considered a normal-for-age finding based on physiological regressive changes in the synchondrosis. Note the proliferative changes on the anterior surface of the manubrium in image **a**. Follow-up proved that the finding was actually a normal variant.

Fig. 3.**103 f, g**
The series of CT scans in Fig.
f1–f11 demonstrate physiologic areas of unsharpness
behind the manubrium sterni
and about the costal incisures
in a 62-year-old woman with
an asymptomatic sternum.
Note the unsharpness in f1
and the slight unsharpness
and spiculation in f2, which
are completely normal findings. Scan f5 cuts a portion of
the synchondrosis. Note the
unsharp areas along the body
of the sternum at the incisures
(f8, f9). Scan f11 shows an
area that is located between
the incisures and displays
smooth contours on both
sides. Note also that the soft-
tissue structures bordering the
manubrium and body of the
sternum appear normal. The
corresponding radionuclide
scan in panel g is normal. The
areas of slightly increased uptake in the right manubrioclavicular joint and in the manubriosternal synchondrosis are
normal for age. The small focus of increased uptake on the
left anterior rib is from a previous known injury.
Note: CT scans f1–f11 are not
contiguous but a cranial-to-
caudal series of selcted scans.

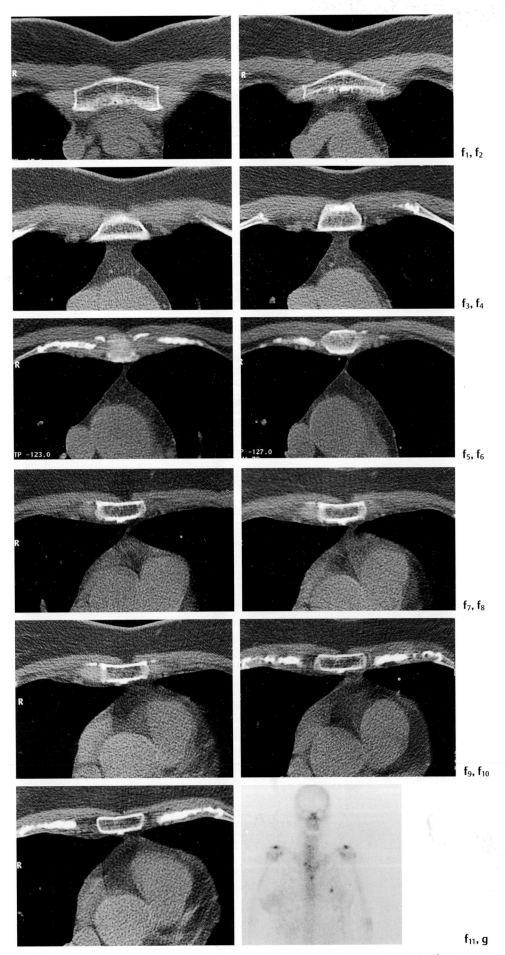

f₁, f₂

f₃, f₄

f₅, f₆

f₇, f₈

f₉, f₁₀

f₁₁, g

Fig. 3.**103 h** ▷

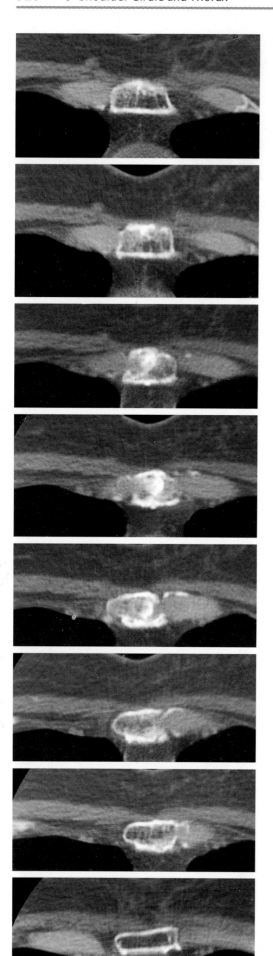

h

Pathological Finding?

Normal Variant or Anomaly?

The morphology of the sternum is so variable that it can be quite difficult in some cases to distinguish normal findings and variants from deformity and disease. An example is shown in Fig. 3.**104**, which demonstrates sternal fissures, notches, and asymmetries in a healthy 14-year-old boy.

Although some works (including the previous edition of this book) advocated that the sternum be used as a test object for detecting skeletal anomalies, we have concluded that this notion is extremely questionable and is contradicted by the radiograph in Fig. 3.**104**.

The **asymmetrical development of the sternal ossification centers**, resulting in irregular and asymmetrical contours of the individual bony elements (Fig. 3.**105**), in itself can make it impossible to distinguish a normal variant or an extreme normal variant from a definite abnormality.

Earlier studies on this subject are of little value today due to the former lack of methods for the accurate depiction of radiographic anatomy. Since the introduction of sectional imaging techniques, very few authors have published any serious work dealing with this problem.

Asymmetrical development of the sternal ossification centers can have various consequences:

- Lateral bowing of the entire sternum or its body
- Unilateral broadening of the manubrium and body of the sternum
- Ribs attaching at unequal levels
- Deviations in the course of the manubriosternal synchondrosis

Delayed median fusion of the ossification centers is difficult to evaluate in terms of distinguishing variants from anomalies and probably can be interpreted only within the context of possible coexisting skeletal changes. Herdner (1947) identified four grades of delayed median fusion according to the degree of ossification that is achieved from below upward (Fig. 3.**106**). Grade 4 appears to be intermediate between delayed fusion and a sternal fissure. Examples of ossification disturbances are illustrated in Figs. 3.**107**–3.**110**.

◁ Fig. 3.**103h**   Supplemental series of 1.5-mm-thick contiguous CT scans through the manubriosternal synchondrosis. The two upper images still show the lower part of the manubrium. The next three images cut the synchondrosis and show central, irregular sclerotic foci (compare with Fig. 3.**125**). The contour defects in the third through sixth images from the top (right side in images 3 and 4, left side in images 4 through 6) coincide precisely with the costal notches, which are cut obliquely by the scans. The bottom two images again show a "solid" sternum with a fully intact cortical boundary. Normal CT findings about the manubriosternal synchondrosis and the synchondroses within the body of the sternum are commonly misinterpreted as tumors (e.g., osteolytic-osteosclerotic metastases), especially when the slice thickness is too thin (1.5–2 mm). Doubts can often be resolved by obtaining reformatted coronal and sagittal images.

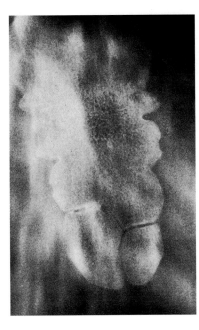

Fig. 3.**104** Coronal tomogram of the sternum of a healthy 14-year-old boy shows numerous fissures, notches, and asymmetries.

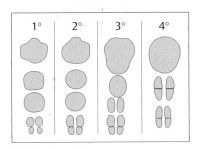

Fig. 3.**106** Schematic diagram of the median fusion of the ossification centers (after Herdner).

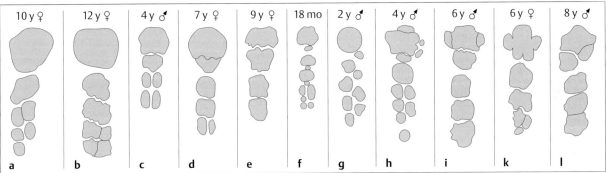

Fig. 3.**105 a–l** Abnormal development of the sternal ossification centers (examples drawn from Zimmer, Herdner, Pfeiffer, Schmid, and Weber). Asymmetrical ossification (**a, g**). Irregular contours of the ossification center (**b, e, i, k**). Stepoffs in the interspaces between ossification centers (**a, g**). Multiple manubrial centers (**c–l**) (after Fischer).

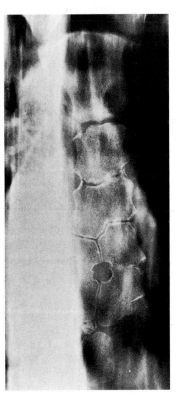

Fig. 3.**107** Sternal foramen with persistent segmentation in a ▷ 22-year-old man.

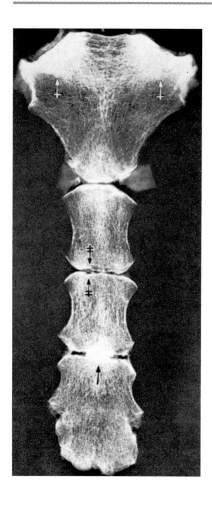

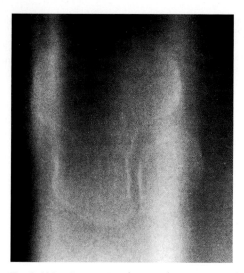

Fig. 3.**109** Conventional coronal tomogram of an abnormal sternal body in an otherwise healthy 12-year-old child. All the ossification centers are fused except for a large distal center on the left side.

◁ Fig. 3.**108** Multipartite sternum in an adult. Subchondral sclerosis is evident along the clavicular notches (arrow). Note also the partial fusion of the inferior body synchondrosis in the median plane (single arrow) and the undulation of the upper and lower rims of the body segments (double arrow). (From Fischer 1968.)

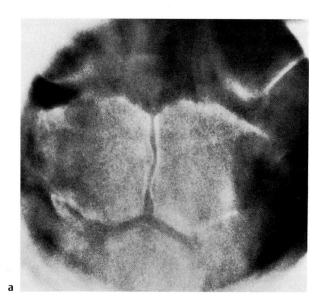

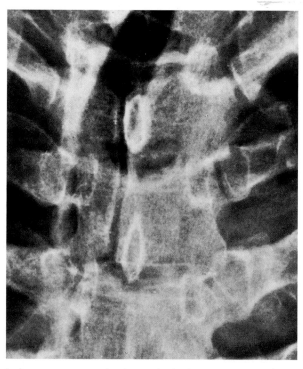

Fig. 3.**110 a, b** Incomplete sternal fissure.
a Tomogram of an incomplete sternal fissure resulting from nonfusion of the manubrium over a fused sternal body.

b On a superimposed radiograph, the fissure is projected over two vertebral bodies to the right of the spinous processes, simulating a vertebral cleft anomaly.

The manubriosternal synchondrosis is preserved in 90% of all persons over 30 years of age. Bony fusion of the synchondrosis occurs in only about 10% and therefore should be classified as a normal variant.

Failure of fusion of the sternal plates results in a **complete sternal fissure**. Gomez et al. (1985) and Sammarai et al. (1985) found an association between sternal fissures and other anomalies involving the diaphragm, abdomen, heart, etc. Many authors also regard an incomplete sternal fissure (Fig. 3.**110**) as a true anomaly. It typically affects the upper part of the sternum and is usually associated with other syndromic abnormalities (partial ectopia cordis, cutaneous fissure with lax jowls, etc.). When a sternal fissure is present, it is extremely common to find persistent segmental clefts, displaced segments, and deformed segments along the unfused sternal plates (Polvar 1951, Ashley 1956).

A special type of fusion anomaly is the **sternal foramen**, which is found in 2–8% of all thoracic CT examinations that include the body of the sternum (Hatfield et al. 1984, Stark 1985, Schratter et al. 1997). In itself, the sternal foramen is a small, harmless, insignificant developmental anomaly. But it can assume major practical importance in sternal aspirations and punctures, including the "KG 17" acupuncture point (Schratter et al. 1997). A needle accidentally passed through the foramen could cause a life-threatening cardiac tamponade or other serious complication.

Schratter et al. (1997) have identified four types of sternal foramen (Fig. 3.**111**).

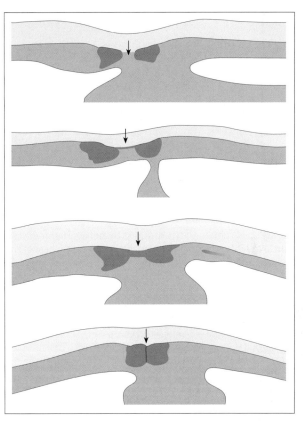

Fig. 3.**111 a–e**   Sternal foramen.
a Diagram illustrating the various types of sternal foramen (after Schratter et al.).

Fig. 3.**111 b–e**   Incidental finding of an incomplete type II sternal foramen, which is bridged by a paper-thin bony plate. The scans also demonstrate a mass lesion in the left anterior mediastinum.

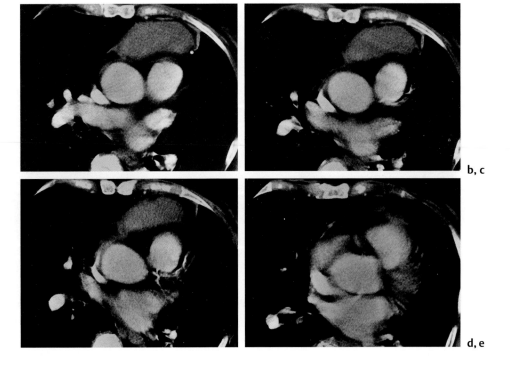

b, c

d, e

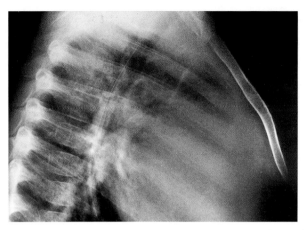

Fig. 3.**112** Premature synostosis of a nonsegmented sternum in a child with complex anomalies involving the rest of the skeleton and the internal organs.

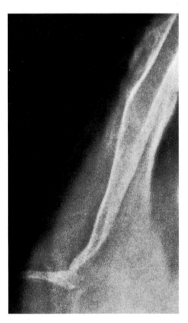

Fig. 3.**113** Failure of segmentation in the lower sternum. The xiphoid process is pronglike and angled forward. This is a normal variant that was detected incidentally.

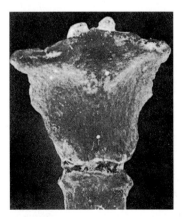

Fig. 3.**114** Manubrium specimen with two suprasternal (episternal) ossicles.

> **Types of sternal foramen defined by Schratter et al.:**
> ➤ *Type I* Complete bony discontinuity on axial CT
> ➤ *Type II* Extremely thin layer of bone bridging the discontinuity in the sternum
> ➤ *Type III* Thicker bone plate composed of three layers (cortex–cancellous bone–cortex)
> ➤ *Type IV* No sternal discontinuity, only a depression in the anterior and/or posterior cortex

Schratter et al. conclude from their observations that whenever an acupuncture or other procedure is planned that requires passing a needle into the body of the sternum, an oblique radiograph of the sternum should be routinely obtained and supplemented if necessary by CT.

In a series of 205 examinations of the sternum, Versé (1910) found only one foramen-like perforation of the manubrium. This author, who based his findings on actual anatomic examinations, found an opening in the body of the sternum in 3% of cases and in the xiphoid process in 5% of cases (Fig. 3.**107**).

Premature synostosis (Fig. 3.**112**) and **failure of segmentation** (Fig. 3.**113**; sternal segmentation does not arise from the metameric centers but precedes ossification in the chondral stage, see above) lead to small, stocky sternum that is angled forward ("pigeon breast").

Suprasternal ossicles (known also as episternal ossicles) represent a true variant. They are usually located slightly **behind** the upper border of the manubrium and result from the fact that the manubrium is derived from two different blastemas during embryological development. They are a harmless incidental finding in approximately 1–7% of all patients (Figs. 3.**114**, 3.**116**, 3.**117**). **Parasternal ossicles** are accessory bone elements, usually triangular in shape, located next to the manubrium in the cartilage of the first ribs (Figs. 3.**115**, 3.**116**).

Isolated or accessory bone elements have also been described in the manubriosternal synchondrosis (Mauch 1956), at the posterosuperior border of the manubrium (Fischer 1968), and at the attachment of the second rib at the level of the superior synchondrosis.

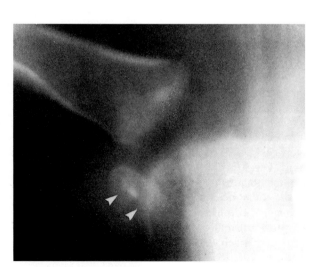

Fig. 3.**115** Tomogram of a parasternal ossicle.

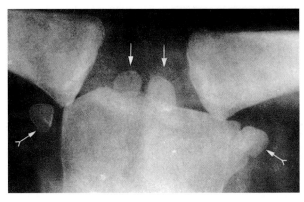

Fig. 3.**116**   Episternal ossicles (arrows) and parasternal ossicles (double arrows).

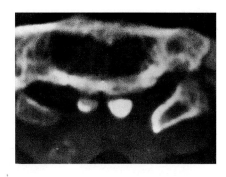

Fig. 3.**117**   CT scan of two suprasternal ossicles located at the posterosuperior border of the manubrium and extending slightly behind the manubrium. (From Elster and Stark 1985.)

The **position of the sternum** relative to the rest of the bony thorax is subject to variations that must be known in order to avoid clinical and radiological diagnostic errors. For example, the angle between the manubrium and body of the sternum increases in many patients with progressive age-related emphysema and progressive kyphosis of the thoracic spine. The sternum may be noticeably "tilted" in children and adolescents, usually due to asymmetries in the curvatures of the costal cartilages (Figs. 3.**118**, 3.**119**).

Often these findings are misinterpreted from their clinical features as **tumors of the anterior chest wall**, especially in young patients who complain of a dull aching pain in the parasternal region. Donnelly et al. (1997) investigated this problem in a series of 51 children examined from 1989 to 1996. They reviewed 27 cross-sectional imaging examinations (13 MRI, 14 CT) to evaluate asymptomatic, palpable, focal anterior chest wall lesions in otherwise healthy children. The palpable lesions were found to be caused by prominent anterior convex ribs in 10 children, a tilted sternum in 6 children, a prominent asymmetric costal cartilage in 4 children, and a bifid rib in 1 child. Based on their findings, the authors conclude that the **low yield of sectional imaging studies in patients with asymptomatic anterior chest wall lesions should be considered in deciding whether to proceed with imaging.** A supplementary cross-sectional imaging technique is warranted only if pain is present or if there is a painful palpable mass, as this may be related to a neoplastic process (e.g., Ewing sarcoma, neuroectodermal tumors, metastatic neuroblastoma, etc.) or an inflammatory disease (osteomyelitis, tuberculosis, Langerhans-cell histiocytosis, etc.).

Funnel chest refers to a funnel-shaped depression in the anterior chest wall. The deepest point of the depression is at the level of the xiphosternal synchondrosis and is usually located off the midline (86% of cases, Hümmer and Rupprecht 1985). The depression occasionally may take the form of a broad hollow rather than a tapered funnel. It is often associated with a complete or partial defect of the pectoralis muscle. Apparent paramedian lung shadows on the chest film are caused by the increased x-ray absorption of the oblique passed anterior medial chest wall (Fig. 3.**120**).

In extreme cases the anterior chest wall may come within a few centimeters of the spinal column.

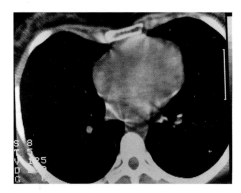

Fig. 3.**118**   "Tilted" sternum. The increased prominence of the upper left parasternal structures can mimic a neoplasm. Slight tenderness of the left thoracic prominence was noted clinically in this 15-year-old girl. Findings are consistent with a harmless anatomic variant. The slight tenderness may result from greater mechanical stresses on the muscle and ligament attachments on the left side. Absence of rest pain is a typical finding.

The heart is usually displaced to the left, rotated clockwise, and is shaped like a pancake. Congenital funnel chest occurs predominantly in males. As an endogenous developmental anomaly, it often occurs in combination with other anomalies such as Marfan syndrome. The syndromic associations of sternal anomalies are listed in Table 3.**5**.

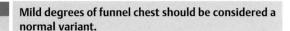
Mild degrees of funnel chest should be considered a normal variant.

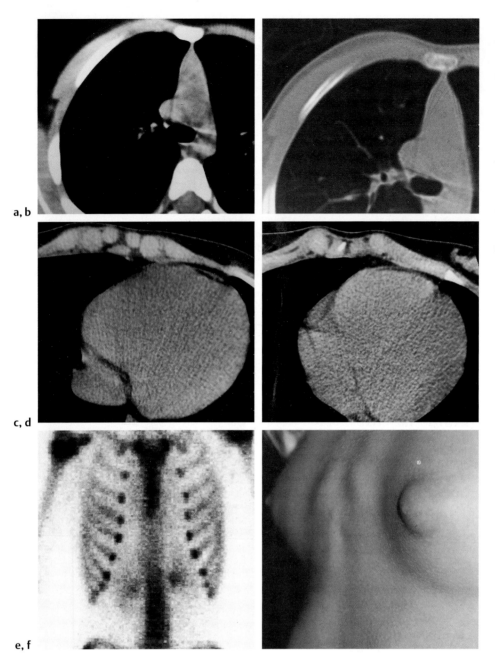

a, b

c, d

e, f

Fig. 3.**119 a–f** Ridgelike prominence of an anterior inferior infrasternal costal cartilage in a 13-year-old girl. The patient had no clinical complaints, but her mother was troubled by the "lump." Radionuclide scan is negative, showing typical increased uptake at the chondro-osseous junctions and throughout the sternum. Note the asymmetrical, somewhat prominent costal cartilage on images **c** and **d**. Note also the presence of normal fatty tissue around the costal cartilage, which rules out a neoplasm.

Table 3.**5** Syndromes associated with sternal anomalies (after Reeder and Felson)

Hypersegmentation
- Trisomy 21 (Down syndrome)

Hyposegmentation (often with hypoplasia and premature fusion)
- Camptomelic dysplasia
- Cornelia de Lange syndrome
- Noonan syndrome
- Trisomy 18 syndrome

Pigeon breast (pectus carinatum)
- Congenital heart defects, especially cyanotic
- Isolated finding
- Morquio syndrome
- Noonan syndrome
- Spondyloepiphyseal dysplasia
- Hyposegmentation, hypoplastic (see above)

Funnel chest (pectus excavatum)
- Congenital bowing of the tibia
- Congenital heart defects
- Ehlers–Danlos syndrome
- Homocystinuria
- Isolated finding; idiopathic
- Marfan syndrome
- Mitral valve replacement syndrome
- Newborns with respiratory distress syndrome
- Osteogenesis imperfecta

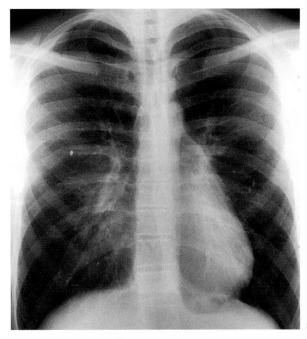

a

Fig. 3.**120 a–c** Typical funnel chest.
a The heart is displaced toward the left side and exhibits a "pancake" shape. It also shows a small degree of clockwise rotation, causing prominence of the pulmonary arterial segment. An inexperienced radiologist might interpret these findings as mitralization.

Fig. 3.**120 b** Lateral chest film clearly demonstrates the posterior displacement of the middle and lower sternum.
c This film was obtained using the Hladik technique. A chain made of lead is placed into the funnel along the anterior chest wall, and the film is doubly exposed at end-inspiration and end-expiration. Thus the nature and amplitude of sternal movements can be directly evaluated on one image. A vertebral and frontosagittal index is used to classify the funnel chest as mild, moderate, or severe and assess the operability of the condition (see Oelsnitz 1983 for a detailed description of the method, surgical indications, and results). Today, of course, funnel chest can also be accurately defined by CT.

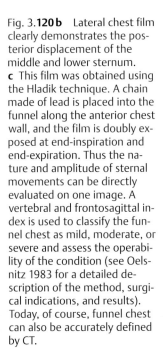

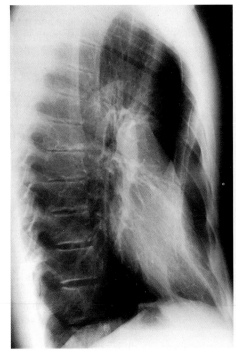

b

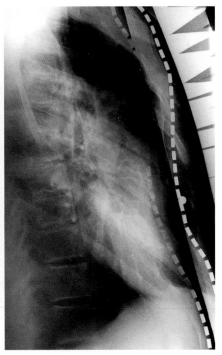

c

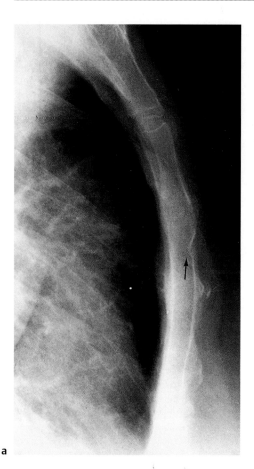

a

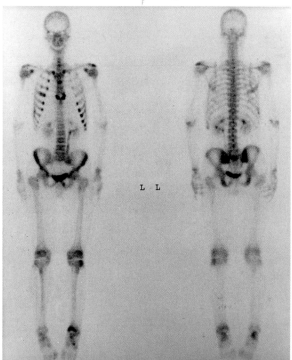

b

Fig. 3.**121 a, b**   Sternal fracture.
a Fresh fracture in the second segment of the body of the sternum in a 62-year-old woman (motor vehicle injury) (arrow).
b Typical radionuclide images of a patient who sustained a severe seatbelt injury to the central anterior right ribs, the lower body of the sternum, and the left hip region.

 ## Fracture, Subluxation, or Dislocation?

Accident statistics indicate that sternal fractures occur in 0.2–0.5% of injuries. Most are caused by direct trauma, as opposed to indirect fractures (e.g., hyperflexion-type vertebral fractures, excessive muscular traction on the sternum during heavy lifting, gymnastic exercises, etc.). The most common injury is a **transverse or oblique fracture near the manubriosternal synchondrosis**. Fractures in the body of the sternum can be particularly difficult to diagnose. They are defined best by a simple lateral chest film or a spot film taken under fluoroscopic guidance (Fig. 3.**121**).

Transverse fractures are very difficult to detect with CT, because generally the axial scan plane runs parallel to the fracture line. Detection is aided by reformatting contiguous scans into multidimensional images. Radionuclide bone scans are excellent for detecting transverse fractures in either a clinical or forensic setting (Fig. 3.**121 b**). Scans generally become positive after about 3–5 days.

The complete, traumatic separation of the sternum from the costal cartilages can be very difficult to diagnose if the displacement does not exceed a few millimeters. Ruptures of the cartilage plates are another rare injury that can also be difficult to detect. Radionuclide scanning is the most sensitive method for detecting ruptures as well as simple contusions of the costal cartilages.

The sternum is a site of predilection for **pathological fractures** in patients with osteoporosis (Fig. 3.**122**). When nondisplaced, this type of fracture can be extremely difficult to diagnose and may even escape detection by CT.

Transverse or oblique areas of increased uptake on bone scans confirm the suspicion of a fracture when corresponding clinical symptoms are present.

Sternal fractures mainly require differentiation from the variants and anomalous clefts of the sternum described above. But given the extreme morphological diversity of the sternum and especially of the xiphoid process, sometimes it is impossible to differentiate a variant from an anomaly or a fracture. It should be reemphasized that radionuclide imaging is the most reliable technique for establishing a diagnosis.

 ## Necrosis?

Presumably, necrosis is as rare in the sternum as in the spinal column because the bone has a relatively good blood supply that supports the early initiation of reparative processes. We know of no published studies on necrosis and its differential diagnosis in the sternum, probably due to the poor imaging conditions in that region and the consequent difficulty of proving necrosis. Necrosis should be differentiated from normal sclerosis about the manubriosternal synchondrosis, from irregular parasternal ossicles, and from sites where individual sternal segments have fused together.

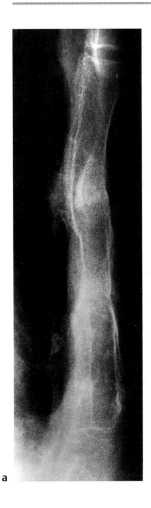

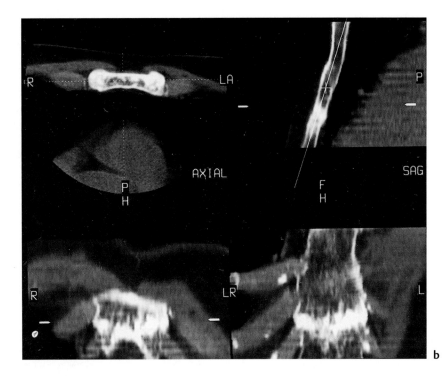

b

a

Fig. 3.**122 a, b** Insufficiency (stress) fracture in an elderly women with osteoporosis. A radionuclide scan showed very intense uptake in the lower body of the sternum.
a Lateral radiograph shows a nonspecific density in the lower body of the sternum.
b Axial CT scan (upper left) shows a nonspecific density. The various reformatted images show an unequivocal transverse zone of increased density across the lower body of the sternum.

 Inflammation?

An **inflammatory process in the manubriosternal region** should be suspected if the patient complains of pain in that area, if the lateral radiograph or CT shows frayed or irregular contours and subchondral sclerosis, and if the radionuclide scan is "hot." True bacterial inflammations, which usually are associated with gross destructive changes, are less common than sternal inflammatory reactions in a setting of **seronegative spondylarthritis**, including **pustulotic arthro-osteitis** (Figs. 3.**91**, 3.**123**).

Table 3.**6** lists the conditions that are most commonly associated with erosion, sclerosis, and/or fusion of the manubriosternal synchondrosis or sternoclavicular joints.

Inflammatory changes in the parasternal costal cartilage are a diagnostic challenge because neither conventional radiographs nor CT can reliably detect changes in the florid stage. We know of no published reports on successful diagnosis with MRI. A radiological diagnosis can be made only in late stages where metaplastic bone formation has occurred (Fig. 3.**124 a, b**), and even then the finding can be difficult to distinguish from chondrosarcoma.

Tietze syndrome is manifested clinically by a tender or spontaneously painful bulging of the parasternal costal cartilage, usually of the second through fourth ribs. We doubt that this syndrome is a separate entity, especially since no reliable, objective diagnostic procedures were

Table 3.**6** Conditions that are associated with erosion, sclerosis, and/or fusion of the manubriosternal synchondrosis or sternoclavicular joints

Common	Unusual
• Ankylosing spondylitis	• Congenital fusion anomaly
• Degenerative changes	• Enteropathic arthritis
• Posttraumatic and post-surgical changes	• Fluorosis
• Psoriatic arthritis (see PAO[1])	• Infectious causes (pyogenic osteomyelitis, tuberculosis)
• Rheumatoid arthritis	• Reiter syndrome
	• Chronic recurring polychondritis

[1] PAO Pustulotic arthro-osteitis (p. 315 ff. and Fig. 3.**123 e–h**)

available at the time it was discovered. It probably represents nothing more than a **nonspecific chondritis-perichondritis of the costal cartilage**, occurring either spontaneously or after trauma, or it may represent an early stage of sternocostoclavicular hyperostosis.

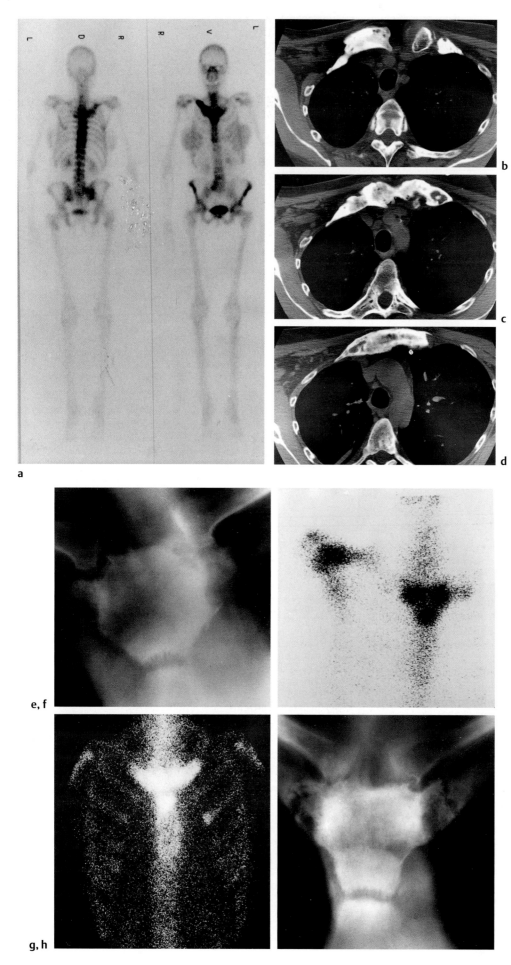

Fig. 3.123 a–h Sternocosto-clavicular hyperostosis and manubriosternal arthritis. Typical cases of sternocostoclavicular hyperostosis in patients with palmoplantar pustulosis (a type of pustular psoriasis).

a–d This 38-year-old woman presented with severe right-sided lumbosacral pain and swelling in the sternocosto-clavicular region. Radionuclide scans show very intense uptake in the sternocostoclavicular region that extends far into the right clavicle (bullhead sign, Freyschmidt and Sternberg 1998). In the CT scans, note the platelike or plaque-like ossifications involving the entire sternum, the clavicles, and the first ribs. Severe inflammatory and destructive changes in the area of the right sacroiliac joint (not shown here) correlate with the radionuclide abnormality (compare this case with Fig. 3.**91** in the chapter on the Sternoclavicular Joint).

e, f Young man with palmo-plantar pustulosis and severe pain in the manubrium and right scapula. The tomogram (**e**) shows extensive destruction of the manubrial portions of the sternoclavicular joints, massive sclerosis throughout the sternum, and ossifications at the attachments of the first ribs. The manubriosternal synchondrosis is widened and has serrated margins. Typical radionuclide scan (**f**) demonstrates a bullhead pattern with additional uptake in the right scapula, which radiologically shows very severe, nonspecific inflammatory changes (not demonstrated here).

g, h Sternocostoclavicular hyperostosis in a young woman with palmoplantar pustulosis. Note the bullhead pattern in the bone scan (**g**) and typical tomographic appearance (**h**). Note also the massive ossification spreading to the attachments of the first ribs. Destructive changes are evident in the manubrioclavicular joints, and there is inflammatory destruction of the manubriosternal synchondrosis.

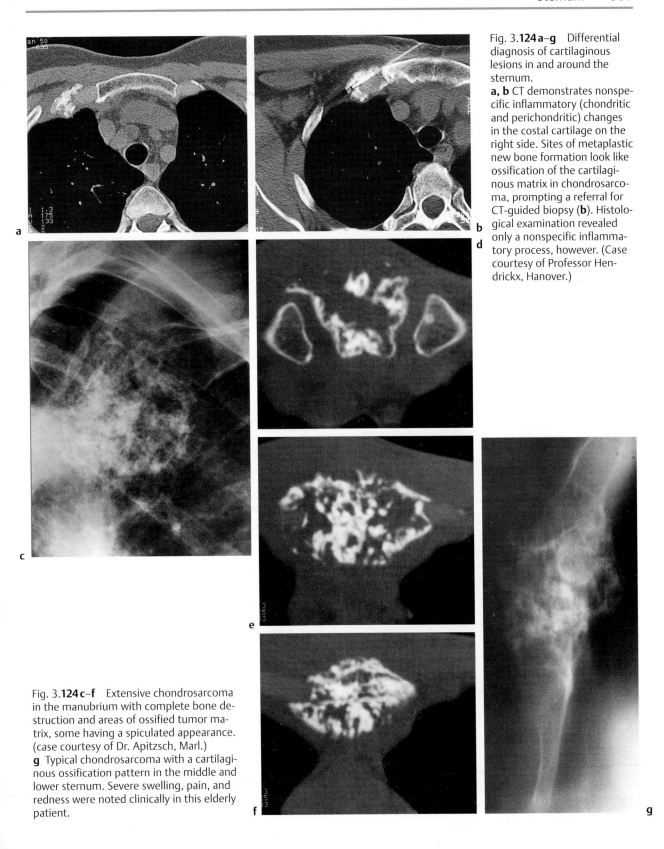

Fig. 3.**124a–g**   Differential diagnosis of cartilaginous lesions in and around the sternum.
a, b CT demonstrates nonspecific inflammatory (chondritic and perichondritic) changes in the costal cartilage on the right side. Sites of metaplastic new bone formation look like ossification of the cartilaginous matrix in chondrosarcoma, prompting a referral for CT-guided biopsy (**b**). Histological examination revealed only a nonspecific inflammatory process, however. (Case courtesy of Professor Hendrickx, Hanover.)

Fig. 3.**124c–f**   Extensive chondrosarcoma in the manubrium with complete bone destruction and areas of ossified tumor matrix, some having a spiculated appearance. (case courtesy of Dr. Apitzsch, Marl.)
g Typical chondrosarcoma with a cartilaginous ossification pattern in the middle and lower sternum. Severe swelling, pain, and redness were noted clinically in this elderly patient.

Tumor?

Reference was made earlier to the **differential diagnosis of physiological unsharpness**, especially in the posterior manubrium and about the costal notches (Figs. 3.**103**, 3.**124a, b**). These ill-defined areas on CT scans should not be interpreted as pathological in themselves unless they are associated with adjacent soft-tissue masses. Tumors can metastasize to the sternum from any organ. The primary bone tumor that most commonly affects the sternum is chondrosarcoma (Fig. 3.**124c–g**). Another common sternal tumor is plasmacytoma, which may consist of an initially solitary lesion or multiple myeloma. The sternum is affected because of its abundant bone marrow (once making it a preferred site for marrow aspiration).

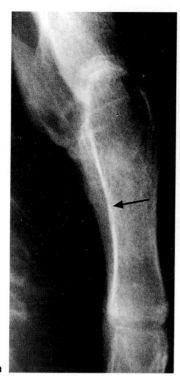

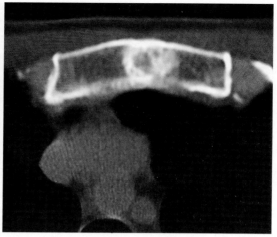

Fig. 3.**125 a, b**   Osteosclerotic metastasis in the body of the sternum (highest segment), originating from a uterine leiomyosarcoma. The lateral radiograph shows nonspecific sclerosis with very slight unsharpness of the posterior cortex (arrow). CT demonstrates a central osteosclerotic metastasis with posterior cortical destruction. This distinguishes the lesion from physiological sclerosis in the central part of the sternal body. Radionuclide imaging showed massive tracer uptake in the affected region.

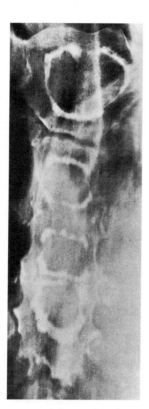

Fig. 3.**126**

Fig. 3.**127** ▷

Fig. 3.**126**   Osteophytes at the margins of the synchondrosis (specimen radiograph).

Fig. 3.**127**   Unusual appearance of the sternum due to osteopetrosis (marble bone disease). The punched-out defects with dense sclerotic borders are most likely simulated defects caused by less dense bone, since marble bone disease is known to be associated with a tree-ring-like ossification pattern. The familiar "sandwich vertebrae" in this disease often appear also as if actual bony defects were present between the sclerotic endplates.

Frequent reference has been made to sites of **physiologic sclerosis** located near the manubriosternal synchondrosis, at the junction of the xiphoid process and body of the sternum, and at the junctions of the fused sternal segments. These relatively dense areas may be mistaken for **osteosclerotic metastases** on CT scans (Fig. 3.**125**).

Radionuclide imaging may be of help in doubtful cases, showing a normal slightly increased uptake near the manubriosternal synchondrosis. Usually it will not display an obvious hot spot as in metastatic disease.

The physiological **fusiform broadening of the parasternal costal cartilages** (Figs. 3.**103**, 3.**118**, 3.**119**) should not be mistaken for soft-tissue tumors. Their bilateral symmetry and smooth margins suggest the correct interpretation. Tumor-mimicking asymmetries in the sternal and parasternal region are discussed on p. 331.

Other Changes?

Degenerative changes with osteophyte formation can occur in the area of the manubriosternal synchondrosis (Fig. 3.**126** and lower row in Fig. 3.**101**). Pronounced osteophyte formation and subchondral sclerosis may result from chronic overloads, but this cannot be proved. The same applies to similar changes in the area of the xiphosternal synchondrosis. At one time, it was claimed that these changes were linked to occupations in which work materials were held against the chest (e.g., locksmiths and cobblers).

The sternum may have a bizarre radiographic appearance in systemic skeletal diseases that are associated with an increase in density (e.g., marble bone disease, Fig. 3.**127**).

References

Ashley, G. T.: The human sternum. J. forens. Med. 3 (1956) 27

Carter, F. R. N.: Congenital absence of the os sternum. J. Indian med. Ass. 18 (1925) 57

Chang, C. H., W. C. Davis: Congenital bifid sternum with partial ectopia cordis. Amer. J. Roentgenol. 86 (1961) 513

Crone-Münzebrock, W., M. Heller, H. Vogel: Computertomographische Befunde bei Brustbeindestruktionen. Fortschr. Röntgenstr. 138 (1983) 703

Currarino, G., F. N. Silverman: Premature obliteration of the sternal sutures and pigeon-breast deformity. Radiology 70 (1958) 532

Dihlmann, W.: Gelenke – Wirbelverbindungen, 2. Aufl. Thieme, Stuttgart 1982 (S. 592)

Donnelly, L. F., C. N. R. Taylor, K. H. Emery et al.: Asymptomatic, palpable, anterior chest wall lesions in children: Is cross-sectional imaging necessary? Radiology 202 (1997) 829

Dziallas, P.: Zur Entwicklung und Histogenese der Sternocostalverbindungen und Sternalfugen. Z. Zellforsch. 37 (1952) 127

Elster, A. D., P. Stark: Episternal ossicles: a normal CT variant. Fortschr. Röntgenstr. 143 (1985) 246

Fischer, E.: Besonderheiten zur Ossifikation des Brustbeins. Fortschr. Röntgenstr. 98 (1963) 151

Fischer, E.: Sternum und Claviculargelenke. In Diethelm, L., O. Olsson, F. Strnad, H. Vieten: Handbuch der Medizinischen Radiologie, Bd. IV/2. Springer, Berlin 1968 (S. 481)

Freyschmidt, J., A. Sternberg: The bullhead sign-scintigraphic pattern of sternocostaclavicular hyperostosis and pustulotic arthroosteitis. Eur. Radiol. 8 (1998) 576

Gassmann, W.: Ungewöhnlich große Osteophytenbildung an der Synchondrosis sterni. Fortschr. Röntgenstr. 86 (1957) 406

Gomez, A. N., L. G. M. Padilla, F. S. Diaz et al.: Fissure sternale complète. Chir. Pédiat. 26 (1985) 44

Goodman, L. R., St. K. Teplick, H. Kay: Computed tomography of the normal sternum. Amer. J. Radiol. 141 (1983) 219

Gugliantini, P., D. Barbuti, D. Rosatti et al.: Histiocytosis X: Solitary localization in the sternum of a 2-year-old child. Pediat. Radiol. 12 (1982) 102

Hatfield, M. K., B. H. Gross. G. M. Glazer et al.: Computed tomography of the sternum and its articulations. Skelet. Radiol. 11 (1984) 197

Herdner, M.: Le sternum de l'enfant. Étude radiologique des anomalies de son dévelopement. Rev. Orthop. 33 (1947) 475

Horns, J., B. J. O'Laughlin: Multiple manubrial ossification centers in mongolism. Amer. J. Roentgenol. 93 (1965) 395

Hümmer, H. P., H. Rupprecht: Die Asymmetrie der Trichterbrust: Beurteilung, Häufigkeit, Konsequenzen. Z. Orthop. 123 (1985) 218

Jurik, A. G., H. Graudahl, A. de Carvalho: Sclerotic changes of the manubrium sterni. Skelet. Radiol. 13 (1985) 196

v. Mauch, D.: Isolierter Knochenkern in der Synchondrosis superior des Sternums. Fortschr. Röntgenstr. 85 (1956) 359

Odita, J.C., A. A. Okolo, J. A. Omene: Sternal ossification in normal newborn infants. Pediat. Radiol. 15 (1985) 165

v. d. Oelsnitz, G.: Die Trichter- und Kielbrust. In Bibliothek für Kinderchirurgie. Hippokrates, Stuttgart 1983

Ogden, J. A., G. J. Conlogue, M. L. Bronson et al.: Radiology of postnatal skeletal development. II. The manubrium and sternum. Skelet. Radiol. 4 (1979) 189

Perez, F. L., R. C. Coddington: A fracture of the sternum in a child. J. pediat. Orthop. 3 (1983) 513

Polvar, G.: Due casi di malformazione sternale. Minerva Chir. (1951) 197

Reeder, M. M.: Reeder and Felson's Gamuts in Bone, Joint and Spine Radiology. Springer, Berlin 1993

Richter, R., W. Nübling, Fr.-J. Krause: Die isolierte Brustbeintuberkulose. Fortschr. Röntgenstr. 139 (1983) 132

Ruge, G.: Untersuchungen über Entwicklungsvorgänge am Brustbein und an der Sternoclavicularverbindung des Menschen. Morph. Jb. 6 (1880) 362

Rush, W. J., L. F. Donnely, A. S. Brody et al.: "Missing" sternal ossification center: Potential mimicker of disease in young children. Radiology 224 (2002) 120

Sammarai, A. W. F., H. A. M. Charmockly, A. A. Atra et al.: Complete cleft sternum: classification and surgical repair. Int. Surg. 70 (1985) 71

Schmitt, H.: Jugendliche Sternumfraktur, durch Muskelzug bedingt. Röntgenpraxis 15 (1943) 395

Schratter, M., M. Bijak, H. Nissel et al.: Foramen sternale: Kleine Anomalie – große Relevanz. Fortschr. Röntgenstr. 166 (1997) 69

Stark, P.: Midline sternal foramen: CT demonstration. J. Comput. assist. Tomogr. 9 (1985) 489

Steiner, R. M., M. E. Kricun, J. Shapiro: Absent mesosternum in congenital heart disease. Amer. J. Roentgenol. 127 (1976) 923

Wolf-Heidegger, G.: Atlas der systemischen Anatomie des Menschen, 2. Aufl. Karger, Basel 1961

Ribs

Normal Findings

During Growth

Ossification centers appear at the costal angles of the sixth and seventh ribs at about the end of the second month of fetal development, followed in rapid succession by centers for the remaining ribs. Ossification proceeds swiftly, although relatively large portions of the ribs are still cartilaginous in newborns and infants. The sternal ends of the ribs are metaphyses. Ossification of the first through tenth ribs starts at the chondro-osseous junction with the appearance of a narrow, more or less elliptical density. Next the superior border ossifies, followed by a slightly narrower area along the inferior border. Finally the intervening cartilage ossifies from below upward and from lateral to medial.

The **epiphyseal centers** appear during puberty (Fig. 3.**128**), one for the head and two for the tubercle. They unite with the shaft between 20 and 25 years of age.

The ossification of the costal cartilages is largely independent of age. There are healthy young people who show pronounced ossification shortly after age 20, and many elderly persons show no appreciable ossification of the costal cartilages. The ossification pattern of the cartilaginous ribs displays gender-specific features. Ossification in males tends to show a fork-shaped pattern along the superior and inferior borders, while a central candlewick pattern is more characteristic in females.

The first pair of ribs is distinctive in that their cartilaginous portion frequently ossifies before all the other ribs, appearing to form bony plates perpendicular to the rib axis.

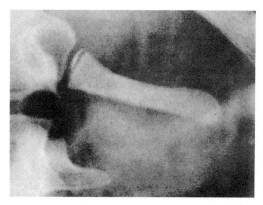

Fig. 3.**128**   Epiphyseal center of the twelfth rib.

In Adulthood

Each rib is composed of a bony part and an anterior cartilaginous part.

The bony portion of the rib consists of three parts: the head, neck, and shaft (Fig. 3.**129**). The head bears an articular surface, which in most ribs (2–10) is separated into two oblique facets by a transverse ridge (crest of the head). The neck is the tapered part of the rib that succeeds the head. The tubercle is located at the junction of the neck with the shaft. In the first 10 ribs, the tubercle bears a small facet that articulates with the transverse process of the corresponding thoracic vertebra. Several centimeters lateral to the tubercle, the rib bends sharply forward at the costal angle. The internal surface of the shaft has a shallow groove along its lower border (the costal groove), which harbors the intercostal nerves and vessels.

The first two and last two ribs exhibit several special features:

- The first rib is shorter, broader, and more curved than the other ribs. It has a well-defined upper and lower surface and an anterior and posterior border. Its cartilaginous part consistently contains transverse ossified bands, even when the remaining costal cartilages show no evidence of ossification. The anterior and inferior chondro-osseous junctions of the first rib generally present spurlike or tuberosity-like features that resemble osteophytes (Fig. 3.**130**). The tubercle is located at the costal angle. A shallow groove in the upper surface of the shaft transmits the subclavian artery, which may be injured when the first rib is fractured. The part of the rib just anterior to the groove bears the tubercle for the anterior scalene muscle (scalene tubercle, Fig. 3.**131**).
- The second rib has a rough area on its anterior outer surface, the tubercle for the serratus anterior muscle, which can be identified on radiographs (Fig. 3.**132**).
- The eleventh and twelfth ribs each have one articular facet on the head. They have no necks, tubercles, grooves, or angles.

Some remarks should be made to the unions of the ribs to the sternum and vertebrae:

The cartilaginous portions of the first through seventh ribs are connected in front to the costal notches of the sternum, as described in the previous chapter (see Fig. 3.**100a, b**). The eighth through tenth pairs of ribs contribute with its cartilage part to the costal arch, and the eleventh and twelfth ribs terminate freely in the abdominal wall. Articulations may exist between the cartilages of the sixth through ninth ribs (intercartilaginous joints).

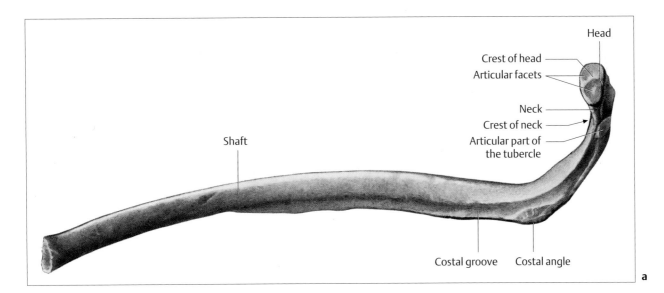

Head
Crest of head
Articular facets
Neck
Crest of neck
Articular part of the tubercle
Shaft
Costal groove
Costal angle

a

Two types of articulation occur between the ribs and the thoracic vertebrae:

- One type connects the heads of the ribs to the bodies of the vertebrae (joints of the heads of the ribs)
- A second type connects the tubercles of the ribs to the transverse processes (costotransverse joints)

Both types are synovial joints, a fact that may be significant in patients with rheumatoid disease. In the joints of the heads of the ribs, the head articulates with a socket formed by the costal facet of the thoracic vertebral body. The first, eleventh, and twelfth ribs each articulate with a single vertebra, while all other ribs articulate with two adjacent vertebrae. The rib corresponds in number to the vertebra with whose upper border it articulates.

Costotransverse joints occur only on the first through tenth ribs. The tubercle of each of these ribs articulates with a socket formed by the costal facet on the transverse process of the corresponding vertebra.

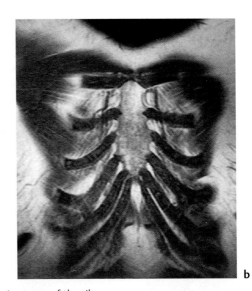

b

Fig. 3.**129** Anatomy of the ribs.
a Specimen photograph of the eighth rib, viewed from the inner aspect.
b Coronal reformatted MR image of the costal arch.

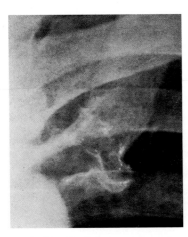

Fig. 3.**130** Typical appearance of the ossified cartilage of the first rib.

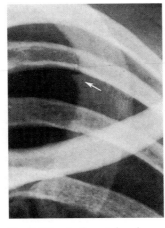

Fig. 3.**131** Scalene tubercle (arrow).

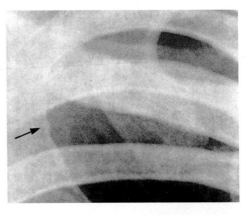

Fig. 3.**132** Tubercle (tuberosity) of the second rib (arrow), where the anterior serratus muscle attaches.

Pathological Finding?

Normal Variant or Anomaly?

The ribs are subject to myriad variants and anomalies that have no pathological significance. In many cases it is impossible to differentiate these innocuous conditions from true deformities. Often this can be done only by checking for coexisting skeletal anomalies (see below). Overall, rib anomalies are noted on 0.15–0.31 % of routine chest radiographs. They show a slight female preponderance and are more common on the right side than on the left (Berner 1944).

Variants

The following are **established variants** that may be encountered in routine practice.

With **asymmetrical development of the first ribs**, one rib may be shorter and broader than the other and may extend only as far as the scalene tubercle. In other cases the first rib may be elongated and exceptionally slender.

Cervical ribs are found in 1–2 % of the healthy population and arise from the transverse process of the last cervical vertebra on one or both sides. They may be partly or completely fused with the first rib, or they may articulate with it (Fig. 3.**133**).

Cervical ribs as well as underdeveloped first ribs can incite neurovascular symptoms (sensory disturbances involving the brachial plexus, thoracic inlet or outlet syndrome), which fall under the heading of **scalenus anticus syndrome**.

Discontinuities in the first rib (Fig. 3.**134**) with pseudarthrosis formation occur as a variant in completely asymptomatic patients with a negative history. Figure 3.**135** shows the case of a 15-year-old girl who had a discontinuity in the right first rib with an interposed bony el-

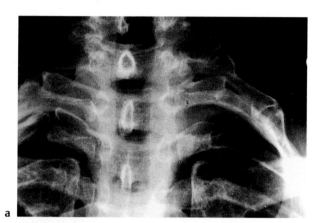

a

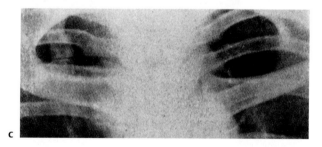

c

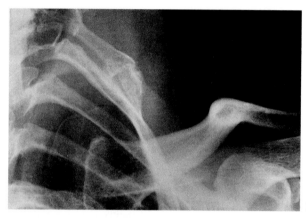

b

Fig. 3.**133 a–c** Cervical ribs.
a, b Left cervical rib with an additional articulation in its lateral portion. The additional joint shows regressive changes. The patient had tingling paresthesias in her left hand, prompting surgery for a presumed carpal tunnel syndrome. Later the cervical rib was removed, eliminating the complaints.
c Right cervical rib, whose anterior portion articulates with the first rib.
b, c Riblike metaplastic-heterotopic new bone formation (Wiens' rib) in the former drainage canal after gastric pull-up operation for oesophageal cancer in the lower third two years before.

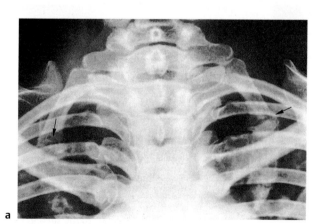

a

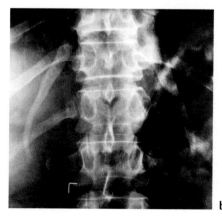

b

Fig. 3.**134 a, b** Rib anomalies.
a Bilateral pseudoarthrosis-like discontinuities in the first rib.

b Supernumerary ribs? (Case courtesy of Professor E. Zeitler, Nuremberg.)

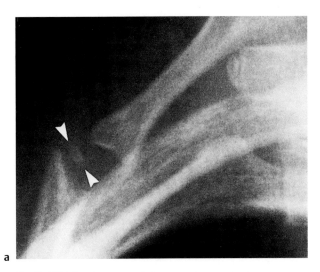
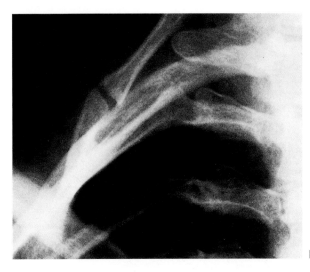

Fig. 3.**135 a, b** Accessory bone.
a Accessory bone located within a rib discontinuity (arrowheads) in a 15-year-old boy.

b Four years later the bone has been assimilated into the pseudarthrosis.

ement that apparently fused with the distal part of the pseudarthrosis over the next four years.

Significant **asymmetries** can also occur in the **twelfth rib**. For example, a rib may be absent on one side or shorter than the opposite rib.

An **intrathoracic rib** is a supernumerary rib that crosses over the other ribs as it projects into the thoracic cavity (Friedrich et al. 1975). It may be extra- or intrapulmonary in its location. An intrapulmonary rib is ensheathed by parietal and visceral pleura and may have a diaphragmatic attachment. The shape is variable:

- A fully developed intrathoracic rib articulates with the anterolateral border of the spinal column and runs laterally downward, passing anterior to the other rib origins.
- A partially developed intrathoracic rib forms a posterior synostosis with a normal rib and also runs laterally downward and anterior to the other ribs (Fig. 3.**136**).

A **bifid rib** is classified as a simple variant (Fig. 3.**137**, no 5). It usually results from the posterior fusion of two ribs.

Intermediary osseous bridges are commonly found between the fourth and fifth ribs and occasionally between the first and second ribs (Fig. 3.**137**, no 6).

The **Srb anomaly** is marked by the presence of hornlike bony structures projecting from one or both sides of the manubrium below the manubrioclavicular joint (Figs. 3.**138**, 3.**139**). Apparently they occur mainly in conjunction with fusions of the first two ribs or the second and third ribs, resulting in deficient or rudimentary development of their anterior portions. By this definition the rudiments correspond to the hornlike projections from the manubrium described above. In some cases they may be located adjacent to the manubrium, as shown in the tomogram in Fig. 3.**139**.

Nearthrosis and fusions may occur between the anterior ends or posterior segments of adjacent ribs (Figs. 3.**140**, 3.**141**).

Bridgelike linkages between ribs and costotransverse joints have also been described as normal variants (Fig. 3.**141**). Of course, these features require differentiation from diseases that are associated with metaplastic bone formation on the spinal column and its joints, such as the large group of seronegative spondylarthropathies.

It is rare for ribs to have a **bifid head**, but this is also classified as a simple variant (Fig. 3.**142**).

Dysplasias and Deformities

As mentioned above, rib anomalies should be interpreted as a malformation or deformity if they are associated with other skeletal anomalies:

- Eleven pairs of ribs (Table 3.**7**)
- Thin, streaklike or tortuous-looking ribs (Table 3.**8**)
- Thin bandlike and streaklike ribs or eroded-looking ribs are also seen in:
  - severe osteoporosis, especially in juveniles
  - angiomatosis (Gorham–Stout disease)
  - basal cell nevus syndrome
  - hyperparathyroidism
  - paraplegia
  - rheumatoid arthritis and scleroderma
- Exceptionally broad or thick ribs (Table 3.**9** and Fig. 3.**145**)
- Unusually broad, thick ribs are also seen in:
  - acromegaly (also with coarsening of the costal cartilage)
  - fluorosis
  - Paget disease
  - storage diseases (e.g., Gaucher disease, Erdheim–Chester disease, etc.)
- Short ribs (Table 3.**10**)
- Symmetrical anterior enlargement, broadening, or cupping of multiple ribs (Table 3.**11**)
- Symmetrical concave defects in the superior aspect of multiple ribs due to subperiosteal resorption (Table 3.**12** and Fig. 3.**143**).
- Rib notching, i.e., pressure erosions in the inferior aspect of ribs (Table 3.**13**, Figs. 3.**144** and 3.**146**).

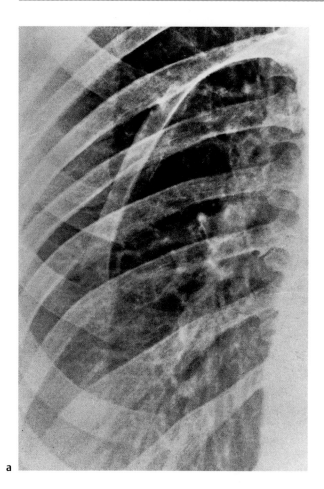

a

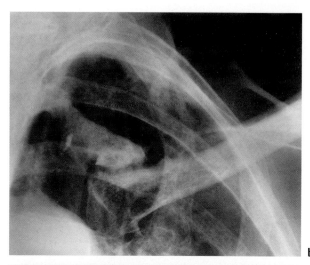

b

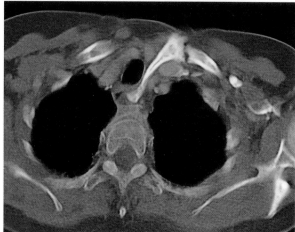

c

Fig. 3.**136 a–c**   Intrathoracic rib and its differential diagnosis.
a True intrathoracic rib. (From Friedrich et al. 1975.)

b, c Riblike metaplastic (heterotopic) new bone formation
(Wien's rib) in the former drainage canal after gastric pull-up
operation for esophageal cancer in the lower third, two years
before.

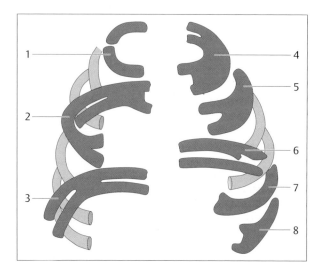

Fig. 3.**137**   Several examples of rib anomalies.
1   Discontinuity in the first rib
2   Partial posterior fusion, anterior bifid rib
3   Localized fusion
4   Anterior fusion
5   Posterior fusion with anterior bifid configuration
6   Suggested fusion dorsal
7   Rudimentary bifid rib
8   Luschka-type bifid rib

Table 3.**7**   Syndromes that are associated with only eleven
pairs of ribs (after Reeder)

- Trisomy 21 syndrome
- Asphyxiating thoracic dysplasia (Jeune syndrome)
- Atelo-osteogenesis
- Camptomelic dysplasia
- Cleidocranial dysplasia
- Short ribs—polydactyly syndrome

Table 3.**8** Syndromes that are associated with thin, streaklike or tortuous-looking ribs (listed in order of frequency) (after Reeder)

- Myotonic dystrophy, myotubular myopathy, Werdnig–Hoffmann disease
- Neurofibromatosis
- Achondrogenesis type I and II
- Aminopterin fetopathy
- Camptomelic dysplasia
- Cockayne syndrome
- Hallermann–Streiff syndrome
- Larsen syndrome
- Metaphyseal chondrodysplasia (Jansen)
- Morquio syndrome (posterior portion)
- Osteodysplastia (Melnick–Needles syndrome)
- Osteogenesis imperfecta
- Progeria
- Spondylocostal dysostosis
- Spondylothoracic dysplasia
- 3-M syndrome
- Trisomy 13 syndrome
- Trisomy 18 syndrome
- Trisomy 21 syndrome
- Turner syndrome

Table 3.**9** Syndromes that may be associated with exceptionally broad or thick ribs (after Reeder)

- Achondroplasia
- Thalassemia and sickle cell disease (Fig. 3.**145**)
- Mucopolysaccharidoses
- Craniodiaphyseal dysplasia
- Dysosteosclerosis
- Endosteal hyperostosis
- Fucosidosis
- Mannosidosis
- Gaucher disease
- Niemann–Pick disease
- Hyperphosphatasia
- Hypochondroplasia
- Melorheostosis
- Pachydermoperiostosis
- Metaphyseal chondrodysplasia, Schmid type
- Metaphyseal dysplasia (Pyle disease)
- Mucolipidosis II and III
- Oculodento-osseous dysplasia
- Osteogenesis imperfecta congenita
- Proteus syndrome
- Trisomy 8 syndrome

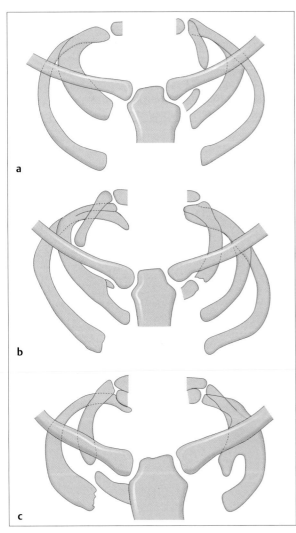

Fig. 3.**138 a–c** Varying degrees of the **Srb anomaly** of the ribs and sternum.

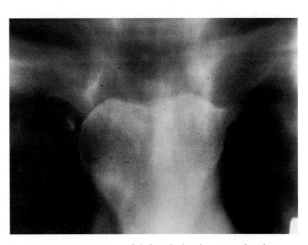

Fig. 3.**139** Tomogram of left-sided Srb anomaly shows a hornlike bony structure projecting from the upper left angle of the manubrium. To the upper right of the manubrium is an isolated bony element that might be classified as an os parasternale were it not for other radiographic and tomographic findings (see p. 330 and Fig. 3.**115**).

Fig. 3.**140** Bridging and nearthrosis formation posteriorly.

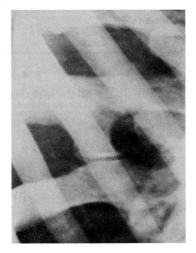

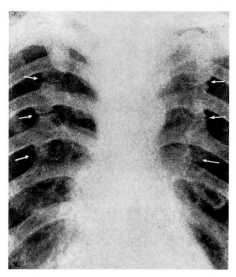

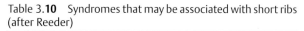

Fig. 3.**141**   Posterior fusions and nearthroses (arrows).

Fig. 3.**142**   Bifurcated head of the twelfth rib (arrows).

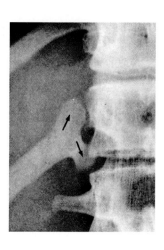

Table 3.**10**   Syndromes that may be associated with short ribs (after Reeder)

- Achondroplasia
- Achondrogenesis type I and II
- Asphyxiating thoracic dysplasia (Jeune syndrome)
- Camptomelic dysplasia
- Cerebrocostomandibular syndrome
- Chondroectodermal dysplasia
- Cleidocranial dysplasia
- Dyssegmental dysplasia
- Enchondromatosis
- Fibrochondrogenesis, hypochondrogenesis
- Hypophosphatasia
- Mandibuloacral dysplasia
- Metatrophic dysplasia
- Mucopolysaccharidoses
- Osteodysplastia (Melnick–Needles syndrome)
- Osteogenesis imperfecta
- Pseudoachondroplasia
- Short ribs—polydactyly syndrome types I, II and III
- Spondylocostal dysostosis
- Spondyloepiphyseal dysplasia (congenital)
- Thanatophoric dysplasia

Table 3.**11**   Syndromes that may be associated with symmetrical anterior enlargement, broadening, or cupping of multiple ribs (after Reeder)

- Achondroplasia
- Asphyxiating thoracic dysplasia and other syndromes with a narrow thorax and short ribs
- Hypophosphatasia
- Menkes syndrome
- Metaphyseal chondrodysplasia (Jansen, McKusick, Schmid)
- Shwachman syndrome
- Short ribs—polydactyly syndrome
- Spondylometaphyseal dysplasia
- Thanatophoric dysplasia

Table 3.**12**   Diseases that may be associated with resorption or notching of the superior rib margins (after Reeder)

- Rheumatoid arthritis
- Collagen diseases (scleroderma, lupus)
- Hyperparathyroidism
- Neurofibromatosis
- Localized pressure effect (e.g., thoracic drainage)
- Coarctation of thoracic aorta (superior and inferior margins)
- Intercostal muscle atrophy in restrictive lung disease
- Marfan-Syndrome
- Osteogenesis imperfecta
- Poliomyelitis, paralysis

Table 3.**13**   Diseases that may be associated with classic rib notching (after Reeder)

- Various forms of coarctation of the thoracic aorta
- Obstruction of vena cava, innominate or subclavian vein
- Pulmonary oligemia
- Obstruction of the superior vena cava, innominate vein or subclavian vein
- AV-fistula of chest wall (intercostal artery-vein)
- Pulmonary A-V fistula
- Intercostal neurofibroma or neurilemoma with or without neurofibromatosis
- Bulbar poliomyelitis; quadriplegia
- Hyperparathyroidism
- Osteodysplasty (Melnick-Needes-S.)
- Thalassemia

Fig. 3.**143** Symmetrical erosions of both seventh ribs (arrows) due to circumscribed bone resorption in scleroderma.

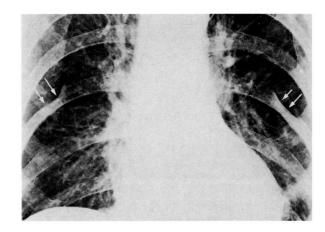

Fig. 3.**144a–c**   Neurofibromatosis.
a Notching of the inferior rib borders in neurofibromatosis. Because of this phenomenon, the costal groove (between the arrows) is broadened while the shaft appears narrowed.
b, c CT scans of the same patient demonstrate multiple neurofibromas with rib erosions (arrows).

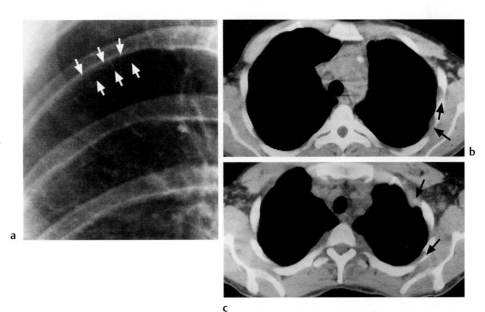

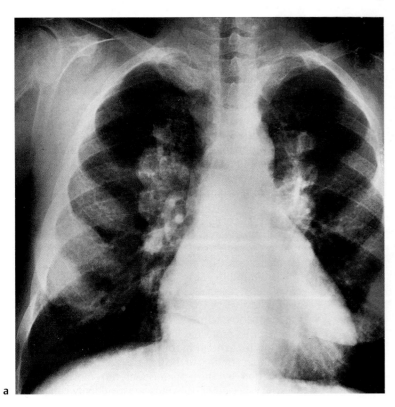

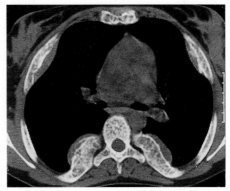

Fig. 3.**145a–c**   Thalassemia.
a, b Chest film in thalassemia shows massive widening and enlargement of the medullary cavities of the ribs, caused by the pathological increase in hematopoiesis. The apparent widening of both hila is caused by broadening of the posterior rib segments and paravertebral soft tissues due to extramedullary hematopoiesis.   Fig. 3.**145c** ▷

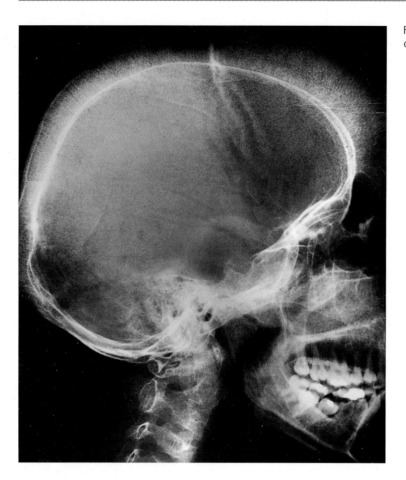

Fig. 3.**145c**   Typical hair-on-end appearance of the skull in thalassemia.

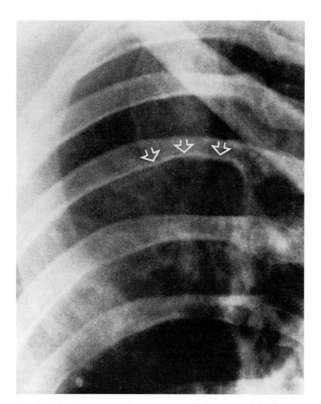

Fig. 3.**146**   Pronounced narrowing of the posterior rib segments in a patient with coarctation of the aorta.

Fracture, Subluxation, or Dislocation?

Fractures

Rib fractures (Figs. 3.**147**, 3.**150**) are best demonstrated on spot radiographs (75–85 kV).

Sites of pain identified by the patient are marked on the skin with small lead markers. It should be noted that superimposed bony structures, pulmonary vessels, pleural boundaries, etc. can easily mimic fracture lines due to superimposition effects or Mach bands (Figs. 3.**148**, 3.**149**).

The key to differential diagnosis in these cases is the clinical presentation. Incomplete fractures or fractures 2–3 weeks old are often undetected on radiographs and require radionuclide imaging. Conversely, radionuclide abnormalities that are detected incidentally often do not correlate with radiographic changes. This can sometimes lead to problems in cancer patients. If there is good reason to suspect metastasis, CT scans should be obtained.

It is often difficult to distinguish fractures from congenital clefts, especially in the **first rib** and especially when the costal cartilage is affected. It should be kept in mind that traumatic fractures of the first rib are relatively rare because of its protected location. It is more common for these injuries to occur in conjunction with clavicular fractures. Indirect trauma to the first rib can result from excessive traction by the scalenus anterior muscle on the tubercle, especially if this muscle is suddenly contracted

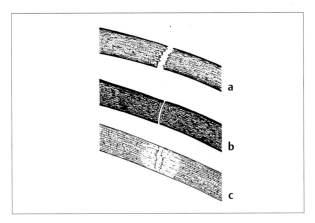

Fig. 3.**147 a–c** Discontinuities in the ribs.
a Typical traumatic rib fracture.
b Smooth break in marble bone disease.
c Cough fracture.

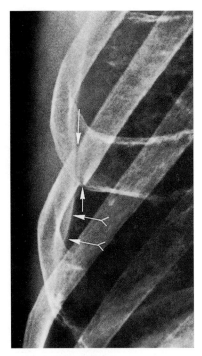

Fig. 3.**148** Posterolateral rib fracture (arrows), not a Mach effect caused by the subpleural fat line (double arrows).

by a brisk turn of the head to one side (e.g., during heavy coughing or sneezing).

Fatigue fractures of the ribs have been observed in golfers (Rasad 1974), surfers (Bailey 1985), and female rowers (Holden and Jackson 1985). Stress fractures can also result from lifting heavy loads (Dietzel and Schirmer 1972), carrying heavy luggage, and from playing baseball or basketball (Sacchetti et al. 1983). A good survey of stress fractures of the ribs can be found in Lankenner and Micheli (1985).

Cough fractures of ribs can occur in persons without bone disease, but cough-induced (insufficiency) fractures are more common in patients with osteoporosis (Fig. 3.**150**).

Figure 3.**151** illustrates an unusually long posterior stress-induced lesion of the right eleventh rib that resulted from crutch use.

Subluxations and Dislocations

Rib dislocations are extremely rare and have been observed only in the eleventh and twelfth ribs.

The **articulation** of the twelfth rib with the vertebra may be so lax that the rib displaces when the patient bends forward. This **slipping rib syndrome** (Machin and Shennan 1983) may be associated with significant pain. When the finger is placed over the rib, crepitus can be felt during flexion-extension of the spine.

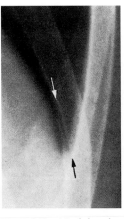

Fig. 3.**149** Mach band effect (arrows).

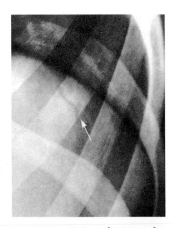

Fig. 3.**150** Fatigue fracture of a rib (arrow).

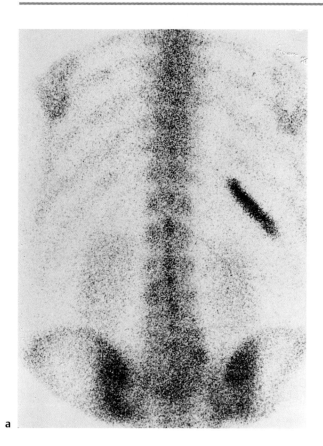

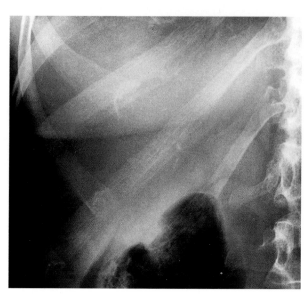

Fig. 3.**151 a, b**   Pronounced, pagetoid structural changes in the eleventh rib on the right side as a result of hyperperfusion due to repetitive stresses. The patient had to use crutches following a motor vehicle accident. She complained of increasing pain in the region of the right eleventh rib. Presumably, the crutch use (the patient was right-handed) caused excessive loads at the insertion of the serratus dorsalis caudalis muscle.

 Necrosis?

There should be no difficulty in distinguishing typical osteonecrosis from a normal variant. It should be noted, however, that collagen diseases in particular can produce more or less extensive osteolytic lesions in ribs, leaving stubby remnants behind. In most cases these lesions are associated with acro-osteolysis involving the clavicles and the bones of the hand.

Radiation necrosis of rib bone is typically manifested on radiographs by discontinuities and fragmentation of the very dense necrotic bone (Fig. 3.**152**).

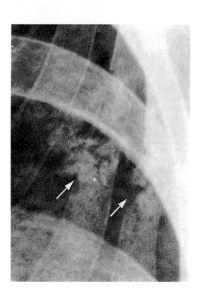

Fig. 3.**152**   Radiation necrosis of the ribs (arrows).

Radiotherapy for breast cancer is the most frequent cause of osteoradionecrosis in the anterior chest wall.

 Inflammation?

Primary hematogenous osteomyelitis is much less common in ribs than contiguous involvement by a pleural empyema. Destructive bone changes and reactive sclerosis should be easily distinguishable from normal findings. Primary chronic osteomyelitis in the form of a Brodie abscess or plasma cell osteomyelitis appears to be very rare in the ribs (Fig. 3.**153**).

Tumor?

Osteomas of the ribs should be considered a normal variant (Fig. 3.**154**), since carefull "reading" of the thoracic skeleton in routine X-rays of the thorax (especially digital) will often reveal their presence in routine imaging studies (especially digital) of the thoracic skeleton.

Unusual oblong osteomas are indistinguishable from melorheostosis (Fig. 3.**155**).

McCarthy et al. (1985) identified painless "**fibro-osseous lesions**" of the rib resembling osteoid osteoma on histological examination. The lesions appeared as hot spots on radionuclide scans and appeared on radiographs as a circumscribed density with a lucent halo. The authors described the foci as reactive. We have not personally encountered such findings and believe that they represent either small foci of fibrous dysplasia with regressive changes or small lipomas with dystrophic calcification.

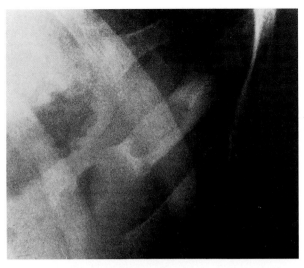

Fig. 3.**153** Primary chronic osteomyelitis, consisting here of plasma cell osteomyelitis or a Brodie abscess, in an anterior rib of a 14-year-old boy. The elliptical lucency with a dense sclerotic border is definitely pathological and not a normal variant. The patient presented clinically with circumscribed swelling and pain.

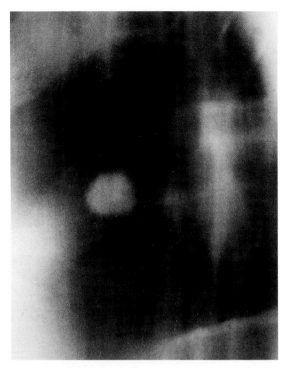

Fig. 3.**154**   Osteoma detected incidentally in a posterior rib.

The most common **true bone tumor of the ribs** is chondrosarcoma, which accounts for approximately 35% of all cases of primary tumorous rib lesions (Fig. 3.**157**). It is followed in frequency (10–14% of all primary bone tumors of the ribs) by Ewing sarcoma, malignant lymphoma, chondroma (Figs. 3.**156**, 3.**157c**), and osteochondroma (Freyschmidt and Spiro 1985).

The series of images in Fig. 3.**158**   show part of the differential diagnostic spectrum of expansile and osteolytic lesions involving the head region of the rib.

Basically there is no need to explore the differential diagnosis of bone tumors within the scope of this monograph, since generally they do not require differentiation from normal variants (see Freyschmidt and Spiro 1985 for a detailed review). It should be noted that the various manifestations of fibrous dysplasia, especially with symmetrical involvement, may occasionally suggest the possibility of a syndrome or extreme normal variant (Figs. 3.**159**–3.**161**).

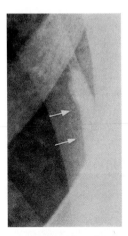

Fig. 3.**155**   Very elongated osteoma or melorheostosis (rare site of occurrence) detected incidentally in a rib (arrows).

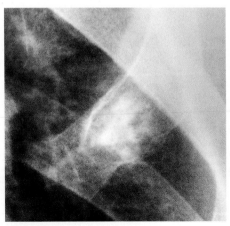

a

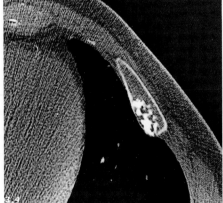

b

Fig. 3.**156a, b**   Calcified enchondroma in an anterior rib (incidental finding).

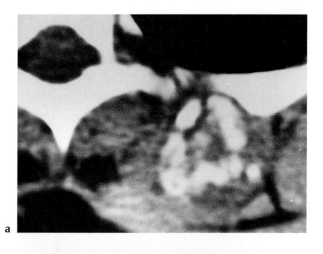

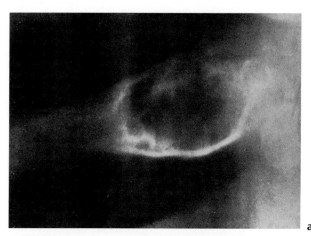

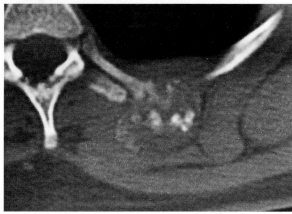

Fig. 3.**157a,b** Exostotic chondrosarcoma in a posterior rib. The discrete foci of matrix ossification in a larger soft-tissue mass demonstrated by the bone-window scan (**b**) are virtually pathognomonic for chondrosarcoma. This type of tumor always requires complete surgical excision with serial histological sections. Here the tumor has penetrated the rib and indented the pleural space.

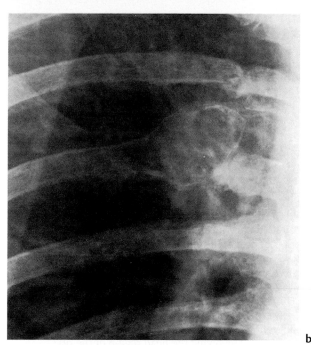

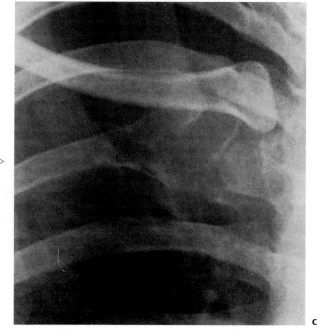

Fig. 3.**158a–c** Morphologically similar but etiologically distinct lesions involving the heads of ribs.
a Focal hematopoietic hyperplasia with regressive bone changes (infarcts) in an otherwise healthy 11-year-old girl. The central bone areas are predominantly affected.
b Giant cell tumor with a relatively broad transition from osteolysis to healthy bone in a 33-year-old woman. The tomogram did not show any calcification within the tumor.
c Chondroma in a 25-year-old woman. Some of the intratumoral calcifications on the tomogram (not demonstrated here) are stellate or crescent-shaped, and some have a stippled appearance. This finding is consistent with a chondroma or grade I chondrosarcoma. (From Freyschmidt and Spiro 1985.)

Fig. 3.**159 a, b** Polyostotic forms of fibrous dysplasia with grotesque transformations of the posterior and lateral portions of the third and fourth ribs on the right side and of the anterior and posterolateral portions of the third, fourth, and fifth ribs on the left side. The left third rib and the posterior portions of the right fourth rib show very little osseous structure because of extensive fibrous replacement. The differential diagnosis of this case should include hemangiomatosis of bone.

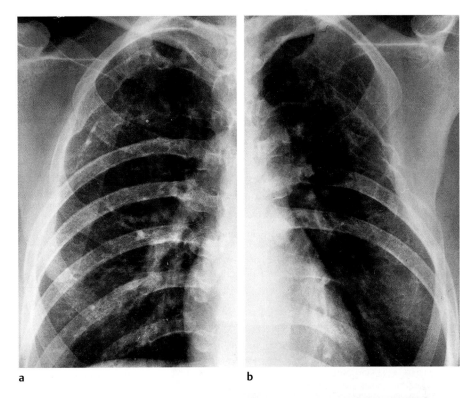

a   b

Fig. 3.**160** Classic fibrous dysplasia of an anterior rib with ▷ massive enlargement (incidental finding). The ground-glass opacity results from ossification of the fibrous tissue and is typical of the ossification stage of this disease.

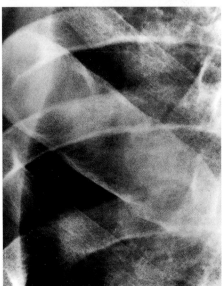

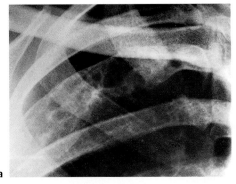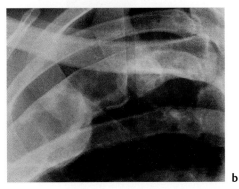

a   b

Fig. 3.**161 a, b** Follow-up of fibrous dysplasia of the posterior fourth rib on the right side (young woman).
a Initial radiograph shows marked enlargement with a soap-bubble appearance. The enlargement is an effective criterion for distinguishing fibrous dysplasia from tumor-associated bone destruction.
b Radiograph eight years later shows rather uniform ground-glass ossification of the woven bone with further expansion.

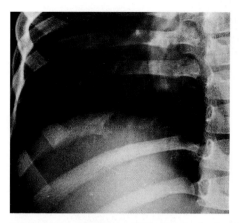

Fig. 3.**162** Langerhans-cell histiocytosis in the posterior tenth rib on the right side, showing a relatively elongated area of complete rib destruction. The only clinical manifestation was a dull aching pain. Additional foci were present in the calvarium.

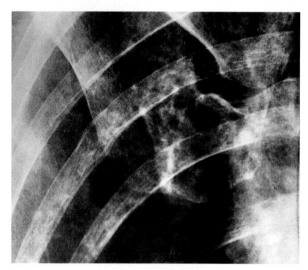

Fig. 3.**163** Very fine, diffuse foci of plasmacytoma in an elderly patient. The lesions are 1–2 mm in size and are visible only on this spot radiograph.

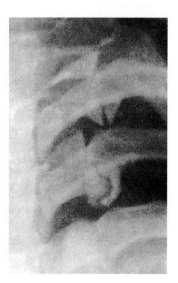

Fig. 3.**164** Costotransverse osteoarthritis.

Circumscribed osteolytic lesions of the ribs in children are most likely due to Langerhans-cell histiocytosis (eosinophilic granuloma) and occasionally can be diagnosed even without biopsy (Fig. 3.**162**). This diagnosis is especially likely when additional foci are found, particularly in the calvarium.

In adults, a more or less nonspecific osteolytic lesion should definitely be investigated by biopsy, as it may represent a metastatic process, plasmacytoma, etc.

While the fully developed presentation of plasmacytoma, marked by 2- to 5-mm osteolytic lesions distributed uniformly throughout all the ribs, is unmistakable and indeed pathognomonic for that disease, early small osteolytic foci are often very difficult to detect, especially in elderly patients with osteoporosis, and can be appreciated only on spot radiographs (Fig. 3.**163**).

 Other Changes?

As in other joints, degenerative changes can develop in the costovertebral and costotransverse joints. They are manifested on radiographs and CT scans by marginal osteophytes, subchondral sclerosis, joint space narrowing, and other typical signs (Fig. 3.**164**).

It is unclear whether pronounced sclerosis at the articulating edges of the sternocostal attachments should actually be termed osteoarthritis. It most likely represents only simple regressive changes that are detected incidentally on radiographs (Fig. 3.**165**).

A strong **increase in the density of the ribs** is seen in congenital conditions that are associated with hyperostosis, most notably:

- Osteopetrosis
- Endosteal hyperostosis
- Osteodysplastia
- Also acquired disorders such as:
  - Osteomyelosclerosis syndrome
  - Fluorosis

Pronounced calcification of the costal cartilages has been reported to occur in adolescents with hyperthyroidism (Senac et al. 1985). The case in Fig. 3.**166** demonstrates that this type of calcification can occur—as an extreme variant—even in young patients with no clinical manifestations of metabolic disease.

Tietze syndrome is discussed on p. 335.

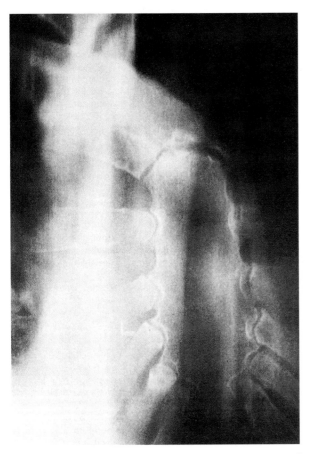

Fig. 3.**165** "Degenerative" changes in the sternocostal joints.

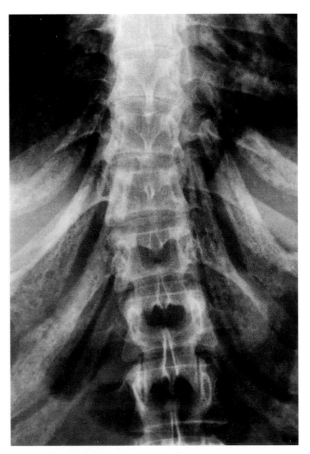

Fig. 3.**166** Extensive bone formation in the costal arch region of a young patient who is clinically healthy except for scoliosis. There was no evidence of metabolic disease.

References

Augustin, V.: Eigenartige Osteolysen der Rippen bei durch Poliomyelits schwer gelähmten Kindern. Fortschr. Röntgenstr. 97 (1962) 771

Bailey, P.: Surfer's rib: isolated first rib fracture secondary to indirect trauma. Ann. Emerg. Med. 14 (1985) 346

Bar-Ziv, J., Y. Barki, A. Maroko et al.: Rib osteomyelitis in children. Early radiologic and ultrasonic findings. Pediat. Radiol. 15 (1985) 315

Berner, F.: Über Rippenanomalien auf Grund von 6 Millionen Reihenbildern. Fortschr. Röntgenstr. 69 (1944) 202

Bernstein, R., J. Isdale, M. Pinto et al.: Short rib—polydaktyly syndrome: a single or heterogeneous entity? A re-evaluation prompted by four new cases. J. med. Genet. 22 (1985) 46

Bertouch, J., T. P. Gordon, D. Henderson et al.: Asymptomatic osteolysis of ribs and clavicles in progressive systemic sclerosis. Aust. N. Z. J. Med. 12 (1982) 627

David, T. J., A. Glass: Hereditary costovertebral dysplasia with malignant cerebral tumor. J. med. Genet. 20 (1983) 441

Derbekyan, V., E. M. Azouz, L. W. Young: Solitary costal erosinophilic granuloma. Amer. J. Dis. Child. 136 (1984) 885

Dietzel, F., H. F. Schirmer: Doppelseitige Ermüdungsfraktur der ersten Rippe. Entstehung unter typischer Belastung. Fortschr. Röntgenstr. 117 (1972) 228

Dihlmann, W.: Gelenke – Wirbelverbindungen, 2. Aufl. Thieme, Stuttgart 1982

Edelstein, G., R. G. Levitt, D. P. Slaker et al.: Computed tomography of Tietze syndrom. J. Comput. assist. Tomogr. 8 (1984) 21

Edelstein, G., M. Kyriakos: Focal hematopoetic hyperplasia of the rib—a form of pseudotumor. Skelet. Radiol. 11 (1984) 108

Eftekhari, F., D. K. Yousefzadeh: Primary infantile hyperparathyreoidism: clinical, laboratory, and radiographic features in 21 cases. Skelet. Radiol. 8 (1982) 201

Fischer, E.: Verkalkungsformen der Rippenknorpel. Fortschr. Röntgenstr. 82 (1955) 474

Fischer, E.: Fehlbildung der knorpeligen Rippen. Fortschr. Röntgenstr. 88 (1958) 687

Fischer, E.: Rippenveränderungen bei der Akromegalie. Fortschr. Röntgenstr. 112 (1970a) 789

Fischer, E.: Der Thoraxumbau nach Armverlust oder Armlähmung und der Einfluß der Schulter-Brust-Muskulatur auf die Form der oberen Thoraxhälfte. Arch. orthop. Unfall-Chir. 67 (1970b) 217

Fischer, E., H. Nowakowski: Gelenkähnliche Spaltbildungen in verkalkten Rippenknorpeln bei adrenogenitalem Syndrom. Fortschr. Röntgenstr. 84 (1956) 57

Fogarty, E. E., T. Beatty, F. Dowling: Spondylocostal dysplasia in identical twins. J. pediat. Orthop. 5 (1985) 720

Freyschmidt, J., T. Spiro: Zur Differentialdiagnose von primären Knochengeschwülsten und geschwulstähnlichen Läsionen an den Rippen. Fortschr. Röntgenstr. 142 (1985) 1

Friedrich, M., E. Gerstenberg, W. Goy: Die intrathorakale Rippe. Fortschr. Röntgenstr. 122 (1975) 438

Ginader, R.: Frei endigende, unterentwickelte 1. Rippe ohne Verbindung mit dem Brustbein. Fortschr. Röntgenstr. 72 (1959) 114

Hoekstra, H. J., L. M. Kingma: Bilateral first rib fractures induced by integral crash helmets. J. Trauma 25 (1985) 566

Holden, D. L., D. W. Jackson: Stress fracture of the ribs in female rowers. Amer. J. Sports Med. 13 (1985) 342

Langeland, P.: Luxation der 12. Rippe im Costo-Vertebral-Gelenk. Fortschr. Röntgenstr. 84 (1956) 645

Lankenner, P. A., L. J. Micheli: Stress fracture of the first rib. J. Bone Jt Surg. 67-A (1985) 159

Machin, D. G., J. M. Shennan: Twelfth rib syndrome: a differential diagnosis of loin pain. Brit. med. J. III (1983) 287

McCarthy, E. F., D. C. Moses, J. W. Zibreg et al.: Painless fibroosseous lesion of the rib resembling osteoid osteoma: a report of six cases. Skelet. Radiol. 13 (1985) 263

Mendl, K., C. J. Evans: Cyst-like and cystic lesions of the rib with special reference to their radiological differential diagnosis based on the discussion of five cases. Brit. J. Radiol. 31 (1958) 146

Moon, B. S., Ch. T. Price, J. B. Campbell: Upper extremity and rib stress fractures in a child. Skelet. Radiol. 27 (1998) 403

Müller, G., W. Dihlmann: Rippenveränderungen bei Leukämie im Kindesalter und ihre Differentialdiagnose. Fortschr. Röntgenstr. 115 (1971) 263

Ontell, F. K., E. H. Moore, J. O. Shepard et al.: The costal cartilages in health and disease. Radiographics 17 (1997) 571

Rasad, S.: Golfer's fractures of the ribs. Report of 3 cases. Amer. J. Roentgenol. 120 (1974) 901

Reeder, M. M.: Reeder and Felson's Gamuts in Bone, Joint and Spine Radiology. Springer, Berlin 1993

Rupprecht, E., A. Gurski: Kurzrippen-Polydaktylie-Syndrom Typ Saldino-Noonan bei zwei Geschwistern. Helv. paediat. Acta 37 (1982) 161

Sacchetti, A. D., D. R. Beswick, St. D. Morse: Rebound rib: stress-induced first rib fracture. Ann. Emerg. Med. 12 (1983) 177

Senac jr, M. O., F . Lee, V. Gilsanz: Early costochondral calcification in adolescent hyperthyroidism. Radiology 156 (1985) 375

Spence, E. K., E. F. Rosato: The slipping rip syndrome. Arch. Surg 118 (1983) 1330

Stark, P., D. D. Lawerence: Intrathoracic rib—CT features of a rare chest wall anomaly. Comput. Radiol. 6 (1984) 365

Sturm jr., A., F. Logan: Rippenusuren ohne Aortenisthmusstenose. Fortschr. Röntgenstr. 97 (1962) 464

Thiemann, H.: Rippenveränderungen bei abszedierender Pneumonie mit eitrigem Pleuraerguß im Kindesalter. Fortschr. Röntgenstr. 105 (1966) 703

Wenz, W., G. Geipert: Röntgenologie und Klinik der Srbschen Rippen-Sternum-Anomalie. Radiologe 7 (1967) 53

Wolf-Heidegger, G.: Atlas der systematischen Anatomie des Menschen, Bd. I, 2. Aufl. Karger, Basel 1961

Woodlief, R. M.: Superior marginal rib defects in traumatic quadriplegia. Radiology 126 (1978) 673

4 Skull

J. Wiens
A. Sternberg

General Aspects

The bony skull, or cranium (Figs. 4.1–4.5), is composed of the cranial vault, or neurocranium, and the facial skeleton, or viscerocranium. The **cranial vault** forms a closed protective capsule for the brain while also enclosing the inner ear and middle ear. The **facial skeleton** is formed by the nasal bones, maxilla, and mandible. From a clinical point of view, the frontal bone of the neurocranium is often considered part of the facial skeleton.

Embryology of the Skull

There are practical reasons for subdividing the skull into the cranial vault and facial skeleton that are unrelated to ontogenic or phylogenic aspects. Embryologically, both the neurocranium and the viscerocranium are initially composed of dense mesenchyme, which later differentiates into membranous bone and cartilage. The cartilaginous elements may persist for life or may undergo endochondral ossification.

Neurocranium

The neurocranium consists of two components: (1) the skull base or chondrocranium, which undergoes endochondral ossification, and (2) the flat membranous bones of the calvarium, which undergo membranous ossification.

Cranial Vault and Membranous Ossification

The flat **membranous bones** of the skull develop directly from the mesenchymal connective tissue that surrounds the primitive cerebral vesicles. This type of ossification is termed membranous (or intramembranous) ossification. It is a process in which the mesenchymal cells condense and differentiate into osteoblasts. After the osteoblasts have been laid down in regular rows, collagen fibers and matrix begin to form. This gives rise to young uncalcified bone, called osteoid, which finally calcifies at some distance from the osteoblasts. Meanwhile, bone formation continues to progress in the ossification center. The entire

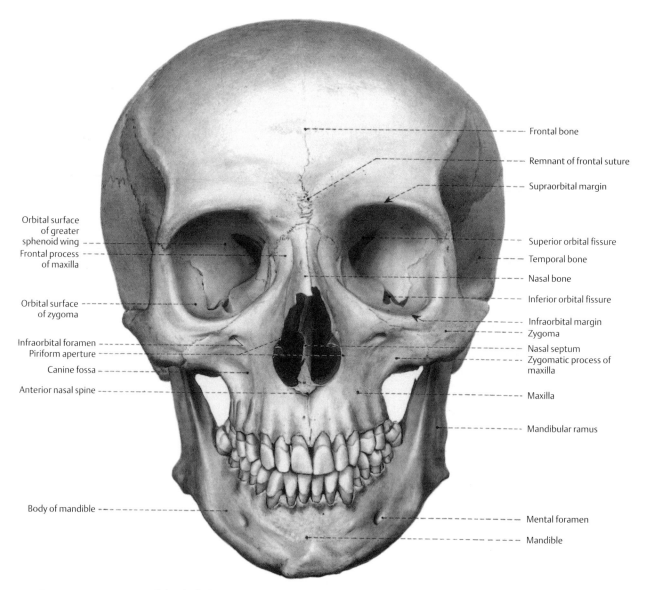

Fig. 4.1   Anterior view of the skull. (From Rauber and Kopsch 1987.)

bony anlage is surrounded by dense mesenchyma, from which the periosteum is formed. Mesenchymal cells deep to this layer differentiate into osteoblasts, which in turn form parallel bony layers on the surface of the original ossification center. The parallel lamellae that are formed by the periosteum are called periosteal bone. The flat membranous bones of the calvarium that are formed by this process enlarge through the apposition of new layers on the outer surface of the bone, while simultaneous osteoclastic bone resorption takes place on the deep surface.

At birth, the flat membranous bones of the skull are still separated from one another by connective tissue along the **cranial sutures**. At sites where more than two bones come together, the sutures are spread open to form **fontanelles**. The anterior fontanelle is located at the junction of the frontal and parietal bones, the posterior fontanelle at the junction of the parietal and occipital bones. The posterior fontanelle closes in about the third postnatal month, the anterior fontanelle in the second year of life.

Development of the Skull Base

The bones of the skull base are derived from cartilaginous elements that subsequently ossify, which is why the skull base is also known as the chondrocranium. The notochord plays a key role in the formation of the chondrocranium. The mesenchyme surrounding the cranial portion of the notochord differentiates into parachordal cartilage. This creates a cartilaginous plate that forms the primitive basal portion of the occipital bone. Another, unsegmented cartilaginous structure forms from three residual sclerotomes that adjoin the parachordal cartilage on the caudal side. That structure finally unites with the parachordal cartilage, lengthening the primitive basal portion of the occipital bone as far as the foramen magnum (Fig. 4.**6a**). Later the cartilaginous anlage of the occipital bone expands dorsally around the neural tube, giving rise to the occipital squama. Only the upper portion of the occipital bone located between the parietal bones undergoes membranous ossification (Fig. 4.**6d**).

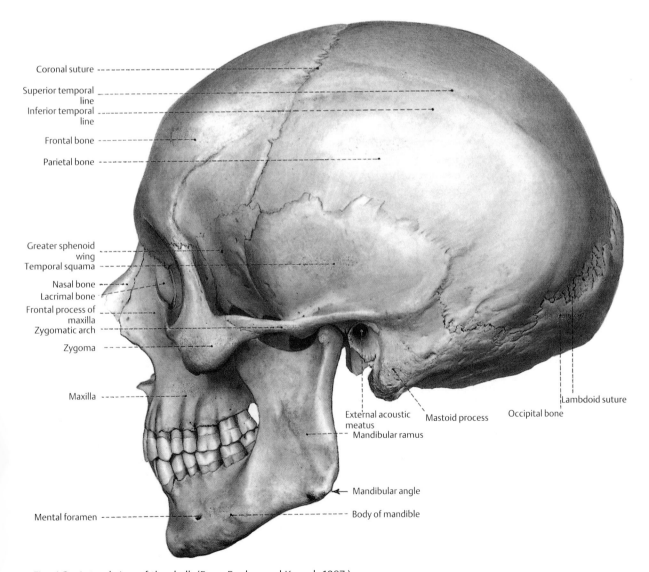

Fig. 4.**2** Lateral view of the skull. (From Rauber and Kopsch 1987.)

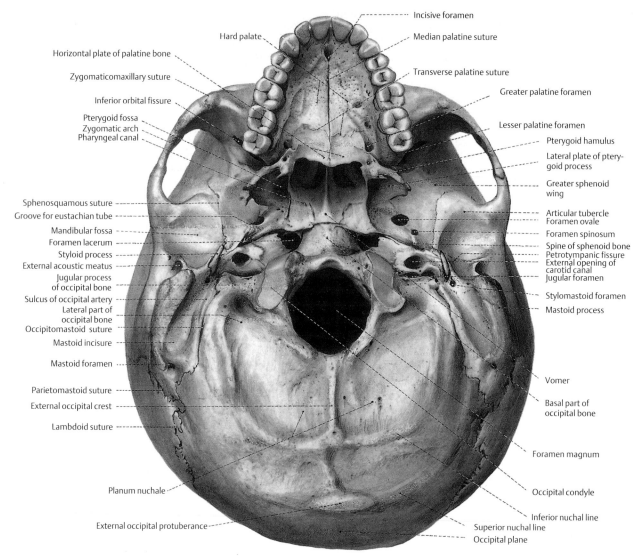

Fig. 4.**3**   External view of the skull base. (From Rauber and Kopsch 1987.)

Rostral to the parachordal cartilage are the pituitary cartilage and the cranial trabeculae. The fusion of these two elements gives rise to the body of the sphenoid bone and the ethmoid bone, resulting finally in an elongated medial cartilaginous plate that extends from the nasal region to the anterior rim of the foramen magnum. Lateral to this cartilaginous plate are additional chondral centers for the lesser sphenoid wing rostrally (from the ala orbitalis) and the greater sphenoid wing caudally (from the ala temporalis). They subsequently fuse with the medial plate, leaving apertures for the emergence of the cranial nerves (Fig. 4.**6a, b**).

The bony labyrinthine capsule, a third component that develops lateral to the parachordal cartilage, becomes the petrous part of the temporal bone. This fuses with the primitive temporal squama to form the definitive temporal bone. The mastoid process of the temporal bone does not

develop until after birth. Finally the original chondrocranium is transformed by endochondral ossification into the bony skull base.

Viscerocranium

The viscerocranium is basically derived from the first two branchial arches. The first branchial arch (mandibular arch) gives rise to the maxilla and mandible. The primitive maxilla arises from the upper portion of the first branchial arch (maxillary process) and the mandible from the lower portion (mandibular process). This includes a cartilaginous bar in the first branchial arch (Meckel cartilage). The rear ends of this cartilage combine with the Reichert cartilage (end of the cartilaginous bar of the second branchial arch) to form the primitive auditory ossicles. Ossification of the auditory ossicles begins in the fourth month of development. The definitive bones of the maxilla and mandible

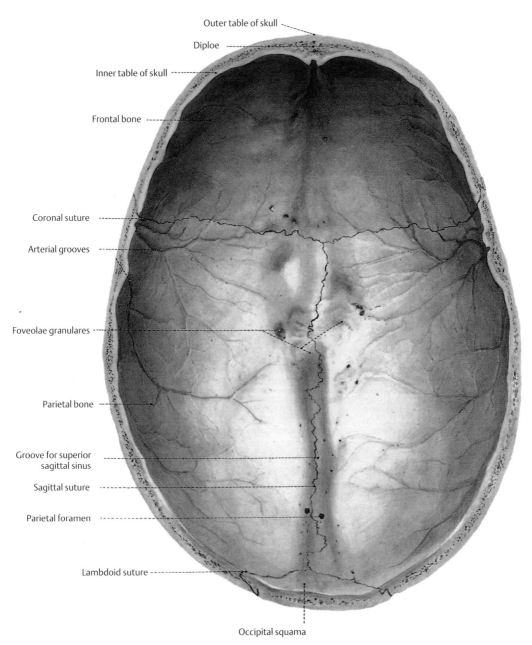

Outer table of skull
Diploe
Inner table of skull
Frontal bone
Coronal suture
Arterial grooves
Foveolae granulares
Parietal bone
Groove for superior sagittal sinus
Sagittal suture
Parietal foramen
Lambdoid suture
Occipital squama

Fig. 4.**4** Internal view of the calvarium. (From Rauber and Kopsch 1987.)

and the temporomandibular joint undergo membranous ossification (Fig. 4.**6c**).

The details described above provide an essential basis for understanding the following simplified classification, which is adequate for routine needs:
The skull develops from chondral centers and from membranous ossification of the flat bones encasing the central nervous system. The chondral centers ossify during ontogenesis and are replaced by bone (chondral bone, replacement bone). Only in the nasal skeleton are chondral elements preserved to form the nasal cartilages. The bones of the neurocranium that are preformed in cartilage are the skull base, the labyrinthine capsules, and a narrow strip around the back of the medulla oblongata, the tectum. Flat bones that are formed by membranous ossification are the cranial vault and portions of the cranial sidewalls. In the facial skeleton, the bones of the jaws and some elements of the nasal skeleton (nasal bone, lacrimal bone, and vomer) develop as flat bones.

Development of Skull Shape

The shape of the skull is determined equally by local intrinsic growth processes and by surrounding forces that shape the cranial bones (brain growth, masticatory apparatus, etc.). The cranial vault and facial skeleton grow at different rates. The growth of the calvarium depends largely on the development of the brain. This is less true of the skull base and the elements of the facial skeleton.

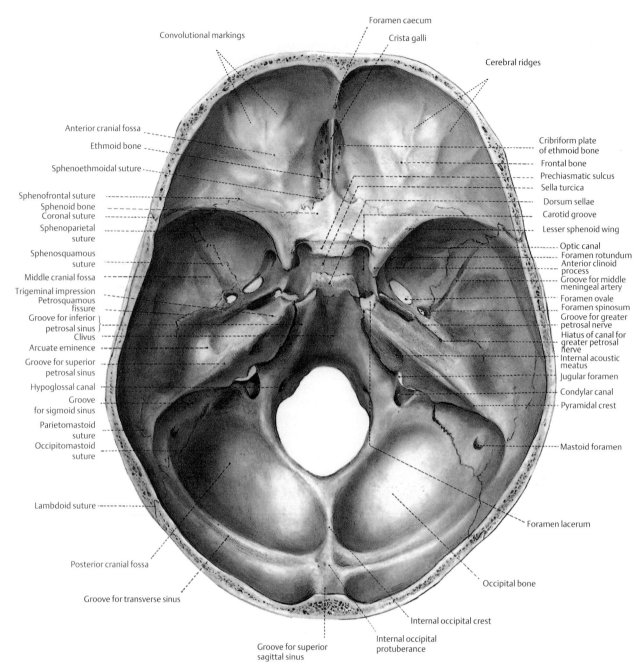

Fig. 4.5 The interior of the skull base. (From Rauber and Kopsch 1987.)

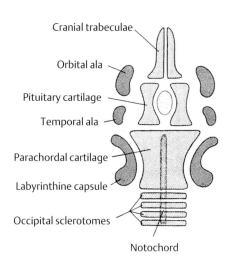

a

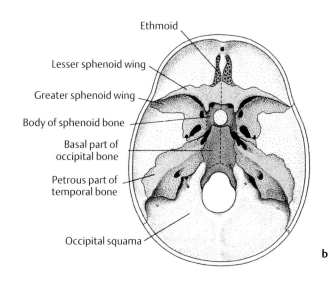

b

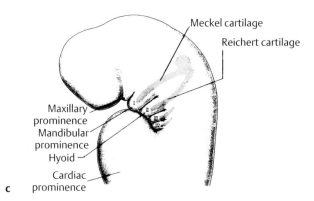

c

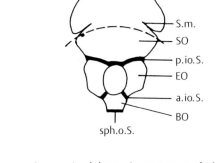

d

Fig. 4.6a–d
a Diagram of rudimentary structures important in the development of the skull base.
b View of the skull base (chondrocranium) in an adult, showing the definitive location of the rudimentary structures pictured in **a**.
c Branchial arches and branchial cartilages during the fourth week of embryonic development. (From Langman 1989.)
d Ossification centers of the occipital bone. (From Schinz 1986) (see Fig. 4.113.)

IP	Interparietal bone (upper part of the occipital squama)
S. m.	Sutura mendosa
SO	Supraoccipital (lower part of the occipital squama)
p. io. S.	Posterior intraoccipital synchondrosis
EO	Exoccipital
a. io. S.	Anterior intraoccipital synchondrosis
BO	Basioccipital
sph. o. S.	Spheno-occipital synchondrosis

The cranial vault is already quite large in newborns, while the facial skeleton still shows relatively little development (Table 4.1 and Fig. 4.7).

The volume of the cranial vault increases rapidly during fetal growth (Table 4.2). By 10 years of age, the brain has al-most reached its definitive volume. The reverse is true for the facial skeleton, as its development is linked to the function of the masticatory apparatus. Growth of the facial skeleton proceeds very slowly during infancy. The viscerocranium reaches approximately 25% of its defini-

Table 4.1   Development of the head: ratio of facial skeleton to cranial vault (from Rauber/Kopsch 1987)

Age	Ratio
Birth	1:8
2 years	1:6
5 years	1:4
10 years	1:3
Mature female	1:2.5
Mature male	1:2 (Fig. 4.7)

Table 4.2   Volume of the cranial vault, development from birth to adulthood (from Rauber/Kopsch 1987)

Age	Volume (cm³)
Birth	360–367
2 months	510–540
1 year	850–900
3 years	1010–1080
10 years	1250–1360
20 years	1300–1450

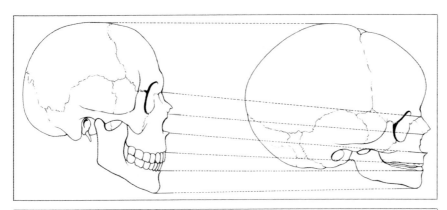

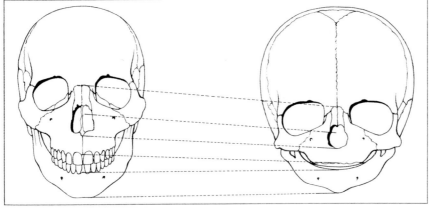

Fig. 4.**7** Changes in the proportions of the skull during growth: lateral and frontal views in an adult (left) and a newborn (right). (From Rauber and Kopsch 1987.)

tive size by one year of age and approximately 50% by 7 years of age. With the eruption of the permanent teeth and the associated development of the alveolar processes of the maxilla and mandible, a second growth spurt occurs. The greater functional demands placed on the masticatory muscles and the increasing pneumatization of the paranasal sinuses lead to a change in the shape and appearance of the facial skeleton. It attains its definite shape only after the teeth have fully erupted.

The Skull as a Whole

The neurocranium and viscerocranium are composed of individual bones that are linked together by sutures (ligament attachments), synchondroses (cartilaginous attachments), or synostoses (bone attachments). Exceptions are the temporomandibular joints connecting the mandible to the skull base, the connections between the auditory ossicles, and the suspension of the hyoid bone.

The bones of the cranial vault are composed of two layers of cortical bone (the outer and inner tables) separated by cancellous bone (the diploe). The **diploe** contains large-caliber venous channels that transmit the valveless diploic veins. These vessels establish a connection between the intracranial veins and the external veins of the head. The bones of the skull base have a comparable structure, but most contain a larger proportion of cancellous bone. The calvarium is ossified from five centers: one for each half of the frontal bone, two for the paired parietal bones, and one for the occipital squama. Initially the ossification centers are widely separated from one another. As the bones grow peripherally, they finally come together to form fontanelles and sutures. These **sutures** function less as growth centers than as seams that increase the elasticity of the skull. Usually the sutural tissue regresses completely in

adulthood, forming synostoses. Premature or asymmetrical closure of the sutures during growth leads to typical, familiar patterns of cranial deformity (p. 375, 389–392).

In addition to the physiological ossification centers of the calvarium, there are isolated ossific centers, rimmed by connective tissue, that are called **sutural bones** (ossa suturalia) because they are located within cranial sutures (Fig. 4.**8**). **Intercalary bones** (ossa intercalaria) are small bones that form an island within a larger cranial bone and are bounded by their own sutures (Fig. 4.**9 d**). These in-

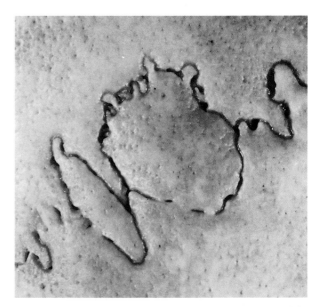

Fig. 4.**8** Sutural bone in the lambdoid suture in an adult. (From Rauber and Kopsch 1987.)

clude the **Inca bone** (os incae, incarial bone; Fig. 4.9 f), although the historical correctness of this term, implying a greater frequency among Inca Indians, is open to dispute. The distinction between sutural bones and intercalary bones is explained further on p. 369.

The sutures are smoother on the inner surface of the cranial vault than on its outer surface. But the inner table of the skull is furrowed and grooved, contrasting with its smooth outer surface (Figs. 4.2, 4.4, 4.5). **Arterial grooves** are most conspicuous in the parietal bones and stem from branches of the middle meningeal artery that run in the epidural space (Figs. 4.4., 4.5, 4.66, 4.112). The groove of the superior sagittal sinus, named for the homonymous dural venous sinus, is deeper occipitally than rostrally (Fig. 4.4). Lateral to this groove are small pits called the **foveolae granulares**; they are variable in size and number and are occupied by the arachnoid granulations (see also p. 369–373). The paramedian foveolae granulares are particularly numerous around the coronal suture. With aging, the calvarium around the foveolae (as elsewhere) thickens. As a result, the pits become deeper but do not increase in number.

The bony skull base is partly composed of sturdy "buttresses" like the petrous temporal bone, while other bony elements of the skull base are quite thin. The structural weak points include the orbital roof, the ethmoid plate, the base of the greater sphenoid wing, the mandibular fossa, the tegmen tympani, the temporal squama, the floor of the sella turcica, the lateral portions of the body of the sphenoid bone, the frequently thin wall between the groove for the transverse sinus and mastoid antrum, and the deepest point of the posterior cranial fossa (Figs. 4.1–4.5).

It should also be noted that the inner skull base can be subdivided into a middle region and paired lateral regions. The boundary between the middle and lateral regions is defined by a line connecting the anterior and posterior clinoid processes. The middle region is an angled area formed by the clivus, the sella turcica, the anterior body of the sphenoid bone, and by the ethmoid bone with the crista galli.

The anterior, middle, and posterior cranial fossae occupy the lateral regions in a multilevel, terraced arrangement (Fig. 4.5). The anterior fossa is the highest of the three and houses the frontal lobe of the cerebrum. Its inner surface bears distinct convolutional markings and cerebral ridges. The middle fossa houses the temporal lobe of the cerebrum. The posterior fossa is the deepest and largest of the three cranial fossae. It is bounded anteriorly by the posterior surface of the petrous temporal bone. The groove for the sigmoid sinus is usually deeper and broader on the

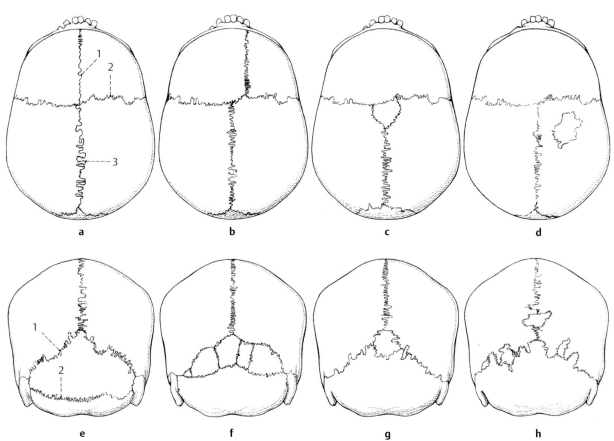

Fig. 4.9 Variants of sutures and accessory bones in the skull of an adult. (From Rauber and Kopsch 1987.) (See Figs. 4.**114**–4.**118**.)
a–d Superior aspect. **e–h** Posterior aspect
a Persistent frontal suture (metopic suture)
  1 Frontal suture
  2 Coronal suture
  3 Sagittal suture
b Asymmetrical location of a persistent frontal suture

c Fonticular bone (os bregmaticum) in the sagittal suture
d Intercalary bone
e Interparietal bone
  1 Lambdoid suture
  2 Transverse occipital suture
f Tripartite Inca bone with two-part center
g Apical bone, os apicis, preinterparietal bone.
h Sutural bones in the lambdoid and sagittal sutures

right side than on the left, corresponding to the width of the venous part of the jugular foramen. The occipital squama forms most of the floor of the posterior fossa.

Dura and Leptomeninges

The interior of the bony cranial cavity is lined by periosteum and the dura mater. The intracranial dura blends with the spinal dura at the foramen magnum, losing its attachment to the periosteum. The dura may be thought of as consisting of two layers: an outer layer (the periosteum lining the inner surface of the skull) and an inner layer (the actual dura mater). The outer layer, then, is adherent to the inner surface of the skull while the inner layer conforms more to the surface of the brain. This creates a number of potential spaces that include the dural sinuses and other expansions (e.g., for the pituitary and trigeminal ganglion).

The dural sinuses are large venous channels that receive the cerebral veins and drain chiefly to the internal jugular veins on both sides. The dura mater also forms septa. A sickle-shaped fold of dura mater, the falx cerebri, dips into the longitudinal cerebral fissure and forms a longitudinal brace. The tentorium is a transverse process that separates the two occipital lobes from the cerebellum and functions as a transverse brace for the skull. The falx cerebelli is a smaller fold that projects into the vallecula of the cerebellum. These three septa, along with the sellar diaphragm, are called the septal dura to distinguish them from the parietal dura. Together they comprise a function unit. The dura is separated from the arachnoid by a narrow space. The pia mater is a delicate layer of connective tissue that covers the surface of the brain and lines all of its sulci and fissures.

References

Skull, General Aspects

Frick, H., H. Leonhardt, D. Starck: Spezielle Anatomie II. Kopf-Hals-Eingeweide-Nervensystem. 2nd ed. Thieme, Stuttgart 1980
Langman, J.: Medizinische Embryologie. Die normale menschliche Entwicklung und ihre Fehlbildungen. 6th ed. Thieme, Stuttgart 1980

Rauber/Kopsch: Bewegungsapparat, Vol. I. Eds. Tillmann, B., G. Töndury. In Rauber/Kopsch: Anatomie des Menschen. Lehrbuch und Atlas, 1st ed. Eds. Leonhardt, H., B. Tillmann, G. Töndury, K. Zilles, Thieme, Stuttgart 1987

Cranial Vault

Normal Findings

 During Growth

The nature and extent of brain development influence the way in which the shape and size of the calvarium change with aging (Fig. 4.**7**). The proportional development of the cranial vault and facial skeleton was reviewed on p. 361–364 (Table 4.**1**), along with the progression of brain volume (Table 4.**2**). The sharpness of the cranial sutures on radiographs reflects the degree of activity of calvarial growth. The sharper the suture margins appear, the less the current growth activity of the adjacent bones. The **cranial index**, which provides information on the shape of the skull, is defined as the ratio of cranial width to cranial length, multiplied by 100. An index between 75 and 84 reflects a normal cranial configuration. An index less than 75 signifies a dolichocephalic skull shape, and an index higher than 84 indicates a brachycephalic pattern (Fig. 4.**10**).

The **Cronqvist index** gives a basic impression of skull size in children up to about 6 years of age. It is measured on standard skull radiographs using a film–focus distance of 80 cm. The index is calculated as the sum of the maximum width, length, and height of the cranial cavity divided by the distance between the inner margins of the necks of the mandibular condyles. The result is multiplied by 10. The normal range is between 51 and 57 with a standard deviation of ±2. Values less than 51 indicate a small neurocranium, and values greater than 57 indicate a large neurocranium (Fig. 4.**10**) (Cronqvist 1968). Additional measurement points on the outer surface of the skull are shown in Fig. 4.**11**. The advent of CT has increased both the practicality and precision of radiological craniometry (Boureks and Lanzieri 1994, Belden 1998). The growth of the ossification centers proceeds along the blood vessels. On radiographs in newborns, the individual bony plates of the cranial vault are separated from one another by spaces that may appear surprisingly broad. The radiographic widths are 3–17 mm for the sagittal suture and 1.5–11 mm for the coronal and lambdoid sutures. Anatomists have been unable to confirm this apparent radiographic variation in suture widths, but microradiographs have revealed thin bony plates that form the boundaries of the "true" normal-width sutures. The margins of the bony plates are not visible on standard radiographs because of their low bone mineral content. The actual postnatal width of the major cranial sutures is approximately 1 mm. The suture widths often increase further during the first month of life, showing a peak at about 2 weeks of age.

As a result of normal brain growth, there is a period from 1 to 3 years of age in which the sutures appear conspicuously wide and often show "fuzzy" margins. This should not be mistaken for abnormal suture spread.

During the first year of life, even standard skull films show the calvarial bone edges growing closer together, narrow-

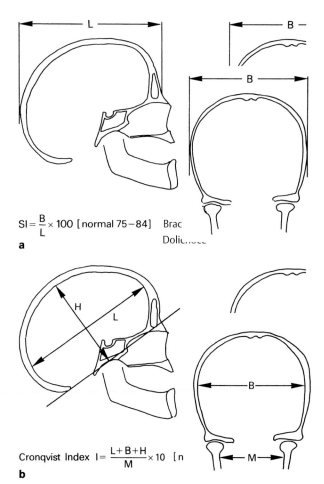

$$SI = \frac{B}{L} \times 100 \; [\text{normal } 75-84]$$

Brac
Dolic......

a

$$\text{Cronqvist Index} \quad I = \frac{L+B+H}{M} \times 10 \; [\text{n}$$

b

Fig. 4.**10 a, b**
a The cranial index (SI) for evaluating the shape of the skull.
b The Cronqvist index (I) for evaluating the size of the skull.
(From Schinz 1986.)

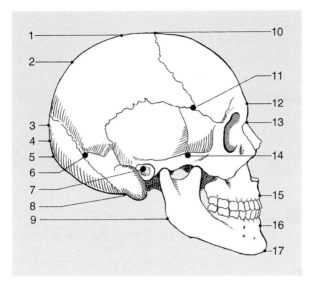

Fig. 4.**11**   Craniometric landmarks on the outside of the skull.

1   Vertex: highest point on the parietal bone
2   Obelion: location of the fontanelle obelia in the parietal bone
3   Lambda: vertex of the angle formed by the lambdoid sutures
4   Opisthocranium: most posterior point on the skull viewed from the side
5   Inion: external occipital protuberance
6   Asterion: point where the mastoid process, parietal bone, and occipital squama intersect
7   Porion: highest point on the roof of the external auditory canal
8   Basion: most anterior point on the rim of the foramen magnum
9   Gonion: most lateral point on the angle of the mandible
10 Bregma: vertex of the obtuse angle formed by the coronal suture
11 Pterion: suture segment located at the anterior lateral fontanelle
12 Glabella: depression in the frontal bone located between the supraorbital tubercles
13 Nasion: point at the root of the nose
14 Zygoma: point over the center of the zygomatic arch
15 Prosthion: point on the alveolar process of the maxilla between the central incisors
16 Infradentale: tip of the mental protuberance between the mandibular central incisors
17 Gnathion: lowest point on the anterior mental protuberance

ing the sutures to a width of 0.5–1 mm. (Normal values for suture widths in children can be found in Schuster and Tamacha, 1996.) During the first months of life, the sutures are straight and smooth or have a slightly wavy configuration. With the development of the diploe at about 12 months of age, the inner and outer tables separate. Both tables retain their sutures, which keep their smooth margins in the inner table but become serrated in the outer table. This process is complete by the third year of life at the latest.

> The suture line in the inner table of the skull is not always centered precisely below the suture line in the outer table. Occasionally this offset can mimic a thin fracture line.

The large anterior fontanelle is about the size of a fingertip from 12 to 18 months of age. The posterior fontanelle is already very narrow at birth and closes in approximately the third postnatal month. The lateral fontanelles (the sphenoidal and mastoid fontanelles) close by the second year of life. In newborns and small children, a step may occur at the boundary between the membranous portion of the occipital squama and the part of the squama that is preformed in cartilage. This step usually disappears during growth.

In Adulthood

> The normal cranial vault measures approximately 18 cm in length, 16 cm in width, and 13 cm in height (outer dimensions).

A skull with these proportions is described as mesocephalic. **Dolichocephaly** describes a skull that is at the long end of the normal range, **brachycephaly** a skull at the short end of the normal range (Fig. 4.**10**). Radiographic skull measurements have little practical importance, because growth abnormalities can be detected more easily and reliably by the clinical measurement of head circumference. If hydrocephalus is suspected, the patient can be referred for appropriate imaging studies (ultrasound, CT, MRI) without delay.

> The morphological variants described above (dolichocephaly and brachycephaly), along with bathrocephaly, are normal variants that do not have pathological significance.

Allocephaly is a general term applied to skulls with an abnormal size and/or shape. It includes macrocephaly, microcephaly, and stenocephaly (craniosynostosis) with their various subforms. The cranial index can provide a general impression of cranial shape (Fig. 4.**10**). The presence of a posterior, steplike projection of the occipital squama past the parietal bones is called **bathrocephaly** (Fig. 4.**12**).

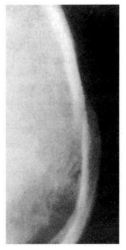

Fig. 4.**12**   Overlapping occipital squama (bathrocephaly)

Cranial Sutures and Sutural Bones/Intercalary Bones

The normal cranial sutures are easily identified by their constant location and their characteristic serrations (in the outer table). The suture lines in the inner table are straighter and are not always centered below the serrated lines in the outer table. As a result, separate radiolucent lines may appear in portions of the inner table and can mimic fracture lines. The temporal suture is occasionally mistaken for a fracture line when viewed in the sagittal projection. In the lateral projection, the serrations of the sagittal suture can sometimes appear as vertical striations near the vertex (Fig. 4.**11**). Again, this is a normal finding that is unrelated to the "hair-on-end" appearance of the skull in anemia, especially thalassemia. Another variant is **sutural hyperostosis** (sutural sclerosis) in adults. This most commonly affects the coronal, temporal, and lambdoid sutures (Fig. 4.**13**). A persistent frontal suture (metopic suture) is found in 5–8% of adults (Figs. 4.**1**, 4.**9a**). A special suture variant with a persistent sutural bone which one could call metopic or preinterfrontal bone is described on p. 405, 406 (Fig. 4.**87**).

Cranial suture variants occur predominantly in the occipital bone. Particularly in children, these variants can cause confusion with skull fractures. **Suture variants** are rooted in embryonic development and are most prevalent in the occiput because that bone develops from four ossification centers grouped around the foramen magnum. The occipital squama itself is formed from a cartilaginous supraoccipital center and from a membranous interparietal center. Between them is the lateral suture (**sutura mendosa**) (Fig. 4.**171**). If this suture is complete, it is called the transverse occipital suture and separates the interparietal bone (Inca bone) from the occiput. Additional ossification centers may appear near the embryonic occiput. If they remain isolated, they can form accessory sutures and sutural bones.

Sutural bones (Figs. 4.**8**, 4.**9h**) are small to medium-size bony structures that are located in the sutures between the cranial bones and are surrounded by connective tissue. Isolated sutural bones can occur in both the inner and outer tables. Sutural bones located in the fontanelles are called **fonticular bones** (Figs. 4.**9c**). An example is the preinter-

parietal bone (os apicis, Fig. 4.**9g**), which is probably a special fonticular type of sutural bone. Sutural bones, called also **wormian bones** after the Danish anatomist O. Wormius, most commonly occur in the lambdoid suture; they are much less common in the sagittal and coronal sutures. Sutural bones occurring in a persistent frontal suture are extremely rare (see Fig. 4.**87**).

> Individual sutural bones have no pathological significance, but multiple sutural bones may signify a generalized ossification disturbance (more than 10 sutural bones at least 4 mm × 6 mm in size and arranged in a mosaic-like pattern are considered pathological). The most frequent causes of multiple sutural bones are listed in Table 4.**3**.

The normal cranial sutures are so variable and distinctive in their individual appearance that they can provide a reliable means of personal identification.

Intercalary bones are small bones that form an island within a larger cranial bone. They arise from independent ossification centers and are rimmed by their own sutures (Fig. 4.**9d**). They are usually located near sutural junction sites, especially between the occiput, mastoid, and parietal squama. There have been rare reports of skulls that consisted predominantly of intercalary bones. The interparietal bone (Inca bone, Fig. 4.**9f**) is a familiar example of an intercalary bone.

Blood Vessels, Vascular Markings, Nutrient Canals, and Vascular Grooves in the Calvarium

The various blood vessels that run on and through the calvarium contribute significantly to the structure of the cranial vault. A large range of variation is encountered. Accentuated vascular markings occur in conditions that are associated with increased perfusion of the vessels, calvarium, meninges, or scalp, including meningiomas, AV malformations, fibrous dysplasia, Paget disease, and collateral flow through meningeal arteries due to arterial occlusions. A unilateral increase in vascular markings is particularly suspicious for a pathological condition.

The "vascular markings" seen on radiographs represent the sum of the vascular grooves in the inner table, the nutrient canals in the diploe, the sinus grooves, and the pacchionian granulations. The prominence of the vascular markings is highly variable, ranging from an almost featureless calvarium to a skull that is heavily permeated by vascular canals (Fig. 4.**14**).

It can be extremely difficult to draw a boundary line between normal and pathological findings.

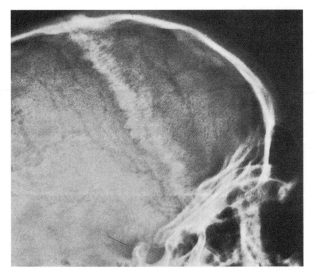

Fig. 4.**13** Very heavy sclerosis of the coronal suture.

Table 4.**3** Principal causes of multiple sutural bones (from Schinz 1986)

Multiple sutural bones
• Idiopathic
• Cleidocranial dysplasia (dysostosis)
• Osteogenesis imperfecta
• Down syndrome
• Hypothyroidism
• Hypophosphatasia
• Hajdu–Cheney syndrome

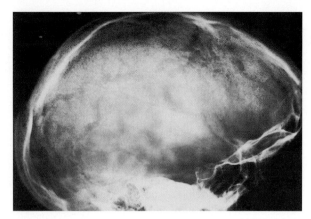

Fig. 4.**14** Venous markings and distinct convolutional markings in the skull.

> A vascular structure typically appears as an elongated, bandlike lucency that runs a straight or tortuous course. Thus, a lucency in the calvarium should be identified as a blood vessel if it exhibits the anatomic course of a vessel.

Several different types of vascular structures may be observed in the calvarium:

Meningeal Vascular Grooves

The extradural meningeal arteries and veins can produce vascular grooves in the inner table of the skull (Figs. 4.**15**, 4.**35**, 4.**52**, 4.**66**, 4.**67**). They first appear during the second or third year of life. They are distinguished from nutrient canals in the diploe by their regularity and the consistency of their course and caliber. Several patterns are seen:

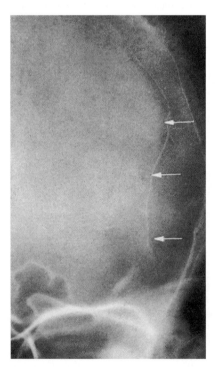

Fig. 4.**15** Groove for the fronto-orbital vein in a child (arrows).

- Straight or slightly curved
- Uniform tapering toward the periphery
- Dichotomous branching

The course of the vascular grooves basically follows the distribution of the middle meningeal artery and its branches, regardless of whether they are caused by the arteries or their accompanying veins.

After entering the skull through the foramen spinosum, the middle meningeal artery ascends along the floor and lateral wall of the middle skull base and divides into a frontal branch and an occipital branch. These branches can be identified after reaching a point above or behind the lateral extension of the lesser sphenoid wing. The frontal branch ascends toward the parietal bone and follows the coronal suture, while the occipital branch runs toward the lambdoid suture, where it divides into additional branches. These vascular grooves are so sharply defined in the thin temporal squama that they may be mistaken for thin fracture lines (Figs. 4.**66**, 4.**67**, 4.**112**). They are distinguished from fracture lines by the presence of increased marginal density at some point along the course of the vascular canal.

Spot films and CT scans can demonstrate another distinguishing feature. Unlike meningeal vascular grooves, fracture lines generally involve the full thickness of the calvarium. The bilateral occurrence of vascular grooves provides another differentiating feature. One additional special feature should also be noted: Between the sphenoid wing and bregma (point at the frontoparietal junction of the coronal and sagittal sutures, see Fig. 4.**11**), the dural vein often runs separate from the artery in its own vascular groove, which is larger than the groove for the meningeal artery (sphenoparietal sinus, bregmatic vein).

Grooves for the Dural Sinuses

The dural sinuses occupy grooves of variable depth and width in the inner table of the calvarium. The grooves for the transverse sinus (Fig. 4.**121 a**) and sigmoid sinus are the most distinct and are usually larger on the right side.

Nutrient Canals and Lacunae in the Diploe

Generally the diploic veins are not visible before the third year of life and are not fully developed until about 15 years of age. They may be very prominent in elderly patients due the associated atrophy of the calvarium. The prominence of the diploic venous system is extremely variable, ranging from almost a complete absence of veins to a very dense and extensive vascular network. The diploic veins communicate with the dural sinuses, the meningeal veins, and the veins of the pericranium. Since they do not have their own bony walls, they appear on radiographs as irregular bandlike or rounded lucencies that correlate with the caliber, course, and branching pattern of the veins.

Four main drainage trunks for the diploic veins can be identified on each side:

- Frontal diploic vein
- Anterior temporal vein
- Posterior temporal vein
- Occipital vein

The diploic veins are most conspicuous in the posterior part of the parietal bones, which is why they are seen with the greatest frequency, where they often show a stellate or radial type of arrangement (Figs. 4.**16**, 4.**17**, 4.**18**). When viewed in an end-on projection, they appear as small

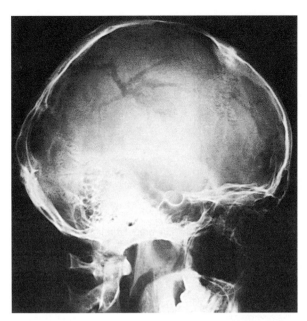

Fig. 4.**16** Stellate venous markings in the parietal bone of an 18-year-old male.

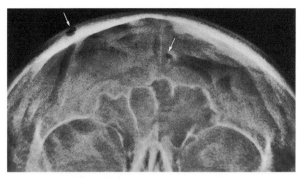

Fig. 4.**17** Frontal bone: venous channels and their "foramina" in the diploe (arrows).

"punched-out" lucencies in the diploe (Fig. 4.**17**). Diploic veins that are unusually broad (varicose?) are called **venous lacunae**.

> Venous lacunae are sometimes difficult to distinguish from foci of bone destruction on conventional radiographs. One differentiating feature is that tumors tend to destroy all layers of the calvarium, whereas venous lacunae are confined to the area within the diploe, exhibit a relatively sharp and slightly lobulated margin, and have a draining vascular canal.

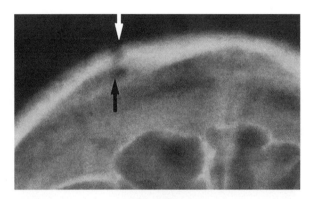

Fig. 4.**18** Venous channel (arrows).

Canals for Emissary Veins

The veins that connect the large dural sinuses with the diploic veins or scalp veins are called emissary veins. They have their own bony walls and traverse the calvarium through short canals. They are highly variable in number and configuration, but the mastoid and occipital emissary veins around the external occipital protuberance are the most consistent (Fig. 4.**19**). The parietal emissary veins pass through the parietal foramen near the midline 3–4 cm above the lambdoid suture (Figs. 4.**99**, 4.**101**). The frontal emissary veins (Figs. 4.**90**, 4.**91**) and condylar emissary veins are rare.

Emissary veins occurring at other sites in the calvarium are considered atypical but still normal anatomic variants.

Pacchionian Granulations (Foveolae granulares, Arachnoid Granulations, Arachnoid Villi, Arachnoid Diverticula)

The cerebrospinal fluid (CSF) is reabsorbed through intradural arachnoid villi or pacchionian granulations and drains into the dural sinuses (Fig. 4.**20**). These arachnoid villi (arachnoid diverticula) or pacchionian granulations form pitlike depressions in the inner table and diploe that can vary greatly in size (Figs. 4.**21**–4.**24**). They range from 10 mm to several centimeters in diameter. The latter can cause extreme thinning of the calvarium with a watch-glasslike bulging of the outer table (Figs. 4.**23**, 4.**120**). Foveolae granulares are most commonly observed in the

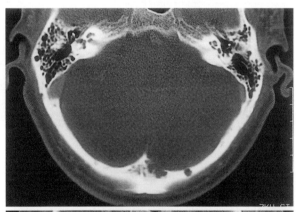

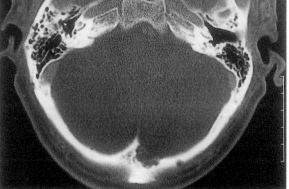

Fig. 4.**19** Typical appearance of an emissary vein near the external occipital protuberance (CT using a high-resolution bone filter).

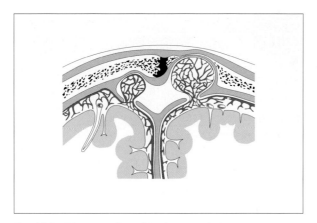

Fig. 4.**20**   Diagram of pacchionian granulations.

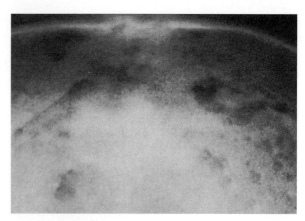

Fig. 4.**21**   Large pacchionian granulations or deep vascular grooves.

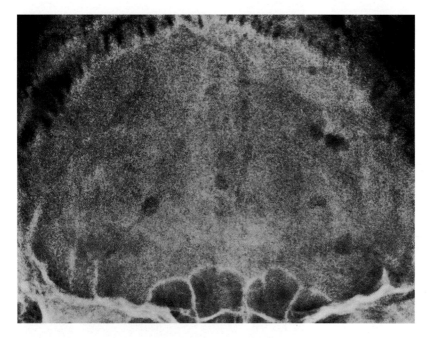

Fig. 4.**22**   Pacchionian granulations with typical inflow and outflow vein and ill-defined margins. The granulations are most commonly found in the frontal bone.

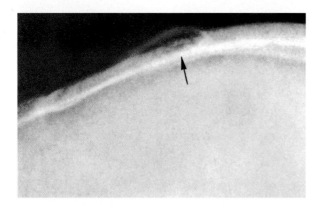

Fig. 4.**23**   Blisterlike bulge in the outer table (arrow) caused by vascular grooves.

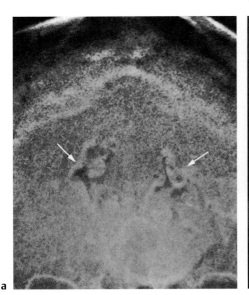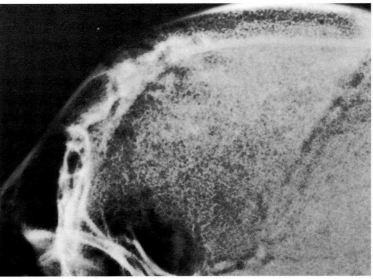

a   b

Fig. 4.**24a, b** Vascular grooves/-pits or pacchionian granulations with coexisting hyperostosis frontalis interna (arrows). They cannot be distinguished by projection radiographs, but this is of no consequence in asymptomatic patients.

frontal region (Fig. 4.**24**). The second most common region is the parietal, where they reportedly are larger. They occur rarely in the occipital region, where they may reach considerable size and are most likely to be mistaken for pathological changes (Fig. 4.**120**). Pacchionian granulations tend to be distributed along the dural sinuses and are rarely located more than 3 cm from them (e.g., from the superior sagittal sinus). They are positively identified on projection radiographs by noting their close relationship to a vascular canal (Fig. 4.**22**). Diagnostic confusion can arise in cases where foveolae granulares are unusually large or are associated with headache, usually in older patients. The differential diagnostic spectrum ranges from metastatic bone destruction to circumscribed osteoporosis in Paget disease. Hamers et al. (2000) used a CSF-suppressing FLAIR sequence to show the relationship of pacchionian granulations to the subarachnoid space (Fig. 4.**120**). CT was unable to show a definite relationship to blood vessels or meningeal structures. This study also explored the clinical aspects of pacchionian granulations (primary and secondary posttraumatic) based on a review of the literature. If an MR imaging unit is unavailable, radionuclide scanning can advance the diagnosis by excluding metastatic bone destruction and Paget disease changes (absence of increased tracer uptake in the area of the foveolae). It is unnecessary to differentiate foveolae granulares from vascular grooves or vascular pits.

Thickness and Density of the Calvarium

The normal subdivision of the calvarium into an inner table, outer table, and intervening diploe is not well developed until about 12 months of age. The inner and outer tables consist of cortical bone, while the diploe is cancellous. The thickness of the calvarium is normally determined chiefly by the diploe, which comprises approximately two-thirds of the total thickness. Calvarial thickness is subject to large interindividual and intraindividual variations, ranging from a few millimeters to more than 1 cm. Certain portions of the calvarium are notably thin, such as the region of the bregma (Fig. 4.**11**), the temporal

squama, and the area between the occipital protuberance and lambdoid suture. The relatively high radiolucency of these areas compared with the thicker surrounding calvarium can mimic osteolysis (Fig. 4.**25a**). We observed one case of extreme "thinning" of the calvarium with fusion of the inner and outer tables in a 15-year-old boy (Fig. 4.**25b–d**). The differential diagnosis includes arachnoid cysts and diverticula that have led to calvarial thinning.

The "**parietal foramina**," which require differentiation from circumscribed atrophic foci in the calvarium, are hereditary bone defects that typically are bilaterally symmetrical and are located 1 cm from the midsagittal plane and 3–4 cm above the lambdoid suture in the parietal bone (see p. 408–410).

The thickest areas of the calvarium are the internal and external occipital protuberances and the parietal tubera. The external occipital protuberance often bears a spurlike prominence (**occipital spur**) located at the attachment of the nuchal ligament. The thickness of the cranial vault often increases with aging.

Convolutional Markings and Cerebral Ridges

The inner surface of the calvarium is marked by depressions corresponding to the gyri of the brain (convolutional markings) and by thicker, intervening bony ridges corresponding to the cerebral sulci (cerebral ridges). The prominence of these features is dependent on constitution and age (Figs. 4.**5**, 4.**26**). Skull radiographs in children consistently demonstrate inner table convolutional markings and cerebral ridges. Their absence at this age may signify a disturbance of normal brain development. The convolutional markings normally disappear around puberty, but traces of them may persist into adulthood and should not be interpreted as abnormal unless there are additional, definite signs of increased intracranial pressure such as suture spreading, changes in the sella turcica, or serial changes. The possible regression of convolutional markings after the surgical removal of tumors causing increased intracranial pressure and their reappearance after tumor recurrence prove that the markings were pathological. One should be careful in interpreting this "symptom," es-

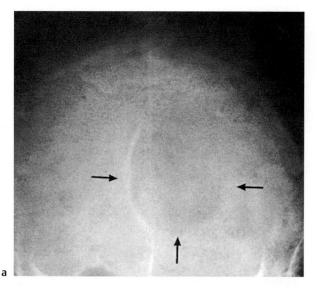

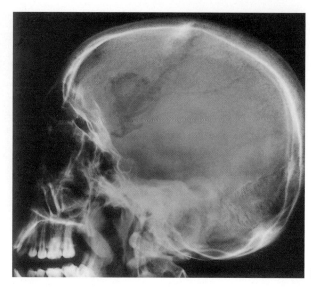

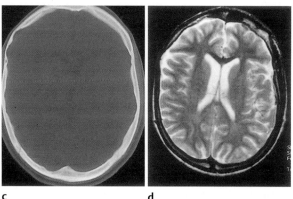

Fig. 4.**25** **a** Localized thinning of the occipital bone (arrows) detected incidentally. When similar thinning was noted in the frontal bone, CT revealed complete "obliteration" of the diploe with apparent fusion of the inner and outer tables.
b–d (different patient from that in **a**)
b Right frontotemporal thinning of the calvarium, resembling osteolysis, detected incidentally in a 15-year-old boy.
c CT shows outward bulging of the outer table with obliteration of the inner table and diploe.
d T2-weighted MRI shows that the "space" contains CSF.

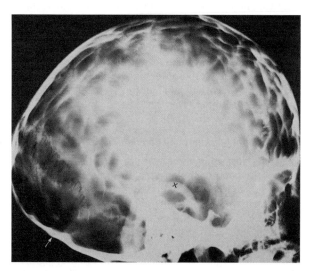

Fig. 4.**26** Premature fusion of the coronal suture and part of the lambdoid suture with accentuated convolutional markings in a 9-year-old boy with severe headaches. Arrow indicates the transverse sulcus.
× Auricle of the ear

pecially in patients under 15 years of age. Unilateral prominence or prominence at a circumscribed site should be considered pathological.

Convolutional markings can be demonstrated throughout life in the skull base (orbital roof, floor of middle fossa) and in basal portions of the calvarium. They appear as round or oval lucencies with indistinct margins, separated by intervening ridges of higher density (Figs. 4.**14**, 4.**26**). The thinner the calvarium, the more prominent the convolutional markings appear on radiographs. They are most commonly observed in the frontal and occipital regions. It has been well established that the convolutional markings and cerebral ridges are a result of brain development and CSF pulsations.

Physiological Calcifications

These are intracranial calcifications that are unaccompanied by any evidence of disease and have no demonstrable pathological cause. They include calcifications of the pineal gland, habenular calcifications, choroid plexus calcifications, meningeal calcifications, as well as certain idiopathic calcifications of the basal ganglia and vessel walls. Falx calcifications can also occur. The frequency with which these calcifications are detected in older patients and their lack of diagnostic, therapeutic, and prognostic significance justify their classification as physiological calcifications. There are exceptions, however. Intracranial calcifications are discussed more fully on p. 380–386.

Pathological Finding?

Normal Variant/Anomaly?

Changes in Size, Shape, Thickness, and Density of the Calvarium

Macrocephaly

The most frequent cause of this condition is hydrocephalus. Other causes consist of diseases that lead to head enlargement due to thickening of the calvarium with no intracranial changes and diseases that cause head enlargement as a result of macroencephaly. In achondroplasia (Fig. 4.**27**), the shortening of the skull base can mimic macrocephaly. The Cronqvist index (Fig. 4.**10**) provides only a general impression of cranial size in children up to about 6 years of age and cannot be used in adults.

Microcephaly

Aside from craniosynostosis, microcephaly almost always results from deficient brain development or microen-

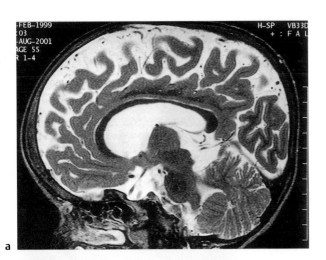

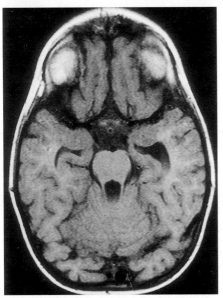

Fig. 4.27 Typical MRI appearance of achondroplasia in a 2.5-year-old child (skull films were not available).

cephaly. The smallness of the cranial vault leads to a disproportion between the viscerocranium and neurocranium. This results in other typical radiographic findings such as a low, sloped forehead; high, rounded supraorbital ridges; thickening of the calvarium with narrow sutures prone to secondary synostosis; and an absence of normal convolutional markings and cerebral ridges on the inner table (Fig. 4.**14**). In a broader sense, microcephaly can be considered to include cranial asymmetries that result from unilateral brain injury in early childhood (see below). As noted under General Aspects, a lack of growth stimulus from the brain causes the affected hemicranium to remain small. The calvarium in that region is thickened and flattened while the skull base, sphenoid wing, and petrous pyramid are elevated. The midline structures (crista galli, pineal calcifications, etc.) may be shifted toward the affected side.

The various causes of macrocephaly and microcephaly are listed in Table 4.**4**.

Asymmetries

Asymmetries and other deformities of the skull in infants and small children can be a result of positioning. This is particularly true in cases where statomotor development is impaired and the child lies predominantly on one side of the head or on the occiput. Accordingly, these deformities most commonly affect the occiput or the parietal bones. The principal causes of cranial asymmetry in children are listed in Table 4.**5**.

Cephalhematomas, which usually result from obstetric trauma, can mimic cranial asymmetry.

Table 4.**4** Macrocranium and microcranium (from Schinz 1986)

Macrocranium
1 Hydrocephalus
2 Diseases associated with thickening of the calvarium and no intracranial changes, such as: – Paget disease – Acromegaly – Mediterranean anemia
3 Diseases associated with macrocephaly such as: – Phacomatoses (especially neurofibromatosis) – Storage diseases
4 Pseudomacrocephaly, as in achondroplasia and other forms of growth retardation
Microcranium
1 Microcephaly due to any cause
2 Craniosynostosis, genetic defects

Table 4.**5** Principal causes of cranial asymmetry in children

• Deformity caused by positioning the infant predominantly on one side (usually combined with infantile scoliosis and a "crooked lie" type of hip deformity) and cranial asymmetry due to torticollis
• Plagiocephaly due to unilateral premature suture closure (see p. 392)
• Unilateral brain atrophy (Fig. 4.**28**)
• Unilateral mass lesion (e.g., tumor, arachnoid cyst, meningioma, large osteoma [Fig. 4.**29**, older patient])
• Neurofibromatosis (usually combined with macrocephaly and hemihypertrophy)
• Progressive facial hemiatrophy (Parry–Romberg syndrome) (literature in Kirchhof et al. 2000)

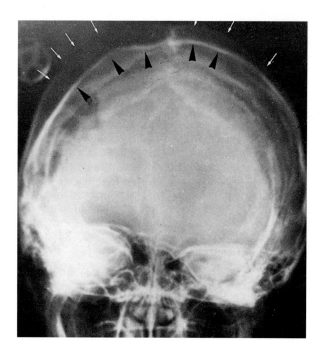

Fig. 4.**28** Cranial asymmetry with right-sided cerebral hemiatrophy and calvarial thickening on the right side (arrows and arrowheads). Note the elevation of the right pyramid and orbital roof and the dilatation of the right frontal sinus.

a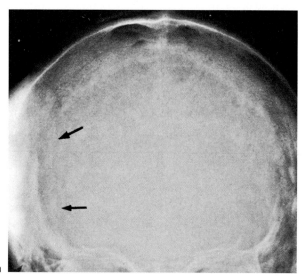

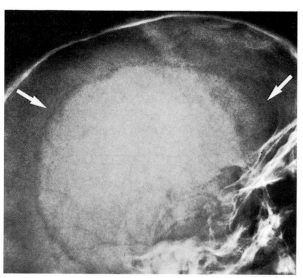 b

Fig. 4.**29 a, b**   Sharply circumscribed osteoma located at the junction of the calvarium and petrous bone (arrows) in an 82-year-old woman. The differential diagnosis would include meningioma en plaque.

Decreased Calvarial Thickness and Density

The radiographic appearance of the calvarium can vary considerably due to variations in the structural pattern and vascular markings of the calvarium and diploe. It can show varying degrees of density, fine or coarse porosity, or even a granular structure (Figs. 4.**30**–4.**32**). Normal growth and aging processes can also significantly affect the thickness and density of the calvarium.

Osteoporosis of the calvarium occurs with aging but is difficult to diagnose without comparison views. The calvarium, unlike the axial skeleton, is not considered a radiographic test region for osteoporosis. **Osteomalacia** is easier to diagnose, as it is distinguished by a more uniform, hazy, ground-glass type of bone structure that has a "rubbed out" appearance on radiographs.

The calvarial changes in **hyperparathyroidism** (Fig. 4.**33**) are characterized by a granular appearance ("salt-and-pepper skull") and loss of the normal three-layered structure. Basilar impression can develop in severe cases. It should be added that a patchy or uniform increase in calvarial density may be seen in atypical forms of primary hyperparathyroidism.

When decalcification of the calvarium occurs, the vascular markings in the diploe stand out more prominently than normal, and the vascular grooves in the inner table often appear more distinct. There are also marked changes in the skull base (Fig. 4.**32**), where a loss of calcium salts can lead to greater lucency of the sella turcica. This should not be misinterpreted as a sign of increased intracranial pressure. A sella that becomes lucent with aging

Fig. 4.**30**   Coarse porous structure of the cal-varium in a 31-year-old man.

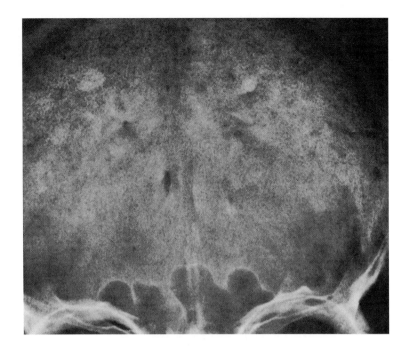

Fig. 4.**31**   Typical age-related changes in the skull of an 81-year-old woman (arrowheads).

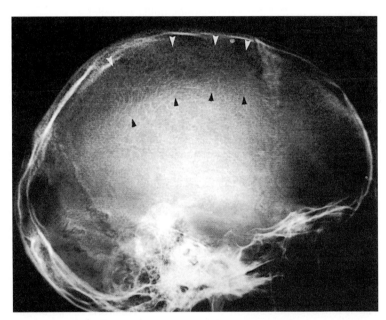

Fig. 4.**32 a, b**   CT of the skull base in a 92-year-old woman who was examined after head trauma. The patchy demineralized areas in the skull base are normal for this age.

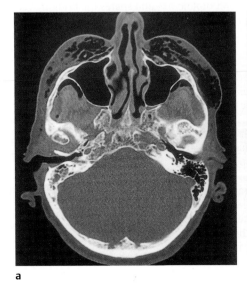
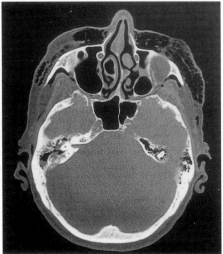

a   b

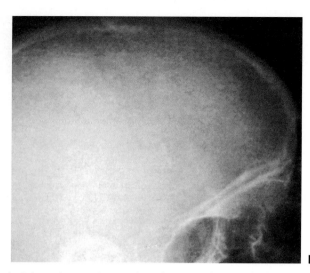

a

b

Fig. 4.**33 a, b** Hyperparathyroidism.
a Skull film shows basilar impression.

b Enlarged view shows salt-and-pepper demineralization of the calvarium with loss of differentiation of the inner and outer tables.

still retains its normal shape and contours, unlike the sellar expansion that occurs as a result of increased pressure.

Circumscribed or **"pitting" atrophy** of the calvarium affects the diploe and outer table of the cranial part of the parietal bones. A frontal view of the skull shows severe thinning and flattening of the parietal bones adjacent to the midline. These changes are symmetrically disposed and are easily identified by their typical location. Differentiation is required from **parietal foramina** bone defects with a familial occurrence that typically show a bilaterally symmetrical distribution (usually about 1 cm from the midsagittal plane and 3–4 cm above the lambdoid suture in the parietal bone). Most are only a few millimeters in size, but occasional **"giant" foramina** reach a diameter of several centimeters (see p. 408–410, Figs. 4.**99**–4.**101**). The parietal foramina provide openings for the passage of emissary veins and have no pathological significance. The adjacent calvarium terminates smoothly at the defects and shows no discontinuities.

The differential diagnosis can be more difficult in patients with spotty or granular atrophy of the calvarium. This is a radiographic sign of osteopenia or osteoporosis that is found in older patients. Patchy calvarial lucencies develop due to increased bone resorption around diploic vessels, causing the vessels to appear more prominent on radiographic films.

Increased Calvarial Thickness and Density

The imaging features of sutural sclerosis were described on p. 369 (Fig. 4.**13**). Fusion of the cranial sutures may be accompanied by bandlike areas of increased density due to perisutural sclerosis of the diploe. This is seen most clearly and frequently in the coronal suture, lambdoid suture, and temporal suture. Because the temporal squama is very thin, bony ridges and hyperostoses are especially conspicuous in that region. They may project over the sella turcica in the lateral view, creating the appearance of calcifications. Conversely, portions of the temporal squama that are very heavily pneumatized may be mistaken for osteolytic lesions in or around the sellar region of the skull base. Various causes of increased calvarial density are reviewed in Tables 4.**12** and 4.**13**.

Hyperostosis frontalis interna

Hyperostosis frontalis interna (hyperostosis cranialis interna) is a thickening of the inner table of the frontal bone that occurs chiefly in women during and after menopause. It is present in almost 40% of women over 50 years of age. In Morgagni–Stewart–Morel syndrome, the frontal hyperostosis may be accompanied by obesity, virilization, headache, and psychoneurological symptoms. It is also considered a part of Troell–Junet syndrome, which consists of acromegaly, diabetes mellitus, and thyrotoxicosis in addition to frontal hyperostosis. The causal connection is disputed, however, due to the overall frequency of inner table hyperostosis of the frontal bone. Hyperostosis frontalis interna is approximately twice as common in diabetics as in nondiabetics. It usually presents radiographically with thickening and increased density of the frontal bone (Figs. 4.**34**, 4.**35**). **Nebula frontalis** is merely a special form of the condition (Fig. 4.**35**). Bone deposition arising from the dura occurs on the deep surface of the inner table. The hyperostosis may also involve the diploe. Skull films are pathognomonic, showing a bilateral, symmetrical hyperostosis that stops at the edge of the superior sagittal sinus and spares the bridging veins that drain into the sinus. The frontal bone is typically affected, but the hyperostosis may also affect the anterior portions of the parietal bone or may even involve the calvarium diffusely (**hyperostosis calvaria diffusa**) (Table 4.**6**).

Table 4.**6** Different radiographic presentations of hyperostosis cranialis interna

- Nodular hyperostosis of the frontal bone (Fig. 4.**34**)
- Patchy hyperostosis in the upper part of the frontal bone (nebula frontalis) (Fig. 4.**35**)
- Frontoparietal hyperostosis with thickening of the affected cranial bone
- Hyperostosis calvaria diffusa

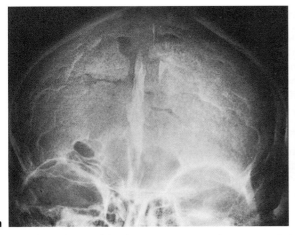
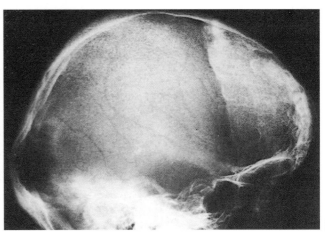

a

b

Fig. 4.**34a, b** Nodular hyperostosis cranialis interna of the frontal bone.
a PA projection additionally shows ossification of the falx.

b Lateral projection shows that the process is confined to the frontal bone.

Fig. 4.**35** Nebula frontalis. Note the grooves for the meningeal vessels.

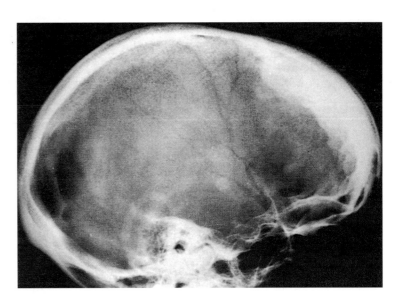

Excessive hematopoietic activity in the blood-forming marrow spaces of the diploe, especially in **thalassemia**, can lead to enlargement of the diploic spaces with thinning of the outer table and a "**hair-on-end**" appearance of the skull (Fig. 4.**36**). Rarely, this finding is also observed in severe secondary anemias (Fig. 4.**37**).

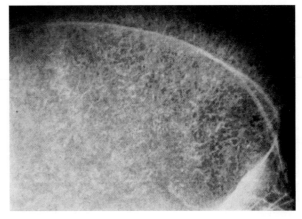

Fig. 4.**36** "Hair on end" appearance of the calvarium (frontal bone) in thalassemia major.

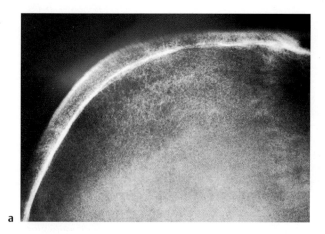

a

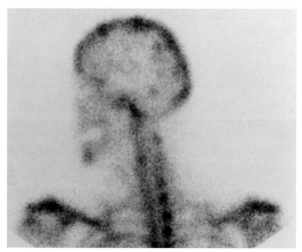

b

Fig. 4.**37 a, b**   "Hair on end" appearance of the calvarium due to lymphoma.
a The bristly changes in the calvarium are a reaction to excessive hematopoietic activity.
b Increased radiotracer uptake in the calvarium.

Physiological Calcifications

These are calcifications that have no demonstrable pathological cause and no pathological significance. They are so common in older patients that it is correct to describe them as physiological. Differentiation is required from calcifications that have a neoplastic or other pathological cause (see p. 384–386).

Pineal Calcifications

Projection radiographs rarely demonstrate pineal calcifications in newborns and small children. These calcifications are found in approximately 25% of patients over age 10 and in some 60–70% of patients over 50 years of age (Fig. 4.**38**, Table 4.**7**).

Table 4.**7**   Age distribution of 80 pineal calcifications based on a review of skull films from 1044 patients (from Helmke and Winkler 1986)

Age group	Number of children	Number of pineal calcifications	Percentage of pineal calcifications
0–1	162	5	3.1
1–2	105	3	2.9
2–3	69	2	2.9
3–4	58	2	3.4
4–5	48	2	4.2
5–6	56	2	3.6
6–7	63	3	4.8
7–8	55	3	5.5
8–9	65	3	4.6
9–10	42	3	7.1
10–11	54	5	9.3
11–12	52	5	9.6
12–13	45	5	11.1
13–14	48	8	16.7
14–15	43	8	18.6
15–16	41	9	22.0
16–17	23	7	30.4
17–18	15	5	33.3
Total	1044	80	

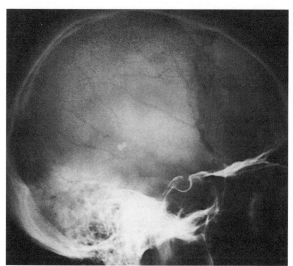

a

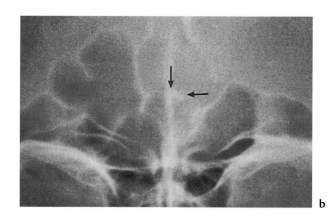

b

Fig. 4.**38 a, b**   Calcification of the pineal gland (arrows).
a Lateral projection.
b Frontal projection.

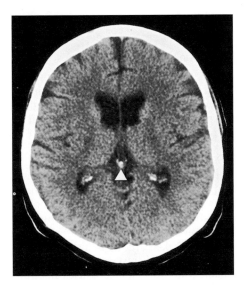

Fig. 4.**39**　Calcification of the pineal gland (arrowhead).

Pineal calcifications are accurately demonstrated by CT (Fig. 4.**39**). A very large pineal calcification in children under 10 years of age is suspicious for a pineal tumor. The displacement of a calcified pineal body away from the median plane may signify an intracranial mass or an atrophic process affecting one side of the brain. A normal pineal calcification has an average diameter of 3–5 mm (maximum of 10 mm) and is projected approximately 3 cm behind and above the dorsum sellae.

Habenular Calcifications

The pineal gland is attached by two pedicles called the habenulae. In approximately 13% of adults they contain striate, curvilinear, or comma-shaped calcifications located several millimeters rostral to the pineal gland itself.

Choroid Plexus Calcifications

Calcifications of the choroid plexus, usually in the lateral ventricles, are a common finding in adults over 40 years of age (Figs. 4.**40**–4.**42**). They are detected in up to 28% of

plain skull films and in approximately 75% of cranial CT scans. Choroid plexus calcifications are rarely found in children under age 10, although sporadic cases have been detected in healthy 2-year-olds. They are more common following toxoplasmosis infection. Cyst-wall calcifications or vascular calcifications in the choroid plexus can develop

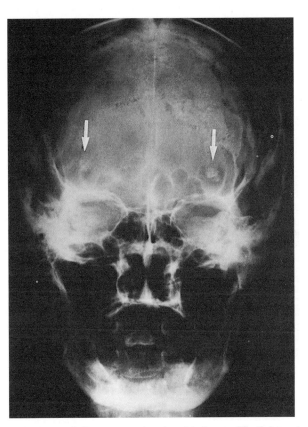

Fig. 4.**41**　Calcifications in the choroid plexus of both lateral ventricles, PA projection (choroid plexus calcifications at different levels, normal finding).

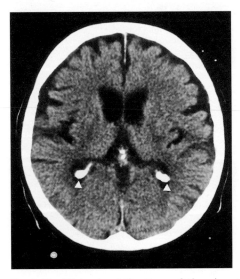

Fig. 4.**40**　Bilateral calcifications of the choroid plexus (arrowheads).

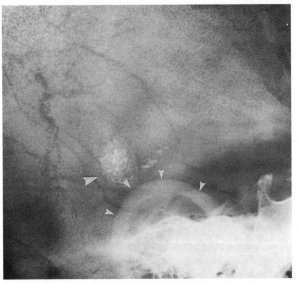

Fig. 4.**42**　Lateral projection demonstrates calcifications in the choroid plexus (large arrowhead). The auricle is also visible (small arrowheads).

as a result of dystrophic changes. They are highly variable in their shape and extent. The areas of the lateral ventricles near the trigone are sites of predilection. Generally the calcifications are arranged symmetrically above the center of each orbital roof in the frontal view (10 mm behind and 5 mm above the level of the pineal gland in the lateral view), but asymmetry may occur (Fig. 4.41). The calcifications may show a mulberry-like pattern on radiographs or they may be amorphous, flaky, or nodular. Choroid plexus calcifications become more common with aging and are more prevalent in men than women. Their presence in children under 15 years of age should raise suspicion of an endocrine disorder.

Sagittal Sinus Calcifications

Convergent, narrow, striate calcific densities below the inner table, situated below the apex of the calvarium in the frontal view, represent dural calcifications of the sagittal sinus (Fig. 4.43). These sinus calcifications may appear V-shaped in the AP projection.

Falx Calcifications

Calcifications of the falx cerebri can be detected in very small children. Falx calcifications, along with calcifications of the superior sagittal sinus, are found in 7–9% of older adults. Falx calcifications are often difficult to distinguish from frontal ossifications that extend from the frontal bone to the falx (Figs. 4.44, 4.45, 4.46). They may also be difficult to distinguish from the **frontal crest**. In many cases they are indistinguishable from isolated **falx ossicles** and from **falx osteoma**. Isolated falx ossicles have sharp, straight margins in the median plane but may form a lateral bulge with a less distinct outline (Fig. 4.47). CT can clearly distinguish an **isolated ossification of the falx** from ossification that has spread to the falx from the frontal bone (Fig. 4.48). **Falx calcifications** occur predominantly in the anterior and middle thirds of the falx and may have a faint linear structure or bonelike appearance ("**falx bones**"). Other dural calcifications can involve the **petrosellar ligament** (approximately 12%), the **sellar diaphragm**, and the interclinoidal ligaments. Massive meningeal calcifications may reflect an endocrine disorder or a disturbance of calcium phosphate metabolism (hypervitaminosis D, chronic renal failure, hyperparathyroidism, etc.).

Tentorial Calcifications

Aside from findings in the parasellar region (p. 447–453), calcifications of the cerebellar tentorium are rare but show a characteristic arrangement (Figs. 4.49, 4.50).

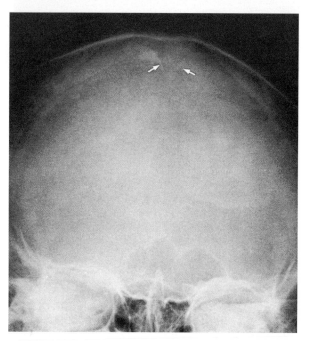

Fig. 4.**43** Dural calcifications of the sagittal sinus (arrows).

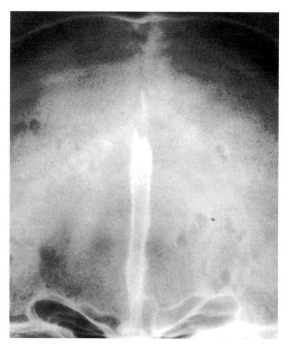

Fig. 4.**44** Very prominent frontal crest.

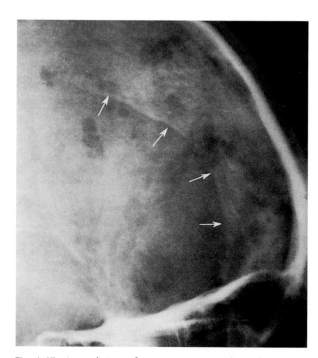

Fig. 4.**45** Lateral view of a very prominent frontal crest (arrows).

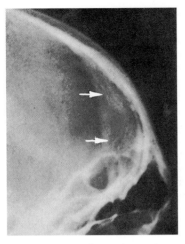

Fig. 4.**46**   Frontal crest (arrows).

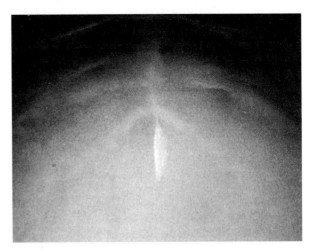

Fig. 4.**47**   Falx ossicle.

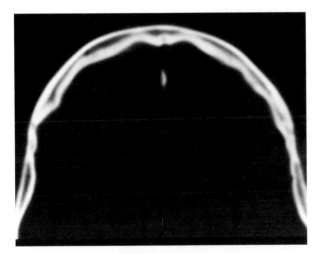

Fig. 4.**48**   Small ossification of the falx. Axial CT, bone window.

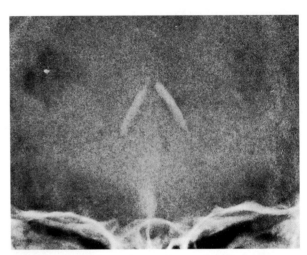

Fig. 4.**49**   Calcific densities outlining the dura mater along the cerebellar tentorium in the PA projection.

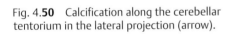

Fig. 4.**50**   Calcification along the cerebellar tentorium in the lateral projection (arrow).

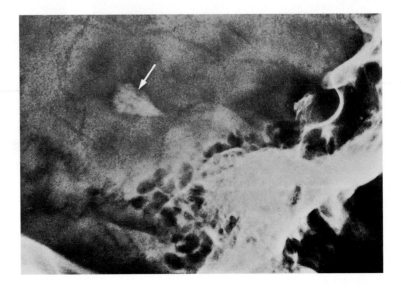

Vascular Calcifications

Physiological calcifications include calcifications in the foveolae granulares (p. 371–373). They are readily identified by their location in the pacchionian granulations on CT scans.

Arterial wall calcifications are most commonly found in the **internal carotid artery**. In the frontal view they appear as ringlike shadows adjacent to the sella, in the lateral view as bandlike, often parallel calcifications projected over the lumen of the sella. They follow the course of the carotid siphon. Arterial wall calcifications are a common finding in older patients but do not correlate with any symptomatic vascular disease (Fig. 4.**51**).

Pathological Calcifications

Calcifications with an Inflammatory Etiology

The most frequent causes of infectious intracranial calcifications are:

- Toxoplasmosis (Fig. 4.**56**)
- Cytomegalovirus infection
- Tuberculosis (Fig. 4.**53**)
- Cryptococcosis
- Cysticercosis (Fig. 4.**52**)
- Coccidiosis
- Echinococcosis

Calcifications in **tuberculosis** appear as dense, well-circumscribed, rounded, stippled tuberculomas with jagged, notched or curved contours. They are rare.

Calcifications following **tuberculous meningitis** generally appear after three months. They occur mainly in the basal cistern region, showing a predilection for the interpeduncular cistern (Fig. 4.**53**). Confluent inflammatory meningeal calcifications may outline individual cerebral convolutions, mimicking the gyral calcifications seen in Sturge–Weber disease.

Neurocysticercosis is the most common parasitic infection of the central nervous system. It is endemic in Central and South America, Africa, and parts of Asia and Eastern Europe. Central nervous system involvement occurs in 60–90% of all infected patients. Lesions occur most frequently at the gray–white matter junction. Intraventricular cysts develop in 20–50% of all cases, usually in the fourth ventricle. Only 10% of cases show isolated involvement of the subarachnoid space. The disease has four stages:

1. Vesicular stage
2. Colloidal vesicular stage
3. Granular nodular stage
4. Nodular calcified stage

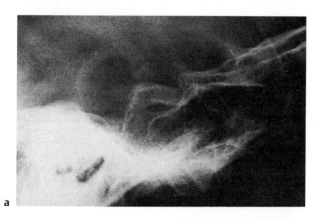

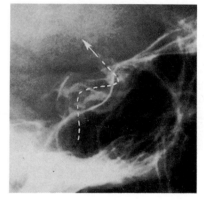

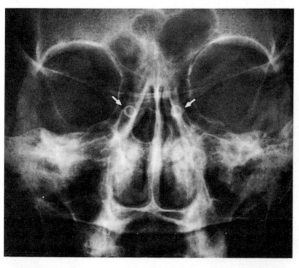

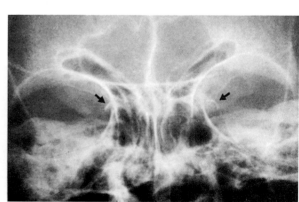

Fig. 4.**51 a–d**   Intimal calcifications of the internal carotid artery.
a Lateral projection: calcifications above the sella turcica.
b Lateral projection, marked to show the course of the internal carotid artery.

c Bilateral ringlike calcifications in the frontal projection (arrows).
d Bilateral shell-like calcifications in the frontal projection (arrows).

Fig. 4.**52** Cysticerci in the brain (arrows) and a coexisting osteoma of the frontal bone (tailed arrow). Note the course of the groove for the middle meningeal artery (black arrow).

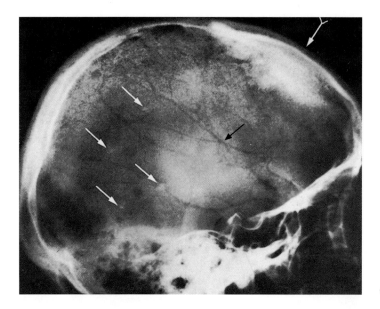

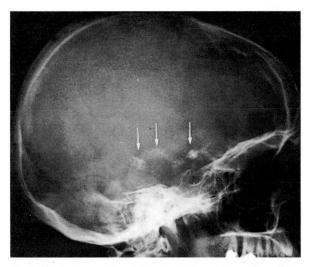

Fig. 4.**53** Intracranial calcifications following tuberculosis (arrows).

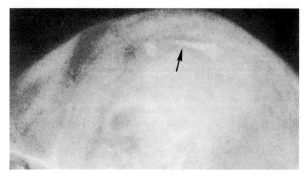

Fig. 4.**54** Calcified hematoma between the dura mater and inner table.

The manifestations on CT and MRI are correspondingly diverse, ranging from nonenhancing cysts to ring-enhancing "target" lesions and calcified nodules (Fig. 4.**52**).

The differential diagnosis should include **calcified intracranial abscesses**.

Tumor-Associated Calcifications

Calcifications occur in a variety of intracerebral tumors: in 70–90% of oligodendrogliomas, in 15–20% of low-grade astrocytomas, rarely in anaplastic astrocytomas and glioblastoma multiforme, and in approximately 10% of pilocytic astrocytomas. Ependymomas calcify in about 50% of cases. Calcifications are found in 20–25% of meningiomas.

Calcifications Due to Other Pathological Processes

Intracranial hemorrhages (e.g., subdural hematomas) can form flocculent or plaquelike calcific densities. Crescent-shaped streaks of calcification can form as a result of epidural hematoma (Fig. 4.**54**).

Plaquelike calcifications of the meninges like those occurring in hemorrhagic pachymeningitis have a characteristic appearance (Fig. 4.**55**).

Intracranial calcifications have been described following hemorrhage due to obstetric trauma in forceps deliveries, in connection with early childhood brain trauma, and as a sequel to space-occupying and neoplastic hemorrhage. Calcifications can also form along the needle track following the puncture of a cerebral ventricle.

Sturge–Weber syndrome, or encephalotrigeminal angiomatosis, is typically associated with a "tram-track" pattern of cortical calcifications. It is produced by calcifications on opposing cerebral gyri that are separated by a widened sulcus. This gyral calcification pattern is particularly well demonstrated by CT. It is often accompanied by a progressive cortical atrophy causing an ipsilateral shift of midline structures. Secondary effects can include ipsilateral thickening of the calvarium, enlargement of the paranasal sinuses, and increased pneumatization of the mastoid.

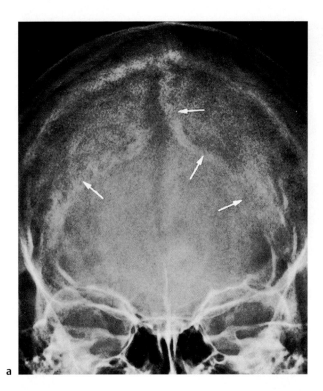

a

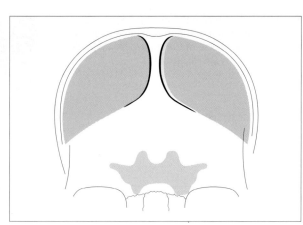

b

Fig. 4.**55a, b** Hemorrhagic pachymeningitis.
a Typical radiographic finding of pachymeningitis with calcifications after skull trauma four years earlier in a 10-year-old child.
b Hemorrhagic internal pachymeningitis ("panzerhirn"), schematic drawing. (From Birkner and Lagemann 1966.)

Tuberous sclerosis (Bourneville–Pringle disease) is an autosomal dominant disease with an incidence of 1 : 10 000 to 1 : 50 000. The classic clinical triad consists of papular facial nevi (adenoma sebaceum), seizures, and mental retardation in less than 50% of cases. Four main categories of intracranial lesions are encountered in tuberous sclerosis:

1 Cortical tubers
2 White matter lesions (histologically benign lesions that probably represent disordered, dysplastic white matter or dysmyelinated foci)
3 Subependymal nodules (hamartomas)
4 Subependymal giant-cell astrocytomas

Subependymal nodules and cortical tubers frequently calcify. In these cases fine cortical, subcortical, and paraventricular calcific foci can be seen even on plain films but are more clearly visualized by CT (Fig. 4.56).

CT has detected intracerebral and cerebellar calcifications in adults who were subjected to decades of excessive lead exposure and had markedly elevated serum levels of lead. These calcifications may be punctate, curvilinear, linear, nodular, or diffuse and are found at subcortical sites, in the basal ganglia, or in the cerebellum.

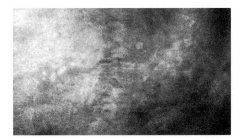

Fig. 4.**56** Fine calcifications anterior and posterior to the coronal suture (tuberous sclerosis? toxoplasmosis?).

Bilateral **basal ganglia calcifications** (Fig. 4.57) are mostly idiopathic and occur in the absence of a detectable endocrine disorder. They are easily demonstrated by CT. Frequent and less frequent causes of basal ganglia calcifications are listed in Table 4.**8**.

Basal ganglia calcifications may also show an asymmetrical or unilateral distribution.

Table 4.**8** Causes of bilateral calcifications of the basal ganglia

Frequent causes
• Idiopathic
• Fahr disease (familial cerebrovascular ferrocalcinosis)
• Postinflammatory (tuberculosis, toxoplasmosis, cysticercosis, congenital HIV infection)
• Encephalitis (e.g., rubella, measles, chickenpox)
• Hypoparathyroidism, pseudohypoparathyroidism

Rare Causes
• Congenital diseases (tuberous sclerosis, Down syndrome, Cockayne syndrome, neurofibromatosis, methemoglobinopathy, MERRF syndrome [mitochondrial encephalopathy with myoclonic epilepsy, muscle weakness, and progressive ophthalmoplegia], MELAS syndrome [mitochondrial myopathy, encephalopathy, lactic acidosis, seizure-like episodes])
• Hyperparathyroidism
• Hemorrhage
• Familial idiopathic basal ganglia calcifications
• Idiopathic lenticulodental calcification (Hastings–James syndrome)
• Lipoid proteinosis (cutaneous hyalinosis)
• Oculo-dento-osseous dysplasia
• Parkinsonism
• Pseudopseudohypoparathyroidism
• Trisomy 21 (Down syndrome)
• Postanoxic or toxic (carbon monoxide intoxication, chemotherapy-induced, radiotherapy-induced, lead intoxicaion, perinatal anoxia, vascular diseases such as atherosclerosis)

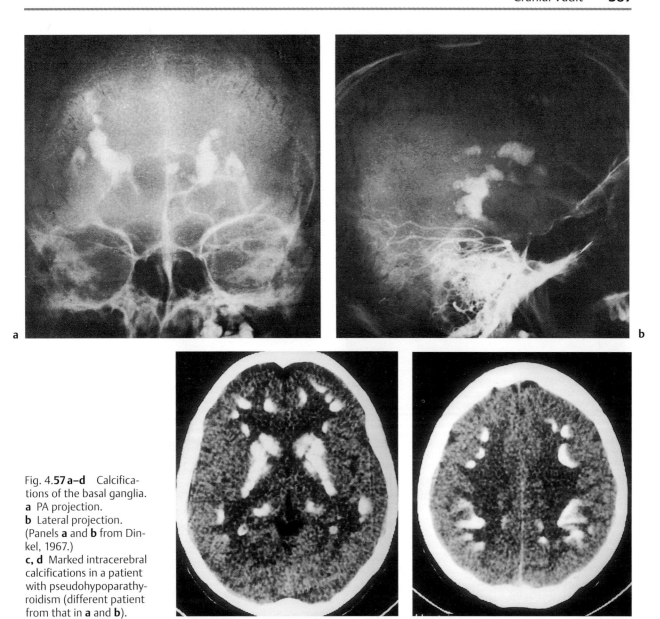

Fig. 4.**57 a–d** Calcifications of the basal ganglia.
a PA projection.
b Lateral projection.
(Panels **a** and **b** from Dinkel, 1967.)
c, d Marked intracerebral calcifications in a patient with pseudohypoparathyroidism (different patient from that in **a** and **b**).

Other Anomalies

Cephaloceles

Cranium bifidum occultum is a bony dysraphic anomaly of the skull that is analogous to spina bifida occulta. It is characterized by a rounded or slitlike cleft in the midline of the calvarium without associated soft-tissue abnormalities. The anomaly is not a true cephalocele, therefore. Cephaloceles (p. 428 and Table 4.**14**) are among the dysraphic anomalies that develop during closure of the neural tube. Malformations of the brain are frequently combined with osseous cranial deformities. Cephaloceles may take the form of encephaloceles, encephalocystoceles, meningoceles, or their combinations depending on whether the protrusion contains brain tissue, portions of the cerebral ventricles, or only a fluid-filled meningeal sac. Cephaloceles occur with a frequency of 1 in 4000 births. In terms of location, occipital cephaloceles are the most common (75%), followed by frontobasal (15%) and parietal (10%). Basal cephaloceles are most commonly located at the junction between the chondrocranium and desmocranium (p. 428). The dura merges with the outer periosteum at the edge of the bony defect through which the sac protrudes, and so the protrusion often does not have a dural covering. External cephaloceles are often recognized at birth (Fig. 4.**58b, c**). Internal or basal cephaloceles may do undetected initially, especially if there are no external signs of dysraphism (broad nasal dorsum, hypertelorism, etc.). Under these circumstances, they are first brought to medical attention during childhood or adolescence because of nasal airway obstruction, CSF rhinorrhea, recurrent bouts of meningitis, or other problems. An unusual case that could be classified as an atretic cephalocele is demonstrated in Figure 4.**58d–g**.

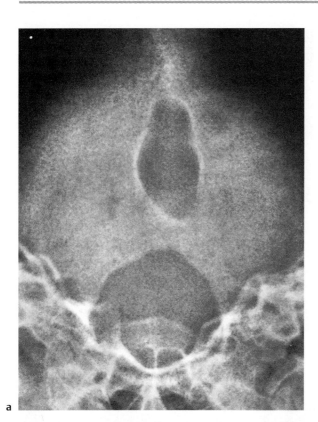

a

Fig. 4.**58 a–g**
a Meningoencephalocele in the occiput of a 24-year-old man.
b, c Different patient: typical MRI appearance of an occipital meningocele in a 2-month-old child.
d Different patient from that in **a–c**. Four weeks earlier, this 26-year-old man noticed a painful swelling in the occipital area that regressed spontaneously. A Towne projection of the occiput shows destruction at the center of the occipital bone.
e, f CT with a high-resolution bone filter and 3-D reconstruction shows an ill-defined defect in the occipital bone with a solid area of ossification.
g T1-weighted MRI after intravenous contrast administration appears to show proliferating meningeal tissue in the defect. Additional MRI sequences (not shown) did not show a CSF collection. The lesion is an atretic occipital cephalocele. We initially considered a meningioma en plaque in the differential diagnosis.

Fig. 4.**58 f** and **g** ▷

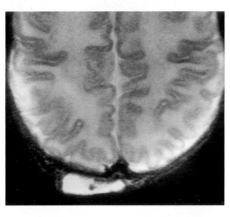

b

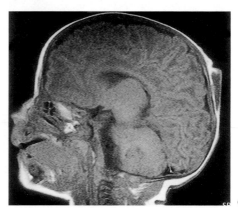

c

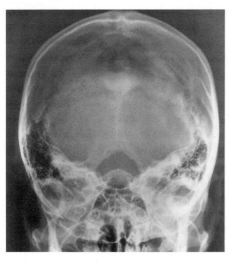

d

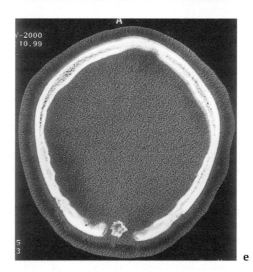

e

Fig. 4.**58 f** and **g**

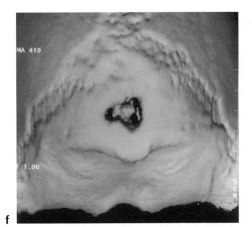

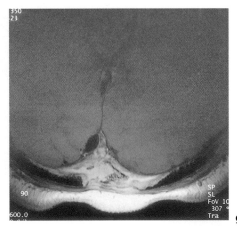

f

g

Lacunar Skull

Lacunar skull (**craniolacunia, lückenschädel**) is characterized by the presence of true defects in the inner table, usually combined with an intact outer table. The dura and periosteum are always preserved. The calvarium exhibits large, rounded areas that are radiolucent due to deficient mineralization and are separated by normal, sharply circumscribed bone areas that resemble ridges. This gives the calvarium a characteristic, honeycomb-like appearance on radiographs. The anomaly is caused by dysplasia of the portions of the calvarium that are preformed in connective tissue. The size and shape of the cranium are normal. Lacunar skull is often associated with other dysraphic anomalies (encephaloceles, myelomeningoceles, Arnold–Chiari malformation). The lacunar changes are confined to the upper portions of the calvarium, predominantly affecting the frontal and parietal region.

Increased Convolutional Markings

A generalized increase in convolutional markings affecting the entire calvarium is easily distinguished from a lacunar skull. The "**beaten brass**" appearance of the skull on radiographs (Fig. 4.**26**) is not seen before about 12 months of age.

Abnormal Suture Widening

Abnormal widening of the cranial sutures may be caused by genetic abnormalities, increased intracranial pressure, traumatic suture dehiscence, or infiltration of the sutural connective tissue. The most frequent cause in children is chronically increased intracranial pressure, which is usually a result of hydrocephalus. If ossification of the suture edges keeps pace with this process, the growth stimulus on the connective tissue leads to lengthening of the sutural interdigitations. If the rising pressure outstrips the ability of the cranial sutures to compensate, suture dehiscence occurs. Rickets is associated with an apparent suture dehiscence, as the defective mineralization does not permit calcification of the newly formed bone at the suture edges. Tumor infiltration of the sutural connective tissue and adjacent bone edges can be seen in children with leukemia, lymphoma, or neuroblastoma and can simulate suture widening. The various types of suture abnormality are reviewed in Table 4.**9**.

Cranial suture abnormalities can have various underlying causes. For example, significant suture spread has been found in infants with congenital heart defects who have

Table 4.**9**   Abnormalities of the cranial sutures (from Schinz 1986)

1 Suture widening
   A Genetic due to delayed suture closure and ossification defects
   - Cleidocranial dysplasia (dysostosis)
   - Hypothyroidism
   - Hypophosphatasia
   - Pyknodysostosis
   - Trisomy 21
   B Increased intracranial pressure
   - Intracranial mass
   - Impairment of CSF circulation
   - Pseudotumor cerebri
   - Deprivation syndrome
   - Lead intoxication
   C Iatrogenic
   - Hypervitaminosis A
   - Tetracyclines
   - Prostaglandin E2
2 Traumatic suture dehiscence
3 Suture destruction
   - Leukemia
   - Lymphoma
   - Neuroblastoma
4 Craniosynostosis (premature suture closure) (see Table 4.**10**)
   - Primary craniosynostosis
   - Secondary craniosynostosis

been treated with **prostaglandin E$_2$** for 100 days. Suture abnormalities have also been described in children with trisomy 21 (Down syndrome). Open sutures and the presence of supernumerary sutural bones in a widened skull with basilar impression characterize **cleidocranial dysplasia (dysostosis)** (**Scheuthauer–Marie–Sainton syndrome**), which has an autosomal mode of inheritance (Fig. 4.**59**). Cleidocranial dysplasia (dysostosis) predominantly affects bone that is preformed in connective tissue. The cranial ossification defects are reflected in a large, wide head with frontal and parietal bossing. Closure of the sutures and fontanelles is delayed. This may be accompanied by median notching of the foramen magnum and other nonspecific cranial findings such as craniofacial hypoplasia with impaired pneumatization and dental anomalies. Other symptoms are moderate growth retardation, funnel chest, scoliosis, genu valgum, and prominent,

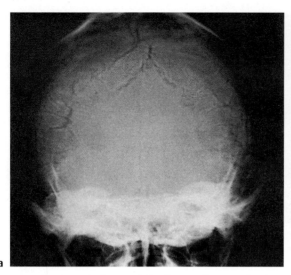
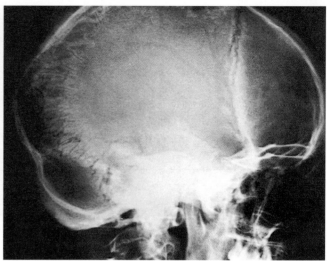

a   b

Fig. 4.**59 a, b**   Cleidocranial dysplasia with unusually distinct sutures, long suture serrations, and basilar impression.

excessively mobile scapulae. Absence or hypoplasia of the clavicle is typical.

Sutural defects are also found in **familial idiopathic hypertrophic osteoarthropathy**. It accounts for less than 5% of all manifestations of idiopathic hypertrophic osteoarthropathy. Enlargement and delayed closure of cranial sutures is characteristic (Reginato 1982). Impairment of calvarial ossification is a cardinal symptom of **hypophosphatasia**. This is an hereditary, autosomal recessive disease characterized by a congenital phosphatase deficiency. The prenatal and neonatal forms are incompatible with life, as there is deficient ossification of the entire skeletal system. The skull base and facial skeleton are at least partially ossified, but there may be no visible calcification of the calvarium. In the early infantile form of hypophosphatasia tarda, ossification of the calvarium and skull base is delayed. The infantile-juvenile form has a better prognosis. The adult form is generally diagnosed after puberty. The cranial skeleton is usually normal, but craniosynostosis may be present.

Craniosynostosis (Premature Suture Closure)

Craniosynostosis is based on the premature closure of one, several, or all of the cranial sutures. This results in a disproportion between the capacity of the cranial vault and its contents. The various forms are reviewed in Table 4.**10**.

Primary premature suture closure is more common than secondary forms. It is probably based on a developmental anomaly of membranous cranial bones, making the closure a secondary phenomenon.

Secondary craniosynostosis in the true sense refers to premature closure in the setting of some other disease (e.g., microcephaly) that tends to reduce the growth stimulus. The pattern of the underlying suture abnormality can usually be inferred from the shape of the skull.

Premature suture closure is observed in 0.6% of cases. It may be a primary or secondary condition (see Tables 4.**10** and 4.**11**). The most frequent combination of cranial de-

Table 4.**10**   Primary and secondary craniosynostosis (premature suture closure) (from Schinz 1986)

Primary craniosynostosis

A Idiopathic craniosynostosis

B Craniosynostosis with craniofacial anomalies:
- Craniofacial dysostosis (Crouzon syndrome)
- Acrocephalosyndactyly syndromes
- Acrocephalopolysyndactyly syndromes
- Cloverleaf skull syndrome
- Craniotelencephalic dysplasia
- Hypotelorism-arhinencephaly malformation syndromes

C Craniosynostosis in a setting of general skeletal dysplasia:
- Hypophosphatasia tarda
- Idiopathic hypercalcemia syndrome
- Vitamin D-resistant rickets
- Mucopolysaccharidosis types I and IV
- Mucolipidosis type III
- Skeletal dysplasias with marked hyperostosis

D Craniosynostosis in patients with endocrine-metabolic disorders:
- Hyperthyroidism
- Vitamin D-deficiency rickets
- Hypervitaminosis D

E Craniosynostosis in anemias (e.g., thalassemia):
- May involve secondary craniosynostosis in microcephaly

Secondary craniosynostosis
- In microcephaly and malformation syndromes
- In patients with shunted hydrocephalus

Table 4.**11**   Idiopathic primary craniosynostosis (from Schinz 1986)

Brachycephaly (short skull)
- Bilateral closure of the coronal and/or lambdoid suture

Acrocephaly (oxycephaly, turricephaly) (steeple skull, tower skull)
- Premature closure of all sutures

Scaphocephaly (long, narrow skull)
- Premature closure of the sagittal suture

Trigonocephaly (triangular skull)
- Premature closure of the frontal suture

Plagiocephaly (crooked skull)
- Unilateral closure of the coronal and/or lambdoid suture

formity and premature suture closure occurs in **turricephaly** (Fig. 4.**60a**). In this condition, known also as tower skull, premature closure of the sagittal and coronal sutures or of all the major sutures causes the top of the skull to acquire a pointed or domelike shape (**acrocephaly, oxycephaly**). Turricephaly is the most severe form of idiopathic craniosynostosis. The results are increased intracranial pressure and exophthalmos. Turricephaly is associated with marked shortening of the anterior skull base and with a steep position of the orbital roof contours that

form the anterior cranial fossa. Shortening of the anterior fossa can occur only if the greater sphenoid wings assume a more transverse position. Normally these structures form an anterior angle of 95°, but this angle averages 115° in turricephaly (Fig. 4.**61**). The more transverse orientation of the greater sphenoid wings leads to **hypertelorism** with consequent dilatation of the intervening ethmoid cells (Fig. 4.**62**). The shallow orbits lead to exophthalmos, and the visual axes may diverge by as much as 18° (divergent strabismus). The hard palate is shortened along with the

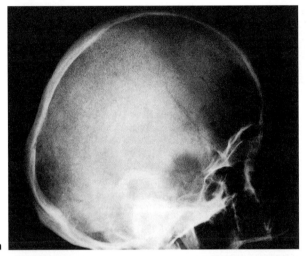
a

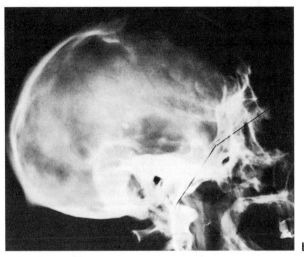
b

Fig. 4.**60a, b**　Frontal dysplasias.
a Turricephaly due to premature fusion of the coronal suture.

b Scaphocephaly due to premature fusion of the coronal and sagittal sutures.

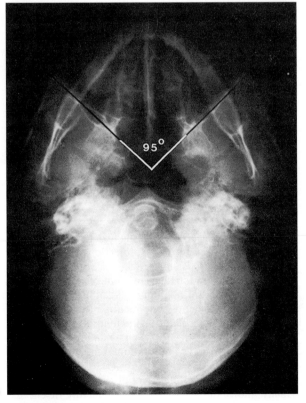
a

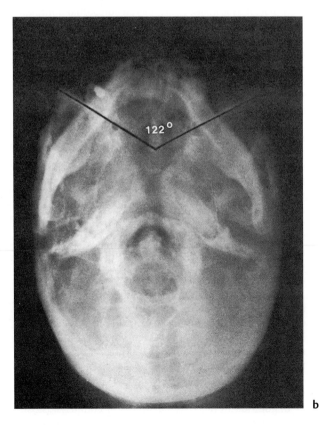
b

Fig. 4.**61a, b**　Facial angles.
a Normal (approximately 95°).

b In frontofacial dysplasia (122°).

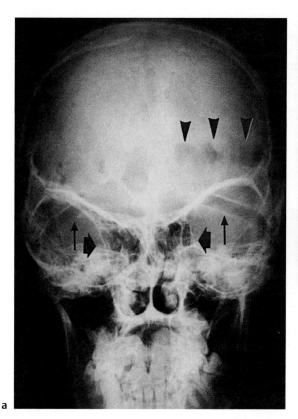

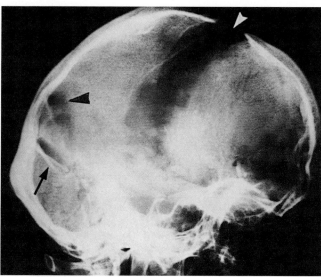

Fig. 4.**62a, b**   Premature closure of cranial sutures (after suturotomy) with frontal dysplasia.
a PA projection shows marked hypertelorism with dilatation of the ethmoid air cells.
b Lateral projection.

Heavy arrows:	Ethmoid air cells
Arrowheads:	Occipital pacchionian granulations
Arrows:	Transverse sinus on each side
White arrowhead:	Surgical defect

frontal skull base, with the result that normal mandibular development leads to prognathism. The facial deformity that coexists with turricephaly is described by the term craniofacial dysostosis, which has an autosomal dominant inheritance or occurs sporadically in 25% of cases. If there are concomitant deformities of the fingers and toes, the condition is classified as one of the various types of acrocephalosyndactyly. If portions of the coronal and sagittal sutures located near the bregma remain open for some time, allowing room for brain expansion, a **pointed skull** (**oxycephaly**) will develop.

A **long, narrow skull** (dolichocephaly or scaphocephaly) results from premature closure of the sagittal suture (Fig. 4.**60b**). The term scaphocephaly is based on the resemblance of the skull to a "skiff" in the sagittal projection. In the lateral view, it is characterized by a greater-than-normal degree of dolichocephaly. If the coronal suture also closes prematurely, as is generally the case, the scaphocephaly is also associated with frontal dysplasia (Fig. 4.**60**). Premature suture closure often leads to a significant increase in convolutional markings (Fig. 4.**26**). This finding is most pronounced in the frontal bone when coronal suture synostosis is present.

A **short skull** (brachycephaly) results from fusion of the coronal and/or lambdoid sutures. Premature ossification of the coronal suture leads to shortening of the anterior skull base with slanted sphenoid wings and elliptical orbits. If both the coronal and lambdoid sutures close during intrauterine development, a cloverleaf skull results.

A **triangular skull** (trigonocephaly) results from premature closure of the frontal suture.

In addition to the classic patterns of craniosynostosis, there are mixed forms, transitional forms, and forms based on the partial obliteration of individual sutures. A typical example is **plagiocephaly**, which results from the premature unilateral fusion of a coronal suture. It is marked by asymmetrical frontal and parietal flattening on the ipsilateral side. An advanced degree of suture obliteration can be detected on radiographs by absence of the suture line or of sutural interdigitations. Early suture closure is more difficult to detect. In these cases the suture line is narrowed and is not bordered by sharp, thin bone edges, as is normally the case, but by blunt or even slightly raised bony margins. Even if the premature fusion is confined to a short segment of the suture, it is tantamount to functional insufficiency of the entire suture.

Secondary changes in the calvarium depend on the degree and duration of the craniosynostosis and include **increased convolutional markings (beaten brass appearance)**, thinning of the calvarium, and deepening of dural sinus grooves.

 Fracture?

Fractures of the calvarium are usually detected on biplane skull radiographs, and a Towne projection may be added if an occipital fracture is suspected. A heavy impact to the skull at low acceleration tends to produce a linear fracture, while an impact from a lighter object at high acceleration often produces a depressed fracture. The calvarium is depressed at the zone of impact but tends to bulge outward at the periphery, causing linear burst fractures of the raised bone. Depression and comminution occur at the center of the trauma zone.

The intracranial complications of a calvarial fracture are usually more important than the fracture itself. Extracranial complications in the region of the calvarium usually have less serious consequences. For this reason, CT has assumed a primary role in the examination of head-injured patients. Linear fractures of the calvarium are often visible only in a certain projection due to the narrowness of the fracture line. The fracture may disappear when the projection is altered by just a few degrees. As a general rule, fractures closer to the film appear sharper than those farther away (imaging geometry!), and this principle can be utilized to identify the affected side. Fracture lines may go undetected on CT scans if they are fine or are directed parallel to the plane of the scan.

The squamous, sphenosquamous, and parietomastoid sutures, which sometimes do not close until the fifth to seventh decade, may occasionally be viewed edge-on in the sagittal projection, causing them to be mistaken for a fracture line or diastatic suture fracture.

Calvarial Fractures in Children

Because the anatomy of the pediatric calvarium differs from that in adults, the nature and appearance of calvarial fractures are also different. Because the pediatric skull is still growing, the calvarium is thinner and more compliant. In many cases the sutures and fontanelles are not yet closed.

Moreover, sutures and synchondroses in the growing skull are apt to be mistaken for fracture lines. For this reason it is important to know the anatomy of the cranial sutures, the timing of their closure, and the lines that can persist in adults. Most of the cranial sutures are paired except for the sagittal suture and the frontal (metopic) suture. A side-to-side comparison is usually sufficient to distinguish suture lines from fractures (Fig. 4.**63**). This comparison requires an accurate radiographic projection. The metopic (frontal) suture is consistently visualized until about the third year of life, and in approximately 10% of cases it persists in the adult (Figs. 4.**1**, 4.**9**). The sutura mendosa is also commonly found in small children. It is usually paired and runs through the occipital bone. It intersects the lambdoid suture near the asterion (Fig. 4.**11**), which marks the junction of the mastoid process, parietal bone, and occipital squama. The sutura mendosa may still be present in adults and may be mistaken for a fracture. Details on the **cranial sutures**, **sutural bones** (p. 364, 365, 375), and abnormal **suture widening** (p. 389–392) were discussed previously.

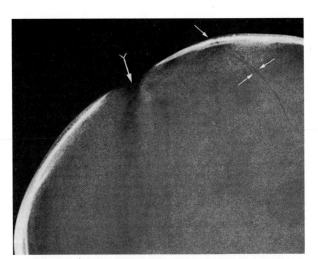

Fig. 4.**63** Typical appearance of a fine calvarial fracture (arrows) located near the anterior fontanelle (tailed arrow) in a one-year-old child. The fracture line is straight and gaping and runs through the inner and outer tables.

The causes of suture abnormalities are reviewed in Tables 4.**9**–4.**11**, and Fig. 4.**9** illustrates important cranial suture variants and accessory bones in adults.

 Diastatic suture fractures can be particularly difficult to recognize if a traumatic intracranial hematoma with no direct bone injury has caused a rise of intracranial pressure leading to generalized spreading of the sutures.

The thinner bony structures of the pediatric skull and the open sutures result in a more compliant skull that absorbs more of the traumatic forces than an adult skull. Because the calvarium is thin, linear fractures in particular are often more difficult to detect.

Depressed fractures in childhood look different than in adulthood.

Depressed fractures in the adult calvarium tend to be comminuted, consisting of multiple fragments. But in newborns and small children, trauma can depress the calvarium without causing a detectable fracture. Fracture healing is significantly more rapid in children than in adults, and fractures in the elderly can often take years to achieve bony union. Fracture lines may even persist for the patients lifetime. Most calvarial fractures in children will heal completely in 6 months.

A "**growing fracture**" is a typical but rare complication of a skull fracture in children. Interposed dura and arachnoid cause widening of the fracture line with the formation of a leptomeningeal cyst. These changes are usually found in the frontal or parietal region. They can also occur in adults but are most common in children under 2 years of age. Their incidence in linear fractures is less than 1%. "Growing fractures," then, are considered a rare, late complication of craniocerebral trauma. Follow-up radiographs should be obtained to exclude the development of leptomeningeal cysts. Asymmetry and a suture width greater than 2 mm are strongly suspicious for a diastatic suture fracture or a posttraumatic progression of initial fracture dehiscence in the form of a "growing fracture." The resulting gaps occasionally become portals for leptomeningeal herniation, which can be clearly demonstrated by CT or MRI. One such "growing" skull fracture has been described as a rare complication following a vacuum extraction delivery.

With few exceptions, depressions of the cranial vault in newborns can be attributed to obstetric trauma and are often associated with fractures. However, the neonatal calvarium may also show conspicuous, localized concavities that do not have a traumatic cause and will regress spontaneously during the first 6 months of life. An isolated lesion of the outer table of the calvarium is considered a rarity.

Ping-pong fractures are depressed fractures of the calvarium in which the periosteum remains intact (greenstick fracture). They may be caused by a forceps delivery or by the skull passing through a relatively narrow birth canal. They can also occur in utero due to pressure on the skull from a fetal extremity, for example.

Calvarial Fractures in Adults

We noted earlier how calvarial fractures can be confused with vascular grooves and how they can be differentiated (p. 370). When linear or patchy densities are seen on plain skull films following a localized flow to the head (stellate or "eggshell" fracture), one should consider the possibility of **overriding fragments** and depression. The extent of this type of injury can be defined by tangential views or preferably by CT (Fig. 4.**64**). Bathrocephaly is an important condition that requires differentiation from fractures. It is characterized by a steplike projection of the occipital squama past the parietal bone along the lambdoid suture. The extent of the projection may equal the width of the cal-

varium. This phenomenon is occasionally noted in lateral views and on CT scans (Fig. 4.**12**). "Indentations" in the parietal bones at the bregma also require differentiation from a traumatic depression of the skull (Fig. 4.**65**).

A fracture extending into the temporal bone from the skull base can be quite difficult to distinguish from an arterial groove (especially the groove for the middle meningeal artery). If doubt exists, CT can establish the identity of the finding in a traumatized patient (Fig. 4.**66**).

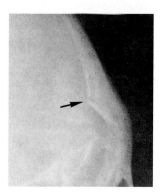

Fig. 4.**64**   Fracture of the inner table (arrow).

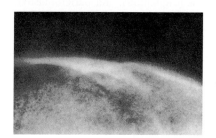

Fig. 4.**65**   Abnormal depression located behind the coronal suture. Not a depressed fracture.

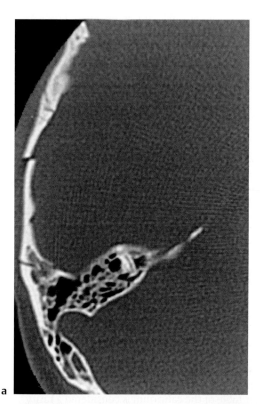

a

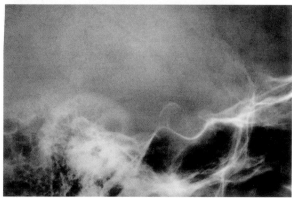

b

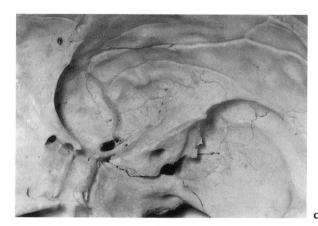

c

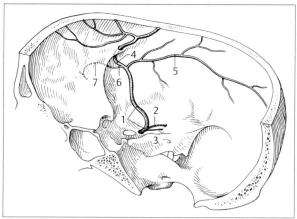

d

Fig. 4.**66 a**   Calvarial fracture in the right temporal area, CT appearance, see Figure 4.**112**.
b The relatively well-defined lucent line in the lateral skull film is a nutrient canal carrying a branch of the middle meningeal artery.
c Branches of the middle meningeal artery traversing the skull. Anatomic specimen.
d Diagram of middle meningeal artery branches. 1 = middle meningeal artery, 2 = petrosal branch, 3 = superior tympanic artery, 4 = frontal branch, 5 = parietal branch, 6 = orbital branch, 7 = anastomotic branch of lacrimal artery.
b–d different patient from that in **a**; **d** from Feneis 1993.

Harmonious linear lucencies that have smooth, often sclerotic margins and a branched configuration are most likely a **vascular groove** (Fig. 4.67), while lucencies with irregular, jagged (not interdigitated) margins suggest a fracture. The diagnosis of a diastatic suture fracture is supported by the presence of additional fracture lines (Figs. 4.68, 4.69).

The introduction of CT has both qualified and expanded the role of the early radiological investigation of calvarial fractures and their therapeutic implications. Besides post-traumatic hernias and their contents mentioned above, intracranial complications can be detected with great sensitivity by CT and MRI. These include the presence of intracranial air (**pneumocephalus**), which is an indirect but definite sign of a penetrating calvarial injury or fractures extending into the paranasal sinuses and/or the nasopharynx (with deep soft-tissue injuries) (Fig. 4.70). A rare complication is concomitant injury to a large intracranial venous sinus from an occipital calvarial fracture (Fig. 4.71).

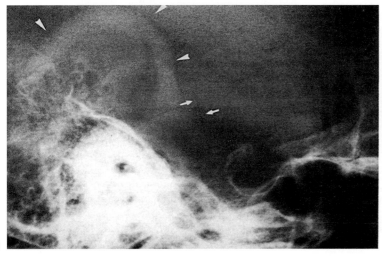
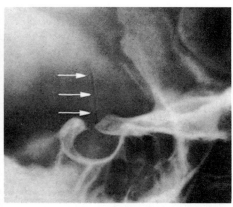

Fig. 4.**67 a, b**   Vascular channel in the temporal bone.
a Vascular channel in the temporal bone projected behind the sella (arrows). Arrowheads = auricle.

b Vascular channel in the temporal bone projected above the sella (arrows).

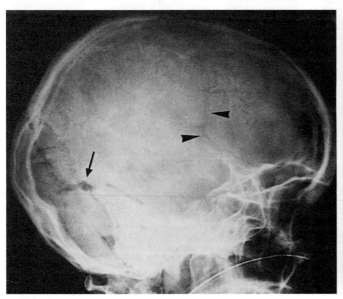
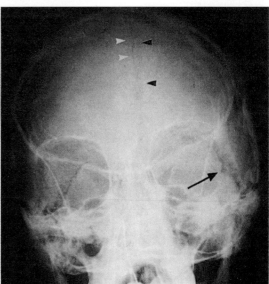

Fig. 4.**68 a, b**   Burst fracture with lambdoid suture dehiscence (arrows) in a 23-year-old woman.
Arrowheads in **a**: Vascular grooves

Arrowheads in **b**: Sagittal suture, outer table
White arrowheads in **b**: Sagittal suture, inner table

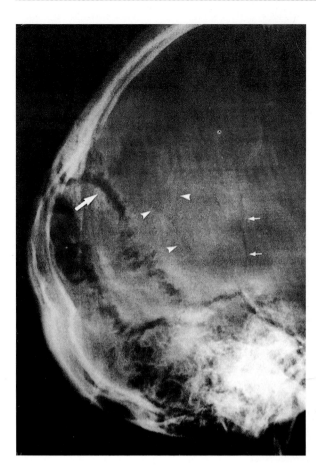

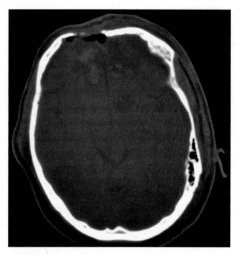

Fig. 4.**70**   CT appearance of intracranial air following a head injury.

◁ Fig. 4.**69**   Dehiscence of the lambdoid suture (arrow) in a 17-year-old woman.
Small arrows: Vertical fracture line
Arrowheads: Arterial grooves

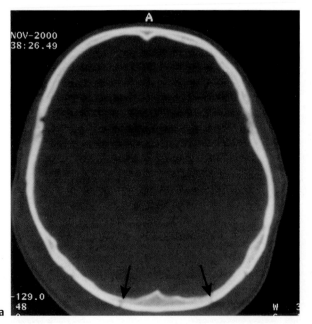

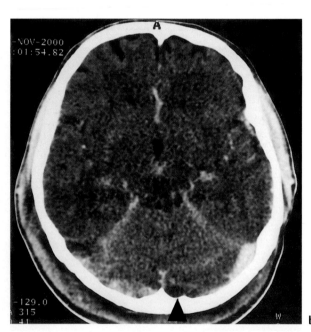

Fig. 4.**71 a,b**   Occipital calvarial fracture (arrow), CT. The fracture has caused an accompanying injury of the transverse sinus, leading to sinus thrombosis (arrowhead).

Necrosis?

The scalp and calvarium are richly vascularized by a network of blood vessels that course in and on the meninges as well as within the scalp: the arterial meningeal vessels (especially the middle meningeal artery), the dural sinuses, the cortical cerebral veins, the small vessels of the meninges and branches of the external carotid artery. For this reason, injuries often lead to profuse bleeding.

 This also explains why necrosis of the calvarium is rare.

Even extensive fractures of the calvarium do not compromise the blood supply to a degree that results in calvarial necrosis. A free calvarial bone flap that has been raised in a bur-hole craniotomy may occasionally become necrotic due to a chronic perfusion deficit, but usually this requires an additional insult to the blood supply. This is illustrated by one of our patients who underwent surgery and radiotherapy in childhood for a malignant left-sided brain tumor. The tumor was exposed through an ipsilateral craniotomy. Radiotherapy was administered during the 1970s. Over time, the reimplanted craniotomy flap became partially necrotic along with the overlying skin and soft tissues (Fig. 4.72). Radiation necrosis of the calvarium is usually marked by patchy decalcification and partially confluent areas of osteolysis. In many cases the changes resemble those of calvarial osteomyelitis. Periosteal reactions are usually absent, and sclerosis rarely occurs. The di-

agnosis is based on the history, no apparent infection, and the location of the changes in the radiotherapy portal. Often the changes progress gradually over a period of years, and resolution may occur.

Inflammation?

Osteomyelitis of the calvarium is characterized by ill-defined lytic areas that may have a moth-eaten appearance. Today it is very rare to find inflammatory calvarial changes aside from foci of osteomyelitis in or on a replaced bone flap following craniotomy. "Bone flap osteomyelitis" may have a septic or aseptic cause. This differentiation must rely on clinical findings. The most frequent cause of aseptic bone flap osteomyelitis appears to be aseptic necrosis based on impaired blood flow. In the case of aseptic osteomyelitis, the bone flap shows patchy decalcification, ill-defined margins, and foci of bone destruction that vary in number and extent. The osseous changes are always confined to the bone flap. The bone edges surrounding the osteotomy are sharply defined and show no abnormalities. The etiology, pediatric aspects, complications, and radiological features of inflammatory diseases of the calvarium and skull base are reviewed on p. 441 and 442.

Tuberculous lesions in the cranial vault appear as punched-out defects rimmed by varying degrees of sclerosis (Fig. 4.73). They may be confused with lesions of Langerhans cell histiocytosis (p. 400).

Osteolytic lesions with a central, buttonlike bone fragment are called "**button sequestrum**" and have been ob-

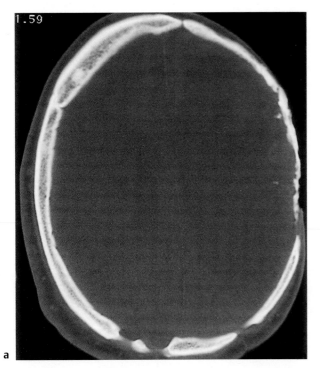

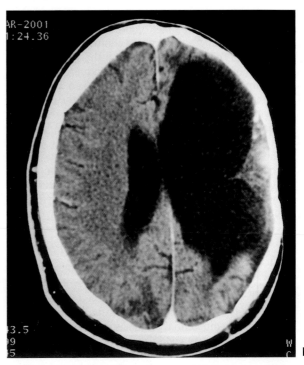

Fig. 4.72 a, b   This patient had surgery and postoperative irradiation in childhood for a malignant left-sided brain tumor. Partial necrosis ensued, causing typical irregular increased density of the left temporal bone flap. The overlying skin also became necrotic, requiring coverage by plastic surgery. The

patient was left with a large parenchymal defect in the left side of the brain. An intensely enhancing meningeal tumor (not yet biopsied) is noted in the left temporoparietal area as an incidental finding.

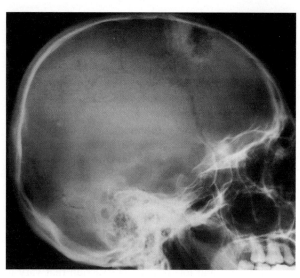

Fig. 4.**73**   Tuberculous lesion in the right frontal bone, observed in a young Indian nurse. The irregular area of osteolysis has a broad sclerotic rim. (Case courtesy of Dr. Bell, Dernbach)

served in eosinophilic granulomas, tuberculous lesions, epidermoid and dermoid cysts, and in neoplastic processes.

Syphilis, caused by the spirochete *Treponema pallidum*, may also be associated with skeletal involvement. Two types of bony changes are observed:

- **Syphilitic periostitis.** This most commonly affects the anterior tibial margins or calvarium and is characterized by an ossifying periostitis with paraosseous calcifications. In advanced stages the calcifying periostitis becomes very dense and eventually fuses with the underlying cortex. The calcifications may be interrupted by lucencies of varying shape (gummatous cavities). In the skull, the changes can lead to confusion with fibrous dysplasia. Differentiation relies on the serological detection of syphilis and histological findings.
- **Gummatous form.** This form is marked by circumscribed, rubbery, elastic nodules either in the medullary cavity or on superficial bone areas such as the frontal bone. These dry, mucinous-appearing, caseating nodules appear radiographically as osteolytic areas at the center of the bone. Sometimes the osteolysis is associated with sequestrum formation, with more peripheral defects, and with ossifying periostitis. The syphilitic calvarial changes regress in response to appropriate antibiotic therapy.

 Tumor?

Increased Structural Density (Sclerosis)

On the whole, it is rare for true neoplasms to arise from the calvarium. The differential diagnosis includes various conditions that can cause a nodular, patchy or more diffuse increase in calvarial density (Tables 4.**12**, 4.**13**).

The outer table may be affected by **plaquelike osteomas** (Fig. 4.**29**, p. 376) or **paraosseous osteomas**, which are very difficult to detect on routine skull films and are recognized by a bulge in the calvarium on spot films or preferably on CT (Figs. 4.**74**, 4.**83 c, d**).

Table 4.**12**   Conditions associated with a nodular or patchy increase in calvarial density

- Irregular sutural sclerosis (p. 369, Fig. 4.**13**)
- Osteosclerotic metastases
- Lymphoma (Fig. 4.**37**)
- Various forms of anemia (e.g., sickle cell anemia) (Fig. 4.**36**)
- Sarcoidosis
- Hyperparathyroidism (Fig. 4.**33**)
- Fibrous dysplasia (see also Fig. 4.**82**)
- Paget disease (see also Fig. 4.**81**)
- Tuberous sclerosis
- Hyperostosis of the inner table (p. 378, 379, Figs. 4.**34**, 4.**35**)
- Multiple osteomas (e.g., in Gardner syndrome) (see also Fig. 4.**29**)

Table 4.**13**   Conditions associated with a more diffuse increase in calvarial density

- Osteopetrosis (Fig. 4.**75**)
- Osteomyelosclerosis
- Endosteal hyperostosis
- Engelmann disease
- Various forms of anemia (Figs. 4.**36**, 4.**37**)
- Extensive fibrous dysplasia (including McCune–Albright syndrome)
- Metabolic disorders (hypoparathyroidism and hyperparathyroidism) (Fig. 4.**33**)
- Generalized hyperostosis of the inner table (Figs. 4.**34**, 4.**35**)

A good example of a condition causing a more or less generalized increase in calvarial density is **osteopetrosis** (Albers–Schönberg disease, marble bone disease). It has at least three different forms that are distinguished by their mode of inheritance and clinical presentation.

The sclerotic changes are more clearly appreciated in the basal portions of the skull than in the calvarium, especially in younger patients. In the AP projection, the dense orbits and sphenoid bones create the appearance of a mask. In many cases the paranasal sinuses are not pneumatized. The calvarium becomes increasingly dense with aging. The autosomal dominant form of osteopetrosis

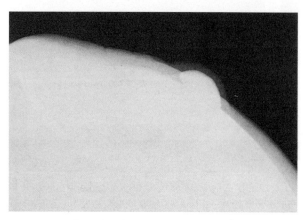

Fig. 4.**74**   Pedunculated osteoma on the outer table of the frontal squama, tangential projection.

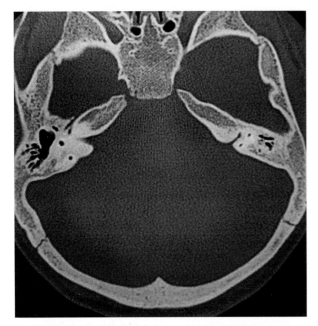

Fig. 4.**75** Generalized thickening and increased density of the cranial bones in osteopetrosis.

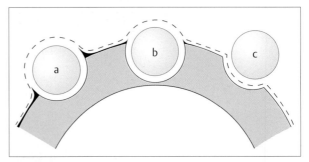

Fig. 4.**76a–c** Simplified diagram of epidermoid cysts in the calvarium. Shaded area indicates diploe; dashed line indicates periosteum.
a Extracranial, subperiosteal epidermoid cyst with typical marginal spurs.
b Intradiploic epidermoid cyst that has eroded through the outer cortex. Small marginal spurs.
c Epiperiosteal epidermoid cyst that has indented the outer table. No marginal spurs.

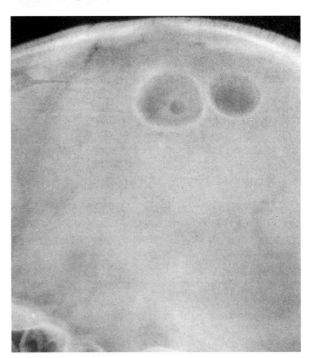

Fig. 4.**77** Dermoid cysts in the parietal bone.

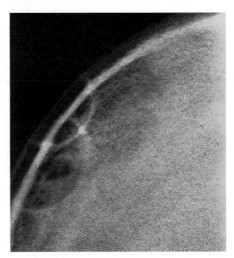

Fig. 4.**78** Tangential projection of dermoid cysts.

has two main forms based on the distribution pattern of the sclerotic changes:

1 Marked sclerosis of the calvarium, usually with a normal spinal column.
2 Pronounced sclerosis of the skull base with thickening of the vertebral endplates and curved areas of sclerosis in the iliac wings.

Figure 4.**75** illustrates the increased density and thickness of the calvarium in osteopetrosis.

Radiolucent Areas (Osteolysis)

Lucent areas in the calvarium have a broad pathoanatomic spectrum that ranges from thinning of the bone by vascular grooves (p. 369–374) and focal thinning of the diploe (Fig. 4.**25**) to the lytic stage of Paget disease and foci of true bone destruction.

Epidermoid cysts develop from dystopic epidermal elements during the third to fifth week of embryonic development. With an overall incidence of 0.9–2%, they rarely occur in bone and tend to occur at paraosseous sites inside or outside the calvarium. Intraosseous or bone-eroding types of epidermoid cyst are shown schematically in Fig. 4.**76**. Their radiographic hallmark is a distinct peripheral rim with destruction of the inner or outer table (Figs. 4.**77**, 4.**78**). Rarely, lobulated lucencies are also found. Epidermoid cysts can occur anywhere in the calvarium.

Dermoid cysts arise from derivatives of all three germ layers and are virtually indistinguishable from epidermoid cysts on radiographs. Sites of predilection besides the skull base and facial bones are:

- The frontal bone
- Near the fontanelles
- The mastoid process

Epidermoid and dermoid cysts in small children may increase in size until about 2 years of age. Thereafter they may resolve without treatment (Fig. 4.**79**).

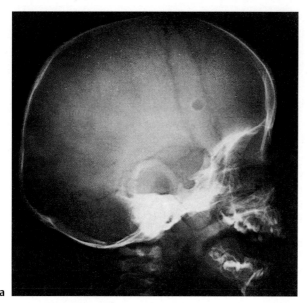

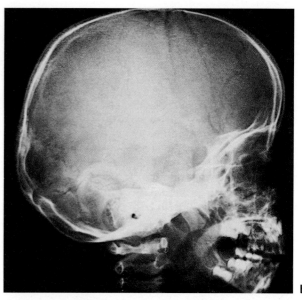

Fig. 4.**79a, b** Apparent epidermoid or dermoid cyst (observation by Holthusen, Hamburg).

a Uniform round lucency, 8 mm in diameter, with a sclerotic rim projected over the posterior part of the frontal bone in a 15-month-old boy (epidermoid or dermoid cyst?).

b Two years later the lesion is no longer visible. The differential diagnosis should include eosinophilic granuloma.

Hemangiomas are usually solitary, occasionally multiple, and may occur in the setting of angiomatous conditions (in various bones, skin, and internal organs). The very rare cavernous form causes circumscribed bean-sized to peanut-sized defects, which may be septated when large. The capillary form presents as a larger, circumscribed area of diffusely scattered millet-sized to lentil-sized lucencies with a very typical radial pattern of trabecular markings (Fig. 4.**80**). Additional features of hemangiomas are:

- Enlarged diploic venous channels
- Emissary veins surrounding the lesion

The most frequent cause of larger calvarial defects in preschool and school-age children is **Langerhans cell histiocytosis**. Pathoanatomically, this disease involve a focal accumulation of proliferating histiocytes accompanied by scattered multinucleated giant cells and varying numbers of eosinophilic granulocytes. Eosinophilic granuloma is a subtype of Langerhans cell histiocytosis, which also includes Hand–Schüller–Christian disease and Abt–Letterer–Siwe disease based on their histological similarities. It is likely that Erdheim–Chester lipoid granulomatosis also belongs to this group of diseases. Eosinophilic granuloma affects the calvarium in approximately 27% of cases, the femur in 17%, the spinal column in 12%, the pelvis in 9%, and the ribs in 8%. It can occur at other sites as well. Osteolytic lesions in the skull have a rounded or oval shape and reach 3 cm or more in diameter.

The morphology of the lesions depends on their age. Lesions in the early stage are sharply demarcated and have a punched-out appearance. The margins of the osteolytic area are occasionally indistinct but never appear motheaten when there is a broad transition from the lesion to normal bone. Usually this is because the lesion has beveled margins due to its different degrees of advancement in the inner and outer tables. Separate lesions may coalesce to form large maplike defects, which may contain sequestra. If the osteolytic lesions coexist with diabetes insipidus (due to sellar destruction) and exophthalmos, a Hand–Schüller–Christian triad is present.

In its healing stage, the lesion develops a sclerotic margin that advances toward the center and leads to a concentric reduction and eventual obliteration of the lesion.

In patients over 50 years of age, the principal cause of larger calvarial defects is **Paget disease** (osteitis deformans, Fig. 4.**81**). Pagetic lesions differ from metastatic lesions in that the matrix of the calvarium is preserved but extremely demineralized (osteoporosis circumscripta, Fig. 4.**81**). This is easily demonstrated on CT scans. Tehranzadeh et al. (1998) may be consulted for a detailed review of the features that distinguish Paget disease from fibrous dysplasia of the calvarium.

Small lucent areas like those normally caused by broad diploic veins (p. 369–373) can be difficult to distinguish from **osteolytic metastases** or foci of **plasmacytoma** if they do not exceed the caliber of large veins. Metastatic lucencies typically have ill-defined margins, which is not always the case with plasmacytoma. In doubtful cases, CT and radionuclide scans can facilitate the diagnosis.

Sarcoidosis can present radiographically with rounded, smoothly marginated lucencies ranging from a few millimeters to several centimeters in size, unaccompanied by significant marginal sclerosis. Cranial involvement is often seen only as an incidental feature of this disease. A correct interpretation is particularly difficult if no other organ manifestations are present.

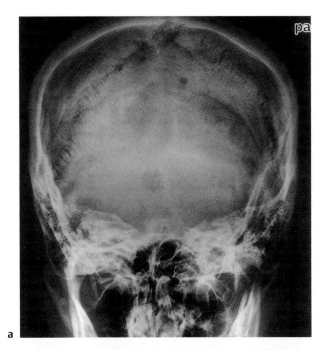

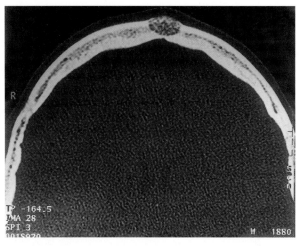

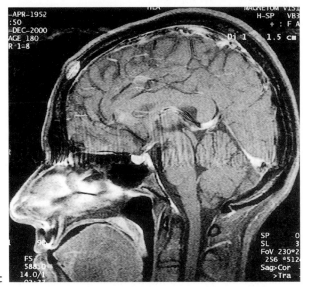

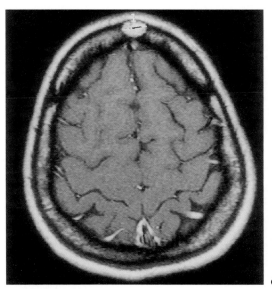

Fig. 4.**80 a–d**   Typical hemangioma in the frontal bone.
a PA skull film demonstrates a small, circumscribed area of osteolysis in the frontal bone.
b Typical CT appearance of calvarial hemangioma, showing characteristic trabecular markings within the lesion (high-resolution bone filter).

c, d Slightly expansile, enhancing lesion in the frontal bone on sagittal and axial MRI (T1 SE sequence with and without fat suppression).

Mixed Lytic and Sclerotic Changes

Paget disease exists in three different manifestations: a lytic stage (stage I), a combined stage (stage II), and a sclerotic stage (stage III).

Stage I is characterized by the appearance of large, sharply circumscribed radiolucent areas. This appearance in the skull is termed osteoporosis circumscripta. In stage II, osteolytic areas coexist with areas of new bone formation (sclerosis). There is an overall increase in bone volume, and the reparative new bone usually shows a streaky, irregularly sclerotic structure. In stage III, the af-

fected area becomes spotty or may have a relatively uniform streaky and sclerotic appearance. The reparative process generally results in thickened and deformed bony structures.

In the skull, the disease begins with one or more rounded or oval, sharply demarcated radiolucent areas that represent the lytic stage. These areas may reach several centimeters in diameter. It is not unusual to find large osteolytic areas involving almost the entire calvarium on one or even both sides. The areas may have serrated, curved, or wavy margins. The most common location is the

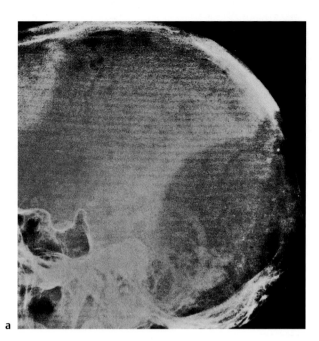

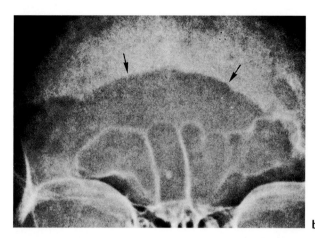

Fig. 4.**81 a, b**   Early stage of Paget disease.
a Osteolytic area in the occiput, lateral projection.
b Osteolytic area in the occiput, PA projection.

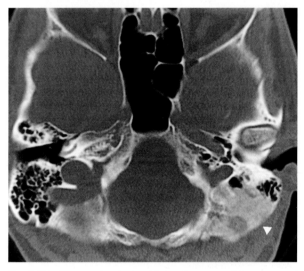

Fig. 4.**82**   Fibrous dysplasia with involvement of the temporal bone and occipital bone on the left side (arrowhead).

frontal region of the calvarium, followed by the occipital region. Ordinarily the process does not spare the cranial sutures. The destruction primarily involves the outer table, leaving the inner table intact. The sclerosis in stage II begins in the inner table, followed by thickening of the diploe and later of the outer table. Focal areas of sclerosis in the diploe give the calvarium a "cotton wool" appearance.

In stage III the sclerosis may be very dense, making it impossible to distinguish the usual three-layered structure of the calvarium. New bone formation may obliterate the paranasal sinuses, and the petrous pyramids appear more dense. Basilar impression is inevitable with occipital involvement due to the consequent weakening of the bone.

The lytic stage of Paget disease may persist for years with no changes, but rapid progression to stages II and III can occur.

Harmless pagetic lesions of the calvarium (osteoporosis circumscripta) as well as rare sarcomatous transformation

mainly require differentiation from metastatic lesions in these mostly older patients. The purely lytic stage of Paget disease requires differentiation from tumors that are known to produce osteolytic metastases, such as renal cell carcinoma. The differential diagnosis of stage II lesions should include metastases from breast carcinoma in women and from prostatic carcinoma in men. The latter metastases are rarely associated with much bone thickening, however, and usually they are smaller and show a more multifocal distribution. Pagetic lesions, by contrast, cover a larger area that is usually very conspicuous on radionuclide images.

Fibrous dysplasia of the skull has three different morphological presentations:

1 Pagetoid type
2 Predominantly sclerotic type
3 Predominantly lytic or cystic type

The pagetoid type is the most common and consists of a mixed pattern of osteolysis and new bone formation. It usually occurs in polyostotic forms. The outer table is expanded outward to form a blister or bulge. The inner table is thickened toward the cranial interior and toward the diploe and shows mottled lucency or mottled increased density.

The lytic or cystic type of fibrous dysplasia is usually solitary but may affect more than one bone if it spreads across the calvarial sutures. The lesions range from 2 to 5 cm in diameter. Often they have a thin, dense border and bulge outward. They are found more commonly in the outer table of the calvarium than in the inner table.

The sclerotic type predominantly affects the skull base, especially the sphenoid bone, and is associated with a diffuse and sometimes homogeneous increase in density. The sclerotic area is expanded and has a broad transition with healthy surrounding bone.

Involvement of the facial bones can cause marked prominence of the paranasal portions of the maxilla and of the frontal region, creating a leonine appearance (facies leontiasis ossea) similar to that in Paget disease. Besides plain radiographs, the changes are accurately demonstrated by CT, which can be important in differentiating the condition from Paget disease (Fig. 4.**82**). Patient age at the time of diagnosis (fibrous dysplasia affecting younger patients, Paget disease affecting older patients) makes a useful differentiating criterion.

Meningioma en plaque can occur in an osteoblastic and/or osteolytic form. The associated changes consist of localized sites of hyperostosis and/or destructive changes in the calvarium, possibly combined with abnormal vessels and calcifications (Figs. 4.**83**, 4.**84a–c**). A **fibrolipoma** of the calvarium is an extremely rare finding (Fig. 4.**84d–g**).

Neurofibromatosis (Recklinghausen disease) is characterized by the combined presence of neurinomas, pressure-induced destructive changes in the skull, and

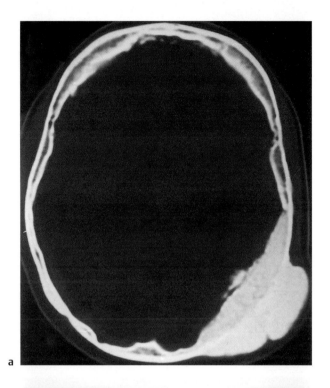

a

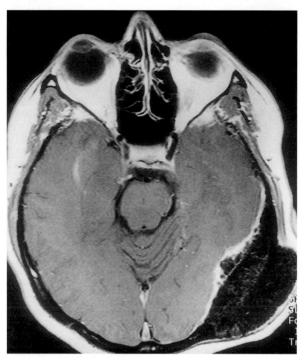

b

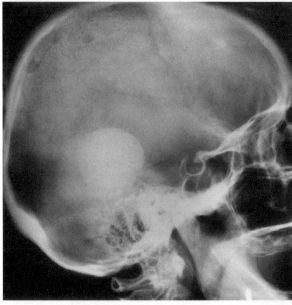

c

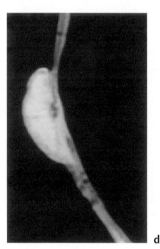

d

Fig. 4.**83 a–d**

a Large meningioma in the left parieto-occipital area. Both the interior and exterior of the skull show hyperostotic changes, and a relatively coarse, hard bony prominence is palpable externally. This CT slice clearly shows that the tumor has grown through the calvarium (apparently from the inside out) without destroying it. The contours of the outer table are still intact.

b T1-weighted MRI after intravenous contrast administration. The dura shows marked enhancement, appearing as a broad hyperintense zone between the hyperostosis and brain structures. Considerable new bone formation has occurred in response to the outward expansion of this meningioma.

c Compare with an eburnated osteoma on the right side of the calvarium of a 55-year-old woman. Clinically there was moderate aching pain, and the exostosis was surgically ablated.

d Magnified CT image using a high-resolution bone filter. The cranial bone below the osteoma shows no structural or morphological changes. Posteriorly, the diploe appears as a conspicuous linear lucency extending into the lesion.

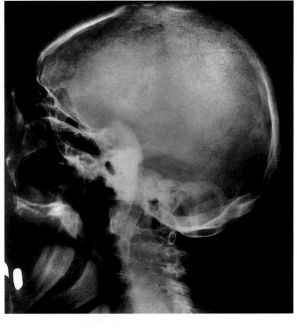

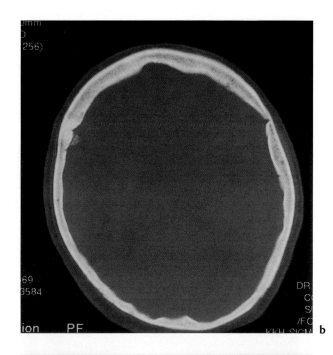

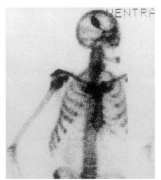

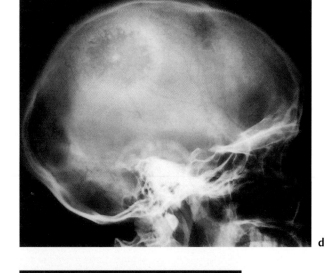

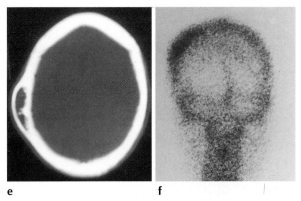

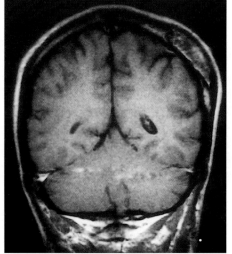

Fig. 4.**84 a–c**   Right frontal meningioma appears as a sclerotic area on the plain radiograph (**a**) and CT scan (**b**). On radionuclide imaging (**c**), the lesion shows high activity. (Histologically confirmed meningioma en plaque)

d–g Different patient than in **a–c**. Histologically confirmed fibrolipoma of the left parietal calvarium. (Case courtesy of Dr. Eising, Recklinghausen.)

d Lateral skull film shows an irregular, almost stellate osteolytic area with central calcifications.

e Bone-window CT shows a localized bulge in the outer table.

f Radionuclide scan shows a patchy area of increased uptake in the parietal region.

g T1-weighted MRI after intravenous contrast administration shows partial, intense enhancement of the mass.

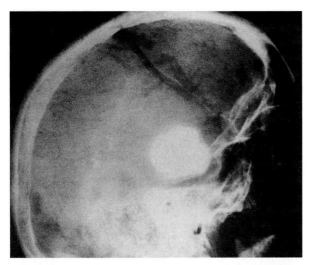

Fig. 4.**85** Large calcific density in an 87-year-old woman represents a calcified atheroma. The tumor was overpenetrated in the frontal projection and could not be identified.

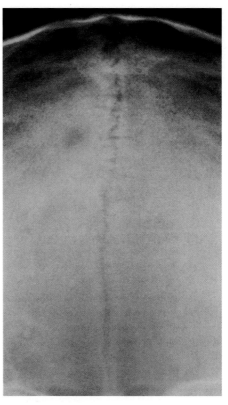

Fig. 4.**86** Frontal (metopic) suture. The parasagittal depressions in the inner table are normal.

meningiomas. Typically there is a defect in the posterosuperior orbital wall caused by a developmental defect involving the sphenoid wing and the orbital part of the frontal bone. This can allow the temporal lobe to come into contact with the orbital soft tissues, sometimes causing a pulsatile exophthalmos. Other cranial anomalies consist of absent or deformed clinoid processes, defects in the calvarium, and enlargement of the middle cranial fossa. Macrocranium is often seen in children (Table 4.**4**).

Hyperparathyroidism is characterized by rarefied or patchy markings with no well-defined trabeculae and loss of normal differentiation between the calvarial tables and the diploe, often accompanied by small sclerotic areas (**salt-and-pepper skull**). Structural weakening of the bone can lead to basilar impression (see Fig. 4.**33**, Table 4.**12**).

Osteolytic areas with a central, buttonlike bone fragment are called "**button sequestrum**" and have been observed in association with eosinophilic granulomas, tuberculous lesions, epidermoid and dermoid cysts, neoplastic processes, and "idiopathically."

A calcified atheroma in the subcutaneous tissue may be encountered as an unusual finding on skull radiographs (Fig. 4.**85**).

Special Aspects of the Frontal Bone, Parietal Bone, Squamous Temporal Bone, and Occipital Bone

Conditions that do not have a proclivity for specific bones of the calvarium were discussed earlier.

Frontal Bone

The frontal bone is a two-part symmetrical bone that is occasionally divided by an extra transverse suture, increasing the number of frontal ossification centers from two to four (Figs. 4.**1**, 4.**9**). Closure of the frontal suture (Fig. 4.**86**) begins in the second year of life. A frontal suture that is still open after 3 years of age is a normal variant called the **metopic suture**. Premature closure of the frontal suture leads to trigonocephaly (p. 390–392 and Table 4.**11**). The frontal suture may be widened in the midportion of its anterior

segment (**metopic fontanelle**), or in the segment above the glabella (**glabellar fontanelle**). The metopic fontanelle sometimes contains a sutural bone (fonticular bone), the os metopicum. This bone might also be called the "preinterfrontal bone" by analogy with the preinterparietal bone (p. 364, 365, Figs. 4.**9**, 4.**87**). The interparietal bone, os incae, in contrast, is an intercalary bone (Fig. 4.**9 f**). Cranium bifidum occultum refers to an increased distance between the frontal ossification centers, which may persist into adulthood.

A persistent and very prominent frontonasal suture is frequently observed on CT scans (Fig. 4.**88**).

Foci of ossification are occasionally found in the area of the normal indentation of the frontal and parietal bones near the bregma (Fig. 4.**65**). The sutural interdigitations in the outer table lengthen as calvarial growth proceeds. Sclerosis of these interdigitations starts at about 10 years of age and is most pronounced in the coronal suture.

Convolutional markings are normally sparse in the inner table of the frontal bone, but the channels for the frontal diploic veins are very prominent (Fig. 4.**89**). The **frontal emissary vein** is found in 0.2–0.3 % of all skull films. It appears as a bandlike lucency with sclerotic margins located one fingerwidth above the orbit and seen more often on one side (Fig. 4.**90**) than on both sides (Fig. 4.**91**). The frontal emissary vein connects the sagittal sinus with the orbital veins.

The sphenoparietal sulcus can form a deep groove, appearing on radiographs as a broad, conspicuous lucency that may terminate in venous lakes near the bregma.

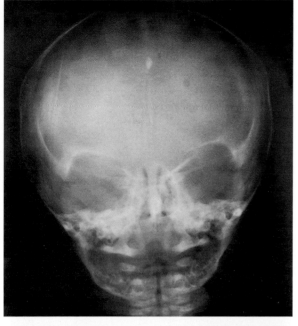

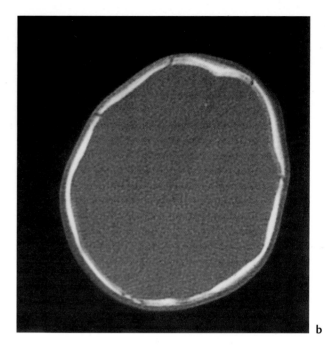

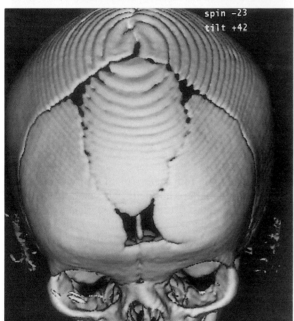

Fig. 4.**87 a–c**　Sutural bone (preinterfrontal bone) detected incidentally in a still-open frontal (metopic) suture. We considered this to be a sutural or fonticular bone of exceptional size. Note the underlying, elongated foci of ossification.
a　The cranial sutures show a "cruciform" pattern in the PA projection.
b　CT appearance using a high-resolution bone filter.
c　Shaded surface display reconstructed from the CT data set.

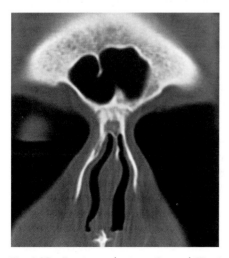

Fig. 4.**88**　Frontonasal suture. Coronal CT using a high-resolution bone filter.

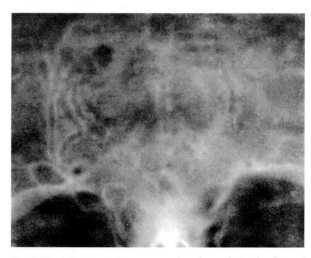

Fig. 4.**89**　Very conspicuous vascular channels in the frontal bone.

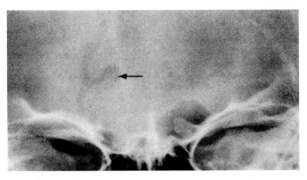

Fig. 4.**90**   Right frontal emissary vein with a saccular protrusion (arrow).

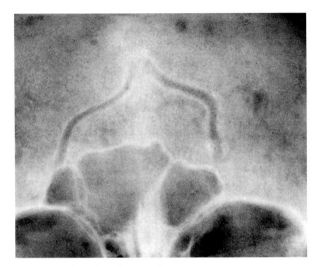

Fig. 4.**91**   Frontal emissary vein.

Parietal Bone

The parietal bone may be subdivided by a horizontal suture, but this is a very rare finding. This suture, which is sometimes incomplete, can mimic a thin fracture line in small children. It disappears with continued growth.

A **sutural bone** (fonticular bone) sometimes develops early within the anterior fontanelle and may completely fill it like an "operculum." It can grow quite large, persist, and in some cases mimic a parietal fracture (p. 364, 365, Table 4.**3** and Fig. 4.**9**).

As noted earlier (p. 373), the cranial vault is thickest at the parietal tubera. Also, sites of increased bone density are found at the attachment of the temporal muscles.

Thickening of the calvarial bone can result from appositional bone formation on the inner table in hyperostosis cranialis interna (p. 378, 379) and also, very rarely, from bone deposition on the outer table of the parietal bones. The latter process creates a typical calvarial deformity in the AP projection (Fig. 4.**92**). The "**asterion process**" is named for its proximity to the **asterion**, or the point where the mastoid process, parietal bone, and occipital squama intersect (see Fig. 4.**11**, no. 6). This process is located behind the mastoid and appears as a bony outgrowth on tangential radiographs.

Thinning of the calvarium may be internal or external. Internal thinning is caused primarily by blood vessels, i.e., by the diploic veins that communicate with the dural sinuses (chiefly the superior sagittal sinus and sphenoparietal sinus), by venous lakes, and by pacchionian granulations. These thinned areas may be unilateral or bilateral, are usually parasagittal at the level of the bregma, and have a characteristic appearance on frontal radiographs (Figs. 4.**93**, 4.**25 b–d**). Vessels, vascular markings, nutrient canals, and vascular grooves that affect the radiographic appearance of the calvarium are discussed on p. 369–373.

Venous lakes that occur on one or both sides of the superior sagittal sinus are called **lateral lacunae** and are extensions of the sagittal sinus. These saccular, blood-filled "**pericranial sinuses**" are found in a subperiosteal location and appear on tangential views as irregularly marginated parasagittal lucencies that are associated with watchglass-like thinning and bulging of the outer table (Figs. 4.**23**, 4.**94**).

Fig. 4.**92 a, b**   Diagram of the radiographic appearance of bony deposits on the outer table of the parietal bones ("crâne natiforme").

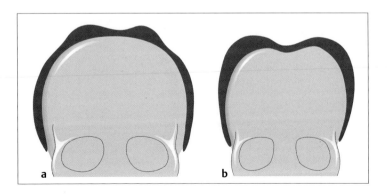

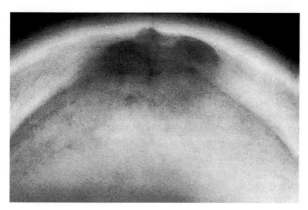

Fig. 4.**93** Normal parasagittal lucency.

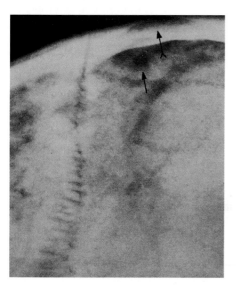

Fig. 4.**94** Parasagittal lucency with a blisterlike bulge of the thinned outer table (tailed arrow). Note the prominent venous plexuses, some appearing as "holes" when projected end-on (arrow). In the upper part of the coronal suture, the straight suture line in the inner table projects over the serrated line in the outer table.

External thinning of the parietal bone results from normal age-related bone resorption in **senile osteoporosis** and tends to flatten the cranial contour (Figs. 4.**95**–4.**98**). Age-related thinning of the calvarium usually occurs in the posterior part of the parietal bone, significantly increases the radiolucency of the bone, and is often combined with increased diploic venous markings, creating a mottled radiolucent pattern. The area of bone loss has straight margins. In the lateral view, the boundary with normal calvarial bone appears as a line or sometimes as two lines located one above the other. The outer table and diploe may even be absent in extreme cases. Figure 4.**96** illustrates an unusual symmetrical thinning of the posterior parietal bone in an anatomic specimen. The diagram in Fig. 4.**95** shows how this may appear on radiographs. These changes and the "pitting" atrophy that accompanies them pose no real problems of differential diagnosis owing to their typical location.

Differentiation is required from **parietal foramina**. These are bone defects with a familial incidence that typically show a bilaterally symmetrical distribution (usually 1 cm from the midsagittal plane and 3–4 cm above the lambdoid suture in the parietal bone). Most are only a few millimeters in size, but occasional "giant" foramina reach several centimeters in diameter (Fig. 4.**100**). The parietal foramina provide openings for the passage of emissary veins and have no pathological significance. The adjacent calvarium terminates smoothly at the defects and shows no discontinuities.

Parietal emissary veins connect the superior sagittal sinus with external soft-tissue veins. They appear as punctate structures in approximately two-thirds of all frontal skull projections (Figs. 4.**99**–4.**101**).

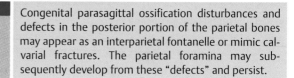

Congenital parasagittal ossification disturbances and defects in the posterior portion of the parietal bones may appear as an interparietal fontanelle or mimic calvarial fractures. The parietal foramina may subsequently develop from these "defects" and persist.

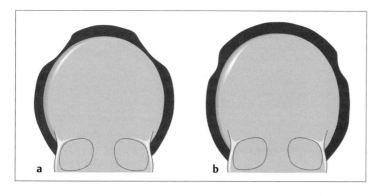

Fig. 4.**95 a, b** Diagrammatic representation of degrees of thinning of the parietal bone.

Fig. 4.**96** Senile atrophy of the skull in an anatomic speci- ▷ men.

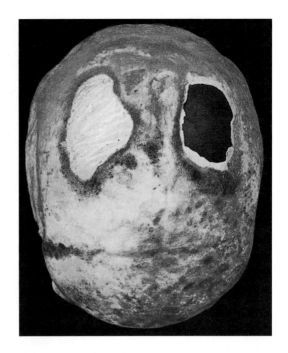

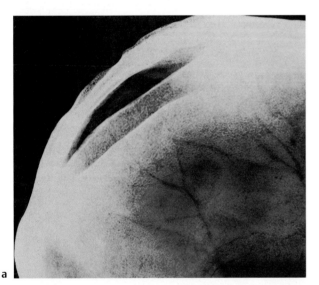

a

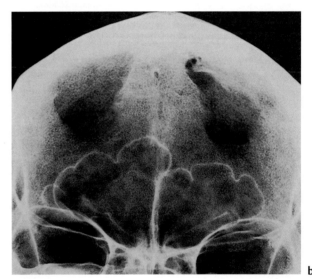

b

Fig. 4.**97 a, b**   Senile atrophy of the skull in a specimen radiograph.

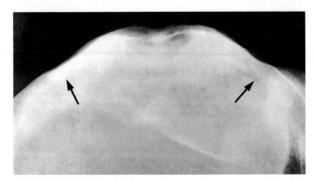

Fig. 4.**98**   Depression of both parietal bones in senile atrophy.

Fig. 4.**99**   Parietal foramina (two-tailed black arrows), lamb- ▷ doid suture (tailed white arrows), sagittal suture (black arrow), showing less serration at the level of the parietal foramina.

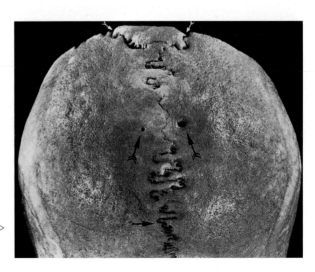

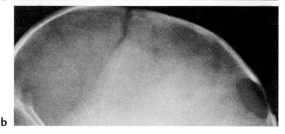

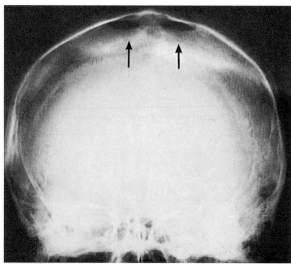

Fig. 4.**100 a, b**   Very large parietal foramina in a 14-month-old child and a defect in the sagittal suture.

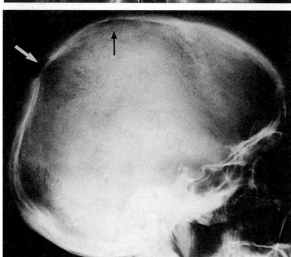

An **abnormal intrauterine lie** has also been identified as a rare cause of circumscribed external thinning of the parietal bone (Fig. 4.**102**).

Cranium bifidum occultum is a bony dysraphic anomaly that is analogous to spina bifida occulta. It is characterized by full-thickness defects in the parietal bone, consisting of rounded or slitlike clefts in the calvarial midline with no associated soft-tissue abnormalities. Thus it is not a true encephalocele, which is among the dysraphic anomalies that can develop during neural tube closure. Of course, cephaloceles (which include encephaloceles, encephalocystoceles, meningoceles, or their combinations) also create portals for the passage of soft tissues through the bony skull (p. 428 and Table 4.**14**).

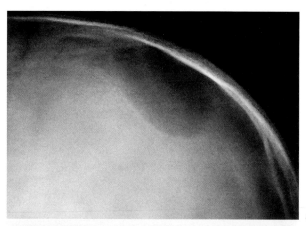

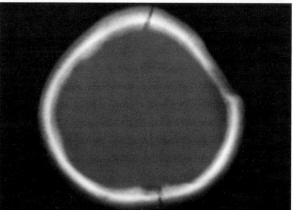

Fig. 4.**102 a, b**   Abnormal intrauterine lie.
Radiograph (**a**) shows an elliptical lucency high in the parietal area. Corresponding CT scan (**b**) shows that the calvarium has been thinned from the outside (bone erosion due to an abnormal intrauterine lie).

◁ Fig. 4.**101 a, b**   Parietal foramen in a 58-year-old man.
a Frontal projection demonstrates normal parasagittal lucencies on both sides (arrows).
b Lateral projection shows typical thinning of the calvarium behind the coronal suture (arrow). Below there is a very large parietal foramen (white arrow).

Squamous Temporal Bone

The temporal squama is the only part of the temporal bone that contributes to the formation of the cranial vault. This flat membranous bone is external to the petrous bone during fetal development, fusing with it only after birth.

Paired lateral fontanelles are present on each side of the calvarium at birth, situated between the frontal and occipital squama and below the parietal bone. The **sphenoidal** **fontanelle** is anterolateral, and the **mastoid fontanelle** is posterolateral (Fig. 4.**103a**). Since they are paired, they account for four of the six fontanelles present at birth, which are located near the skull base, petrous temporal bone, and greater sphenoid wing. In some cases these fontanelles can persist far into adulthood and may be mistaken for sites of pathological bone destruction (Fig. 4.**103b, c**).

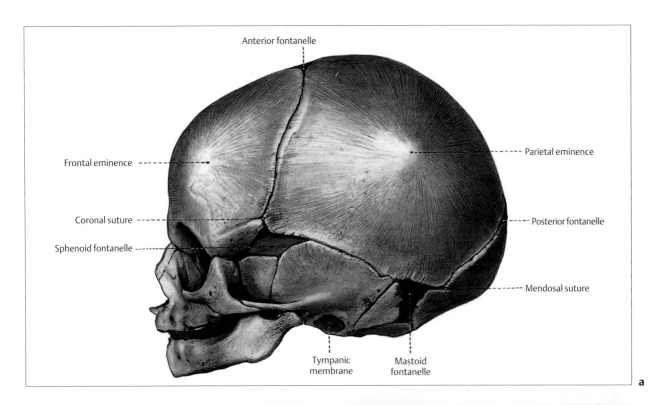

a

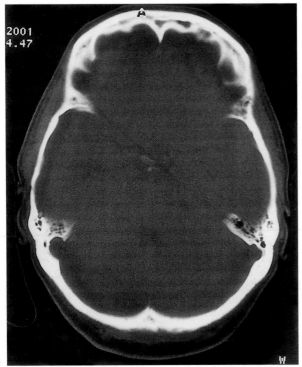

b

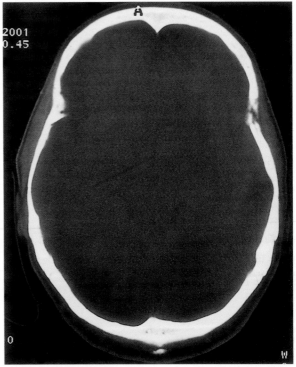

c

Fig. 4.**103a–c**
a Lateral view of the skull of a newborn. (From Rauber and Kopsch 1987.)

b, c Cranial CT in a 56-year-old woman who was examined for exclusion of intracranial hemorrhage. The scans show extensive structural irregularities in the area of the former left sphenoid fontanelle.

As elsewhere, atypical sutures can also occur in the temporal squama (p. 364, 365). A lateral skull projection with 30° of craniocaudal tube angulation is best for demonstrating the temporal squama, like the tube position used for a Schüller view of the petrous bone (p. 459, 460). Because of its thinness, the temporal squama often appears more radiolucent than the other cranial bones in the lateral projection. Besides the roof of the mandibular fossa, the temporal squama is the weakest part of the lateral skull wall.

The **senile atrophy** mentioned in the section on the parietal bone (p. 408, 409) may extend to the squamous part of the temporal bone. The temporal muscle attachments may be outlined in these cases by a sclerotic rim (Fig. 4.**104**).

It is sometimes difficult in the temporal squama to distinguish fracture lines from vascular grooves (p. 369–373, Figs. 4.**66**, 4.**67**).

> A vascular structure typically appears as an elongated, bandlike lucency that runs a straight or tortuous course. A lucency in the calvarium should therefore be identified as a blood vessel if it exhibits the anatomic course of a vessel. Unlike a fracture line, a vascular groove will usually show a slight increase in density somewhere along its margin (Figs. 4.**66**, 4.**67**). Also, vascular grooves generally show a symmetrical arrangement. Another difference can be appreciated on spot films and CT scans: unlike meningeal vascular grooves, fracture lines generally involve the full thickness of the calvarium.

Figures 4.**105** and 4.**106** show the radiographic anatomy and appearance of the squamous suture in a specimen, along with other structures located about the temporal squama. The **petrotympanic fissure** (glaserian fissure), located posteromedial to the mandibular fossa, is projected anterior to the external porus acusticus over the posterior margin of the temporomandibular joint (Figs. 4.**107**, 4.**108a**). CT provides a much clearer view of the petrotympanic fissure than projection radiographs (Fig. 4.**108b**).

In the axial view, the **petrosquamous fissure** is visible between the tegmen tympani and the petrous pyramid (Figs. 4.**107**, 4.**109**). Projection effects between the tegmen, a thin bony layer that forms the roof of the tympanic cavity, and other superimposed, denser bony structures such as the styloid process can cause apparent string-of-beads densities in the axial projection (Fig. 4.**110**). More details on the anatomy of the tegmen tympani are given on p. 457, 466 and Fig. 4.**221**.

The **sphenosquamous suture** is projected over the petrous apex in the Stenvers view of the petrous temporal bone. Normally it extends beyond the petrous apex (Figs. 4.**5**, 4.**111**).

The **groove for the middle meningeal artery** runs along the inner wall of the squamous temporal bone and may project over the upper margin of the petrous bone in the Stenvers view (Figs. 4.**66**, 4.**112**, 4.**268**). The groove may be bridged by bone, transforming it into a tunnel. In the lateral projection (and the Schüller projection), the auricle appears as a semicircular shadow of cartilaginous density above the petrous bone (Figs. 4.**35**, 4.**42**, 4. **50**, 4.**52**). It may contain calcifications, especially after frostbite, chronic trauma, and chronic recurring polychondritis.

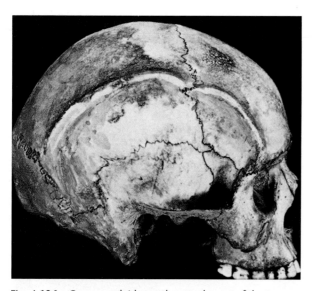

Fig. 4.**104**   Groove and ridge at the attachment of the temporal muscle.

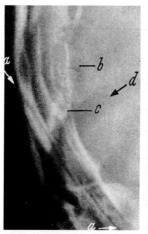
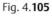
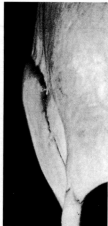

Fig. 4.**105**   Fig. 4.**106**

Fig. 4.**105**   Cranial sidewall in the frontal projection.
a In the direction of the arrow: squamous suture (between the temporal squama and parietal bone).
b Coronal suture in the outer table.
c Coronal suture in the inner table.
d Groove for the transverse sinus (transverse sulcus, arrow).

Fig. 4.**106**   Temporal squama in a specimen, showing the typical oblique suture line entering the squama.

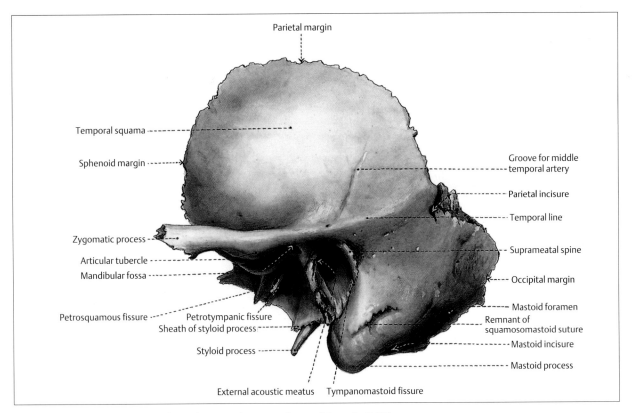

Fig. 4.**107**   Left temporal bone, lateral aspect. (From Rauber and Kopsch 1987.)

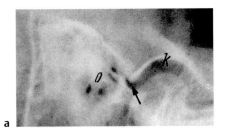

a

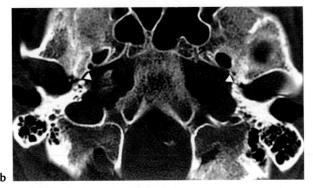

b

Fig. 4.**108 a, b**
a Schüller projection. Petrotympanic fissure (of Glaser). Arrow projected between the anterior wall of the auditory canal (O) and the glenoid fossa of the temporomandibular joint (K).
b Petrotympanic fissure on each side (arrowheads). CT with high-resolution bone filter.

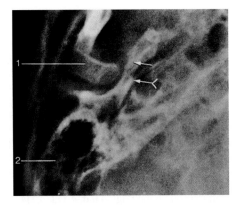

Fig. 4.**109**   Petrosquamous fissure (tailed arrow) and orthograde projection of the tegmen ("crista tegmentalis," arrow) in an axial view.
1   Mandibular condyle
2   Mastoid

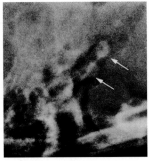

Fig. 4.**110**   String-of-beads pattern in the region of the tegmen in an axial view (arrows). The pattern is produced by superimposed bony prominences (in this case the styloid process).

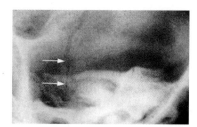

Fig. 4.**111**   Sphenosquamous suture (arrows) on a Stenvers view of the petrous bone.

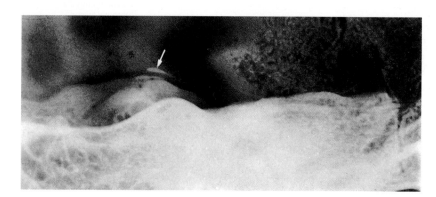

Fig. 4.**112**   Stenvers view of the petrous bone. A middle meningeal artery groove is visible above the petrous ridge (arrow). See also Figures 4.**66** and 4.**67**.

Occipital Bone

Only the portion of the occipital squama located above the transverse sinus (the upper part of the squama) is included in the cranial vault. This part is membranous bone that ossifies from paired centers (Figs. 4.**2**–4.**6**).

The membranous bones appear shortly after the formation of the first unpaired ossification center for the lower part of the squama (the supraoccipital), which is preformed in cartilage. The occipital squama is formed from the cartilaginous supraoccipital and the membranous interparietal (Fig. 4.**6d**). The upper and lower parts of the squama unite early across the intervening fissure, first through bridging of their outer and inner margins by periosteal trabeculae and later through direct fusion. A **lateral incisure** 1–3 cm long and 0.5–1 mm wide ("**mendosal suture**") persists on each side of the squama in the newborn to mark the line of union between the upper and lower parts. Each incisure is still located entirely within the membranous bone (Figs. 4.**6 d**, 4.**113**, 4.**114**). It is still open by 5–8 years of age in 10% of cases, by age 9–10 in 4%, and by age 15 in 1%.

The fissure itself may persist as the **transverse suture**, separating both parts of the squama just above the transverse sinus on each side. The portion of the upper squama that extends to the lambdoid suture is called the **interparietal bone** or Inca bone (Figs. 4.**9e, f**, 4.**115**, 4.**116**).

Subdivision of the interparietal bone by additional, sagittally directed sutures gives rise to a bipartite or multipartite Inca bone (Fig. 4.**9f**). The median suture is called the biinterparietal suture; the lateral sutures are called the lateral interparietal sutures (Fig. 4.**114**).

Not to be confused with the interparietal bone is the **preinterparietal bone** or **apical bone**, which is located above the lambdoid suture in the area of the posterior fontanelle and may be multipartite (Figs. 4.**9g**, 4.**117**). Radiographs show one or more sutural bones that can usually be seen until about 10 years of age and then disappear. Sutural bones of varying size are also occasionally found in the

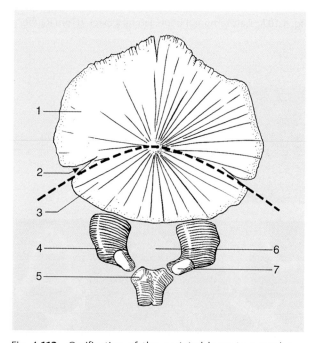

Fig. 4.**113**   Ossification of the occipital bone in a newborn. The dashed line marks the boundary between membranous bone and chondral bone. Posterior aspect. (After Theiler). See also Figure 4.**6d**

1   Upper part of the occipital squama (interparietal bone)
2   Lateral incisure
3   Lower part of the occipital squama (supraoccipital)
4   Exoccipital
5   Basioccipital
6   Foramen magnum
7   Occipital condyle

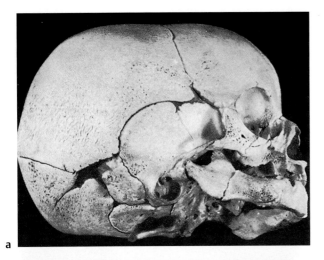

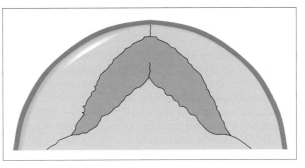

Fig. 4.**115** Lambdoid suture with interparietal bone and transverse suture (persistent). See radiograph in Fig. 4.**116** and Fig. 4.**9 e, f** (diagram).

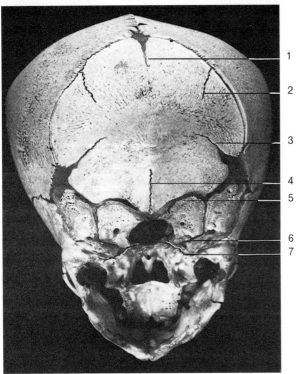

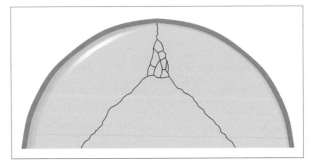

Fig. 4.**116** Interparietal bone (Inca bone) detected incidentally in a one-year-old child.

Fig. 4.**114 a, b**   Cranial sutures in an anatomic specimen.
a Lateral aspect. Intercalary bone in the posterolateral (mastoid) fontanelle between the occipital squama, parietal squama, temporal squama, and mastoid.
b Sutures in and adjoining the occipital squama. See Figures 4.**9** and 4.**113**.
1   Biinterparietal suture
2   Lateral interparietal suture
3   Mendosal suture
4   Median cerebellar synchondrosis
5   Posterior interoccipital synchondrosis
6   Basioccipital synchondrosis
7   Anterior interoccipital synchondrosis

Fig. 4.**117** Lambdoid suture with multipartite preinterparietal bone (see also Fig. 4.**9 g**) (apical bone), which is a fonticular bone.

sagittal and lambdoid sutures (Figs. 4.**117**, 4.**118**). General aspects of sutural bones and intercalary bones are reviewed on p. 364, 365, 369.

When foramen-like, bandlike, or honeycomb-like lucencies are found in the area of the transverse sinus, it can be extremely difficult to distinguish between venous lakes and pacchionian granulations (arachnoid diverticula) on projection radiographs (Figs. 4.**20**, 4.**119**). The differential diagnosis of calvarial lucencies in general covers a broad spectrum ranging from cephaloceles (p. 387, 388, 428, Fig. 4.**58**) and lacunar skull (p. 389) to other conditions such as tumor-associated bone destruction, eosinophilic granuloma, epidermoid/dermoid cysts (Figs. 4.**76**–4.**79**) or hemangioma (Fig. 4.**80**). Another important differential diagnosis is shown in Fig. 4.**120**, though it is rarely as conspicuous as in the figure.

The **grooves for the transverse sinuses** are usually easy to identify on a Towne projection of the occiput (Fig. 4.**121 a**). It is rare to find complete or partial absence of the initial portion of the sinus due to partial or complete aplasia (Fig. 4.**122**). Reportedly, the right transverse sinus is consistently somewhat larger than the left sinus. The transverse sinus may appear as a "hole" when viewed in an end-on projection. When the cerebellomedullary cistern is enlarged, the groove for the transverse sinus on each side may show a bell-shaped upward extension into the area of the sinus confluence to encompass the enlarged cistern. In the axial projection, the condylar fossae (canales) may appear above the petrous ridges on each side (Fig. 4.**121 b**). The occipital squama is particularly thick in the area of the internal and external **occipital protuberances** (Fig. 4.**123**). A spurlike bony process is often found on the external protuberance and may be of considerable size; this is the **occipital spur** at the attachment of the nuchal ligament (Fig. 4.**124 a, c**). It may be evidence for the presence of acromegaly. In other cases, rounded ossifications that are separate from the skull may form in the nuchal ligament and establish a jointlike connection with the occiput (Fig. 4.**124 b**).

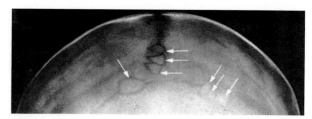

Fig. 4.**118**   Sutural bones in the sagittal and lambdoid sutures (arrows).

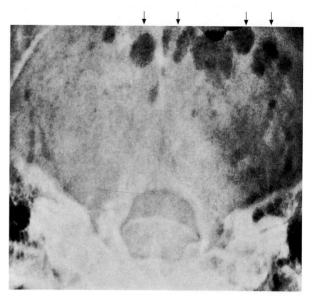

Fig. 4.**119**   Pacchionian granulations (or venous lacunae) near the transverse sinus on each side (arrows).

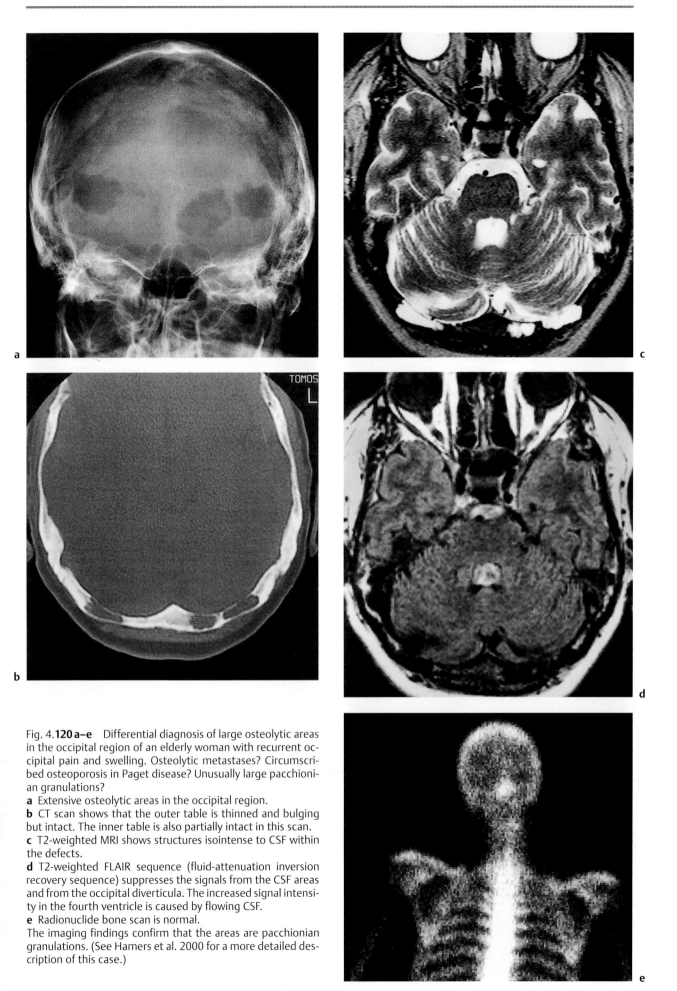

Fig. 4.**120 a–e** Differential diagnosis of large osteolytic areas in the occipital region of an elderly woman with recurrent occipital pain and swelling. Osteolytic metastases? Circumscribed osteoporosis in Paget disease? Unusually large pacchionian granulations?

a Extensive osteolytic areas in the occipital region.

b CT scan shows that the outer table is thinned and bulging but intact. The inner table is also partially intact in this scan.

c T2-weighted MRI shows structures isointense to CSF within the defects.

d T2-weighted FLAIR sequence (fluid-attenuation inversion recovery sequence) suppresses the signals from the CSF areas and from the occipital diverticula. The increased signal intensity in the fourth ventricle is caused by flowing CSF.

e Radionuclide bone scan is normal.

The imaging findings confirm that the areas are pacchionian granulations. (See Hamers et al. 2000 for a more detailed description of this case.)

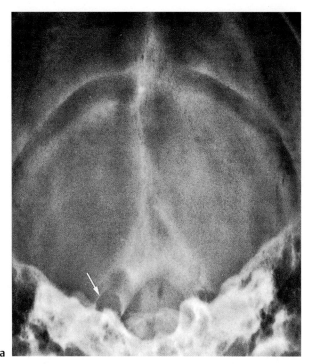

a

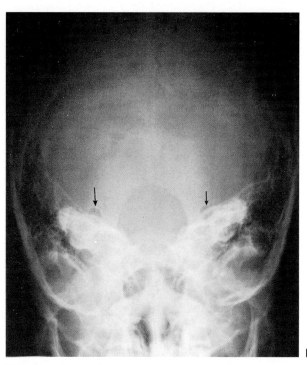

b

Fig. 4.**121 a, b**   Lucencies caused by vascular structures.
a The transverse sinus is very well developed and is larger on the right side than on the left. A large jugular foramen is visible on the right side (arrow).

b Fossa of the condylar canal on each side (arrows).

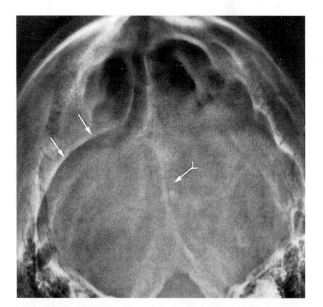

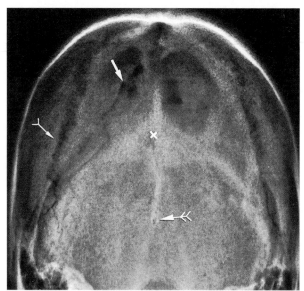

Fig. 4.**122**   Very prominent groove for the transverse sinus on the right side (arrows) merging with the groove for the superior sagittal sinus. A transverse sinus groove is not visible on the left side, probably due to aplasia of the left transverse sinus. A tailed arrow marks the occipital crest.

Fig. 4.**123**   Thickening of the bone by the external and internal occipital protuberances (×).
Arrow: pacchionian granulation
One-tailed arrow: lambdoid suture
Two-tailed arrow: internal occipital crest

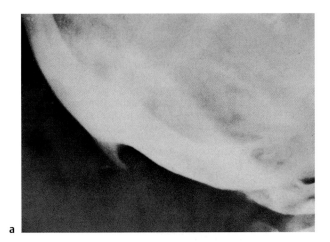

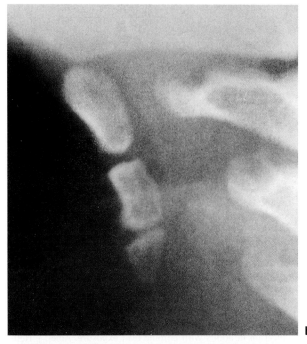

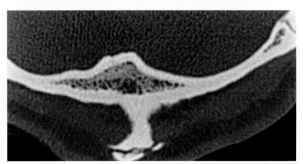

Fig. 4.**124 a–c**   Occipital spur and ligamentous ossification.
a Occipital spur.
b Foci of ossification in the nuchal ligament.
c Prominent occipital spur in a different patient.

References

"Cranial Vault"

Andersen, P. E., J. Bollerslev: Heterogeneity of autosomal dominant osteopetrosis. Radiology 164 (1987) 223

Belden, C. J.: The skull base and calvaria. Adult and pediatric. Neuroimaging Clin. N. Amer. 8 (1998) 1

Bergerhoff, W.: Metrische Untersuchungen an der Basis des Skelettschädels. Fortschr. Röntgenstr. 82 (1955 a) 505

Bergerhoff, W.: Messungen von Winkeln und Strecken am submento-vertikalen Röntgenbild der Schädelbasis. Fortschr. Röntgenstr. 82 (1955 b) 509

Bergerhoff, W.: Statistische Untersuchungen der Schädelbasis am submento-vertikalen Röntgenbild. Acta Neurochir. Suppl. 3 (1955 c) 67

Bergerhoff, W., W. Hübler: Messungen von Winkeln und Strecken am Röntgenbild von Kindern und Jugendlichen. Fortschr. Röntgenstr. 78 (1953) 190

Bergerhoff, W., R. Martin: Messungen von Winkeln und Strecken am Röntgenbild des Schädels von Säuglingen und Kleinkindern. Fortschr. Röntgenstr. 80 (1954) 742

Boureks, E. C., C .F. Lanzieri: The calvarium. Semin. Ultrasound 15 (1994) 424

Cohen, C. R., P. M. Duchesneau, M. A. Weinstein: Calcification of basal ganglia as visualized by computed tomography. Radiology 134 (1980) 97

Cronqvist, S.: Roentgenologic evaluation of cranial size in children. Acta Radiol. 7 (1968) 97

Dinkel, L.: Symmetrische Verkalkungen des Hirnstammes und ihre Differentialdiagnose. Fortschr. Röntgenstr. 106 (1967) 407

Dolan, K. D.: Cervico-basilar relationships. Radiol. Clin. N. Amer. 15 (1977) 155

Du Boulay, G., H.: Principles of X-Ray Diagnosis of the Skull. Butterworths, London 1980

Eising, E. G., A. Roessner, F. Brandt: Fibrolipom der Schädelkalotte, eine Erstbeschreibung? Osteologie 5 (1996) 231–236

Feneis, H.: Pocket Atlas of Human Anatomy 4. Aufl. Thieme, Stuttgart–New York 2000

Fischer, E.: Processus asteriacus des Scheitelbeines. Fortschr. Röntgenstr. 88 (1958) 69

Freyschmidt, J.: Skeletterkrankungen. Klinisch-radiologische Diagnose und Differentialdiagnose. 2. Aufl. Springer, Berlin–Heidelberg–New York 1997

Freyschmidt, J., H. Ostertag, G. Jundt: Knochentumoren. 2. Aufl.. Springer, Berlin–Heidelberg–New York 1998

Frick, H., H. Leonhardt, D. Starck: Spezielle Anatomie II. Kopf-Hals-Eingeweide-Nervensystem. 2. Aufl. Thieme, Stuttgart 1980

Furuya, Y., M. S. B. Edwards, C. E. Alpers, B. M. Tress, D. K. Ousterhout, D. Norman: Computed tomography of cranial sutures. Part I: Comparison of suture anatomy in children and adults. J. Neurosurg. 61 (1984) 53

Hamers, S., J. Freyschmidt, B. Terwey: Diagnostik tumorsimulierender intraossärer Arachnoidaldivertikel mittels flüssigkeitssensitiver MR-Sequenzen, ein Fallbericht. Fortschr. Röntgenstr. 172 (2000) 850

Helmke, K., P. Winkler: Die Häufigkeit von Pinealisverkalkungen in den ersten 18 Lebensjahren. Fortschr. Röntgenstr. 144 (1986) 221

Hoevels-Guerlich, H., L. Haferkorn, M. Persigehl, R. Hofstetter, G. von Bermuth: Widening of cranial sutures after long-term prostaglandin E 2 therapy in 2 newborn infants. J. Pediat. 105 (1984) 72

Jinkins, J. R.: Atlas of Neuroradiologic Embryology, Anatomy, and Variants.
Lippincott Williams and Wilkins, Philadelphia 2000

Kirchhof, K., T. Welzel, K. Ziegel: Neuroradiologische Befunde bei der Hemiatrophia facialis progressiva (Parry–Romberg-Syndrom). Fortschr. Röntgenstr. 172 (2000) 785

Osborn, A. G.: Diagnostic Neuroradiology.
Mosby, St. Louis, Baltimore, Boston, Chicago 1994

Rauber/Kopsch: Bewegungsapparat, Bd. I. Hrsg. von Tillmann, B., G. Töndury. In Rauber/Kopsch: Anatomie des Menschen. Lehrbuch und Atlas. 1. Aufl.. Hrsg. Leonhardt, H., B. Tillmann, G. Töndury, K. Zilles.
Thieme, Stuttgart 1987

Reeder, M. M., W. G. Bradley Jr.: Reeder and Felsons's Gamuts in Radiology. Comprehensive lists of Roentgen Differential Diagnosis. 3rd ed.
Springer, New York–Berlin–Heidelberg 1993

Reginato, A. J., Schiapachasse, V., Guerrero, R. Familial Idiopathic Hypertrophic Osteoarthropathy and Cranial Suture Defects in Children. Skeletal Radiol. 8 (1982) 105–109.

Reyes, P., C. F. Gonzales, M. K. Zalewsky, A. Besarab: Intracranial calcification in adults with chronic lead exposure. Amer. J. Neuroradiol. 6 (1985) 905

Schinz, H. R.: Schädel—Gehirn. In: Schinz: Radiologische Diagnostik in Klinik und Praxis, Bd. V, Teil 1. 7. Aufl. Hrsg. Frommhold, W., W. Dihlmann, H.-St. Stender, P. Thurn.
Thieme, Stuttgart 1986

Schultze, J., E. Kraus: Wachsende Fraktur im Kindesalter. Fortschr. Röntgenstr. 151 (1989) 112

Schuster, W., L. A. Tamacha: Das Verhalten der Schädelnähte beim Neugeborenen und Säugling unter physiologischen und pathologischen Bedingungen. Ann.Radiol. 9 (1996) 232

Som, E. M., H. D. Curten: Head and Neck Imaging. 3rd ed., Mosby, St. Luis 1996

Swartz, J. D., H. R. Harnsberger: Imaging of the Temporal Bone. 3rd ed., Thieme 1998

Tehranzadeh, J., Y. Fung, M. Donohue, A. Anavim, H. W. Pribram: Computed tomography of Paget disease of the skull versus fibrous dysplasia. Skelet. Radiol. 27 (1998) 664

Thelen, M., G. Ritter, E. Bücheler: Radiologische Diagnostik der Verletzungen von Knochen und Gelenken.
Thieme, Stuttgart–New York 1993

von Torklus, D., W. Gehle: Die obere Halswirbelsäule, 3. Auflage Thieme, Stuttgart 1987

Voigt, K., M. Schumacher, C. Ostertag, B. Kraft: Röntgenologische Diagnose und Differentialdiagnose der Stammganglienverkalkungen. Radiologe 18 (1978) 113

Zimmermann, R.A.: Evaluation of head injury: Supratentorial. In Taveras, J. M., J. T. Ferrucci: Radiology: Diagnosis—imaging—intervention, Vol. III.
Lippincott, Philadelphia 1987

Skull Base

Various criteria can be used in subdividing the skull base into parts. We prefer an anatomic subdivision that also takes into account functional aspects.

We divide the internal skull base into a **median cranial region** that is flanked by paired **lateral cranial regions**. The line connecting the anterior and posterior clinoid processes marks the boundary between the middle and lateral regions.

The median cranial region is formed by the clivus, the sella turcica, the anterior part of the body of the sphenoid bone, and by the ethmoid bone with the crista galli. The region as a whole has an angled shape. The lateral cranial regions contains the anterior, middle, and posterior fossae, which are arranged in a tiered configuration (Fig. 4.**5**). The anterior fossa is the highest of the three and houses the frontal lobe of the cerebrum. The middle fossa contains the temporal lobe of the cerebrum. The posterior fossa is the lowest of the three fossae and also the largest. It is bounded rostrally by the posterior surface of the petrous bone. The groove for the sigmoid sinus is usually deeper and broader on the right than on the left, as is the diameter of the venous part of the jugular foramen. The occipital squama forms most of the floor of the posterior fossa. The development of the skull base was discussed on p. 359.

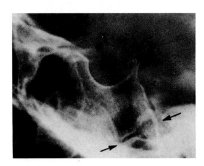

Fig. 4.**125**   Spheno-occipital synchondrosis (arrows).

posterior intraoccipital synchondroses each close between the second and third year of life. The sphenooccipital synchondrosis does not close until the 16th to 20th year and appears radiographically as a transverse lucent band in the clivus at the level of the petrous apex (Fig. 4.**125**).

The **temporal bone** consists of the temporal squama and tympanic part, which are preformed in membranous tissue, and the petrous part, which is preformed in cartilage.

The **sphenoid bone** is ossified from numerous centers in a very complex process (Fig. 4.**6a**), accounting for the many developmental variants that can occur in the sphenoid bone itself and in the foramina of the middle skull base, the optic canal, and the sella turcica.

The most anterior portion of the skull base reaches its approximate definitive length by the third year of life and undergoes no significant further growth thereafter. The clivus reaches about half of its definitive length during the first two years of life.

Anterior, Middle, and Posterior Cranial Fossae

Normal Findings

 During Growth

The bones of the skull base are preformed in cartilage, and so this part of the skull is also termed the **chondrocranium**. The cartilaginous structures of the skull base begin to form during the second month of fetal development. Ossification commences shortly thereafter. Only portions of the sphenoid bone and occipital bones and the sphenooccipital and petrooccipital synchondroses are still cartilaginous at birth. Most of the **occipital bone** is preformed in cartilage and is ossified from four centers located around the foramen magnum:

- A ventral basioccipital
- Two lateral exoccipitals
- A dorsal supraoccipital

The interparietal part of the occipital bone is preformed in connective tissue (Fig. 4.**6d**). It combines with the supraoccipital to form the occipital squama. The anterior and

 In Adulthood

Unlike the calvarium, the skull base does not show sex differences in adults. The depth of the posterior fossa increases with aging, as do the width of the skull base and the transverse diameter of the cranial vault.

Constants in the Architecture of the Skull Base

- The anterior skull base has a relatively constant internal length of 60 mm.
- The location of the important structural supports of the skull base does not depend at all on the shape of the cranial vault. The principal support columns in the skull base are the petrous pyramids and the greater wings of the sphenoid bone. Based on the statistical analysis of submentovertex views of the skull, the petrous pyramids enclose a posterior angle of approximately 120° while the greater sphenoid wings form an anterior angle of approximately 90° (Fig. 4.**126**).

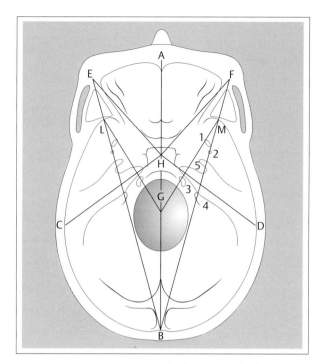

Fig. 4.**126**   Drawing of the angles formed by the basal support structures (after Bergerhoff).
CHD 119°
EBF 36°
EHF 90°
LGM 70°
1   Foramen ovale
2   Foramen spinosum
3   Condylar canal
4   Jugular foramen
5   Carotid canal

- Measurements in skulls with a wide range of configurations have shown no significant differences in the location of the basal support structures. This consistency is important, as it provides a way to differentiate normal variants from anomalies (Fig. 4.**61**).
- The relatively constant sphenoid angle (nasion–tuberculum sellae–basion = basal angle = Welcker angle) averages 132° (126–138°) and provides a way to measure skull base angulation in adults. It is still 144° in newborns and thus decreases by an average of 12° during growth. An obtuse basal angle is suggestive of basilar impression. In this case the posterior surface of the clivus, which is normally flat or slightly concave, is frequently convex.
- The anterior rim of the foramen magnum (basion) is slightly higher than the posterior rim (opisthion) in relation to the canthomeatal plane, i.e., the plane of the posterior rim is inclined slightly upward from backward to forward. The slope of the foramen magnum can be described by several angles, e.g.: the angle between the plane of the foramen magnum and the clivus slope, which normally measures 136 ± 12°. The basal angle (opisthion-basion angle, Fig. 4.**149**) is important in the detection if **basilar impression**. It measures approximately 163°.
- The length of the basal part of the occipital bone at the clivus normally measures 31 mm in specimens and approximately 32 mm on radiographs. The radiographic

measurement (subject to significant errors) is made from the petrous apex near the sphenooccipital synchondrosis to the inferior border of the clivus. The shape of the clivus is highly variable (Fig. 4.**127**). A small "exostosis" (shape 7 in Fig. 4.**127**) marks the former closure site of the sphenooccipital synchondrosis (see Fig. 4.**5**).
- The width of the lateral part of the occipital bone, measured between the occipitomastoid sutures past the foramen magnum, is 80 mm in specimens and 84 ± 4 mm on radiographs.
- The length and width of the foramen magnum average 36 mm and 31 mm, respectively.

Besides standard radiographic views of the skull in the lateral and frontal projections, the semiaxial view (Towne projection) is particularly important for demonstrating the posterior fossa and skull base. It permits a comparative evaluation of the mastoid processes and petrous bones. The occipital squama is also visualized along with the grooves for the transverse sinus. The calvarium above the sinus grooves is thinner and more radiolucent on both sides. The axial submentovertex projection is considered the standard view for demonstrating the skull base. Although this projection gives the best view of the skull base as a whole, it is of limited value in the diagnosis of skull base lesions. Pathological processes must reach considerable size before they are visible in the submentovertex view. This has to do both with the complex anatomy of the skull base and with interference from the superimposed facial bones and cervical spine. For these reasons, CT and MRI have become the primary tools for examinations of the skull base. CT clearly defines all the bony structures, while MRI gives an excellent view of the soft-tissue structures in and around the skull base.

It is still important, however, to review some important principles in conventional radiographic examinations. The axial (submentovertex) view is best for demonstrating the **foramen ovale** (Figs. 4.**3**, 4.**5**) and is still requested by many oral surgeons. An undistorted unilateral view of the foramen ovale can be obtained by extending the head back at a 45° angle on the anthropological line, similar to the Waters projection, rotating the head 10° toward the opposite side with the mouth open, and directing the central ray perpendicular to the plane of the table and the cassette. This view is mainly used to locate sites for ganglion blockade. Normally the foramina are not symmetrical in their size and

Shape	1	2	3	4
Prevalence in %	37	5	8,5	10
Shape	5	6	7	8
Prevalence in %	6	20	9	4,5

Fig. 4.**127**   Diagram showing the normal shapes of the basal part of the occipital bone.

shape. The wall separating the foramen ovale from the foramen spinosum may be absent, as may the bony boundary between the foramen ovale and the foramen lacerum. The variants are most clearly demonstrated by CT (Fig. 4.**128**). Unilateral enlargement of the foramen ovale may be a result of tumor destruction. Duplication of the **vidian canal** may occur as a very rare normal variant (Fig. 4.**129**). Ossification of the pterygospinal ligament can mimic a bipartite foramen ovale.

Large air cells located in the sphenoid bone and pterygoid process, like a pneumatized clinoid process, can lead to unusual findings in the axial projection. Usually these findings have no clinical significance, but sometimes they may be mistaken for areas of tumor destruction. Soft-tissue structures like the uvula (Fig. 4.**130**) or enlarged tonsils may be projected into the middle fossa on axial radiographs (Fig. 4.**131**). The foramina lacera (Fig. 4.**132**) and carotid canals (Fig. 4.**133**) are also occasionally visible in the axial projection. Very rarely, the site of emergence of the carotid artery may be enlarged on one side, simulating destruction by tumor.

The complex anatomy and embryology of the **posterior fossa** also give rise to some notable features with which the radiologist should be familiar. The **foramen of the hypoglossal nerve** is best visualized in the occipital condyle

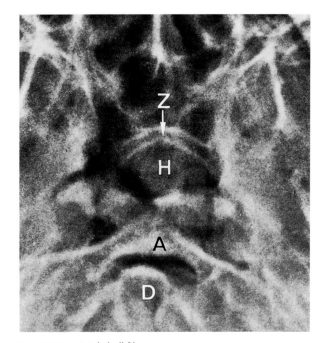

Fig. 4.**130**   Axial skull film.
A   Anterior arch of the atlas   H   Uvula
D   Dens of the axis   Z   Hyoid bone

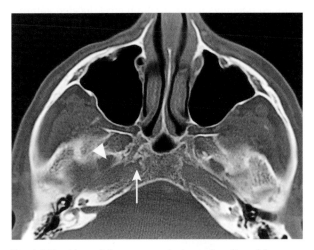

Fig. 4.**128**   Normal foramen ovale (arrowhead) and foramen lacerum (arrow) on the right side. Axial CT using a high-resolution bone filter.

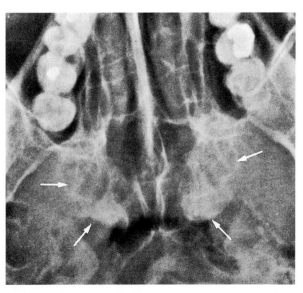

Fig. 4.**131**   Swelling of both tonsils (arrows). Axial skull film.

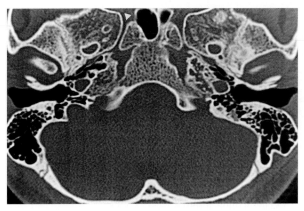

Fig. 4.**129**   Vidian canal (pterygoid canal). The complete course of the canal is shown (arrowhead).

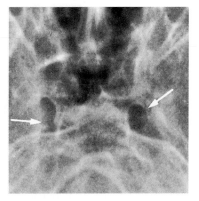

Fig. 4.**132**   View of the foramen lacerum (arrows) on each side of the clivus in a 9-year-old child. Axial skull film.

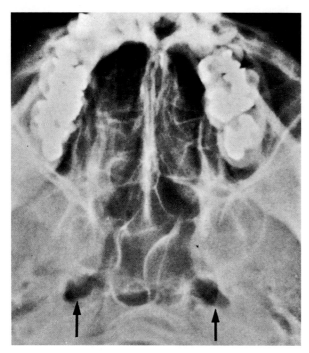

Fig. 4.**133** Carotid canal on each side (arrows). Axial skull film.

by positioning the head as for a Stenvers view of the petrous bone but with the beam centered at a slightly lower level (Figs. 4.**134c, d**, 4.**135a**). The hypoglossal canal can also be seen on conventional tomograms (Fig. 4.**135b**), but this modality has become obsolete. The foramen of the hypoglossal nerve and the nerve itself can be accurately

defined by CT and MRI (Fig. 4.**135c, d**). The **occipital condyles** are located at the sides of the foramen magnum on the inferior aspect of the occipital bone. Normally the condyles are larger medially than laterally. With increasing flattening of the occipital condyles, the articular surfaces incline laterally. In about 5 % of cases the articular surfaces of the condyles are divided into two parts (Fig. 4.**134b**). Behind each occipital condyle is a condylar fossa. The floor of the fossa may be perforated by the posterior opening of the **condylar canal**, which terminates anteriorly at the sigmoid sinus (Fig. 4.**134c**). Located above each condyle is the hypoglossal canal. The jugular notch bears a prominence, the intrajugular process, that may partially or completely divide the jugular foramen into a medial and lateral part (Fig. 4.**134a**). A condylar emissary vein—not to be confused with the mastoid emissary vein—passes through the condylar canal, linking the sigmoid sinus with the external vertebral venous plexus. This canal is located posterior to the occipital condyle (Fig. 4.**136**) and is occasionally visible on radiographs (Fig. 4.**137**). In one of our trauma patients, the condylar canal and the venous sinus were visible on CT scans obtained to exclude a traumatic carotid and/or vertebral artery dissection. Initially we had some difficulty in interpreting this finding (arteriovenous malformation? variant?) (Fig. 4.**138**).

Canals for the **occipital emissary veins** that connect the sinus confluence with the occipital vein appear as small, rounded openings in the occipital crest, located approximately midway between the internal occipital protuberance and the posterior rim of the foramen magnum (Fig. 4.**139a, b**). The **occipital crest** may appear as a curved, eccentric ridge but is readily identified by its descending path from the external occipital protuberance to the foramen magnum (Fig. 4.**139c**).

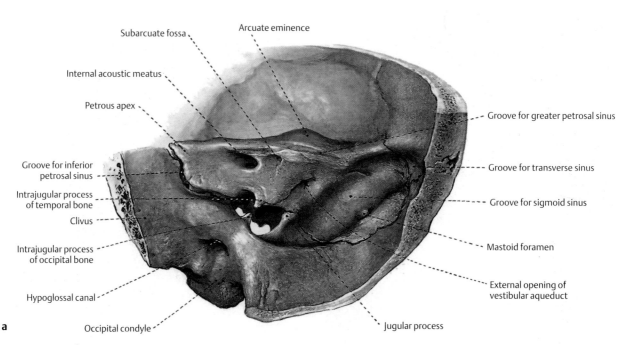

Fig. 4.**134a–d**

a Posterior surface of the temporal bone with the adjacent part of the occipital bone on the right side. Medial aspect.
b Occipital bone, posteroinferior aspect.

c Occipital bone, internal aspect.
d Occipital vertebra with the formation of a tertiary condyle. (From Rauber and Kopsch 1987.)

Fig. 4.**134b–d** ▷

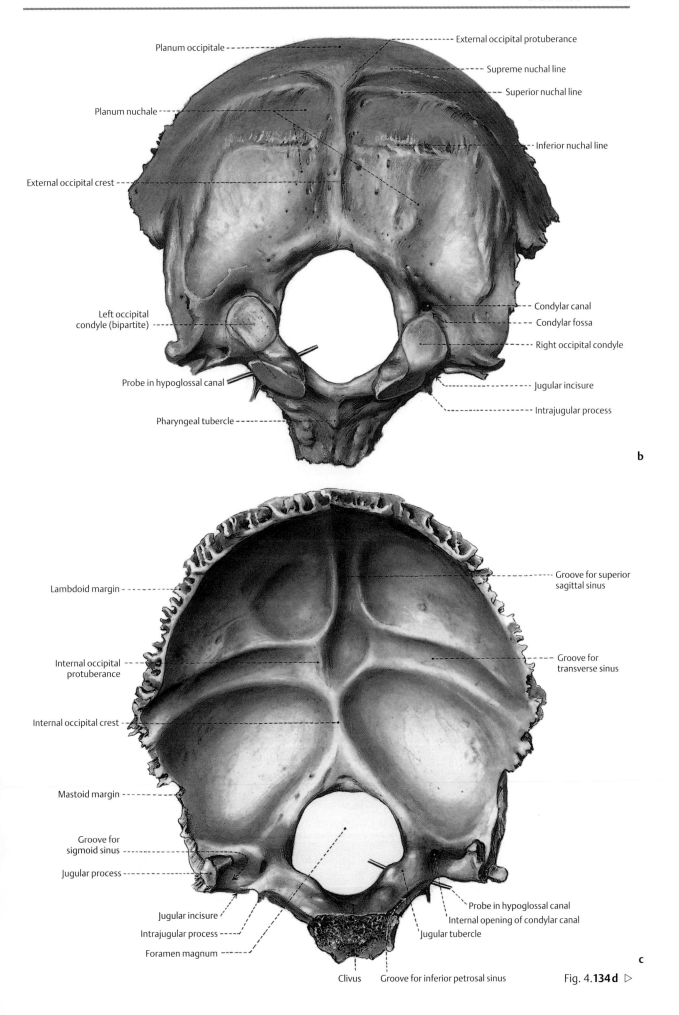

Planum occipitale

External occipital protuberance

Supreme nuchal line

Superior nuchal line

Planum nuchale

Inferior nuchal line

External occipital crest

Condylar canal

Condylar fossa

Left occipital condyle (bipartite)

Right occipital condyle

Probe in hypoglossal canal

Jugular incisure

Intrajugular process

Pharyngeal tubercle

b

Lambdoid margin

Groove for superior sagittal sinus

Internal occipital protuberance

Groove for transverse sinus

Internal occipital crest

Mastoid margin

Groove for sigmoid sinus

Jugular process

Probe in hypoglossal canal

Internal opening of condylar canal

Jugular incisure

Intrajugular process

Jugular tubercle

Foramen magnum

Clivus   Groove for inferior petrosal sinus

c

Fig. 4.**134 d** ▷

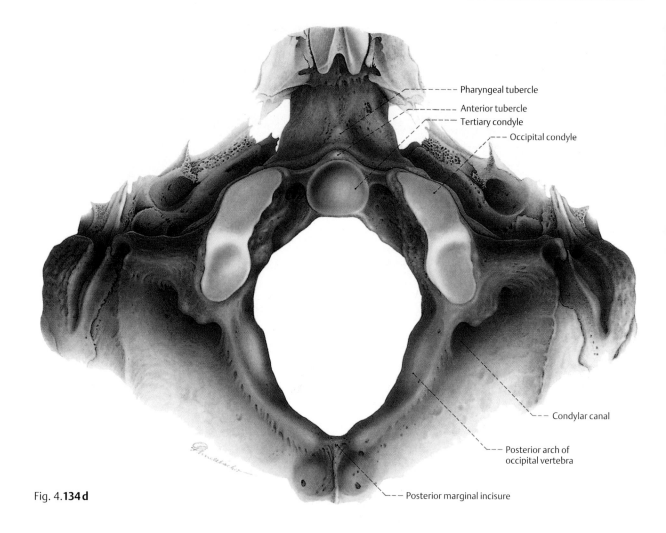

Pharyngeal tubercle

Anterior tubercle

Tertiary condyle

Occipital condyle

Condylar canal

Posterior arch of
occipital vertebra

Posterior marginal incisure

Fig. 4.**134 d**

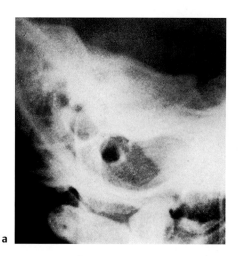

a

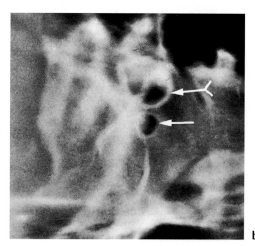

b

Fig. 4.**135 a–d**
a Hypoglossal canal in the Stenvers projection.
b Hypoglossal canal (arrow) and jugular foramen (tailed arrow) in a tomogram. Different patient from that in panel **a**.
c Hypoglossal canal (arrowhead). CT using a high-resolution bone filter.
d T2-weighted turbo SE image demonstrates the course of the hypoglossal nerve (arrowhead). 3-D imaging sequence.

Fig. 4.**135 c–d** ▷

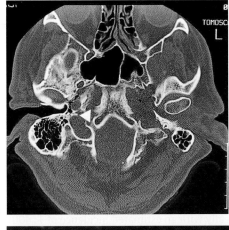

c

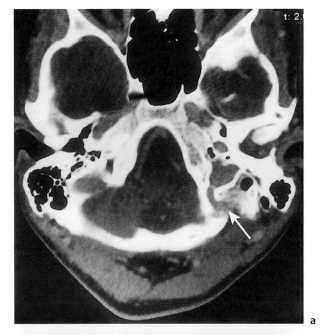

a

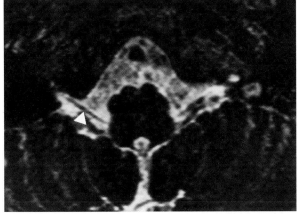

d

Fig. 4.**135 c–d**

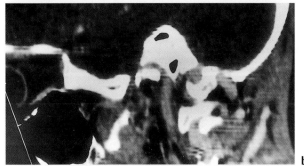

b

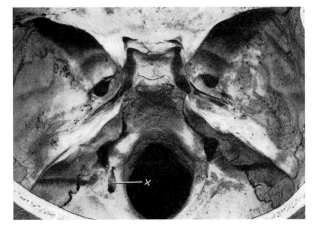

Fig. 4.**136**   Condylar emissary vein (×). Interior view of the skull base.

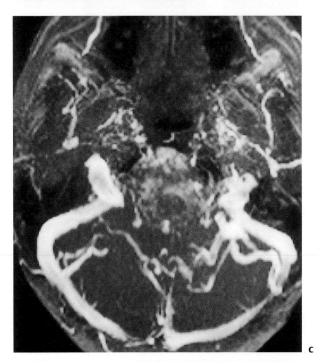

c

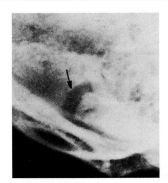

Fig. 4.**137**   Condylar emissary vein in the occiput (arrow).

Fig. 4.**138**
a Typical condylar canal (arrow). Axial CT using a high-resolution bone filter.
b Secondary reconstruction of axial CT scans demonstrates the course of the condylar canal through the skull.
c Contrast-enhanced MRI confirms the presence of a transcranial vein.

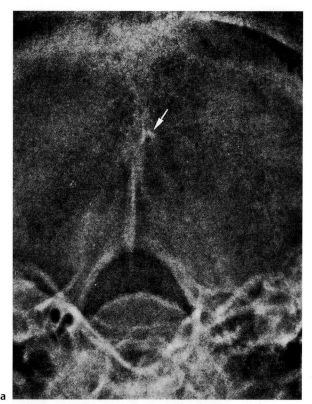

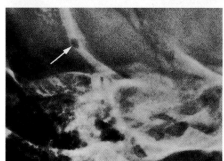

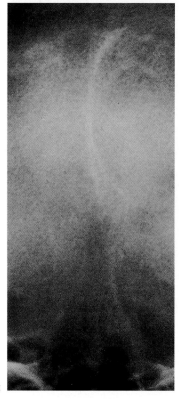

Fig. 4.**139**
a Occipital emissary vein at the center of the occipital squama (arrow).
b Occipital emissary vein in the occipital crest. Stenvers view.
c Asymmetrical curvature of the occipital crest.

Pathological Finding?

 ### Normal Variant/Anomaly?

Cephaloceles

A cephalocele is caused by the protrusion of intracranial structures through a defect in the skull. The dura may be thinned or dehiscent. A protrusion that contains only meninges and subarachnoid space with CSF is called a **meningocele**. If the sac contains brain tissue, it is called an **encephalocele**. Meningoceles can occur anywhere in the skull but are most common in the midline. Most cases occur sporadically with an estimated incidence of 1:4000 births. Only about 20% of all encephaloceles are located in the anterior or central skull base, and most of these are anterior. One possible classification is shown in Table 4.**14**.

Sphenoethmoidal encephaloceles may enter the posterior nasal cavity or the anterior nasopharynx. If an encephalocele extends into the sphenoid sinus but does not perforate the floor and enter the nasopharynx, it is classified as a transsphenoidal form. Transethmoidal encephaloceles are located farther anteriorly and pass through the anterior ethmoid and cribriform plate into the anterior sinonasal system. Of the laterobasal encephaloceles, the sphenoorbital form extends through the superior orbital fissure into the orbit, leading to proptosis. This form is frequently associated with neurofibromatosis and with anomalous development of the greater and lesser sphenoid wings. This developmental abnormality is manifested by an "**empty orbit**" on PA skull radiographs. Sphenomaxillary encephaloceles are extremely rare. They extend into the pterygopalatine fossa and farther laterally into the infratemporal fossa. Today, CT and MRI are the primary tools for the diagnostic imaging of meningoencephaloceles. Patients with basal encephaloceles often have coexisting anomalies such as agenesis of the corpus callosum and midfacial anomalies (hypertelorism, cleft lip and palate).

Arachnoid Cysts

Arachnoid cysts are benign, congenital cysts that are filled with CSF. Their precise etiology is unknown but is based on an abnormality of meningeal development. Males predominate by a 3:1 ratio. The cysts occur at the following locations:

- Middle fossa: 50–65%
- Suprasellar cistern: 5–10%
- Quadrigeminal cistern: 5–10%
- Posterior fossa (with cerebellopontine angle and cisterna magna): 5–10%
- Brain surface: 5%

Table 4.**14** Classification of skull-base encephaloceles based on the location of the defect and the sac

1 Transethmoidal	Midline encephalocele
2 Sphenoethmoidal	Midline encephalocele
3 Sphenoorbital	Laterobasal encephalocele
4 Transsphenoidal	Midline encephalocele
5 Sphenomaxillary	Laterobasal encephalocele

Extensive cysts may be associated with cranial asymmetries and thinning of the compressed portion of the skull base or calvarium (Fig. **25 b–d**), for while arachnoid cysts can occur at any age, 75% are present during childhood and therefore can affect growth.

Compensatory Changes and Mass Effects

Masses that occur during growth and are associated with a rise in intracranial pressure lead to thinning or bossing of the skull. In other cases there may be reactive thickening of the cranial bone due to decreased growth pressure from the brain, filling the gap by a compensatory "ex vacuo" mechanism. The most pronounced changes occur as a result of cerebral hemiatrophy that is congenital or acquired in early childhood. They consist of:

- Unilateral bony thickening of the skull base (Fig. 4.**140**)
- Abnormally high position of the skull base and pyramid
- Dilatation of the paranasal sinuses (Fig. 4.**141**)
- Increased air cells in the temporal bone

Asymmetry of the Skull Base

In approximately 2% of cases, skull radiographs show an asymmetry in the level of the petrous pyramids (Fig. 4.**142**). This is almost always an incidental clinical finding. Skull base asymmetry can also result from the causes of asymmetrical calvarial development discussed earlier, such as congenital or acquired torticollis or placing an infant predominantly on one side of the head. This involves a purely bony deformity that is not based on a neural dysplasia. Some narrowing of the cranial fossae may also occur (Fig. 4.**143**).

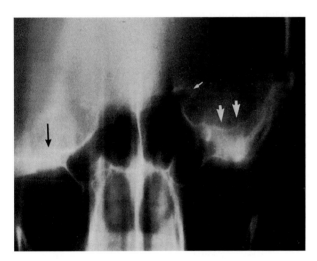

Fig. 4.**140** Thickened bone (white arrows) in the floor of the left middle fossa due to "cerebral hemiatrophy" following a left hemispherectomy. Tomogram shows normal height of the middle fossa on the right side (black arrow). Pneumatization of the left anterior clinoid process is noted as an incidental finding (small white arrow).

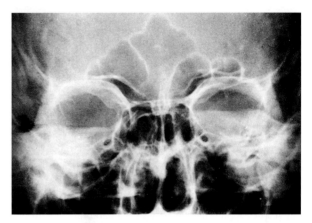

Fig. 4.**142** High position of the pyramid on the left side—a clinically unimportant variant.

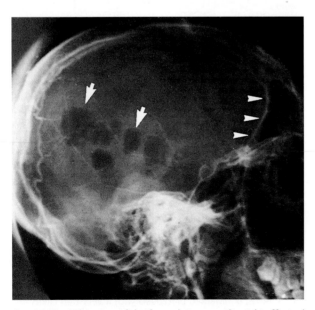

Fig. 4.**141** Dilatation of the frontal sinus on the side affected by cerebral hemiatrophy (arrowheads). Post-pneumoencephalography air bubbles are also visible (arrows).

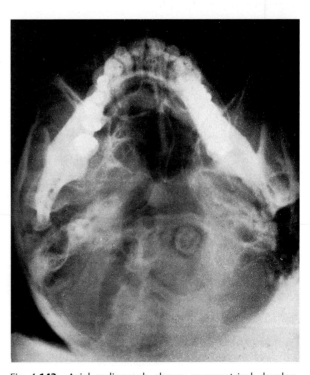

Fig. 4.**143** Axial radiograph shows asymmetrical development of the cranial fossa in a patient with basal scoliosis convex to the left.

In contrast to cranial changes associated with hemiatrophies (Fig. 4.**144**), the altered growth influences lead to deformity of the entire skull (Fig. 4.**145**). The effects of neurofibromatosis should also be considered, however, in the differential diagnosis of cranial asymmetries.

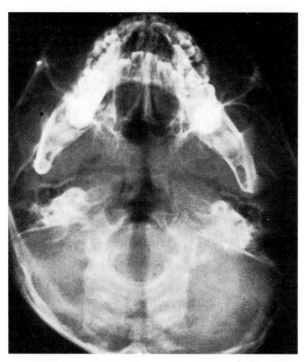

Fig. 4.**144** Axial skull film shows right cerebral hemiatrophy in a patient without scoliosis.

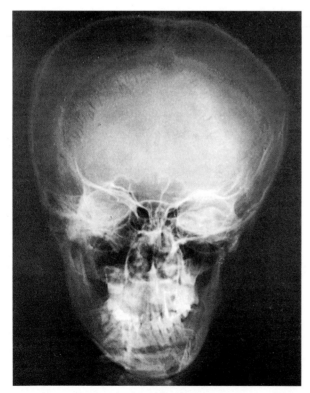

Fig. 4.**145** Asymmetrical development of the skull in a patient with congenital torticollis. PA projection.

Platybasia, Basilar Impression

Although platybasia and basilar impression may coexist, they represent different changes in the skull base.

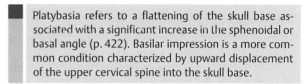

Platybasia refers to a flattening of the skull base associated with a significant increase in the sphenoidal or basal angle (p. 422). Basilar impression is a more common condition characterized by upward displacement of the upper cervical spine into the skull base.

The main causes are diseases that alter the mechanical properties of the craniovertebral joints and skull base, such as osteomalacia, hyperparathyroidism, and storage diseases such as mucopolysaccharidosis. Secondary basilar impression can result from generalized osteoporosis or from injuries and inflammatory processes of the skull base (e.g., rheumatoid arthritis). Basilar impression can also develop as a result of congenital defects of the craniovertebral junction, and rarely it may be caused by tumors or tumorlike lesions such as skull base involvement by fibrous dysplasia.

Platybasia can develop in various situations. Typically it occurs in entities that are characterized by the deformation of abnormal bone that can no longer bear the weight of the skull and brain, as in Paget disease, osteogenesis imperfecta, and osteomalacia. Virchow redefined platybasia to mean a flattening of the basal angle due to elevation of its posterior line, appearing as a more horizontal inclination of the clivus (Fig. 4.**146**). In cases of frontal dysplasia, which is usually associated with turricephaly and sometimes with the dysplasia of facial bones, the angle is again flattened but

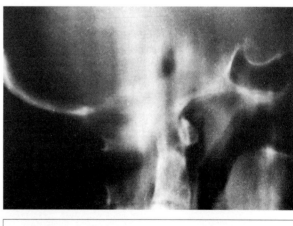

a

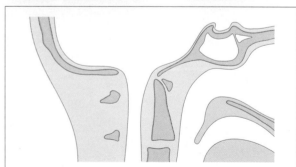

b

Fig. 4.**146 a, b** Marked platybasia with a very thin clivus and extremely shallow posterior fossa. This rules out true basilar impression. Lateral tomogram in the median plane (**a**) and correlative drawing (**b**).

the anterior line is elevated rather than the posterior line. This deformity is not actually referred to as platybasia (p. 390, Fig. 4.**60a**). In true cases of platybasia, the anterior rim of the foramen magnum is elevated while the posterior rim almost always remains in a normal position. This leads to (1) a more vertical orientation of the plane of the foramen magnum and (2) an apparent indrawing of the central skull base at the level of the clivus. This deformity is associated with an upward displacement of the upper cervical spine into the skull base and is therefore classified as a true basilar impression (Fig. 4.**149**). The horizontal position of the clivus is not necessarily the sole cause of a higher position of the basion. The same process occurs when the basilar part of the occipital bone is underdeveloped, causing the clivus to remain too short (Fig. 4.**147**).

A variety of **craniometric measurements** can be used in the diagnosis of basilar impression. The most common reference lines and measuring techniques are shown in Figs. 5.**17** and 5.**18**.

> Basilar impression can be diagnosed and measured only if the reference points for the measurements are in a normal location. This is not always the case.

Besides the internal measurement of an enlarged **sphenoidal angle** (basal angle = Welcker angle: normal value

132 ± 6°), the high position of the cervical spine due to the impression of the skull base is measured in relation to reference points on the skull.

A frontal skull projection can be used to measure the distance from the upper cervical spine (the dens of C2) to the bimastoid line, a line of variable length connecting the tips of the mastoid processes. The position of this line is somewhat uncertain, however, due to variations in the lengths of the mastoid processes. A better reference line is the digastric line that interconnects the digastric groove. Normally the tip of the dens does not project above the digastric line (Fig. 5.**17**).

Other important measurements are listed below (Fig. 5.**18**):

- Palato-occipital line (Chamberlain line): in the lateral projection, a line connecting the posterior end of the hard palate to the posterior rim of the foramen magnum. The tip of the dens lies an average of 1 ± 3.6 mm below this line (Fig. 4.**148**).
- McGregor line: drawn from the posterior margin of the hard palate to the inferior margin of the occipital squama. The tip of the dens should not extend more than 6.4 mm above this line (Fig. 4.**148**).
- Basal angle: measured as the angle between the plane of the foramen magnum (opisthion–basion) and a line connecting the basion and nasion (Fig. 4.**149**). The normal value is 163°. As the basion moves upward, the basal angle becomes flatter and may even go past 180° (negative basal angle).
- Condylar angle (normal = 125 ± 2°). This angle is increased by upward displacement of the medial portions of the occipital condyles, like that occurring in the medial form of basilar impression or with flattened, hypoplastic condyles. Angles greater than 150° are measured in occipital dysplasia (Fig. 4.**150**).
- Foramen magnum–clivus angle (Boogaard angle). The normal range is from 119° to 135°, averaging 122°. An increased Boogaard angle in platybasia reflects the more vertical orientation of the plane of the foramen magnum and the more horizontal orientation of the clivus. Angles of 138–156° (average 151°) are measured in occipital dysplasia.

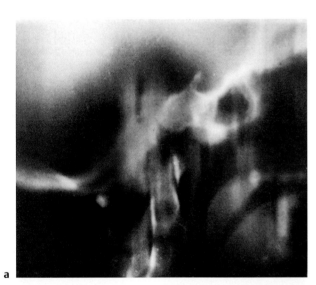

a

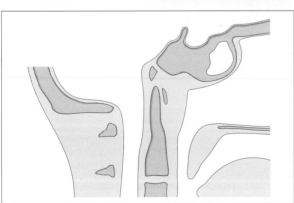

b

Fig. 4.**147a, b** Severe hypoplasia of the stumplike basilar part of the occipital bone, with a basal transverse cleft and no platybasia. Lateral tomogram in the median plane (**a**) and correlative drawing (**b**).

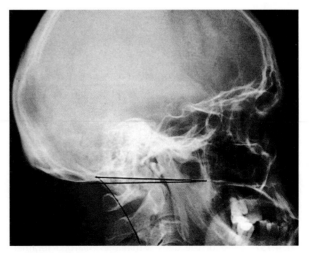

Fig. 4.**148** Palato-occipital lines of Chamberlain and of McGregor. A curved line has also been drawn along the posterior boundary of the spinal canal, making it easier to locate the posterior rim of the foramen magnum.

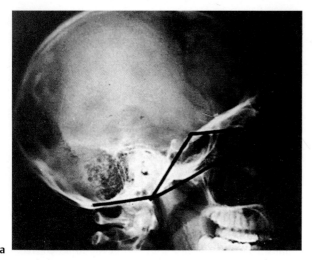 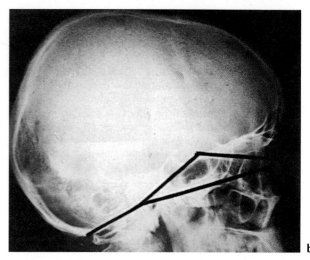

Fig. 4.**149 a, b**   Basal angle (lines connecting the opisthion with the basion and the basion with the nasion) and sphenoidal angle (nasion–sellar tubercle–basion = base angle).
a Normal findings.

b Platybasia and basilar impression. The basal angle is negative due to basilar impression.
(From Schmidt et al. 1978.)

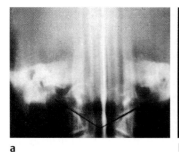 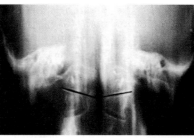

a   b

Fig. 4.**150 a, b**   Axial angles of the craniovertebral joints.
a Normal findings.
b Findings with condylar hypoplasia and medial basilar impression.
(From Schmidt et al. 1978.)

- Foramen magnum line (McRae line). Normally the tip of the dens does not extend past this line. If it does, it compromises the lumen of the foramen magnum (Figs. 4.**151**, 4.**152**).
- Klaus height index. A line connecting the tuberculum sellae and the endinion (cruciform eminence of the internal occipital protuberance) is largely unaffected by structural changes in the skull base at the foramen mag-

num. The distance from the tip of the dens to this line normally averages 40–41 mm. A value between 30 and 36 mm is borderline, and less than 30 mm signifies basilar impression.
- Distance from the TMJ to the arch of the atlas. This distance normally ranges between 22 and 39 mm, averaging 30 mm.
- Boogaard line. The basion should be below this line.

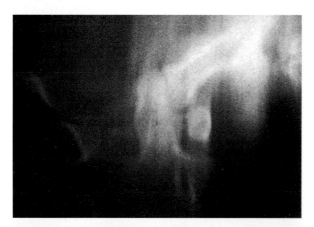 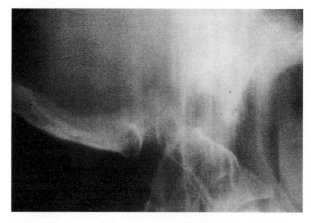

Fig. 4.**151**   Apex of the dens within the enlarged foramen magnum. A pseudoarticulation exists between the dens apex and the anterior rim of the foramen magnum. The dens projects above the McRae line. Lateral tomogram in the median plane. (From Schmidt et al. 1978.)

Fig. 4.**152**   Apex of the dens above the McRae line. The dens apex is within 8 mm of the posterior rim of the foramen magnum. Assimilation of the anterior arch of the atlas with the skull base. The trauma patient presented clinically with tetraplegia.

A very useful technique for detecting asymmetries is to locate the intervestibular midline (between the vestibular structures of the inner ear) and drop a perpendicular from its midpoint. Normally the perpendicular will pass through the tip of the dens and the apex of the condylar angle. The line will bypass those points if asymmetry is present. Underdevelopment of the central, occipital part of the skull base will become apparent if the surrounding bones are normally developed. Basilar impression is characterized by an upward displacement of lateral and posterior structures toward the center in relation to normal surrounding structures. Accordingly, we can distinguish both a medial and an anterior form of basilar impression. The anterior form is somewhat more difficult to recognize on skull films, since most of the upslope of the median skull base occurs within the void of the foramen magnum (Fig. 4.**147**).

Figure 4.**153** shows the upslope of normally developed lateral structures that occurs in the medial form of basilar impression. This form is very difficult to detect if it is bilateral and symmetrical. But it is easier to detect than an anterior basilar impression if it affects only one side, as this creates a lateral-to-medial asymmetry of the petrous pyramids. This can be one cause of asymmetry in the height of the petrous ridges (Fig. 4.**154**).

If the lateral parts of the occipital bone are also elevated as part of the developmental anomaly of the skull base, this will reduce the relative prominence of the basilar impression (Fig. 4.**155**).

In the case shown in Fig. 4.**154**, a paramedian "step" in the lateral rim of the foramen magnum is a sign that the lateral part of the occipital bone is included in the plateau of the basilar impression. It is common for a basilar impression to involve the lateral parts of the occipital bone in varying degrees. Thus, it is common to encounter an "asymmetrical" type of basilar impression in which one side of the occipital bone or one of the petrous pyramids is higher than the other. While that appears to be the unaffected side, it actually shows a higher degree of developmental abnormality (Fig. 4.**155**).

As Fig. 4.**146** illustrates, platybasia may be associated with an extremely flat and shallow posterior fossa. This case involves an extreme developmental deficiency of the skull base.

> If the dens crosses the plane of the foramen magnum and impinges upon the medulla oblongata, it can cause potentially life-threatening neurological deficits (Figs. 4.**151**, 4.**152**).

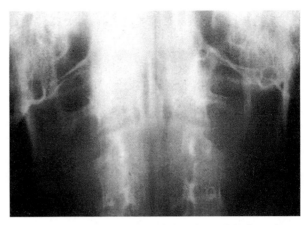

Fig. 4.**153** Ipsilateral steep medial upslope of the lateral part of the occipital bone in a patient with medial basilar impression.

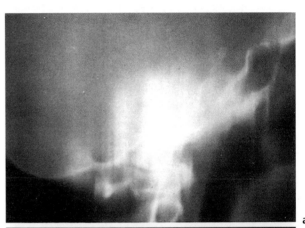

a

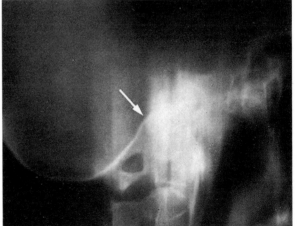

b

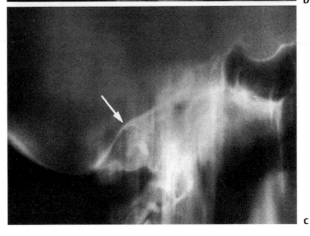

c

Fig. 4.**154a–c** Paramedian tomograms show different degrees of basilar impression on the right and left sides with a "step" in the lateral rim of the foramen magnum. The basilar (anterior) impression extends posteriorly past the basion.
a Normal appearance.
b Anterior step (arrow).
c Posterior step (arrow).

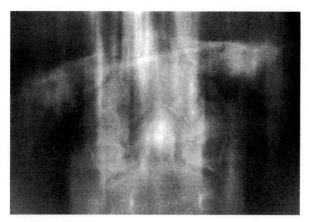

Fig. 4.**155**   Asymmetry of the lateral portions of the occipital bone. On the right side, the contour of the lateral pars rises medially: medial basilar impression. On the left side, the contour does not rise but the pyramid is higher than on the right, indicating a more severe developmental abnormality on the left side.

Variants of the Occipital Bone and Posterior Fossa

It is not unusual to encounter anatomic variants around the foramen magnum. Some of the processes, clefts, and deformities covered in this section are clinically unimportant variants. Most of them have a high association with minor or more serious anomalies.

The **retromastoid process** (Fig. 4.**156**) is a clinically unimportant variant that may be mistaken for an osteoma or cartilaginous exostosis. The **processus asteriacus** is a bony prominence arising from the asterion (Fig. 4.**11**). It is located behind the mastoid and appears as an exostosis on tangential radiographs and CT scans. A rare bony variant may be seen on the medial aspect of the occipital squama above the opisthion (Fig. 5.**18**). It is a bony process called the **suboccipital process** (Fig. 4.**157**). **Basilar processes** appear as small, budlike bony prominences at the anteroinferior border of the clivus (Figs. 4.**158**, 4.**159**).

A shift of the craniovertebral junction can occur as a craniovertebral developmental anomaly. It can lead to an

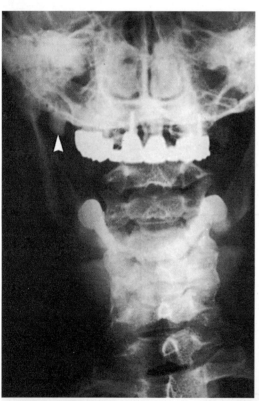

a

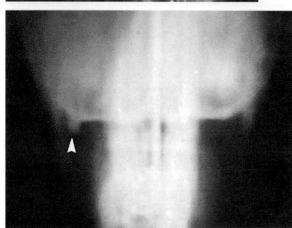

b

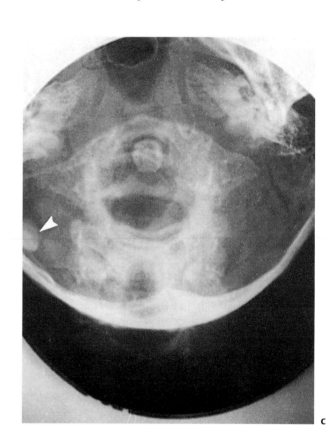

c

Fig. 4.**156 a–c**
a Right retromastoid process (arrowhead). PA projection of the cervical spine.
b Retromastoid process in a sagittal tomographic plane behind the foramen magnum (arrowhead). (The process appears slightly blurred because it is just outside the tomographic plane.)
c Right retromastoid process (arrowhead) in an axial projection of the skull base.

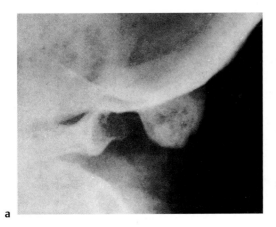

a

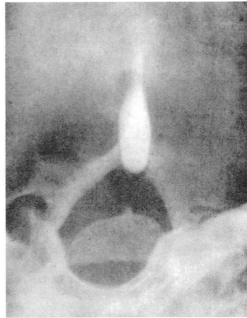

b

Fig. 4.**157 a, b**   Suboccipital process (observation by Gassmann, Hamburg).

Fig. 4.**158**   Paired arrangement of the basilar processes (arrows) in a specimen photograph.

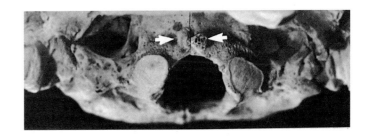

occipital vertebra (Fig. 4.**134 d**) or to **atlas assimilation**, in which all or part of the atlas is fused with the occipital bone. An asymmetrical atlanto-occipital synostosis that involves a forced rotation of the atlas can result in congenital torticollis. Asymmetrical atlas assimilation is almost always seen with a small, deformed foramen magnum and can result in neurological abnormalities.

Some variants are remnants of embryological segmentation. They include the paracondylar process (paramastoid process), the tertiary condyle (Fig. 4.**134 d**), the terminal ossicle (Bergmann ossicle), subdivision of the hypoglossal canal, and ponticle formation on C1.

The **paracondylar process** is a bony prominence that arises from the lateral part of the occipital bone and extends to the transverse process of C1. Located at the attachment of the rectus capitis lateralis muscle, this process can be demonstrated in a modified Stenvers projection centered on the hypoglossal foramen (Fig. 4.**160 a**). An accessory paracondylar fissure may be located medial to this process. These features may or may not be accompanied by other occipitovertebral dysplasias (Figs. 4.**160 b**, 4.**161**). A process arising from the transverse process of C1 and extending toward the paracondylar process is called the epitransverse process of the atlas. A short bony element may be interposed between both processes and may have joint-like connections with them (Fig. 4.**162**). The paracondylar process may be pneumatized.

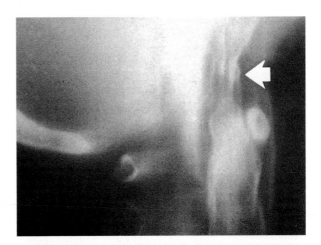

Fig. 4.**159**   Basilar process (arrow) in a lateral tomogram.

A small notch, the **posterior occipital incisure**, is found consistently at the posterior rim of the foramen magnum in infants and occasionally in adults (Fig. 4.**163 a**), along with a handlelike protuberance called the **Kerckring process** (Fig. 4.**163 b**). The Kerckring process is not a variant that is combined with other anomalies, but an ossicle that arises from the lower part of the occipital squama in the

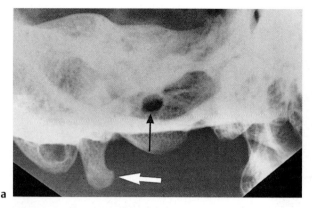

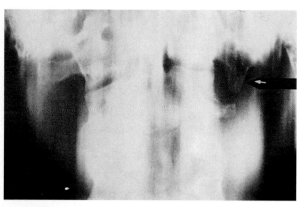

Fig. 4.**160a, b**   Paracondylar process.
a Right paracondylar process (white arrow) in a specimen radiograph. Stenvers-like projection centered on the hypoglossal foramen (black arrow).

b A bony process below the assimilated transverse process of C1 (arrow), resembling the paracondylar process. Sagittal tomogram.

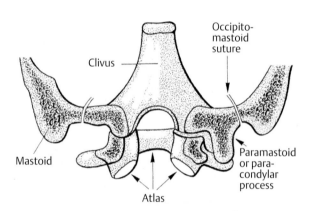

Fig. 4.**161**   Diagram of a left paracondylar process. Occipitomastoid suture.

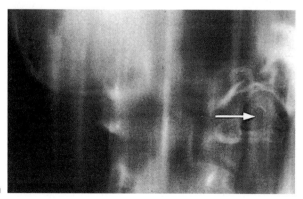

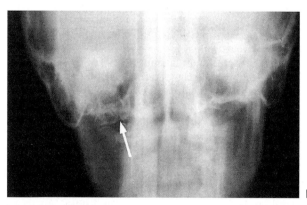

Fig. 4.**162a, b**   Segmented paracondylar process.
a Segmented paracondylar process located between the transverse process of C1 and the lateral part of the occipital bone (arrow). Tomogram. (From Schmidt et al. 1978.)

b Segmented right paracondylar process with paracondylar fissure in a sagittal tomogram (arrow indicates the paracondylar synchondrosis).

Fig. 4.**163 a, b** Posterior rim of the foramen magnum.
a Posterior occipital incisure.
b Kerckring process (arrow).

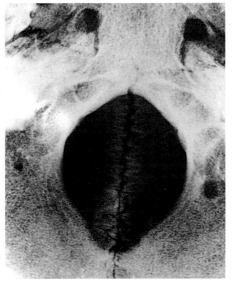
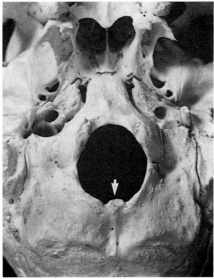

a   b

fourth month of fetal development and fuses with the lateral parts of the occiput in the second year of life.

A number of isolated ossific foci occur in the soft tissues surrounding the craniovertebral junction. They have various sources:

- Variants in the complex embryological development of the craniocervical junction
- Foci of ossification in tendon attachments and ligaments, often secondary in nature

The **tertiary condyle** is located at the anterior rim of the foramen magnum and articulates with the anterior arch of the atlas, the tip of the dens, or both (Figs. 4.**134 d**, Fig. 4.**164**, Fig. 4.**165**). Very rarely, misshapen bony structures are found on one or both sides of the anterior rim of the foramen magnum and may narrow the anterior part of

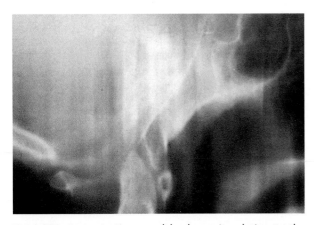

Fig. 4.**164** Large tertiary condyle shown in relation to the apex of a very long dens and to the hypoplastic anterior arch of the atlas.

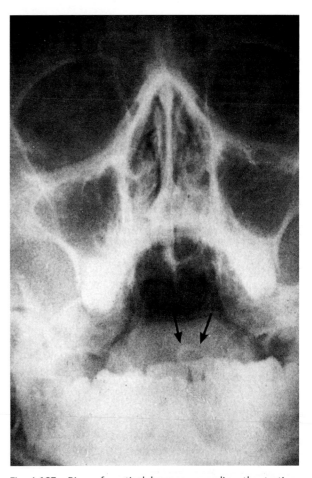

Fig. 4.**165** Ring of cortical bone surrounding the tertiary condyle (arrows), seen in an open-mouth occipitomental projection. (From Schmidt et al. 1978.)

a large foramen in a saddle-shaped configuration (Fig. 4.**166**). The shape of the foramen magnum can also be distorted as a result of condylar dysplasia (Fig. 4.**167**). With their cortical boundaries, these bony structures have a characteristic appearance in the submentovertex projection and also in the semiaxial projection. Combinations of various processes can also occur at the anteroinferior border of the clivus in connection with marked osseous dysplasia of the occipital bone.

The **terminal ossicle** (Bergmann's ossicle) is an isolated bony element located on the dens of C2. It constitutes the body of the proatlas and develops as a separate bone when the apical center of the dens does not undergo bony fusion with the rest of the dens. The terminal ossicle may come into contact with the occipital bone. This situation and the issue of ponticle formation on C1 are discussed in the section on anomalies of the axis (p. 584).

Complete or incomplete **transverse basilar clefts in the clivus** are occasionally seen as incidental findings on radiographs of the paranasal sinuses (Figs. 4.**168**, 4.**169**). The differential diagnosis of sutures, persistent synchon-droses, and fracture lines about the foramen magnum is reviewed on p. 440. There may be several coexisting basioccipital clefts that, like the sphenooccipital synchondrosis, persist well beyond the growth period.

Figure 4.**114b** illustrates a **median cerebellar suture** (more accurately termed a median cerebellar synchondrosis). The persistence of a continuous suture appears to be extremely rare and has been described as a "midline occipital fissure" only in connection with an occipital encephalocele. A superimposed persistent frontal suture should be excluded before this diagnosis is made.

Cephaloceles were discussed on pp. 387 and 428.

Occipital dysplasias may occur separately or in association with other malformations of the axial skeleton. It is assumed that the skeletal malformation precedes or precipitates the neural anomaly (as in Arnold–Chiari malformation).

Finally, it should be noted that an abnormally small foramen magnum can occur in the setting of achondroplasia. An abnormally large foramen magnum has been described in Rubinstein–Taybi syndrome.

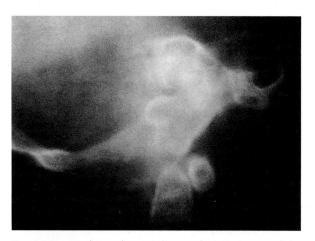

Fig. 4.**166**   Misshapen bony masses at the anterior rim of the foramen magnum. Lateral tomogram.

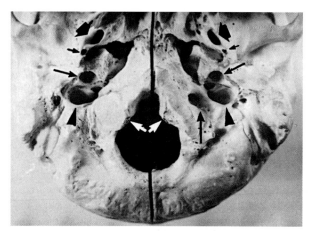

Fig. 4.**167**   Skull base in an anatomic specimen, inferior aspect.
Large arrows: foramina ovalia.
Small arrows: foramina spinosa.
Long arrows: carotid canals.
Arrowheads: jugular foramina.
White arrows: condylar dysplasia.

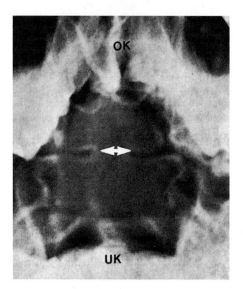

Fig. 4.**168**   Bilateral, incomplete basilar transverse cleft (double arrow). Open-mouth view in the submento-occipital projection.
OK Maxilla
UK Mandible
(From Schmidt et al. 1978.)

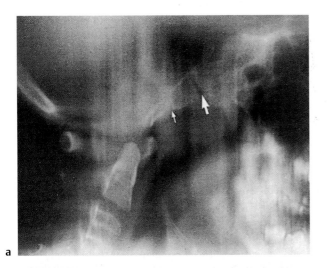

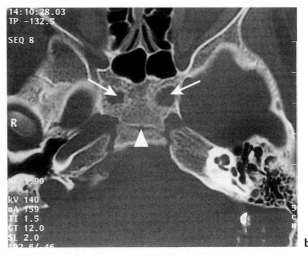

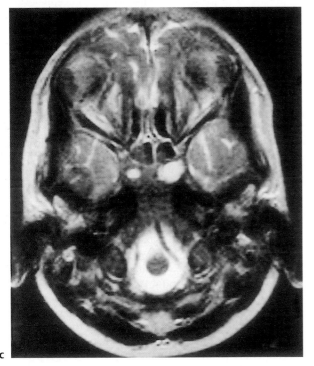

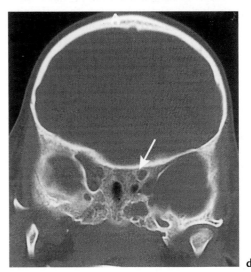

Fig. 4.**169 a–d**

a Clivus of an adolescent in a lateral tomogram. Spheno-occipital synchondrosis (large arrow). Another synchondrosis is visible in the basilar part of the occipital bone (small arrow) (basilar transverse cleft?). (From Schmidt et al. 1978.)

b Two "spaces" (arrows), almost symmetrical, located anterior to the spheno-occipital synchondrosis (arrowhead) in a 4-year-old girl (different patient than in **a**). Both areas have irregular sclerotic margins that lie directly in the path of an embryonic suture line, the intersphenoidal synchondrosis. Rostral to that, at the same level, are portions of the sphenoid sinus, which is already pneumatized.

c The features appear hyperintense on T2-weighted axial MRI, suggesting mucosal niches in portions of the sphenoid sinus that are not yet pneumatized. This interpretation is supported by contrast enhancement at the periphery of the changes on T1-weighted MRI (not shown here).

d Coronal CT scan clearly defines the relationship of the features to the rest of the sphenoid sinus (arrow). They probably represent a developmental variant of the sphenoid sinus. The differential diagnosis includes a harmless developmental variant of the embryonic intersphenoidal synchondrosis. MR tomography ruled out a meningocele or meningoencephalocele, as there was no "connecting stalk" leading to brain structures or extra-axial CSF spaces.

Fracture?

Plain skull films are a cumbersome and imprecise tool for the diagnosis of **basal skull fractures**. Only 50% of laterobasal fractures can be detected on standard radiographs. Today only the lateral and PA projections and the Towne occipital projection are considered to have diagnostic value. Important structures like the posterior wall of the frontal sinus, the cribriform plate, and the planum sphenoidale are not adequately depicted on plain skull radiographs. Intracranial air, sinus clouding, and traumatic intrasinus hemorrhage provide indirect signs of basal skull fracture, although these findings are usually indistinguishable from clouding due to inflammatory disease.

CT has assumed a major role in examinations of the skull base. Fracture lines that run along the scan plane can occasionally escape detection. But thin CT slices using single-slice or multislice spiral technique with overlapping image reconstruction and secondary multiplanar reformatting have largely solved this problem. These techniques are also useful in defining soft-tissue and vascular injuries (using contrast administration for the latter). MRI can be added in selected cases to advance the soft-tissue diagnosis.

For the reasons stated above, CT should be used in the primary evaluation of head-injured patients, largely eliminating the need for conventional radiographic films in the detection of basal skull fractures.

The fracture lines that occur in bending and burst fractures of the calvarium can extend into the skull base and along its major support structures (petrous pyramids, sphenoid wings). If they extend into the skull base foramina, they may be associated with vascular injuries or cranial nerve palsies (Fig. 4.**170**).

The diagnosis of basal skull fractures in **children** presents a special challenge. Besides the features and conditions described above, the differential diagnosis should include areas of incomplete ossification and unfused sutural lines that can mimic fractures. Cranial sutures that are still open in children, like the sphenosquamous suture, can almost always be distinguished from fracture lines on CT scans by their harmonious course and their sclerotic margins.

Fractures of the occipital squama are easily detected on a Towne projection that covers the posterior half of the foramen magnum.

The **differential diagnosis** of fractures in the lower part of the occipital squama in the posterior fossa should include the following features:

- The median occipital fissure, an extremely rare persistent suture in the occipital midline that has only been described in association with occipital encephalocele (and whose existence is controversial).
- The median cerebellar synchondrosis, which almost always closes during the first year of life (see Fig. 4.**114b**) and may be identical with the median occipital fissure.
- The posterior occipital incisure, a notch consistently present in the posterior rim of the foramen magnum in infants and occasionally present in adults (Fig. 4.**163a**).
- A diploic vein perforating the occiput in the sagittal plane (Fig. 4.**19**).
- The human fetus in the third month has one ossification center for the basilar part of the occipital bone, one for each lateral part, and one for the squamous part. In the newborn, these four centers are separated by broad cartilages that reduce to narrow synchondroses as cartilaginous growth progresses during the first year of life. These synchondroses close between the second and tenth years of life, the posterior synchondrosis closing somewhat later than the anterior one. Like the mendosal suture, they may be misinterpreted as fracture lines (see Figs. 4.**113** and 4.**114** for ossification centers, Figs. 4.**171** and 4.**172** for radiographic findings).
- Before it is assumed that a linear lucency on skull films is one of the above sutures or a fracture, the possibility of other superimposed sutures should be considered. This effect is most commonly seen with a persistent frontal (metopic) suture.

In the past, fractures of the **occipital condyle** have been described in only a few isolated cases. We feel that this is due entirely to the historical difficulties of recognizing these fractures on traditional skull films. The occipital condyles can be accurately evaluated by CT, and we have seen several cases of occipital condyle fractures in brain-injured patients (Fig. 4.**173**).

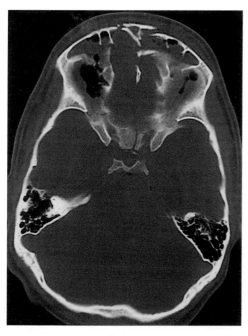

Fig. 4.**170**   Fracture of the anterior to middle skull base in a patient who sustained a severe head injury. Axial CT using a high-resolution bone filter.

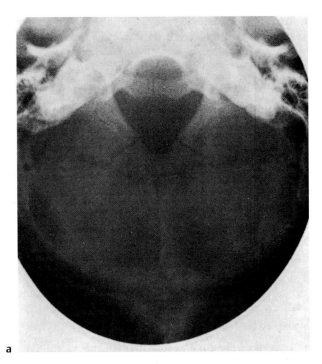

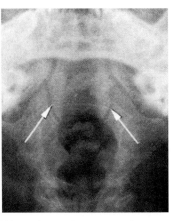

Fig. 4.**172** Pediatric skull film in the axial projection shows an anterior synchondrosis (arrows).

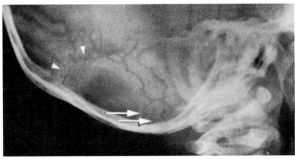

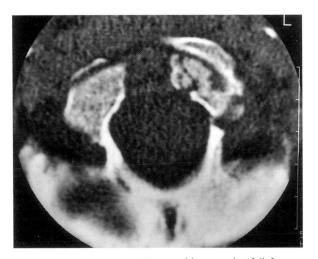

Fig. 4.**171 a, b** Pediatric skull films demonstrate a posterior synchondrosis (arrows) and mendosal suture (arrowheads).
a Axial projection.
b Lateral projection.

Fig. 4.**173** CT scan in a 60-year-old man who fell from a height demonstrates a fracture of the left occipital condyle with numerous displaced fragments.

 Necrosis?

Radiotherapy in the medical history of a patient is the most frequent cause of osteonecrosis of the skull base. Radiographs in these cases show patchy demineralization, partially confluent zones of osteolysis, and fragmentation of the bone. Some cases also show slight to moderate thickening of the affected bone (p. 397, Fig. 4.**72**). As elsewhere in the skeletal system, it is not unusual for 10–20 years to pass before signs of radiation osteitis become evident in the calvarium and skull base. CT can accurately demonstrate demineralization, osteolytic changes, fragmentation, sclerotic changes, and sequestration, including superficial sequestrum formation in the overlying soft tissues.

 Inflammation?

Nonspecific Forms of Osteomyelitis

As described on p. 369, the diploe is heavily vascularized and has numerous venous connections with the dural sinuses, the meningeal veins, and the veins of the scalp. While the dura resists the spread of infection to intracranial structures, there are no anatomic barriers to the spread of infection in the bone. Untreated osteomyelitis of the calvarium or skull base can spread swiftly and extensively, leading to serious complications that may include subdural and epidural empyema, meningitis, brain abscess, and septic venous thrombosis. Calvarial osteomyelitis can arise directly or indirectly through the spread of septic venous thrombosis or by the hematogenous route.

Calvarial osteomyelitis has the following main causes:

- Sinogenic or otogenic infections
- Other infections spreading from nearby tissues (open fractures, infected wounds, surgery), septic venous sinus thrombosis
- Primary hematogenous osteomyelitis

Osteomyelitis caused by the local spread of infection is most commonly detected near the frontal sinus. This is explained clinically by the frequent inflammatory disorders of this sinus and anatomically by the fact that purely cancellous bony walls, rather than cortical walls, enclose portions of the frontal sinus.

With osteomyelitis of the heavily vascularized calvarium, radiographs do not show marked sequestrum formation or periosteal reactions. Sclerotic changes are absent or develop at a very late stage. Radiographs in the early stage are normal. The first visible changes consist of focal lucencies in the bone. Later these coalesce to form larger defects and areas of bone destruction, which often still contain residual islands of intact bone. These patchy osteolytic areas have ill-defined margins and blurred trabecular markings, creating a very disordered appearance on radiographs. Marginal sclerosis is absent or may be greatly delayed in chronic osteomyelitis of long duration. The **frontal bone**, however, shows conspicuous sclerotic and hyperostotic changes in patients with chronic sinusitis or chronic subdural empyema.

Specific Forms of Osteomyelitis

Tuberculous or **syphilitic** bone changes in the skull base are rarely encountered in present-day medicine. **Actinomycosis** still has some significance. Tuberculous osteomyelitis develops as a result of hematogenous spread. Children and adolescents are chiefly affected, and the frontal and parietal bones are sites of predilection. Isolated tuberculosis is extremely rare in the skull base. Like syphilis, tuberculosis in that region most commonly affects the body of the sphenoid bone, the sphenoid sinus, and the sella turcica. A circumscribed, perforating form of the disease is distinguished from a progressive, diffuse form. The circumscribed form is characterized by one or more foci that are usually well demarcated. They completely permeate the calvarium and can mimic eosinophilic granuloma. The adjacent calvarium may react with mild sclerosis or may remain unaffected. The diffusely progressive form is seen either with a very virulent infecting organism or in patients with impaired host resistance (or both). This form mimics the course of a nonspecific, aggressive pyogenic osteomyelitis. Skeletal involvement by syphilis was discussed in a previous section (p. 398). Here we note that syphilitic involvement of the skull base is characterized by hyperostosis of the body of the sphenoid bone and obliteration of the sphenoid sinus, which can mimic the productive bony changes that occur with meningioma.

 Tumor?

CT and MRI have revolutionized the diagnosis of skull base tumors. In some cases the combination of clinical findings, history, pattern of involvement, lesion type, and characteristic imaging features point to a definitive diagnosis. In other cases only a differential diagnosis can be made despite precise anatomic localization of the lesion. Sphenoid wing meningioma is a prime example of a bone-destroying tumor of the skull base that can be diagnosed from the clinical and imaging findings. Similarly, clivus chordoma is associated with typical findings that provide a high level of diagnostic confidence.

Some tumors are associated with **increased intracranial pressure**. Besides changes in the sella turcica (p. 454), the pressure increase can produce the following signs:

- Expansion of the internal auditory canals
- Destruction of the petrous apices
- Enlargement of the skull base foramina

- Progressive thinning of the lesser sphenoid wing with loss of its posterior portions, creating a visible discontinuity between the anterior clinoid process and the orbital roof (sphenofrontal suture, Fig. 4.**5**).

Soft-tissue structures that are superimposed over the skull base can simulate tumors on plain radiographs. Examples are the **uvula** (Fig. 4.**130**) and enlarged **tonsils** (Fig. 4.**131**).

Normally the shape and size of the **foramen ovale** are not symmetrical. The wall separating the foramen ovale and foramen spinosum may be absent. Large **air cells** located in the sphenoid bone and pterygoid process, like a pneumatized clinoid process, can lead to unusual findings on axial radiographs. Generally they have no clinical significance, but they should not be mistaken for sites of bone destruction. CT is helpful in equivocal cases.

The **foramina lacera** (Fig. 4.**132**) and **carotid canals** (Fig. 4.**133**) are occasionally visible in the axial projection and can mimic sites of bone destruction by tumor. Very rarely, the site of emergence of the internal carotid artery is larger on one side.

Unilateral **enlargement of the foramen ovale** is caused mainly by the following disorders:

- Trigeminal neurinoma of the mandibular nerve (Fig. 4.**174**)
- Adenoid cystic carcinoma arising from the epipharynx
- Chordoma, meningioma, nasopharyngeal tumors (rare)
- Marginal erosions due to inflammation
- Systemic diseases (lymphoma, plasmacytoma)
- Traumatic lesions

A foramen ovale that has been enlarged by a neurinoma is distinguished by its sharply defined margins.

Narrowing of the foramen ovale has been described in association with fibrous dysplasia, Paget disease, osteopetrosis, and osteoplastic metastases (Fig. 4.**175**).

A rare cause of diffuse osteosclerosis of the skull base is **diaphyseal dysplasia (Camurati–Engelmann disease)** (Fig. 4.**176**). This autosomal dominant bone disease with varying penetration is characterized by thickening of the diaphyses of the long tubular bones due to periosteal and endosteal bone formation. The radiographic changes are highly variable and range from slight hyperostosis in the skull base region and mild cortical thickening of the diaphyses to marked sclerosis of the skull and all the tubular bones. Cranial nerve deficits with blindness and sensorineural hearing loss can occur in pronounced cases.

Differentiation is mainly required from **craniodiaphyseal dysplasia**, which is characterized by craniofacial deformities and absence of the muscle weakness that is typical of Engelmann disease. Differentiation is also required from **endosteal (cortical) hyperostosis** of the **van Buchem** type.

Diffuse osteosclerosis of the skull base is demonstrated very clearly by CT using a high-resolution bone filter. It occurs in diffuse osteopetrosis (Fig. 4.**175**) and in the following disorders:

- Craniometaphyseal dysplasia: an autosomal dominant (rarely autosomal recessive) disorder characterized by marked sclerosis of the entire skull and widening of the metaphyses, especially of the long tubular bones. The cranial sclerosis is more pronounced than in metaphyseal dysplasia. The main difference is in the clinical presentation, which includes a large skull, prognathism, and asymmetry along with marked dental irregularities, prominence of the paranasal sinus region (es-

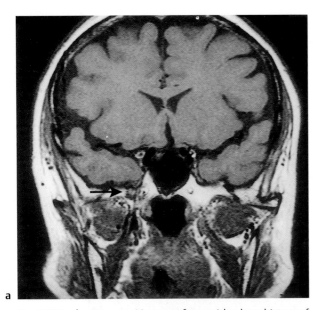

a

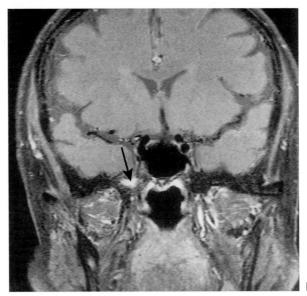

b

Fig. 4.174a, b Woman 63 years of age with a long history of classic trigeminal neuralgia on the right side.

a MRI of the skull base. T1-weighted SE sequence before contrast administration shows a hypointense mass in the right foramen ovale (arrow).

b Fat-saturated image after intravenous contrast injection shows a circumscribed, 6-mm intraosseous area of intense enhancement in the course of the mandibular nerve in the foramen ovale (arrow). This finding is typical of an intraosseous trigeminal neurinoma.

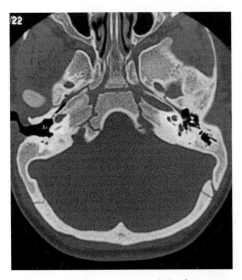

Fig. 4.175 Slight narrowing of the foramen ovale by diffuse osteopetrosis. Axial CT with a high-resolution bone filter.

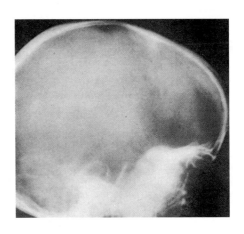

Fig. 4.176 Marked sclerosis of the skull base in Camurati-Engelmann disease (diaphyseal dysplasia).

pecially the maxillary sinuses), and cranial nerve dysfunction predominantly affecting the facial and vestibulocochlear nerves.

- Craniodiaphyseal dysplasia: an autosomal recessive disorder that presents radiographically with massive periosteal and endosteal sclerosis of the diaphyses of the tubular bones, sparing the epiphyses and metaphyses. There are also sclerotic skull changes that may be associated with cranial nerve deficits (especially of nerves II and VIII). In contrast to Camurati–Engelmann syndrome, the dominant features are marked cranial sclerosis and facial skeletal changes that are already conspicuous in childhood (prominent paranasal sinus region, flat nose, cranial nerve deficits).

- Metaphyseal dysplasia (Pyle disease): an autosomal recessive disorder characterized by a peculiar flaring of the metaphyses of the long tubular bones. Cranial changes consist of mild sclerosis of the calvarium and skull base. Clinically palpable expansion of the medial ends of the clavicles appears to be a characteristic feature. Another clinical sign is genu valgum.
- Other less common syndromes.

Fibrous dysplasia (Jaffe–Lichtenstein disease) and **Paget disease** also lead to sclerotic areas in the skull base accompanied by structural changes. The differential diagnosis was reviewed on p. 401. Important differentiating criteria are listed in Table 4.**15**.

Table 4.**15** Criteria for differentiating between fibrous dysplasia and Paget disease on cranial CT (Tehranzadeh et al. 1998)

	Paget's Disease	Fibrous Dysplasia
1. "Groundglass" appearance	0/8	17/18
2. Symmetry of cranial involvement:		
a. Symmetrical cranial involvement	7/8	0/10[a]
b. Asymmetrical cranial involvement	1/8	10/10[a]
3. Sinus involvement:		
Ethmoid	1/7[b]	15/18
Sphenoid	2/7[b]	16/18
Maxillary	1/7[b]	7/18
Frontal	1/7[b]	9/18
4. Appearance of cortical tables:		
a. Thin cortical tables	0/8	9/13[c]
b. Thick cortical tables	8/8	4/13[c]
5. Sphenoid bone involvement	3/7[b]	15/18
6. Orbital involvement	0/8	7/18
7. Nasal cavity involvement	0/8	6/18
8. Soft tissue involvement	0/8	3/18
9. Maxillary involvement	0/8	2/18
10. Cystic changes of cranial wall	1/8	7/18

[a] Includes the 13 patients with cranial involvement; five of 18 cases lacking skull CT were excluded

[b] One of eight cases lacked images of sinus and base of skull

[c] Of the 18 patients, 13 had cranial CT and involvement. Of these, 10 of 13 cases had bilateral cranial involvement

Occasionally it can be difficult to differentiate among fibrous dysplasia, Paget disease, meningioma en plaque, and intraosseous meningiomas that are associated with skeletal hyperostosis. Differentiation is aided by the clinical presentation and, if necessary, by CT and MRI.

Changes in the **carotid canal** and in the horizontal carotid segment in the foramen lacerum are best demonstrated by MRI and CT. This particularly applies to soft-tissue masses such as glomus tumors (Fig. 4.**177**).

Two special features should be noted in the **posterior fossa**:

The **jugular tubercles** (Fig. 4.**134c**), which overlie the hypoglossal canals next to the jugular foramina, may be eroded and flattened by cerebellopontine angle tumors that extend posteriorly.

Chordomas are derived from remnants of the primitive notochord. They show a slow, progressive type of growth but are locally aggressive. Sites of predilection are the extremities of the spinal column, i.e., the spheno-occipital and sacrococcygeal regions. Approximately 35% of chordomas occur on the skull base near the clivus, and 15% are located in the cervical spine. While the tumor is demarcated from surrounding soft tissues by a pseudocapsule, it is not demarcated from adjacent bone. Clivus chordoma is characterized on CT scans by marked destructive changes and a soft-tissue mass, which often contains calcifications. A mucogelatinous material can be obtained at biopsy. The tumor often reaches considerable size and tends to recur after surgical removal.

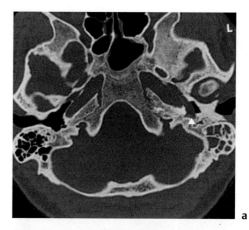

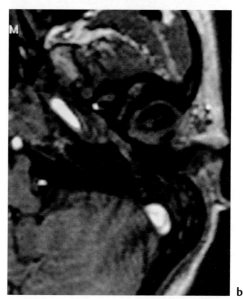

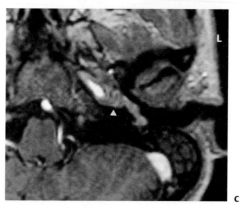

Fig. 4.**177a–c** Glomus tumor that has destroyed the posterior portions of the foramen lacerum.

a Axial CT with a high-resolution bone filter shows circumscribed expansion of the foramen lacerum in the left side of the skull base with a soft-tissue density in the hypotympanum (arrowhead) and partial clouding of the mastoid air cells.

b T1-weighted gradient-echo MRI shows a hypointense soft-tissue mass around and behind the left internal carotid artery.

c Axial T1-weighted gradient-echo MRI after intravenous contrast injection shows intensely enhancing soft tissue surrounding the left internal carotid artery (arrowhead).

Sella turcica

The sphenoid bone develops essentially through the re-placement of the chondrocranium by bone. The sphenoid complex ossifies in two parts, an anterior and a posterior, separated by the intersphenoidal suture. The posterior part develops from the initially paired centers of the ba-sisphenoid and from the alae temporales, which when ossified form the greater wings. The anterior part develops from three basal ossification centers that fuse to form the presphenoid. The anterior and posterior parts of the sphe-noid begin to fuse into a single body before birth.

The sella turcica is a hollow located within the sphenoid bone. It is bounded by the following structures:

- The anterior clinoid processes of the lesser wings
- The tuberculum sellae of the sphenoid body
- The floor of the sella
- The dorsum sellae with the posterior clinoid processes

Just anterior to the tuberculum sellae is the **prechiasmatic sulcus**, a transverse groove that interconnects the right and left optic canals. Anterior to the groove is the **jugum sphenoidale**, which radiologists call the **planum sphe-noidale**. It is separated from the cribriform plate of the eth-moid bone on the cerebral surface by the sphenoethmoidal suture. A sphenoid limbus (unofficial nomenclature) sepa-rates the prechiasmatic sulcus from the planum sphe-noidale (Fig. 4.**178**). The roof of the sphenoid sinus usually forms a portion of the sellar boundary (Fig. 4.**5**, Fig. 4.**179**).

Because CT demonstrates the sella and adjacent bony structures with much greater precision than projection ra-diography, CT of the skull base has largely replaced plain films in the detection of bony abnormalities. MRI is cur-rently used to evaluate the soft-tissue structures in and around the sella (Fig. 4.**180**).

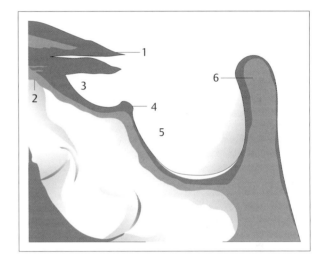

Fig. 4.**178**   Diagram of a sella turcica with a pronounced pre-chiasmatic sulcus.
1   Anterior clinoid process
2   Planum sphenoidale
3   Prechiasmatic sulcus
4   Tuberculum sellae
5   Floor of sella
6   Dorsum sellae

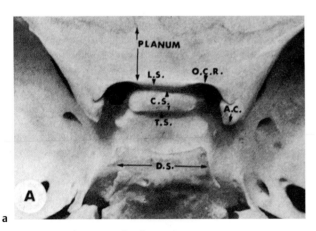

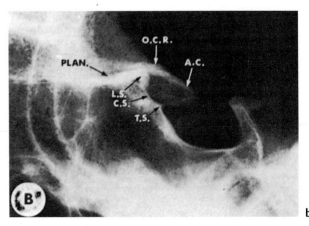

Fig. 4.**179 a, b**   Normal sellar region.
a Superior aspect (anatomic specimen).
b Lateral radiograph. (From Kier 1968.)
A.C.   Anterior clinoid process
C.S.   Chiasmatic sulcus
D.S.   Dorsum sellae
L.S.   Sphenoid limbus
O.C.R. Roof of optic canal
PLAN   Planum sphenoidale
T.S.   Tuberculum sellae

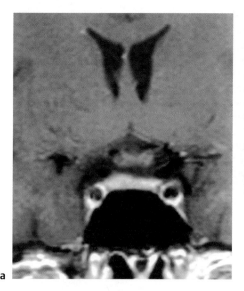
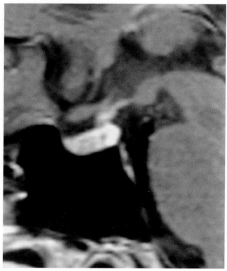

a

b

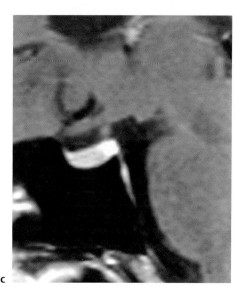

c

Fig. 4.**180 a–c**   MRI appearance of the normal pituitary.
a Coronal image after contrast administration.
b, c Sagittal images after contrast administration.

Normal Findings

During Growth

The **tuberculum sellae** can be defined radiographically as the anterosuperior boundary of the sella in 98% of newborns. The dorsum sellae and planum sphenoidale are not yet ossified. The **interspenoidal synchondrosis** (Fig. 4. **181**) is still visible in 15% of cases but is more frequent in premature infants and infants with hydrocephalus. It should not be confused with the **craniopharyngeal canal**, which starts at the deepest part of the sellar floor, runs obliquely downward, and normally is no longer visible in newborns.

The ossification center of the **dorsum sellae** appears shortly after birth. By the third to eighth year of life, expansion of the sphenoid sinus tends to flatten the presellar region where it borders the planum sphenoidale and prechiasmatic sulcus. If the sinus is very large, it can even alter the slope of the jugum sphenoidale, giving it an anterior upslope or shaping it into a kind of hillock. The shape of the sella in adults follows from its infantile shape. Differences in the demarcation between the prechiasmatic sulcus and the tuberculum sellae lead to different sellar configurations. The extent of the sphenoid sinus also affects the shape of the sella. The term "**rucksack sella**" is a purely descriptive term applied to dilatation of the sphenoid sinus with a high planum sphenoidale and a bulging prechiasmatic sulcus. The small ossification center for the mostly cartilaginous sella in the newborn (Fig. 4.**182**) grows rapidly during the first year of life. For the next year or so the sella grows at a slower rate, increasing mostly in length, and continues to enlarge until about 11 years of age. From 11 to 14 years of age, the sella grows faster in girls than in boys.

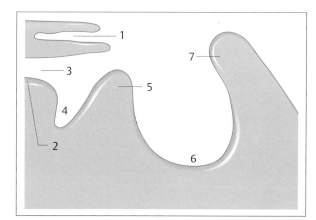

Fig. 4.**181**   Persistent interspenoidal synchondrosis (after Mayer).
1   Anterior clinoid process
2   Planum sphenoidale
3   Sphenoid limbus
4   Persistent interspenoidal synchondrosis
5   Tuberculum sellae
6   Floor of sella
7   Dorsum sellae (pediatric shape)

Fig. 4.**182 a, b**   Specimen radiographs of a mature newborn (observation by Richter, Hamburg).
a Lateral projection of the intact skull.
b Intracranial surface with the skull opened and the brain removed. Note the relatively thick cartilage layer between the contrast material and the relatively small bony sella turcica. The sella is partially filled with contrast material.

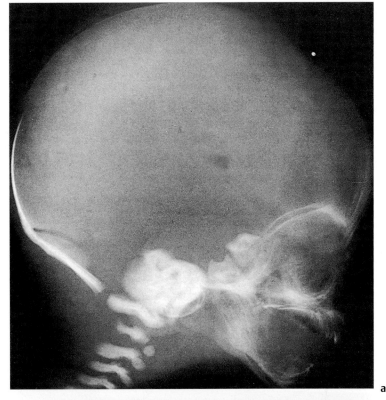

a

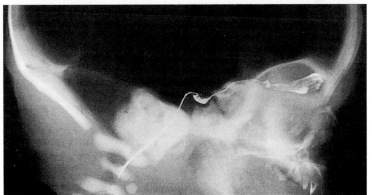

b

In Adulthood

The sella turcica has an oblong shape in almost two-thirds of cases and is round in the remaining third. A variety of sellar configurations have been described (Fig. 4.**183**). The two **anterior clinoid processes** overhang the sella, and the roots of the processes where they unite with each lesser wing are projected over the planum sphenoidale in the lateral view (Fig. 4.**184**). The **dorsum sellae** is variable in its length, thickness, and position (Fig. 4.**183**). The **posterior clinoid processes** at the angles of the dorsum sellae are also of variable size and may appear hyperostotic when large. In the frontal view, an occipital Towne projection with the tube angled about 35° toward the foot of the table gives a clear projection of the dorsum sellae within the foramen magnum (Fig. 4.**185**). Modern CT and MRI techniques have almost entirely replaced plain films of the sella, however. The mineralization of the dorsum sellae decreases after 45 years of age. CT densitometry has shown a sharp decline in both sexes after 50 years of age, correlating with the bone mass of the axial skeleton.

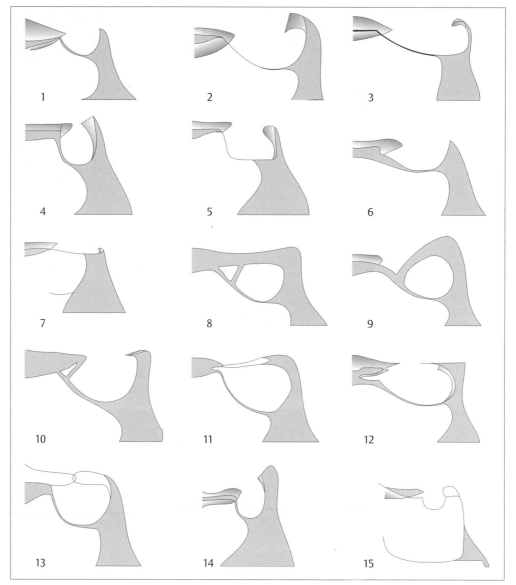

Fig. 4.**183**   Sellar configurations. The most common shapes are shown in 1–6.

1   Round
2   Elliptical
3   Shallow
4   Deep
5   Quadrangular
6   Distorted (contracted)
7   This shape lacks a real fossa and dorsum, resulting in a very small sellar cavity.

8–12 These shapes are characterized by various types of bridging. The bridging in 12 is incomplete.
13   Apparent bridging ("pseudo-bridging") is caused by the superimposed terminal portions of the anterior and posterior clinoid processes.
14   Variant with a tall, stocky dorsum.
15   Variant with a small, rounded fossa and a broad, low dorsum, which is often pneumatized. The posterior clinoid processes may be present or absent.

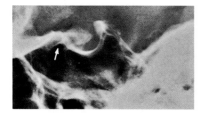

Fig. 4.**184**   Bulky anterior clinoid processes and a small sella turcica over a well-developed sphenoid sinus. The arrow indicates the groove for the internal carotid artery on the undersurface of the anterior clinoid process.

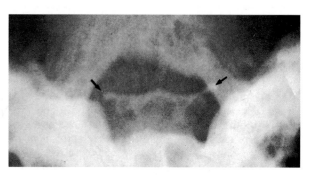

Fig. 4.**185**   Osteophytes on the dorsum sellae (arrows) in an occipital radiograph.

Pathological Finding?

Normal Variant/Anomaly?

When the paranasal sinuses are heavily pneumatized ("pneumatosinus dilatans"), air cells may also be present in the anterior clinoid processes (Fig. 4.**186**). In another variant, the anterior processes may appear thickened and sclerotic (Fig. 4.**187**). In other cases they may be absent or underdeveloped.

If the dorsum sellae has a buttonlike appearance in the lateral view, this is usually caused by **osteophytes** on the posterior clinoid processes (Fig. 4.**185**). It is somewhat common to find a strandlike calcification (Fig. 4.**188**) or horsetail-like calcification (Fig. 4.**189**) extending posteriorly from the dorsum sellae.

Calcifications at the attachment of the tentorium extend horizontally and posteriorly. Calcifications in the **petrosellar ligament** (medial petroclinoid ligament) extend obliquely downward and laterally to the petrous apex, and calcifications in the sphenopetrosal ligament are located between the lateral margin of the dorsum sellae and the anteromedial tip of the petrous bone (anatomy in Fig. 4.**5**). The **sphenopetrosal ligament** passes over the abducens nerve ("abducens bridge") and the petrosal sinus on both sides, forming a canal ("Dorello's canal"). It can also cross over the trigeminal nerve ("trigeminal bridge") if it arises from the trigeminal impression. In this case it may run horizontally or ascend slightly in the medial direction, inserting either on the lower part of the posterior clinoid process lateral to the clivus or on the lesser alar process as the lateral petroclinoid ligament. This alar process can be explained phylogenetically but has no clinical importance. An exostosis-like bony protuberance has also been observed posterior to the base of the dorsum sellae (Fig. 4.**190**).

It is not uncommon to see a small **medial clinoid process (tertiary clinoid process)** located below the tuberculum sellae, the "knob of the saddle" (Fig. 4.**191**). This process may be present only on one side (Fig. 4.**192**). The morphological variants of the sella were described previously (p. 447, Fig. 4.**183**).

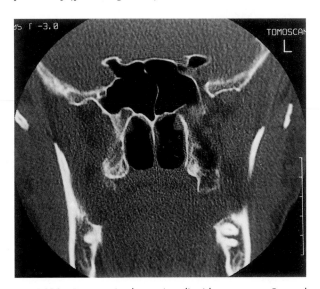

Fig. 4.**186** Pneumatized anterior clinoid processes. Coronal CT with a high-resolution bone filter.

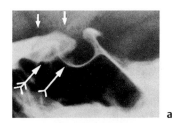

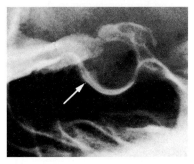

Fig. 4.**187 a, b** Clinoid processes.
a Very broad anterior clinoid processes (arrows). Sella turcica (tailed arrow). Groove for the internal carotid artery (two-tailed arrow).
b Hyperostotic anterior clinoid processes. Medial clinoid process (arrow).

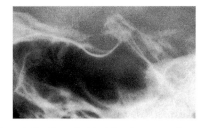

Fig. 4.**188** Streaklike calcifications behind the dorsum sellae.

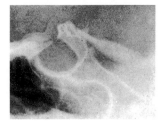

Fig. 4.**189** Horse-tail-like calcifications behind the dorsum sellae.

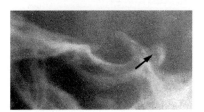

Fig. 4.**190** This dorsum is angled forward, and a fluffy bony prominence is visible behind its base.

Ossification across the entrance to the sella is called a **sellar bridge**. This term can be misleading, however. In a strict sense it refers to arched clinoid processes on each side of the sella, which are present in up to 8% of the population. A delicate, vertical calcific spicule has been found in the lumen of the sella and interpreted as a "calcification" in the connective tissue between the adenohypophysis and neurohypophysis. Sellar bridges may form a carotico-clinoid foramen owing to their proximity to the internal carotid artery. The clinical significance of sellar bridges is uncertain. They have been observed in the pediatric age group. They can form between the dorsum sellae and anterior clinoid process (Fig. 4.193) and between the dorsum sellae and medial (tertiary) clinoid process (Figs. 4.194, 4.195). Ossification can also occur between the medial clinoid process and the anterior clinoid processes (Fig. 4.196). The bridge need not form a complete arch (Fig. 4.197), and bridges between the anterior and medial clinoid processes may cross one another (Figs. 4.198, 4.199). In other cases a gap may persist within a broad sellar bridge (Fig. 4.200). Figure 4.201 illustrates a combination of sellar bridges and other dural calcifications.

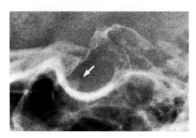

Fig. 4.**191** Medial (tertiary) clinoid process (arrow).

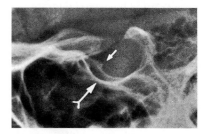

Fig. 4.**192** The sellar floor bulges outward on one side (tailed arrow). There is a unilateral medial (tertiary) clinoid process (arrow), and the anterior clinoid processes are prominently developed.

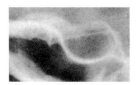

Fig. 4.**193**

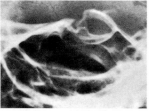

Fig. 4.**194** ▷

Fig. 4.**193** Ossification of the sellar inlet between the dorsum sellae and the anterior clinoid processes on both sides.

Fig. 4.**194** Bone formation between the posterior clinoid process and medial clinoid process.

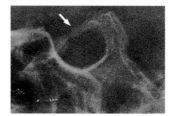

Fig. 4.**195** "Sellar bridge" caused by bone formation between the posterior and medial clinoid processes. A relatively high planum sphenoidale is noted as an incidental finding.

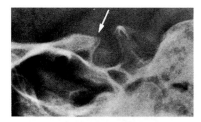

Fig. 4.**196** Bone formation between the anterior and medial clinoid processes (arrow).

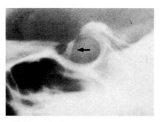

Fig. 4.**197** Bony projection arising from the medial clinoid process (arrow). Note the streaklike calcification behind the dorsum sellae.

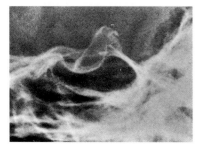

Fig. 4.**198** Upper and middle "sellar bridges" overlap, making a cruciform pattern.

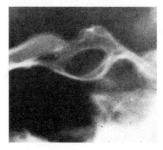

Fig. 4.**199** Upper and middle sellar bridges over a strongly pneumatized sphenoid sinus.

Calcifications of the internal carotid artery usually appear as typical ringlike opacities at a suprasellar and/or parasellar location. They are rarely visible on plain films (Fig. 4.**51**), but vessel wall calcifications are a common finding in thin CT slices of the skull base. Calcifications in the wall of the basilar artery are located posterior to the clivus along the course of the vessel, and calcifications of the ophthalmic artery are located in the prechiasmatic sulcus.

A notch in the undersurface of the anterior clinoid processes represents an incomplete bony canal for the internal carotid artery (Figs. 4.**202**, 4.**187 a**). An incisure may persist at the site where the **intersphenoidal synchondrosis** (Fig. 4.**181**) reaches the sphenoid bone anterior to the sella at the level of the anterior clinoid processes (Fig. 4.**203**). The associated areas of increased bone density and bone thickening should not be mistaken for meningiomas.

The **craniopharyngeal canal**, which originally connects the pituitary with the pharyngeal roof, arises from the deepest part of the sellar floor and may persist in 0.5% of the population. The point from which the remnant of Rathke's pouch extends from the sellar floor to the pharyngeal roof may be marked by a small bony protuberance on the sellar floor (Figs. 4.**204**, 4.**205**). A close relationship exists between this canal and transsphenoidal meningoencephaloceles.

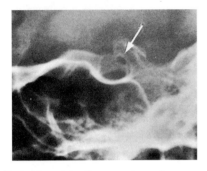

Fig. 4.**200**   Broad sellar bridge with a foramen (arrow).

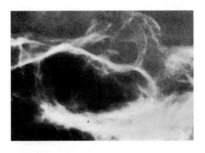

Fig. 4.**201**   Sellar bridges combined with irregular dural calcifications.

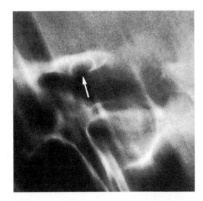

Fig. 4.**202**   Tomogram shows a notch for the internal carotid artery (arrow) in the inferior border of the anterior clinoid process. The sphenoid sinus is heavily pneumatized, especially in its basal portion.

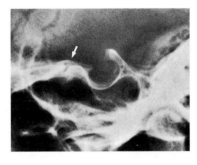

Fig. 4.**203**   Persistent intersphenoidal synchondrosis (arrow) in a 36-year-old woman.

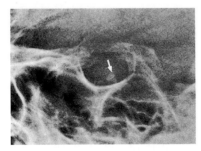

Fig. 4.**204**   Bony eminence at the origin of the craniopharyngeal canal (pharyngeal tubercle).

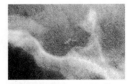

Fig. 4.**205**   Pharyngeal tubercle.

"**Sellar spine**" refers to a midline bony prominence that juts obliquely upward from the anterior margin of the dorsum sellae toward the interior of the sella. It has no known clinical significance.

An unusually high dorsum sellae is called a **dorsum elongatum**. Turretlike bony processes are interpreted as remnants of an embryological cord of the meninges and especially of the dura mater.

A **persistent chordal canal**, the median basilar canal (Fig. 4.**206**), runs obliquely downward within the bone along the posterior edge of the dorsum sellae. When viewed in an end-on projection, the inlet to this canal may appear as a hole in the posterior contour of the dorsum sellae (Figs. 4.**207**–4.**211**). While this is a common finding, it may resemble an isolated air cell in the cancellous bone of the dorsum sellae if the sphenoid sinus is large and the

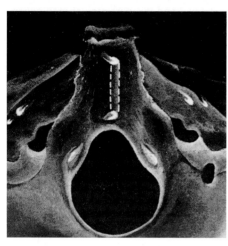

Fig. 4.**206**   Chordal canal (median basilar canal) on the dorsal aspect of the clivus. (From Neiss 1964.)

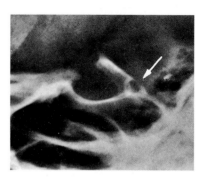

Fig. 4.**207**   The orifice of the median basilar canal appears as a foramen-like opening in the posterior border of the dorsum sellae (arrow).

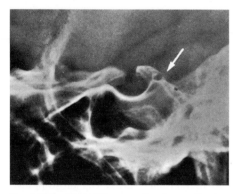

Fig. 4.**208**   Typical foramen for the median basilar canal (arrow).

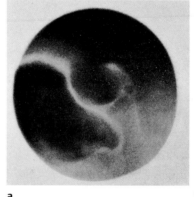

a   b

Fig. 4.**209a, b**   Foramen for the median basilar canal in a tomogram.

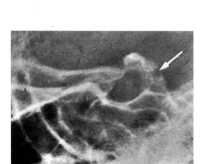

Fig. 4.**210**   Discontinuity in the broad, irregular, indistinct posterior border of the dorsum sellae (arrow). Median basilar canal.

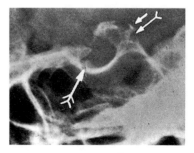

Fig. 4.**211**   Dorsum sellae with a small exostosis (arrow), below which is the median basilar canal (one-tailed arrow). Medial clinoid process (two-tailed arrow).

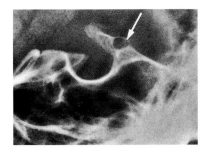

Fig. 4.**212**   Blisterlike expansion of the initial part of the median basilar canal (arrow). Below is a large pneumatized sphenoid sinus.

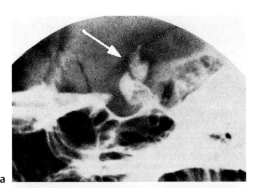

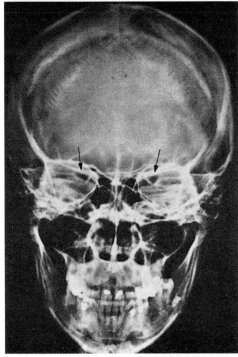

Fig. 4.**213 a, b**   Suprasellar calcification. (From Neutsch and Cramer 1967.)
a Special sellar view shows an angel-wing-shaped calcification (arrow) projected over and above the posterior clinoid processes.
b Frontal skull film shows typical small, symmetrical, ringlike calcifications projected over the orbits (lipoproteinosis, Urbach–Whiete syndrome).

posterior border of the dorsum is thinned and bulging (Fig. 4.**212**).

Pituitary dwarfism with primary aplasia or hypoplasia of the pituitary may be associated with a very small sella ("**microsella**"). In other cases an extremely small sella that is heavily bridged may have no clinical significance from an endocrinological standpoint. Children with untreated hypothyroidism or athyrosis are often found to have a large, rounded, ballooned sella turcica that must be distinguished from a primary pituitary neoplasm, especially pituitary adenoma, by MRI (p. 454).

Characteristic symmetrical calcifications in the parahippocampal gyrus are found in **lipoid proteinosis (Urbach–Wiethe syndrome)**. This is an autosomal recessive disorder of lipid metabolism that, while rare, should be included in the differential diagnosis of suprasellar and parasellar calcifications. The calcifications in Urbach–Wiethe syndrome are projected over the dorsum sellae in the lateral view, and in frontal views they appear in the area where carotid calcifications are also found ("angel wing syndrome," Fig. 4.**213**).

Fracture?

Fractures of the skull base often extend into the sella and the sphenoid sinus. They can show varying degrees of displacement and may be associated with hemorrhage. CT is currently used for primary evaluation. An example is shown in Fig. 4. **214**. More information on basal skull fractures can be found on pp. 440, 508 and 537. Differentiation from open cranial sutures is particularly important in children and can be accurately accomplished with CT.

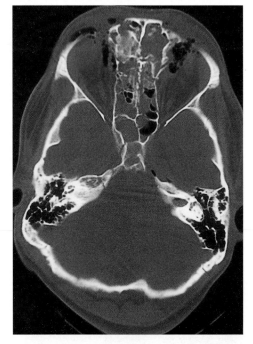

Fig. 4.**214**   Basal skull fracture extending into the sphenoid sinus.

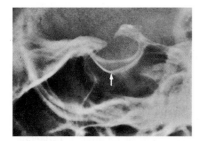

Fig. 4.**215**   Unilateral deepening of the sellar floor (arrow).

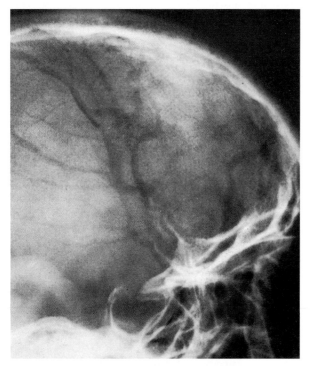

Fig. 4.**216**   Enlarged sella with destructive changes in the dorsum sellae and posterior clinoid processes. Wide diploic veins are noted as an incidental finding.

 Tumor?

Today, MRI is most commonly used for the imaging investigation of the pituitary, the sella, and their surroundings while CT is preferred for imaging bony structures and extraosseous calcifications. Conventional radiographs could occasionally show direct or indirect sellar changes caused by intrasellar or extrasellar tumors or increased intracranial pressure ("**pressure sella**"). The signs were very uncertain and nonspecific. In the interpretation of plain films, asymmetrical erosions or notches in the anterior and posterior clinoid processes or sellar floor suggest an intrasellar tumor and, in principle, can identify the affected side. Some unilateral deepening of the sellar fossa can occur as a normal variant, however (Fig. 4.**215**). A classic rule in radiography is that the angle between the planum sphenoidale and the anterior wall of the sella tends to be acute with intrasellar tumors and obtuse with suprasellar tumors. The "pressure sella" is caused by increased pressure in the third ventricle or surrounding basal cisterns. As the dorsum sellae and posterior clinoid processes are progressively thinned, and as the anterior clinoid processes decrease in volume due to the rise in pressure, the walls of the sella turcica expand and the sella becomes enlarged (Fig. 4.**216**). In other pressure-related effects, the anterior clinoid processes may appear sharply tapered while the dorsum sellae appears straightened or angled forward. MRI can accurately define the various forms of pituitary adenomas, even in the case of small tumors that are unaccompanied by bony changes (Fig. 4.**217**). The "**empty sella**" is also demonstrated most clearly by MRI (Fig. 4.**218**).

Langerhans cell histiocytosis was described on p. 400. In the skull, slightly more than half the lesions are asymptomatic and are detected on skull radiographs obtained after trauma. Lesions that involve the sphenoid wings may infiltrate the orbit and produce exophthalmos. Involvement of the sella may be associated with symptoms of diabetes insipidus.

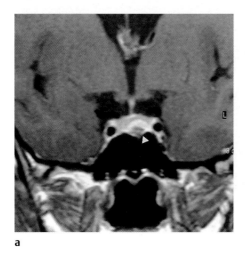

a

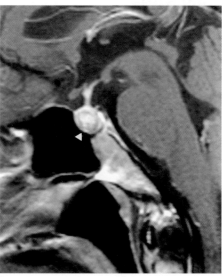

b

Fig. 4.**217 a, b**   Pituitary adenoma with intratumoral hemorrhage.
a Coronal MRI. T1-weighted SE sequence after intravenous contrast injection shows a predominantly hyperintense mass in the pituitary (arrowhead), representing a pituitary adenoma with intratumoral hemorrhage.
b Sagittal MRI. T1-weighted SE sequence after intravenous contrast injection again shows the hemorrhagic pituitary adenoma as a predominantly hyperintense mass (arrowhead).

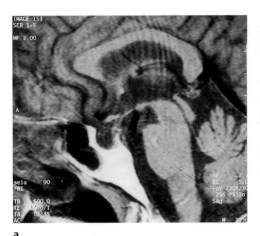 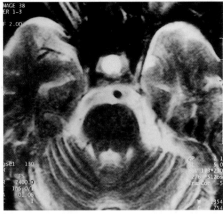

a   b

Fig. 4.**218 a, b**   "Empty sella" on sagittal and axial MRI.

With bony and sphenoid sinus lesions that are destroying the walls of the sella, the following entities should mainly be considered:

- Chordomas of the dorsum sellae or clivus
- Epipharyngeal tumors that are destroying the skull base
- Rare mucoceles of the sphenoid sinus

Optic glioma and **optic sheath meningioma** are examples of tumors that are associated with a characteristic pattern of destruction. The tuberculum sellae is occasionally eroded. This leads to enlargement of the sellar fossa along the area where the prechiasmatic sulcus has been destroyed. The bone destruction may extend farther rostrally, causing the entire sellar cavity to assume the shape of a "J" lying on its side: **J-shaped sella.**

Various other primary or secondary intracranial tumors, which may or may not obstruct the ventricular system (malignant glial tumors, meningiomas, tumors of the third ventricle, metastases, pseudotumors, etc.), can produce sellar abnormalities that are detectable by plain radiographs.

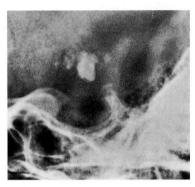

Fig. 4.**219**   Suprasellar craniopharyngioma (histologically confirmed) located by the floor of the third ventricle (observation by Cottier, Bern).

> Plain film examination of the sella has become obsolete in this context and has been superseded by MRI and CT.

Intratumoral calcifications, especially in craniopharyngiomas, provide indirect evidence of the location of an intrasellar or juxtasellar tumor. The calcifications are usually nodular or stippled. A suprasellar, midline location is typical in most young patients (Fig. 4.**219**). Some calcifications are suprasellar and intrasellar, and a small number are entirely intrasellar. Small granular or linear calcifications are occasionally seen at the periphery of pituitary adenomas. Suprasellar optic nerve gliomas and hypothalamic tumors may also calcify. The nature of the calcifications found in parasellar meningiomas (e.g., cavernous sinus meningioma) and in dermoids or epidermoids is highly variable. Today these lesions are diagnosed with MRI and sometimes with CT (Fig. 4.**220**).

Calcified **aneurysms of the internal carotid artery** produce a typical, ringlike suprasellar or parasellar density that may be continuous or disrupted. Calcifications of the carotid artery were discussed previously. Calcifications in aneurysms should always be included in the differential diagnosis of tumor-associated calcifications and variants (p. 451).

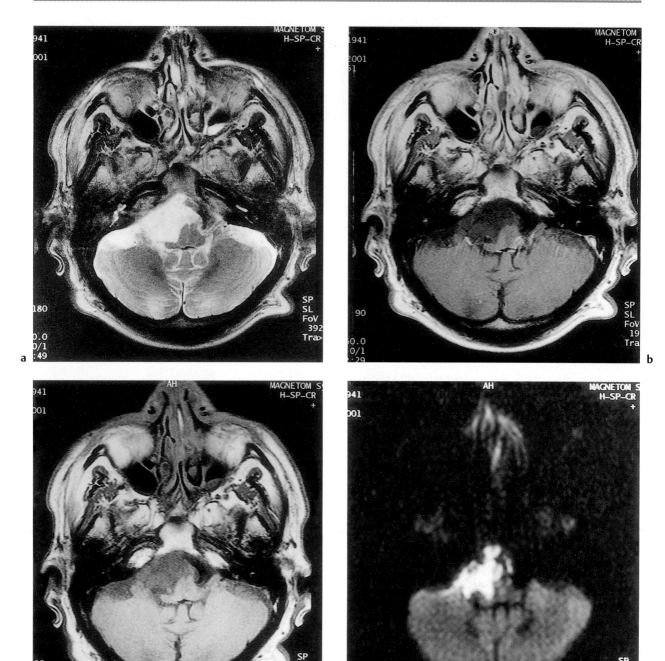

Fig. 4.**220 a–d** Typical epidermoid/dermoid of the skull base.

a T2-weighted axial SE sequence shows a hyperintense mass in the right cerebellopontine angle.

b T1-weighted axial SE sequence without contrast medium.

c T1-weighted axial SE sequence after intravenous contrast injection.

d Diffusion-weighted EPI sequence demonstrates characteristic high contrast.

Temporal Bone

Development and Anatomy

The temporal bone helps to form the base and lateral wall of the skull. It consists of several parts:

- Petrous part
- Tympanic part
- Squamous part

Embryologically, all three parts of the temporal bone have a different origin. The petrous part develops from the chondrocranium. The squamous part is a flat membranous bone, and the tympanic part develops as part of the branchial arches.

The **inner ear** is formed from thickened patches of superficial ectoderm, the auditory placodes. The surface of each placode invaginates to form the auditory vesicles, which differentiate further to form the saccule and the cochlear duct with the organ of Corti (ventral component) and the utricle, semicircular canals, and endolymphatic duct (dorsal component). This complex epithelial tubular system is called the membranous labyrinth. The surrounding mesenchyme is transformed into a cartilaginous capsule, which finally ossifies to form the bony labyrinth of the inner ear.

The various components of the temporal bone unite shortly before birth. The **petrous part** (petrous bone) is located in the skull base and encloses the inner ear. The **squamous part** (temporal squama) forms a portion of the

cranial sidewall between the sphenoid bone and occipital bone, its base articulating with the mandibular condyles. The **tympanic part** of the temporal bone forms the floor, anterior wall, and posterior wall of the bony external auditory canal. The petrous part forms the **mastoid process** located behind the external auditory canal. The squamous part also contributes to this process. The mastoid process is pneumatized from the tympanic cavity and contains the mastoid cells.

The **petrous pyramid** refers to the medial portion of the petrous and tympanic parts located in front of the mastoid process, including the styloid process. The pyramid, with its superior margin or ridge, projects into the cranial cavity (Figs. 4.**3**, 4.**5**, 4.**221 a–d**). The **tegmen tympani** is a thin bony plate that forms the roof of the tympanic cavity. This area is located between the arcuate eminence (prominence marking the superior semicircular canal of the vestibular apparatus) and the lateral petrosquamous fissure (Fig. 4.**5**).

In contrast to these anatomical considerations it is helpful clinically to subdivide into inner, middle, and outer ear.

The **inner ear** harbors the auditory and vestibular apparatus. The **middle ear** is formed by the tympanic cavity, air cells, and eustachian tube. The tympanic cavity contains the auditory ossicles: the malleus, incus, and stapes. The handle (manubrium) of the malleus, which inserts on the tympanic membrane, is followed by the rest of the ossicular chain that transmits sound through the incus to the stapes. The footplate of the stapes is fixed in the oval window below the horizontal segment of the facial nerve. This portion of the facial nerve is discussed here because it

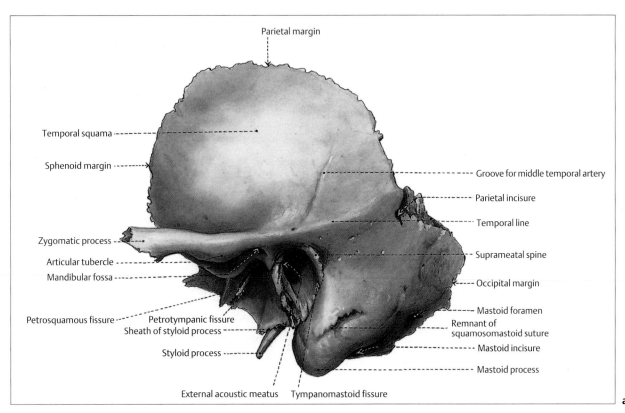

Parietal margin

Temporal squama

Sphenoid margin

Zygomatic process

Articular tubercle

Mandibular fossa

Petrosquamous fissure
Petrotympanic fissure
Sheath of styloid process

Styloid process

External acoustic meatus   Tympanomastoid fissure

Groove for middle temporal artery

Parietal incisure

Temporal line

Suprameatal spine

Occipital margin

Mastoid foramen

Remnant of squamosomastoid suture

Mastoid incisure

Mastoid process

a

Fig. 4.**221 a–d**
a Left temporal bone, lateral aspect.
b Left temporal bone, medial aspect.
c Left temporal bone, lateral aspect with the medial, superior and inferior wall of the middle ear.

d Left temporal bone, lateral aspect. Medial wall of the middle ear, course of the facial canal, mastoid antrum. (From Rauber and Kopsch 1987.)

Fig. 4.**221 b–d** ▷

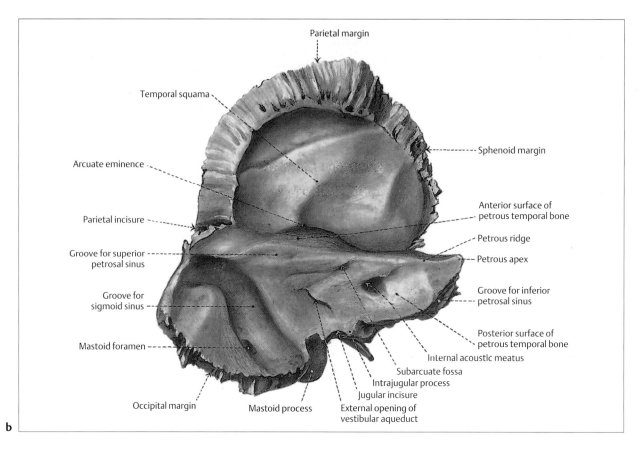

Parietal margin

Temporal squama

Arcuate eminence

Parietal incisure

Groove for superior
petrosal sinus

Groove for
sigmoid sinus

Mastoid foramen

Sphenoid margin

Anterior surface of
petrous temporal bone

Petrous ridge

Petrous apex

Groove for inferior
petrosal sinus

Posterior surface of
petrous temporal bone

Internal acoustic meatus

Subarcuate fossa

Intrajugular process

Jugular incisure

External opening of
vestibular aqueduct

Occipital margin

Mastoid process

b

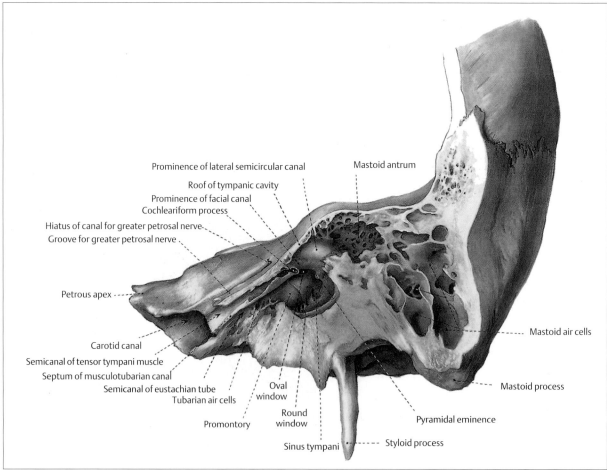

Prominence of lateral semicircular canal

Mastoid antrum

Roof of tympanic cavity

Prominence of facial canal

Cochleariform process

Hiatus of canal for greater petrosal nerve

Groove for greater petrosal nerve

Petrous apex

Mastoid air cells

Carotid canal

Semicanal of tensor tympani muscle

Septum of musculotubarian canal

Semicanal of eustachian tube

Tubarian air cells

Oval
window

Mastoid process

Promontory

Round
window

Pyramidal eminence

Sinus tympani

Styloid process

c

Fig. 4.**221 b–c**

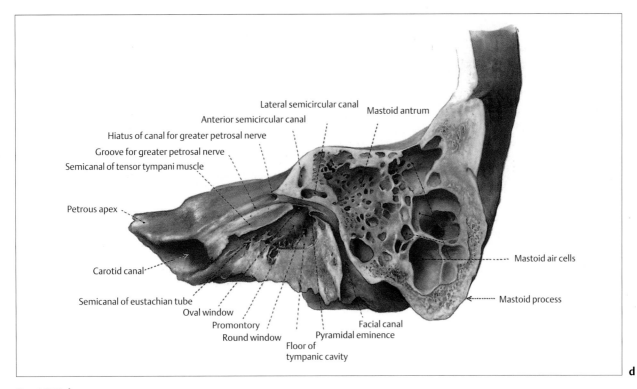

Fig. 4.**221 d**

passes through the middle ear, and it is important to know its course in order to evaluate damage to the nerve. The facial nerve is the motor nerve for the muscles of facial expression and other muscles. It leaves the brain at the cerebellopontine angle, enters the facial canal through the internal auditory canal, passes through the petrous bone in an anterolateral direction, then makes a 90° turn in the posterolateral direction, forming the external genu of the facial nerve. It continues through the tympanic cavity, traverses the mastoid, and exits the skull base through the stylomastoid foramen. A second part of the facial nerve is termed the intermediate nerve (nervus intermedius). The geniculate ganglion is located at the genu of the facial nerve. The bony canal between the internal auditory canal and external genu is called the **facial canal (fallopian canal)**.

The **external ear** consists of the external auditory canal and the auricle. The lateral two-thirds of the external auditory canal is composed of cartilage, the medial third of bone. The length of the auditory canal is approximately 2.5 cm. The bony part is directed medially and anteriorly and is narrower than the cartilaginous part. In two-thirds of cases the bony canal is narrowed from both the anterior and posterior walls, and this constriction is defined most clearly on axial CT scans.

Radiographic Projections

The usual standard skull views in the frontal, lateral or axial projections yield very little information on the petrous bone, and it is customary to obtain special petrous views. But even special views provide only a crude impression of temporal bone anatomy compared with CT and cannot detect most pathological processes.

The three standard temporal bone projections—still used by many radiologists—are as follows:

- The **Schüller** projection (Fig. 4.**222**)
- The **Stenvers** projection (Fig. 4.**223**)
- The **Mayer** projection (Fig. 4.**224**)

Only CT or MRI can permit a detailed evaluation of the petrous bones (Fig. 4.**225**). The main application of MRI is in visualizing the inner ear structures, the internal auditory canal, and the cerebellopontine angle owing to its superlative definition of soft-tissue structures (Fig. 4.**226**).

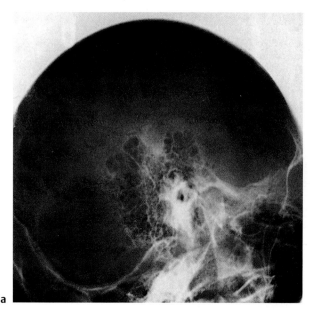

a

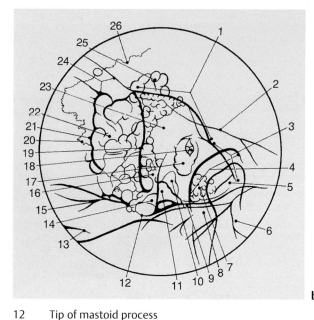

b

Fig. 4.**222a, b**   Lateral Schüller projection of the petrous bone.
a Radiographic appearance.
b Explanatory drawing (after Mayer).

1	Superolateral border of pyramid with arcuate eminence
2	Superior border of zygomatic process
3	Superior border of petrous apex
4	Glenoid fossa
5	Mandibular condyle
6	Petro-occipital synchondrosis
7	Sphenoid sinus
8	Peritubal cells
9	Contralateral pyramid
10	Jugular fossa
11	Jugular foramen
12	Tip of mastoid process
13	Bony ridge around the foramen magnum
14	Epibulbar or terminal cells
15	Bony ridges at the mastoid notch
16	Retrofacial cells
17	External auditory canal and tympanic cavity
18	Internal auditory canal and vestibule
19	Posterior border of petrous pyramid
20	Occipitomastoid suture
21	Posterior border of air cell system
22	Marginal or emissary cells
23	Bony center of the labyrinth
24	Transverse and sigmoid sinus grooves
25	Cells at petrous apex
26	Parietomastoid suture

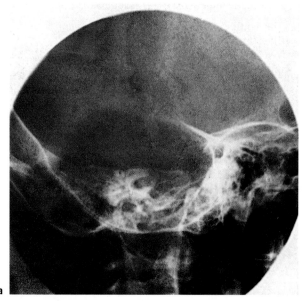

a

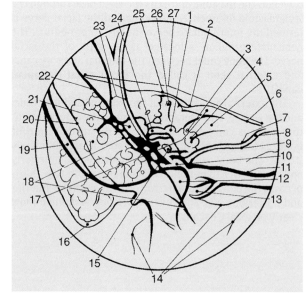

b

Fig. 4.**223a, b**

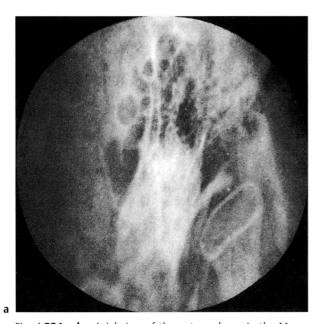

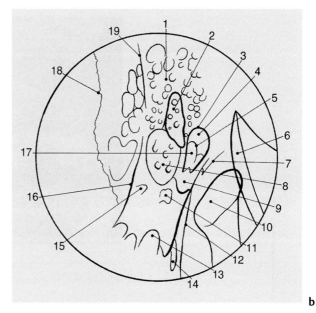

a

b

Fig. 4.**224 a, b**   Axial view of the petrous bone in the Meyer projection.
a Radiographic appearance.
b Explanatory drawing (after Mayer).

1	Mastoid cells
2	Mastoid antrum
3	Lateral border of the attic
4	Lateral attic wall
5	Tympanic ring
6	Zygomatic process
7	Tympanic bone
8	Labyrinthine capsule
9	Medial wall of tympanic cavity
10	Mandibular condyle
11	Cochlea
12	Posterior border of greater sphenoid wing
13	Carotid canal
14	Styloid process
15	Internal auditory canal
16	Posterior border of pyramid
17	External auditory canal and tympanic cavity
18	Occipitomastoid suture
19	Posterior contour of pyramid, marking the site of the superior genu of the sinus

◁ Fig. 4.**223 a, b**   Frontal Stenvers view of the petrous bone.
a Radiographic appearance.
b Explanatory drawing (after Mayer).

1	Vestibule
2	Subarcuate fossa
3	Facial canal
4	Cochlea
5	Internal auditory canal
6	Trigeminal notch
7	Lower contour of petrous pyramid
8	Petro-occipital synchondrosis
9	Border of clivus
10	Temporomandibular joint space
11	Floor of middle cranial fossa
12	Mandibular condyle
13	Hypoglossal canal
14	Vertebral body contours (especially of C1) below the skull base
15	Tympanic cavity
16	Mastoid process
17	Bony center of labyrinth
18	Zygomatic process and temporal line
19	Lateral wall of skull
20	Lateral border of sigmoid groove
21	Mastoid antrum
22	Medial border of sigmoid groove
23	Sagittal crest
24	Lateral semicircular canal
25	Arcuate eminence
26	Superior (anterior) semicircular canal
27	Petrous ridge

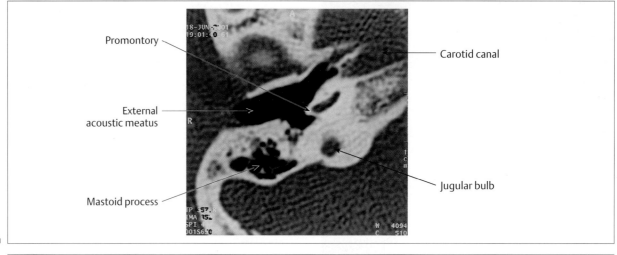

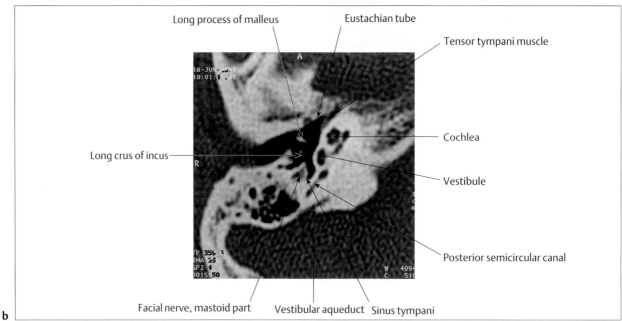

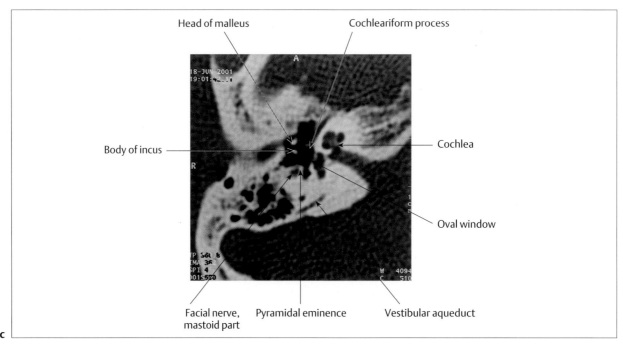

Fig. 4.**225 a–f**   Normal anatomy of the right petrous bone on axial CT using a high-resolution bone filter.

Fig. 4.**225 d–f** ▷

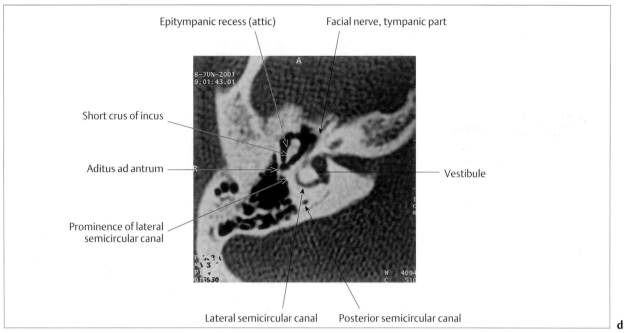

Epitympanic recess (attic)

Facial nerve, tympanic part

Short crus of incus

Aditus ad antrum

Vestibule

Prominence of lateral
semicircular canal

Lateral semicircular canal   Posterior semicircular canal

d

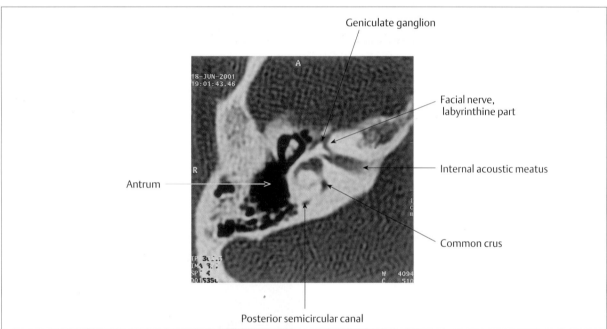

Geniculate ganglion

Facial nerve,
labyrinthine part

Internal acoustic meatus

Antrum

Common crus

Posterior semicircular canal

e

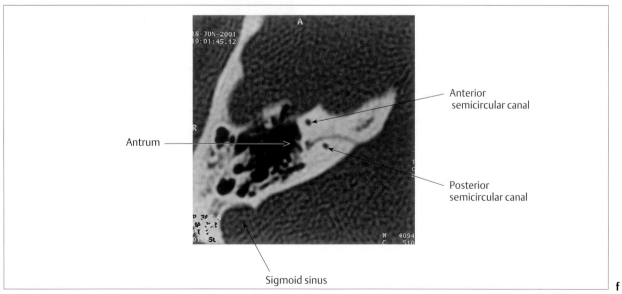

Anterior
semicircular canal

Antrum

Posterior
semicircular canal

Sigmoid sinus

f

Fig. 4.**225 d–f**

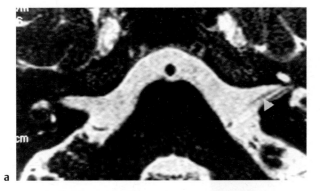
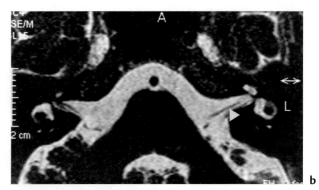
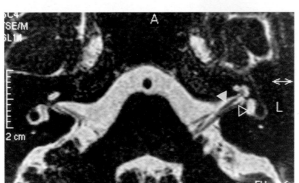
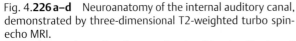
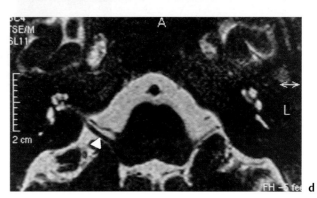

Fig. 4.**226 a–d**   Neuroanatomy of the internal auditory canal, demonstrated by three-dimensional T2-weighted turbo spin-echo MRI.
a Facial nerve (arrowhead). Note also the clear visualization of the cochlea and vestibular apparatus on both sides.
b Course of the facial nerve in the internal auditory canal (arrowhead).

c Cochlear nerve (arrowhead) and inferior vestibular nerve (open arrowhead). Note also the very clear definition of the inner ear structures on both sides.
d Course of the vestibulocochlear nerve (arrowhead) in the area of cerebellopontine angle.

Middle Ear, Air Cells, and External Auditory Canal

Normal Findings

 During Growth

In the newborn and during the first year of life, air is present only in the epitympanic recess (attic) and eustachian tube. Some degree of pneumatization has been occasionally found in the fetus as well. The air cell system develops during the first and second years of life.

Little or no pneumatization of the mastoid by 3 years of age is abnormal and signifies inhibition of air cell development.

The mastoid process should have a full complement of air cells by 4 years of age at the latest. The mastoid air cells should be regularly shaped and uniformly arranged, and the central cells are usually smaller than the more peripheral ones. The cells vary considerably in number, form, and size in different individual (Fig. 4.**227**). In boys 2 to 7 years of age, the air cells occupy a significantly smaller area than in girls.

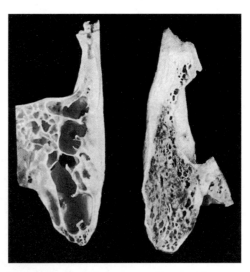

Fig. 4.**227**   Typical patterns of mastoid pneumatization in anatomic specimens.

In Adulthood

Conventional radiographs can define the extent of mastoid pneumatization in the Schüller projection (Fig. 4.**222**). CT can do this more accurately, however, and can demonstrate normal mastoid pneumatization, extreme pneumatization, inhibition of air cell development in various portions of the mastoid, and the pneumatization of the petrous bone (Figs. 4.**228**, 4.**229**). The aeration of the middle ear can also be accurately assessed by CT.

> The air cells in adults form a honeycomb-like arrangement of thin-walled cells of varying size. Normally the mastoid process, the basal portions of the petrous pyramid, and portions of the adjacent temporal squama are pneumatized.

The air cells lateral to and behind the sigmoid sinus are called the **marginal cells** or **emissary cells** (because they are adjacent to the mastoid emissary vein). Air cells located behind the wall of the auditory canal but in front of the mastoid process are called **retrofacial cells** because of their proximity to the facial canal. Cells near the jugular fossa are called **peribulbar cells**. Air cells located below the petrous ridge in close proximity to the superior petrosal sinus and its groove (Fig. 4.**5**) are known as petrous apex cells. Other air cells of varying size like those already described are known to occur in the anterior and posterior root of the zygoma and thus close to the zygomatic process of the temporal bone (Fig. 4.**221 a**). Air cells projected over the lower part of the petrous pyramid in the Schüller view, behind the mandibular condyle, are called **peritubal cells** (Figs. 4.**230**, 4.**231**).

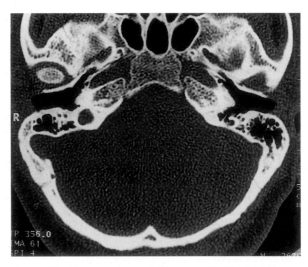

Fig. 4.**228**   Very sparse mastoid pneumatization, with even fewer air cells on the right than on the left. A high right jugular bulb is noted as an incidental finding (same case as in Fig. 4.**235**).

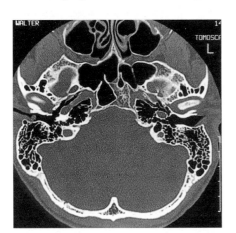

Fig. 4.**229**   Very pronounced pneumatization of the temporal bone on both sides. Axial CT with a high-resolution bone filter.

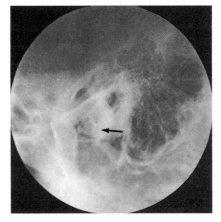

Fig. 4.**230**   Schüller view shows heavy pneumatization of the mastoid and the peritubal cell complex (arrow).

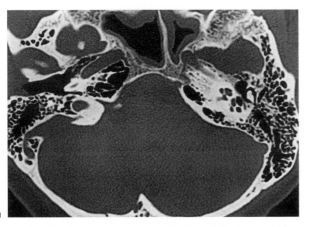

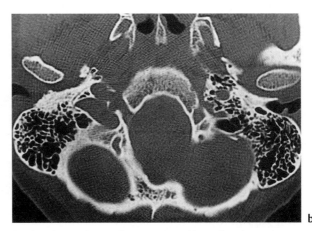

a
b

Fig. 4.**231 a, b**   Extreme pneumatization of the temporal bone on both sides, with air cells anterior and lateral to the temporomandibular joint.

▌ *Pathological Finding?*

Normal Variant/Anomaly?

The variable pneumatization of the air cells of the temporal bone was discussed on p. 465. Variants range from very sparse aeration to extensive pneumatization of the entire temporal bone including large portions of the skull base: **pneumatosinus dilatans** (Figs. 4.228–4.231). Differentiation is required from inhibition of air cell development due to childhood infection, which can lead to marked obliteration of the mastoid and petrous air cells (Fig. 4.232).

The **tympanic bone** correlates in size and form with the dimensions and configuration of the tympanic cavity. The cranial wall of the tympanic cavity is formed by the **tegmen tympani**, a very thin bony plate that may be partially absent. This finding should not be mistaken for bone destruction in coronal projections (Fig. 4.233). The anatomy of the tegmen tympani is reviewed on p. 457 and in

Fig. 4.**221 c**. A **low position of the tegmen** may affect all or part of the tegmen plate. A posterior extension of the superior border of the zygomatic arch provides a reference line that is approximately parallel to the orbitomeatal line. Normally the posterior part of the tegmen tympani is 5–10 mm above the reference line. If the tegmen is level with the line or below it, it is too low. The anterior part of the tegmen tympani is located just below the orbitomeatal line. If the tegmen is so oblique that its outline is not visible on plain films, its position can be determined from the **Citelli angle**, which is decreased when the tegmen is low. Also, a low tegmen line does not cross the sigmoid groove at the superior genu of the sinus as it normally does, but lower in the area of its vertical portion (cf. Fig. 4.**222**).

Bulging of the bony wall of the sigmoid sinus toward the posterior wall of the auditory canal (anteposition) or laterally toward the outer cortex of the mastoid process (lateral position) influences the route that must be used for surgical access to the mastoid and middle ear. The same applies to the variable level of the jugular bulb, since a **high jugular bulb** is a risk factor for serious hemorrhagic complica-

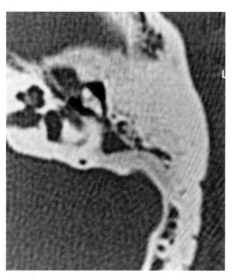

Fig. 4.**232**   Almost complete inhibition of air cell development on the left side. Axial CT with a high-resolution bone filter.

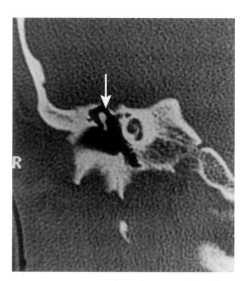

Fig. 4.**233**   Coronal CT of the right petrous bone shows an extremely thin tegmen tympani, portions of which are not defined.

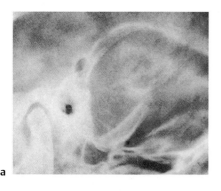

a

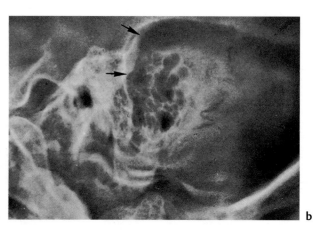

b

Fig. 4.**234 a, b**   Schüller projections.
a High position of the transverse sinus.
b High transverse sinus showing marked curvature (arrows).

tions (Figs. 4.**234**, 4.**235**). Normally the anterior wall of the sigmoid sinus is 10–15 mm from the posterior wall of the auditory canal. An anteposition and lateral position of the sinus may coexist, and the sinus can also show various forms of diverticula, hypoplasia, and aplasia. Plain films have been relegated to a minor role since the advent of axial and coronal CT scanning of the temporal bone. Abnormalities of the tegmen, such as a perforated tegmen with intracranial complications, can be accurately demonstrated by CT or MRI. These modalities are also excellent for dural sinus imaging (Fig. 4.**236**).

Usually the **mastoid emissary vein** is clearly visualized on radiographs (Fig. 4.**237**). Normally it is only 2–3 mm wide but may enlarge to the width of the small finger if the dural sinuses are underdeveloped. The superior petrosal sinus may be embedded deeply in the petrous pyramid before entering the sigmoid sinus. It appears most clearly in the Schüller projection as a 3-mm-wide lucent band that runs obliquely backward and upward just below the petrous ridge and is bounded inferiorly by the floor of the groove for the superior petrosal sinus (see Fig. 4.**221b** for

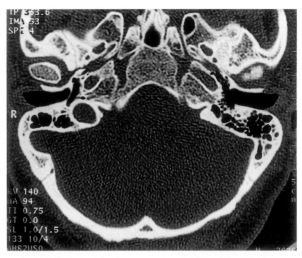

Fig. 4.**235**   High position of the jugular bulb on the right side. Axial CT with a high-resolution bone filter.

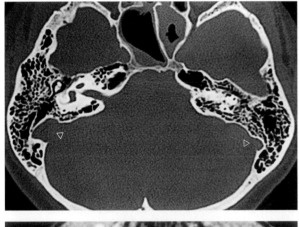

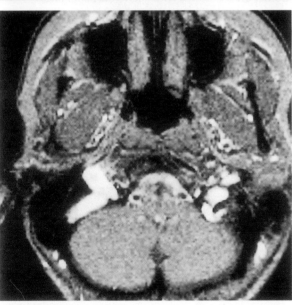

Fig. 4.**236a, b**
a CT with a high-resolution bone filter defines the course of the sigmoid sinus on both sides (arrowheads). A large venous channel and large sigmoid sinus are visible on the right side. Some clouding of the sphenoid sinus is noted as an incidental finding.
b Venous TOF angiography (single slice) shows a normal-appearing sigmoid sinus in a different patient.

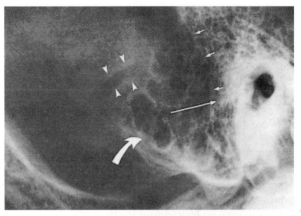

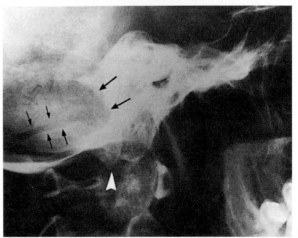

Fig. 4.**237a, b**   Mastoid emissary vein.
a Mastoid emissary vein (arrowheads), emissary cells (marginal cells, curved arrow), and retrofacial cells (long arrow). Bony sinus shell (small arrows).
b Straight horizontal mastoid emissary vein (small arrows). Bony sinus shell (arrows). Complete inhibition of air cell development in the mastoid and petrous bone (arrowhead).

anatomy). The inferior petrosal sinus rarely exhibits blind pouches that arise from the corresponding sulcus (Fig. 4.**221 b**).

Atresia of the external auditory canal (Fig. 4.**238**) generally coexists with microtia or anotia. With very few exceptions, severe auricular anomalies are associated with atresia of the external auditory canal. This atresia, in turn, is associated with malformations of the middle ear. Moderate deformities may be accompanied by a narrow antrum.

The **middle ear cavity** may contain septa. The auditory ossicles are subject to hypoplasia and deformity, interosseous fusion (Fig. 4.**239**), or the absence of one or all of the

ossicles. The middle ear cavity is of variable size and may be absent in extreme cases (Fig. 4.**240**). Narrowing of the tympanic cavity by a high jugular bulb (Fig. 4.**235**) or low tegmen tympani has been described.

The **oval** and **round windows** can be demonstrated by axial and/or coronal CT. This applies to the depiction of normal anatomy as well the detection of variants and congenital or acquired abnormalities such as fenestral otosclerosis (Fig. 4.**241**). When the tympanic part of the temporal bone is hypoplastic, the distance between the mastoid and temporomandibular joint is decreased. The facial canal is shifted anteriorly in these cases along with the mastoid process.

The **otocraniofacial syndromes** include mandibulofacial dysostosis (Treacher–Collins syndrome), craniofacial dysostosis (Crouzon syndrome), acrocephalosyndactyly (Apert syndrome), and hemifacial-microsomia syndrome. Mandibulofacial dysostosis and hemifacial-microsomia syndrome have special importance as developmental abnormalities of the first two branchial arches. Mandibulofacial dysostosis is characterized by varying degrees of stenosis or atresia of the external auditory canal, deformities or absence of auditory ossicles, a small middle ear cavity, underdevelopment of the mastoid, or an abnormal course of the facial nerve, which is usually shifted anteriorly. Craniofacial dysostosis is marked by stenosis or atresia of the external auditory canal, a small tympanic cavity, and fused elements of the ossicular chain (e.g., the malleus to the attic wall or the stapes to the promontory). The external and internal ear show no malformations in acrocephalosyndactyly syndrome, but there is abnormal fixation of the stapes footplate. Hemifacial-microsomia syndrome is associated with microtia and with atresia or stenosis of the external auditory canal, which also may be directed vertically. Other features are a low tegmen and absent or deformed auditory ossicles. Inner ear anomalies are absent in this syndrome. The four otocraniofacial syndromes are associated with additional anomalies.

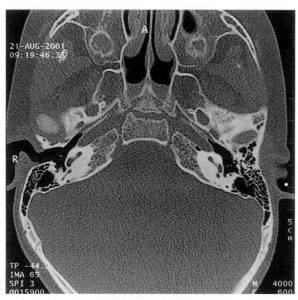

Fig. 4.**238** Bony atresia of the left ear canal in a 12-year-old girl. There were no concomitant malformations of the inner ear.

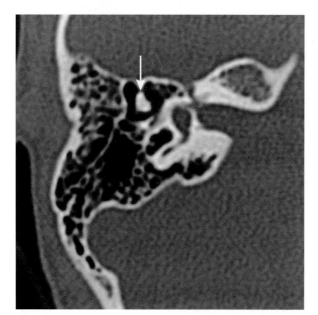

Fig. 4.**239** Middle ear anomaly with fusion of the malleus and incus (arrow). Axial CT with a high-resolution bone filter.

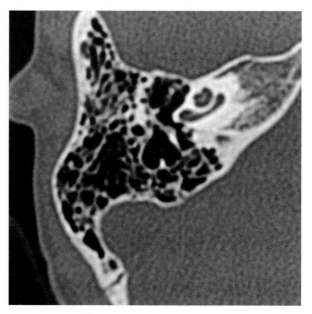

Fig. 4.**240** Small tympanic cavity in a patient with anomalies of the middle ear and ossicular chain. Axial CT with a high-resolution bone filter.

Fig. 4.**241 a–d**   Slight ossification in the oval window area in fenestral otosclerosis (clinically confirmed).

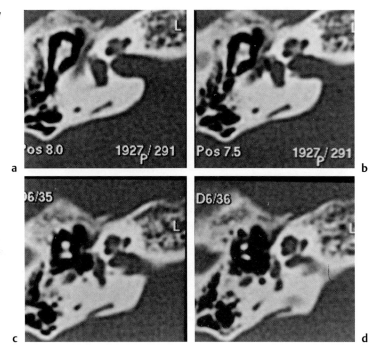

 Fracture?

Linear fractures of the squamous part of the temporal bone are well visualized on plain skull films or large-format Schüller views. They occasionally extend into the tympanic part and external auditory canal, in which case that portion of the fracture usually cannot be seen on projection radiographs. Like fractures of the petrous bone, however, these fractures are accurately defined by CT (Fig. 4.**242**). Differentiation is required from the **petrotympanic fissure** (Glaser fissure) (Figs. 4.**107**, 4.**108**), which indeed may be dehiscent due to involvement by a fracture. Injuries of the petrous bone are more apt to be burst fractures caused by indirect violence rather than a direct blow.

A laterally directed traumatizing force tends to produce a **longitudinal fracture of the petrous bone**. An **anterior** longitudinal petrous fracture extends from the anterior part of the temporal squama through the tegmen tympani and anterior facial nerve genu to the petrous apex. A **posterior** longitudinal petrous fracture runs through the posterior parietal bone, the mastoid, and the posterosuperior portion of the pyramid. The auditory ossicles and the external genu of the facial nerve are typically involved. Longi-

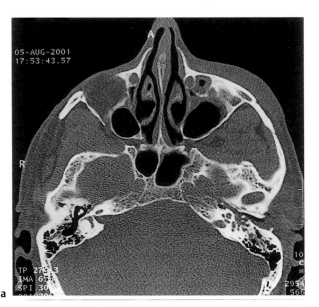

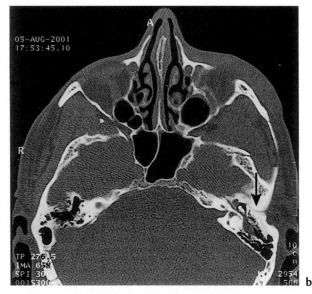

Fig. 4.**242**   Left temporal skull fracture extending into the petrous bone (arrow). The fracture also runs through the anterior wall of the external auditory canal and close to the temporomandibular joint.

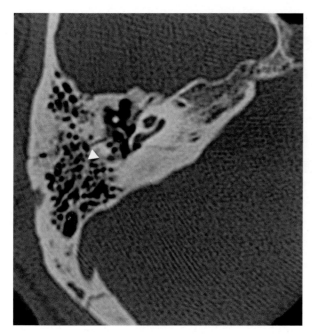

Fig. 4.**243**   Transverse fracture lines through the air cell system of the temporal bone (arrowhead).

Transverse fractures of the petrous bone are only about one-fifth as common as longitudinal fractures and are caused by sagittally directed violence to the petrous bone. The fracture runs perpendicular to the long axis of the bone. A **lateral** type of transverse fracture with possible involvement of the inner ear is distinguished from a less common **medial** type with involvement of the internal auditory canal. Transverse fractures are also associated with hematotympanum, but the tympanic membrane and external auditory canal are intact. Common symptoms are sensorineural hearing loss due to frequent involvement of the inner ear, also dizziness or spontaneous nystagmus. Up to 50% of patients have facial nerve palsy as a result of direct nerve injury. CSF rhinorrhea through the eustachian tube is not uncommon with transverse fractures. The lateral and medial types may be combined (Fig. 4.**243**).

Trauma to the petrous bone can also cause **rupture, displacement, dislocation, or subluxation** of the auditory ossicles. The ossicular chain is most frequently ruptured at the incudostapedial joint. With an isolated or concomitant dislocation of the incudomalleolar joint, there can be considerable displacement of the incus. The malleus is the most securely anchored of the auditory ossicles. The best method for examining the ossicles is single-slice or multislice spiral CT scanning using a thin slice thickness and high-resolution bone filter (Fig. 4.**244**). Avulsions of the mastoid process may involve the external auditory canal, the lateral and posterior semicircular canals, and perhaps even the tympanic segment of the facial nerve, leading to facial paralysis.

tudinal fractures of the petrous bone are associated with hematotympanum due to tearing of the middle ear mucosa. Rupture of the tympanic membrane leads to bleeding from the external auditory canal. Both types of fracture are typically extralabyrinthine. The cardinal symptom is conductive hearing loss caused by bleeding in the tympanic cavity and by frequent disruption of the ossicular chain, which is irreversible without surgery. Twenty percent of cases develop facial nerve palsy, which is usually caused by perineural edema near the geniculate ganglion.

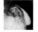 **Necrosis?**

Necrosis of the calvarium and skull base was discussed in the sections on the Cranial Vault (p. 397) and the Skull Base (p. 441). Inokuchi et al. (1990) described a case of temporal bone necrosis following the irradiation of a maxillary carcinoma.

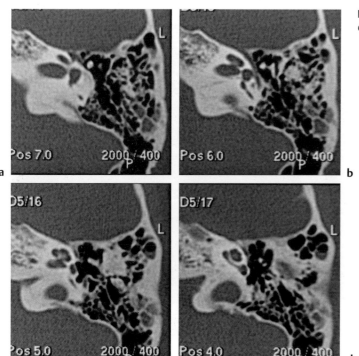

Fig. 4.**244 a–d**   Ossicular dislocation (malleus, incus) on the left side.

Inflammation?

The quality of the middle ear mucosa affects pneumatization. Poor-quality mucosa inhibits pneumatization and predisposes to infection. A link exists, therefore, between acquired inflammations and congenital anomalies.

Decreased pneumatization may be caused by external factors such as inflammatory diseases in early childhood, including neonatal otitis. These conditions lead to loss of the mucosa, which has a formative effect on the degree of pneumatization of the air cell system. Genetic factors also influence the development of mastoid and petrous pneumatization.

Conversely, the size and extent of the petrous air cells serve as indicators for the quality of the mucosa and its competence in resisting infection (Figs. 4.**232**, 4.**245**). Early **mucosal hyperplasia** can promote the formation of bony cavities around hyperplastic islands of mucosa. Because the mucosa does not completely regress, it continues to exert a growth stimulus on the bone, which eventually becomes thickened and sclerotic with widened intercellular septa. **Mucosal atrophy** (fibrosis) can lead to a complete or partial absence of pneumatization (Fig. 4.**251**). The complete inhibition of air cell development can lead, for example, to a mastoid process with normal cancellous bone but with no air cells and no sclerosis. In cases of **mucosal hypotrophy**, pneumatization is slowed in varying degrees.

> When air cell development is asymmetrical, chronic unilateral otitis always affects the ear with the smaller air cells. Acute unilateral otitis generally affects the ear with the smaller air cells.

Clouding of the air cells means only that the air in the cells has been replaced by a denser medium. This may consist of mucosal swelling, exudate, granulation tissue, or even blood (after trauma). With acute suppuration in the middle ear, the clouding rarely disappears before clinical resolution and usually clears gradually after the clinical symptoms have subsided. Persistent clouding is a sign of osseous involvement.

While acute inflammations of the middle ear such as otitis media and middle ear effusion usually do not require radiographic examination, complications such as **mastoiditis** or **otomastoiditis** often necessitate a detailed CT evaluation. This will demonstrate any bony changes that would require surgical treatment. Otomastoiditis usually presents with total or subtotal opacification of the tympanic cavity and mastoid air cells. In suppurative mastoiditis with osseous involvement, the bony boundaries initially become indistinct and later undergo varying degrees of destruction as the disease progresses. It is common to find air–fluid levels in acute inflammations with incomplete clouding of the middle ear spaces. Air–fluid levels are also found in chronic forms of otitis.

Projection radiographs can be misleading, as in cases where a Schüller view is obtained without turning the auricle forward due to simple oversight or auricular pain (Fig. 4.**246**).

Petrous apicitis (petrositis, Gradenigo syndrome) occurs when an inflammatory process spread to involve the apex of the petrous pyramid. This usually develops as a complication of acute otomastoiditis. Theoretically, this can occur only in cases where the petrous apex is pneumatized (30–35% of the population). If an inflammation of the otomastoid spreads into a nonpneumatized petrous apex, it is more accurately described as osteomyelitis. The classic triad of otomastoiditis, abducens paralysis, and pain in the distribution of the trigeminal nerve rarely occurs. Patients often present clinically with retro-orbital pain and otorrhea. CT shows destructive changes in the petrous apex combined with fluid in the middle ear and mastoid. MRI shows a poorly marginated lesion with increased T2 signal intensity. Postgadolinium MRI shows enhancement around the bony defects that may extend to the meninges and perhaps to the gasserian ganglion (see Figs. 4.**247** and 4.**248**).

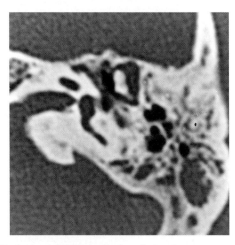

Fig. 4.**245**   Moderate inhibition of air cell development on the left side, with clouding of a relatively large mastoid cell. The malleus and incus show normal position and articulation. Axial CT with a high-resolution bone filter.

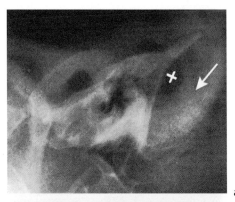

a

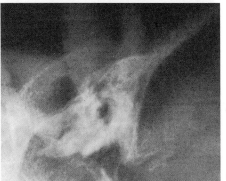

b

Fig. 4.**246 a, b**   Temporal bone.
a Schüller view of the temporal bone. Leaving the auricle in place (arrow) creates a superimposed lucency that mimics a defect (×).
b When the auricle is properly reflected forward, the position of the lucency is shifted accordingly.

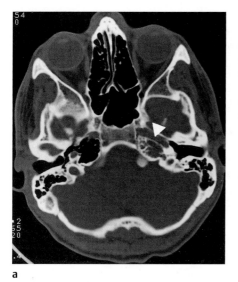

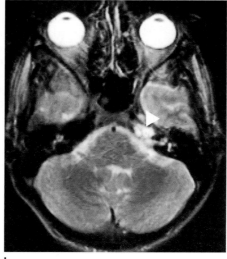

Fig. 4.**247 a, b**   Clouding in the area of the petrous apex.
a Bone-window CT shows clouding in the area of the left petrous apex (arrowhead).
b T2-weighted turbo SE image shows a hyperintense structure in the area of the left petrous apex (arrowhead) that correlates with the CT opacity. The finding is interpreted as a nonspecific inflammation.

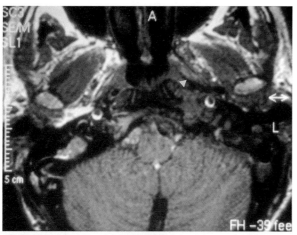

Fig. 4.**248 a–c**   Petrous apicitis (Gradenigo syndrome).
a T1-weighted SE image shows a focus with irregular margins at the left petrous apex (arrowhead).
b T1-weighted SE image after contrast administration shows pathological enhancement of the inflamed tissue at the left petrous apex (arrowhead).
c T1-weighted coronal SE after intravenous contrast administration shows enhancing parasellar tissue at the left petrous apex, corresponding to inflammatory granulation tissue (arrowhead).

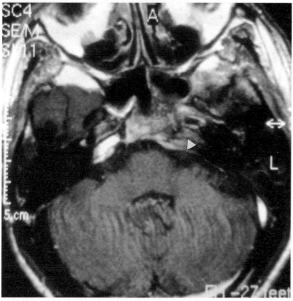

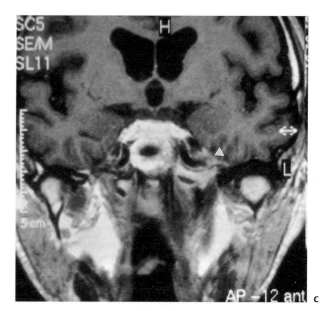

Cholesteatomas may be congenital or acquired. The congenital lesions, which are the same as epidermoids, arise from embryonic ectodermal rests and occur in all cranial bones, showing a predilection for the petrous bone. They comprise 2 % of all cholesteatomas in the middle ear. Acquired cholesteatomas are far more common. They result from a chronic inflammation with progressive destruction of the adjacent bone (the term "chronic bone suppuration" is also used). In order for a cholesteatoma to form, there must be direct contact between the keratinizing squamous epithelium in the external ear canal and the inflamed middle ear mucosa. Middle ear cholesteatomas are classified as follows according to their site of formation:

- Pars flaccida cholesteatomas
- Pars tensa cholesteatomas
- Cholesteatomas behind an intact tympanic membrane

Unusual sites of occurrence of cholesteatomas (Fig. 4.**249**) are:

- Mastoid process
- Petrous apex
- External auditory canal (Fig. 4.**250**)

If a cholesteatoma or mastoiditis penetrates into the epidural space, it can lead to epidural and eventual subdural or subarachnoid pneumocephalus. Brain abscess and venous sinus thrombosis take a dramatic clinical course. The complications of acute and chronic otomastoiditis and acquired cholesteatomas are reviewed in Table 4.**16**. CT often shows typical findings after radical surgery or modified radical surgery, which should be differentiated from pathological postoperative findings (Figs. 4.**251**, 4.**252**, 4.**253**, 4.**254**).

Table 4.**16** Complications of acute and chronic inflammation of the middle ear

Complications of acute otomastoiditis
• Coalescence (enzymatic absorption of the mastoid cell septa and empyema formation in the mastoid)
• Subperiosteal abscess
• Labyrinthitis
• Gradenigo syndrome, petrous apicitis
• Sigmoid sinus thrombosis
• Intracranial complications (meningitis, subdural abscess, epidural abscess, brain abscess)
Complications of chronic otomastoiditis
• Middle ear effusion
• Tympanic membrane retraction
• Granulation tissue
• Cholesterol granuloma
• Acquired cholesteatoma
• Ossicular fixation
• Ossicular erosion
Complications of acquired cholesteatomas
• Bone erosions near the pars flaccida or pars tensa
• Labyrinthine fistula
• Facial nerve lesion
• Destruction of the tegmen tympani
• Destruction of the sinus plate
• Intracranial and extracranial infections

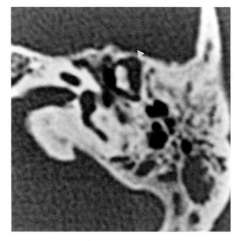

Fig. 4.**249**   Small cholesteatoma in Prussak's pouch on the left side (arrowhead). Axial CT with a high-resolution bone filter.

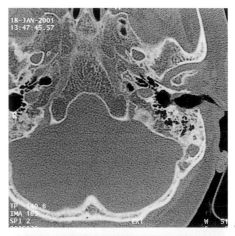

a

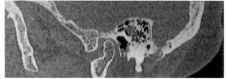

b

Fig. 4.**250a, b**   Histologically confirmed cholesteatoma of the external auditory canal. Foci of bone destruction are more pronounced on the anterior and posterior walls of the canal.
a Axial CT with a high-resolution bone filter.
b Sagittal reformatted image.

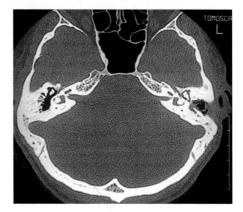

Fig. 4.**251**   Almost complete lack of air cell development on the right side in a patient who underwent a previous left-sided mastoidectomy. Axial CT with a high-resolution bone filter.

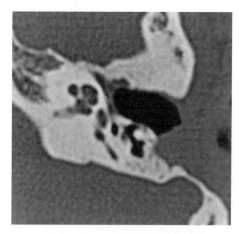

Fig. 4.**252** Normal postoperative findings after middle ear surgery. CT shows only a narrow layer of soft tissue within the surgical cavity. Axial CT with a high-resolution bone filter.

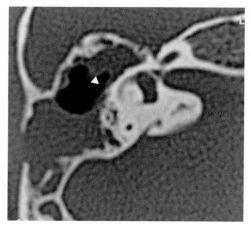

Fig. 4.**253** Recurrent cholesteatoma (arrowhead) following right middle ear surgery. Axial CT with a high-resolution bone filter.

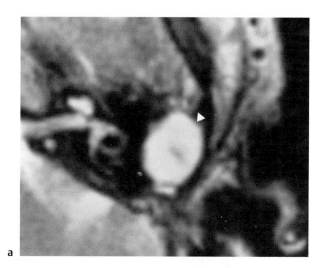

a

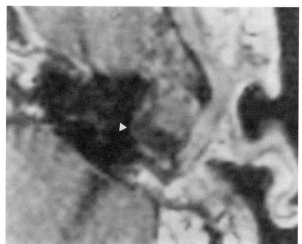

b

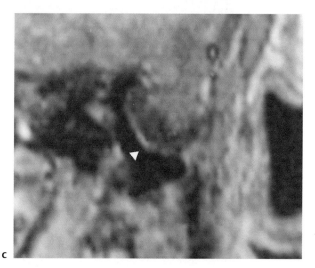

c

Fig. 4.**254 a–c** Meningoencephalocele.
a Axial T2-weighted MRI following middle ear surgery: meningoencephalocele (arrowhead).
b Axial T1-weighted image shows a postoperative meningoencephalocele with isointense and hypointense components (arrowhead).
c Coronal T1-weighted image after intravenous contrast injection demonstrates the postoperative meningoencephalocele on the left side (arrowhead).

Osteomyelitis develops when an inflammation of the air cells penetrates the cortical boundaries and reaches the diploe. The most frequent causes are surgery and trauma. Hematogenous spread is less common. Osteomyelitis may be seen at any age. It typically takes an acute to peracute course in small children. The imaging features are the same as those described for calvarial osteomyelities. Basically this also applies to the extremely rare cases of tubercular or syphilitic involvement of the petrous and mastoid air cells.

Otitis externa maligna is an infectious necrotizing disease that arises from the external auditory canal, spreads to adjacent soft-tissue structures, and sometimes leads to destruction of the petrous bone. It predominantly affects older patients with diabetes mellitus but can also occur in immunosuppressed patients or patients immunocompromised due to AIDS. The causative organism in the great majority of cases is *Pseudomonas aeruginosa*, an aerobic Gram-negative rod bacterium. The disease often takes an atypical course in AIDS patients, and other organisms such as aspergilli are often causative. Patients present clinically with severe otalgia, otorrhea, and persistent granulation tissue in the lower part of the ear canal at the junction of the bony and cartilaginous portions. Untreated, the disease typically spreads from the ear canal to the soft-tissue structures on the temporal bone, around the stylomastoid foramen, and into the infratemporal fossa. Other, less common routes of spread are posteriorly into the mastoid, anteriorly into the temporomandibular joint, and medially into the middle ear and petrous apex. Downward spread can lead to facial nerve palsy. Posteromedial spread of infection into the jugular foramen leads to paralysis of cranial nerves IX–XII (jugular foramen syndrome). Middle ear involvement is usually secondary via bony destruction of the mastoid, since the tympanic membrane appears to be an effective barrier to the spread of the disease. Intracranial spread leads to meningitis, intracranial abscess formation, or thrombosis of the sigmoid sinus or other venous sinuses. Advanced cases may show more or less extensive spread to the skull base with the development of osteomyelitis.

CT and MRI demonstrate abnormal soft-tissue structures in the external auditory canal, fluid in the mastoid or middle ear, and abnormal soft tissue around the eustachian tube. There may also be involvement of the cranial soft-tissue structures named above, including the parapharyngeal space, carotid artery, venous sinuses, and jugular bulb.

Besides CT and MRI, **radionuclide imaging** with $^{99\,m}$Tc-methylene diphosphonate, gallium citrate, or ^{111}In leukocyte scanning continues to have a role in the detection of bony changes. SPECT can provide sectional images for more accurate localization.

A malignant tumor is difficult to distinguish from otitis externa maligna by CT and MRI. For this reason, biopsy is often necessary to establish the diagnosis and identify the infecting organism.

 Tumor?

Exostoses and **osteomas** of the temporal bone are usually located in the medial portion of the external auditory canal. A small number arise from the promontory of the medial, labyrinthine wall of the tympanic cavity and spread into the ear canal (Fig. 4.**255**). Osteomas are also occasionally found in the mastoid air cells.

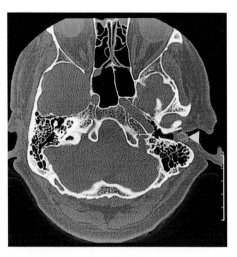

Fig. 4.**255** Osteoma (arrowhead) in the left external auditory canal. The lesion was confirmed at operation.

As noted earlier, **fibrous dysplasia** has three distinct morphological presentations:

1 Pagetoid type
2 Predominantly sclerotic type
3 Predominantly lytic or cystic type

Involvement of the petrous bone and mastoid by **fibrous dysplasia** is rare. Involvement of the squamous part of the temporal bone is more common in the setting of calvarial fibrous dysplasia.

The most common true neoplasms of the middle ear are **glomus tumors**. After acoustic neurinomas, they are the second most common tumor of the temporal bone. Carcinoma and other tumors such as osteoblastoma are rare. In terms of location, glomus jugulare tumors, which arise from nonchromaffin cells in the area of the jugular foramen, are distinguished from glomus tympanicum tumors, which are derived from the tympanic plexus. Patients may present clinically with pulsatile tinnitus, hearing loss, and pressure in the ear, depending on the size of the tumor and its site of origin. Dysequilibrium and cranial nerve deficits also develop in advanced stages. On otoscopic examination, a bluish-red mass can be seen in the tympanic cavity behind the intact eardrum. MRI, CT, and arterial angiography can confirm the diagnosis with high confidence. Conventional radiographs are now considered obsolete. Contrast administration is an essential diagnostic adjunct, especially when time–density curves are plotted (Fig. 4.**256**). CT can accurately define the extent of the tumor and the associated sites of bone destruction. The fact that glomus tumors follow the path of least resistance is important in differential diagnosis. This means that since glomus jugulare tumors and glomus tympanicum tumors can each grow into the area typically occupied by the other, some can be differentiated only by noting where the greatest tumor extension has occurred. This also means that glomus tumors can spread into the hypotympanum, the eustachian tube, and the vascular canals and neural foramina in the skull base. By contrast, **malignant tumors** such as carcinomas, sarcomas, and metastases cause irregular bone destruction as their growth progresses. This also applies to tumors that occur in the setting of systemic diseases, such as plasmacytoma, lymphoma, etc. Neurinomas generally do not affect the middle ear, and mening-

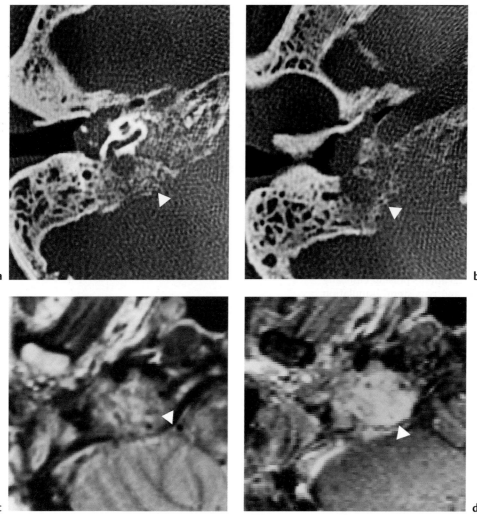

Fig. 4.**256 a–d**   Petrous bone destruction.
a CT with a high-resolution bone filter shows petrous bone destruction (arrowhead).
b CT shows extensive petrous bone destruction (arrowhead) with a soft-tissue structure extending into the hypotympanum.
c T2-weighted turbo SE image shows a nonhomogeneous, predominantly hyperintense mass (arrowhead) permeated by small flow voids (salt-and-pepper pattern) in the jugular foramen of the right petrous bone.
d T1-weighted SE image after contrast administration shows a very hyperintense mass (arrowhead) with small hypointense and signal void areas representing intravascular flow. The mass was identified as a glomus jugulare tumor.

iomas frequently contain calcifications and are associated with hyperostosis.

Glomus tumors mainly require otoscopic and CT differentiation from vascular anomalies in the **middle ear**, specifically:

- An intratympanic segment of the internal carotid artery
- A high superior jugular bulb (Figs. 4.**228**, 4.**235**)

Contrast administration can confirm the vascular nature of these anatomic structures. They have smooth margins and are not associated with bone destruction. Upward extension of the jugular bulb to the level of the internal auditory canal is not unusual and should not be mistaken for osteolysis. A diverticulum-like protrusion into the internal auditory canal causing auditory disturbance is very unusual. It should also be noted that the jugular foramina are usually asymmetrical, the foramen on the right being slightly larger than the one on the left. Finally, it should be mentioned that chronic inflammatory changes in the middle ear can be confusing at otoscopic examination if they appear as a bluish-red retrotympanic mass. This finding can be differentiated from a glomus tumor by CT.

Benign tumors of the middle ear, such as adenomas, are uncommon. There have also been rare reports of dermoids and epidermoids of the middle ear and mastoid process (Fig. 4.**220**). The differential diagnosis of bone destruction

in the middle ear should include inflammatory changes in chronic otitis media and congenital/acquired cholesteatoma.

Massive bone destruction, possibly combined with cranial nerve lesions, should raise the possibility of a rare embryonic rhabdomyosarcoma when detected in children. **Osteosarcoma** of the petrous bone is another rare entity (Fig. 4.**257**).

Another rare differential diagnosis is an **aneurysmal bone cyst** arising from the external auditory canal. This lesion is typically associated with rarefaction and increased lucency of the cancellous bone between the upper part of the ear canal and the temporomandibular joint margin, with the formation of fluid-filled cavities that are typical of aneurysmal bone cysts. Radiographs show mottled, honeycomb-like lucencies surrounded by an eggshell-like layer of periosteal new bone.

Foreign bodies in the external auditory canal also require differentiation from neoplasms. Rarely they may work their way into the tympanic cavity or even the eustachian tube. They are clearly demonstrated by CT, but the history is paramount in making a diagnosis.

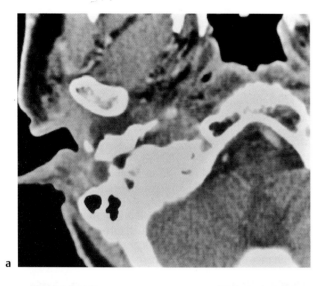

a

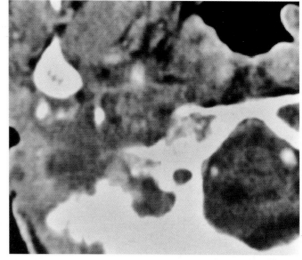

b

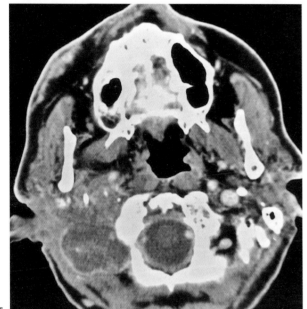

c

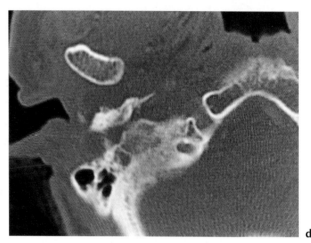

d

Fig. 4.**257 a–d**   Osteosarcoma of the petrous bone.
a–c Axial CT after contrast administration shows a rim-enhancing mass with central necrosis located in the right petrous bone and mastoid.
d Axial CT with a high-resolution bone filter shows extensive petrous bone destruction by the osteosarcoma.

Petrous Temporal Bone and Inner Ear

Embryology

The cartilaginous labyrinthine capsule develops lateral to the parachordal cartilage (see Fig. 4.6 a). It encloses the auditory vesicle and gives rise to the petrous part of the temporal bone. The inner ear is of ectodermal origin and develops from a thickening of the superficial ectoderm (otic placode), which invaginates near the rhombencephalon to form an auditory vesicle. This vesicle, or otocyst, is surrounded by the cartilaginous labyrinthine capsule. With further development, the auditory vesicle differentiates into a ventral component (from which the saccule and cochlear duct are formed) and a dorsal component (from which the utricle, semicircular canals, and endolymphatic duct are formed). The resulting epithelial tubules constitute the membranous labyrinth. Initially this structure is embedded in mesenchyme. Later the mesenchyme is transformed into a cartilaginous capsule, which finally ossifies to form the bony labyrinth that completely encloses the membranous labyrinth.

Ossification of the ectodermal otic capsule starts between weeks 16 and 20 of fetal development, when the cartilage has reached its maximum size and maturity. The bony labyrinth undergoes no further changes in size or shape and, like the auditory ossicles, is devoid of haversian canals, being composed entirely of cortical bone. A narrow rim of cartilage remains around the oval window.

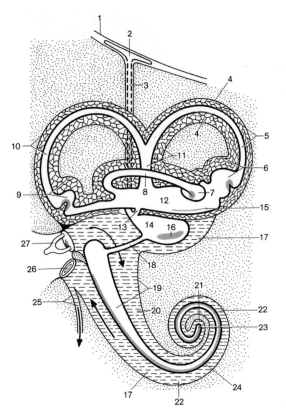

Fig. 4.**258** Diagram of the membranous and bony labyrinth viewed from the lateral side. (From Frick et al. 1980.)

 1 Dura mater
 2 Endolymphatic sac
 3 Endolymphatic duct
 4 Perilymphatic tissue
 5 Anterior semicircular canal and duct
 6 Anterior bony ampulla and anterior membranaceous ampulla
 7 Lateral membranaceous ampulla
 8 Lateral semicircular duct
 9 Posterior bony ampulla and posterior membranaceous ampulla
10 Posterior semicircular canal and duct
11 Common bony crus and common membranaceous crus
12 Utricle
13 Utriculosaccular duct in vestibule
14 Saccule
15 Macula utriculi
16 Macula sacculi
17 Perilymph
18 Ductus reuniens
19 Spiral canal of cochlea and cochlear duct
20 Scala vestibuli
21 Helicotrema
22 Scala tympani
23 Cecum cupulare
24 Spiral organ
25 Cochlear canaliculus and perilymphatic duct
26 Secondary tympanic membrane in round window
27 Stapes and footplate in oval window

Normal Findings

During Growth

At birth, the auditory and vestibular apparatus are fully developed except for the bony portion of the external auditory canal. The internal auditory canal has almost reached its normal diameter, which increases by no more than 1 mm on average as the child grows. The length of the internal auditory canal, on the other hand, increases considerably along with the dimensions of the skull base.

During childhood and early adolescence, periosteal bone and cancellous bone are laid down around the bony labyrinthine core. Air cells may even form around the oval window, in the oval window niche, and over the lateral prominence of the lateral semicircular canal.

In Adulthood

Anatomy and Imaging Appearance

The bony labyrinth consists of three parts:

● The vestibule
● The semicircular canals
● The cochlea

The **vestibule** (Fig. 4.**258**) measures approximately 4 mm diagonally. It is posterior to the cochlea and anterior to the semicircular canals. It is connected to the stapes of the middle ear by the oval window, to the endolymphatic sac by the endolymphatic duct, and to the cochlea by the ductus reuniens. The vestibule consists basically of the **utricle** and **saccule**. The three **semicircular canals** arise from the utricle, each describing about two-thirds of a circle. They are situated in three mutually perpendicular planes that are arranged in space to form a laterally open "corner" whose apex is toward the center. The planes of the semicircular canals do not conform to the cardinal planes of the body. The anterior and posterior "walls" of the corner each form a 45° angle with the median plane of the body, and the "floor" of the corner lies approximately on the transverse plane. The anterior semicircular canal is placed vertically in the plane of the anterior "wall," and the lateral semicircular canal is placed horizontally in the plane of the "floor."

The **cochlea** is located in the anterior part of the labyrinth and forms a spiral with a diminishing lumen that winds around a central axis called the **modiolus**. It normally consists of $2^{1}/_{2}$ to $2^{3}/_{4}$ turns. The membranous and bony portions of the cochlea cannot be distinguished by CT. The perilymphatic duct arises near the round window, the cochlear aqueduct forming its bony boundary. It opens posteriorly into the subarachnoid space at the medial border of the petrous bone. A thin bony plate separates the cochlear aqueduct from the jugular foramen. The orifice or medial third can almost always be visualized, but the entire duct can rarely be defined (Fig. 4.**260**).

The facial nerve leaves the brain at the cerebellopontine angle and enters the facial canal above the vestibulocochlear nerve in the internal auditory canal. It first traverses the petrous bone in an anterolateral direction and then makes a right-angle turn in the posterolateral direction, forming the external genu of the facial nerve. In

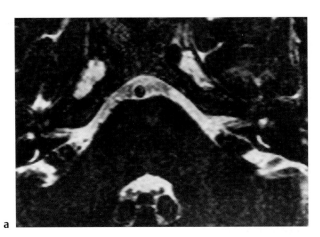

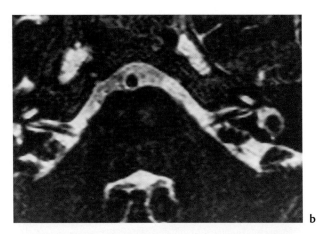

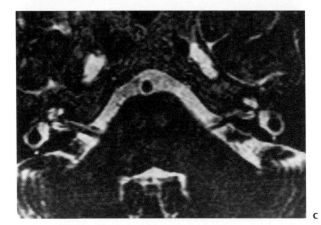

Fig. 4.**259 a–c** Three-dimensional T2-weighted turbo SE images of the cerebellopontine angle, the internal auditory canal, the nerves traversing the canal, and the inner ear. Image **c** defines the vestibulocochlear nerve and inferior vestibular nerve within the internal auditory canal and after their emergence from the cerebellopontine angle.

its course through the petrous bone, the nervus intermedius leaves the facial nerve first as the greater petrosal nerve and second as the chorda tympani. A small motor branch is distributed to the stapedius muscle in the tympanic cavity. All other motor fibers leave the skull base through the stylomastoid foramen and ramify outside the skull (Figs. 4.**259**, 4.**261**, 4.**262**).

The vestibulocochlear nerve carries afferent fibers whose vestibular part begins at the sensory cells of the vestibular apparatus and whose cochlear part begins at the sensory cells of the auditory apparatus. Both parts of the vestibulocochlear nerve course together through the internal auditory canal, exit the petrous bone below the facial nerve through the internal porus, and enter the rhombencephalon with a vestibular root and a cochlear root (Fig. 4.**259 c**).

The vestibular part contains the vestibular ganglion. A superior part and an inferior part, nerve fibers from the receptor cells, pass toward this ganglion in two portions.

The cochlear part contains the cochlear ganglion. Nerve fibers pass from the receptor cells of the spiral organ (of Corti) to the cochlear ganglion.

A horizontal bony ridge arising from the fundus in the medial part of the **internal auditory canal** (the transverse crest) separates the canal into a superior compartment for the facial nerve and the upper part of the vestibular nerve and an inferior compartment for the cochlear nerve and the lower part of the vestibular nerve. A physiological expansion of the internal auditory canal at its upper and lower boundaries is sometimes noted on coronal CT scans and should not be mistaken for expansive tumor growth.

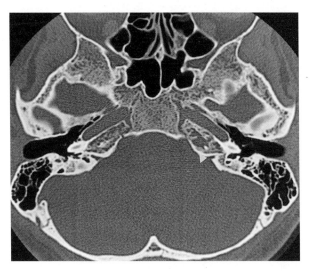

Fig. 4.**260** Cochlear aqueduct (arrowhead). Axial CT with a high-resolution bone filter.

The structures of the internal auditory canal cannot be differentiated by high-resolution CT, even after contrast administration. MRI can distinguish the intrameatal nerves and vascular structures, especially looping vessels such as the anterior inferior cerebellar artery (Figs. 4.**263**, 4.**264**).

Conventional radiographs of the petrous bone and inner ear have become largely obsolete and therefore will be discussed only briefly. While the Schüller projection and possibly the Mayer projection yield the most useful in-

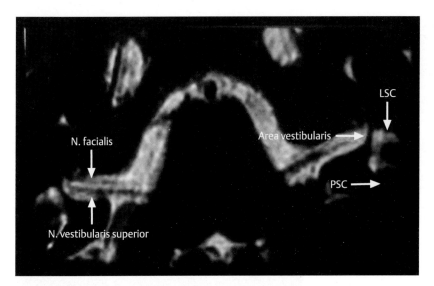

Fig. 4.**261**   MRI appearance of the nerves of both internal auditory canals and the structures of the inner ear. Three-dimensional T2-weighted turbo SE technique.
LSC   Lateral semicircular canal
PSC   Posterior semicircular canal

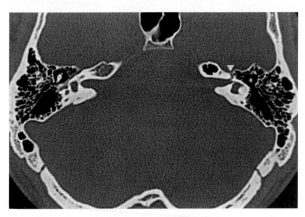

Fig. 4.**262**   View of the labyrinthine segment of the facial nerve canal. The arrowhead points to a slight dilatation of the canal by the geniculate ganglion. Axial CT with a high-resolution bone filter.

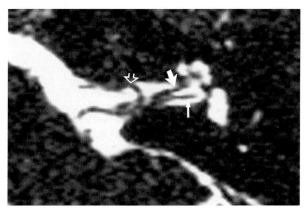

Fig. 4.**263**   Vascular loop in the internal auditory canal. Three-dimensional T2-weighted turbo SE image defines the course of the vascular loop (open arrow) within the canal. Note also the clear visualization of the cochlear nerve (large arrow) and inferior vestibular nerve (arrow).

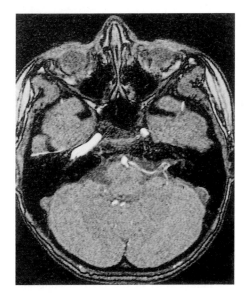

Fig. 4.**264**   Single slice of an MRI TOF angiogram. A loop of the AICA extends into the internal auditory canal on the left side. Incidental finding.

formation on the middle ear, the Stenvers view is best for visualizing the petrous pyramid (Figs. 4.**222**–4.**224**). Conventional tomograms have become obsolete. The lateral semicircular canal is only occasionally visible in the Stenvers view (Fig. 4.**265**). The anterior (superior) semicircular canal is occasionally visible as a lucent band with dense tramline borders extending downward below the arcuate eminence (Figs. 4.**265**, 4.**266**). The vestibule can sometimes be recognized at the base of the semicircular canals (Fig. 4.**265**). Below the vestibule, directed toward the petrous apex, is the cochlea (Fig. 4.**223**). The internal porus and internal auditory canal are easily identified. Only high-resolution MRI using high-resolution, thin-slice technique can define cranial nerves VII and VIII as separate structures in the internal auditory canal (Fig. 4.**267**).

The petrous ridge typically shows a wavy contour. Located between the arcuate eminence and a tubercle near the petrous apex is the subarcuate fossa (Figs. 4.**221 b**, 4.**268**), which is particularly deep in children. A double outline between the subarcuate fossa and arcuate eminence may be caused by the groove for the superior petrosal sinus, which may form a tunnel (Fig. 4.**221 b**, 4.**269**). Oblique groovelike or fissurelike linear lucencies

Fig. 4.**265 a, b** Streaky opacities at the petrous apex on each side (arrows). The anterior and lateral semicircular canals and vestibule are clearly visible.

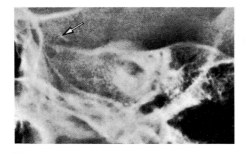

a

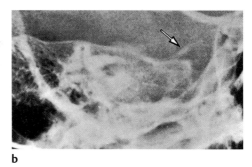

b

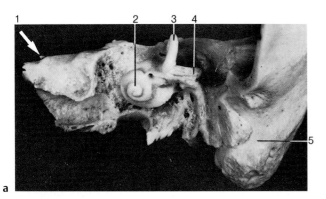

a

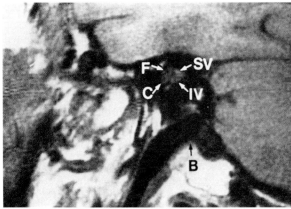

b

Fig. 4.**266 a, b**

a Petrous bone specimen, opened to demonstrate the middle ear structures.
1   Petrous apex
2   Cochlea
3   Anterior semicircular canal
4   Posterior semicircular canal
5   Mastoid process

b Gross anatomic section, anterior aspect.
1   Petrous apex
2   Internal auditory canal
3   Vestibule (utricle and saccule)
4   Anterior semicircular canal
5   Posterior semicircular canal
6   Sigmoid sulcus
7   Petro-occipital fissure

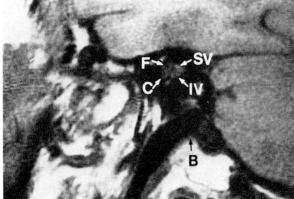

Fig. 4.**267** T1-weighted parasagittal MRI of the internal auditory canal. Each nerve has two signal intensities. The central zone of low signal intensity (most apparent in the cochlear nerve) may represent the actual nerve while the slightly more intense ring is the nerve sheath. (From Swartz 1985.)
B   Jugular bulb
F   Facial nerve
C   Cochlear nerve
IV Inferior vestibular nerve
SV Superior vestibular nerve

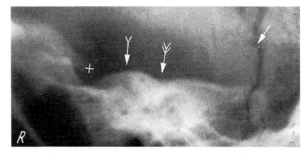

Fig. 4.**268** Sphenosquamous suture (arrow) crossing over the petrous apex. Note the deep groove (×) between the arcuate eminence (one-tailed arrow) and cranial sidewall. Subarcuate fossa (two-tailed arrow). Compare with Fig. 4.**221 b**.

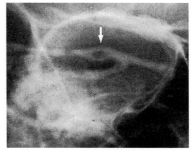

Fig. 4.**269** The lucent area at the center of the petrous ridge (arrow) may represent the groove for the superior petrosal sinus or air cells located below the petrous ridge.

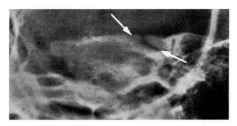

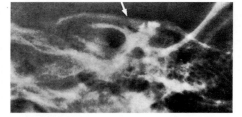

Fig. 4.**270**

Fig. 4.**271**

Fig. 4.**270** Groove (facial canal?) medial to the anterior semicircular canal (arrows).

Fig. 4.**271** Groove (facial canal?) medial to the anterior semicircular canal (arrow).

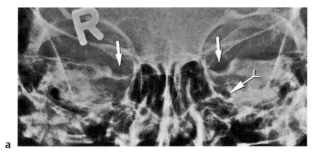

a

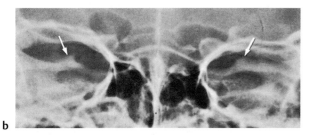

b

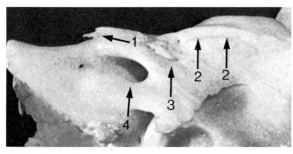

c

Fig. 4.**272 a–c** Trigeminal impression.
a Trigeminal impression on both sides (arrows) in the frontal projection.
b Knoblike protuberances are visible at the lateral margins of the trigeminal impression on both sides in the frontal projection (arrows).
c Petrous ridge in an anatomic specimen.
1 Exostosis at the attachment of the cerebellar tentorium (after bridging the trigeminal impression)
2 Groove for superior petrosal sinus
3 Subarcuate fossa
4 Internal porus acusticus

that interrupt the petrous ridge medial to the anterior semicircular canal are sometimes visible and in the past have been interpreted as facial canals. Their origin is not fully understood (Figs. 4.**270**, 4.**271**).

The trigeminal impression of the temporal bone is a depression of variable depth located at the lateral border of the petrous apex (Fig. 4.**5**). It is seen more clearly on the PA radiograph than in the Stenvers view (Fig. 4. **272**).

Pathological Finding?

Normal Variant/Anomaly?

A unilateral **high petrous pyramid** may be noted in conventional radiographs and ordinarily has no clinical significance (see Fig. 4.**142**). CT may rarely demonstrate rotation of the pyramid as a normal variant.

The lateral border of the **trigeminal impression** (Fig. 4.**272 a**) may be raised or exostosis-like (Fig. 4.**272 b, c**). Small, isolated foci of ossification sometimes adjoin the exostosis (Fig. 4.**273**). Rarely, similar ossific foci may be seen on the petrous ridge near the petrous apex. They probably represent calcifications of the petrosellar ligament (see p. 449).

There are also isolated bony elements that abut the petrous bone. **Petrosphenobasilar ossicles** are located in the petrooccipital synchondrosis (Fig. 4.**274**). This synchondrosis unites the posterior margin of the petrous bone (which separates the posterior and inferior surfaces of the pyramid) with the basilar part of the occipital bone. The **jugular notch** of the petrous bone interrupts the petrooccipital synchondrosis. It combines with the jugular notch of the occipital bone to form the jugular foramen. The jugular notch may be subdivided by an intrajugular process, resulting in a bipartite jugular foramen. Suprapetrosal bones may directly adjoin the petrous bone below the dura mater.

Peculiar hyperostoses are occasionally found at the lateral border of the trigeminal notch (Fig. 4.**273 b**). Bony outgrowths cranial to the petrous ridge are more often unilateral than bilateral.

The petrous bone may be heavily pneumatized, with air cells extending into the petrous apex, in a variant that should not be mistaken for bone destruction (Figs. 4.**275**, 4.**276**).

The **transverse crest** is a normal feature that is best demonstrated by coronal CT (p. 479). Above this ridge are the facial nerve quadrant (anteromedial) and superior vestibular quadrant (lateral); below it are the cochlear quadrant (medial) and inferior vestibular quadrant (lateral).

Lack of development of the bony structures about the **carotid canal** can lead to a higher, more lateral and posterior position of the canal. This moves it closer to the middle ear and may cause pulsatile tinnitus. Extension of the carotid canal to the hypotympanum is a variant in which the bony boundaries of the canal are often absent or partially absent.

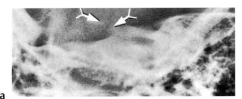
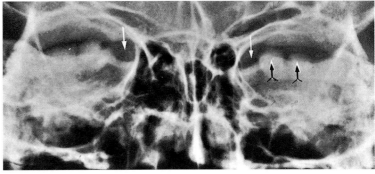

Fig. 4.**273 a, b**   Trigeminal impression.

a Exostosis-like bony projection on the petrous ridge (tailed arrows) pointing toward the petrous apex. An oblong calcific density appears as a continuation of the bony projection (arrow); it may be a dural calcification, a trigeminal bridge, or a petrosellar ligament.

b Trigeminal impression on both sides (arrows). Nodular hyperostoses (tailed arrows) are visible along the petrous ridge on each side.

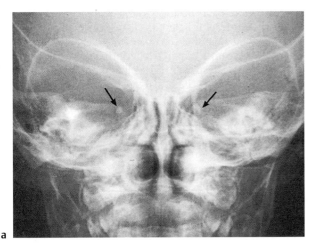
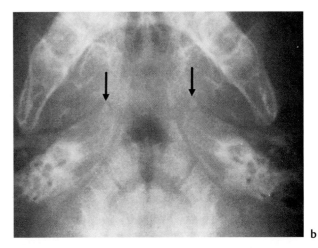

Fig. 4.**274 a, b**   Bilateral petrosphenobasilar ossicles (arrows) in a one-year-old girl.

a AP projection.
b Near-axial projection.

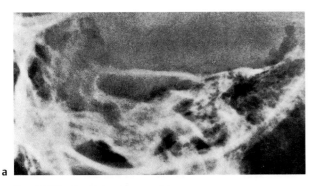
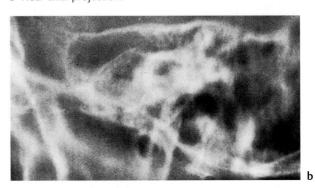

Fig. 4.**275 a, b**   Petrous pyramid.
a Large air cell below the petrous ridge.

b Enlargement of the petrous bone due to pronounced pneumatization (pneumatosinus dilatans?).

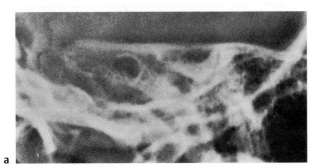
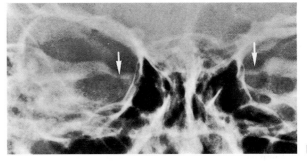

Fig. 4.**276 a, b**   Pneumatization.
a Pea-size air cell, rimmed by sclerosis, in the right petrous bone at the internal auditory canal.

b Pronounced pneumatization of the petrous bone on both sides. The trigeminal impression is clearly visible on both sides (arrows). There is possible enlargement of the internal auditory canal on the right side.

Defects can also occur in the wall between the hypotympanum and jugular foramen. A high jugular bulb may reach the middle ear and cause pulsatile tinnitus, and it may be mistaken for a glomus tumor at otoscopy. Diverticula-like protrusions of the jugular bulb can erode the internal carotid artery, displace the vestibular aqueduct upward, and cause tinnitus or hearing loss.

The bony canal of the **cochlea** typically makes from $2^1/_2$ to $2^3/_4$ turns around the modiolus, its diameter gradually diminishing from a normal value of 9 mm at the cochlear base. There are variants in which the cochlea makes only two turns or a full three turns.

Malformations of the inner ear may affect the bony and membranous structures alone or in various combinations. A severe anomaly is complete aplasia of the labyrinth (**Mi-chel deformity**), resulting in failure of development of the inner ear (Fig. 4.**277**). The normal inner ear structures are replaced by a single, small, cystlike cavity or several smaller cavities. Michel deformity is caused by an early developmental error during the third week of gestation. Aplasia of the inner ear is an essential feature of this disease. The middle ear and external ear are normally developed.

The classic **Mondini malformation** (Fig. 4.**278**) is characterized by a small cochlea with deficient turns combined with incomplete or absent intrascalar septa. This anomaly of the cochlear skeleton with lack of development of the modiolus results in only $1^1/_2$ cochlear turns instead of the normal $2^1/_2$ to $2^3/_4$. The basal turns of the cochlea show a variable degree of thickening, and there is expansion of the endolymphatic duct and sac, which CT shows as dilatation of the vestibular aqueduct. Dysplasia of the vestibule with involvement of the lateral semicircular canal may also be present. The anomaly occurs in the seventh week of gestation. The radiographic hallmark is an "empty cochlea."

While total aplasia of the inner ear (Michel type) is indistinguishable from acquired labyrinthine sclerosis based on CT findings, dysplasia of the membranous labyrinth alone is associated with normal radiographic findings.

A side-to-side difference of more than 2 mm in the diameter of the internal auditory canal is usually considered abnormal. Bone-window CT alone is inadequate for evaluating the petrous bones, because (1) even larger tumors may not cause expansion of the internal auditory canal, and (2) the internal porus may be larger than 1 cm as a normal finding, and the two poruses may be of unequal size. **Acoustic neurinomas** can be reliably detected with MRI (p. 489). Anomalies of the internal auditory canal, which may appear as definite sites of narrowing on CT, are often associated with hypoplasia or aplasia of the nerves that traverse the internal auditory canal (Figs. 4.**279**, 4.**280**). The only technique at present that can detect hypo-

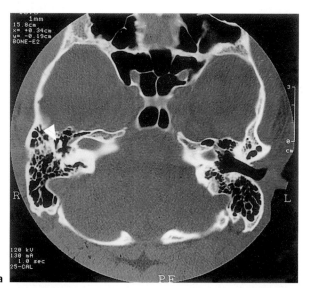

a

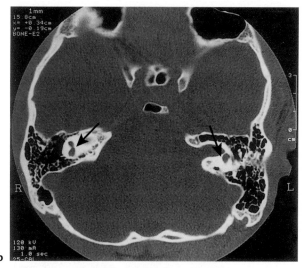

b

Fig. 4.**277 a, b** Typical appearance of Michel deformity in a 21-year-old man. The normal inner ear structures are replaced by a small, cystlike cavity (arrows). Normal middle ear structures (arrowhead). (Images courtesy of Dr. A. Aschendorff, Department of Otorhinolaryngology, University of Freiburg, Germany.)

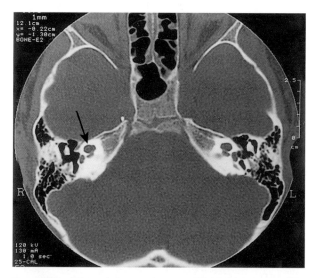

Fig. 4.**278** Bilateral incomplete partition (classic Mondini malformation) in a 7-year-old child, characterized by a small, stout, "empty" cochlea (arrow) and incomplete intrascalar septa. Vestibular dysplasia is also present. Scans from the same patient at the level of the dilated vestibular aqueduct are shown in Fig. 4.**281**. (Image courtesy of Dr. A. Aschendorff, Department of Otorhinolaryngology, University of Freiburg, Germany.)

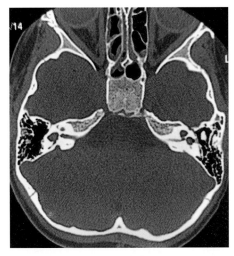

Fig. 4.**279**   Severe, bilateral dysplasia of the inner ear structures accompanied by a very narrow internal auditory canal. Axial CT with a high-resolution bone filter.

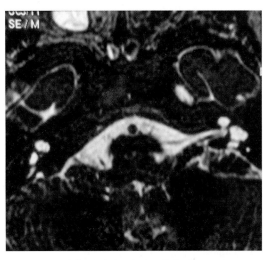

Fig. 4.**280**   Severe, bilateral dysplasia of the inner ear structures with almost complete nonvisualization of the left cochlear nerve. Axial MRI, 3-D T2-weighted turbo SE sequence.

plasia or aplasia of neural structures in the internal auditory canal is high-resolution, thin-slice MRI with heavy T2 weighting, aided if necessary by multiplanar reconstructions perpendicular to the internal meatus.

CT can detect narrowing or atresia of the **vestibular aqueduct** if the affected site is distal to the isthmus. The vestibular aqueduct has a normal width of 0.5–1 mm. Smaller values have been cited as a possible cause or predisposing deformity for Ménière's disease. For the otosurgeon planning a shunt procedure to relieve endolymphatic hydrops, it is important to visualize the postisthmic segment of the vestibular aqueduct and the endolymphatic sac, define their relationship to the jugular bulb and internal auditory canal, and assess the pneumatization of the petrous bone.

CT and MRI can clearly demonstrate enlargement of the vestibular aqueduct and marked dilatation of the endolymphatic sac with no other visible anomalies of the ear or inner ear region (Fig. 4.**281**). This condition, known as **large vestibular aqueduct syndrome** (LVAS), has been described as a cause of congenital hearing loss.

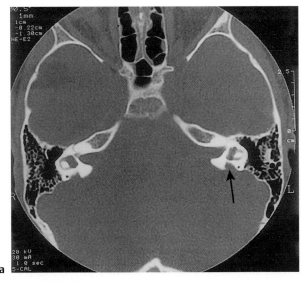

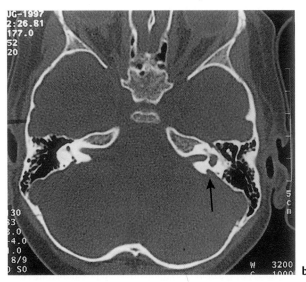

Fig. 4.**281 a, b**   Two different patients (**a** 7 years, **b** 4 years) with different degrees of expansion of the vestibular aqueduct in the setting of LVAS (arrows). The second patient has an inner ear anomaly. (Images courtesy of Dr. A. Aschendorff, Department of Otorhinolaryngology, University of Freiburg, Germany.)

Fracture?

Fractures of the petrous bone were discussed on p. 469. CT is necessary for an accurate diagnosis. Petrous fractures are classified as longitudinal or transverse.

A longitudinal fracture runs parallel to the long axis of the petrous bone. A transverse fracture is perpendicular to the long axis of the pyramid. Frequently, both fracture types are combined (Fig. 4.**282**). Fractures of the external auditory canal are also easily detected by CT, which will also show any concomitant involvement of the temporomandibular joint. While the cochlea, vestibule, semicircular canals, and internal auditory canal are usually easy to distinguish from fracture lines by their solid bony margins, there are some common pitfalls. Normal anatomic structures such as cranial sutures or the petromastoid canal (Fig. 4.**283**) can mimic fractures in their course and appearance.

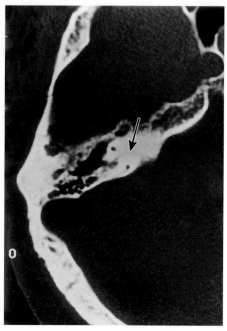

Fig. 4.**283**   Typical appearance of the petromastoid canal (arrow) on axial CT. This feature is easily mistaken for a fracture.

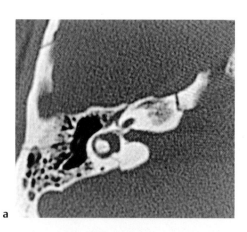

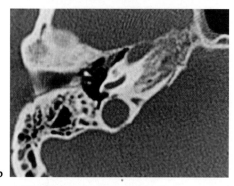

Fig. 4.**282 a, b**   Temporal bone fractures.
a Axial CT with a high-resolution bone filter demonstrates longitudinal and transverse petrous bone fractures and a temporal bone fracture on the right side.
b Axial CT with a high-resolution bone filter shows the longitudinal petrous fracture.

 Necrosis?

Necrosis of the calvarium and skull base was discussed on p. 397 and 441. Basically the same phenomena can occur in the petrous bone, although necrotic changes in that region are very rare.

Necrotizing otitis externa is synonymous with malignant otitis externa. This is a necrotic condition that does not originate in the bone but spreads from a very aggressive soft-tissue inflammation of the external auditory canal to involve the bony ear canal and skull base, in some cases leading to osteomyelitis. Additional details can be found on p. 475.

 Inflammation?

Inflammation of the membranous labyrinth, or **labyrinthitis**, usually has a viral etiology but may also have a bacterial, autoimmune, syphilitic, or tuberculous cause. Labyrinthitis of the inner ear can be classified as follows according to its pathogenesis:

- Tympanogenic
- Meningogenic
- Hematogenous
- Posttraumatic (or postoperative)

Tympanogenic cases result from otitis media in which infection has spread to the labyrinth through the round or oval window. A labyrinthine fistula, usually located at the level of the lateral semicircular canal, most commonly results from destruction by a cholesteatoma and can also lead to labyrinthitis. **Meningogenic labyrinthitis** results from the spread of inflammation along CSF pathways and is usually bilateral. The vestibular portion of the labyrinth is most commonly affected in these cases due to the direct proximity of the lateral wall of the internal auditory canal to the vestibule. Inflammation can also spread from the subarachnoid CSF spaces into the membranous labyrinth of the inner ear through the cochlear aqueduct.

Hematogenous labyrinthitis usually has a viral etiology, mumps and measles being a frequent cause. Other cases result from the hematogenous spread of syphilis, tuberculosis, or other infectious bacterial diseases.

Posttraumatic labyrinthitis can result from a previous injury with fracture involvement of the inner ear or from prior surgery on the middle ear or inner ear.

A **perilymph fistula** is an abnormal communication between the middle ear and inner ear. These fistulas may be iatrogenic (usually following stapedial surgery) or may be caused by direct or indirect trauma. CT shows an unexplained middle ear effusion, air in the labyrinth, or both. On MRI, T1-weighted images before and after intravenous contrast administration show enhancement of the membranous labyrinth. The images must be closely scrutinized to detect this finding (Fig. 4.**284**).

The concomitant presence of facial nerve palsy with thickening and enhancement of cranial nerve VII should prompt a search for "blisters" in the external ear canal, as this combination is suspicious for **herpes zoster oticus (Ramsey–Hunt syndrome)**. Cranial nerve VIII may also

show contrast uptake in this condition. It should be noted that the facial nerve may also be involved by labyrinthitis due to other causes, especially in syphilis.

When acute labyrinthitis progresses to a chronic stage, the membranous labyrinth is gradually replaced by fibrous tissue. Finally, in **end-stage labyrinthitis**, the membranous labyrinth ossifies in a condition termed labyrinthitis ossificans (Fig. 4.**285**). The fibrotic changes can be demonstrated by CT and by thin-slice T2-weighted MRI. When MRI is used, T1-weighted images should be acquired before intravenous contrast administration to check for intralabyrinthine hemorrhage, which is occasionally seen in labyrinthitis. More often, however, it is a sign of coagulopathy, a neoplasm, or trauma. Contrast enhancement of the membranous labyrinth or of granulation tissue on MRI can have other causes as well, such as an intralabyrinthine schwannoma, which has been described most often in the vestibule. This type of tumor shows relatively intense contrast enhancement.

Cholesteatomas were discussed on p. 473. Bone erosion by cholesteatomas that reach the medial wall of the tympanic cavity can break through into the labyrinth (Fig. 4.**286**).

Although otosclerosis is not an inflammatory disorder, we include it in this chapter in order to have a more

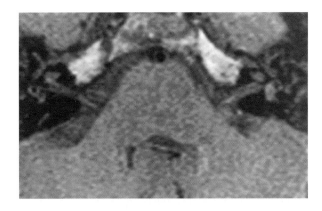

Fig. 4.**284** Bilateral increased enhancement of the membranous labyrinth in labyrinthitis. The finding is more pronounced on the left side than on the right. Axial MRI, T1-weighted SE sequence after intravenous contrast administration.

Fig. 4.**285 a, b** Ossifying labyrinthitis.
a Axial CT with a high-resolution bone filter shows sclerosis of the cochlea due to ossifying labyrinthitis.
b 3-D axial T2-weighted turbo SE sequence in the same patient shows decreased signal intensity of the cochlea in ossifying labyrinthitis.

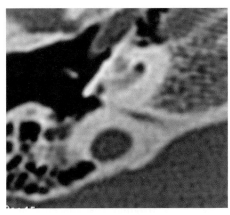

a

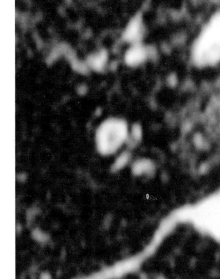

b

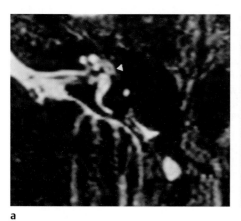
a

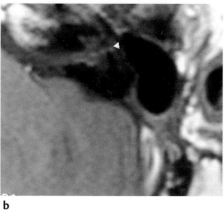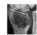
b

Fig. 4.**286 a, b** Invasion of the cochlea by a cholesteatoma.
a 3-D axial T2-weighted turbo SE sequence shows a small hyperintense mass (arrowhead) that has invaded the cochlea on the left side.
b T1-weighted axial SE sequence after contrast administration shows a mass of soft-tissue density on the left cochlea: a cholesteatoma that has invaded the cochlea from the middle ear (arrowhead).

complete differential diagnosis. **Otosclerosis** (otospongiosis) is a noninflammatory condition, bilateral in about 75% of cases, affecting the endochondral portion of the labyrinthine capsule (Figs. 4.**241**, 4.**287**). First the affected bone areas are transformed into spongy bone (otospongiosis, active foci) and later undergo sclerosis (otosclerosis, inactive foci). The process can spread to inner ear structures through the endosteal part of the bony labyrinth. Spread via the periosteum is more common, however, producing changes in the round window and especially the oval window that can lead to fixation and bony ankylosis of the stapes. Three types of hearing loss can occur:

- Middle ear type with conductive hearing loss (approximately 80%)
- Mixed type with combined conductive and sensorineural hearing loss (approximately 15%)
- Inner ear type with pure sensorineural hearing loss (approximately 5%)

Subjectively, the disease presents with slowly progressive hearing loss and unremitting tinnitus with no pain, otorrhea, or vestibular symptoms. The imaging procedure of choice is high-resolution CT. The oval window changes leading to conductive hearing loss can always be detected if they go beyond simple fixation of the stapes. CT is diagnostic only if there is also thickening of the stapes footplate, otosclerotic plaques, or otospongiotic changes. A site of predilection for otosclerotic bone formation is the **fissula ante fenestrum**, a small cartilaginous space located at the anterior oval window margin between the middle and inner ear.

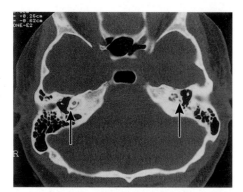

Fig. 4.**287** Typical appearance of bilateral capsular otosclerosis (arrows). The 41-year-old woman presented with combined conductive and sensorineural hearing loss.

The differential diagnosis of otospongiotic labyrinthine foci should include osteogenesis imperfecta. Usually this disease is indistinguishable from otospongiosis based on CT findings. Otosclerosis/otospongiosis also requires differentiation from Paget disease. Coexisting decalcification of nonlabyrinthine areas of the petrous bone are suggestive of Paget disease. Progression can lead to increasing sclerosis and concomitant involvement of the membranous labyrinth, causing obliteration of the perilymphatic and endolymphatic spaces.

With otosclerotic lesions that narrow the oval window, the differential diagnosis should also include **tympanosclerosis** due to inflammatory disease. Both conditions are associated with otosclerotic deposits. Tympanosclerosis occurs in the setting of chronic otitis media and is characterized by conductive hearing loss caused by fixation of the ossicular chain. There is hyaline degeneration of the middle ear mucosa with the formation of submucosal sclerotic plaques. If the tympanosclerotic plaques are located on the medial wall of the tympanic cavity near the oval window, they are indistinguishable from otosclerotic foci by CT. But they can be distinguished from other chronic inflammatory processes by their high attenuation values.

Tumor?

Primary intraosseous **epidermoids** of the petrous bone can lead to bone destruction in the inner ear and internal auditory canal. Dermoids or epidermoids located outside the petrous bone can be accurately defined by MRI. They account for 6–7% of cerebellopontine angle tumors. The lesions appear hyperintense on diffusion-weighted MR (see Fig. 4.**220**). Differentiation is required from cerebellopontine meningiomas and cerebellar meningoencephalocele. **Cerebellopontine meningiomas** typically have broad contact with the petrous bone and can erode its bony structures, especially the petrous apex. The internal auditory canal often retains its normal width. Meningiomas (like angiomas) may contain small intratumoral calcifications that can have a broad, shell-like configuration near the pyramid. The adjacent bone may become decalcified due to infiltration or pressure, or it may show a reactive hyperostosis. Sometimes the internal auditory canal is expanded due to the obstruction of CSF drainage. A **cerebellar meningoencephalocele** can lead to the pressure erosion of both petrous apices. The bony changes in this case may extend to the osseous labyrinth.

The appearance of glomus tumors on CT and MRI was covered on p. 475.

Neurinomas of the facial nerve can occur anywhere in the course of the nerve and are detectable by the presence of bone destruction and by the direct CT or MRI visualization of an enhancing tumor. Differentiation is required from intraneural hemorrhage (often posttraumatic) (Fig. 4.**288**). Trigeminal neurinomas can cause deepening of the trigeminal notch in the superior border of the petrous bone. Neurinomas typically show marked enhancement on CT and MRI after intravenous contrast administration. Multiple neurinomas or neurofibromas can develop in neurofibromatosis (Recklinghausen disease). An **acoustic neurinoma** inside or outside the internal auditory canal can be reliably detected by MRI and in many cases by CT (Fig. 4.**289**).

Various benign skeletal abnormalities of the petrous bone, such as Langerhans cell histiocytosis (Fig. 4.**290**), as well as petrous involvement by carcinoma, sarcoma, plasmacytoma, or metastases have no typical characteristics and appear as osteolytic lesions. Primary malignant tumors of the petrous bone are very rare.

The osseous changes that occur in Paget disease, fibrous dysplasia, and osteopetrosis were described on pp. 398, 401 and 443. The radiographic signs of petrous bone involvement by these diseases do not differ significantly from those in the remainder of the skull. CT is a particularly valuable tool in the diagnosis of these diseases.

Unlike the rare entities mentioned above, **cholesterol cyst (cholesterol granuloma)** is the most common primary cause of destructive changes in the petrous apex. In most cases the contralateral petrous apex is well pneumatized, suggesting that cholesterol cysts develop in a pneumatized apex. Presumably the pathogenesis involves an interruption in the pneumatization of cells in the petrous apex and recurrent intra-apical hemorrhages that

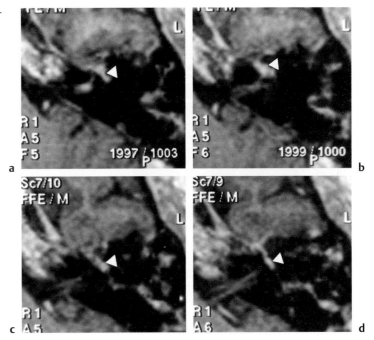

Fig. 4.**288a–d**   Intraneural hemorrhage of the left facial nerve (arrowheads). Axial T1-weighted gradient-echo MRI sequence.

Fig. 4.**289a, b**   Man 41 years of age with progressive hearing loss.
a Very heavily T2-weighted CISS sequence demonstrates a rounded mass in the right internal auditory canal.
b T1-saturated coronal MRI after contrast administration shows an intensely enhancing tumor in the internal auditory canal.
(Case courtesy of Professor Terwey, Bremen.)

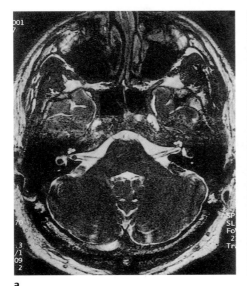

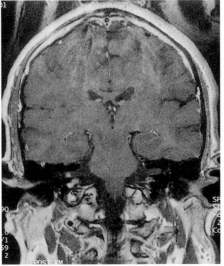

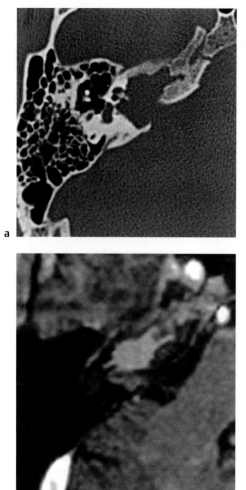

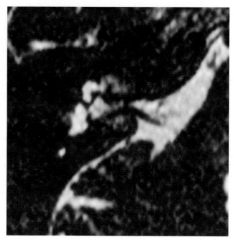

Fig. 4.**290 a–c**   Langerhans cell histiocytosis in the petrous bone.
a Axial CT with a high-resolution bone filter shows extensive destruction of the right petrous bone involving the cochlea and portions of the vestibular apparatus.
b 3-D axial T2-weighted turbo SE sequence shows a hyperintense mass in the right petrous bone with extension to the labyrinth.
c 3-D axial T1-weighted gradient-echo sequence shows the postcontrast appearance of the right petrous bone mass with invasion of the cochlea.

incite a granulation tissue reaction. Cholesterol cysts contain a brownish fluid with cholesterol crystals and are surrounded by fibrous tissue. Embedded in the fibrous capsule are giant cells with cholesterol crystals, blood vessels, erythrocytes, hemosiderin, and inflammatory cells. Cholesterol cysts occur in young and middle-aged patients and affect both sexes equally. Cholesterol cysts enlarge within the petrous apex, are located behind the horizontal segment of the carotid canal, and average 3 cm in diameter at the time of diagnosis. Clinical symptoms are hearing loss, tinnitus, and hemifacial spasms. There may be concomitant involvement of cranial nerves V, VI, IX, X, XI, and XII. The clinical symptoms often persist for years. Cholesterol granulomas exhibit smooth, sharp margins on CT. They arise from the petrous apex and can erode or destroy the bony boundaries of the carotid canal, foramen lacerum, and jugular foramen. The lesions are very hyperintense on T1-weighted MRI. They may also contain nonhomogeneous, hypointense tissue that represents hemosiderin from prior hemorrhages. The lesion margins often appear hypointense on T1- and T2-weighted images. In gradient-echo sequences, susceptibility artifacts and chemical shift artifacts lead to a reduction of signal intensity. Except for a thin peripheral rim, the lesion does not enhance after intravenous contrast administration.

Styloid Process, Hyoid Bone, Larynx

Normal Findings

During Growth

The styloid process is derived from the second branchial arch (Reichert cartilage), like the stylohyoid ligament that connects the styloid process to the hyoid bone. Because of this arrangement, the larynx and hyoid bone form a **functional unit** with the skull base. This complex develops embryologically from the following components (Fig. 4.**291**):

- The base of the styloid process is formed from the tympanohyoidal component.
- The actual styloid process develops from the stylohyal component.
- The stylohyoid ligament develops from the ceratohyal component.
- The direct connection between the stylohyoid ligament and hyoid bone corresponds to the hypohyal component.

Fig. 4.**291** Ossification of the stylohyoid ligament (modified from Augier). The various elements of the stylohyoid chain are labeled.

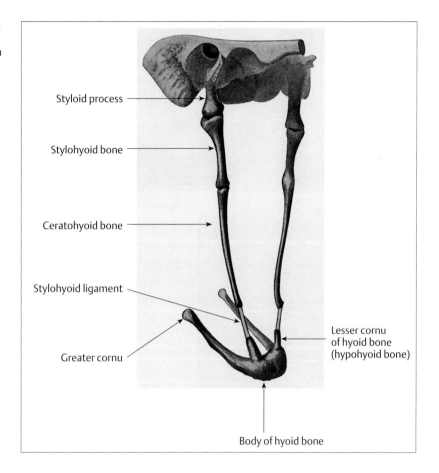

Styloid process

Stylohyoid bone

Ceratohyoid bone

Stylohyoid ligament

Greater cornu

Lesser cornu of hyoid bone (hypohyoid bone)

Body of hyoid bone

The **styloid process** is ossified from two centers. The upper center is thought to appear shortly before birth, and the lower center afterward. While the upper center soon fuses with the petrous and tympanic parts of the temporal bone, it does not fuse with the lower center until puberty.

The **hyoid bone** develops from the first and second branchial arches. Calcifications may appear in the fifth month of embryonic development. Calcification is detectable in 75% of newborns. The greater and lesser cornua unite with the hyoid bone between the 6th and 10th years of life. It is very rare to observe calcifications in the laryngeal cartilage before age 15 on conventional radiographs, but foci of ossification are sometimes seen even earlier on CT scans. Calcifications in the laryngeal skeleton vary greatly in different individuals. Most are asymmetrical, and the inner and outer layers often show different degrees of ossification. The extent of the intervening medullary cavity is also highly variable (Fig. 4.**292**).

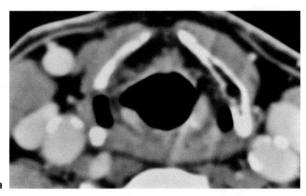

a

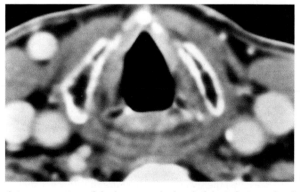

b

Fig. 4.**292 a–e** Appearance of the thyroid cartilage and larynx on axial CT (soft-tissue filter in **a–d**, high-resolution bone filter in **e**)
a Upper portion of the thyroid cartilage and larynx.
b Midportion of the larynx above the vocal cord.
c Mid- to lower portion of the larynx at the level of the crico-arytenoid joint.

d Lower portion of the larynx at the level of the inferior pole of the thyroid cartilage and upper part of the cricoid.
e Normal thyroid cartilage. Note the varying width of the cortical boundaries and the variable extent of the medullary space of the thyroid cartilage. Aside from cancellous and cortical ossifications, there are no significant calcifications.

Fig. 4.**292 c–e** ▷

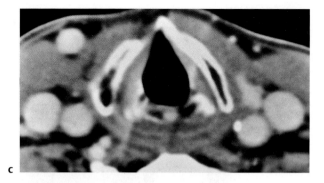

c

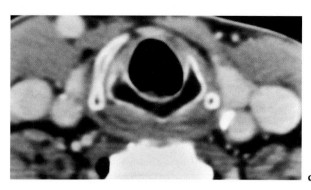

d

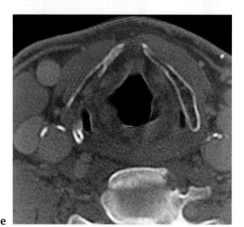

e

Fig. 4.**292 c–e**

(Fig. 4.**291**). Development of the lesser cornua is subject to extreme individual variations (Fig. 4.**293**). They may be absent or very small, or they may reach considerable size. Often the greater cornua are clearly visible on both sides of the C3 vertebra in AP radiographs and should not be mistaken for the transverse processes of that vertebra (Figs. 4.**294**, 4.**295**). On axial views the hyoid bone is projected in front of the anterior arch of the atlas. CT can provide detailed visualization of the bone (Fig. 4.**296**).

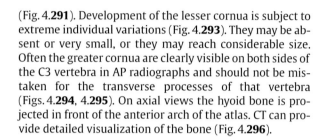

 In Adulthood

The styloid process extends downward, forward, and medially from the skull base. Ossifications in the stylohyoid ligament may be isolated or may form jointlike connections with the styloid process and/or hyoid bone. Single or multiple **ceratohyal bones** may be present within the stylohyoid ligament. They may be isolated or may be in contact with the lower portion of the styloid process (stylohyal bone) or with the lesser cornu of the hyoid bone (hypohyal bone). The stylohyal bone at the bottom of the styloid process also may occur in isolation or may have a jointlike connection with portions of the styloid process near the skull base. Complete fusion between the ceratohyal bone and the lesser cornu of the hyoid bone can also occur (Fig. 4.**291**).

> In extreme cases the entire stylohyoid ligament may be ossified, forming a bony connection between the skull base and hyoid bone.

> The normal length of the styloid process measured from the skull base to its tip is 25 mm. Elongation is present if the styloid process and/or the adjacent stylohyoid ligament is ossified, exceeding a total length of 25 mm.

The hyoid bone consists of the body and the paired greater and lesser cornua on the right and left sides. The lesser cornu gives attachment to the stylohyoid ligament

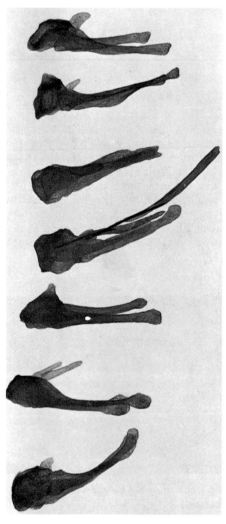

Fig. 4.**293**   Lateral radiographic images of the hyoid bone. Note the variable development of the body of the bone and its lesser cornua. The center image shows ossification in the stylohyoid ligament.

The calcified **thyroid cartilage** is projected over the transverse processes of the C4–C6 vertebrae in the AP projection. The inner and outer cortices may create a tram-track figure several centimeters long (Fig. 4.**297**). CT and MRI have become the preferred modalities for examining the soft-tissue and bony structures of the **larynx** (Fig. 4.**292**).

The **cricoid cartilage** is sometimes visible on AP projections of the cervical spine, usually appearing as a very delicate, slightly curved, linear calcific density located just medial and caudal to the calcified thyroid cartilage (Fig. 4.**297**). CT or MRI is used to examine the cricoid cartilage for any adjacent soft-tissue processes or infiltration by tumor (Fig. 4.**292**). The paired, pyramid-shaped **arytenoid cartilages** abut the superior border of the cricoid cartilage. They ossify after 20 years of age in 90% of cases (autopsy findings). The arytenoid cartilages are poorly visualized on conventional radiographs. Calcifications in the **tracheal rings** (Fig. 4.**298**) are often detected incidentally in older individuals and have been termed tracheobronchopathia calcerea. Figure 4.**299** shows a conventional AP tomogram of the larynx, and Fig. 4.**300** gives a schematic view of the lateral radiographic appearance of the cervical soft tissues and bony structures, noting the relationship of air-filled spaces to the osseous structures.

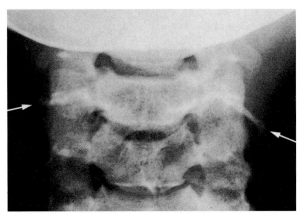

Fig. 4.**294**   Parts of the hyoid bone are projected lateral to the cervical spine (arrows) in the frontal view.

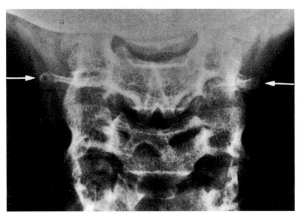

Fig. 4.**295**   Portions of the hyoid bone are displayed on an AP projection of the cervical spine (arrows).

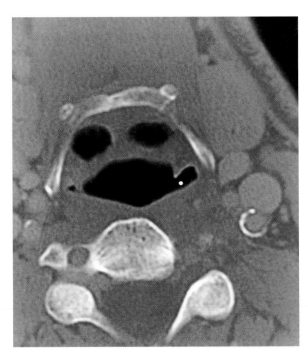

Fig. 4.**296**   Appearance of the hyoid bone and its lesser cornua on axial CT with a high-resolution bone filter. Note the variable cortical width of the hyoid.

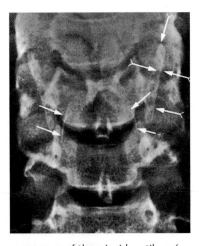

Fig. 4.**297**   Streaklike appearance of the cricoid cartilage (arrows). Ossifications of the thyroid cartilage appear above the cricoid cartilage on both sides. Tailed arrows: plaquelike calcifications of the thyroid cartilage on the left side.

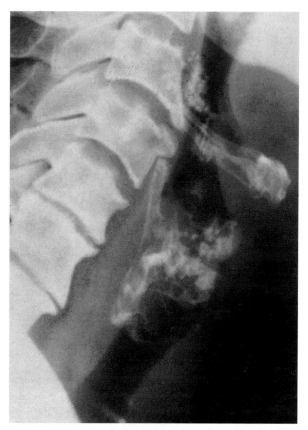

Fig. 4.**298**   Lateral cervical radiograph shows extensive calcifications in cervical lymph nodes, some of which mimic or even obscure laryngeal ossification. Calcified tracheal rings are visible at the lower edge of the film.

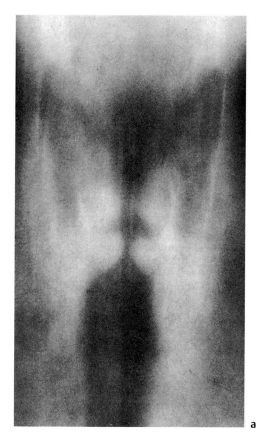

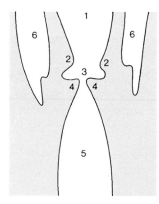

Fig. 4.**299 a, b**   Tomographic appearance of soft-tissue structures.
a Frontal tomogram of the larynx.
b Explanatory diagram.
1   Laryngeal vestibule
2   Ventricular fold
3   Sinus of Morgagni
4   Vocal cord
5   Trachea
6   Piriform recess

◁ Fig. 4.**300**   Diagram of the cervical soft tissues.
1   Mandible
2   Base of tongue
3   Epiglottis
4   Hyoid bone
5   Hypopharynx
6   Thyroid cartilage, anterior part
7   Thyroid cartilage, posterior part
8   Sinus of Morgagni
9   Cricoid cartilage
10   Trachea
11   Calcified tracheal cartilage
12   Calcified goitrous nodule
13   Triticeal cartilage

Pathological Finding?

 ## Normal Variant/Anomaly?

A **triticeal cartilage** is occasionally found in one or both free margins of the thyrohyoid ligament below the hyoid bone and above the laryngeal skeleton. These cartilaginous structures may ossify, appearing as calcific densities. Several millimeters in size, they are projected in front of the C3 or C4 vertebral body on lateral radiographs of the cervical spine (Fig. 4.**301**).

Elongation of the styloid process and ossification of the stylohyoid ligament (see p. 492 and Fig. 4.**291**) may be associated with pain in the tonsillar area on chewing and swallowing, dysphagia, foreign-body sensation and temporal headache due to pressure on the external carotid artery, or orbital and parietal pain due to compression of the internal carotid artery. Clinical complaints are particularly common in cases where the tip of the styloid process is directed inward. The clinical manifestations of the **styloid process syndrome** (classic **Eagle syndrome**) (Fig. 4.**302**) can be divided into two categories:

- An elongated styloid process or an abnormal superior stylohyoid segment with pain predominantly in the neck, pharynx, and occipital area.
- Ossification in the midportion of the stylohyoid ligament, with complaints on head movement and TMJ discomfort

When these variants are associated with the aforementioned clinical symptoms, with paresthesias and coughing fits, or with a carotid artery syndrome, surgical treatment should be considered.

Progressive ossification occurs along the stylohyoid chain from birth to 20 years of age. Isolated ossification in the upper stylohyoid segment predominates in adolescence and early adulthood. With aging, there is increased ossification of the middle and lower segments and more numerous and varied combinations of ossification variants. More than 30% of the population show variants in the

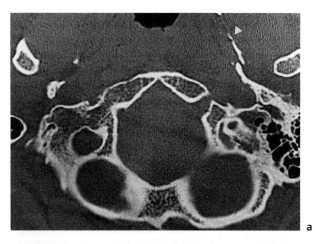

a

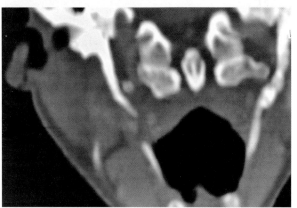

b

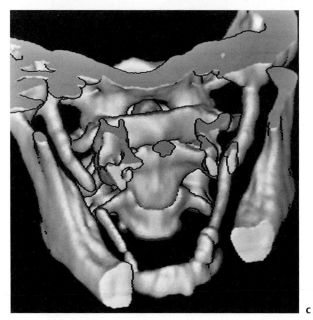

c

Fig. 4.**302 a–c** CT views of the styloid process.
a Axial CT shows a markedly elongated left styloid process (arrowhead).
b Coronal reconstruction from axial slices shows considerable elongation of the styloid process on both sides.
c 3-D reconstruction shows bilateral elongated styloid processes connected to the hyoid bone.

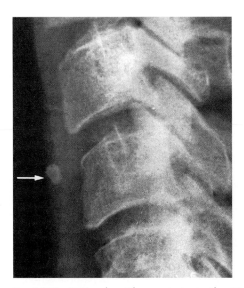

Fig. 4.**301** Triticeal cartilage anterior to the C4 vertebra (arrow).

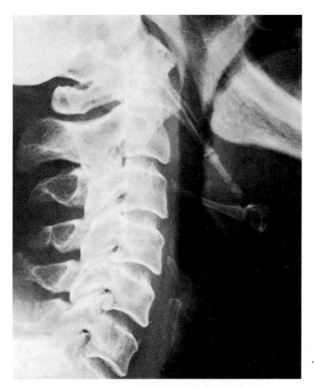

ossification of the stylohyoid complex, typically consisting of an elongated styloid process and/or ossifications of the stylohyoid ligament. This frequency of variants should be considered in interpreting clinical complaints and correlating them with radiographic findings.

Typical **ossification variants** in the stylohyoid complex are illustrated in Figs. 4.**303** to 4.**305**. Other variants and explanations can be found in Figs. 4.**291**, 4.**293–298**, 4.**301**, and 4.**302**.

At the posterior end of the greater cornu of the hyoid bone are isolated bony elements that may be projected into the intervertebral foramen on oblique radiographs (Figs. 4.**306**, 4.**307**).

◁ Fig. 4.**303**   Ossified area in the stylohyoid ligament with a jointlike connection.

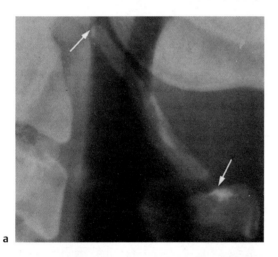

a

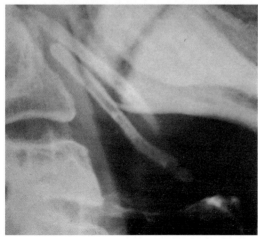

b

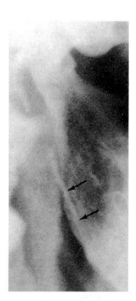

Fig. 4.**305**   Ossification in the stylohyoid ligament (arrows).

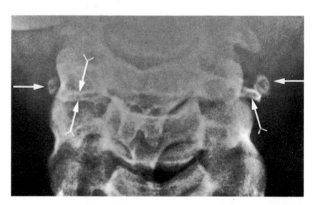

Fig. 4.**304 a, b**   Calcifications.
a Extensive calcification of the stylohyoid ligament with jointlike connections (arrows).
b Bilateral calcification of the stylohyoid ligaments.

Fig. 4.**306**   The hyoid bone is projected over the upper cervical spine as a narrow bony strip that extends past the vertebral contour on the left side. Tailed arrows indicate the right and left greater cornua. An isolated ossification center adjoins each of the cornua (arrows).

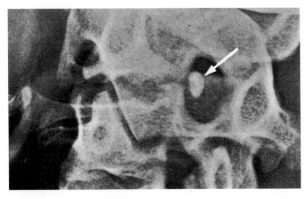

Fig. 4.**307**   An isolated ossification center adjacent to the left greater cornu is projected within the C2–C3 intervertebral foramen (arrow).

 ## Fracture?

Fractures of the hyoid bone may be caused by direct violence or muscle traction. They may or may not be accompanied by a mandibular fracture. CT is best for evaluating injuries of the hyoid bone. MRI is used to investigate presumed soft-tissue injuries or fractures of the cartilaginous framework in children.

The larynx in children is located higher in relation to the mandible than in adults, which offers it greater protection from external injuries. When the cartilage is calcified to a substantial degree, fractures can sometimes be detected on plain radiographs. The imaging modality of choice is CT, however. MRI can be used in selected cases to investigate concomitant soft-tissue injuries and mucosal lacerations (Fig. 4.**308**). It is particularly important to detect bone or cartilage fragments that are compromising the airways or have perforated the mucosa. Fractures of the larynx may involve the thyroid cartilage, cricoid cartilage, or both. Isolated or coexisting cartilage dislocations are accessible to CT diagnosis.

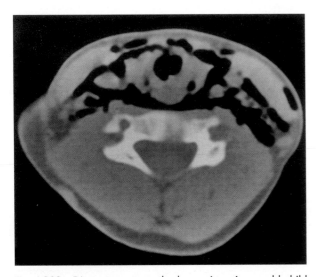

Fig. 4.**308**   Direct trauma to the larynx in a 4-year-old child has caused asymmetry of the laryngeal skeleton. A fracture of the cartilaginous laryngeal skeleton was confirmed at operation. The trauma caused a deep mucosal laceration with marked soft-tissue emphysema.

 ## Necrosis?

Necrosis of the larynx and hyoid bone is most commonly seen after radiation therapy. The initial response is mucositis. Higher radiation doses incite a deep edema and fibrosis, often associated with perichondritis or chondronecrosis. Nearly all patients who are treated at 60–65 Gy will develop radiation-induced soft-tissue changes in the larynx. Clinical examination reveals thickening of the epiglottis and swelling of the arytenoid cartilage. CT may show thickening of the epiglottis or aryepiglottic folds, the false vocal cords, and the soft-tissue structures about the arytenoid cartilage. The preepiglottic and paraglottic fatty tissue typically shows streaky congestion. The true vocal cords and subglottic larynx are usually normal. High radiation doses incite an initial perichondritis, followed by necrosis and collapse of the cartilaginous laryngeal skeleton, which may culminate in true fragmentation of the bony and cartilaginous structures.

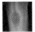 ## Inflammation?

The various inflammatory conditions of the larynx include croup, epiglottitides, the local spread of inflammatory processes to the larynx (e.g., from a neck abscess or peritonsillar abscess), and superinfected laryngocele (laryngopyocele). Tuberculosis and other granulomatous diseases of the larynx are rare. In years past, it was more common to encounter perichondritis and abscesses of the larynx or laryngeal skeleton in the setting of typhus, measles, scarlet fever, erysipelas, anthrax, and mycoses. Tuberculosis of the larynx has also become rare. In the past, it was usually associated with pulmonary tuberculosis. The earliest clinical finding is mucosal edema. Spread of the inflammation leads to ulcerations and necrosis, which may be accompanied by multinodular enlargement of the epiglottis. With involvement of the cricoarytenoid joint, which is a true synovial joint, fixation of the joint may occur in addition to perichondritis.

Wegener granulomatosis can also affect the larynx in rare cases. Sarcoidosis can lead to diffuse thickening of the larynx or small nodular or circumscribed infiltrative lesions. Imaging findings are nonspecific, and other system disease manifestations are usually present.

Because the cricoarytenoid and cricothyroid joints are true synovial joints, they are occasionally involved by **rheumatic disease**. The initial stage consists of synovial swelling with decreased motion in the cricoarytenoid joint. With further progression, the disease can lead to fixation of the cricoarytenoid and cricothyroid joints. CT in these cases may demonstrate irregular sclerosis or periarticular erosions. The soft tissues bordering the arytenoid joint are often swollen.

Polychondritis is a rare, nonbacterial inflammation of uncertain etiology. It involves the articular cartilage in addition to the auricular and nasal cartilages. The laryngeal cartilage may also be affected, and laryngeal edema can develop. The imaging features are increased sclerosis, thickening of the cartilage, or diffusely increased calcifications in the affected cartilage areas.

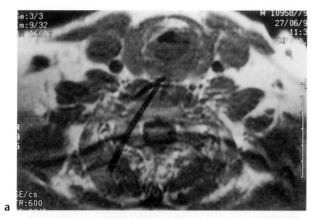

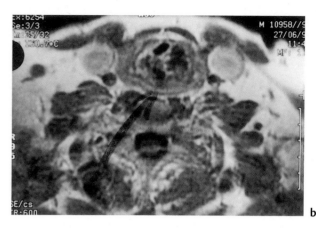

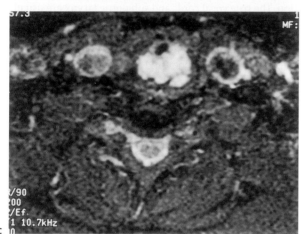

Fig. 4.**309**   A 69-year-old man was evaluated for slowly progressive hoarseness. T1-weighted axial MRI was performed before (**a**) and after contrast administration (**b**). The study shows an enhancing mass arising from the posterior and left portions of the cricoid cartilage. Proton-density image (**c**) demonstrates the very hyperintense mass. Histology identified the lesion as a cricoid chondrosarcoma.

 ## Tumor?

The familiar tumors of the larynx and pharynx need not be discussed here. Chondral tumors that originate from the cartilaginous laryngeal skeleton, such as laryngeal **chondrosarcoma**, are rare lesions that can be diagnosed by CT and especially by MRI. A definitive diagnosis requires histological confirmation, however (Fig. 4.**309**).

 ## Other Changes?

The bony changes that accompany diseases of the hyoid bone and larynx usually cannot be diagnosed on conventional radiographs. But there are other calcifications in the cervical soft tissues that can be identified and differentiated:

- Lymph node calcifications following tuberculosis
- Calcifications of gravitation abscesses
- Vascular calcifications
- Calcified goitrous nodules

The diagnosis can be made with greater accuracy and confidence by CT (see also Fig. 4.**298**). Smaller calcifications of the tracheal rings can also be detected more reliably with CT and often are not visible on conventional radiographs.

References

Ahlgren, P., J. Dahlerup: Fractura condylus occipitalis. Fortschr. Röntgenstr. 101 (1964) 202

Ahlgren, P., Th. Mygind, B. Wilhjelm: Eine selten vorkommende Fractura Basis cranii. Fortschr. Röntgenstr. 97 (1962) 388

Aimi, K.: Role of the tympanic ring in the pathogenesis of congenital cholesteatomas. Laryngoscope 93 (1983) 1140

Aremdaroglou, A.: Os suprapetrosum of Meckel: CT appearance. J. Comput. Assist. Tomogr. 10 (1986) 164

Ballinger, P. W.: Merill's Atlas of Radiographic Positions and Radiographic Procedures, 5th ed. Mosby, St. Louis 1982

Banna, M., J. A. J. Ferris, L. Mc Lean, P. Thomson: Anatomico-radiological study of the borderline sella. Brit. J. Radiol. 56 (1983) 1

Basset, J. M., A. Perrin: Un faux osteome obstructif du donduit auditive externe (Dysplasie fibreuse du tympanal). J. franc. Oto-rhino-laryngol. 33 (1984) 353

Bergerhoff, W.: Metrische Untersuchungen an der Basis des Skelettschädels. Fortschr. Röntgenstr. 82 (1955) 505

Bergerhoff, W.: Messungen von Winkeln und Strecken am submento-vertikalen Röntgenbild der Schädelbasis. Fortschr. Röntgenstr. 82 (1955) 509

Bergerhoff, W., R. Stilz: Die Beugung der Schädelbasis im Röntgenbild. Fortschr. Röntgenstr. 80 (1954) 618

Bergeron, R. Th.: Embryology and developmental anatomy. In Bergeron, R. Th., A. G. Osborn, P. M. Som: Head and Neck Imaging. Mosby, St. Louis 1984 a (pp. 728–733)

Bergeron, R. Th.: Normal anatomy. In Bergeron, R. Th., A. G. Osborn, P. M. Som: Head and Neck Imaging. Mosby, St. Louis 1984 b (pp. 733–744)

Bergeron, R. Th.: Temporal bone imaging. In Bergeron, R. Th., A. G. Osborn, P. M. Som: Head and Neck Imaging. Mosby, St. Louis 1984 c (pp. 744–754)

Bergeron, R. Th.: Inflammatory disease. In Bergeron, R. Th., A. G. Osborn, P. M. Som: Head and Neck Imaaging. Mosby, St. Louis 1984 d (pp. 791–804)

Bergeron, R. Th.: Disorders of growth, metabolism, and aging. In Bergeron, R. Th., A. G. Osborn, P. M. Som: Head and Neck Imaging. Mosby, St. Louis 1984 e (pp. 804–813)

Bergeron, R. Th., R. S. Pinto: Anatomic variations and developmental anomalies. In Bergeron, R. Th., A. G. Osborn, P. M. Som: Head and Neck Imaging. Mosby, St. Louis 1984 (pp. 778–791)

Bergeron, R. Th., A. E. George, R. S. Pinto: Tumors. In Bergeron, R. Th., A. G. Osborn, P. M. Som: Head and Neck Imaging. Mosby, St. Louis 1984 (pp. 813–842)

Bewermeyer, H., H. A. Dreesbach, B. Hünermann, W. D. Heiss: MR imaging of familial basilar impression. J. Comput. Assist. Tomogr. 8 (1984) 953

Bird, C. R., A. N. Hasso, B. P. Drayer, D. B. Hinshaw, J. R. Thompson: The cerebellopontine angle and internal auditory canal: neurovascular anatomy on gas CT cisternograms. Radiology 154 (1985) 667

Bliesener, J. A., R. Schmidt: Normal and pathological growth of the foramen occipitale magnum showing in the plain radiograph. Pediat. Radiol. 10 (1980) 65

Bonneville, J. F., J. L. Dietemann: Radiology of the Sella Turcica. Springer, Berlin 1981

Brogan, M., D. W. Chakeres: Computed tomography and magnetic resonance imaging of the normal anatomy of the temporal bone. Semin. Ultrasound 10 (1989) 178

Campana, L., G. C. Schubert: Ausgedehnte Schädeldeformitäten bei den subarachnoidalen und porencephalen Zysten. Fortschr. Röntgenstr. 117 (1972) 165

Chakeres, D. W., D. J. Weider: Computed tomography of the ossicles. Neuroradiology 27 (1985) 99

Chakeres, D. W., A. Kapila, D. La Masters: Soft-tissue abnormalities of the external auditory canal: subject review of CT findings. Radiology 156 (1985) 105

Charachon, R.: Temporal bone cholesteatoma. Amer. J. Otolaryngol. 6 (1985) 233

Charachon, R., G. Dumas, R. Chastang, O. Roux: Meningoencephalocele de l'apex petreux associe a une craniostenose a type de scapocephalie. J. franc. Oto-rhino-laryngol. 34 (1985) 123

Chilton, L. A.: The volume of the sella turcica in children. New standards. Amer. J. Roentgenol. 140 (1983) 797

Chintapalli, K., J. M. Unger, K. Schaffer, St. J. Millen: Otosclerosis. Comparison of complex-motion tomography and computed tomography. Amer. J. Neuroradiol. 6 (1985) 85

Chong, V. F., Y. F. Yan: Radiology of the jugular foramen. Clin. Radiol. 53 (1998) 405

Conocer, G. L., R. J. Crammond: Tympanic plate fracture from mandibular trauma. J. Oral Max.-fac. Surg. 43 (1985) 292

Courtheoux, P., D. C. da Silva, J. P. Houttevielle, A. Valdazo. L. Chevalier, J. Theron: Schwannome du formamen jugulaire. J. Radiol. 63 (1992) 557

Cremers, C. W. R.: Osteoma of the middle ear. J. Laryngol. 99 (1985) 383

Currarino. G., K. R. Maravilla, K. E. Salyer: Transsphenoidal canal (large craniopharyngeal canal) and its pathological implications. Amer. J. Neuroradiol. 6 (1985) 39

Curtis, D. J., R. M. Allmann, J. Brion, G. S. Holborow, Sh. L. Brahman: Calcification and ossification in the arytenoid cartilage: incidence and patterns. J. Forens. Sci. 30 (1985) 1113

Daniels, D. L., I. L. Williams, V. M. Haughton: Jugular foramen: anatomic and computed tomographic study. Amer. J. Neuroradiol. 4 (1983) 1227

Daniels, D. L., J. F. Schenck, Th. Foster, H. Hart Jr., St. J. Millen, G. A. Meyer, et al.: Surface-coil magnetic resonance imaging of the internal auditory canal. Amer. J. Neuroradiol. 6 (1985) 487

DeFilipp, W. A. Buchheit: Magnetic resonance imaging of acoustic neuromas. Neurosurgery 16 (1985) 763

Dieckmann, H.: Basilare Impression, Atlasassimilation und andere Skelettfehlbildungen der Zerviko-okzipital-Region. Hippokrates, Stuttgart 1966

Diemel, H.: Über eine ungewöhnliche Tentoriumverkalkung. Fortschr. Röntgenstr. 104 (1966) 116–119

Dietemann, J. L., J. F. Bonnevell, F. Cattin, D. Poulignot: Computed tomography of the sellar spine. Neuroradiology 24 (1983) 173

Dietrich, H.: Ein seltener Fall von medianer Längsnaht der Hinterhauptsschuppe bei okzipitaler Schädellücke. Fortschr. Röntgenstr. 76 (1952) 600

Dihlmann, W., G. Ling, G. Nebel: Das Dorsum sellae als Indikator der Stammskelettosteoporose. Fortschr. Röntgenstr. 139 (1983) 531

Disbro, M. A., H. R. Harnsberger, A. G. Osborn: Peripheral facial nerve dysfunction: CT evaluation. Radiology 155 (1985) 659

Djupersland, G., K. F. Nakken, C. Müller, F. Skjorten, T. Rohrt, P. Eldevik: Bone scintigraphy in the diagnosis of fracture and infection of the temporal bone. Acta Otolaryngol. 95 (1983) 670

Dudley, J. P., A. A. Mancuso, W. Fonkalsrud: Arytenoid dislocation and computed tomography. Arch. Otolaryngol. 110 (1984) 483

Feneis, H.: Anatomisches Bildwörterbuch. 8. Aufl. Thieme, Stuttgart 1998

Fischer, E.: Über Verknöcherungen in der Nachbarschaft der Felsenbeinspitze. Fortschr. Röntgenstr. 100 (1964) 236–241

Fochem, K., F. Gschnait, J. Klumair: Die röntgenologische Symptomatik des Urbach–Wiethe-Syndroms. Fortschr. Röntgenstr. 138 (1983) 376

Franken, E. A.: The midline occipital fissur: diagnosis of fracture versus anatomic variants. Radiology 93 (1969) 1043

Frankel, M., D. Fahey, G. Alker: Otogenic pneumencephalus secondary to chronic otitis media. Arch. Otolaryngol. 106 (1980) 437

Frick, H., H. Leonhardt, D. Starck: Spezielle Anatomie II. Kopf-Hals-Eingeweide-Nervensystem. 2. Auflage, Thieme Stuttgart 1980

Fried, M. P., D. M. Vernick: Dermoid cyst of the middle ear and mastoid. Otolaryngol. Head Neck Surg. 92 (1984) 594

Grewal, D. S., N. L. Hiranandi, J. S. Kalgutkar: Congenital absence of the palatine tonsil associated with congenital malformation of the external ear. A congenital anomaly. J. Laryngol. Otol. 96 (1985) 285

Gordon, H.: Lipoid proteinosis in an inbred Namaqualand community. Lancet I (1969) 1032

Grote, W., B. Hoffmann, V. John-Mikolajewski: Aktueller Stand der Diagnose und Behandlung laterobasaler Schädelfrakturen. HNO 34 (1986) 496

Haaga, J. R., R. J. Alfidi: Computed Tomography of the Brain, Head and Neck. Mosby, St. Louis 1995

Han, J. S., R. G. Huss, J. E. Beson, B. Kaufmann, Y. S. Yoon, St. C. Morrison et al: MR imaging of the skull base. J. Comput. Assist. Tomogr. 8 (1984) 944

Hanafee, W., A. Mancuso: Introductory Workbook for CT of the Head and Neck. Williams and Wilkins, Baltimore 1985

Harwood-Nash, D. C.: Fractures of the petrous and tympanic parts of the temporal bone in children: a tomographic study of 35 cases. Amer. J. Roentgenol. 110 (1970) 598

Heller, M., M. Wöhrl, H.-H. Jend, K. Hörmann, K. Helmke: Aussagekraft der CT in der Diagnostik von Tumoren der Kleinhirnbrückenwinkelregion. Fortschr. Röntgenstr. 139 (1983) 48

Holland, B. A., M. Brant-Zawazki: High-resolution CT of temporal bone trauma. Amer. J. Neuroradiol. 5 (1984) 291

Howard, J. D., A. D. Elster, J. S. May: Temporal bone: three-dimensional CT. Part I. Normal anatomy, techniques, and limitations. Radiology 177 (1990) 421

Imhoff, H., G. Caninigiani, P. Hajek, W. Kumpan, H. Schratter, E. Brunner, et al.: CT in der Mittelohrdiagnostik—ein Vergleich mit konventionellen Methoden. Radiologe 24 (1984) 502

Inokuchi, T., K. Sano, M. Kaminogo: Osteonecrosis of sphenoid and temporal bone in a patient with maxillary sinus carcinoma: a case report. Oral. Surg. 70 (1990) 278

Irnberger, Th.: Diagnostische Möglichkeiten und Wertigkeit der konventionellen Radiographie, Röntgentomographie und hochauflösende Computertomographie beim komplexen orbitalen Trauma. Fortschr. Röntgenstr. 142 (1985) 146

Jend, H. H.: Mittelgesichtsverletzungen. In Heller, M., H. H. Jend: Computertomographie in der Traumatologie. Thieme, Stuttgart 1984

Jend, H. H., I. Jend-Rossmann: Sphenotemporal buttress fracture. Neuroradiology 26 (1984b) 411

Jend, H. H., I. Jend-Rossmann, D. Borchers, M. Heller: Die Analyse der Gesichtsschädelfrakturen im CT. Fortschr. Röntgenstr. 137 (1982) 379

Jend, H. H., I. Jend-Rossmann, W. Crone-Münzebrock, E. Grabbe: Die Computertomographie der Schädelbasisfrakturen. Fortschr. Röntgenstr. 140 (1984) 147

Jinkins, J. R.: Atlas of Neuroradiologic Embryology, Anatomy, and Variants. Lippincott, Williams and Wilkins, Philadelphia, 2000

Jurik, A. G., U. Pedersen, A. Norgard: Rheumatoid arthritis of the cricoarytenodid joints: a case of laryngeal obstruction due to acute and chronic joint changes. Laryngoscope 95 (1985) 846

Juslyn, J. N., S. E. Mirvis, B. Markowitz: Complex fractures of the clivus: diagnosis with CT and clinical outcome in 11 patients. Radiology 166 (1988) 817

Kadori, S., Cl. Limberg: Unfallbedingte Läsionen des N. facialis in Abhängigkeit vom Ausmaß der Pyramiden-Pneumatisation. HNO 33 (1985) 534

Kapila, A., D. W. Chakeres, E. Blanco: The Meckel cave: computed tomographic study. Part I: Normal anatomy. Part II: Pathology. Radiology 152 (1984) 425

Kavanagh, K. T., J. E. Salazar, R. W. Babin: Bone marrow extension of the thyroid cartilage: a source of confusion with malignant invasion in CT studies. J. Comput. Assist. Tomogr. 9 (1985) 170

Kier, E. L.: The infantile sella turcica; new roentgenologic and anatomic conceps based on a developmental study of the sphenoid bone. Amer. J. Roentgenol. 102 (1968) 747

Klaus, E.: Röntgendiagnostik der Platybasie und basilaren Impressionen. Weitere Erfahrungen mit einer neuen Untersuchungsmethode. Fortschr. Röntgenstr. 86 (1957) 460

König, H., B. Kurtz: Hochauflösende Computertomographie der Felsenbeine. Fortschr. Röntgenstr. 141 (1984) 129

Krennmair, G., F. Lenglinger, H. Lugmayr: Ossifikationsvarianten der stylohyoidalen Kette. Fortschr. Röntgenstr. 173 (2001) 200

Kullwig, G.: Peristierender offener Ductus craniopharyngicus. Fortschr. Röntgenstr. 79 (1953) 127

Kuta, A. J., F. J. Laine: Imaging the sphenoid bone and basiocciput: anatomic considerations. Semin. Ultrasound 14 (1993) 146

Laine, F. J., L. Nadel, I. F. Braun: CT and MR imaging of the central skull base. Part I: Techniques, embryologic development, and anatomy. Radiographics 10 (1990) 591

Lamothe, A., L. Brazeau-Lamontagne, D. Bergeron, J. F. Poliquin, B. G. Strom. High-resolution CT scan of the temporal bone. J. Otolaryngol. 12 (1983) 119

Lang, J.: Strukture and postnatal organization of heretofor univestigated and infrequent ossification of the sella turcica region. Acta Anat. (Basel) 99 (1977) 121

Lang, J., Ch. Hack: Über die Länge und Lagevariationen der Kanalsysteme im Os temporale. Teil I: Kanäle der Pars petrosa zwischen Margo superior und Meatus acusticus internus. Teil II: Kanäle der pars petrosa zwischen Meatus acusticus internus und Facies inferior partis petrosae. HNO 33 (1985) 176, 279

Latack, J. T., M. D. Graham, J. L. Kemink, J. P. Knake: Giant cholesterol cysts of the petrous apex. Amer. J. Neuroradiol. 6 (1985) 409

Lenz, M., H. König, R. Sauter, M. Schrader: Kernspintomographie des Felsenbeins und Kleinhirnbrückenwinkels. Fortschr. Röntgenstr. 143 (1985a) 1

Lenz, M., H. König, R. Sauter, M. Schrader: Kernspintomographie bei Erkrankungen im Bereich des Felsenbeins. Fortschr. Röntgenstr. 143 (1985b) 623

Lorman, J. G., J. R. Briggs: The Eagle syndrome: Amer. J. Roentgenol. 140 (1983) 881

Lustrin, E. S., R. L. Robertson, S. Tilak: Normal anatomy of the skull base. Neuroimag. Clin. N. Amer. 4 (1994) 465

Madeira, J. T., G. W. Summers: Epidural mastoid pneumatocele. Radiology 122 (1977) 727

Mafee, M. F., J. A. Schild, A. Kumar, G. E. Valvassori, S. Pruzansky: Radiographic features of ear-related developmental anomalies in patients with mandibulofacial dysotosis. Int. J. Pediat. Otorhinolaryngol. 7 (1984a) 229

Mafee, M. F., E. L. Singleton, G. E. Valvassori, G. A. Espinos, A. Kumar, K. Aimi: Acute osteomyelitis and its complications. Role of CT. Radiology 155 (1985) 391

Marin-Padilla, M., T. M. Marin-Padilla: Morphogenesis of experimentally induced Arnold-Chirai malformation. J. Neurosurg. Sci. 50 (1981) 29

Meyer, J. E., R. F. Oot, K. K. Lindfors: CT appearance of clival chordoma. J. Comput. Assist. Tomogr. 10 (1986) 34–38

McDonald, Th. J., D. Thane, R. Cody, R. E. Bryan: Congenital cholesteatoma of the ear. Ann. Otol. 93 (1984) 637

Nager, G. T.: Epidermoid (Congenital Cholesteatomas) Involving the Temporal Bone. Cholesteatoma and mastoid surgery. Proceedings 2nd International Conference. Kugler, Amsterdam 1982 (pp. 41–51)

Neiss, A.: Nachweis des Canalis Chordae (Canalis basilaris medianus) im Röntgenbild. Fortschr. Röntgenstr. 84 (1956) 206

Neiss, A.: Die Bedeutung des Canalis basilaris medianus (Canalis chordae). Morphol. Jb. 106 (1964) 541–544

Neutsch, W. D., H. J. Cramer: Typische intrakranielle Verkalkungen bei Hyalinosis cutis et mucosae (Lipoidproteinose) Fortschr. Röntgenstr. 107 (1967) 131

Noyek, A., H. S. Shulman, M. I. Steinhardt, J. Zizmor, P. M. Som: The larynx. In Bergeron, Th., A. G. Osborn, P. Som: Head and Neck Imaging. Mosby, St. Louis 1984 (pp. 427–440)

Oehler, M. C., P. Schmalbrock, D. Chakeres, S. Kuracay: Magnetic susceptibility artifacts on high-resolution MR of the temporal bone. Amer. J. Neuroradiol. 16 (1995) 1135

Osborn, A. G.: Diagnostic Neuroradiology. Mosby, St. Louis, Baltimore, Boston, Chicago 1994

Paaske, P. B., E. Tang: Tracheopathia osteoplastica in the larynx. J. Laryngol. Otol. 99 (1985) 305

Palva, T., H. Virtan, J. Mäkin: Acute and latent mastoiditis in children. J. Laryngol. 99 (1985) 127

Pestalozza, G.: Otitis media in newborn infants. Int. J. pediat. Otorhinolaryngol. 8 (1984) 109

Platzer, W.: Zur Anatomie der "Sellabrücke" und ihre Beziehung zur A. carotis interna. Fortschr. Röntgenstr. 87 (1957) 613

Rauber/Kopsch: Bewegungsapparat, Bd. I. Hrsg. von Tillmann, B., G. Töndury. In Rauber/Kopsch: Anatomie des Menschen. Lehrbuch und Atlas. 1. Aufl.. Hrsg. Leonhardt, H., B. Tillmann, G. Töndury, K. Zilles. Thieme, Stuttgart 1997

Reisser, C., O. Schubert, H. Weidauer: Three-dimensional imaging of temporal bone structures using spiral CT. Initial results in normal temporal bone anatomy I. HNO 43 (1995) 405

Roberto, M., R. Zito: Ossicular chain interruption with present acoustic reflex. J. Laryngol. 99 (1985) 85

Rogers, L. F.: Radiology of Skeletal Trauma. Churchill-Livingstone, New York 1982 (p. 307)

Schaaf, J., G. Wilhelm: Über den Canalis craniopharyngeus. Fortschr. Röntgenstr. 86 (1957) 748

Schade, A., A. Wadinsky: Einsatz und Problematik der hochauflösenden Computertomographie des Felsenbeines. HNO 33 (1985) 171

Schellhas, K. P., Ch. Wilkes, H. M. Fritts: MR of osteochondritis dissecans and avascular necrosis of the mandibular condyle. Amer. J. Neuroradiol. 10 (1989) 3

Schellhas, K. P., Ch. Wilkes: Temporomandibular joint inflammation: comparison of MR fast scanning with T1- and T2-weighted imaging techniques. Amer. J. Roentgenol. 153 (1989) 93

Schinz, H. R.: Schädel–Gehirn. In: Schinz: Radiologische Diagnostik in Klinik und Praxis, Bd. V, Teil 1. 7. Aufl.. Hrsg. Frommhold, W., W. Dihlmann, H.-St. Stender, P. Thurn. Thieme, Stuttgart 1986

Schmidt, H.: Röntgenologische Darstellung eines Processus retromastoideus. Fortschr. Röntgenstr. 88 (1958) 66

Schmidt, H.: Occipitale Dysplasien. I. Mitteilung: Die Manifestation des Occipitalwirbels im Röntgenbild. Fortschr. Röntgenstr. 90 (1959a) 691

Schmidt, H.: Occipitale Dysplasien. II. Mitteilung: Die occipitale Hypoplasie. Fortschr. Röntgenstr. 91 (1959b) 207

Schmidt, H.: Occipitale Dysplasien. III.Mitteilung: Begleitende Entwicklungsstörungen und Folgen der occipitalen Dysplasie. Fortschr. Röntgenstr. 91 (1959c) 221

Schmidt, H.: Über die Besonderheiten des Cranio-cervikalen Überganges und seiner knöchernen Dysplasien. Radiologe 18 (1978) 49

Schmidt, H., E. Fischer: Über zwei verschiedene Formen der primären basilaren Impression. Fortschr. Röntgenstr. 88 (1958) 60

Schmidt, H., E. Fischer: Die occipitale Dysplasie. Thieme, Stuttgart 1960

Schmidt, H., E. Fischer: Über die Bedeutung knöcherner Varianten des Okzipito-zervikalen Überganges. Fortschr. Röntgenstr. (1962) 479

Schmidt, H., K. Sartor, R. W. Heckl: Bone malformations of the craniocervical region. In: Congenital Malformations of the Spine and Spinal Cord, red. v. N. C. Myrianthopoulos (in collab.). In: Handbook of Clinical Neurology. Vinken, P. J., G. W. Bruyn. North-Holland Publishers, Amsterdam 1978 (pp. 1–97)

Schratter, M., G. Canigiani, F. Karnel, H. Imhof, W. Kumpan: Maskierte Frakturen im Schädelbereich. Radiologe 25 (1985) 108

Schultze, J., E. Kraus: Wachsende Fraktur im Kindesalter. Fortschr. Röntgenstr. 151 (1989) 112

Schumaker, H. M., P. E. Doris: Radiographic parameters of an adult epiglottis. Ann. Emerg. Med. 13 (1984) 588

Schwartz, R. H., N. Mossavaghi, E. D. Marion: Rhabdomyosarcoma of the middle ear: a wolf in sheep's clothing. Pediatrics 65 (1980) 1131

Shaffer, K. A.: The temporal bone. In: Latchaw, R. E.: Computed Tomography of the Head, Neck and Spine. Year Book, Chicago 1985

Shapiro, R., F. Robinson: The formina of the middle fossa: a phylogenetic, anatomic and pathologic study. Amer. J. Roentgenol. 101 (1967) 779

Shapiro, R., F. Robinson: Embryogenesis of the human occipital bone. Amer. J. Roentgenol. 126 (1976) 1063

Som, E. M., H. D. Curten: Head and Neck Imaging. 3rd ed., Mosby, St. Louis 1996

Spector, G. J.: Developmental temporal bone anatomy and its clinical significance. In: Schuknecht, H. F.: Variations on themes. Ann. Otol. 93, Suppl. 112 (1984) 101

Stein, G., J. Wappenschmidt: Lokalisation der röntgenologisch erfaßbaren, intrakraniell gelegenen Veränderungen bei der Hyalinosis cutis et mucosae. Fortschr. Röntgenstr. 100 (1964) 778

Swartz, J. D.: The facial nerve canal: CT analysis of the protruding tympanic segment. Radiology 153 (1984) 443

Swartz, J. D., H. R. Harnsberger: Imaging of the Temporal Bone, 3rd ed., Thieme 1998

Swartz, J. D., A. Lensman, F. I. Marlowe, G. L. Popky, A. S. Berger: High-resolution computed tomography; part 3: The larynx and hypopharynx. Head Neck Surg. (1985a) 231

Swartz, J. D., Margaret L. Bazarnie, T. P. Naidich, L. D. Lowry, H. T. Doan: Aberrant internal carotid artery lying within the middle ear. Neuroradiology 27 (1985b) 322

Swartz, J. D., E. N. Faerber: Congential malformations of the external and middle ear. Amer. J. Neuroradiol. 6 (1985c) 71

Swartz, J. D., Deline W. Mandell, E. N. Faerber, G. L. Porky, J. M. Ardito, St. B. Steinberg, Ch. L. Rojer: Labyrinthine ossification: etiologies and CT Findings. Radiology 157 (1985d) 395

Swartz, J. D., Delaine W. Mandell, R. J. Wolfson, F. J. Marlowe, G. L. Porky, H. D. Silberman, H. Wilf, Nancy G. Swartz, A. S. Berger: Fenestral and cochlear otosclerosis: computed tomographic evaluation. Amer. J. Otol. 6 (1985e) 476

Swartz, J. D., Nancy G. Swartz, Holly Korswick, R. J. Wolfson, A. Hampel, M. L. Ronos, L. D. Lowry: Computerized tomographic evaluation of the middle ear and mastoid for posttraumatic hearing loss. Ann. Otol. (St. Louis) 94 (1985f) 263

Swartz, J. D., R. J. Wolfson, G. L. Porky, A. J. Mauriello, F. L. Marlowe, G. V. Vernose, A. Hampel: External auditory canal dysplasias: CT evaluation. Laryngoscope 95 (1985g) 841

Swartz, J. D., Ph. S. Yussen, Delaine M. Mandell, D. O. Mikaelian, A. S. Bergr, R. J. Wolfson: The vestibular aqueduct syndrome: computed tomographic appearance. Clin. Radiol. 36 (1985h) 241

Swischuk, L. E.: Radiology of the Newborn and Young Infant, 2nd ed. Williams and Wilkins, Baltimore 1980

Taiby, H.: Radiologie der Syndrome. Thieme, Stuttgart 1982

Tänzer, A.: Die Veränderungen am Tuberculum jugulare bei raumbeschränkenden Prozessen im Kleinhirnbrückenwinkel. Radiologe 9 (1969) 484

Teodori, J. B., M. J. Painter: Basilar impression in children. Pediatrics 74 (1984) 1097

Thelen, M., G. Ritter, E. Bücheler: Radiologische Diagnostik der Verletzungen von Knochen und Gelenken. Thieme, Stuttgart-New York, 1993

Tos, M., S.-E. Stangerup: The causes of asymmetry of the mastoid air cell system. Acta Otolaryng. (Stockh.) 99 (1985a) 564

Tos, M., S.-E. Stangerup: Secretory otitis and pneumatization of the mastoid process. Amer. J. Otolaryng. 6 (1985b) 199

Valavanis, A., S. Kunik, M. Oguz: Exploration of the facial nerve canal by high-resolution computed tomography: Anatomy and pathology. Neuroradiology 24 (1983) 139

Valvassori, G. E., G. D. Dobben: Multidirectional and computerized tomography of the vestibular aqueduct in Ménière's disease. Ann. Otol. (St. Louis) 93 (1984) 547

Valvassori, G. E., G. D. Potter, W. N. Hanafee, Barbara L. Carter, R. A. Buckingham: Radiologie in der Hals-Nasen-Ohrenheilkunde, deutschsprachige Ausgabe, hrsg. v. G. Canigiani, G. Wittich. Thieme, Stuttgart 1984 (1 S. 6; 2 S. 36; 3 S. 75–77; 4 S. 108–111; 5 S. 111–113; 6 S. 47; 7 S. 52; 8 S. 50; 9 S. 114; 10 S. 116)

Valvassori, G. E., G. D. Dobben: CT Densitometry of the cochlear capsule in otosclerosis. Amer. J. Neuroradiol. 6 (1985)

Vignaud, J., M. Bouquet, M. L. Aubin, M. T. Iba Zizen, C. Stoffels: IRM des tumeurs intra-axiales de la fosse posterieure. NMR Imaging of intra-axial tumours of the posterior fossa. J. Neuroradiol. 11 (1984) 249

Virapongse, Ch., St. L. G. Rothmann, E. L. Kier, M. Sarwar: Computed tomographic anatomy of the temporal bone. Amer. J. Neuroradiol. 3 (1982) 379

Virapongse, Ch., M. Sarwar, C. Sasaki, E. L. Kier: High-resolution computed tomography of the osseous external auditory canal. I. Normal anatomy. JCAT 7 (1983a) 486

Virapongse, Ch., M. Sarwar, C. Sasaki, E. L. Kier: High-resolution computed tomography of the osseous external auditory canal. II Pathology. JCAT 7 (1983b) 493

Wackenheim, A.: Hypoplasia of the basi-occipital synchondrosis in a patient with transitory supplementary fissure of the basi-occipital. Neuroradiology 27 (1985) 226

Weidner, W. A., J. E. Wenzl, L. E. Swischuk: Roentgenographic findings in lipoid proteinosis: a case report. Amer. J. Roentgenol. 110 (1970) 457

Wiley, C. J.: Lipoid proteinosis: a new roentgenologic entity. Amer. J. Roentgenol. 89 (1963) 1220–1221

Zimmer-Brossy, M.: Lehrbuch der röntgendiagnostischen Einstelltechnik. 4. Auflage (1992) Springer-Verlag, Berlin, Heidelberg, New York.

Facial Skeleton

Orbit

Each orbit has the approximate shape of a pyramid with the apex pointing posteromedially and the base directed anterolaterally (Fig. 4.**310**). If the axes of the two pyramids are extended posteriorly, they intersect at the internal occipital protuberance. The entrance to the orbital cavity, the orbital opening, is bounded by the supraorbital and infraorbital margins. The medial orbital wall consists of the orbital plate of the ethmoid bone and is located approximately on the sagittal plane. It is bounded anteriorly by the lacrimal bone and the frontal process of the maxilla, posteriorly by the medial border of the optic canal. The lateral wall of the orbital cavity consists of the orbital surface of the greater sphenoid wing and the orbital surface of the zygoma. The orbital roof is formed by the orbital part of the frontal bone. It relates posteriorly to the lesser sphenoid wing. The orbital floor consists mostly of the orbital process of the maxilla, and the zygoma forms much of its anterior portion. It is continuous posteriorly with the orbital process of the palatine bone. The orbital floor is separated from the lateral wall of the orbital cavity by the inferior orbital fissure, a cleft located between the greater sphenoid wing and the orbital surface of the maxilla (Figs. 4.**1**, 4.**310**). The superior orbital fissure starts below the optic canal and runs between the greater and lesser sphenoid wings. The superior and inferior orbital fissures intersect at the posterior end of the orbital floor.

Normal Findings

 ### During Growth

The ossification of the orbital skeleton begins in the second month of embryonic development. In the third embryonic month, the greater portion of the eyeball (globe) protrudes from the shallow orbital cavity. Despite deepening of the orbit during fetal growth (partly to accommodate the retrobulbar fat), the superior margin of the orbital cavity has not yet attained its definitive shape in the newborn, and more time is needed to develop a projecting supraorbital rim.

The orbital cavities in small children are large in relation to the rest of the skull. By the end of the second postnatal month, they have attained three-fourths of their definitive adult size. The orbit has a transverse elliptical shape in newborns and a more circular shape in adults.

 ### In Adulthood

The anatomy of the orbits is illustrated in Figs. 4.**1** and 4.**310**.

In standard frontal radiographs of the skull, the petrous pyramids are projected at approximately the center of the

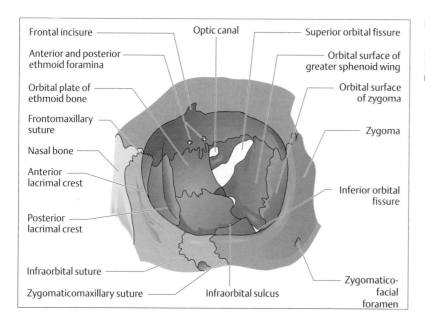

Frontal incisure
Anterior and posterior ethmoid foramina
Orbital plate of ethmoid bone
Frontomaxillary suture
Nasal bone
Anterior lacrimal crest
Posterior lacrimal crest
Infraorbital suture
Zygomaticomaxillary suture
Optic canal
Infraorbital sulcus
Superior orbital fissure
Orbital surface of greater sphenoid wing
Orbital surface of zygoma
Zygoma
Inferior orbital fissure
Zygomatico-facial foramen

Fig. 4.**310**   View of the left orbit, anterior aspect. (From Sobotta: *Atlas of Human Anatomy*, 18th Ed., Urban and Schwarzenberg, Munich, Vienna, Baltimore, Fig. 116.)

Fig. 4.**311 a, b**   Normal appearance of the optic canal in the Rhese–Goalwin view.

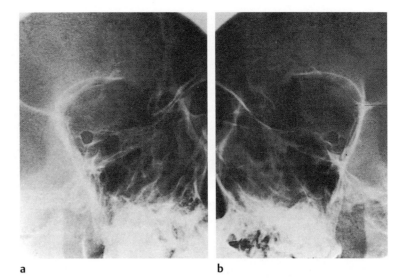

orbits. The **Rhese–Goalwin view** gives a cross-sectional view of the optic canal, projecting it over the upper lateral quadrant of the orbit. For this view the head is turned so that a line from the external occipital protuberance to the mastoid process, running parallel to the axis of the optic canal, forms a 40–45° angle with the median plane. The chin, nasal tip, and lateral orbital rim should rest against the cassette or table surface (Fig. 4.**311**). The orbital specimen in Fig. 4.**312** is helpful in interpreting the structures that are seen in this projection. However, only high-resolution axial and coronal thin-slice CT scanning can provide an accurate and anatomically precise view of the orbits (Figs. 4.**313**, 4.**314**).

In the Rhese projection of the skull, ethmoid air cells are seen medial to the optic canal. The septa of these cells are thinner than the marginal ridge of the optic canal (Figs. 4.**311**, 4.**312**). The lumen of the optic canal is usually circular, rarely reniform or triangular, and occasionally almost rectangular. By 3 years of age it has reached its definitive diameter of 4.3–5 mm (extreme range 3.3–5.5 mm).

Frontal radiographs of the skull show a straight, oblique linear density that runs medially downward in the lateral part of the orbit. This feature, called the **innominate line**, is a tangential projection of the cortical bone of the temporal fossa, especially its anteromedial portion formed by the greater sphenoid wing where it meets the frontal bone anteriorly at the frontosphenoidal suture (Fig. 4.**2**). In its lower portion, the innominate line deviates medially where the inferior border of the temporal fossa adjoins the infratemporal fossa (Figs. 4.**320**, 4.**322**).

The **lacrimal fossa** and **nasolacrimal duct** are clearly defined by CT (Fig. 4.**314**). Today the orbital apex is also imaged with CT or MRI, which can demonstrate not only the anatomic relationships of the optic nerve and cranial nerves III–VI but also their relationship to changes in the ethmoid labyrinth (Fig. 4.**315**).

Below the orbital roof is a crescent-shaped zone of increased radiolucency caused by intraorbital fat. This zone may be more conspicuous in older individuals (Figs. 4.**316**, 4.**324**). The palpebral fissure may appear as a lucent line crossing the orbit, especially in patients with enophthalmos and on radiographs taken during upward gaze.

The superior orbital margin often presents a double contour due to the normal vaulted shape of the orbit. The double contour is given by the thick anterior rim and the

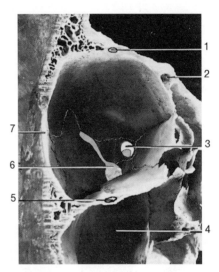

Fig. 4.**312**   Anatomic specimen of the orbit.
1   Supraorbital foramen
2   Marginal air cell belonging to the frontal or ethmoid sinus
3   Optic canal
4   Maxillary sinus
5   Infraorbital canal
6   Superior orbital fissure
7   Lateral wall of orbit

tangential projection of the overlying orbital roof. Within the supraorbital margin is the **frontal notch**, sometimes converted to a foramen, which transmits the medial branch of the supraorbital nerve with the concomitant vessels. Lateral to it, in the middle third of the supraorbital margin, is the **supraorbital foramen** (frontal foramen), often present only as a notch, which transmits the lateral branch of the supraorbital nerve and the concomitant vessels. The supraorbital foramen is often very conspicuous on radiographs, especially in children (Figs. 4.**317**–4.**319**). It marks the location of the pressure point for the first division of the trigeminal nerve. The **infraorbital foramen** (Figs. 4.**320**, 4.**321**) forms the anterior opening of the infraorbital canal, which transmits the infraorbital nerves and vessels. It is the pressure point for the second division of the trigeminal nerve.

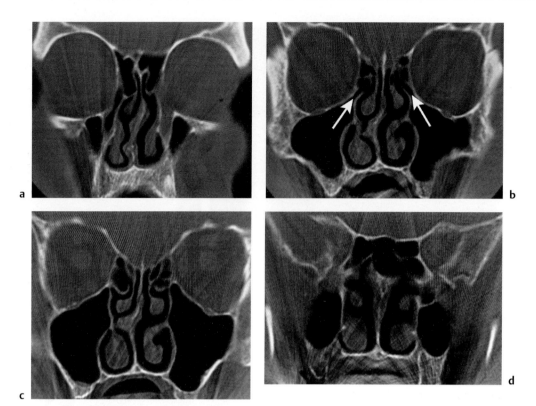

Fig. 4.**313 a–d**   Orbital imaging.
a Coronal CT with a high-resolution bone filter. The scan demonstrates the anterior portions of the orbit and the adjacent paranasal sinuses.
b, c Coronal CT with a high-resolution bone filter shows the central portions of the orbit and adjacent paranasal sinuses in the area of the ethmoid infundibulum (arrows).

d Coronal CT with a high-resolution bone filter demonstrates the posterior portions of the orbit, ethmoid labyrinth, and both maxillary sinuses.

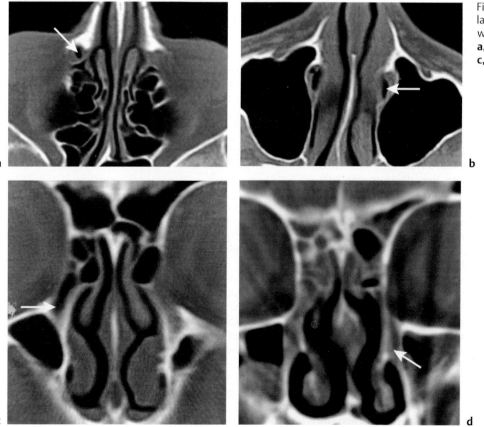

Fig. 4.**314 a–d**   The nasolacrimal duct (arrow). Bone-window CT.
a, b Axial scans.
c, d Coronal scans.

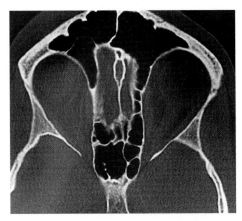

Fig. 4.**315** Relationship of the orbital apex to the ethmoid labyrinth. Axial CT with a high-resolution bone filter.

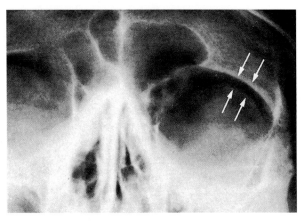

Fig. 4.**316** Physiological fat pad between the orbital roof and the globe (arrows) in a 54-year-old woman.

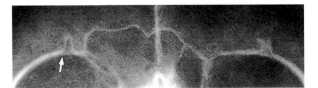

Fig. 4.**317** Supraorbital foramen (supraorbital canal) (arrow).

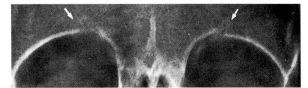

Fig. 4.**318** Supraorbital foramen (arrow) in a 6-year-old child (projected obliquely in the radiograph).

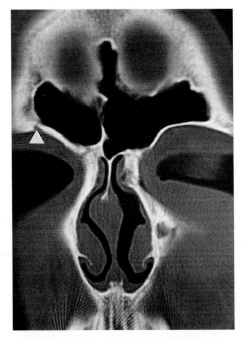

Fig. 4.**319** CT appearance of the right supraorbital foramen (arrowhead). Coronal CT with a high-resolution bone filter.

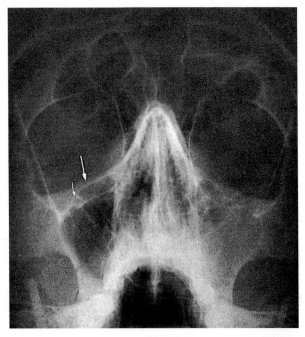

Fig. 4.**320** Right infraorbital foramen (infraorbital canal) in the occipitonasal projection.
Small arrow: infraorbital foramen
Large arrow: periorbital air cells

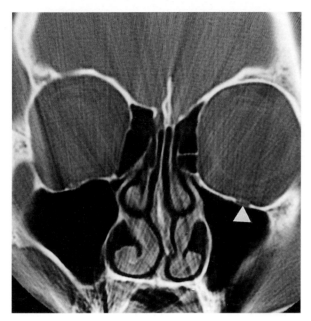

Fig. 4.**321**   Course of the infraorbital canal (arrowhead). Coronal CT with a high-resolution bone filter.

The **meningo-orbital foramen** is an inconstant feature on radiographs, sometimes appearing as a small opening in the posterior portion of the lateral orbital wall below the lesser sphenoid wing. It transmits an arterial connection that links the lacrimal artery with the middle meningeal artery. In the anterior third of the lateral orbital wall are vascular foramina and canals belonging to the zygoma. One such foramen, the zygomatico-orbital, is sometimes visible on paranasal sinus radiographs as an opening 1–2 mm in diameter.

The anterior clinoid process may project into the optic canal, resembling an exostosis. When pneumatized, it can closely resemble an ethmoid air cell in radiographs (Figs. 4.**312**, 4.**379**). Occasionally the dorsum sellae is also projected over the inferior border of the optic canal.

The **temporozygomatic suture**, which unites the anterior border of the zygomatic arch with the zygoma (Fig. 4.**2**), may be very conspicuous on frontal radiographs. It normally appears as a slightly gaping line projected into each of the orbits. The structure of the orbital roof depends to a large degree on the prominence of the inner-table convolutional markings, which may appear as large, superiorly concave curvilinear densities, especially in the lateral third of the orbital roof.

▌ Pathological Finding?

Normal Variant/Anomaly?

Variants

When the sphenoid sinus is heavily pneumatized, the bony walls of the optic canal are particularly thin. The innominate line (Fig. 4.**346**) may be partially or completely absent, depending on the shape of the temporal fossa. An unusual radiographic projection can also produce this phenomenon.

Various morphological variants of the optic canal may be encountered, as described below:

● A relatively broad optic canal may present a figure-of-eight configuration.
● With ossification of the dural layer between the optic nerve and ophthalmic artery, the optic canal may appear to be divided into two compartments.
● A bony apposition at a muscle attachment may extend laterally into the optic canal from the lower part of the orbital opening of the canal. It is present in 87% of the population but is rarely visible on radiographs due to its small size.

> Projection-related changes in the shape of the optic canal should not be considered a variant. For example, the optic canal appears more elliptical when it is projected into the upper outer quadrant of the orbit in the Rhese view.

Anomalies

In our previous discussion of craniosynostosis, we reviewed the frontal deformities that can result from premature closure of the cranial sutures (p. 390–392 and Table 4.**10**). **Craniofacial dysostosis** (**Crouzon disease**) is an autosomal dominant disease that is quite variable in its expression. **Acrocephalosyndactyly syndrome type I** (**Apert disease**) is also an autosomal dominant disease that has similar craniofacial manifestations. It is associated with brachycephaly, hypertelorism, bilateral exophthalmos, maxillary hypoplasia, relative prognathism, and orbital malformations. Crouzon disease is associated with various other deformities such as oxycephaly, scaphocephaly, or trigonocephaly. Apert syndrome may exhibit various craniosynostoses that are combined with syndactylies of the hands and feet and other skeletal anomalies such as ankylosis of the elbow, hip, and shoulder as well as cardiovascular, gastrointestinal, and urogenital malformations.

The orbital anomalies in craniofacial dysostosis and acrocephalosyndactyly syndrome type I are caused by premature synostosis of the coronal suture. The orbit shows a range of typical deformities: it is shortened in its sagittal diameter. The short orbital roofs appear to be located high above the level of the skull base. They show a steep posterior downslope (in the lateral view) and increased convolutional markings. The lesser sphenoid wings show a steep lateral upslope. The planum sphenoidale is very low (Fig. 4.**322**). The distance between the medial orbital walls is increased (**hypertelorism**). The ethmoid cells may be enlarged. Hypoplasia of the maxilla leads to exophthalmos and relative prognathism. The optic canal is usually narrow in both diseases, and this predisposes to optic nerve atrophy.

In unilateral coronal synostosis with plagiocephaly, the ipsilateral half of the forehead is flattened and the floor of the anterior fossa presents a steep lateral upslope. The frontal orbital view shows a linear density running above and parallel to the superior orbital fissure. The horizontal orbital diameter is slightly decreased, while its vertical diameter is unaffected (Fig. 4.**323**).

Narrowing of the optic canal can also occur in various other dysplasias:

1   **Metaphyseal dysplasia (Pyle disease)** is an autosomal recessive condition whose dominant features are widening of the metaphyses of the long tubular bones, especially the distal femurs, and severe cortical thinning. The metaphyses of the proximal humerus, distal forearm, and proximal tibia and fibula may also be very broad and stout. Skull radiographs show slightly increased sclerosis of the calvarium and skull base. Additional signs are widening of the medial portions of the clavicles and genu valgum.

2   **Craniometaphyseal dysplasia** is a rare disease with an autosomal dominant and occasionally autosomal recessive mode of inheritance. It is associated with marked, generalized sclerosis of the skull and with widening of the metaphyses, especially in the long tubular bones (distal femurs). Cranial sclerosis is more pronounced than in Pyle disease, and the widened metaphyses (especially in the femurs) are more club-shaped than Erlenmeyer-flask-shaped. Perhaps the main differentiating feature from Pyle disease is the clinical presentation, which is marked by a large skull, prognathism, craniofacial asymmetry, marked dental irregularities, and prominence of the paranasal sinuses (especially the maxillary sinuses). Also, the marked sclerosis of the skull base leads to cranial nerve palsies predominantly affecting the facial and vestibulocochlear nerves.

3   **Craniodiaphyseal dysplasia** is apparently an autosomal recessive disease that has been described only sporadically in the literature. The dominant radiographic signs are massive periosteal and endosteal sclerosis involving the diaphyses of the long tubular bones while sparing the epiphyses and metaphyses. Again, the skull exhibits sclerotic changes that may be accompanied by cranial nerve deficits, particularly of nerves II and VIII. The disease takes a progressive course, and most cases are diagnosed during childhood. In contrast to **Camurati–Engelmann syndrome (diaphyseal dysplasia)**, patients exhibit a greater degree of cranial sclerosis and early changes in the facial skeleton with prominent paranasal sinuses, a flat nose, and cranial nerve deficits.

4   **Frontometaphyseal dysplasia (Hart syndrome)** is characterized by pronounced hyperostoses in the frontal region, predominantly affecting the supraorbital ridges, and frequent lack of pneumatization of the frontal sinuses. Only a few cases have been described to date. Other anomalies include deformities of the auditory ossicles, cochlear anomalies, micrognathism, and increased sclerosis of the calvarium, causing potential confusion with Paget disease. Underconstriction of the metaphyses of the long tubular bones with posterolateral bowing of the tibia and fibula, underconstriction of the phalanges in the hand, platyspondylisis, and bilateral protrusio acetabuli have also been described. The extremity bones in this case were disproportionately long in relation to the trunk.

5   **Hereditary optic atrophy (Leber disease)** is also associated with narrowing of the optic canal.

The foregoing anomalies and dysplasias of the optic canal require differentiation from apparent narrowing of the optic canal due to projection-related effects (e.g., in the Rhese view). The dimensions of the optic canal can be accurately measured on CT scans.

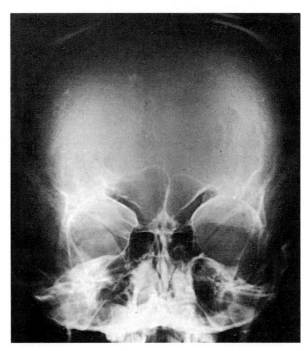

Fig. 4.**322**   Frontal dysplasia of the orbits, sagittal projection.

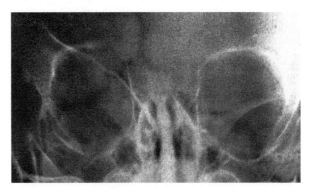

Fig. 4.**323**   Left frontal dysplasia. (From Beutel and Tänzer 1963.)

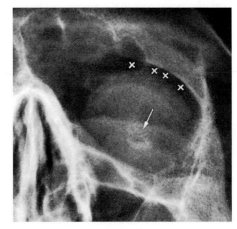

Fig. 4.**324**   Calcification in the left globe (arrow) of a cataract patient. The crescent-shaped lucency below the orbital roof (++++) results from atrophy of the fat pad and inward displacement of the globe in this elderly patient.

Cephaloceles are covered on pages 387, 388, 428 and in Table 4.**14**.

As noted earlier, **meningoencephaloceles** that reach the orbit may herniate through the superior orbital fissure, causing proptosis. They can also enter the orbit through a bony gap in the lower part of the frontal squama or through a gap in the frontonasal suture. Other potential sites of access to the orbit are the rostral ethmoidolacrimal suture (an anterior basal portal), the superior orbital fissure, and congenital bony defects in the orbit. These defects may involve the sphenoid wings, the orbital floor, the orbital roof, and rarely the lateral orbital wall or the apex of the orbital pyramid.

There are numerous routes for the herniation of cephaloceles in the frontoethmoid region. Frontoethmoid cephaloceles can be classified by their location as follows:

1 Nasofrontal cephaloceles (50–60%)
2 Nasoethmoid cephaloceles (approximately 30%)
3 Naso-orbital cephaloceles (6–10%)

Serous cysts composed of heterotopic mucosa may be observed in the globe immediately after birth. Large cysts can erode the orbital walls.

Small orbits (often with compensatory paranasal sinus dilatation) and small orbital canals develop as a sequel to enucleation or orbital exenteration when these surgical procedures are carried out during skeletal growth.

Enlargement of the orbits may accompany hypoplasia of the paranasal sinuses, especially the maxillary sinus. Orbital enlargement may also be caused by angiomas and other mass lesions that develop during growth.

 Fracture?

Fifty percent of multiple-trauma patients have midfacial injuries, and 40% of these patients have ocular complications. Orbital injuries are commonly associated with injuries of the facial skeleton.

CT is the current modality of choice for investigating injuries of the facial skeleton including the orbits. Axial CT should be done as a primary examination in patients with multiple injuries, preferably using spiral technique. With spiral CT, a small reconstruction increment can be selected to allow for secondary reformatted coronal images. Another option is direct coronal scanning. With some patients, pseudocoronal scanning can be performed by hyperextending the head and tilting the gantry in the opposite direction. CT can also detect the soft-tissue injuries that accompany skeletal trauma.

Classification of orbital fractures
➤ Fractures of the orbital floor
  – Lateral fractures involving the inferior orbital margin
  – Medial fractures not involving the inferior orbital margin
➤ Fractures of the medial wall
➤ Fractures of the roof and lateral orbital margin
➤ Fractures of the optic canal

The **blow-out fracture** is a burst fracture caused by a blow to the eye from a blunt object. Orbital soft tissues usually herniate through the orbital floor, occasionally through the medial orbital wall (in about 30% of cases), and rarely through the orbital roof. Complications are often present:

- A fragment impinging on the neck of the hernia sac, hampering or preventing reduction of the herniated orbital contents. Typically, intraorbital fat or extraocular muscles (especially the inferior rectus muscle) are entrapped in the fracture line in the orbital floor or remain herniated in the maxillary sinus.
- An exceptionally large hernial opening compounds the difficulty of surgical repair.

The Le Fort classification of midfacial fractures (Fig. 4.**325**)

➤ **Le Fort I** (Fig. 4.**325**). The maxilla is separated from the rest of the facial skeleton. The fracture line runs through the base of the maxillary sinuses, the basal portion of the nose, and the pterygoid process of the sphenoid bone. Typical clinical findings are dental malocclusion, epistaxis, and cutaneous emphysema. CT defines the path of the fracture in coronal scans. This fracture is distinguished from a Le Fort II fracture by the presence of an intact nasoethmoid complex.

➤ **Le Fort II** (4.**325**). This is a transverse, pyramid-shaped fracture across the central facial skeleton that extends through the nasal bone, the nasoethmoid complex, the medial borders of the orbit, the frontal process of the maxilla, and the nasolacrimal canal, descending through the orbital floors and the anterior orbital margin near the zygomatic–maxillary junction (Fig. 4.**1**). The fracture also involves the lateral walls of the maxilla, and thus the maxillary sinuses, along with the pterygoid processes. Typically the zygomas remain attached to the skull. In a classic Le Fort II fracture, the fracture line runs through the frontonasal suture. The fracture can be classified as "high" or "low" depending on whether the fracture line is above or below the suture. The injury is caused by a direct blow to the center of the facial skeleton from the front or side (Fig. 4.**326**). Displacement of the pyramidal fragment can be demonstrated by lateral radiographs or, preferably, by axial CT.

➤ **Le Fort III** (Fig. 4.**325**). The facial skeleton is completely separated from the neurocranium. The fracture extends transversely from the nasal root area through the ethmoid cells, lacrimal bone, and medial orbital wall back to the inferior orbital fissure. There the fracture divides into two limbs:
  1 The upper limb runs laterally upward through the zygomatic arches and lateral orbital walls into the frontozygomatic suture.
  2 The lower limb runs downward and backward through the roots of the pterygoid processes. The Le Fort III fracture is caused by a very heavy impact to the facial skeleton from above.

Conventional radiographs can be used to evaluate the lateral wall of the orbit, the roof, the anteroinferior orbital margin, and also the orbital floor to a limited degree. Only CT can detect additional fractures, especially of the orbital apex, which are commonly associated with injuries of the optic nerve and other neurovascular structures.

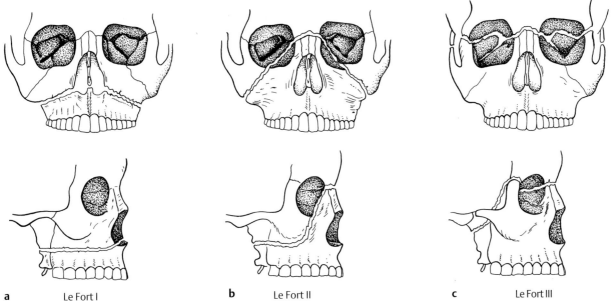

| a | Le Fort I | b | Le Fort II | c | Le Fort III |

Fig. 4.325 a–c Le Fort classification of midfacial fractures. Le Fort I: transverse fracture through the base of the maxillary sinuses, the lower portions of the nose, and the pterygoid processes of the sphenoid bone.

Le Fort II: "pyramid fracture" separating the central portions of the facial skeleton from the rest of the skull.
Le Fort III: complete separation of the facial skeleton from the neurocranium. (From Thelen et al. 1993)

Direct fracture signs on conventional radiographs
➤ Bony discontinuities
➤ Stepoffs
➤ Displaced fragments
➤ Suture diastasis (especially of the frontozygomatic suture)

Indirect fracture signs on conventional radiographs
➤ Circumscribed soft-tissue densities at the fracture site (periosteal/subperiosteal hematoma or herniation of soft tissues such as intraorbital fat, entrapped extraocular muscles).
➤ Partial or complete opacification of adjacent paranasal sinuses (hematosinus) and/or orbital emphysema (present in 90% of fractures of the medial wall and orbital floor)

The imaging workup of facial fractures includes frontal projections of the orbit and paranasal sinuses, lateral projections of the facial skeleton, and especially CT scans. Special radiographic views of the optic canal and ultrasonography to detect blow-out fractures may be omitted, as they cause loss of time that might jeopardize the patient. Blow-out fractures may not be directly visualized on plain radiographs, even if orbital muscle or fat is entrapped in the fracture line.

 Inflammation?

Primary inflammatory processes rarely involve the bony structures of the orbits. Osteitis that spreads to the orbit from the adjacent paranasal sinuses is often associated with visible foci of inflammatory destruction and, in chronic cases, with sclerotic changes. Because the bony boundaries of the orbit (especially the lamina papyracea)

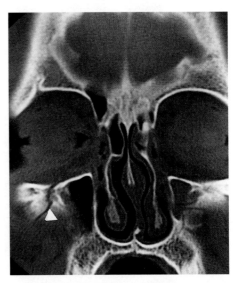

Fig. 4.326 Fracture line running through the inferior rim of the right orbit (arrowhead) in a Le Fort II fracture. Coronal CT with a high-resolution bone filter.

are so thin that sometimes parts of the bone cannot be visualized even with CT, there are cases in which even CT cannot detect bone destruction originating from the ethmoid labyrinth. Tuberculous osteitis or periostitis of the orbit, which may be associated with very small sequestra and usually involves the inferolateral orbital wall, is rarely seen in current practice. It is also rare to encounter orbital manifestations of syphilis, which may also be associated with small sequestra.

Paget disease requires differentiation from chronic inflammatory bacterial infections of the paranasal sinuses that adjoin the orbit.

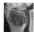 Tumor?

Localized expansion of the orbital boundaries by erosions or defects initially affect the natural openings: the optic canal, superior orbital fissure, and inferior orbital fissure. A general **rise in intracranial pressure** leads to circular enlargement of the optic canal, which is unilateral if the pressure increase is confined to one side. **Optic sheath meningioma**, **optic glioma**, and **optic neuroma** are tumors that can expand the optic canal through pressure erosion. **Vascular tumors** and **meningiomas** can expand the superior orbital fissure. The lower part of the fissure may be expanded due to enlargement of the cavernous sinus by a **carotid–cavernous fistula**, for example.

Expansion of the ophthalmic vein by a carotid–cavernous fistula can cause notching of the orbital roof. **Cavernous hemangioma** is often located posterolateral to the globe and can cause local pressure erosion in addition to orbital enlargement (if it occurs during skeletal growth). Again, this can result in expansion of the superior orbital fissure.

An infraclinoidal aneurysm of the internal carotid artery can also lead to expansion of the superior orbital fissure. Calcifications are sometimes visible within the aneurysmal sac or in its wall.

The rest of the orbital structures may be deformed or destroyed by a variety of tumors and tumorlike lesions. Causes are epidermoid and dermoid cysts, neurofibromas, aneurysmal bone cysts, fibrous dysplasia, and Paget disease. Additionally, there are many malignant neoplasms that can occur in the orbit, e.g., lymphoma, plasmocytoma, rhabdomyosarcoma, or metastasis.

Turning the eyes to one side during a CT examination can produce a **thickening of the eye muscles** that **mimics a tumor** (Fig. 4.**327**).

 Other Changes?

Spiral CT is used for the diagnosis of intraorbital or intraocular **foreign bodies**. This study can detect even small foreign bodies, including wood splinters.

Calcifications

Calcifications due to amyloid or hyaline degeneration in the **conjunctiva of the eyelids** are rarely seen on conventional radiographs. Metaplastic calcifications following tarsitis and calcifications in chalazions and dermoids are larger. Calcifications in the lower eyelid have been described in chalazions and fibromas and in the form of phleboliths. Ectopic intraorbital teeth have also been described, and teeth have been found inside dermoid cysts within the orbit and lower eyelid. Calcifications of the lacrimal glands are located in the upper outer quadrant of the orbit.

Calcification of the lens of the eye may develop after injuries (Fig. 4.**324**) or inflammations. Punctate calcifications may also form around the lens. A calcified lens has a diameter less than 1 cm. A larger calcific density may reflect calcification of the vitreous body.

Rarely, retrolenticular calcifications are found in the setting of **retrolenticular fibroplasia** in underweight preterm infants who have been on oxygen ventilation for a period of days or weeks.

Retinal calcifications are located in the posterior part of the globe. They may also accompany lenticular calcifications in cataract patients.

CT can clearly demonstrate calcifications located within a calcium-containing **retinoblastoma** (retinal glioma [Virchow]). This is the most common ocular tumor in children under 5 years of age. It occurs mainly in children during the first months and years of life. It is characterized by fine, speckled calcifications, which are seen in 75% of these cases.

Phleboliths are sometimes observed in **chronic adhesive retrobulbar thrombophlebitis**, also in hemangiomas and other vascular malformations.

X-ray-absorbing eyelid shadows are a common pitfall in differential diagnosis and can mimic pathological calcifications. They are accessible to visual inspection.

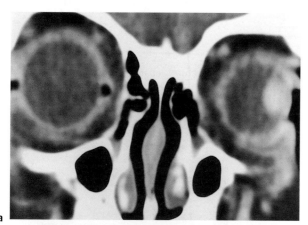

a

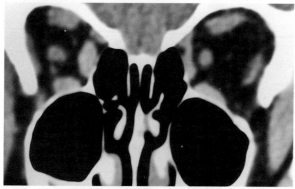

b

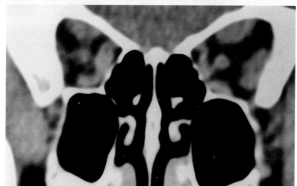

c

Fig. 4.**327 a–c**   Thickening of the eye muscles as a function of gaze direction (patient looking to the left).
a Left lens in gaze toward the left.
b Right medial rectus muscle is contracted and therefore thickened.
c Left lateral rectus muscle in a contracted state.

Nose: Nasal Bone, Cartilaginous Nasal Skeleton, and Nasal Cavity

Normal Findings

The **nasal cavity** is subdivided into two approximately symmetrical cavities by an oblique partition, the **nasal septum**, which is often located slightly off the midline. The septum is formed anterosuperiorly by the perpendicular plate of the ethmoid bone and posteroinferiorly by the vomer. The anterior part of the septum is cartilaginous. The inferior nasal turbinates are usually clearly visible on frontal skull radiographs (Fig. 4.**328**) along with the nasal fossa on each side and the nasal septum. The lateral projection shows the frontonasal suture, the nasomaxillary suture, and a structure called the ethmoid sulcus located at the junction of the nasal bone with the perpendicular plate of the ethmoid (Figs. 4.**329**, 4.**330**). Today, however, CT and MRI can provide a more accurate evaluation of the nasopharyngeal structures.

The superior and middle nasal turbinates are part of the ethmoid bone. The inferior turbinate is a separate bone. Coronal CT is best for defining the nasal turbinates and tracking the circadian fluctuations in their shape and size (Fig. 4.**331**). The radiologist should be familiar with these normal changes to avoid misinterpreting "thick" turbinates as hyperplasia. It is known that in about 80% of the population, the turbinates swell and shrink over a cycle of

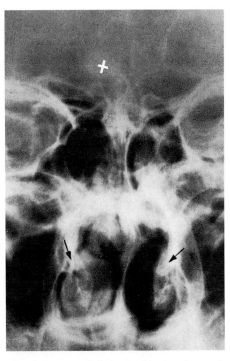

Fig. 4.**328** Deviated septum. Inferior turbinates (arrows), frontal sinus osteoma (+).

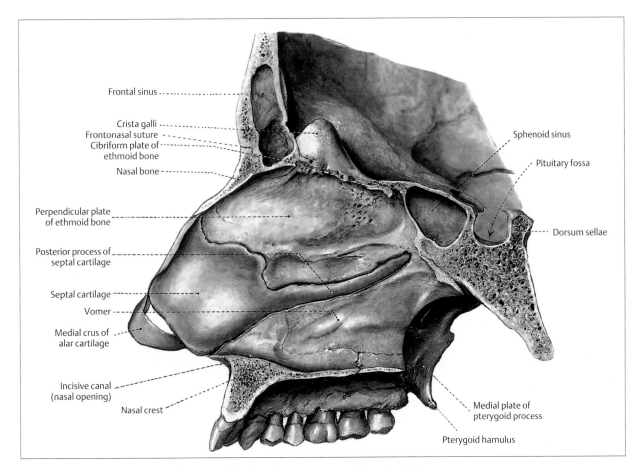

Fig. 4.**329** Nasal septum viewed from the left side. (From Rauber and Kopsch 1987.)

Labels on figure:
- Frontal sinus
- Crista galli
- Frontonasal suture
- Cibriform plate of ethmoid bone
- Nasal bone
- Perpendicular plate of ethmoid bone
- Posterior process of septal cartilage
- Septal cartilage
- Vomer
- Medial crus of alar cartilage
- Incisive canal (nasal opening)
- Nasal crest
- Sphenoid sinus
- Pituitary fossa
- Dorsum sellae
- Medial plate of pterygoid process
- Pterygoid hamulus

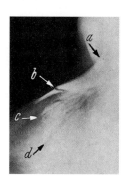

Fig. 4.**330** Nasal skeleton.
a Frontonasal suture
b Nasal fracture
c Ethmoid sulcus
d Nasomaxillary suture

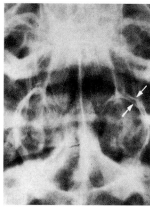

Fig. 4.**332** "Double contours" of the nasal wall.

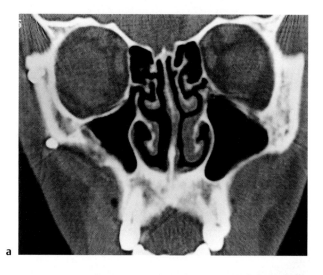

a

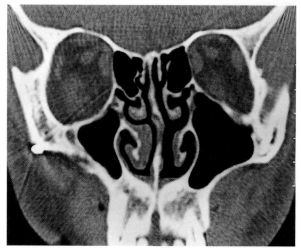

b

Fig. 4.**331 a, b** The turbinate cycle.
a Image taken at 0849 shows swelling of the left inferior turbinate.
b Image taken at 0911 shows swelling of the right inferior turbinate and shrinkage of the left turbinate. Both **a** and **b** were taken on the same plane.

1–5 hours, regardless of external stimuli. This **turbinate cycle** is subject to very large interindividual and intraindividual variations. While the amount of airflow through the right or left nasal cavity varies with the turbinate cycle, the total nasal airflow remains approximately constant.

An apparent double contour of the lateral nasal wall is often seen on radiographs. It is usually caused by an air-filled space between the nasal turbinate and the medial wall of the maxillary sinus or occasionally by pneumatization of the inferior turbinate (Fig. 4.**332**).

Pathological Finding?

Normal Variant/Anomaly?

Variants

Deviation of the nasal septum is a common finding (Figs. 4.**328**, 4.**333**). The etiology is diverse and ranges from a normal variant to the result of chronic inflammatory changes or trauma.

The detection of a unilateral or bilateral **bullous turbinate (concha bullosa)** is best accomplished with CT. The diagnosis of concha bullosa is of major importance in functional endoscopic sinus surgery (FESS, Fig. 4.**334**).

Anomalies

Choanal atresia or **choanal stenosis** is the most common congenital abnormality of the nasal cavity, occurring in approximately 1 in 5000 to 1 in 8000 live births. Although bony atresia is more common than membranous atresia, both forms are usually combined. Most atresias and stenoses are unilateral and go undetected until the child is older. Patients with unilateral choanal atresia usually present with a chronic, unilateral, purulent nasal discharge. The main differential diagnosis in these older children is a foreign body lodged in one side of the nasal cavity (Fig. 4.**341**). Because newborns are obligate nose breathers, bilateral choanal atresia can cause serious respiratory compromise. This life-threatening respiratory insufficiency and the inability to pass a nasogastric tube deeper than 3–4 cm into the nose despite the presence of air in the trachea and lungs provide clinical confirmation of the diagnosis.

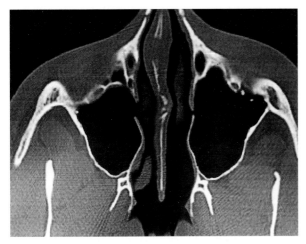

Fig. 4.**333**   Deviation of the nasal septum toward the left. CT with a high-resolution bone filter.

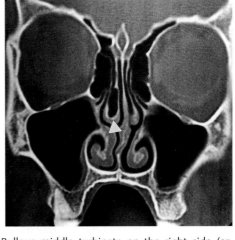

Fig. 4.**334**   Bullous middle turbinate on the right side (arrowhead). Coronal CT with a high-resolution bone filter.

The examination of choice is CT, which can accurately define the bony and/or membranous components of the anomaly. The critical component of all bony atresias is abnormal thickening of the vomer. Typically the posteromedial portions of the maxilla are bowed medially and extend to the vomer or are fused to its lateral margin. The average width of the posterior choanal airway in newborns is 0.67 cm, increasing to 0.86 cm by the 6th year of life and 1.13 cm by the 16th year. In children under 8 years of age, the vomer diameter is generally less than 0.23 cm and should not exceed 0.34 cm. In children over 8 years of age, the average width of the vomer is 0.28 cm and should not exceed 0.55 cm. The thickness of the bony plate causing the atresia should be documented, as it is an important guide for the surgeon. The stated measurements are based on the narrowest point of the posterior choana and the maximum width of the posteroinferior vomer.

Meningoencephaloceles may appear as a solid and/or fluid-filled mass in the median plane of the nasal cavity, depending on their contents. A nasofrontal type is distinguished from a nasoethmoid type, and each is associated with significant pressure erosion of the displaced bones. Meningoencephaloceles are discussed further on pp. 387, 388, 428 and in Table 4.**14**.

Rare **dermoid cysts** can enter the upper nasal cavity through median clefts, causing bony defects below the frontonasal suture or soft-tissue expansion within the nasal septum.

Nasopalatine cysts are the most common form of intermaxillary fissural nonodontogenic cysts. The cysts probably arise from epithelial rests within the **incisive canal**. They can occur at any age but are most common in the fourth to sixth decades. The cysts are usually asymptomatic but some may cause palatal swelling, especially when located in the incisive papilla. Most of these cysts are small and are detected on routine radiographs. Differentiation from a cyst in the incisive canal is based on an enlarged incisive fossa. An incisive canal cyst is always located on or very near the midline and is usually round or elliptical, occasionally lobulated. It is usually surrounded by a solid cortical rim (Fig. 4.**335**).

Congenital hypoplasias of the nasal bone occur in achondroplasia, congenital syphilis, mucopolysaccharidoses, and other malformation syndromes.

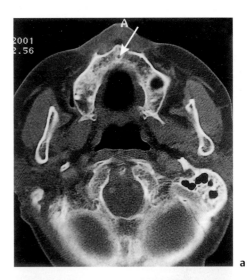

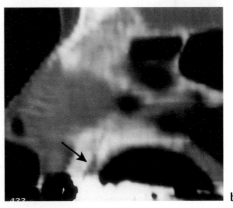

Fig. 4.**335a, b**   Typical appearance of an incisive canal (arrow) without a nasopalatine cyst.
a Axial CT with a bone filter.
b Reformatted sagittal image.

A fluid collection caused by retained secretions in the main nasal cavity can mimic meningocele or encephalocele, but in the typical case it lacks the bony defect that is often found in association with encephaloceles.

Fracture?

Fractures of the nasal bones are often best appreciated in the lateral view. The axial view can also be helpful, since some nasal fractures are not depressed and are manifested only by a lateral offset of the nose, which can be seen only in the axial projection. If differentiation from sutures, vascular grooves, and neural grooves proves difficult, it should be noted that the fracture line is sharper and more distinct and that the normal structures do not extend into the bony nasal dorsum (see Figs. 4.**330** and 4.**336**). When CT is used, it should be considered that any angulation of the nasal skeleton parallel to the scan plane may be missed. Multiplanar reconstructions can be helpful in these infrequent cases.

An avulsion fracture of the **anterior nasal spine** often accompanies fractures of the nasal bones. If the presence of a fracture is uncertain during evaluation of the nasal skeleton, attention should be given to the anterior nasal spine, and therefore this structure should be depicted in lateral views of the nasal skeleton. "Boxer's nose" is a condition resulting from multiple healed fractures with permanent impression of the nasal bones and typical secondary deformity (Fig. 4.**336**).

The nasal fractures that are part of Le Fort II and III midfacial fractures are illustrated in Fig. 4.**325**.

 Necrosis?

Necrosis of the cartilaginous and bony nasal septum, caused in many cases by cocaine abuse, is diagnosed clinically or with CT. Cocaine induces a necrotizing vasculitis followed by granuloma formation in the nasal septum. If the abuse is continued, erosions of the nasal septum will result. There may also be an accompanying, nonspecific in-flammation of the mucosa that is induced not by the cocaine itself but by talcum that has been added to "cut" the drug. Necrosis can have other causes as well:

- Trauma
- Polychondritis
- Chronic inflammatory processes (see also under "Inflammation?" below)
- Irradiation

A typical radiographic sign is fragmentation with very radiodense fragments.

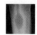 **Inflammation?**

Today the principal tool for evaluating inflammatory changes in the nasal cavity—besides mirror examination by an otolaryngologist—is CT. Coronal CT scans are also excellent for defining the extent of nasal polyposis, which may be associated with changes in the bony structures of the paranasal sinuses (Figs. 4.**337**, 4.**362**, 4.**363**).

Wegener granulomatosis (Fig. 4.**338 a–c**) is a necrotizing, granulomatous vasculitis that most commonly affects the upper and lower respiratory tract and incites a glomerulonephritis. In the limited form, only the sinonasal system is affected. The dominant feature is a chronic, nonspecific inflammation of the nose and paranasal sinuses lasting for 1–2 years. The nasal septum is affected first. The disease may spread, causing ulcerations of the nasal septum and perforations that create a saddle-nose deformity. Additional spread past the nasal septum may occur.

Sarcoidosis (**Boeck disease**) is a systemic disorder marked by the development of noncaseating, epithelioid-cell granulomas. From 3% to 20% of patients show nasal involvement, with multiple small granulomas appearing in the nasal septum and turbinates. Clinical manifestations include nasal airway obstruction, dysesthesia, or epistaxis.

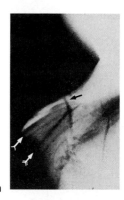
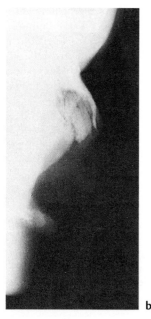

a

b

Fig. 4.**336 a, b**   Fractures of the nasal skeleton.
a Fracture in the nasal skeleton (arrow). Compare with the normal lucent lines of the ethmoid sulcus (tailed arrow) and nasomaxillary suture (two-tailed arrow).
b Repetitive, healed fractures (boxer's nose).

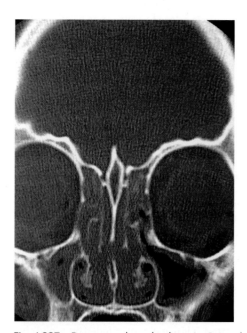

Fig. 4.**337**   Pronounced nasal polyposis. Coronal CT of the paranasal sinuses using a high-resolution bone filter.

The paranasal sinuses are rarely involved. Sarcoidosis generally does not cause destructive changes in the sinonasal system, although portions of the nasal septum or turbinates may occasionally be destroyed (Fig. 4.**338 d–g**). Osteolytic lesions may also develop in the facial skeleton and calvarium.

Several other inflammatory diseases are known:

- Chronic intranasal granulomas caused by beryllium exposure
- Tuberculosis

- Leprosy
- Exposure to chromium salt compounds

Fungal infections of the nose, which often emanate from the paranasal sinuses, can destroy the skeletal portions of the nasal cavity. The cause is a fungus-induced vasculitis that culminates in necrosis of the bone. The most common forms are:

- Aspergillosis (Fig. 4.**364**)
- Mucormycosis (Fig. 4.**364**)
- Candidiasis

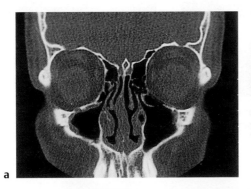
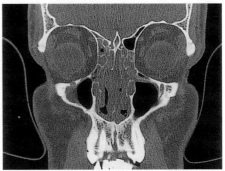
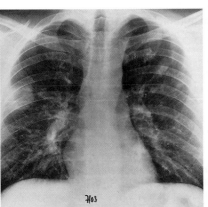
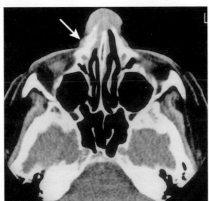
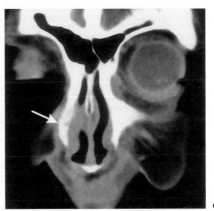
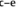
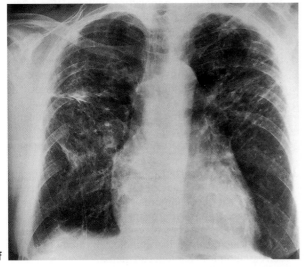
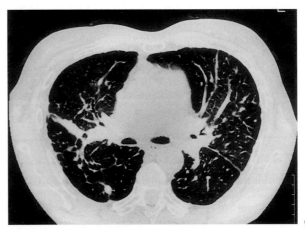

Fig. 4.**338 a–g**   (a–c Wegener's granulomatosis, d–g Sarcoidosis).
a Early Wegener's granulomatosis: only subtle changes within the nasal cavity and paranasal sinuses. At this time, diagnosis could not be determined by histology. Coronal CT with high resolution bone filter.
b Three weeks later without therapy, CT confirmed extensive changes due to Wegener's granulomatosis.
c At the time of b, chest radiograph shows rounded opacities, some with circumscribed cavitations.
d, e Histologically confirmed nasal involvement by sarcoidosis: nonspecific thickening of the nasal soft tissues and in the lateral part of the nasal cavity spreading to the septum. Foci of nasal bone destruction (arrows).
f, g Typical granulomatous and fibrotic pulmonary changes in the same woman as in d and e.

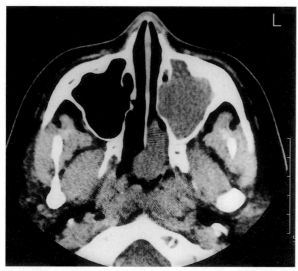
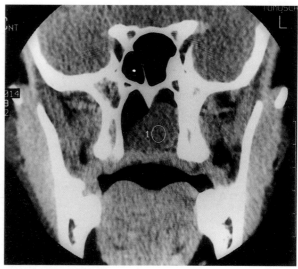

Fig. 4.**339** Nasal airway obstruction in a 12-year-old boy. Axial (**a**) and coronal CT (**b**) demonstrate a choanal polyp on the left side and complete obliteration of the left maxillary sinus.

- Histoplasmosis
- Cryptococcosis
- Coccidioidomycosis
- Blastomycosis
- Rhinosporidiosis

> **Four types of mycotic sinonasal disease** can occur in fungal infections, especially aspergillosis. They are classified as follows based on clinical and pathological criteria:
> 1 Acute, invasive, fulminating disease
> 2 Chronic invasive disease
> 3 Noninvasive fungal colonization (fungus ball)
> 4 Allergic mycotic sinusitis

A **choanal polyp** usually extends from the excretory duct of an opacified maxillary sinus into the nasal cavity and from there into the nasopharynx. It may destroy the lateral wall of the nasal cavity. Most of these polyps can be distinguished from true benign or malignant tumors by their teardrop configuration. If the polyp is not yet fully developed, it may still fill the maxillary sinus and extend into the lateral nasal cavity through an enlarged infundibulum, but at this stage it may be confused with hypertrophic, polypoid antral mucosa. Antrochoanal polyps account for approximately 4–6% of all nasal polyps (Fig. 4.**339**).

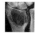 **Tumor?**

Juvenile nasopharyngeal angiofibroma is a benign but aggressive vascular lesion that occurs exclusively in males 5 to 25 years of age. The main clinical symptoms are unilateral nasal obstruction and recurrent spontaneous epistaxis. Plain radiographs show a "mass" in the nasal cavity and nasopharynx, expansion of the pterygopalatine fossa, anterior displacement of the rear wall of the maxillary sinus, erosion of the medial plane of the pterygoid process, and soft tissue in the sphenoid sinus. Sites of bone destruction and enhancing soft-tissue masses are accurately defined by CT and MRI.

The following benign tumor entities occur in the nasal cavity of adults:

- Hemangioma
- Meningioma
- Neurofibroma
- Lipoma
- Osteochondroma

Papilloma is another tumor entity, which occurs in the following forms:

1 **Fungiform papilloma** (50% of all papillomas). This lesion predominantly affects men 20–50 years of age. The nasal septum is affected in 95% of cases. Some 75% of the lesions are solitary, and 95 % are unilateral.
2 **Inverted papilloma** (endophytic papilloma) (Fig. 4.**340**) comprises approximately 45% of all papillomas and occurs predominantly in men 40–70 years of age. These tumors typically develop on the lateral nasal wall near the middle turbinate and usually extend secondarily into the maxillary sinus and ethmoid cells and less commonly into the sphenoid sinus and frontal sinuses. The most common clinical symptoms are nasal airway obstruction, epistaxis, and anosmia. Tumor extension into the sinuses and orbit can cause increasing pain, purulent nasal discharge, proptosis, diplopia, and hypernasal speech.
3 **Carcinoma—exinverted papilloma** is reported in approximately 10–15% of cases. The carcinoma may coexist with inverted papilloma or may develop from it. Most of the tumors are squamous cell carcinomas, but there are also reports of verrucous carcinoma, mucoepidermoid carcinoma, spindle cell carcinoma, clear cell carcinoma, and adenocarcinoma.
4 **Cylindrical cell papillomas** comprise only 3–5% of all papillomas.

Inverted papilloma (Fig. 4.**340**) mainly requires differentiation from chronic polypous pansinusitis (Fig. 4.**337**). But the two entities may be indistinguishable in some cases, even by CT.

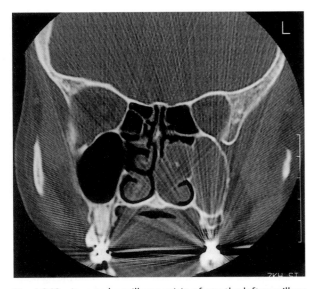

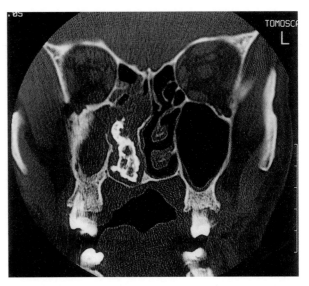

Fig. 4.**340** Inverted papilloma arising from the left maxillary sinus. Coronal CT with a high-resolution bone filter shows complete opacification of the left maxillary sinus, also destruction of the medial sinus wall and spread of the soft-tissue mass to the left nasal cavity.

Fig. 4.**341** Large rhinolith in the right nasal cavity. On histological examination, the original foreign body could no longer be identified.

Other Changes?

Various kinds of foreign bodies are found in the nasal cavity and paranasal sinuses. A **rhinolith**, which in extreme cases may occupy the entire lumen of the main nasal cavity or a paranasal sinus, is produced by a foreign body that has been retained in the nose for a prolonged period. This foreign body serves as a crystallization nucleus, becoming encrusted with mineral salts. The calcified mass may be termed a rhinolith or **sinolith**, depending on whether it is located in the nasal cavity or in a paranasal sinus (Fig. 4.**341**). Differentiation is required from infectious-inflammatory calcifications caused, for example, by *Aspergillus* or *Mucor* species (p. 515, 516, 527 and Fig. 4.**364**).

Paranasal Sinuses

During Growth

Fetal development of the paranasal sinuses begins in the second month of intrauterine life. The paranasal sinuses develop through outgrowth and evagination of the nasal epithelium, starting from the lateral nasal wall. From there the sinuses expand into the maxilla, ethmoid bone, frontal bone, and sphenoid bone. They expand into areas that can accommodate the sinuses—areas where the bone is subject to relatively low functional demands. Postnatal development of the paranasal sinuses proceeds slowly until the sixth or seventh year of life, and then more rapidly until puberty. It is during puberty that the sinuses reach their definitive size.

Imaging the Paranasal Sinuses

To obtain a PA projection of the paranasal sinuses in the prone or sitting patient, the central ray is angled toward the canthomeatal plane so that the petrous ridge is projected at or below the level of the orbital floor. This can be accomplished with the **Caldwell view**, in which the tube is angled 23° caudad and the canthomeatal plane is perpendicular to the film plane (occipitofrontal projection). This affords an extended view of the frontal sinus and ethmoid cells (Fig. 4.**342**). It also gives the best view of the ethmoid–maxillary plate, a diagnostically important curved bony plate that separates the maxillary sinus from the ethmoid.

In the **Waters view** (occipitomental or occipitonasal projection), the beam is horizontal and the head is dorsiflexed so that the petrous ridges are projected into the upper dental arch just below the alveolar recess of the maxilla. This gives an overview of the maxillary sinus, but the ethmoid cells and frontal sinuses are considerably foreshortened (Fig. 4.**342**).

Lateral radiographs are useful for determining the depth of the maxillary and frontal sinuses, localizing polyps and unerupted teeth, and evaluating the hard palate and the posterior soft tissues of the nasopharynx.

> Conventional radiographs, however, cannot exclude even relatively large traumatic and neoplastic processes in the paranasal sinuses, and this casts doubt on their value. The anterior ethmoid cells and the sphenoid sinus are virtually inaccessible to plain film examination.

For this reason, CT or MRI is currently used for evaluating the paranasal sinuses. CT usually begins with coronal scans, supplemented if necessary by axial scans. Next, a high-resolution bone filter is used. Many investigations may also require a soft-tissue filter and window, if necessary with additional intravenous contrast. Spiral CT using thin slices and a small reconstruction increment is particularly useful for reconstructing secondary multiplanar images from the axial scans (Fig. 4.**343**).

With MRI, the paranasal sinuses can be imaged in any desired plane. Options include T1-weighted spin-echo sequences before and after contrast administration and T2-weighted sequences with and without fat suppression, depending on the nature of the study (Fig. 4.**344**).

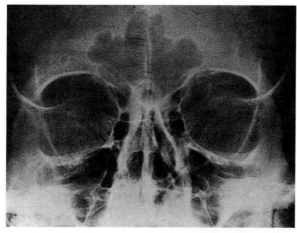

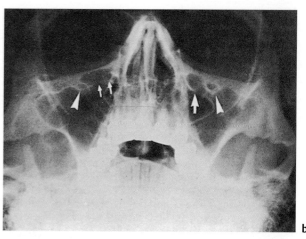

Fig. 4.**342 a, b**   Occipitofrontal and occipitonasal projections. **a** Occipitofrontal projection. The petrous ridges are projected below the infraorbital margin and orbital floor (Caldwell's view).

b Occipitonasal projection with the mouth open. The petrous ridges are projected below the alveolar process of the maxilla (Waters view). Note also the periorbital air cell on the right side (small arrows), the left infraorbital recess (large arrow), and the infraorbital foramen on each side (arrowheads).

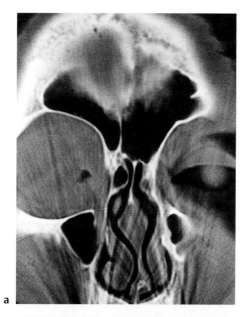

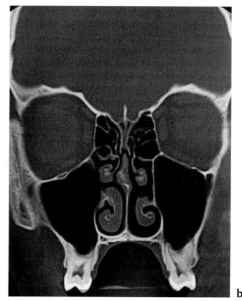

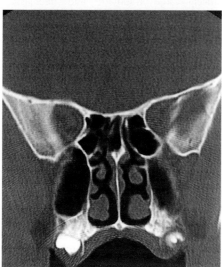

Fig. 4.**343 a–c**   Frontal sinuses, ethmoid labyrinth, maxillary sinuses, and anterior portions of the sphenoid sinus. Coronal CT with a high-resolution bone filter.

Fig. 4.**344** T1-weighted coronal MRI at the level of the posterior margin of the globe.
1 Globe
2 Ethmoid cells
3 Middle turbinate and nasal septum
4 Inferior turbinate
5 Maxillary sinus
6 Polyp on lateral wall of maxillary sinus

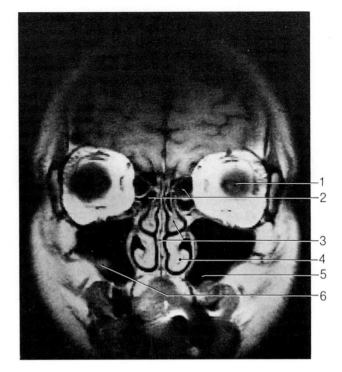

Maxillary Sinus

Normal Findings

During Growth

The maxillary sinuses, which are mere slits adjacent to the lateral nasal wall after birth, develop within several months into small triangular cavities. They are always demonstrable by 12 months of age, and by 5 years they extend approximately to the infraorbital foramen. They reach their definitive size at 15–18 years of age (Fig. 4.**345**).

In Adulthood

Except for the alveolar recesses, the maxillary sinuses show little individual variation in size and shape compared with the rest of the paranasal sinuses, and they tend to be fairly symmetrical between the two sides.

Axial and especially coronal CT scans provide nonsuperimposed views of the paranasal sinuses that depict their anatomy and relationships more clearly than conventional radiographs. Because of sinus anatomy, it is often impossible for projection radiographs to demonstrate even gross mucosal and bony changes. A normal-appearing conventional radiograph of the maxillary sinuses does not exclude a pathological process.

The lateral recess of the maxillary sinus is narrow posteriorly and widens anteriorly to form the **zygomatic recess**. Because of the variable width of the lateral recess, the lateral boundary of the maxillary sinus appears in the frontal projection as a pair of vertical ridges with a dense intervening area (Fig. 4.**346**). This normal finding is apt to be misinterpreted as mucosal opacity on the sinus wall.

The medial superior recess of the maxillary sinus may contain a chamber, extending from the upper part of the sinus, called the **infraorbital recess**. Located at the junction of the sinus with the ethmoid labyrinth, this recess is difficult or impossible to distinguish from an ethmoid cell on plain radiographs (Figs. 4.**342**, 4.**347**). CT greatly facilitates or enables the differentiation of the various air cells and variants in this region.

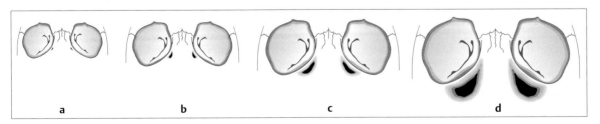

Fig. 4.**345 a–d** Development of the maxillary sinuses.
a 16 days.
b 9 months.
c 5 years.
d 12 years.

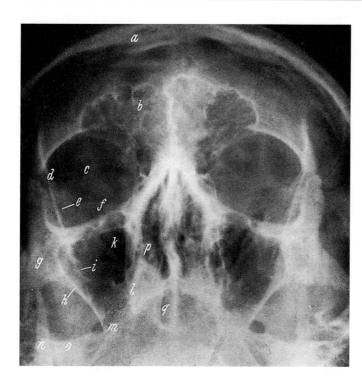

Fig. 4.**346**   Occipitonasal projection.
a   Superimposed convolutional markings in the frontal bone and/or hyperostosis frontalis interna
b   Frontal sinus: mottled opacification in chronic sinusitis
c   Orbit
d   Frontozygomatic suture
e   Innominate line
f   Infraorbital foramen
g   Zygoma
h   Lateral wall of anterior maxillary sinus
i   Lateral wall of posterior maxillary sinus
k   Inferior orbital fissure
l   Foramen rotundum
m   Foramen ovale
n   Coronoid process of mandible
o   Petrous bone
p   Ethmoid cells
q   Sphenoid sinus

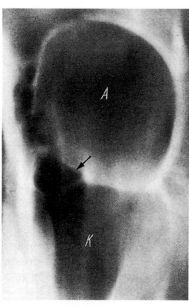

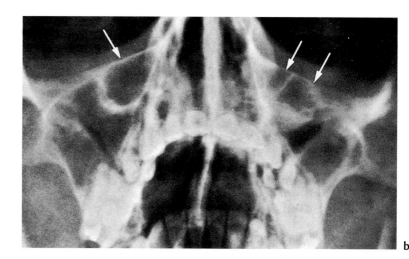

Fig. 4.**347 a, b**   Periorbital air cells.
a   Conventional tomogram. The air cell between the ethmoid and maxillary sinus (arrow) may be an ethmoid bulla or a Haller cell. This differentiation can be accomplished with CT.
A   Orbit
K   Maxillary sinus

b   Maxillary sinus with periorbital cells, which show inflammatory changes on the left side (arrows).

Although most **variant air cells** arise from the ethmoid system, they are discussed here because of their proximity to other paranasal sinuses, including the maxillary sinus. Some of these cells are relevant in the planning of surgical procedures.

The ethmoid cells are subdivided into an anterior and a posterior group. The anterior ethmoid cells drain into the middle meatus of the nasal cavity, the posterior cells into the superior meatus. The **ethmoid bulla** (Fig. 4.**348 d**) is the most commonly encountered anterior ethmoid cell and is also the largest. The **agger nasi** is a bony ridge or promi-

nence arising from the frontal process of the maxilla. It may be pneumatized in varying degrees by **agger nasi cells** that arise from the anterior ethmoid. As a result, its wall may be thick or thin. The most anterior cells of the ethmoid are called agger nasi cells, and the most posterior cells are called **Onodi cells** (Fig. 4.**348 c**). They may extend posteriorly and laterally to the optic nerve or may even encase the nerve. They may migrate into the body of the sphenoid bone and may even reach the anterior wall of the sella turcica.

Haller cells are ethmoid cells that extend in the orbital floor to a point near the ostium of the maxillary sinus.

Fig. 4.**348 a–d**
a Superior orbital fissure (arrows) and periorbital cells or Haller cells (tailed arrows) at the infraorbital foramen (two-tailed arrow). Conventional radiograph.
b Pneumatization of the left orbital floor extending to the infraorbital foramen, Haller cell (arrow). High-resolution coronal CT.
c Large posterior ethmoid cells have developed posterolaterally and are larger on the right side than on the left (Onodi cell, arrow). Dorsally, other slices showed a direct relation of this cell to the optic canal. High-resolution coronal CT.
d Ethmoid bulla (arrow). High-resolution coronal CT.

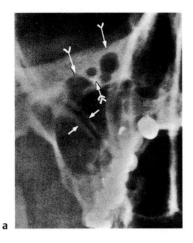
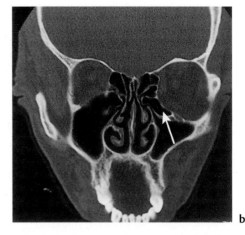
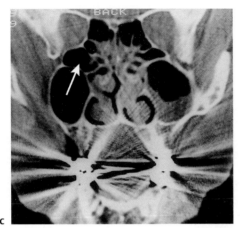
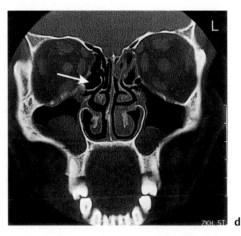

When enlarged, they can narrow the ethmoid infundibulum and maxillary sinus outlet. The cells are clearly visualized by coronal CT (Fig. 4.**348 b**). The origin of Haller cells is uncertain. Most of these cells open into the middle meatus, and so they can be classified by their origin as ethmoid cells. Haller cells may pneumatize the orbital floor to a variable degree, and some of the cells may be grouped around the infraorbital canal.

The **ostiomeatal complex** consists of the following structures:

- **Ostium of the maxillary sinus**
- **Ethmoid infundibulum**
- **Semilunar hiatus**
- **Frontal recess**
- **Ethmoid bulla**
- **Uncinate process**

> The ostiomeatal complex forms a common end-path for drainage from the frontal and maxillary sinuses and the anterior ethmoid cells.

During growth, the superomedial portion of the **maxillary antrum** directly adjoins the infraorbital foramen, which moves laterally with increasing pneumatization of the maxillary sinus until it reaches its definitive adult position. The roof of the maxillary sinus is the floor of the orbit (Fig. 4.**310**). Three horizontal contour lines are often seen at this level:

- The soft-tissue line above the orbital floor
- The infraorbital margin and anterior orbital floor

- The deepest part of the orbital floor (seen in tangential view)

The lateral wall of the maxillary sinus sometimes contains a **posterior superior alveolar canal**, whose foramen may appear in an end-on view (Fig. 4.**349**).

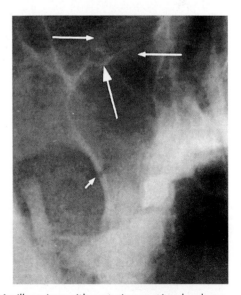

Fig. 4.**349** Maxillary sinus with posterior superior alveolar canal (small arrow on outer wall of maxillary sinus), infraorbital canal and infraorbital foramen (long arrow with larger head pointing upward and outward), periorbital cells (horizontal arrows).

The alveolar recess of the maxilla is separated from the dental alveoli by a layer of cancellous bone. The thickness of this bone is highly variable, ranging from a bulging sinus floor that extends far into the alveolar process to a shallow alveolar recess that is separated from the dental alveoli by a thick layer of cancellous bone. In children who still have permanent tooth buds, this normal finding can easily be misinterpreted as an abnormal density.

A soft-tissue shadow from the upper lip or mustache is occasionally superimposed over the alveolar recess, maxillary sinus, or both (Fig. 4.**350**).

The soft tissues of the nasal alae can mimic polyps arising from the medial wall of the maxillary sinus. In the lateral view, the coronoid process of the mandible can also be mistaken for an intrasinus polyp.

The **foramen rotundum** has a characteristic appearance on radiographs (Fig. 4.**351**). In some projections the foramina ovale and spinosum can occasionally be seen above the petrous ridge (Figs. 4.**346**, 4. **352**). The pterygoid canal (Vidian canal) can additionally be identified on axial and coronal CT scans (Fig. 4.**353**).

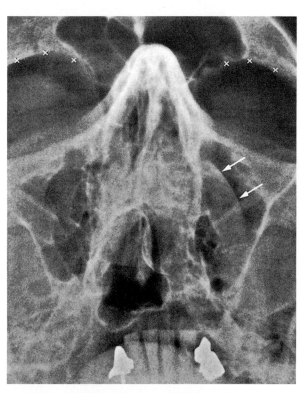

Fig. 4.**350**   Partial opacification of the left maxillary sinus by a raised lip (arrows) pressed against the edentulous maxilla. Intraorbital fat pad (×) appears as a crescent-shaped lucent zone below the orbital roof.

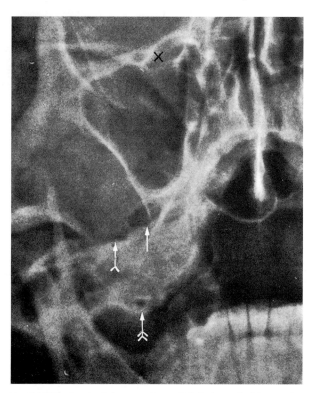

Fig. 4.**352**   Semiaxial projection, slightly lateral oblique, demonstrates the foramen ovale (arrow), foramen spinosum (tailed arrow), and hypoglossal nerve canal (two-tailed arrow) below the petrous bone. Periorbital air cell (×).

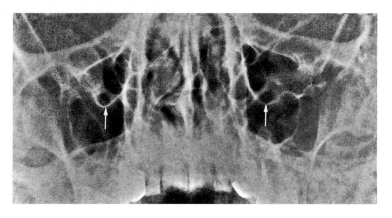

Fig. 4.**351**   Foramen rotundum on both sides (arrows).

Fig. 4.**353**   Vidian canal (arrowhead) in the floor of the sphe- ▷
noid sinus. Coronal CT with a high-resolution bone filter (see
also Fig. 4.**129**).

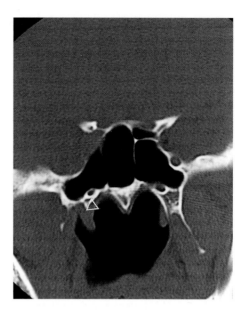

▌ Pathological Finding?

Normal Variant/Anomaly?

Variants

The bony walls of the maxillary sinus, especially the facial
or medial wall, may bulge into the sinus interior, reducing
the size of the cavity. When this occurs unilaterally, or when
there is unilateral deficient pneumatization of a maxillary
sinus, facial asymmetry can result. A small maxillary sinus
that contains little air appears darker on radiographs compared with the normal side, and its floor is elevated
(Figs. 4.**354**, 4.**355**). The complete **absence** of one or both
maxillary sinuses is still considered a normal variant. It is
much less common than absence of one or both frontal
sinuses and should not be misinterpreted as the total opacification of an air space. **Hypoplasia** of the maxillary sinuses
represents deficient pneumatization, that normally begins
near the antrum, the degree of which is proportional to the
degree of medialization of the infraorbital foramen.

  Pneumosinus dilatans (Fig. 4.**367**) of the maxillary
sinus refers to an externally visible bulging of the nasal
recess. It is a harmless variant whose cause is not fully understood. The pneumosinus dilatans may be the result of
inhibition of growth of neighboring structures (e.g. the
frontal cerebrum, Fig. 4.**354**). Partial or complete subdivision of the maxillary sinuses into one or more chambers by
bony ridges or **septa** is very difficult to detect on conventional radiographs but is clearly demonstrated by CT. Septa
are a common finding, particularly in the alveolar recess.

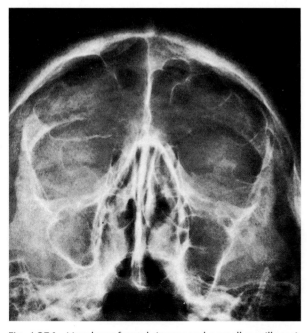

Fig. 4.**354**   Very large frontal sinuses and a small maxillary sinus on the right side.

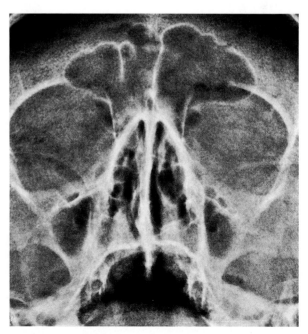

Fig. 4.**355**   Underdevelopment of both maxillary sinuses in a
patient with normal-size frontal sinuses.

The presence of septa in the paranasal sinuses can be an important factor in surgical planning.

Heterotopic tooth buds in the maxillary sinus usually consist of dystopic molars and premolars.

Anomalies

Maxillonasal dysplasia (Binder syndrome) is an anomaly that is transitional with arhinencephaly. Radiographs show a premaxillary hypoplasia with basal flattening of the maxilla, aplasia or hypoplasia of the anterior nasal spine, hypoplasia of the frontal sinuses, and pseudoprognathism. These anomalies are often associated with malformations of the cervical spine and concomitant deformities of the facial bones, especially the jaws. Other combinations of typical facial anomalies with spinal malformations are found in hemifacial microsomia, mandibulofacial dysplasia, and the craniofacial dysplasias.

Palatal clefts result from faulty development of the embryonic frontonasal process or its failure to fuse with adjacent structures. A variety of developmental anomalies of the nasomedial process and nasolateral process culminate in the various forms of cleft lip and palate. Associated deformities of the facial skeleton, including hypoplasias of the nose and paranasal sinuses, are frequent and are best demonstrated by CT.

 Fracture?

Midfacial fractures and the Le Fort classification were covered on p. 508, 509 and in Fig. 4.**325**. As the figure indicates, all the Le Fort fractures may involve the pterygoid process.

Two special types of midfacial fracture warrant separate discussion:

The **palatoalveolar fracture** (Fig. 4.**356**) involves both the alveolar process and the palatine process of the maxilla. Extension of the fracture into the alveoli often causes tooth displacement.

The **zygomaticomaxillary fracture** (tripod fracture, trimalar fracture, "three-pillar fracture") is the most common type of midfacial fracture. By definition, this zygomatic fracture involves the bony separation of all the pillars of the zygoma (frontal process, infraorbital process, alveolar and temporal processes) (Fig. 4.**357**). (The fracture lines in the infraorbital and alveolar processes are often considered as one, accounting for the term "three-pillar fracture.") The usual causal mechanism is localized trauma to the body of the zygoma. Primary evaluation of the injury is assisted by Waters and Caldwell views. CT accurately defines the fracture pattern and gives information on associated injuries. It should be added that the fracture line in the lateral orbital wall does not necessarily pass through the frontozygomatic suture. The fracture may also run above it (through the orbital process of the frontal bone) or below it (through the frontal process of the zygoma). If

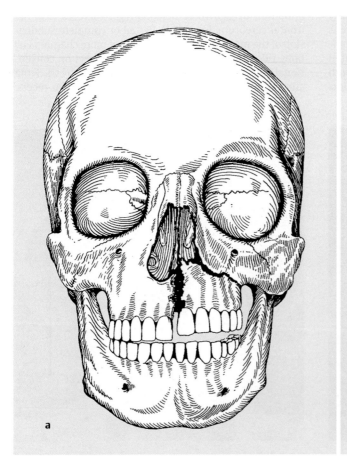

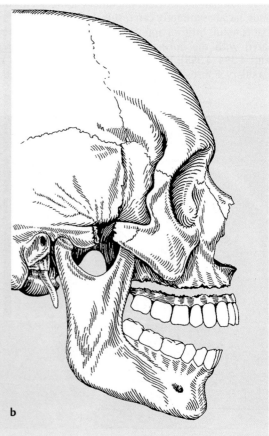

Fig. 4.**356 a, b**   Palatoalveolar fracture (after Birzle et al.).

Fig. 4.**357** Zygomaticomaxillary (tripod) fracture (after Rogers).
1 Dehiscence of the frontozygomatic suture
2 Fracture of the zygomatic arch
3 Fracture of the infraorbital margin extending through the anterior and lateral walls of the maxillary sinus

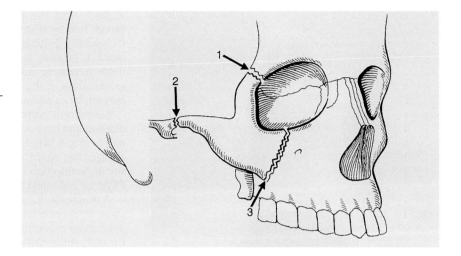

forces are transmitted through the medial or lateral orbital wall when the injury is sustained, the fracture may extend to the orbital apex and cause orbital nerve complications. The clinical features consist of periorbital and subconjunctival hemorrhage with edema, crepitus, and paresthesia in the cheek.

Teeth may become displaced in maxillary fractures that involve the alveolar process. With fractures involving the maxillary sinuses, radiographs generally show sinus clouding due to intrasinus hematoma and swelling of the overlying soft tissues.

Inflammation?

Inflammatory secretions and thickening of the maxillary sinus mucosa produce the radiographic findings of **maxillary sinusitis**. When sinus radiographs are taken in an acute stage in the supine patient, the exudate in the affected maxillary sinus causes homogeneous sinus clouding due to the paucity of air (Fig. 4.**358**). When radiographs are taken in an upright posture, an air–fluid level appears (as with a posttraumatic hematoma) as the fluid layer gravitates below the air (Figs. 4.**358**, 4.**359**).

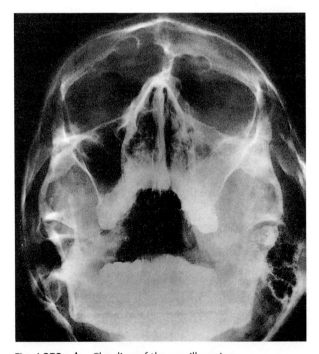

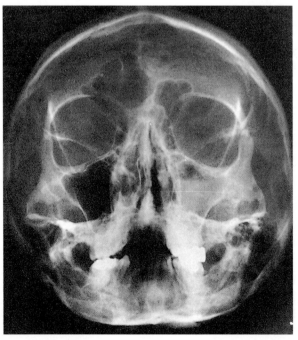

Fig. 4.**358 a, b** Clouding of the maxillary sinus.
a Homogeneous clouding of the left maxillary sinus in the supine patient.

b Fluid level in the left maxillary sinus of the same patient filmed in an upright position.

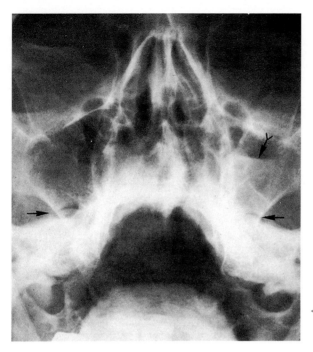

Aside from the air–fluid level sign, plain radiographs cannot reliably discriminate among acute and chronic inflammatory, polypous, or neoplastic changes in the sinus mucosa. In many cases this can be accomplished much more accurately with CT (Figs. 4.360–4.363). Ultrasound examination of the paranasal sinuses is also mentioned, but only as an adjunct.

Submucous, serous cysts may persist following inflammations and have much the same radiographic features as polyps (Fig. 4.361). Unlike polyps, however, the cysts may change their shape when the patient is repositioned. The site of predilection is the floor of the maxillary sinus. The CT density of solid cysts is close to water attenuation.

A **mucocele** is a somewhat rare entity in the maxillary sinus. When infected, it is called a pyocele. Typically it appears as an expansile mass that "balloons" the bone, thins the bony sinus walls, and may cause bone erosion.

◁ Fig. 4.**359** Left maxillary sinusitis with a fluid level (tailed arrow). The small crescents (arrows) above the petrous bones (projected into the maxillary sinuses) are Mach effects.

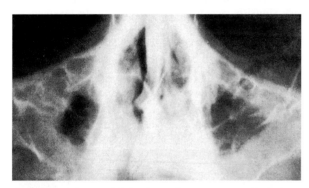

Fig. 4.**360** Chronic, bilateral maxillary sinusitis with thickening of the mucosa.

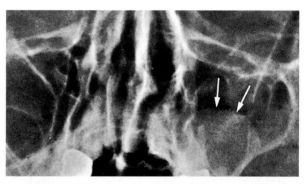

Fig. 4.**361** Mucosal polyp on the floor of the left maxillary sinus (arrows).

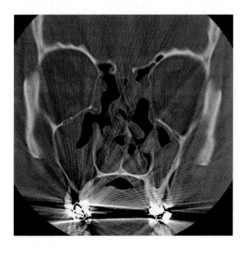

Fig. 4.**362** Recurrent polyposis following endoscopic paranasal sinus surgery. Coronal CT with a high-resolution bone filter.

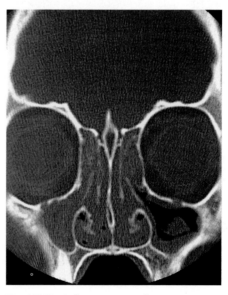

Fig. 4.**363** Inflammatory polyps appear as soft-tissue opacities within the paranasal sinuses. Coronal CT with a high-resolution bone filter.

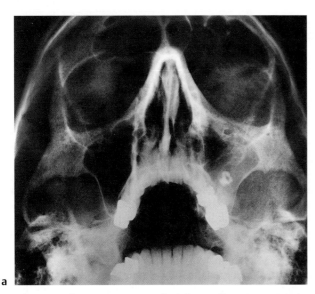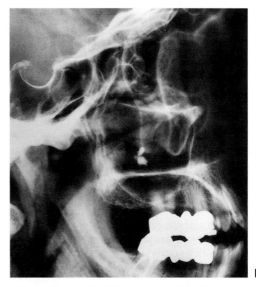

a   b

Fig. 4.**364a, b**　Typical mucormycosis in the left maxillary sinus with deposits of metallic density. The patient is diabetic.

Surgical procedures on the paranasal sinuses leave behind typical CT findings. The radical **Caldwell–Luc operation** leaves a typical defect in the medial wall of the maxillary sinus. Functional paranasal sinus surgery causes expansion of the ostiomeatal unit (Fig. 4.**362**).

Chronic inflammatory processes often incite a reactive sclerosis of the maxillary sinus walls that is detectable even on conventional radiographs. With aggressive inflammations that involve the zygomatic recess and/or the roof of the maxillary sinus (orbital floor), cortical bone is lost and replaced by osteomyelitic lesions with sequestra.

Like chronic inflammatory changes, severe iron deficiency anemia of long duration leads to deficient pneumatization of the paranasal sinuses with broadening and thickening of the bone.

While granulomatous diseases such as tuberculosis, Langerhans cell histiocytosis, and sarcoidosis very rarely affect the maxillary sinus walls and are indistinguishable from nonspecific inflammations on radiographs, **Wegener granulomatosis** (Fig. 4.**338**) is associated with rapidly progressive destruction of the sinus walls. Clouding of the maxillary sinuses is often the only initial finding, however.

In **mucormycosis**, extremely dense opacities may be seen in the basal portions of the maxillary sinuses. They are caused by opportunistic fungi of the order Mucorales, ubiquitous organisms that are inhaled into the nasopharynx with environmental dust. Rhinocerebral mucormycosis occurs predominantly in diabetics. Metabolic products from the fungi account for the high density of the opacities (Fig. 4.**364**). Comparable findings are seen in **Aspergillus** infections of the paranasal sinuses.

 Tumor?

Primordial cysts that develop from enamel cells prior to tooth development as well as odontogenic, follicular **dental cysts** that contain tooth crowns occur toward the end of the secondary dentition. They may occupy part or all of the maxillary sinus and may cause pressure erosion of its walls

(Fig. 4.**365**). The more common **radicular cysts**, seen mainly in older patients and at multiple sites, arise from apical root granulomas.

Osteomas are recognized by their very high density.

In **fibrous dysplasia**, the normal bone is generally replaced by deformed fiber bone showing a ground-glass or honeycombed osseous structure (see pp. 401–403 and Tables 4.**13**, 4.**15**). Fibrous dysplasia of the facial skeleton mainly require differentiation from Paget disease (see pp. 401–403, 443, 444).

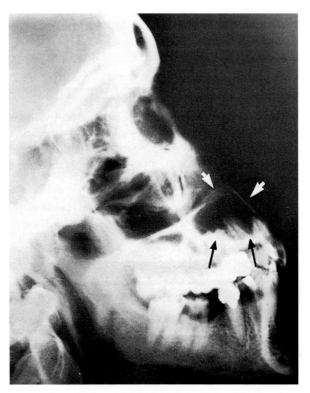

Fig. 4.**365**　Large cyst in the anterior portion of the maxillary sinus (arrows).

Frontal Sinus

Normal Findings

During Growth

Embryologically, the frontal sinus is a specialized anterior ethmoid cell that drains directly into the middle meatus or indirectly into the upper part of the semilunar hiatus. It is not present at birth. It begins as an outpouching of the nasal mucosa into the diploe of the frontal bone between the 2nd and 4th years of life. It extends half the height of the orbit in the 4th year, reaches the level of the orbital roof by the 8th year, and transcends it through vertical growth into the frontal bone at 10 years of age. The frontal sinus attains its definitive size by 20 years of age. Small frontal sinus cavities in children, especially at the level of the orbital margin, may represent well-developed ethmoid cells or an initial stage of frontal sinus development.

In Adulthood

The frontal sinuses show marked individual differences in their development. They can range in size from barely perceptible spaces to extremely large cavities in **pneumosinus dilatans** (Fig. 4.**367e**). Asymmetries, asymmetrical septations, and a very thin or absent fibrous septum located off the midline may be encountered. With age-related atrophic changes, the bony structures separating the frontal sinus and orbit may seem to disappear, creating an apparent communication between the two cavities.

Pathological Finding?

Normal Variant/Anomaly?

Variants

A large **supraorbital recess** that extends into the orbital roof (Fig. 4.**366**) is considered a normal finding, as is extension of the frontal sinus into the frontal squama (Fig. 4.**367a**). Pneumatization that arises from the frontal sinus and extends beyond the anatomic boundaries of the frontal bone into adjacent bones is considered a normal variant in the pneumatization of this paranasal sinus.

The detection of **septa** that compartmentalize the frontal sinus in varying degrees is an important factor in the planning of endoscopic sinus surgery (Fig. 4.**367b–d**). The best modality for defining these septa is CT, which will also show any opacities within loculated spaces (Fig. 4.**368**).

Anomalies and Deformities

Unilateral or bilateral absence of the frontal sinus is still within the borderline-normal range. Hypoplasia or aplasia of the frontal sinus can also occur in several syndromes:

- **Kartagener syndrome (dyskinetic cilia syndrome):** dyskinesia of the ciliated respiratory epithelium with underdevelopment of the paranasal sinuses, usually cylindrical bronchiectasis, and other anomalies such as visceral transposition with dextrocardia and cardiovascular anomalies.
- **Cystic fibrosis.** Chronic sinusitis is one manifestation of this systemic disease (which may also involve the pancreas, liver, bowel, respiratory tract, and sweat glands). Aplasia or hypoplasia of the frontal sinus is not uncommon. Mucoceles are also relatively common due to the impaired drainage of secretions.
- Marfan syndrome.
- Trisomy 21.

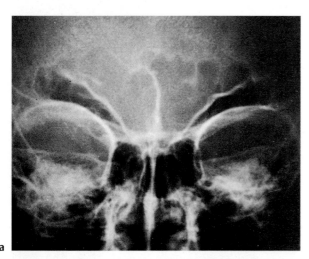
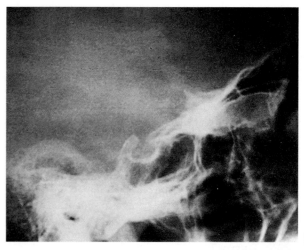

Fig. 4.**366**   Supraorbital recess.
a PA projection.
b Lateral projection.

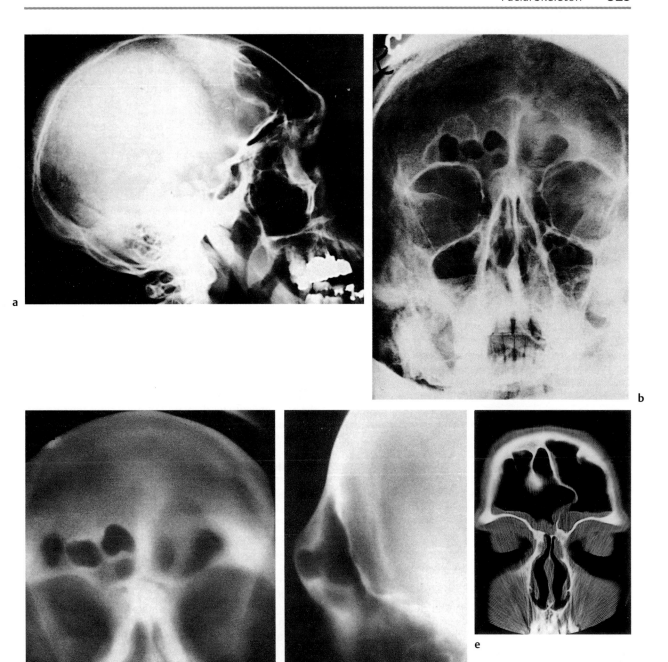

Fig. 4.**367 a–e**
a Lateral skull radiograph. The pneumatization of the frontal sinuses extends into the frontal squama.
b PA radiograph. The considerable extension of the frontal sinus in depth, especially toward the right side, accounts for the increased radiolucency.

c, d Conventional biplane tomograms define the depth of the frontal sinus.
e Pneumosinus dilatans of the frontal sinus is detected incidentally by coronal CT in a different patient. Basal mucosal swelling is also noted.

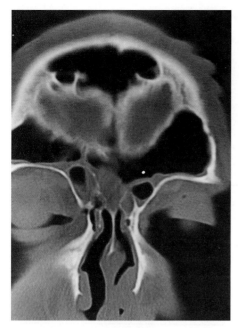

Fig. 4.**368**   Large frontal sinus with soft-tissue densities in its basal portions. Accessory bony septa produce distinct loculations within the frontal sinus. Some are filled with solid tissue. Coronal CT with a high-resolution bone filter.

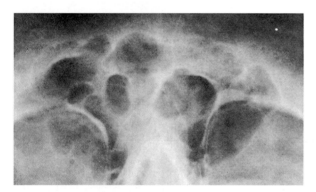
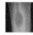

Fig. 4.**369**   Multiloculated frontal sinus in chronic frontal sinusitis.

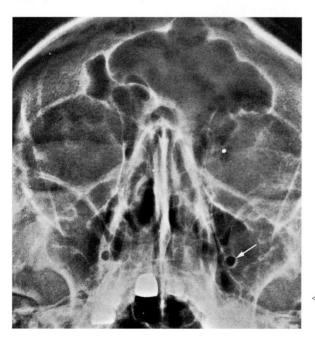

Hyperpneumatization (Fig. 4.**368**) can occur in the following syndromes, anomalies, and diseases:

- **Cerebral hemiatrophy** (see Fig. 4.**28**) may be associated with unilateral enlargement of the frontal sinus. This is a secondary phenomenon caused by compensatory dilatation of the sinus to fill the empty space.
- A compensatory, space-occupying hyperpneumatization of the facial skeleton and skull base in microcephaly can lead to abnormally large, symmetrical frontal sinuses.
- Acromegaly.
- Sturge–Weber syndrome.

Fracture?

Isolated fractures of the frontal sinus usually occur as **linear fractures** of the anterior sinus wall. **Combined fractures** of the anterior and posterior sinus walls are not uncommon, however. The anterior and/or posterior sinus walls are also commonly involved in injuries of the anterior cranial fossa, orbit, or nasoethmoid complex. Bleeding into the frontal sinus appears radiographically as an air–fluid level in the sitting patient and as sinus clouding in the supine patient. The differential diagnosis should include retained secretions due to an inflammatory condition. CT is the best modality for detecting a frontal sinus fracture and defining its extent.

Inflammation?

Swelling of the mucosa in frontal sinusitis may appear as mucosal thickening along the sinus wall or along septa within the sinus or as hemispherical or polypous soft-tissue swellings, which are usually demonstrated much better by CT than conventional radiographs. CT can also define the air–fluid level of exudate in acute frontal sinusitis with greater clarity than plain radiographs.

A special form of acute frontal sinusitis is **Pott's puffy tumor** (named for the famed eighteenth century English surgeon). The lesion consists of a soft-tissue swelling at the center of the forehead caused by a subgaleal abscess secondary to frontal sinusitis. Septic thrombosis of the perforating veins can apparently cause the abscess. Osteomyelitis is not necessarily present in the frontal bone itself.

With chronic frontal sinusitis that develops in the setting of a very slowly progressive osteitis, the margins of the frontal sinus become denser and less distinct, and a distinctive mottled pattern can develop (Fig. 4.**369**).

A thick, sclerotic anterior wall can occur as a normal variant in the frontal sinus and can mimic an inflammatory density on plain radiographs. Differentiation is required from a previous, unnoticed episode of sinusitis that incited a reactive hyperostosis of the surrounding bone. A confident differentiation cannot be made from plain radiographs, but CT scans showing mixed resorptive and reactive hyperostotic changes, possibly combined with small bony sequestra, provide evidence of a prior inflammation. A **mucocele** or **pyocele** of the frontal sinus is often very difficult to detect on conventional radiographs (Fig. 4.**370**).

◁ Fig. 4.**370**   Mucocele of the left frontal sinus, manifested only indirectly by expansion of the sinus contour, especially on the right side. Arrow: foramen rotundum.

Tumor?

Polypous densities can occur in the frontal sinus as in other paranasal sinuses and are easily identified on CT scans.

Classic **osteoma** of the skull occurs almost exclusively in cranial bones that have been preformed in connective tissue, particularly the outer table of the calvarium and the frontal and ethmoid sinuses. Very rarely it is found in the sphenoid sinus. Osteoma is a round, oval, or lobulated tumor that usually is extremely dense due to the newly formed bone, which contrasts sharply with its surroundings (Figs. 4.**371**, 4.**372**). Some tumors also show an annular configuration with mostly peripheral ossification. Tumors in the frontal sinus region that are associated with extensive sclerosis require differentiation from reactive hyperostosis due to meningioma and from chronic sclerosing osteomyelitis. The osteoma and its origin in one of the paranasal sinuses are generally well depicted on axial and coronal CT scans. Also, MRI can demonstrate the "tail sign" of reactive hyperostosis that is associated with a bone-infiltrating meningioma.

Two main types of osteoma are distinguished:

- Primary spherical osteomas no larger than pea-size (Fig. 4.**372**).
- Large, lobulated osteomas that arises from remnants of the ethmoid cartilage and invade the frontal sinus from the ethmoid. Occasionally this type may also show intraorbital extension.

Ethmoid Cells

Normal Findings

 During Growth

Slitlike ethmoid cells are already present in the newborn. They are detectable on radiographs at 6 months of age, and by one year they reach twice their size at parturition. The system of ethmoid air cells, called the ethmoid labyrinth, continues to develop swiftly and is fully developed by 16 years of age.

 In Adulthood

The ethmoid cells are highly variable in size and number and are often asymmetrical between the sides. Generally the cells become larger in the anterior-to-posterior direction. The ethmoid bone is divided into two halves by the **perpendicular plate** and is situated between the orbits. Its cribriform plate fits into the ethmoid notch of the frontal bone. The ethmoid labyrinth is bounded medially by the lateral wall of the nasal cavity and laterally by the medial boundaries of the orbit. These laminae papyraceae diverge slightly posteriorly and inferiorly.

The semiaxial Waters view can give a clear projection of the anterior part of the laminae papyraceae and the anterior ethmoid cells.

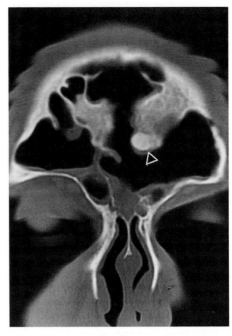

Fig. 4.**371**   Small osteoma (arrowhead) of the left frontal sinus. Coronal CT with a high-resolution bone filter.

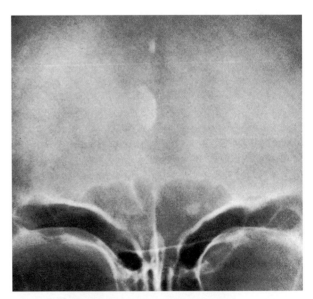

Fig. 4.**372**   Osteoma of the left frontal sinus. Orthograde projection of the supraorbital recess of both frontal sinuses. Typical ossification of the falx cerebri is noted on the midline above the frontal sinuses.

Pneumatization of the following structures can proceed from the ethmoid labyrinth:

- The middle turbinate may be pneumatized in its anterior or posterior portion. The resulting air cell is called the **concha bullosa** (Fig. 4.**373**).
- The **agger nasi** is a bony ridge or protuberance in the frontal process of the maxilla (Fig. 4.**1**). It is located in front of the anterior base of the middle turbinate. The agger nasi may be pneumatized in varying degrees by agger nasi cells of the anterior ethmoid, and consequently its wall may be thick or thin.

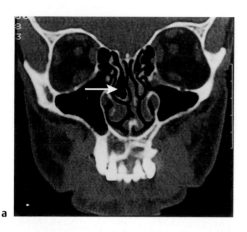
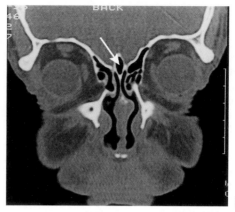

Fig. 4.**373 a, b**   Coronal CT of the paranasal sinuses using a high-resolution bone filter to exclude sinusitis.
a Concha bullosa (bullous middle turbinate) (arrow).
b Pneumatized crista galli (arrow).

- The **uncinate process** is a delicate bony layer located directly behind the agger nasi.
- The **crista galli** projects upward from the cribriform plate into the cranial cavity in the median plate. It is frequently pneumatized (Fig. 4.**473 b**). The bony process gives attachment to the falx cerebri.
- Portions of the lesser sphenoid wing are also frequently pneumatized, especially the **anterior clinoid process** (Fig. 4.**186**). The ethmoid bulla is the largest of the anterior ethmoid cells and is often detectable on radio-

graphs. It shows varying degrees of pneumatization (Fig. 4.**348 d**). It may be so small that it is replaced by a mere bony ring.

Other aspects of ethmoid pneumatization (Haller cells, Onodi cells) were reviewed on p. 520 and in Fig. 4.**348 a–d**. Axial and/or coronal CT can provide detailed, nonsuperimposed views of the ethmoid labyrinth (Fig. 4.**374**). Plain radiographs are wholly inadequate for this purpose, and conventional tomograms are obsolete by current standards.

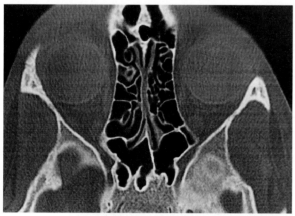
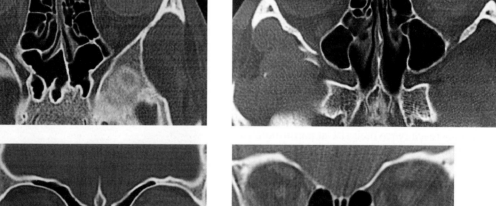
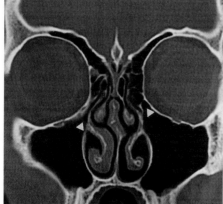
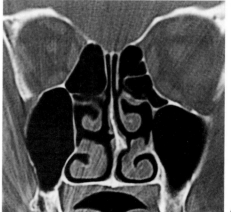

Fig. 4.**374 a–d**   CT imaging of the ethmoid labyrinth.
a Axial CT with a high-resolution bone filter. Cranial portion of the ethmoid labyrinth.
b Axial CT with a high-resolution bone filter. Basal portions of the ethmoid labyrinth.

c Coronal CT with a high-resolution bone filter. Anterior to central portions of the ethmoid labyrinth. The ethmoid infundibulum is visible on both sides (arrowheads).
d Coronal CT with a high-resolution bone filter. Posterior portions of the ethmoid labyrinth. The nasal septum is deviated toward the left side.

Pathological Finding?

Normal Variant/Anomaly?

Variants

Of all the paranasal sinuses, the ethmoid labyrinth is most rarely hypoplastic or aplastic. Complete **aplasia** of all the paranasal sinuses including the ethmoid is extremely rare. On the other hand, given the large number of ethmoid cells and the diversity of their size and shape, the variability of the ethmoid labyrinth is greater than that of any other paranasal sinus. Variants in the pneumatization of the agger nasi, middle turbinate, crista galli, special cells (Onodi, Haller), and the lesser sphenoid wing were discussed on pp. 520, 534.

Changes in the size of the ethmoid cells can result from changes in nearby structures during growth. For example, the dilatation of ethmoid cells occurs in cerebral hemiatrophy (Fig. 4.**28**) and also following enucleation or orbital exenteration in a growing patient.

Anomalies and Deformities

Bilateral dilatation of the ethmoid labyrinth with hypertelorism can result from abnormalities of cranial development. A small ethmoid labyrinth with hypotelorism is much less common, occurring for example in trisomy 13 or trisomy 20.

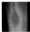

Fracture?

Le Fort II and III midfacial fractures extend through the ethmoid bone. The current diagnostic modality of choice for these injuries is CT. **Posttraumatic CSF leak** can be detected and localized by CT or occasionally by CSF radionuclide imaging.

Inflammation?

At one time, isolated inflammatory disease of the ethmoid labyrinth went undetected in conventional radiographic studies, but today they are detected with high sensitivity by CT (Fig. 4.**375**). In many cases even CT is unable to distinguish between a mucocele and pyocele (Fig. 4.**376**).

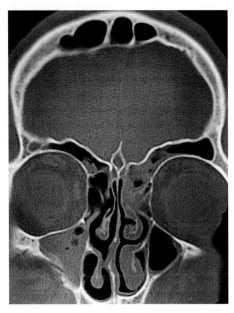

Fig. 4.**375**   Opacities in the ethmoid labyrinth, more conspicuous on the left side, are caused by inflammatory exudate and inflammatory swelling of the mucosa. Coronal CT with a high-resolution bone filter. There is also extensive clouding of the right maxillary sinus including the ethmoid infundibulum.

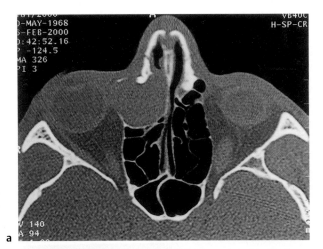

a

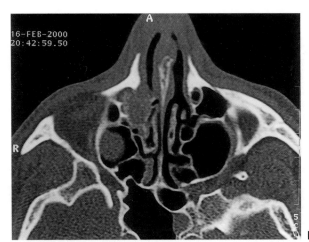

b

Fig. 4.**376 a–d**   Woman 31 years of age with right-sided epiphora due to a right ethmoid mucocele obstructing the nasolacrimal duct. Note the eggshell-like expansion of the adjacent nasal bone.

a, b Axial CT with a high-resolution bone filter.
c Axial CT with a soft-tissue filter confirms a solid mass.
d Reformatted image demonstrates the relationship of the ethmoid to the nasolacrimal duct.

Fig. 4.**376 c–d** ▷

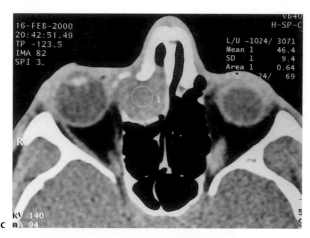
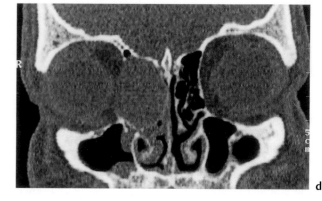

Fig. 4.**376 c–d**

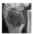

Tumor?

Osteomas of the ethmoid (Fig. 4.**377**) are less common than osteomas arising from the frontal sinus (see p. 531). Figure 4.**378** illustrates **hyperostosis of the planum ethmoidale and sphenoidale.**

Plain radiographs can detect malignant tumors of the ethmoid labyrinth only in advanced stages. CT and MRI can detect these lesions earlier and with greater clarity.

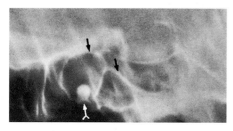

Fig. 4.**377**   Large posterior ethmoid cells (arrows). A small osteoma (tailed arrow) is also visible.

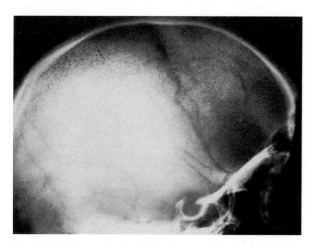

Fig. 4.**378**   Hyperostosis of the planum ethmoidale and planum sphenoidale. The cause may be a type I osteopetrosis, but in itself the finding could just as well be endosteal hyperostosis (van Buchem) or diaphyseal dysplasia (Camurati–Engelmann).

Sphenoid Sinus

Normal Findings

During Growth

The sphenoid sinus in newborns is either absent or only a few millimeters in size. Generally it cannot be seen on radiographs until the 4th to 8th year of life. Pneumatization of the sphenoid sinus, with varying amounts of air in the body of the sphenoid bone, is usually complete at puberty or by 25 years of age at the latest.

In Adulthood

There is a great range of normal variation in the size and aeration of the sphenoid sinus, ranging from very small cavities beneath the anterior sellar floor to extensive pneumatization of the sphenoid bone, including the dorsum sellae and clinoid processes (Figs. 4.**186**, 4.**379**). In

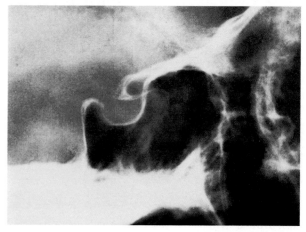

Fig. 4.**379**   Pneumatization of the dorsum sellae and clinoid processes in a lateral spot radiograph (compare with Fig. 4.**186**).

most cases the sinus consists of two cavities separated by a median septum that is often oblique or curved. Additional accessory bony septa are also common. The lateral walls of the sphenoid sinus may bear sigma-shaped vascular grooves for the internal carotid arteries.

Pathological Finding?

Normal Variant/Anomaly?

Variants of sphenoid pneumatization range from aerated anterior and/or posterior clinoid processes to pneumatization of the greater sphenoid wing via a **pterygoid recess** (Fig. 4.**380**). The shape of the bony boundaries of the sphenoid sinus varies with its degree of pneumatization. Greater sinus pneumatization ("ballooned sinus") is associated with a shallow sella (Fig. 4.**381**) or a higher planum sphenoidale (Fig. 4.**382**). The morphology of these variants differs gradually, and in its most heavily pneumatized form is called **pneumosinus dilatans** (Fig. 4.**383**). Large sinuses tend to displace neighboring structures from their normal anatomic position, and this may lead to clinical symptoms, especially when there is encroachment on neurovascular structures. The symptoms are basically the same as those caused by other space-occupying lesions. For example, extreme ballooning of the posterior ethmoid cells (large Onodi cell, Fig. 4.**348c**) and the sphenoid sinus can lead to optic nerve compression.

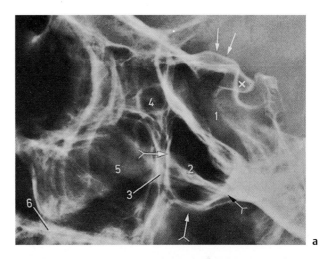

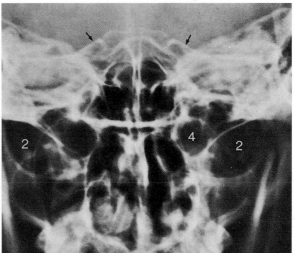

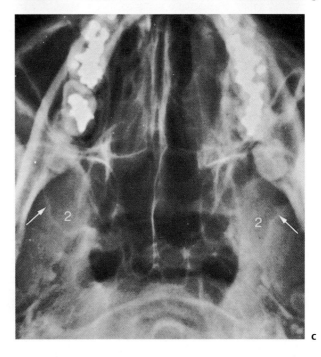

Fig. 4.**380a–c** Extensive dilatation of the sphenoid sinus. The 24-year-old woman complained of recurrent, severe generalized headaches for several years.
a Lateral projection. The frontal and sphenoid sinuses are of normal size. The planum sphenoidale shows a convex bulge (arrows), and heavily pneumatized anterior clinoid processes (×) are visible below it. The dorsum sellae is pneumatized. The numbers indicate the large, pneumatized sphenoid sinus (1), the pterygoid recess (2), the pterygoid process (3), a junction cell between the roof of the maxillary sinus and the sphenoid sinus (4), the posterior wall of the maxillary sinus (5) and floor of the sphenoid sinus (tailed arrows), and the hard palate (6).
b Occipitofrontal projection shows the pneumatized anterior clinoid processes (arrows) with the superiorly convex planum sphenoidale between them and the posterior clinoid processes above.
c Axial projection shows the far lateral extension of the pterygoid recess on both sides (arrows).

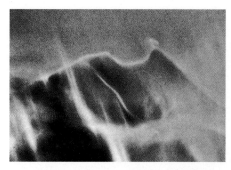

Fig. 4.**381**   Large pneumatized sphenoid sinus extends far anteriorly and also posteriorly to the clivus. Shallow sella (lateral tomogram).

The presence of multiple septa creates separate aerated spaces. Isolated air cells located at the junction between the posterior ethmoid cells and sphenoid sinus generally cannot be localized to a specific sinus on radiographs, so they are simply called **junction cells** (Figs. 4.**384**–4.**386**).

Whether an asymmetrically enlarged sphenoid sinus (Fig. 4.**387**) represents unilateral ballooning or hyperpneumatization is a matter of how these terms are defined. Lateral radiographs in these cases show an oblique position of the planum sphenoidale or a double contour due to the asymmetry of the sinus cavities. This variant, as well as very small sphenoid sinuses and the various intrasinus septa that may occur, are best demonstrated by CT (Fig. 4.**388**), as are all variants and deformities of the sphenoid sinus.

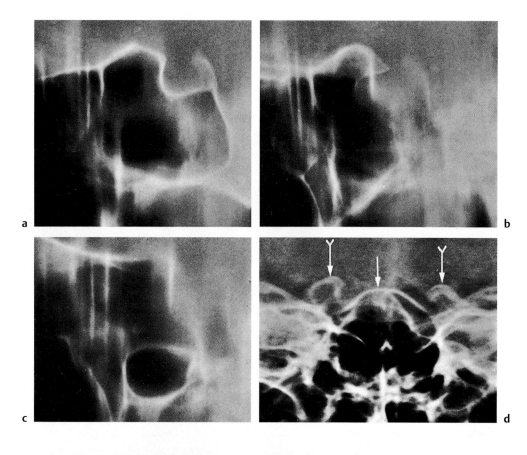

Fig. 4.**382 a–d**   Extensive dilatation of the sphenoid sinus.
a Elevation of the planum sphenoidale (median tomogram).
b Pneumatized anterior clinoid process (paramedian tomogram).
c Basal chamber separated from the sphenoid sinus (far paramedian tomogram).
d Superior convexity of the planum sphenoidale (arrow), pneumatized anterior clinoid process on both sides (tailed arrows).

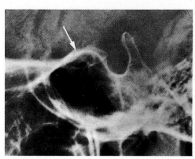

Fig. 4.**383**   Extensive anterior pneumatization of the sphenoid sinus in a 9-year-old girl. Note the relatively small posterior extent of the sinus cavity, the small sella turcica, and the high planum sphenoidale (arrow).

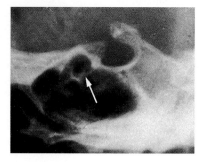

Fig. 4.**384**   Isolated air cell at the junction between the sphenoid sinus and posterior ethmoid cells (arrow).

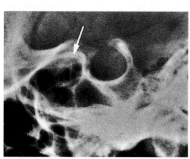

Fig. 4.**385**   Elevation of the planum sphenoidale by isolated air cells located between the relatively small sphenoid sinus and the posterior ethmoid cells (arrow).

Fracture?

Fractures of the walls of the sphenoid sinus generally occur in the setting of complex basal skull fractures. It is common to mistake the superimposed lines of multiple loculations for sinus fractures on conventional radiographs. Fluid levels in the sphenoid sinus that are trauma-related are an important radiographic sign and may signify a hematosinus. Fractures of the sella turcica have a reported incidence of 1–20% among all skull fractures. Extensive injuries may be associated with avulsion fractures of the posterior clinoid process or fractures of the dorsum sellae. Rare spontaneous fractures of the dorsum sellae can occur after prolonged hydrocephalus, radiotherapy, or pituitary apoplexy.

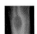

Inflammation?

Areas of mucosal thickening in the sphenoid sinus are a relatively common incidental finding in CT examinations (Fig. 4.**389**). It is reasonable to assume, then, that sphenoid sinusitis is not as rare as traditionally believed. With its paucity of symptoms, however, it rarely has much clinical importance.

Classic **retention cysts** are caused by the obstruction of a mucous gland in the paranasal sinus mucosa, resulting in the formation of a cyst filled with mucoid material. The cyst wall is composed of ductal or glandular epithelium. Retention cysts in any of the paranasal sinuses can be detected incidentally in approximately 10% of the population. Often the affected sinus has some residual aeration. It is rare for retention cysts to expand the sinus or alter its bony wall.

In contrast, **mucoceles** are caused by obstruction of the ostium or one compartment of a septated paranasal sinus. The wall of the lesion is formed by the paranasal sinus mucosa. The affected sinus is completely filled with mucoid material, and the affected cavity is no longer aerated. Typically the sinus shows expansile enlargement with eggshell-like thinning of its bony wall. Mucoceles are most commonly found in the frontal sinus (60–65% of all cases), followed by the ethmoid sinus (20–25%), maxillary sinus (10%), and sphenoid sinus (only 1–2%). If infection supervenes, the lesion is classified as a pyocele or mucopyocele.

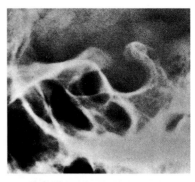

Fig. 4.**386**   Isolated, thick-walled air cell located between a small sphenoid sinus and the posterior ethmoid cells.

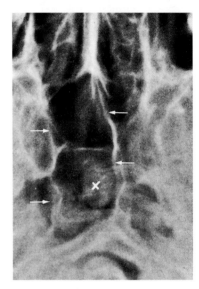

Fig. 4.**387**   Larger sphenoid sinus on the right side (arrows). Orthograde projection of the uvula (×).

While a classic mucocele produces symptoms due to enlargement of the affected sinus, such as proptosis, a feeling of pressure in the forehead, unilateral or bilateral nasal obstruction, hypernasal speech, and a mass in the superomedial orbit, the development of a pyocele is marked by increasing pain and the systemic symptoms of an infectious disease.

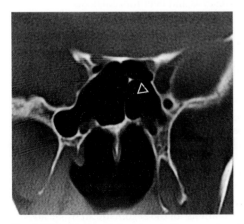

Fig. 4.**388**   Horizontal septum in the upper portion of the left sphenoid sinus (open arrowhead). Coronal CT with a high-resolution bone filter.

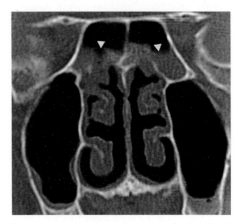

Fig. 4.**389**   Inflammatory changes (arrowheads) in both sphenoid sinuses. Coronal CT with a high-resolution bone filter.

Tumor?

The sphenoid sinus is among the cranial regions that may be affected by **osteomas** (see preceding sections). Pituitary tumors and other intracranial masses can affect the sphenoid bone and especially the sella turcica, leading to changes such as sellar expansion or erosion of the sphenoid sinus roof. The radiographic findings can be very subtle. Some signs are described in the section on the sella turcica.

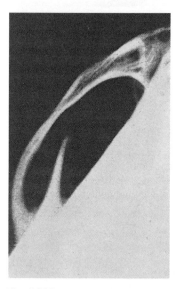
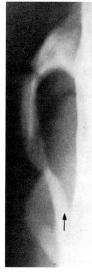

Fig. 4.**390**   Fig. 4.**391**

Fig. 4.**390**   Zimmer projection of the zygomatic arch.

Fig. 4.**391**   Depressed fracture of the zygomatic arch. The posterior fracture site is obscured by the coronoid process of the mandible (arrow).

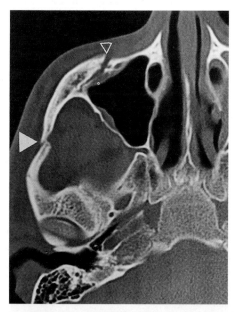

Fig. 4.**392**   Fracture of the right zygomatic arch (arrowhead) and facial wall of the right maxillary sinus (open arrowhead). A third fracture is present at the origin of the zygomatic process from the temporal bone close to the articular tubercle. Axial CT with a high-resolution bone filter.

Zygomatic Arch

Normal Findings

 During Growth

The zygomatic arch is formed by the zygomatic process of the temporal bone and the temporal process of the zygoma. Both bony processes meet at the temporozygomatic suture. This diagonal suture is directed obliquely downward and backward and is approximately 1.5 cm long. The zygomatic arch tapers from anterior to posterior.

 In Adulthood

The zygomatic arch spans the temporal fossa, through which the temporal muscle passes to the coronoid process of the mandible. The **Zimmer view** affords a clear axial projection of the zygomatic arch (Fig. 4.**390**), which "frames" the coronoid process of the mandible behind it.

Pathological Finding?

 Normal Variant/Anomaly?

Indentations of the zygomatic arch that have a slightly W-shaped configuration can occur as a normal variant when bilaterally symmetrical. A tubercle located behind the temporozygomatic suture sometimes projects from the zygomatic arch toward the temporal fossa. It appears as a kind of exostosis arising from the arch. This tubercle is very rare and may have a connection with the mandibular condyle, best demonstrated by CT.

Incomplete fusion of the temporal process of the zygoma with the zygomatic process of the temporal bone can lead to a **bipartite zygoma** or, very rarely, a tripartite zygoma. The **os interzygomaticum** is an accessory bone that is sometimes present in the zygomatic arch.

Hypoplasia of the zygomatic arch occurs in mandibulofacial dysostosis and neurofibromatosis.

 Fracture?

Fractures of the zygomatic arch may occur in the setting of complex facial fractures or as isolated injuries caused by direct violence to the arch itself. Three fracture lines are present in classic zygomatic arch fractures. The most posterior fracture line runs through the temporal end of the zygomatic arch, the most anterior through the zygoma. The third is located at about the center of the zygomatic arch. Significant depression of the central fragment can lead to entrapment of the coronoid process of the mandible, causing limitation of jaw opening (Figs. 4.**391**, 4.**392**). Broad sutures and "indentations" of the zygomatic arch (see above) should not be mistaken for fractures.

Inflammation?

Inflammatory changes can spread from adjacent regions to the zygomatic arch, leading to osteitis.

 ## Tumor?

The zygomatic arch may be eroded by osteomas and osteochondromas of the coronoid process of the mandible. Decalcification and moth-eaten destruction of the zygoma due to tuberculosis can spread to the zygomatic arch (Fig. 4.**393**). The zygomatic arch may also be affected, eroded, or destroyed by malignant or benign processes in neighboring tissues (e.g., rhabdomyosarcoma, schwannoma, neurinoma, etc.).

Mandible

Normal Findings

 ## During Growth

The mandible is still divided into right and left halves in the newborn (Fig. 4.**394**). Small ossicles are sometimes incorporated into the **symphysis menti**. The two halves of the mandible fuse across the midline, with disappearance of the symphysis, during the first or second year of life.

Further development of the mandible is subject to the rules governing the development of the facial skeleton, which in turn are determined in large part by the masticatory function of the jaws. Thus, growth of the facial skeleton is episodic, with alternating periods of rapid and slow growth, following a pattern that is quite different from that of the neurocranium. Without going into details, we point to the mandibular angle as a particularly striking feature of the mandible. This angle becomes more acute by 10–20° from the neonatal period to adulthood, then becomes more obtuse in old age with loss of the dentition (Fig. 4.**395**).

A characteristic sex difference exists in the pattern of mandibular growth. While the female mandible reaches its maximum height during the 15th year of life, the male mandible undergoes an additional significant gain in height between the 15th and 20th years. After the teeth are lost in old age, the diminished stress transfer to the mandible leads to a progressive atrophy of the alveolar crest, and up to one-third of the facial height may eventually be lost (Fig. 4.**395**).

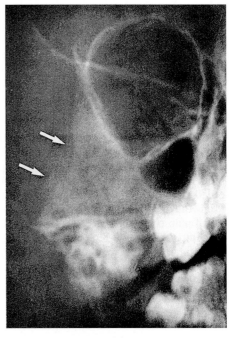

Fig. 4.**393**   Moth-eaten destructive changes in the right zygoma caused by hematogenous skeletal tuberculosis in childhood (arrows). Turkish boy 6 years of age (observation by Holthusen, Hamburg).

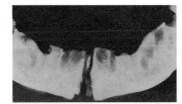
a

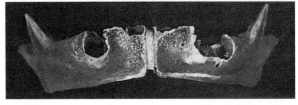
b

Fig. 4.**394a, b**   Mandible of a newborn, showing the symphysis menti.
a Radiograph.
b Anatomic specimen.

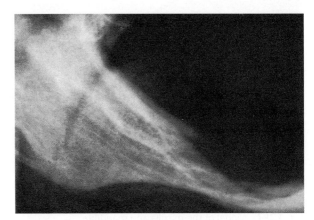

Fig. 4.**395**   Atrophy of the alveolar process and flattening of the mandibular angle in old age. Air in the pharynx appears as a bandlike lucency projected over the mandibular angle.

In Adulthood

To better understand the nature of pathological findings in the mandible, it is necessary to know the normal anatomy of the tooth and some details of its histological structure. Figure 4.**396** shows the structure of a normal tooth. It consists of **dentin, enamel,** and **cementum.** The tooth is composed mostly of dentin. Its crown is covered by enamel, its root by cementum. The root extends into the alveolus of the jaw, where it is anchored by the transverse fibers of the **periodontium** (periodontal ligament). The portion of the tooth between the enamel border and the alveolar arch is called the neck of the tooth and is covered by the gingiva. Inside the tooth is a cavity whose coronal end is expanded into a pulp chamber, from which narrow root canals extend into each root. Each root canal opens at its tip into an apical foramen. Canals may also divide and open to the left and right of the apex.

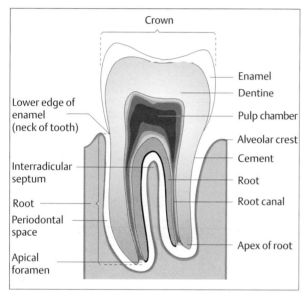

Fig. 4.**396**   Diagram of the structure of a tooth.

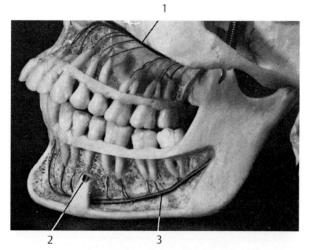

Fig. 4.**397**   Model of the maxilla and mandible.
1   Neurovascular supply (superior dental plexus)
2   Mental foramen
3   Mandibular condyle with inferior alveolar nerve

The mandible consists of a **body** and two **mandibular rami** (vertical rami). Each ramus projects laterally upward and backward and terminates in two processes:

- The **coronoid process** anteriorly (which gives attachment to the temporalis muscle)
- The **condylar process** posteriorly, consisting of a neck and head (condyle)

Between the two processes is the mandibular notch, which may be very shallow or quite deep. At the center of the medial surface of the ramus is the mandibular foramen, which is the opening of the **mandibular canal**. Surrounded by thin cortical bone, this canal runs forward through the cancellous bone of the mandible to open at the mental foramen (Fig. 4.**397**).

On the lingual surface of the body of the mandible, the area above the anterior part of the **mylohyoid line** (origin of the mylohyoid muscle) bears a depression for the sublingual salivary gland, the **sublingual fossa**. The bone below the posterior part of the mylohyoid line bears a hollow for the submandibular salivary gland, the **submandibular fossa**. On the lateral surface of the mandible, the oblique line runs from the anterior border of the ramus to the external surface of the body at the level of the molar roots.

For patients who can be examined in an upright position, **panoramic radiographs** are best for demonstrating the maxilla and mandible, although spot radiographs of individual teeth can provide more accurate information for selected clinical problems.

The standard **lateral radiograph** superimposes the two halves of the mandible but is the only projection for measuring the mandibular angle. The lateral oblique projection ("hanging jaw" view) displays the horizontal rami separately. For lateral tomography, the skull should be rotated 20–30° toward the affected side to allow for the natural posterolateral extension of the mandibular body. Just 10–15° of rotation is adequate for lateral tomography of a single vertical ramus.

The standard frontal projection of the skull shows both mandibular rami and occasionally defines the temporomandibular joints. Frontal tomography can be used to visualize the anterior part of the mandible.

The **Clementschitsch view** is used for conventional studies of mandibular abnormalities. The **Towne projection** is also available.

In the axial projection, a **mental tubercle** arises lateral to the mental protuberance on each side. The area between the tubercles may be slightly indrawn. On the internal surface of the mandible, the **mental spine** arises on the midline from the symphysis menti and gives attachment to the genioglossus and geniohyoid muscles (Fig. 4.**398a**). This area also contains the **medial mental foramen** along with smaller foramina (Fig. 4.**398 b**).

> It is normal to find relatively lucent, rarefied areas at the center of the mandible at the location of the former symphysis menti.

High-resolution CT with the capacity for multiplanar reconstructions (**dental CT**) has established itself as a valuable adjunct in dental imaging. Panoramic and orthoradial sections can provide a detailed, full-scale anatomic map of the jaw with no distortions. This technique has proved particularly valuable in the preoperative planning of implants

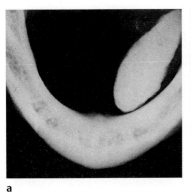
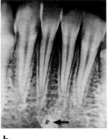

b

a

Fig. 4.**398 a, b** Mental spine and medial mental foramen.
a Mental spine. A large salivary stone is also visible on the left side.
b Medial mental foramen in the incisor region of the mandible (arrow).

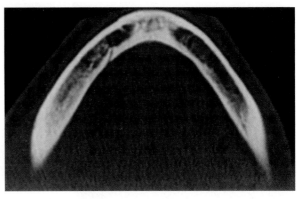

Fig. 4.**399** Lateral lingual nutrient canal in the mandible. Axial CT with a high-resolution bone filter.

(Rothmann 1998). Dental CT will disclose any unexpected abnormalities of the bones and soft tissues, making it excellent for preoperative studies (Swartz et al. 1985). It has also become important in the preoperative visualization of key anatomic details. This includes the mapping of vascular canals (Fig. 4.**399**) to avoid intraoperative bleeding complications (Gahleitner et al. 2001). Dental CT can also provide essential cephalometric data for orthognathic surgeons, but these techniques are too specialized for discussion in this book.

Pathological Finding?

Normal Variant/Anomaly?

The air–soft tissue interface of the nasopharynx may be superimposed on the mandibular ramus when the head is tilted (Fig. 4.**395**). The mandibular angle may be broad and stout and may show lateral bulges in the frontal projection. The median cartilaginous plate may persist in the body of the mandible. Various forms of a **bifid mandibular canal**, present in about 0.9% of cases, have been described. Both canals contain nerves and may be associated with accessory mandibular foramina. Occasionally the mandibular canal extends anterior to the mental foramen, with an elongated but very narrow lumen extending as far as the incisor teeth. Projection-related artifacts, especially in the panoramic radiograph, can mimic lesions (Figs. 4.**400**, 4.**401**).

A bony concavity in the lingual cortex is relatively common in the area of the mandibular angle and may appear as a cystic lesion on panoramic radiographs. This normal variant, known as a **Stafne cyst** (pseudocyst), can be positively identified by CT (Fig. 4.**402**). The Stafne cyst appears as a round or elliptical area of increased lucency and is usually located in the posterior mandible, often close to the mandibular angle below the mandibular canal. Found predominantly in males, the lesion is usually asymptomatic and detected incidentally. As Fig. 4.**402** shows, the bony defect opens onto the lingual surface of the mandible. The Stafne cyst is generally 1–2 cm in size, has well-defined margins, and is often associated with mild sclerosis. Differentiation is required from other benign or malignant skeletal abnor-

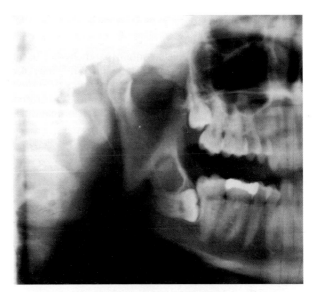

Fig. 4.**400** Panoramic radiograph (right half) shows an apparent cyst posterior to the lower right third molar. This phenomenon is caused by the prominent superior cortex of the mandible, the roof of the mandibular canal, and the posterior border of the tooth follicle of the unerupted third molar.

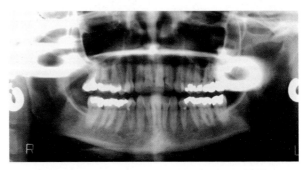

Fig. 4.**401** Panoramic radiograph shows "ring artifacts" projected over both mandibular rami. Each artifact is caused by the contralateral earring.

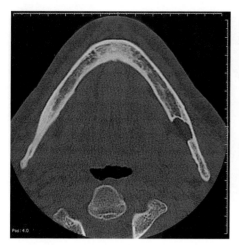

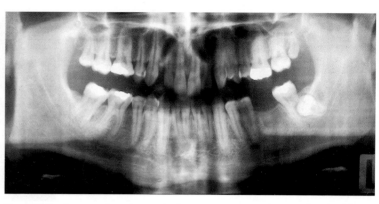

Fig. 4.**404**   Panoramic radiograph shows an unerupted, mesially tilted lower third molar that has caused complete distal root resorption in the adjacent molar.

Fig. 4.**402**   Stafne cyst in the area of the left mandibular angle (third molar) appears as a sharply circumscribed bone defect in the lingual cortex. Usually the cyst is filled with salivary gland components, fat or muscle tissue.

malities. Some Stafne cysts contain parenchymal tissue from the submandibular gland (Fig. 4.**403**). They may also contain aberrant or ectopic salivary glandular tissue like that found at other sites such as the middle ear, external auditory canal, lower neck, upper neck, anterior mandible, and cerebellopontine angle.

Tooth malposition is the most common cause of abnormalities in the mandibular region. In particular, the lower wisdom teeth may be impacted, tilted, or displaced in varying degrees. A tooth that directly abuts an adjacent root can lead to resorption (Fig. 4.**404**).

Hypoplasia of the mandible may occur in isolation but is more often combined with other skeletal anomalies. More than 49 syndromes have been described that may be associated with mandibular hypoplasia due to various causes (Taybi 1982). The most familiar are anomalies involving derivatives of the first brachial arch such as **mandibulofacial dysostosis** (Treacher–Collins syndrome, Franceschetti–Zwahlen syndrome) (Fig. 4.**405**), **cleidocranial dysplasia (dysostosis)** (see p. 389), **hemifacial microsomia**, and many other clinically important syndromes. When combined with medial cleft palate, the mandibular hypoplasia leads to a glossoptosis that can cause life-threatening respiratory difficulties in newborns. This condition, known as **Pierre–Robin syndrome**, can occur in isolation but more often occurs in the setting of numerous malformation syndromes and skeletal dysplasias. The bony expansion that occurs in infantile cortical hyperosto-

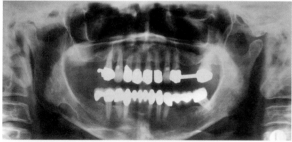

a

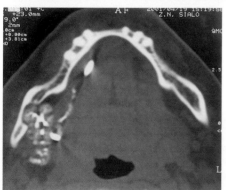

c

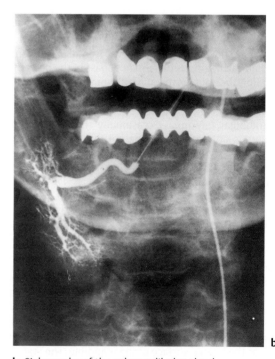

b

Fig. 4.**403 a–c**   Typical Stafne cyst detected incidentally.
a Panoramic radiograph shows a sclerosis-rimmed defect in the right mandibular angle.

b Sialography of the submandibular gland.
c CT sialography. Glandular tissue within the Stafne cyst.

sis is manifested initially and most commonly in the mandible.

Anomalies of the mandible (and of the mandibular teeth and tooth buds) occur in several metabolic diseases and dysplasias, such as the following.

- **Pyknodysostosis** is a rare autosomal recessive disease characterized by osteopetrosis and dwarfism. Its radiographic signs are generalized osteosclerosis, lack of aeration of the paranasal sinus, a large anterior fontanel that remains open in adulthood, micrognathism, spool-shaped vertebral bodies, hip dysplasia, and fractures with malunion.
- **Mucopolysaccharidosis** type VI (Maroteaux–Lamy syndrome) is an autosomal recessive disorder of mucopolysaccharide metabolism marked by the intralysosomal accumulation of dermatan sulfate and its increased excretion in the urine. Skull radiographs show moderate enlargement of the calvarium, mandibular deformities, and dental follicular cysts. There may be pronounced deformities of the vertebral column, and pelvic involvement is marked by hypoplasia of the ilium with steep acetabular roofs. The dominant clinical features are short stature, joint contractures, kyphosis, thoracic deformities, coarse facial features, corneal opacities, hepatosplenomegaly, macroglossia, hearing loss, and cutaneous thickening. Patients show marked general debilitation with normal intelligence. Hydrocephalus can lead to increased intracranial pressure, however.

Fracture?

Approximately 80% of all jaw fractures affect the mandible, and 80% of these injuries are caused by direct violence such as a fist blow or motor vehicle accident. Facial fractures are rare in children and account for just 5% of all facial fractures. This relates to the different anatomy and biomechanics of the forces that act on the facial skeleton in children. Also, children under 5 years of age are less susceptible to trauma than older children as a result of parental supervision. Fractures of the nasal bones account for 60% of facial fractures in children. Next come mandibular fractures, which account for 21%. Bicycle accidents are a frequent cause. If undetected, these fractures can lead to growth disturbances. The affected mandibular regions are listed below in order of frequency:

- Body of the mandible (20–40%, with weak points in the canine and premolar regions)
- Mandibular angle (20–30%)
- Symphyseal area (10–15%)
- Vertical ramus (2–9%)
- Coronoid process (2–9%)
- Alveolar process (1.5–4%)

Fractures of the condylar process of the mandible (15–30%) are discussed on p. 550.

Concomitant fractures of dental roots or alveolar process fractures accompanying dental fractures are usually located in the canine region.

Fractures of the mandible tend to be multiple. Since double and triple fractures (symphysis and both condylar processes) are present in 50–60% of cases, the detection of one fracture line warrants a meticulous search of the entire mandible for additional fractures.

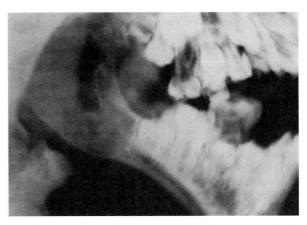

Fig. 4.**405**   Absence of the mandibular angle in mandibulofacial dysostosis.

While any combination of fractures can occur in the mandible, the fractures are rarely unilateral, and the majority are multiple and bilateral. Fractures of the mandibular angle are often combined with contralateral fractures of the mandibular body.

Since **wisdom teeth** located in the fracture line are extracted, it is important to make this diagnosis on radiographs. All other teeth in fracture lines are left alone whenever possible. It is difficult for the oral surgeon to immobilize an edentulous mandible, as there are no intact teeth that are available for interdental wiring of the jaw in an occluded position.

Dental CT must be used to localize and define the extent of **monocortical mandibular fractures**.

A **fracture of the alveolar process** can be considered an avulsion type of fracture in which the roots of the involved teeth protrude from the detached fragment in varying degrees. Shear fractures of the coronoid process are very rare and easily overlooked. The avulsed coronoid fragment is displaced upward by the pull of the temporalis muscle. These fractures are always associated with a fracture of the zygoma or condylar neck.

Dental fractures may be caused by trauma or endodontic treatment (root procedure, post crown) (Youssefzadeh 1999). Whereas traumatic dental fractures are usually horizontal and are easily detected on conventional dental radiographs, endodontic fractures are usually vertical and are detected more easily by dental CT (Fig. 4.**406**) (White 1999).

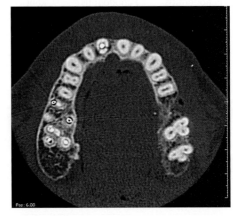

Fig. 4.**406**   Dental CT of the maxilla shows a filled pulp canal and a vertical mesiodistal root fracture of the upper right central incisor.

Necrosis?

Necrosis of the mandible following radiotherapy, termed **osteoradionecrosis**, usually occurs when doses higher than 60 Gy have been administered. The mandible is probably the bone that is most often affected by radiotherapy for carcinoma of the tongue or tongue base. In patients who receive radiation for paranasal sinus carcinoma, post-radiogenic osteitis more often leads to swelling and inflammation over the zygoma or maxilla, which may raise clinical suspicion of a recurrent tumor. Clinical symptoms are sometimes improved by the removal of bony sequestra. Osteoradionecrosis or osteoradiodystrophy can also result from occupational exposure to phosphorus.

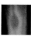 ## Inflammation?

Because the teeth are embedded in the mandible and maxilla, the jaws are exposed to a greater frequency and variety of diseases than other skeletal regions. Even if we disregard dental and periodontal conditions, we still must consider inflammatory processes—**osteitis** and osteomyelitis—that may be caused by acute periodontal infections and may spread to the jaws via the alveolar process and teeth. The diagrams in Fig. 4.**407** illustrate the great variety of odontogenic lesions that can occur.

Periodontal infections are a common starting point for inflammatory bone destruction in the mandible. In cases with an acute onset, one or more weeks may pass before

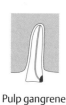

Pulp gangrene after silicate filling (not visible on radiographs)

Focus of osteitis (arrow); e.g., carious defect, trauma (arrowhead)

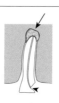

Granuloma (arrow); e.g., carious defect, trauma (arrowhead)

Inner granuloma, barely visible on radiographs (arrow). Filling (arrowhead)

Focus of osteitis with a widened periodontal space (arrow). Caries (arrowhead)

Persistent deciduous tooth surrounded by a zone of osteitis (arrow). Filling (arrowhead)

Periodontal abscess

Hypoplastic tooth

Tooth in a fracture

Subluxated tooth

Apical root fracture

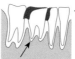

Projecting fillings with vertical periodontal bone resorption (arrow)

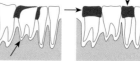

Projecting crown (arrow), post crown (arrowhead) with periodontal bone resorption

Periodontal pocket (arrow) caused by tooth angulation (e.g., due to early extraction of the first molar)

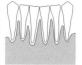

Periodontitis

Periodontitis with extreme horizontal bone resorption

Root remnant (arrow)

Root tip extending into the maxillary sinus (arrow)

Excess cement expelled into the maxillary sinus (arrow)

Root canal perforation in a curved root apex

Foreign body (extirpation needle) in the canal protrudes from the apical foramen. (Metal pins driven into the bone, arrows)

Unerupted dentition (arrow)

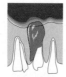

Cyst in the maxilla

Cyst in the mandible

Unerupted, displaced canine tooth (arrow)

Foreign body inclusions

Fig. 4.**407**   Radiographic appearance of odontogenic lesions.

osteolytic changes can be seen on radiographs. Hematogenous osteitis was once common in children and tended to form sequestra, but this disease has become rare since the advent of antibiotics. **Submandibular abscess** is still relatively common in small children, however, and occasionally it incites a lamellar periosteal reaction in the adjacent horizontal ramus. This does not signify osteomyelitis of the mandible itself or even an odontogenic cause.

Chronic osteomyelitis, whether primary or secondary, may run a course of years or decades and is associated with typical sclerotic changes in the bone and possible sequestration and fistulation (Fig. 4.**408**). Chronic sclerosing osteomyelitis, which arises from the infection of necrotic dental roots in children and adolescents, can produce a typical shell-shaped pattern of periosteal bone formation along the inferior border of the mandible (Fig. 4.**409**).

All forms of **osteopetrosis** (Albers–Schönberg disease) predispose to mandibular osteomyelitis. In **Gaucher disease**, involvement of the mandible has been seen in very rare cases, appearing on radiographs as a large radiolucent zone.

Specific forms of osteitis (actinomycosis, syphilis, tuberculosis) occur rarely as nonspecific inflammations of the mandibular bone and are indistinguishable from other forms by radiography. Leprosy typically leads to foci of tooth and bone destruction in the medial portion of the mandible.

 ## Tumor?

Fibrous dysplasia is among the tumorlike lesions that can occur in the mandible (special form: **cherubism**). Other skeletal lesions of the jaw can originate from the cementum or other dental tissues or from the periodontal ligaments. When sclerotic changes are present, the differential diagnosis should include **Paget disease**, **melorheostosis**, and **osteopetrosis**.

Multiple foci of increased density in a rapidly thickening mandible are characteristic of **juvenile fibromatosis**.

The basic problems that are encountered in the differential diagnosis of sclerotic lesions due to inflammatory, neoplastic, and systemic diseases apply equally in differentiating the various causes of radiolucent areas. This is particularly true with cysts, especially those that lack a well-defined cortical boundary (Fig. 4.**410**), have a honeycomb or multilocular structure, or occur in clusters (polycystic lesions).

Ameloblastoma is classified as an odontogenic epithelial tumor without odontogenic ectomesenchyma. It is the most common odontogenic tumor, accounting for 13–18% of cases if odontomas are disregarded (see below). It can occur at any age, but about half occur in the third and fourth decades. Ameloblastomas have a locally aggressive growth potential and tend to recur but almost never metastasize. Three histological types are distinguished:

- Follicular type
- Plexiform type
- Unicystic type

More than three-fourths of all cases affect the mandible, and half of these occur in the premolar and molar regions. Desmoplastic ameloblastoma is a rare variant that is found predominantly in the anterior incisor region of the maxilla. Sporadic ameloblastomas may also occur in the extraos-

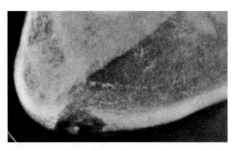

Fig. 4.**408** Mandibular osteomyelitis with a sequestrum, histologically confirmed.

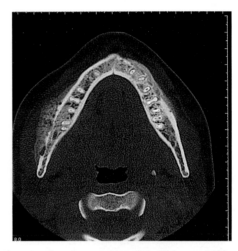

Fig. 4.**409** Chronic sclerosing osteomyelitis of the mandible in dental CT. Note the sites of pronounced periosteal bone formation.

seous submucous connective tissues. The clinical signs are nonspecific and usually include a painless swelling. The loosening of teeth, pain, and inflammation are occasionally seen. With superficial tumors, erosion of the mandibular mucosa may occur due to bite injuries or tension from the tumor itself. Lesions of the maxilla may cause nasal airway obstruction.

The radiographic signs are not specific for ameloblastoma. Radiographs show a unilocular or multilocular soap-bubble-like or honeycomb-like osteolytic lesion with more or less sharply defined margins. An irregular, rounded peripheral bulge is seen with some tumors. There may be re-

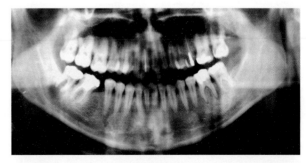

Fig. 4.**410** Panoramic radiograph shows a radicular cyst in the lower right third molar. The margins of the cyst are indistinct because the lesion is located just outside the tomographic plane. The lesion is verified by the mandibular canal, which has been displaced downward by local cyst growth.

sorption of the roots of neighboring teeth, but neither this sign nor the inclusion of an unerupted tooth are specific for ameloblastoma.

Root resorption also occurs in association with other benign and malignant tumors. An unerupted tooth is typical of a **follicular cyst**, for example. MRI appears to aid in differentiating this type of lesion, especially from keratocysts. A mixed solid-cystic pattern with irregular wall thickening, intense contrast enhancement of the solid components, intraluminal papillary structures, and significantly prolonged T2 relaxation times are typical of ameloblastoma and help to distinguish it from a keratocyst. The rare desmoplastic ameloblastoma, which probably has osteoinductive potential, usually does not show a typical unilocular or multilocular structure on radiographs. It has more the appearance of a fibro-osseous lesion with coarse, usually peripheral, zones of increased density, frequent ill-defined margins, and the tilting of adjacent teeth.

Most authors regard **odontomas** as developmental anomalies, classifying them as hamartomas. Two types of odontoma are distinguished according to their structure: complex and compound. Both types are diagnosed mainly in the first two decades of life, with no apparent sex predilection. Odontomas can occur at any age, however. Complex odontomas tend to occur in the postcanine region, while compound odontomas are more common in the anterior region. Both types generally present clinically with painless swelling.

Complex odontoma appears radiographically as a mass of bone or enamel density that is frequently associated with an unerupted tooth and often located above its crown. **Compound odontoma** often appears as a collection of very small denticles. Odontomas are also occasionally found between the roots of teeth. The lesions are surrounded by a narrow lucent border (Figs. 4.**411**, 4.**412**). The radiographic findings are definitive in most cases, but in early stages the mineralization may be so subtle that it cannot be distinguished from other cystlike lesions. A complex odontoma that is fully mature may be mistaken for an osteoma or focal sclerosing osteomyelitis. Differential diagnosis is aided, however, by the clinical manifestations and patient age.

Trauma was discussed earlier as a potential cause of **bone cysts**.

Hemangiomas of the mandible, **hemangiomatosis** (marked radiologically by osteolytic lesions), and Gorham–Stout hemangiomatosis have been reported in isolated cases.

Osteomas of the mandible occur below the molars, where they may be broad-based or pedunculated and tend to spread downward, rarely causing symptoms. Whenever they are detected, the possibility of Gardner syndrome should be considered (cutaneous tumors, intestinal polyps, mandibular osteoma, odontomas, supernumerary teeth). Differentiation is required from **mandibular tori**

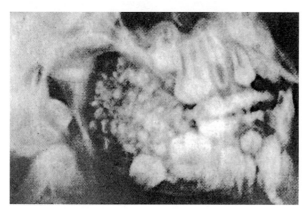

Fig. 4.**411**   Odontoma with innumerable tooth germs in the mandibular ramus.

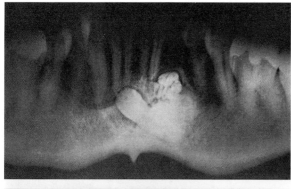

a

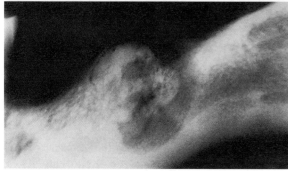

b

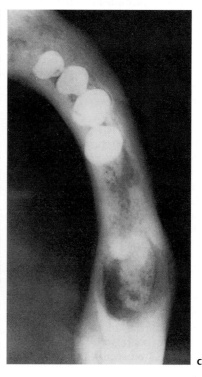

c

Fig. 4.**412 a–c**   Odontomas (observation by Selle, Göttingen).
a "Condensed" odontoma with typical displacement of adjacent teeth and sharply marginated sclerosis.
b, c Complex odontoma.

(Fig. 4.**413**). These are innocuous bony prominences on the lingual surface of the mandible that usually show a bilateral symmetrical arrangement in the canine region above the mylohyoid line.

Broadening of the coronoid processes occurs at an early age, is sometimes found in siblings, and is more likely a congenital hyperplasia than an osteochondroma. The resulting impairment of temporomandibular joint function often requires surgical treatment.

Carcinomas of the mandible are most common in the region of the alveolar processes. They usually arise in the soft tissues of the lateral oral cavity (oral floor, tonsillar fossa, peritonsillar region, gingiva, alveolar mucosa) and can spread to the adjacent bone. Some carcinomas arise secondarily from intraosseous, epithelium-lined cysts. The earliest radiographic signs are ill-defined bone margins and blurring of the trabecular structure. Osteosarcoma, chondrosarcoma, and Ewing sarcoma rarely occur in the mandible. The jaws are not a site of predilection for plasmacytoma. The appearance of mandibular metastases is basically the same as in other skeletal regions.

Expansion of the **alveolar canal** may be caused by a neurinoma or neurofibroma of the inferior alveolar nerve or its sheath or by an angioma of the inferior alveolar artery.

Langerhans cell histiocytosis involves the calvarium in approximately 27% of cases and the mandible in approximately 6%. Smaller lesions, especially when solitary, do not produce clinical complaints and are therefore detected incidentally. Calvarial lesions are sometimes associated with a circumscribed, painless swelling that correlates with a bony defect on radiographs. More aggressive, fast-growing granulomas can cause local pain and soft-tissue swelling but do not cause significant hyperemia or local warmth. **Eosinophilic granuloma** of the mandible may present clinically with pain, swelling, and tooth loss. "Floating teeth" are a frequent clinical finding.

Several differentiating criteria can be helpful in the interpretation of radiographic findings in the mandible:

- **Patient age:** Odontomas, dental cysts, and primordial cysts develop in young patients, usually accompanied by normal development of the teeth. Tumors and inflammatory lesions, including ameloblastomas, radicular cysts, and residual cysts, usually form in adults over 30 years of age.
- **Configuration:** Most radiolucent changes in the mandible (92% of all mandibular lesions) are unifocal. This may not apply to lesions such as ameloblastoma, aneurysmal bone cyst, and odontogenic myxoma, which have some distinctive characteristics.
- **Ameloblastoma** may contain smaller lytic cavities arranged around a larger osteolytic area. The septa in an ameloblastoma are typically curvilinear. A uniform size and straight septa (honeycomb-like) are more consistent with odontogenic myxoma. There are no pathognomonic signs for ameloblastoma.
- **Location:** Lesions located anterior or posterior to the mandibular canal typically do not arise from the dental tissues. Ameloblastomas are located more in the posterior tooth-forming jaw areas, while giant cell granulomas and cysts due to trauma usually occur anterior to the roots of the first molars. Primordial cysts and odontogenic keratocysts appear as more posterior lucencies. As for lesions that cause increased density, 90% of periapical cement dysplasias are located in the anterior mandible. Multiple teeth are usually involved.

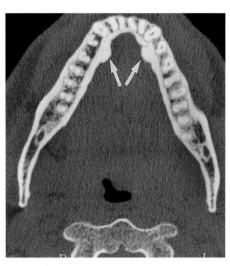

Fig. 4.**413** Mandibular tori (arrows). Axial CT with a high-resolution bone filter.

 ## Other Changes?

Bony changes in the mandible are rare in all forms of **rickets**, including the vitamin D-resistant form. Progressive systemic sclerosis (**scleroderma**) not only causes enlargement of the periodontal spaces but often leads to deep erosions in the outer bony contour of the mandibular angle. In **hyperparathyroidism**, the giant cell tumors (**epulis**) mentioned above are accompanied by a disproportion between the reduced calcium content of the jaw bones and the normal density of the teeth on radiographs. **Acromegaly** shows a typical disproportion between the enlarged jaw bones and interdental spaces and the normal-size teeth. The mandible may also be involved in **sickle cell anemia**. The changes in the medullary spaces can lead to generalized osteopenia with cortical thinning.

Soft-tissue examinations of the oral cavity should include a search for **salivary stones** (sialoliths). They are best demonstrated in a frontal projection with the mouth open, the head turned to the affected side and the chin drawn inward, or in an axial projection of the oral floor (Figs. 4.**398**, 4.**414**).

Fig. 4.**414** Salivary stone.

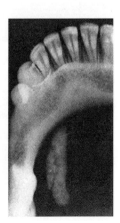

Temporomandibular Joint

Normal Findings

During Growth

The **mandibular condyle** does not possess an epiphyseal plate. Its growth proceeds from the articular cartilage. The shape of the mandibular condyle, glenoid fossa, and articular disk (which corrects for the incongruity of the articular surfaces) and the condylar neck angle are determined both by constitutional factors and by functional stimuli that are active during growth. This growth continues until the subchondral zone of calcification is ossified.

In Adulthood

The adult mandibular condyle has an average mediolateral width of 15.6–26.6 mm. The anteroposterior diameter is 13.0–20.0 mm in its lateral portion and 14.0–22.9 mm in its medial portion. The articular surface of the condyle (including the articular disk) varies considerable in shape (Fig. 4.**415**) and undergoes secondary changes throughout life.

The **temporomandibular joint (TMJ)** consists of the articular surface of the mandibular condyle and the glenoid fossa. Formed by the squamous part of the temporal bone, the glenoid fossa is bounded anteriorly by the articular tubercle of the temporal bone. The lateral skull base is excavated by the glenoid fossa in varying degrees. A small portion of the fossa is formed by the inferior surface of the zygomatic arch and projects past the lateral aspect of the skull base. The tympanic part of the temporal bone helps to form the posterior boundary of the glenoid fossa.

In **plain film examinations**, the Schüller view, lateral oblique view, and Clementschitsch view are most commonly used to demonstrate the TMJ and mandibular condyle. The panoramic radiograph is a primary tool in the diagnosis of TMJ fractures. Conventional tomography is rarely used today. High-resolution CT with multiplanar reconstructions is the most precise technique for examining the bony structures of the TMJ. MRI is used mainly to evaluate the integrity and position of the articular disk (Fig. 4.**416**).

"Snapshot" views of the open and closed jaw can assess the basic **function of the TMJ**. Only a few examiners still use cineradiography to provide a seamless record of jaw movements for stomatological investigations. Today, MRI LOLO (local look) sequences are the diagnostic tool of choice for TMJ function studies.

Since open-mouth images also have applications other than TMJ function studies, it should be kept in mind that when the mouth is opened, the mandibular condyle not only rotates in the glenoid fossa but also slides forward and downward. In the process, it may slip out of the glenoid fossa below the articular tubercle and enter the infratemporal fossa. The rotating-gliding movements of the TMJ are extremely complex, and their nuances are not yet fully understood.

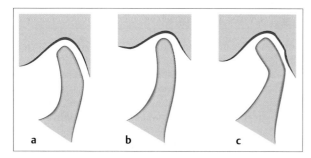

Fig. 4.**415**   Variable shape of the normal temporomandibular joint in the Schüller projection (after Doub and Henny).
a Normal shape.
b Flat type.
c Convex type.

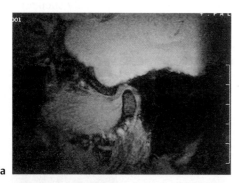

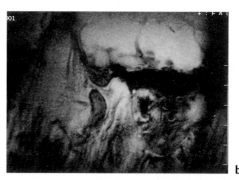

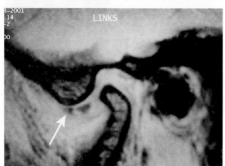

Fig. 4.**416 a–c**   MR images of the temporomandibular joint.
a Sagittal T1-weighted gradient-echo image of a normal temporomandibular joint with the mouth closed.
b Sagittal T1-weighted gradient-echo image of a normal temporomandibular joint with the mouth open.
c Sagittal T1-weighted gradient-echo image shows the typical appearance of anteriorly dislocated and torn articular disk (arrow) with the mouth closed.

▌ *Pathological Finding?*

Normal Variant/Anomaly?

The normal anatomy of the TMJ is best defined by CT with a high-resolution bone filter and by MRI, which is used mainly in coronal and sagittal planes (Fig. 4.**416**). Given the great range of variation in the bones that comprise the TMJ (Fig. 4.**415**), we cannot draw a precise dividing line between normal variants and anomalies. Indeed, there are some cases in which a growth variant cannot be confidently distinguished from a childhood injury (Fig. 4.**417**).

In **hypoplasia of the mandibular condyle**, the underdeveloped condyle is diminished in size but displays a normal shape (Fig. 4.**418**).

Hypoplasias of the mandible in length and height are usually associated with condylar hypoplasia. Mandibular hypoplasia occurs in hemifacial microsomia, in mandibulofacial dysostosis, in other auricular and zygomatic arch dysplasias, and in Robin syndrome. The cartilage covering the condylar process of the mandible may be partially or completely absent. The TMJ and/or the condylar process may be absent, ankylosed, or aplastic. The glenoid fossa and articular disk may also be absent. **Duplication of the condylar process** (Fig. 4.**419**) and zygomaticocoronoid ankylosis have been described along with many other mandibular anomalies.

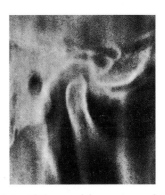

Fig. 4.**418** Unilateral hypoplasia of the condylar process of the mandible.

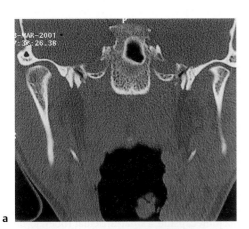

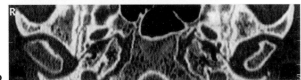

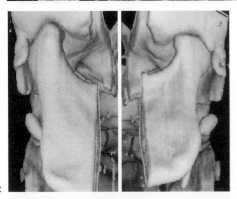

Fig. 4.**417** The mandibular condyle on the right side appears somewhat enlarged relative to the opposite side. The accompanying expansion of the glenoid fossa suggest a growth disturbance, but this cannot be reliably distinguished from an old fracture.
a Coronal CT with a high-resolution bone filter.
b Axial reconstruction from the volume data set.
c Three-dimensional surface reconstruction. Right image: expanded right mandibular condyle. Left image: normal mandibular condyle.

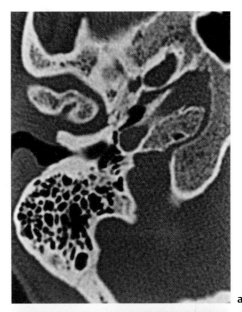

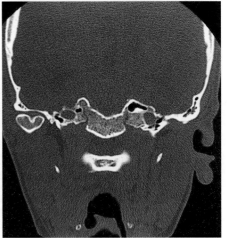

Fig. 4.**419a, b** Duplication of the mandibular condyle. CT with a high-resolution bone filter.
a Axial CT.
b Coronal CT.

Bite abnormalities can cause asymmetric functional stresses in the mandible and lead to mandibular dysfunction. During growth, these abnormalities can lead to condylar hyperplasia on one side (with or without dysmorphia) and to condylar hypoplasia on the opposite side. Hyperplasia is sometimes difficult to distinguish from an **osteoma**. It cannot be determined in retrospect how a congenital hyperplasia may have contributed to bite abnormalities or how the latter may have contributed to enlargement of the mandibular condyle.

Flattening or concavity of the articular surface of the mandibular condyle, as well as hyperplasia, are typical manifestations of mucopolysaccharidosis type I and II (Pfaundler–Hurler disease).

 ## Fracture, Subluxation, or Dislocation?

Widening of the temporomandibular joint space by an intra-articular hematoma provides an indirect imaging sign of TMJ injury.

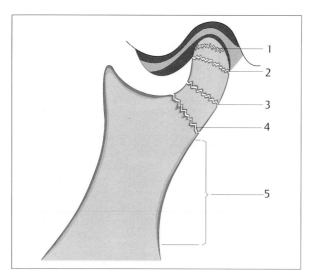

Fig. 4.**420**   Condylar fractures of the mandible (after Dihlmann).
1   Diacapital fracture
2   Subcapital fracture
3   Mid-neck fracture
4   Basal neck fracture
5   Subcondylar fractures

A fall onto the chin in children can produce **microfractures** at the chondro-osseous junction, which is functionally equivalent to a growth center. The resulting growth disturbance can have serious consequences, but functional treatment often has excellent results owing to the copious blood supply and cartilage cells in the mandibular condyles of adolescents. Conventional radiographs, including panoramic views, often fail to detect fractures that are defined clearly by CT using a high-resolution bone filter.

Fractures of the **glenoid fossa** may be caused by the impaction mechanism noted above (central mandibular dislocation) or by the extension of calvarium fractures into the mandibular fossa. Fractures of the **mandibular condyle**, which are more often unilateral than bilateral, should prompt a thorough examination of the entire mandible (and skull base) for the presence of additional bony injuries. Often the radiologist is unable to answer the clinical question of whether the fracture is intracapsular or extracapsular. **Diacapital and subcapital fractures** (Figs. 4.**420**, 4.**421**) are usually intracapsular and nondisplaced, whereas extracapsular mid- and basal **neck fractures** are very often displaced medially and anteriorly by the pull of the lateral pterygoid muscle (in 60% of cases) (Fig. 4.**422**). There may be persistent limitation of jaw opening unless the fractures are reduced (Fig. 4.**423**).

Displacement of the articular disk behind the mandibular condyle restricts jaw closure, while displacement in front of the condyle limits jaw opening. This can be documented by functional radiographs or preferably by MRI in the resting position and various functional positions (examination with the mouth closed and opened to various degrees).

With an anterior **dislocation** of the TMJ (e.g., caused by opening the mouth too widely), the mandibular condyle slides forward over the articular tubercle and up its anterior surface. The masticatory muscles tend to retain the condyle in its dislocated position. Any combination of factors such as a lax joint capsule, a small articular tubercle, or a shallow glenoid fossa can promote recurrent dislocations. TMJ dislocations are termed "habitual" if they are frequent and easily reducible. Posterior dislocations below the external auditory canal are very rare and almost always occur in the setting of fracture-dislocations. It is very unusual for a posterior inferior dislocation to occur in the absence of a fracture. Dislocation of the mandibular condyle into the middle cranial fossa is also very rare.

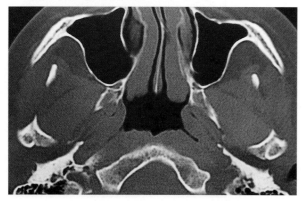

Fig. 4.**421**   Bilateral fractures of the mandibular condyles. Axial CT with a high-resolution bone filter.

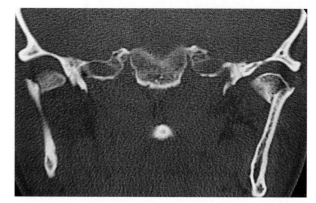

Fig. 4.**422**   Bilateral subcapital mandibular fractures with medial displacement of the condyle. Coronal CT with a high-resolution bone filter.

Fig. 4.**423 a, b** Consolidated fracture of the mandibular condyle.
a CT with a high-resolution bone filter shows a consolidated condylar fracture.
b Coronal CT with a high-resolution bone filter shows bony consolidation of a left condylar fracture.

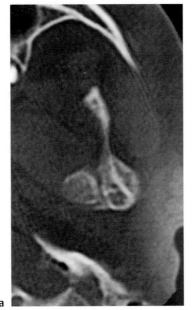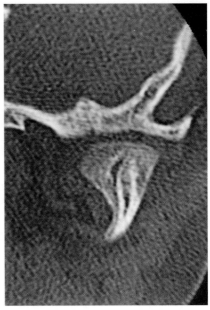

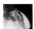

Necrosis?

The TMJ is almost never affected by **juvenile aseptic necrosis**, presumably due to the absence of an epiphyseal growth plate. While predisposing factors for avascular necrosis of the femoral head are steroid use, immunosuppressive therapy, alcoholism (with or without pancreatitis), and diseases such as sickle cell anemia, avascular necrosis of the mandibular condyle is attributed to local trauma due to an intrinsic derangement of the TMJ. In the case of fractures, fragments of the mandibular condyle may become necrotic. This is most common with fragments that have been displaced some distance from other main fragments and deprived of their blood supply.

Inflammation?

Acute **pyogenic arthritis** of the TMJ is rarely encountered in modern practice. Several etiological forms are distinguished:

- Hematogenous
- Posttraumatic
- Local spread of osteomyelitis from the mandibular ramus or otitis media

The diagnosis is made clinically. The role of imaging studies (usually CT or MRI) is to define the extent of the changes.

Chronic arthritis of the TMJ can also result from the diseases listed above, but it occurs predominantly in patients with **rheumatoid arthritis** (Fig. 4.**424**) (including the juvenile form) and **seronegative spondylarthritis**, including psoriatic osteoarthropathy and Reiter disease.

The cardinal imaging signs are erosions of the mandibular condyle and joint space narrowing. The effects can range from limited motion to ankylosis. Involvement of the TMJ by **gout** has also been described.

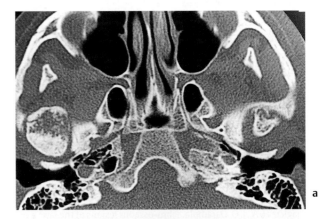

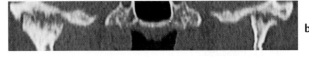

Fig. 4.**424 a, b** Severe degenerative changes in the TMJ.
a Axial CT with a high-resolution bone filter shows very severe, bilateral osteoarthritic changes in the TMJ.
b Coronal image reformatted from axial CT scans with a high-resolution bone filter. The image shows very severe degenerative changes in both TMJs with destruction of the mandibular condyles and inflammatory erosions.

Tumor?

Osteochondromas of the condylar process of the mandible are of special significance because of their ability to alter facial features and cause TMJ dysfunction. They are rare tumors that can be difficult to distinguish from the more common thickening of the mandibular condyle that occurs in **osteoarthritis**.

Other tumors may affect the TMJ, including **osteosarcoma**, but they are very rare. Imaging evaluation relies on CT, MRI, or both.

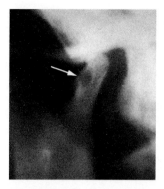

Fig. 4.**425** Subchondral degenerative cyst in the condylar process of a 44-year-old man with degenerative arthritis of the mandibular condyle (arrow).

 ## Other Changes?

Osteoarthritis of the TMJ is characterized by joint dysfunction and pain that can radiate to the temporal and occipital areas. It is one of the most common diseases in dentistry, oralogy, and stomatology. Crepitus in the TMJ is a frequent sign of osteoarthritis. Conventional radiographs can detect erosions, sclerosis, and bony morphological changes. The latter consist of decreased depth of the glenoid fossa along with flattening and broadening of the mandibular condyle. **Subchondral degenerative cysts** (Fig. 4.425) and **marginal osteophytes** can also be detected. Asymmetrical mastication and occlusion that favor muscle groups on one side often lead to a lateralization of jaw opening movements, imposing excessive stresses on one TMJ. CT shows increased bone density of the mandibular condyle in the af-

fected joints. While unilateral hyperplasia of the mandibular condyle can occur during **growth**, condylar enlargement and displacement in **adults** can result from degenerative osteophytes.

Pigmented villonodular synovitis is a usually monoarticular disease characterized by pronounced villus formation and synovial proliferation, which may cause bone destruction. The proliferation is accompanied by intense hemosiderosis in the deeper portions of the synovial membrane. Basically the disease is not an inflammatory process, and so the term "synovitis" is misleading. Pigmented villonodular synovitis of the TMJ with nonpainful preauricular swelling is very rare. As the disease progresses, there are increasing complaints due to changes in the joint capsule, progressive bone destruction, and secondary osteoarthritis. MRI has greatly facilitated the detection of pigmented villonodular synovitis, which is commonly misdiagnosed on radiographs.

Synovial chondromatosis is another rare disease that is monoarticular in the great majority of cases. The rare biarticular form tends to affect symmetrical joints. The knee is most commonly involved, followed by the elbow, hip, shoulder, ankle, wrist, and the phalangeal joints of the hand. The TMJ is very rarely affected. Synovial chondromatosis is manifested clinically by a painful limitation of motion or even a complete loss of joint motion. Chondromas that have undergone ringlike or nodular calcification can be detected on plain radiographs or CT scans. Micronodular chondromas that do not calcify cannot be detected on standard radiographs. They appear as filling defects on arthrography, and they are often detectable with CT owing to the high contrast resolution of that modality. They can also be demonstrated by MRI. Synovial chondromatosis is a potent preosteoarthritic condition. Treatment consists of surgery.

References

Ajaglee, H. A., J. O. Daramola: Fibro-osseous lesions of the jaw: a review of 133 cases from Nigeria. J. Nat. Med. Ass. 75 (1983) 593

Alexandridis, E., H. Weidauer: Medial blow-out fracture. Orbit 4 (1985) 81

Anneroth, G., B. Johansson: Peripheral ameloblastoma. Int. J. Oral Surg. 14 (1985) 295

Antonyshyn, O., J. S. Gruss: Complex of orbital trauma: the role of rigid fixation and primary bone grafting. Adv. Ophthal. Plast. Reconstr. Surg. 7 (1987) 61

Barbrel, Ph., D. Laniel, J. Serieye, P. Gros: Difficultés de diagnostic radiologique des fractures mandibulaires monocorticales. Rev. Stomatol. Chir. max.-fac. 85 (1984) 469

Beighton, P., Cremin, B. J.: Sclerosing Bone Dysplasias. Springer, Berlin–Heidelberg–New York 1980

Bellavoire, A., J. Suleau, F. Jouen, J. Pons: Considérations statistiques á propos des fractues sinusales de la face. Rev. Stomatol. Chir. max.-fac. 85 (1984) 414

Berg, O., Ch. Carenfelt: Etiological diagnosis in sinusitis. Ultrasonography as clinical complement. Laryngoscope 95 (1985) 851

Bernstein, L., F. Bruce: Bilateral hyperplasia of the coronoid process of the mandible. Arch. Otolaryngol. 110 (1984) 480

Beutel, A., A. Tänzer: Röntgendiagnostik der Orbitae, der Augen und der Tränenwege. In Röntgendiagnostik des Schädels, Part 2, Ed. by L. Diethelm, F. Strnad. In Olsson, O., F. Strnad, H. Vieten, A. Zuppinger: Handbuch der Medizinischen Radiologie, Vol. VII. Springer, Berlin 1963

Bierny, I.-P., R. Dryden: Orbital enlargement secondary to paranasal sinus hypoplasia: Amer. J. Roentgenol. 128 (1977) 850

Birzle, H., R. Bergleitner, E. H. Kuner: Traumatologische Röntgendiagnostik, 2nd Ed. Thieme, Stuttgart 1985

Blanc, J. L., J. P. Lagier, R. Gras, D. Bremond, D. Beloni: Les séquelles des fracutes condyliennes á travers l'expérience du service et l'experitise médical. Rev. Stomatol. Chir. max.-fac. 86 (1985) 29

Blaschke, D. P.: The temporomandibular joint. In Bergeron R. Th., A. G. Osborn, P. Som: Head and Neck Imgaging, Mosby, St. Louis 1984 (pp. 251–278)

Blaschke, D. T., A. G. Osborn: The mandible and teeth. In Bergeron, R. Th., A. G., Osborn, P. M. Som: Head and Neck Imaging. Mosby, St. Louis 1984 (pp. 283–298)

Boland, Th., O. R. Beirne: Zygomatic exostosis. Int. J. Oral. Surg. 12 (1983) 124

Bomalaski, J. S., S. A. Jimenez: Erosive arthritis of the temporomandibular joint in Reiter's syndrome. J. Rheumatol. 11 (1984) 400

Bryan, R. N., R. A. Lewis, St. L. Miller: Choroidal osteoma. Amer. J. Neuroradiol. 4 (1983) 491

Bryan, R. N., J. A. Craig: The eye. Section one: CT of the orbit. In Bergeron, R. Th., A. G. Osborne, P. M. Som: Head and Neck Imaging. Mosby, St. Louis 1984 (pp. 575–618)

Cadin, P.: Le syndrome oculo-auriculo-vertébral de Goldenhar. Ann. Pédiat. 29 (1982) 413

Canigiani, G.: Das Panorama-Aufnahmeverfahren. Thieme, Stuttgart 1976

Canigiani, G., C. W. Czech: Fibröse Dysplasie der Mandibula. Fortschr. Röntgenstr. 119 (1973) 492

Carter, B. L.,: Computertomographie. In Valvassori, C. E., G. D. Potter, W. N. Hanafee, B. L. Carter, R. A. Buckingham: Radiologie in der Hals-Nasen-Ohren-Heilkunde. Hrsg. G. Canigiani, G. Wittich. Thieme, Stuttgart 1984

Carter, B. L., V. S. Runge: Imaging modalities for the study of the paranasal sinuses and nasopharynx. Otolaryngol. Clin. N. Amer. 21 (1988) 395

Cobb, St. R., J. W. Weakley, K. F. Lee, C. M. Mehringer, V. S. Grinnell: Computed tomographic evaluation of ocular trauma. Comput. Radiol. 9 (1985) 1

Coker, N. J., B. Brooks, T. el Gammal: Computed tomography of orbital medial wall fractures. Head Neck Surg. 5 (1983) 383

Constans, J. P., J. F. Meder, P. Justiniano, M. Michalski, D. Fredy: Ostéome frontal à extension orbitaire. J. Fr. Ophthalmol. 7 (1984) 381

Costa, L. S., L. A. L. Resende: Sphenoid sinus mucocele. Arch. Neurol. 41 (1984) 897

Crysdale, W. S., P. Cole., P. Emery: Cephalometric radiographs, nasal airway resistance and the effect of adenoidectomy. J. Otolaryngol. 14 (1985) 92

Curtin, H. D., P. Wolfe, L. Gallia, M. May: Unusually large nasopalatine cyst: CT-findings. J. Comput. Assist. Tomogr. 8 (1984) 139

Daffner, R. H., J. S. Apple, J. A. Gehweiler: Lateral view of facial fractures. Amer. J. Roentgenol. 141 (1983) 587

Dammann, F., E. Momino-Traserra, C. Remy, et al.: Strahlenexposition bei der Spiral-CT der Nasennebenhöhlen. Fortschr. Röntgenstr. 172 (2000) 232

Daniels, D. L., P. Pech, M. C. Kay, K. Pojunas, A. L. Williams, V. M. Haughton: Orbital apex. Amer. J. Neuroradiol. 6 (1985) 705

Dihlmann, W.: Gelenke, Wirbelverbindungen, 2nd Ed. Thieme, Stuttgart 1982 (S. 440–451)

Dolan, K. D.: Paranasal sinus radiology: part 2 A: Ethmoidal sinuses. Head Neck Surg. Jul./Aug. (1982 a) 486

Dolan, K. D.: Paranasal sinus radiology: part 2 B: Ethmoidal sinuses. Head Neck Surg. Sept./Oct. (1982 b) 53

Dolan, K. D.: Paranasal sinus radiology: part 3 A: Sphenoidal sinus. Head Neck Surg.. Nov./Dec. (1982 c) 1

Dolan, K. D.: Paranasal sinus radiology: part 3 B: Sphenoidal sinus. Head Neck Surg.. Nov./Dec. (1982 d) 237

Dolan, K. D.: The ethmoid sinus. Plain-film and tomographic radiology. Otolaryngol. Clin. N. Amer. 18 (1985) 1

Dolan, K. D., W. R. K. Smoker: Paranasal sinus radiology: part 4 B: Maxillary sinuses. Head Neck Surg. 5 (1983) 428

Doub, H. P., F. A. Henny: Radiological study of the temporomandibular joints. Radiology 60 (1953) 666

Düker, J.: Röntgendiagnostik mit der Panoramaschichtaufnahme. Hüthig, Heidelberg 1992

Eggert, J. H., J. Dumbach, E. W. Steinhäuser: Zur Ätiologie und Therapie der Osteoradionekrose des Unterkiefers. Dtsch. zahnärztl. Z. 40 (1985) 2

Engelmayer, E.: Ringförmige Verkalkungen des Augapfels. Fortschr. Röntgenstr. 119 (1973) 482

Eriksson, L., M. Rohlin, P.-L. Westesson: The correlation of temporomandibular joint sounds with joint morphology in fifty-five autopsy specimens. J. Oral Max.-fac. Surg. 43 (1985) 194

Eversole, L. R., D. Strub: Radiographic characteristics of cystogenic ameloblastoma. Oral Surg. 57 (1984) 572

Farkas, L. G., J. C. Kolar, I. R. Munro: Cranofacial disproportions in Apert's syndrome: an anthropometric study. Cleft Palate J. 22 (1985) 255

Feneis, H.: Anatomisches Bildwörterbuch. 8th Ed. Thieme, Stuttgart 1998

Fischer-Brandies, H., E. Fischer-Brandies, E. Dielert: Der Unterkieferwinkel auf dem Orthopantomogramm. Radiologe 24 (1984) 547

Fitz, C. R., S. H. Chuang, D. C. Harwood-Nash: Computed tomography diagnoses of eye tumors and anomalies in early childhood and infancy. Ann. Radiol. 28 (1985) 235

Forbes, G., D. Gehring, C. A. Gorman, M. D. Brennan, I. T. Jackson: Volume measurements of normal orbital structures by computed tomographic analysis: Amer. J. Neuroradiol. 6 (1985) 419

Freyschmidt, J.: Skeletterkrankungen. Klinisch-radiologische Diagnose und Differentialdiagnose. 2nd Ed., Springer, Berlin, Heidelberg, New York 1997

Freyschmidt, J., H. Ostertag, G. Jund: Knochentumoren. 2nd Ed., Springer, Berlin, Heidelberg, New York 1998

Frick, H., H. Leonhardt, D. Starck: Spezielle Anatomie II. Kopf-Hals-Eingeweide-Nervensystem. 2nd Ed., Thieme, Stuttgart 1980

Gahleitner, A., U. Hofschneider, G. Tepper, M. Pretterklieber, S. Schick, K. Zausa, G. Watzek: Lingual vascular canals of the mandible: Evaluation with dental CT. Radiology 220 (2001) 186

Gardner, D. G.: The mixed odontogenic tumors. Oral Surg. 58 (1984) 166

Geist, E. T., J. N. Kent, R. F. Carr, St. Super: Multiloculated radiolucency of the left mandible. Clinico-pathologic conferences, Case 52. J. Oral Max.-fac. Surg. 43 (1985) 205

Gentry, L. R., W. F. Manor, P. A. Turski, Ch. M. Strotter: High-resolution CT analysis of facial struts in trauma: 1. Normal anatomy. Amer. J. Roentgenol. 140 (1983) 533

Georgi, M., H. Betz, R. Günther: Röntgendiagnostik der Orbitafrakturen unter besonderer Berücksichtigung der Aufnahmetechnik. Radiologe 14 (1974) 517

Gilbard, St. M., M. F. Mafee, P. A. Lagouros, B. G. Langer: Orbital blow-out fractures. The prognostic significance of computed tomography. Ophthalmology 11 (1985) 1523

Gornig, H., W.-E. Goldhahn, F. Schmidt, A. Arendt: Fibröse Dysplasie der knöchernen Orbita mit "Neuritis retrobulbaris". Opthalmologica 190 (1985) 91

Gutin, P. H., W. G. Cushard jr., C. B. Wilson: Cushing's disease with pituitary apoplex leading to hypopituitarism, empty sella, and spontaneus fracture of the dorsum sellae: Case report. J. Neurosurg. 51 (1979) 866

Guyon, J. H., M. Brant-Zawadzkj, St. R. Seiff: CT demonstration of optic canal fractures. Amer. J. Neuroradiol. 5 (1984) 575

Halimi, Ph., D. Doyon, Ph. Madoule, M. T. Iba-Zizen, A. Lopez: L'imagerie par resonance magnétique du massif facial/nuclear magnetic resonance imaging of facial structures. J. Neuroradiol. 11 (1984) 274

Hall, M. B., R. W. Brown, R. A. Baughman: Gaucher's disease affecting the mandible. J. Oral Max.-fac. Surg. 43 (1985) 210

Han, J. S., R. G. Huss, J. E. Benson: MR imaging of the skull base. J. Comput. Assist. Tomogr. 8 (1984) 944

Harris, J. H., R. D. Ray, E. N. Rauschkolb, N. H. Rappaport: An approach to midfacial fractures. Crit. Rev. Diagn. Imag. 21 (1984) 105

Haschim, A. S. M., T. Asakura, H. Awa, K. Yamashita, K. Takasaki, F. Yuhi: Giant mucocele of paranasal sinuses. Surg. Neurol. 23 (1985) 69

Helms, C. A., R. B. Morrish jr., L. T. Kurcos, R. W. Katzberg, M. F. Dolwick: Computed tomography of the meniscus of the temporomandibular joint: preliminary observations. Radiology 145 (1982) 719

Helms, C. A., J. B. Vogler, R. B. Morrish, St. M. Goldman, R. E. Capra, E. Proctor: Temporomandibular joint internal derangements: CT diagnosis. Radiology 152 (1984) 459

Hoffmeister, B.: Die parodontale Reaktion im Bruchspalt stehender Zähne bei Unterkieferfrakturen: Dtsch. zahnärztl. Z. 40 (1985) 32

Hollmann, K.: Traumatische Veränderungen der Kiefer und Zähne. In Röntgendiagnostik des Schädels, Part 2, Ed. by L. Diethelm, F. Strnad. In: Olsson, O., F. Strnad, H. Vieten, A. Zuppinger: Handbuch der Medizinischen Radiologie. Springer, Berlin 1963 (S. 111)

Holt, G. R., J. E. Holt: Nasoethmoid complex injuries. Otolaryngol. Clin. N. Amer. 18 (1985) 87

Hosten, N.: Auge und Orbita. Radiologische Differentialdiagnostik. 1st Ed., Thieme, Stuttgart-New York 1995

Hüls, A., E. Walter, W. Schulte: Konventionelle Röntgendiagnosik und CT der Kiefergelenke bei Myoarthopathien. Radiologe 24 (1984) 360

Hüls, A., E. Walter, W. Schulte, W. B. Freesmeyer: Computertomographische Stadieneinteilung des dysfunktionellen Gelenkkopfumbaus. Dtsch. zahnärztl. Z. 40 (1985) 37

Irnberger, T.: Diagnostische Möglichkeiten und Wertigkeit der konventionellen Radiographie, Röntgentomographie und hochauflösenden Computertomographie beim komplexen orbitalen Trauma. Fortschr. Röntgenstr. 142 (1984) 146

Jend, H.-H., I. Jend-Rossmann: A systematic approach to the diagnosis of transethmoidal fractures in CT. Europ. J. Radiol. 5 (1985) 8

Judisch, G. F., St. P. Kraft, J. A. Bartley, Ch. G. Jacoby: Orbital Hypotelorism. Arch. Ophthalmol. 102 (1984) 995

Katzberg, R. W., R. W. Bessette, R. H. Tallents, D. B. Blewes, J. V. Manzione, J. F. Schenck et al.: Hart: Normal and abnormal temporomandibular joint: MR imaging with surface coil. Radiology 158 (1986) 183

Katzberg, R. W., J. Schenck, D. Roberts, R. H. Tallents, J. V. Manzione, H. R. Hart, et al.: Magnetic resonance imaging of the temporomandibular joint meniscus. Oral Surg. 59 (1985) 332

Kojima, T., Sh. Waga, F. Masakazu: Fracture of the sella turcica. Neurosurgery 16 (1985) 225

Komisar, A., C. Silver, Sh. Kalnicki: Osteoradionecrosis of the maxilla and skull base. Laryngoscope 95 (1985) 24

Kotscher, E.: Die Röntgendiagnostik der Schädeltraumen. I. Traumatische Veränderungen. In: Röntgendiagnostik des Schädels, Part 2, Ed. by L. Diethelm, F. Strnad. In: Olsson, O., F. Strnad, H. Vieten, A. Zuppinger: Handbuch der Medizinischen Radiologie, Vol. VII. Springer, Berlin 1963

Kudryk, W. H., G. L. Baker, J. S. Persy: Ankylosis of the temporomandibular joint from psoriatic arthritis. J. Otolaryngol. 14 (1985) 336

Laine, F. J., W. F. Conway, D. M. Laskin: Radiology of maxillofacial trauma. Curr. Probl. Diagn. Radiol. 22 (1993) 145

Langlais, R. P., R. Broadus, B. Junfin Glass: Bifid mandibular canals in panoramic radiographs. Amer. Dent. Ass. 110 (1985) 923

Langmann, J.: Medizinische Embryologie. 8th Ed. Thieme, Stuttgart 1989

Leyder, P., R. Rue, J. Texier, J. Laufer: Tumeurs osseuses mandibulaires. Les difficultes du diagnostic. Rev. Stomatol. Chir. max.-fac. 85 (1984) 320

Li, K. C., P. Y. Poon, P. Hinton, R. Willinsky, C. J. Pavlin, J. J. Hurwitz et al.: MR Imaging of orbital tumors with CT and ultrasound correlations. J. Comput. Assist. Tomogr. 8 (1984) 1039

Lloyd, G. A. S.: Radiology of the Orbit. Saunders. London 1975

Lörinc, P., J. E. Rosengren: Über die Röntgendiagnose der Schleimhautzyste der Kieferhöhle. Radiologe 23 (1983) 553

Lombardi, G., A. Passerini, A. Cecchini: Pneumosinus dilatans. Acta Radiol. Diagn. 7 (1968) 535

Mafee, M. F., S. Pruznansky, M. M. Morales, M. G. Phatak, G. E. Valvassori, G. D. Dobbenc et al.: CT in the evaluation of the orbit and the bony interorbital distance. Amer. J. Neuroradiol. 7 (1986) 265

Marks, R. B., D. M. Carlton, R. F. Carr: Osteochondroma of the mandibular condyle. Oral Surg. 58 (1984) 30

Marsot-Dupuch, K.: Facial sinuses. Inflammation. Ann. Radiol. 34 (1991) 28

Masing, H., G. Wolf: Der Nachweis des Nasenmuschelzyklus mit Hilfe des Röntgenschichtverfahrens. Z. Laryng. Rhinol. 48 (1969) 684

Matschke, R. G.: Die Bewertung der Sonografie bei Erkrankungen der Nebenhöhlen. HNO 32 (1984) 502

Mattox, D. E., G. Delaney: Anatomy of the ethmoid sinus. Otolaryngol. Clin. N. Amer. 18 (1985) 3

Mendelsohn, D. B., Y. Hertzanu: Hypoplasia of the maxillary antrum. S. Afr. Med. 63 (1983) 496

Merville, L. C., E. Gitton: Une forme inhabituelle de fracture isolée du plancher orbitaire: "La fracture en clapet". Rev. Stomatol. Chir. max.-fac. 86 (1985) 165

Mizuno, A., T. Nakamura, K. Motegi, H. Shirasawa: Osteochondroma of the mandibular condyle. Int. J. Oral Surg. 12 (1983) 221

Mosesson, E. E., P. M. Som: The radiographic evaluation of sinonasal tumors: an overview. Otolaryngol. Clin. N. Amer. 28 (1995) 1097

Neiss, A.: Über wenig bekannte Skelettvariationen. Fortschr. Röntgenstr. 94 (1961) 227

Novak, D., W. Bloss: Röntgenologische Aspekte des Basal-Zell-Naevus-Syndroms, Gorlin-Goltz-Syndrom. Fortschr. Röntgenstr. 124 (1976) 11

Olow-Nordenham, M. A. K., C. T. Radberg: Maxillo-nasal dysplasia (Binder syndrome) and associated malformations of the cervical spine. Acta. Radiol. Diagn. 25 (1984) 353

Osaki, T., K. Ryoke, T. Nagami, T. Ogawa, T. Hamada: Ameloblastoma with hypoproteinaemia due to protein leakage. Int. J. Oral Surg. 14 (1985) 302

Osborn, A. G.: Diagnostic neuroradiology. Mosby, St. Louis, Baltimore, Boston, Chicago 1994

Osborn, A. G.: The nose. In: Bergeron, R. Th., A. G. Osborn, P. M. Som: Head and Neck Imaging. Mosby, St. Louis 1984 a (pp. 143–171)

Osborn, A. G.: The pterygopalatine (sphenomaxillary) fossa. In: Bergeron, R. Th., A. G. Osborn, P. M. Som: Head and Neck Imaging. Mosby, St. Louis 1984 b (pp. 172–185)

Osborn, A. G., W. H. Hanafee, A. A. Mancuso: Normal and pathologic CT anatomy of the mandible. Amer. J. Roentgenol. 139 (1982) 555

Osborn, A. G., E. B. McIff: Computed tomography of the nose. Head Neck Surg. 4 (1982) 182

Paatero, Y. V.: Pantomography and orthopantomography. Oral Surg. 14 (1985) 947

Pandolfo, I., M. Gaeta, M. Longo, A. Blandino, M. Longo: The radiology of the pterygoid canal: normal and pathologic findings. Amer. J. Neuroradiol. 8 (1987) 479

Pandolfo, I., M. Gaeta, M. Longo, A. Blandino, E. G. Russi, S. Volta et al.: Computed tomography of the pterygopalatine fossa. Normal anatomy and neoplastic pathology. Radiol. Med. 76 (1988) 340

Parizel, P., R. Kets, A. de Schepper, R. Geerts: Sarcoidosis of the nasal bones. Fortschr. Röntgenstr. 139 (1983) 103

Pepper, L., M. F. Zide: Mandibular condyle fracture and dislocation into the middle cranial fossa. Brit. J. Oral Surg. 14 (1985) 278

Pincock, J. L., S. K. El-Mofty: Recurrence of cystic central mucoepidermoid tumor of the mandible. Int. J. Oral Sug. 14 (1985) 81

Pöschl, M: Juvenile Osteochondronekrosen. In: Röntgendiagnostik der Skeletterkrankungen, Part 4, Ed. by L. Diethelm, L. Olsson, F. Strnad, H. Vieten, A. Zuppinger. Handbuch der Medizinischen Radiologie, Vol. V. Springer, Berlin 1971

Potter, G. D.: Röntgendiagnostik der Nasennebenhöhlen und des Gesichtsschädels. In Valvassory, G. E., G. D. Potter, W. N. Hanafee, B. L. Carter, R. A. Buckingham: Radiologie in der Hals-Nasen-Ohrenheilkunde. Hrsg. V. G. Canigiani, G. Wittich. Thieme, Stuttgart 1984

Rao, V. M., K. I. el Noueam: Sinonasal imaging. Anatomy and pathology. Radiol. Clin. N. Amer. 36 (1998) 921

Rauber/Kopsch: Bewegungsapparat, Bd. 1. Hrsg. von Tillmann, B., G. Töndury. In Rauber/Kopsch: Anatomie des Menschen. Lehrbuch und Atlas. 1st Ed. Ed. by Leonhardt, H., B. Tillmann, G. Töndury, K. Zilles. Thieme, Stuttgart 1997

Rauch, St. D.: Medial orbital blow-out fracture with entrapment. Arch. Otolaryngol. 111 (1985) 53

Raustia, A., M. J. Phytinen, K. K. Virtanen: Density of the caput mandibulae in computed tomography compared with clinical findings related to TMJ dysfunctions. Fortschr. Röntgenstr. 143 (1985) 408

Reinhardt, K., Linsenverkalkung. Fortschr. Röntgenstr. 126 (1977) 275

Reyes de la Rocha, S., T. J. Pysher, J. C. Leonard: Dyskinetic cilia syndrome: clinical, radiographic and scintigraphic findings. Pediat. Radiol. 17 (1987) 97

Rhea, J. T., A. L. Weber: Giant-cell-granuloma of the sinuses. Radiology 47 (1983) 135

Rice, D. H.: Benign and malignant tumors of the ethmoid sinus. Otolaryngol. Clin. N. Amer. 18 (1985) 113

Reeder, M. M., W. G. Bradley Jr.: Reeder and Felsons's Gamuts in Radiology. Comprehensive Lists of Roentgen Differential Diagnosis. 3rd. Ed., Springer, New York–Berlin–Heidelberg 1993

Robert, Y., M. Provost, J. P. Francke, L. Lemaitre: Normal imaging of facial structures. Ann. Radiol. 34 (1991) 18

Roberts, M. W., N. W. Barton, G. Constantopoulos, D. P. Butler, A. H. Donahne: Occurence of multiple dentigerous cysts in a patient with the Maroteaux-Lamy syndrome (mucopolysacharidosis type VI). Oral Surg. 58 (1984) 169

Rogers, L. F.: Radiology of Skeletal Trauma. Churchill-Livingstone, New York 1982

Ronner, H. J., I. Snow Jones: Aneurysmal bone cyst of the orbit: a review. Ann Ophthalmol. 15 (1983) 626

Rothmann L. G.: Dental Applications of Computerized Tomography: Surgical Planning for Implant Placement. Quintessence 1998

Russel, E. J., L. Czervionke, M. Huckmann, D. Daniels, D. McLachlan: CT of the inferomedial orbit and the lacrimal drainage apparatus. Amer. J. Neuroradiol. 6 (1985) 759

Sartor, K. J., M. P. Ward, F. J. Hodges, H. S. Glazer: Current state of ENT radiology. Curr. Probl. Diagn. Radiol. 14 (1985) 1, 28

Schatz, S. L., H. R. Cohen, M. J. Ryvicker, A. M. Deutsch, J. V. Manzione: Overview of computed tomography of the temporomandibular joint. J. Comput. Tomogr. 9 (1985) 351

Schinz: Schädel–Gehirn. In: Schinz: Radiologische Diagnostik in Klinik und Praxis, Vol. V, Part 1. 7th Ed. Edited by Frommhold, W., W. Dihlmann, H.-St. Stender, P. Thurn. Thieme, Stuttgart 1986

Schneider, G., E. Tölly: Radiologische Diagnostik des Gesichtsschädels, Thieme, Stuttgart 1984

Schwickert, H. C., H. Cagil, H. U. Kauczor, F. Schweden, H. Riechelmann, M. Thelen: CT and MRT of the paranasal sinuses. Akt. Radiol. 4 (1994) 88

Shankar, L., K. Evans, M. Hawke, H. Stommberger: Atlas der Nasen-nebenhöhlen. Chapman and Hall, London-Glasgow-Weinheim-New York-Tokio-Melbourne-Madras 1994

Shanmugham, M. S.: Cementifying fibroma of the ethmoidal sinus. J. Laryngol. Otol. 98 (1984) 639

Sherk, H. H., L. A. Whitaker, P. S. Pasquariello: Facial malformations and spinal anomalies: a predictate relationship. Spine 7 (1982) 526

Sherman, N. H., V. M. Rao, R. E. Brenna, J. Edeiken: Fibrous dysplasia of the facial bones and mandible. Skelet. Radiol. 8 (1982) 141

Shields, J. A., B. Bakewell, J. J. Augsburger, J. C. Flanagan: Classification and incidence of space-occupying lesions of the orbit. Arch. Ophthalmol. 102 (1984) 1606

Sjöberg, S., P. Lörine: Intracranial supernumerary tooth. Radiologe 24 (1984) 561

Slowis, Th. L., B. Renfro, F. B. Watts, L. R. Kuhns, W. Belenky, J. Spoylar: Choanal atresia: precise CT evaluation. Radiology 155 (1985) 345

Smahel, Z.: Cephalometric and morphologic changes associated with unilateral cleft lips and palate in adults. Acta Chir. Plast. 24 (1982) 1

Sobotta-Becher: Atlas der Anatomie des Menschen. Hrsg. Ferner, H., J. Staubesand. 18th Ed., Urban und Schwarzenberg, Munich-Vienna-Baltimore 1972

Sollberg, W. K., T. L. Hansson, B. Nordström: The temporomandibular joint in young adults at autopsy: a morphologic classification and evaluation. J. Oral Rehabil. 12 (1985) 303

Som, P. M.: The paranasal sinuses. In Bergeron, T., A. G. Osborn, P. M. Som: Head and Neck Imaging. Mosby, St. Louis 1984 (pp. 1–142)

Som, P. M.: CT of the paranasal sinuses. Neuroradiol. 27 (1985) 189

Som, P. M., H. D. Curten: Head and Neck Imaging. 3rd Ed., Mosby, St. Louis 1996

Sonesson, A.: Die Röntgendiagnostik der Kiefer und Zähne. In Röntgendiagnostik des Schädels, Part 2, Ed. by L. Diethelm, F. Strnad. In Olsson, O., F. Strnad, H. Vieten, A. Zuppinger: Handbuch der Medizinischen Radiologie, Vol. VII. Springer, Berlin 1963

Sonnabend, E., W. Hielscher,: Zähne und Kiefer. In Schinz: Radiologische Diagnostik, 7th Ed. Schädel, Gehirn, Vol. V/1, Edited by W. Dihlmann, H.-St. Stender, Thieme, Stuttgart 1986

Staloff, R. Th., Ch. B. Grossmann, C. Gonzales, M. H. Naheedy: Computed tomography of the face and paranasal sinuses: Part I. Normal anatomy. Head Neck Surg. 7 (1984) 110

Stammberger, H.: Zur Entstehung röntgendichter Strukturen bei Aspergillus-Mykosen der Nasennebenhöhlen. HNO 33 (1985) 62

Stammberger, H., R. Jaske, F. Beaufort: Aspergillus-Mykosen der Nasennebenhöhlen. Münch. Med. Wschr. 125 (1983) 815

Stewart, G., D. G. Young, A. F. Azmy: Das sog. Charge-Mißbildungssyndrom bei Neugeborenen mit Choanalatresie. Z. Kinderchir. 42 (1987) 12

Stewart, R. E., A. E. Poole: The orofacial structures and their association with congenital abnormalities. Pediat. Clin. N. Amer. 29 (1982) 547

Stobel, D. F., C. Mills, D. Charr, D. Norman, M. Bratzawadzki, L. Kaufmann, et al.: NMR or the normal and pathologic eye and orbit. Amer. J. Neuroradiol. 5 (1984) 345

Süsse, H. S.: Nerven- und Gefäßkanäle am Os zygomaticum und am Sinus maxillaris. Fortschr. Röntgenstr. 95 (1961) 505

Swartz, J. D., N. A. Abaza, B. H. Hendler, O. Tielwell, G. L. Popky: High-resolution computed tomography; Part 4: Evaluation of odontogenic lesions. Head Neck Surg. 7 (1985) 409

Syrjänen, S. M.: The temporomandibular joint in rheumatic arthritis. Acta Radiol. Diagn. 26 (1985) 235

Szalay, B.: Ein die rechtsseitige Nasenhöhle völlig verlegender Rhinolith. Fortschr. Röntgenstr. 108 (1968) 687

Tadmor, R., M. Ravid, D. Millet, G. Leventon: Computed tomographic demonstration of choanal atresia. Amer. J. Neuroradiol. 5 (1984) 743

Tanizaki, Y., S. Kobayashi, N. Kobayshi, K. Sugita: Salaam fracture of the dorsum sellae. Neurosurgery 10 (1982) 748

Taybi, H.: Radiologie der Syndrome: Thieme, Stuttgart 1982

Terrier, F., W. Weber, D. Ruefenacht, B. Procellini: Anatomy of the ethmoid. Amer. J. Neuroradiol. 6 (1985) 77

Thelen, M., G. Ritter, E. Bücheler: Radiologische Diagnostik der Verletzungen von Knochen und Gelenken. Thieme, Stuttgart-New York, 1993

Thompson, J. R., E. Christansen, A. N. Hasso, D. B. Hinshaw: Temporomandibular joints: high-resolution computed tomographic evaluation. Radiology 150 (1984) 105

Tucker, M. R., W. Bonner Guilford, C. W. Howard: Coronoid process hyperplasia causing restricted opening and facial asymmetry. Oral Surg. 58 (1984) 130

Unger, J. M., K. Shaffer, J. A. Duncavage: Computed tomography in nasal and paranasal sinus disease. Laryngoscope 94 (1984) 1319

Valvassori, G. E., M. F. Mafee, B. L. Carter: Imaging of the Head and Neck. Thieme, Stuttgart 1995

Vogl, Th. J., D. Eberhard: MR-Tomographie Temporomandibulargelenk: Untersuchungstechnik, klinische Befunde, diagnostische Strategien. Thieme, Stuttgart, New York 1993

Waldron, Ch. A.: Fibro-osseous lesions of the jaw. J. Oral Max.-fac. Surg. 43 (1985) 249

Walter, A., O. Kleinsässer: Intranasale extradurale Meningeome. Z. Laryngol. Rhinol. Otol. 64 (1985) 198

Weber, A. L., A. Rodriguez-DeVelasquez, M. J. Kucarelli, H. M. Cheng: Lymphoproliferative disease of the orbit. Neuroimag. Clin. N. Amer. 6 (1996) 199

Welfare, R. D.: Paget's disease. Case report. Brit. Dent. J. 158 (1985) 90

Wells, R. G., J. R. Sty, A. D. Landers: Radiologic evaluation of Pott puffy tumor. J. Amer. Med. Ass. 255 (1986) 1331

White, S. C., M. J. Pharoah: Oral Radiology, Principles and Interpretation, 4rd Ed. Mosby-Year Book, St. Louis 1999

Young, L. W.: Radiological imaging of Pott puffy tumor and other frontal sinusitis complications. Amer. J. Dis. Child. 410 (1986) 197

Youssefzadeh, S., A. Gahleitner, R. Dorffner, T. Bernhard, F. M. Kainberger: Dental vertical root fractures: value of CT in detection. Radiology 210 (1999) 545

Zachariades, N., I. Koundouris: Maxillofacial symptoms in two patients with pyknodysostosis. J. Oral Max.-fac. Surg. 42 (1984) 819

Zachariades, N., D. Papavassiliou, D. Triantafyllou, E. Vairaktaris, I. Papademetriou, M. Mezitis et al.: Fractures of the facial skeleton in the edentulous patient. J. Max.-fac. Surg. 12 (1984) 262

Zanella, F. E., U. Mödder, G. Benz-Bohm, F. Thun: Die Neurofibromatose im Kindesalter. Fortschr. Röntgenstr. 141 (1984) 498

Zanella, F. E., U. Mödder, B. Kirchhof: Computertomographie der Orbita Teil I: Traumatisch bedingte Veränderungen. Fortschr. Röntgenstr. 142 (1985) 670

Zhilka, A.: Computed tomography of blow-out fracture of the medial orbital wall. Amer. J. Roentgenol. 134 (1981) 963

Zhilka, A.: Computed tomography in facial trauma. Radiology 144 (1982) 545

Zimmer-Brossy, M.: Lehrbuch der röntgendiagnostischen Einstelltechnik. 4th Ed. (1992) Springer Verlag, Berlin, Heidelberg, New York.

5

Spinal Column

J. Brossmann

The spinal column forms the axial skeleton of the trunk and in humans is normally composed of 24 free or pre-sacral vertebrae. The free spinal column consists of 7 cervical vertebrae (C1–C7), 12 thoracic vertebrae (T1–T12), and 5 lumbar vertebrae (L1–L5). The first and second cervical vertebrae, called the atlas and axis, have special morphological and functional features that distinguish them from the other free vertebrae. They combine with the occiput to form the cranioverterbral joints. The fifth lumbar vertebra articulates with the sacrum, which is formed by the synostotic fusion of five vertebrae. The boundary between the free vertebral column and sacrum is variable: 24 presacral vertebrae exist in 92–95% of cases, while in 5–8% of cases lumbarization of the first sacral vertebra or sacralization of the fifth lumbar vertebra can be found. Often the sacralization exists on one side only. The coccyx extends downward from the apex of the sacrum. The rudimentary coccygeal vertebrae vary in number from four to six (Rauber and Kopsch 1998).

The spinal column of adults in the upright posture presents a double S-shaped curve in the sagittal plane. The physiological curvatures consist of a cervical lordosis from C1 to C6, a lumbar lordosis from T9 to L5, a thoracic kyphosis from C6 to T9, and a sacral kyphosis spanning the sacrum and coccyx. A mild degree of scoliosis in the region from T3 to T5 is considered normal. The physiological curves of the spinal column are already present, though mildly pronounced, in newborns.

Basic Anatomy of the Vertebrae and Ligaments

Vertebrae

Except for the atlas, each vertebra consists of a **vertebral body** and a posterior **vertebral arch** (neural arch). The body and arch enclose a central opening, the **vertebral foramen**. The upper and lower surfaces of the vertebral body are covered by a **cartilaginous end plate** that is bounded by a curved, bony **marginal ridge**.

The vertebral arch consists of two symmetrical hemiarches, which join together posteriorly and fuse in the midline with the **spinous process**. The vertebral arch is composed of an anterior **pedicle** and a posterior **lamina**. Projecting from each pedicle are a **superior and inferior articular process**. The superior and inferior vertebral notches of adjacent vertebrae form the **intervertebral foramen**, which links the **vertebral canal** with the paravertebral soft tissues. The **transverse processes** of the vertebral bodies project laterally from the pedicles. They are powerfully developed in the thoracic spine and rudimentary in the cervical and lumbar spine. The vertebrae in different regions of the spine have characteristic features that are discussed more fully in the sections on specific vertebrae.

The **intervertebral disks** are composed of fibrocartilage and are attached to the upper and lower surfaces of the vertebrae by a thin layer of hyaline cartilage. The central **nucleus pulposus**, located slightly toward the posterior side of the disk, is composed of soft fibrocartilage with irregular strands of connective tissue and degenerative remnants of the embryonic notochord. It is surrounded by the **anulus fibrosus**, a firm outer layer of connective-tissue fibers arranged in layers.

Ligaments

The **anterior longitudinal ligament** extends from the anterior tubercle of the atlas to the first sacral vertebra (Fig. 5.**1**). It becomes broader and thicker as it descends.

The collagen fibers of the anterior longitudinal ligament are attached to the superior and inferior margins of the vertebral bodies. The ligaments are not firmly fixed to the intervertebral disks (Rauber and Kopsch 1998).

The **posterior longitudinal ligament** runs along the posterior surface of the vertebral bodies inside the vertebral canal (Fig. 5.**1**). It is narrower and thinner than the anterior longitudinal ligament. It extends from the body of the axis to the sacral canal and is broader superiorly than inferiorly. At the thoracic and lumbar levels, the posterior longitudinal ligament covers only a narrow portion of the vertebral bodies but widens intermittently to form lateral extensions over the intervertebral disks. The posterior longitudinal ligament is attached to the margins of the vertebral bodies and to the intervertebral disks, lacking a firm attachment to the midportions of the vertebral bodies.

The **ligamenta flava** connect the laminae of adjacent vertebral arches (Fig. 5.**1**). They consist largely of elastic fibers and, together with the capsules of the apophyseal joints, help to enclose the vertebral canal.

The **interspinous ligaments** are located just posterior to the ligamenta flava and stretch between adjacent thoracic spines. The **intertransverse ligaments** are between the transverse processes. The **supraspinous ligaments** connect the apices of the thoracic spines from C7 to the sacrum. This ligament is replaced in the cervical spine by the **nuchal ligament**, which is also composed of elastic fibers and extends from the spinous process of C7 to the external occipital protuberance.

Development of the Spinal Column

The antenatal development of the spinal column goes through three distinct stages.

> **Stages in the development of the spinal column**
> - Initial **mesenchymal stage**
> - **Chondrification stage** in the second month of embryonic development
> - **Ossification stage** in the third month of fetal development

A brief description of this development is useful at this point, as it will help us in understanding the pathogenesis of several types of spinal anomaly.

Mesenchymal Stage

The **notochord** is a nonsegmental axial rod located ventral to the neural tube of the embryo. It functions as a supportive framework. Together with the neural tube, it is responsible for the metameric organization of the dorsal axial organs. The notochord is a flexible rod composed of water-rich, pressure-elastic cells and enclosed by a membranous sheath. It runs the entire length of the spinal column, being situated slightly dorsal to the center of the vertebral bodies (Fig. 5.**2**).

Early in embryonic development the notochord regresses almost completely, leaving as its only remnants the **nucleus pulposus** and the **apical ligament of the dens**. The notochord provides a support around which the mesenchymal spinal column is formed. Mesenchymal cells migrate venteromedially from the sclerotomes, enclose the notochord, and form a mesenchymatous column that establishes the segmental organization of the somites in the form of intersegmental gaps.

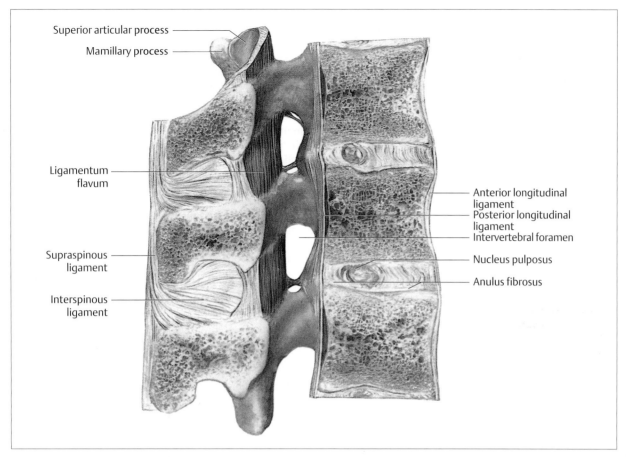

Fig. 5.**1** Midsagittal section through the first three lumbar vertebrae, showing the ligaments and intervertebral disks. (From Rauber and Kopsch, 1998.)

Within the segments are transverse **intrasegmental gaps** or sclerotomic fissures, which subdivide the individual sclerotomes into cranial and caudal halves. The intrasegmental gaps are the precursors of the future intervertebral disks. With further development, one cranial and one caudal half of adjacent sclerotomes fuse together to form the mesenchymal anlage of the vertebral bodies. Each vertebra thus contains components of two segments. Consistent with the origin of the spinal blastema from paired somites, the mesenchymal anlages of the vertebral bodies are also paired. They are separated by a **perichordal septum** derived from the perichordal tube (Fig. 5.**3**).

The **vertebral arches** themselves do not arise from the vertebral bodies but form separately at their anatomic location, establishing a connection with the primitive vertebral body secondarily.

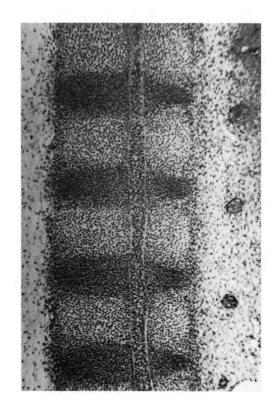

Fig. 5.**2** Embryonic spinal column in the mesenchymal stage, ▷ viewed in sagittal section. The notochord runs through the entire specimen in a slightly eccentric position. (From Rauber and Kopsch, 1998.)

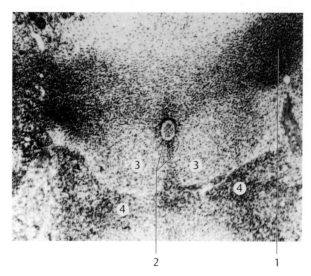

Fig. 5.**3**   Oblique section through the paired anlages of the spinal column in an embryo. (From Rauber and Kopsch, 1998.)
1   Anlage of vertebral arch
2   Notochord and perichordal septum
3   Anlage of vertebral body
4   Anlage of intervertebral disk

Chondrification Stage

This stage is characterized by the **chondrification** of the mesenchymal vertebral components. This process starts in the second month of embryonic development with the appearance of paired **chondral centers** in the primitive cervical vertebrae. It proceeds in the caudal direction and is completed in the vertebral bodies during the second month of embryonic development. The chondrification of the **vertebral arches** starts symmetrically in the pedicles and continues until the fourth month of fetal development. The chondrification of the mesenchymal vertebral body tissue presses the notochord cells into the primitive intervertebral disks, where "chordal segments" are formed. These are located at the center of the intervertebral disks and serve as precursors for the **nucleus pulposus**. Vestiges of the notochord sheath can still be detected in the vertebral bodies for some time (Fig. 5.**4**).

Ossification Stage

Osteogenesis is the final stage in the development of the spinal column. Starting in the third month of fetal development, each vertebra is generally **ossified from three centers**, one each located in the anterior portion of the vertebral arch and one at the center of the vertebral body (Fig. 5.**5**).

Ossification at the upper and lower ends of the spinal column deviates from this scheme. The varying origins of the cervical, thoracic, lumbar, and sacral vertebrae are shown schematically in Fig. 5.**6**.

The first **ossification centers** appear in the **arches** of the **lower cervical and upper thoracic vertebrae**, followed quickly by the centers in the upper cervical vertebrae. From there, ossification progresses in the caudal direction. The first **ossification center**s for the **vertebral bodies** appear in the **lower thoracic spine**. From there, ossification of the vertebral bodies continues in the cranial and caudal directions. While ossification of the vertebral bodies is principally enchondral and occurs from a central nucleus that may appear bipartite on radiographs (Fig. 5.**7**), primary ossification of the vertebral arches is perichondral and starts on the inner surface of the arches.

The shape of the ossification centers is particularly variable in the lower thoracic and lumbar vertebral bodies and depends on the ingrowth of blood vessels. If the posterior and anterior vessels remain separate, two separate ossification centers may form and then fuse together at a later stage.

In newborns, all primary ossification centers are fully developed except for the anterior arch of the atlas and the coccyx. Table 5.**1** reviews the stages in the postnatal development of the spinal column.

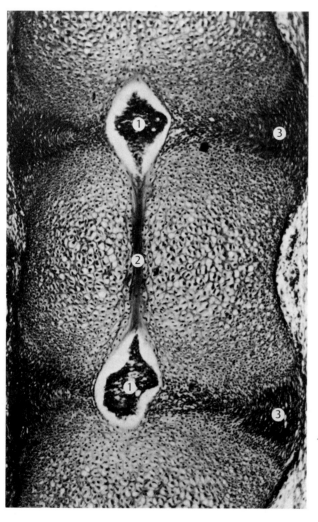

◁ Fig. 5.**4**   Spinal column of an embryo, viewed in sagittal section. Note the eccentric position of the notochordal segments and the lateral funiculus of the notochord.
1   Notochordal segment
2   Lateral funiculus of notochord
3   Intervertebral disk

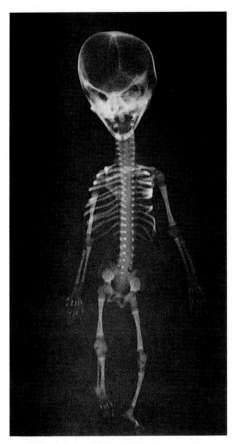

Fig. 5.**5** Four-month-old fetus showing a typical arrangement of three ossification centers in each vertebra (radiograph of an embryo from the collection of the Anatomical Institute of Tübingen University).

Fig. 5.**6a–d** Origin of the individual segments of the cervical, thoracic, lumbar, and sacral vertebrae (after Rauber, Kopsch and Schinz).
a Cervical vertebra.
b Thoracic vertebra.
c Lumbar vertebra.
d Sacral vertebra.
Dark gray   Anlage of rib
Lined   Anlage of vertebral body
Light gray   Anlage of vertebral arch

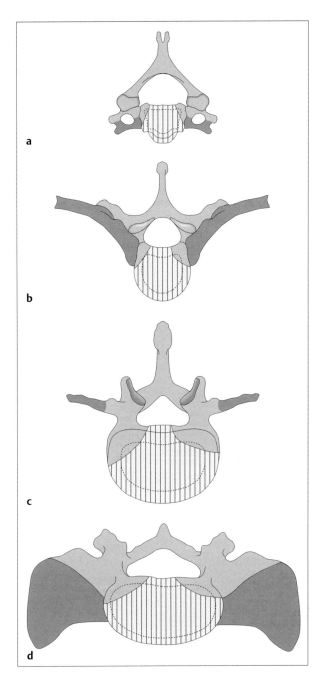

Fig. 5.**7** Sagittal section through the second lumbar vertebral body of a fetus. Note the hourglass-shaped ossification center, which is traversed by the lateral funiculus of the notochord. (From Rauber and Kopsch 1998.)

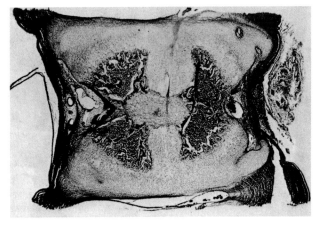

Table 5.**1**   Stages in the postnatal development of the spine (after Schinz)

Primary ossification centers

• Time of appearance	Prenatal (present at birth) Exceptions: • Anterior arch of atlas: first year of life • Coccyx: variable
• Bony closure of the vertebral arch	First to second year of life (starts at lumbar level, reaches cervical level by 4th year of life)
• Epiphyseal closure of the vertebral arch (neuro-central synchondrosis)	Third to seventh year of life (starts at thoracic level, ends at lumbosacral level); fusion may be asymmetrical
• Fusion of dens and axis	Third to seventh year of life
• Fusion of sacral vertebrae	Start and finish are highly variable; fusion may continue for more than 10 years

Secondary ossification centers

Marginal ridge

• Appearance	Around the 10th year of life (highly variable; first ossification centers may appear in 7th year or earlier)
• Complete marginal ridge	14th–15th year of life
• Fusion	Around the 20th year of life (starts at the lumbar level)

Apophyses of the vertebral processes:

• Appearance	Around puberty (usually before the start of puberty in girls, afterward in boys)
• Fusion	15th–25th year of life, about 5–10 years after time of appearance (persistence may occur)

Ossiculum terminale (dens)

• Appearance	Second through sixth year of life
• Fusion	Around 12th year of life

By the time the child is born, the ossification centers have reached the anterior and posterior surfaces of the vertebral bodies. The ossification centers of the vertebral body and neural arch are separated from each other by cartilaginous septa called the **neurocentral synchondroses** (Figs. 5.**8**, 5.**131**, 5.**264**, 5.**265**). Above and below the ossification center for the vertebral body are the **cartilaginous end plates**, which enable the vertebral body to grow in height through chondral proliferation. These cartilaginous plates form the boundaries of the intervertebral space and become thinner as growth progresses. Meanwhile, the rim of the cartilaginous plate develops into a sturdy ring that encloses the ossification center of the vertebral body: the **cartilaginous marginal ridge**. This feature appears on lateral radiographs as a steplike notch in the anterior borders of the vertebral bodies. Small ossification centers develop in the marginal ridge between the 10th and 12th years of life. These centers progressively fuse together and form a closed bony ring by the 12th year of life (Figs. 5.**132**, 5.**214**, 5.**216**). Ossification starts at the anterior border and gradually spreads posteriorly. The **ossified marginal ridge**, or **apophyseal ring**, fuses with the vertebral body between the 14th and 24th years of life. The marginal ridges do not contribute to the growth of the vertebral bodies in height. Their purpose is to provide a site of attachment for the anulus fibrosus of the intervertebral disk and the anterior longitudinal ligament.

Fusion of the **bony arch centers** probably occurs during the first two years of life, commencing in the lumbar spine. Fusion of the **neurocentral synchondroses** starts at the thoracic level in about the third year of life and is completed by the seventh year. The transverse, spinous, and articular processes may have **secondary ossification centers**, designated by their location as the apophyses of the transverse, spinous or articular processes. These secondary ossification centers generally fuse with the corresponding processes but also may persist in later life (see discussion below and Fig. 5.**8**).

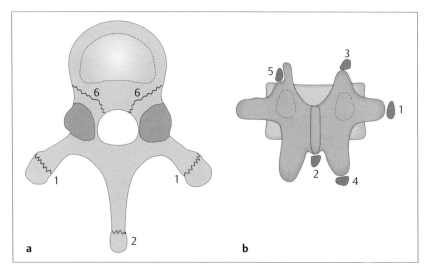

Fig. 5.**8 a, b**   Secondary ossification centers of a vertebral body.
a Superior aspect.
b Posterior aspect.
1   Apophysis of transverse process
2   Apophysis of spinous process
3   Apophysis of superior articular process
4   Apophysis of inferior articular process
5   Apophysis of mamillary process
6   Neurocentral synchondrosis

References

Rauber/Kopsch: Bewegungsapparat, Bd. 1. In: Rauber/Kopsch: Anatomie des Menschen. Lehrbuch und Atlas, 2. Aufl. Hrsg. Leonhardt, H., B. Tillmann, G. Töndury, K. Zilles. Thieme, Stuttgart 1998

Schinz, H. R.: Wirbelsäule–Rückenmark. In: Schinz: Radiologische Diagnostik in Klinik und Praxis, Bd. V/2, 7. Aufl. Hrsg. Frommhold, W., W. Dihlmann, H.-St. Stender, P. Thurn. Thieme, Stuttgart 1986

Atlas and Axis

▌ *Normal Findings*

The first and second cervical vertebrae, called the atlas and the axis, have evolved into rotatory vertebrae. The **atlas** (C1) does not have a vertebral body. It consists of two lateral masses interconnected by an anterior arch and a posterior arch (Fig. 5.**9**).

The lateral masses bear the superior articular facets that articulate with the occipital condyles and the inferior articular facets that articulate with the superior articular processes of the axis. On the dorsal aspect of the posterior arch is a bony protuberance of variable prominence, the posterior tubercle, which represents a rudimentary

spinous process. Just dorsal to the superior articular facet on each side is a groove for the vertebral artery, which may be surmounted by a bony bar (see discussion below). Lateral to the lateral mass is the transverse process, which encloses the transverse foramen (foramen transversarium) that transmits the vertebral artery. On the back of the anterior arch is a facet for articulation with the dens of the axis.

The **axis** (C2) reveals the characteristic **dens** (odontoid process), a peglike process that juts upward from the body and forms a pivot on which the atlas can rotate (Fig. 5.**10**). On the anterior surface of the dens is the anterior facet that articulates with the anterior arch of the atlas. Posteriorly,

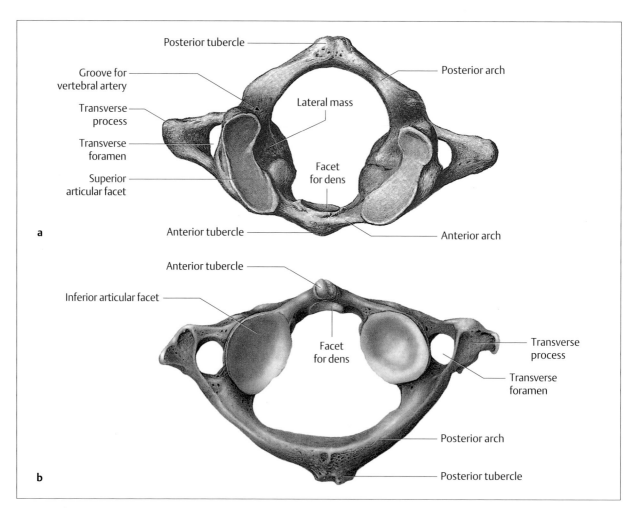

Fig. 5.**9 a, b**   Anatomy of the atlas. (From Rauber and Kopsch 1998.)

a Superior aspect.
b Inferior aspect.

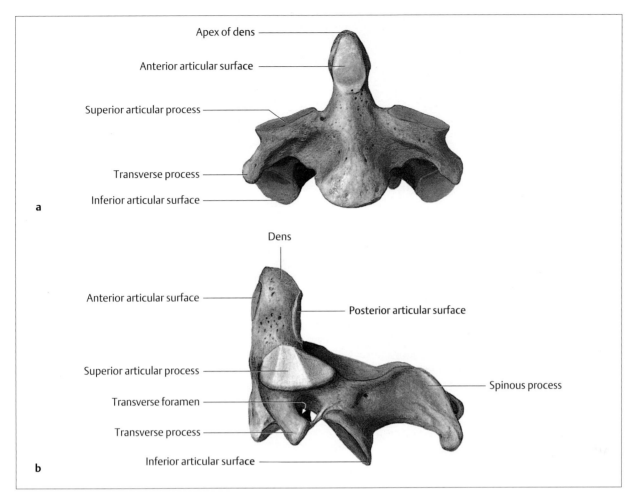

Fig. 5.**10 a, b**   Anatomy of the axis. (From Rauber and Kopsch 1998.)   **a** Anterior aspect.
b Lateral aspect.

the dens bears a facet for contact with the transverse ligament of the atlas. The superior articular processes articulate with corresponding facets on the inferior surface of the atlas. The inferior articular processes are like those of the other cervical vertebrae. The vertebral arch ends in a powerful spinous process, which frequently is bifid. The transverse process of the axis, like that of most cervical vertebrae, is pierced by a transverse foramen that is traversed by the vertebral artery on each side. The radiographic anatomy of the first two cervical vertebrae is illustrated in Fig. 5.**11**.

 ## During Growth

The first and second cervical vertebrae differ from the other vertebrae in their osseous development. The **atlas** is ossified from **three centers**. Ossification begins in the lateral masses, comparable to the ossification of the vertebral arches at other spinal levels. In newborns, only these two ossification centers are visible on radiographs. They are responsible for forming the posterior arch of the atlas and the lateral masses. Bony closure of the posterior arch is completed by the end of the fourth year (Fig. 5.**12**).

The third ossification center of the atlas is located in the anterior arch and is already present at birth in about 20% of

cases (Odgen 1984). In 80% of cases this center develops during the first year of life. Its ossification is nonuniform and occasionally involves several paramedian centers that form the anterior arch during the first year. The ossification centers of the atlas fuse together between the fifth and ninth years.

The development of the body and arch of the **axis** corresponds to that of the thoracic and lumbar vertebrae. At birth, the arch of the axis has two symmetrical ossification centers, which fuse together by the fourth year (Odgen 1984). The **dens** is ossified from a paired center that is pierced centrally by the notochord (Fig. 5.**13**). Newborns have two ossification centers for the vertebral body and dens (Fig. 5.**14**). Occasionally two ossification centers are still found in the dens.

The ossification centers of the dens and body fuse together between the third and seventh years. Until then, a horizontal synchondrosis with a rudimentary notochordal segment is interposed between the two centers (Fig. 5.**15**). After bony union occurs, a sclerotic band, notch, or partial cleft may persist in this area (Fig. 5.**16**).

As the ossification centers fuse together, the center for the dens appears to sink into the center for the body (Ogden 1984) (Fig. 5.**15 c**). Another, separate ossification center may already be present in the apex of the dens at birth (von Torklus and Gehle 1987) but usually does not ap-

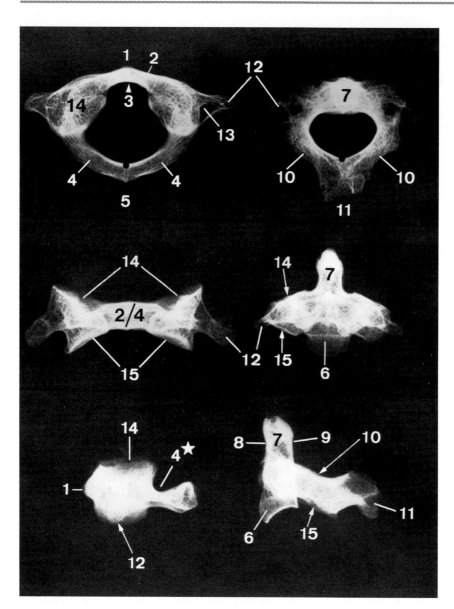

Fig. 5.**11**   Radiographic views of the atlas (left) and axis (right) in the craniocaudal, AP, and lateral projections (from top to bottom). (From Schinz 1986.)

1 Anterior tubercle
2 Anterior arch
3 Facet for dens
4 Posterior arch with groove for vertebral artery
5 Posterior tubercle
6 Body of axis
7 Dens
8 Anterior articular surface of dens
9 Posterior articular surface of dens
10 Lamina
11 Spinous process
12 Transverse process
13 Transverse foramen
14 Superior articular surface
15 Inferior articular surface

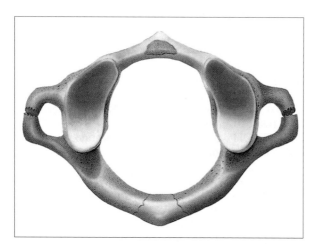

Fig. 5.**12**   Bone formation in the atlas of a one-year-old child. Ossification centers appear in the anterior arch and at the bases of the posterior arch. (From Rauber and Kopsch 1998.)

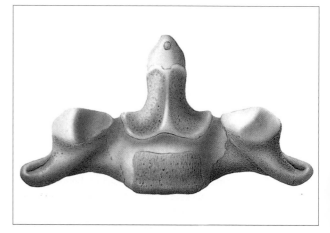

Fig. 5.**13**   Bone formation in the axis in a newborn. There is a single ossification center in the dens, deeply cleft by cartilage, plus ossification centers in the body and vertebral arch. Note the terminal ossicle in the apex of the dens. (From Rauber and Kopsch 1998.)

pear until the second year. This apical center for the dens, also called the proatlas or ossiculum terminale, occasionally remains isolated but generally fuses with the center for the dens by the twelfth year. The ossiculum terminale, which may lie in a V-shaped cleft in the apex (Figs. 5.**15**, 5.**16**), forms the apex of the dens and can account for certain changes in this region (Figs. 5.**27**, 5.**28**; see discussion below).

The interosseous distance between the posterior aspect of the anterior arch of the atlas and the anterior aspect of the dens, called the **atlantodental distance**, is up to 4 mm wide in children. When the neck is flexed in children, slight anterior displacement of the atlas can occur and the interosseous interval may widen (Jirout 1967).

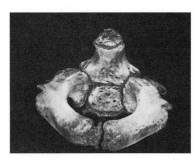

Fig. 5.**14**   Ossification centers of the axis in an anatomic specimen.

Fig. 5.**15 a–c**   Synchondroses in children.
a Center for the dens (arrow) and center for the anterior arch of the atlas (double arrow) in a 5-month-old child.
b Persistent synchondrosis between the centers for the dens and body of the axis (broad arrow). Apical center for the dens (arrow) (observation by Holthusen, Hamburg). Five-year-old child.
c Synchondrosis at the base of the dens in a child.

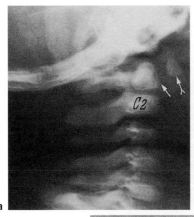
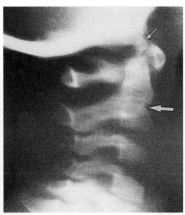

In Adulthood

While radiographic visualization of the first two cervical vertebrae presents few difficulties in the lateral projection, an open-mouth projection is necessary to obtain a satisfactory AP view.

The principal craniometric techniques used in the occipitoatlantoaxial region are reviewed in Figs. 5.**17** and 5.**18**.

In the **AP view** of the craniocervical junction, the apex of the dens should cross the bimastoid line by no more than 10 mm and should not cross the biventer line (Dolan 1977). In the **lateral view**, the apex of the dens should not extend past a line connecting the anterior and posterior margins of the foramen magnum (the McRae line). The dens should extend no more than 5 mm past the Chamberlain line (connecting the posterior end of the hard palate to the posterior rim of the foramen magnum) and no more than 7 mm past the McGregor line (connecting the posterior end of the hard palate to the lowest point of the occipital squama) (Dolan 1977). Today, CT and MRI have replaced the special views that were formerly used to define the craniovertebral junction (see Fig. 5.**75**). The atlantoaxial distance in adults normally does not exceed 2 mm measured at the inferior articular margin (Weissman 1983). The average height of the dens is 18 mm in men and 16.9 mm in women (McManners 1983).

The arch of the atlas is quite variable in its prominence. **Hypertrophy** of the anterior arch and tubercle is virtually indistinguishable from apparent enlargement due to

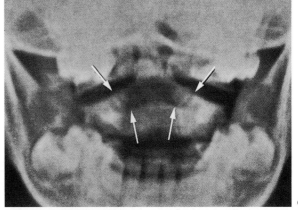
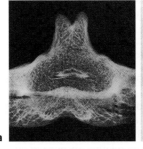
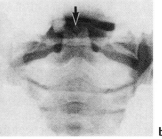

Fig. 5.**16 a, b**   Specimen and radiograph of apical notch in dens axis.
a Specimen shows an apical notch in the dens and a persistent synchondrosis between the body and dens.
b Ossification center within a V-shaped notch in the apex of the dens (arrow) (observation by Holthusen, Hamburg). Five-year-old girl.

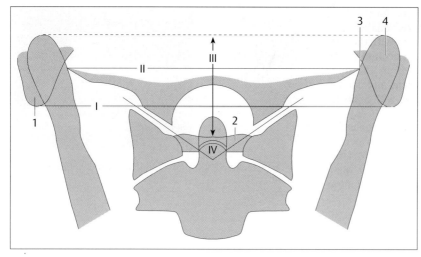

Fig. 5.**17**   AP craniometry. (From von Torklus and Gehle 1987.)

I   Bimastoid line (apex of dens should be no more than 10 mm above it; usually passes through the center of the atlanto-occipital joints)

II   Biventer line (should be above apex of dens)

III   Distance from temporomandibular joint to arch of atlas (22 to 39 mm)

IV   Angle of atlanto-occipital joint axes (124–127°)

1   Apices of the mastoid processes
2   Anterior arch of atlas
3   Mastoid notch
4   Mandibular condyle

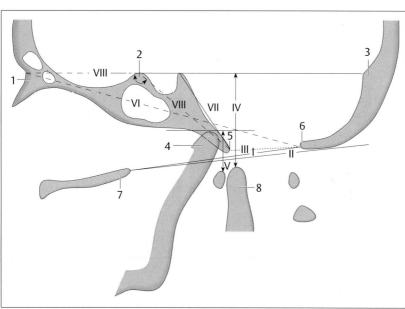

Fig. 5.**18**   Lateral craniometry with landmarks. (From von Torklus and Gehle 1987.)

I	Chamberlain line (on average, apex of dens should be 1 ± 3.6 mm below the line)
II	McGregor line (apex of dens should be no more than 6.4 mm above the line)
III	McRae line (apex of dens should not cross the line)
IV	Height index of Klaus (averages 40–41 mm; 36–30 mm may be pathological, less than 30 mm suggests basilar invagination)
V	Distance from temporomandibular joint to arch of atlas (22–39 mm; averages 30 mm)
VI	Boogard line (basion should be below the line)

VII + III	Boogard angle (119–135°; averages 122°)
VIII	Welcker angle (averages 132°)
1	Nasion
2	Tuberculum sellae
3	Cruciform eminence of internal occipital protuberance
4	Mandibular condyle
5	Basion
6	Opisthion
7	Hard palate
8	Apex of dens

degenerative osteophytosis or ossification of the attached ligaments (Fig. 5.**19**).

By contrast, the variable size of the posterior arch of the atlas and its tubercle and the relatively common **asymmetries** of the posterior hemiarches are easily evaluated in the lateral projection owing to the relative absence of superimposed structures (Figs. 5.**20**–5.**22**).

An oblique projection of the atlas may create the erroneous impression of a posterior arch fracture (Fig. 5.**23**).

Notch-shaped lucencies at the medial border of the superior articular facets of the atlas are caused by bony depressions adjacent to the articular facets (Viehweger

1956). They may be accentuated by a medial tubercle (Ogden 1984) (Fig. 5.**24**).

Asymmetrical widths of the **transverse foramina** are occasionally seen and result from congenital asymmetries of the vertebral arteries (Fig. 5.**25**).

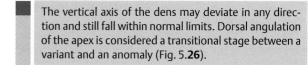

The vertical axis of the dens may deviate in any direction and still fall within normal limits. Dorsal angulation of the apex is considered a transitional stage between a variant and an anomaly (Fig. 5.**26**).

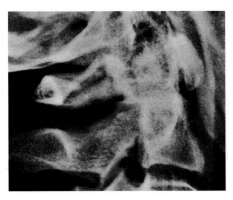

Fig. 5.**19**   Large anterior arch of atlas.

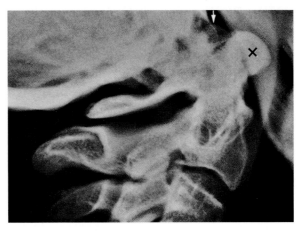

Fig. 5.**20**   Slender posterior arch and a normally developed anterior arch of atlas (×). A persistent terminal ossicle is visible above the dens (arrow).

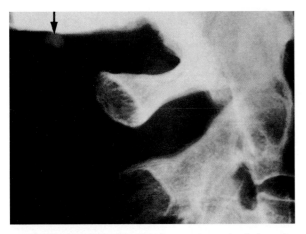

Fig. 5.**21**   Powerfully developed posterior arch of the atlas. An isolated accessory ossicle appears below the occiput.

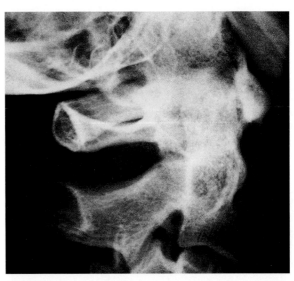

Fig. 5.**22**   Asymmetrical development of the posterior arch of the atlas.

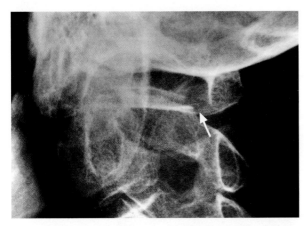

Fig. 5.**23 a, b**   Pseudofractures of the posterior arch of the atlas in an oblique projection.
a Apparent posterior arch fracture of the atlas (arrow) in an oblique projection of the upper cervical spine.

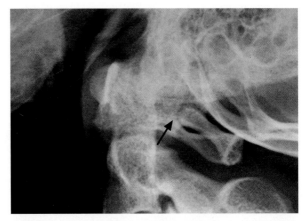

b Another pseudofracture with an apparently rounded fracture line (arrow).

The apex of the dens is generally hemispherical, but it may be conical or may taper to a sharp point (Figs. 5.27, 5.28). The dens itself may be peg-shaped or balloon-shaped, or it may be narrow and elongated and extend past the anterior arch of the atlas (Fig. 5.29). An area of increased density is occasionally seen in the apex where the ossiculum terminale has fused to the dens (Fig. 5.30).

On an oblique projection of the cervical spine, the posterior part of the transverse process of the axis may be projected as a comma-shaped figure within the intervertebral foramen (Fig. 5.31).

The transverse foramen of the axis can simulate a variant when oriented at a steep angle (Figs. 5.32, 5.33).

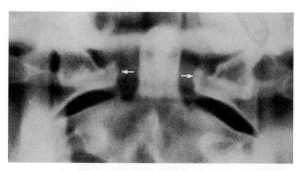

Fig. 5.**24** Radiographic view of notches medial to the superior articular facets of the atlas. The notches are accentuated by medial tubercles (arrows).

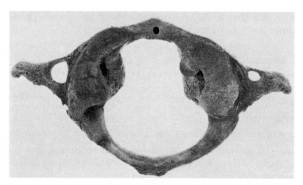

Fig. 5.**25** Marked asymmetry of the transverse foramina of the atlas.

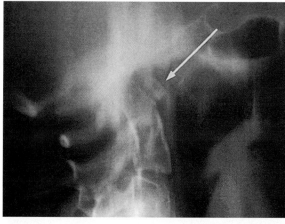

Fig. 5.**26** Dorsal angulation of the dens apex in basilar invagination and platybasia.

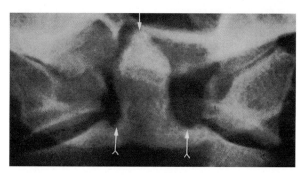

Fig. 5.**27** Budlike protuberance on the apex of the dens (straight arrow). The dens is displaced to the right, with asymmetrical development of the dentolateral grooves (double arrows).

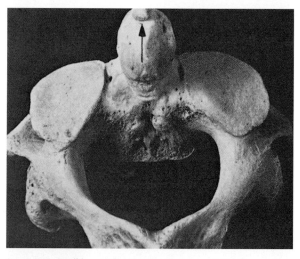

Fig. 5.**28** Budlike ossification on the apex of the dens.

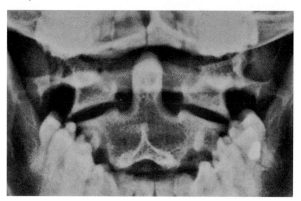

Fig. 5.**29** Atypical long dens axis.

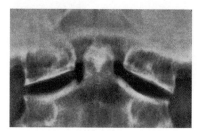

Fig. 5.**30** Zone of increased density at the center of the dens apex.

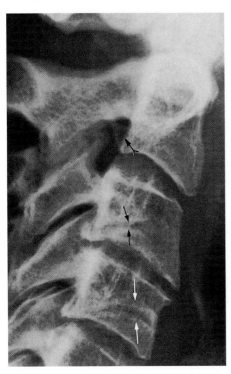

Fig. 5.**31** Projection of the posterior root of the transverse process of C2 (double arrow). The streaklike lucency projected in the body of C3 is caused by the superimposed uncovertebral joint at C2/C3 (arrows) and is even more pronounced at C3/C4 (white arrows).

Fig. 5.**33** AP open-mouth view showing the transverse foramina of the axis on each side. ▷

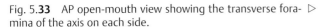

Summation effects from the dens and the posterior arch of the atlas can produce a Mach effect that mimics a fracture line (Figs. 5.**34**, 5.**35**).

The projection of the space between the upper central incisors onto the dens can also simulate a fracture (Fig. 5.**36**). A similar effect is produced by the projection of a gap in the anterior or posterior arch of the atlas onto the dens (Fig. 5.**49**) (Tänzer 1957, Chapman et al. 1991). Occasionally the lips in an open-mouth AP projection can produce a ringlike shadow around the dens (Bohrer and Brody 1992). The apices of the **styloid processes** of the sphenoid bone are often projected onto or in front of the anterior tubercle of the anterior arch of the atlas (see Fig. 5.**178**).

A cartilaginous disk can persist between the dens and body of the axis until advanced age (Figs. 5.**16**, 5.**37**). It is extremely common to find a sclerotic band or notch on the anterior surface of the vertebra at this location (Odgen 1984) (Fig. 5.**38**).

Cleftlike or occasionally foramen-like grooves of variable prominence are located medial to the borders of the superior articular facets of the axis and mark the junction of the former cartilaginous zones with the ossification centers of the dens and body of the axis (Figs. 5.**27**, 5.**39**).

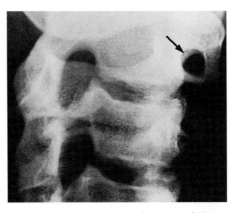

Fig. 5.**32** Right transverse foramen of the axis viewed in an oblique projection.

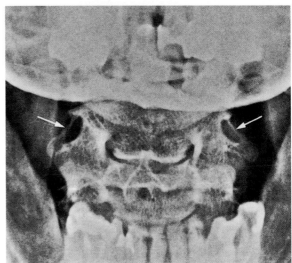

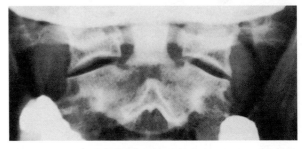

Fig. 5.**34** Summation effect from the posterior arch of the atlas. The posterior arch produces a transverse density along the base of the dens. This should not be mistaken for a healed dens fracture.

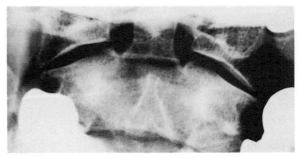

Fig. 5.**35** Mach effect simulates a transverse cleft through the base of the dens.

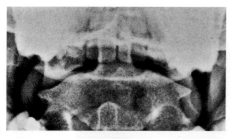
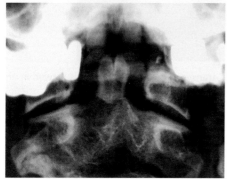

Fig. 5.**36 a, b**   Projection of the space between the upper central incisors onto the dens.
a   The projected features mimic vertical and transverse fracture lines through the dens.
b   Apparent bicornuate dens.

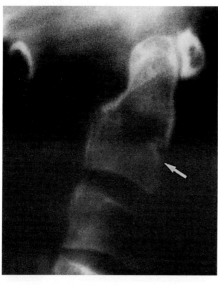

Fig. 5.**38**   Vestigial synchondrosis appears as a sclerotic stripe between the centers for the dens and body of the axis. The unusually prominent but otherwise typical notch in the anterior contour of the axis (arrow) should not be mistaken for a healed fracture. Lateral tomogram.

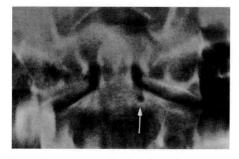

Fig. 5.**39**   Deep notch (dentolateral groove) at the base of the dens on the left side.

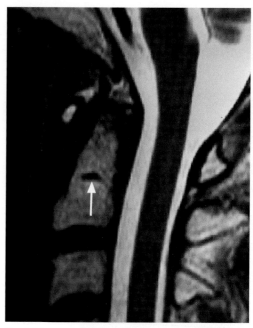

Fig. 5.**37**   Persistent cartilaginous disk at the junction of the dens and body of the axis (arrow). Sagittal T2-weighted MRI of a 40-year-old man.

Normal Movements

Flexion and Extension

Flexion of the head occurs at the atlanto-occipital joint. Flexion and extension can be evaluated on lateral radiographs taken at the limits of these movements (Schmidt 1964, Wackenheim 1969). The following reference lines are used (Cramer 1958, Lewit and Krausová 1963, Schmidt 1964, Endler et al. 1984):

- Foramen magnum line (McRae line)
- Atlas plane (line connecting the center of the anterior arch to the posterior tubercle, or a tangent to the superior borders of the anterior and posterior arches)
- Axis plane (line connecting the inferior border of the transverse process to the inferior border of the posterior arch).

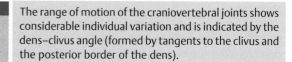

The range of motion of the craniovertebral joints shows considerable individual variation and is indicated by the dens–clivus angle (formed by tangents to the clivus and the posterior border of the dens).

Published values for the range of motion of the atlanto-occipital joint range from 8.8° to 15.2° (Schmidt 1964, Levine 1983). It should be added that the angle formed by the foramen magnum line with the atlas plane shows varying degrees of anterior divergence and especially posterior divergence through flexion-extension, and that by studying this angle in different head positions we can appreciate the positional changes that occur between the occiput and the atlas during function (Fig. 5.**40**).

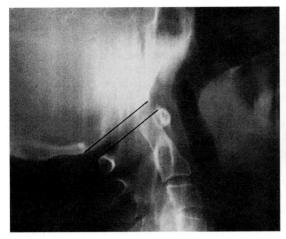

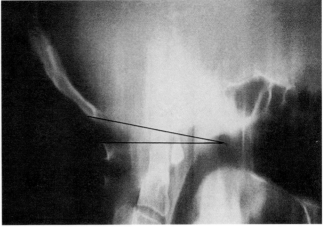

a   b

Fig. 5.**40a, b**   Functional views during flexion-extension of the head. The atlas line and foramen magnum line have been drawn on the midsagittal tomograms.

a Atlas and foramen magnum lines are parallel in extension of the head.
b When the head is flexed forward, the angles diverge posteriorly.

> On a lateral view of the head in the neutral position, the atlas plane is roughly parallel to the foramen magnum line. With a *high atlas* (atlas superior), the angle between the McGregor line and atlas plane is greater than 24° in the neutral head position. With a *low atlas* (atlas inferior), the angle is less than 10° (Fig. 5.**41**).

In the absence of a deformity in nearby structures and without range-of-motion testing of the cervical spine in flexion-extension, the observation of a high or low atlas has no clinical significance. Atlanto-occipital motion is considered normal if the posterior arch of the atlas moves closer to the occiput during extension and away from it during flexion. If atlanto-occipital joint motion is restricted, the posterior arch has the same relationship to the occiput during flexion as it does in the neutral position (Kamieth 1983). In children up to 8 years of age, the anterior arch of the atlas may overlie the apex of the dens by more than two-thirds of its width when the head is extended (Cattell and Filtzer 1965) (Fig. 5.**108**).

Lateral Bending

With a normal range of lateral bending, the average angulation of the foramen magnum relative to the axis plane is 5.6° (1–14°) (Lewit and Krausová 1964). When the neck is bent laterally, the body of C2 immediately rotates in the direction of the bend. As lateral bending increases, the other cervical vertebrae start to rotate as well, the degree of rotation decreasing in the craniocaudal direction. The atlas can rotate with the axis. Besides rotating and tilting in the direction of the bend, the axis also undergoes a transverse shift in that direction (Kamieth 1986). The vertebral bodies below the axis undergo a similar shift, but to a considerably lesser degree.

The rotation, tilting, and transverse displacement of the axis are closely interrelated.

> The greater the rotation of the axis, the greater its degree of tilting and transverse displacement.

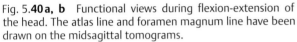

Atlas superior   Atlas inferior

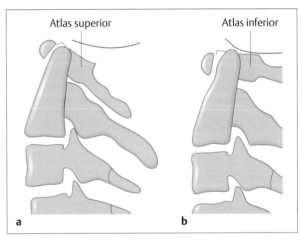

a   b

Fig. 5.**41 a, b**   High and low variants in the position of the atlas (after Dihlmann).
a   Atlas superior.
b   Atlas inferior.

When the neck is bent toward one side, the spinous process of the axis moves toward the opposite side (El-Khoury et al. 1985) (Fig. 5.**42**).

Lateral bending also causes the articular surface of the axis to project past that of the atlas on the concave side of the bend. The occipital condyles generally move toward the opposite side in relation to the atlas (Jirout 1968). Even in the neutral position, a small degree of "lateral offset" may be observed (Ono et al. 1985).

Rotation

Rotation involves a synchronous rotation of the head and the atlas. Rotation about the long axis of the dens takes place in the lateral atlantoaxial joints. When the head begins to turn, the atlas rotates approximately 10° (intrinsic atlas rotation) before the axis and the other cervical vertebrae join in the rotation (Kamieth 1983), the degree of rotation decreasing in the craniocaudal direction. As the

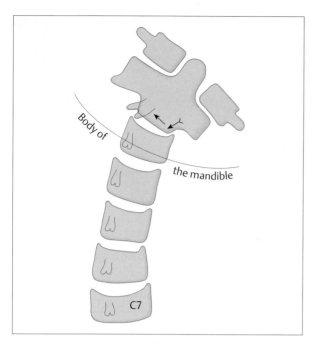

Fig. 5.**42**   Functional views of lateral cervical flexion. The axis is rotated and tilted in the direction of the head tilt (double arrow). It is also displaced transversely toward the side of the tilt (arrow) (after Dihlmann).

head continues to turn, the difference between the rotation of the atlas and axis increases to approximately 30°. Structures important in analyzing the position of the atlas on conventional radiographs are the **lateral mass triangles** (Kamieth 1983), which are formed by the lower contour of the posterior arch superimposed over the lateral masses (Fig. 5.**43**).

When the atlas is in a neutral position, both triangles are symmetrically displayed. When the atlas rotates, the base of the lateral mass triangle appears broadened on the side toward which the atlas is rotated (Fig. 5.**43**). When the axis starts to rotate along with the rotating atlas, several effects are noted on the AP radiograph:

- A decrease in the lateral atlantodental distance on the side of the rotation
- Narrowing of the lateral mass on the side of the rotation, or broadening of the lateral mass on the opposite side
- Narrowing of the radiographic atlantoaxial joint space on the side of the rotation (Fig. 5.**43**)

The increased rotation of the atlas relative to the axis leads to a **rotational offset** in which the articular contour of the nonrotated or less rotated vertebra laterally overlaps that of the rotated or more rotated vertebra on the side of the rotation (Fig. 5.**43**). When the head is rotated by more than 40–45°, a small offset is also visible on the opposite side.

The spinous process of the axis is an indicator of axis rotation, but due to its frequent asymmetries it is not useful for detecting small degrees of rotational malalignment. This can be done more accurately by analyzing the recesses between the body and transverse processes of the axis and the bases of its vertebral arch (Fig. 5.**43**) (Kamieth 1983).

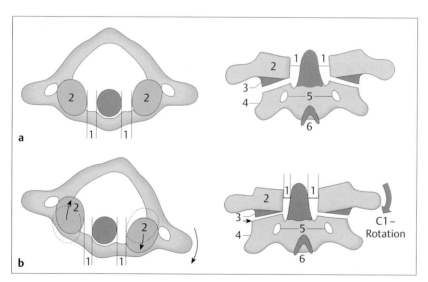

Fig. 5.**43 a, b**   Rotational analysis of the atlantoaxial joint (after Dihlmann).

a Neutral position without rotation. The lateral atlantodental distance, the lateral masses of the atlas, and the lateral mass triangles are equal on both sides. The recesses between the body and transverse processes of the axis and the elliptical bases of the vertebral arch of the axis are symmetrical.

b Rotation of the atlas to the right. This causes a narrowing of the atlantodental distance, the lateral mass, and the radiographic atlantoaxial joint space on the right side, while the lateral mass on the opposite side appears broadened. Note the rotational offset on the right side (arrow), the articular contour of the nonrotated or less rotated vertebra overlapping the con-

tour of the more rotated vertebra. Note also the asymmetry of the recesses between the body and transverse processes of the axis, the asymmetric elliptical bases of the vertebral arch of the axis, and the movement of the spinous process toward the left side with slight concomitant rotation of the axis.
1   Lateral atlantodental distance
2   Lateral mass
3   Lateral mass triangle
4   Recesses between body and transverse processes of axis
5   Elliptical base of the vertebral arch
6   Spinous process of articular facet of nonrotated vertebral body (arrow)

With even slight rotation of the axis, the recess between the body and transverse process appears to flatten on the side of the rotation, while the bases of the vertebral arch shift toward the opposite side.

> ■ Rotational malalignments of the axis can be detected by noting that the atlas is in a neutral position while the axis shows signs of rotation (normally the axis starts to rotate only after the atlas has moved through about 10° of independent rotation).

Before diagnosing a malposition of the first two cervical vertebrae, the radiologist must rule out congenital morphological asymmetries as well as congenital or acquired ligamentous weakness. Atlantoaxial rotation can be analyzed with much greater accuracy on CT scans (Penning and Wilmink 1986, Dvorak et al. 1987 a, b).

▌ Pathological Finding?

 ## Normal Variant or Anomaly?

The craniocervical junction develops from the anlage of four primitive vertebrae. The first primary vertebra and the anteproatlas give rise to the basiocciput. The third primary vertebra (proatlas) contributes to the formation of the dens apex. The atlas develops from the fourth primary vertebra (Muller and O'Rahilly 1994), and finally the axis develops from the fifth primary vertebra.

Abnormalities in the differentiation and development of the vertebral bodies in this region result in various anomalies (Chandraraj and Briggs 1992, Smoker 1994, Menezes 1997, Prescher 1977). Anomalies of the craniocervical junction can affect the occipital bone (q.v.) as wll as the atlas and axis. While anomalies of the occipital bone (tertiary condyle, condylar hypoplasia, basal occipital hypoplasia, atlanto-occipital assimilation) are associated with changes in the skull base and basilar invagination, this does not apply to most anomalies of the atlas and axis.

Abnormalities of the craniovertebral junction are diagnosed on routine radiographs and special views. Conventional tomography can provide a more accurate evaluation, but CT and especially MRI are significantly better owing to their multiplanar capabilities (Sharma et al. 1991, Ellis et al. 1991, Schweitzer et al. 1992, Smoker 1994) (Fig. 5.75).

Anomalies of the Atlas

As a rule, isolated anomalies of the atlas are not associated with abnormalities of the craniovertebral junction. The most frequent anomalies and variants of the atlas are:

- Hypoplasias
- Anomalous clefts
- Aplasias of the vertebral arch

A knowledge of the ossification centers of the atlas make it easy to understand these changes. Given the frequent coexistence of variants and anomalies, both will be discussed together.

Posterior Arch

The posterior arch of the atlas may be very narrow (Fig. 5.**20**), it may be notched at its base (Fig. 5.**44**), or it may have a superiorly directed bony process (Fig. 5.**45**).

Hypoplasia of the posterior arch has been observed with increased frequency in retrognathic and dolicofacial individuals (Huggare and Kylämarkula 1985, Huggare 1995) and may be associated with neurological abnormalities (Menezes 1997, Phan et al. 1998, Yamashita et al. 1997). A rare anomaly is **atlas stenosis** caused by a narrow sagittal diameter of the posterior arch (Fig. 5.**46**). It may be associated with impairment of CSF circulation and cord compression.

Occasionally an **accessory joint** forms between the posterior arch of the atlas and the vertebral arch of the axis (Fig. 5.**47**).

Posterior arch clefts and defects have an incidence of approximately 3–4% (Geipel 1955, von Torklus and Gehle 1987, Gehweiler et al. 1983). The most frequent anomaly is a **posterior arch cleft** (spina bifida), which is located on the midline in 97% of cases (Figs. 5.**48**, 5.**49**). In just 3% of cases the cleft involves the area of the groove for the vertebral artery behind the lateral mass (Fig. 5.**50**). The affected half of the vertebral arch is often hypoplastic (von Torklus and Gehle 1987). In the **lateral view**, the spinolaminar line is typically absent.

In the **AP projection**, spina bifida of the atlas can mimic a fracture of the dens or body of the axis. CT can establish the diagnosis in questionable cases (Fig. 5.**51**).

When a posterior cleft anomaly is present, the ends of the posterior arch bordering the cleft may show bulbous thickening.

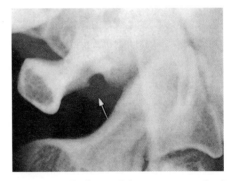

Fig. 5.**44**   Inferior notch at the base of the posterior arch of the atlas.

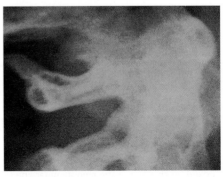

Fig. 5.**45**   Posterior arch of the atlas with upward angulation of an elongated posterior tubercle.

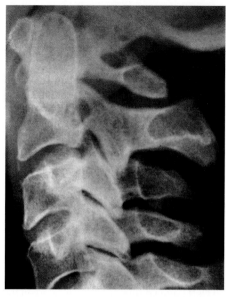

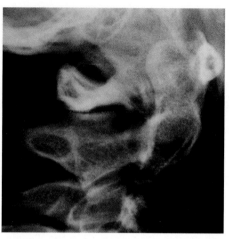

Fig. 5.**47**   Accessory joint formation between the vertebral arches of C1 and C2.

Fig. 5.**46**   Atlas stenosis. In the lateral view, the spinolaminar line of the atlas shows a steplike offset relative to C2–C5. A ponticulus posterior is noted as an incidental finding. (From von Torklus and Gehle 1987.)

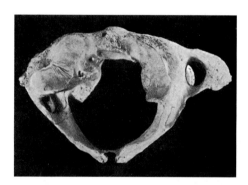

Fig. 5.**48**   Spina bifida of the atlas in an anatomic specimen.

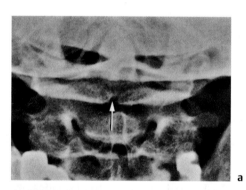

a

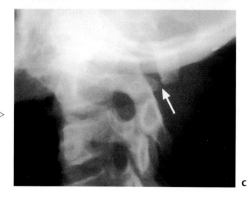

b

c

Fig. 5.**49 a–c**   Spina bifida of the atlas.   ▷
a Transoral projection.
b In the lateral projection, the vertebral arch defect is characterized by absence of the spinolaminar line (arrow). Note the
unilateral hypoplasia of the vertebral arch.
c Posterior arch cleft in the oblique projection (arrow).

Posterior arch clefts of the atlas frequently coexist with craniocervical dysplasias. Spina bifida of the posterior arch is often associated with a cleft in the arch of the axis (Fig. 5.**71**) (Stolze 1969, Kirschbichler 1972).

Larger defects of the posterior arch are associated with unilateral or bilateral partial or complete aplasia (Fig. 5.**52**). Figure 5.**53** illustrates the types of posterior arch defect that may be encountered.

The spectrum ranges from partial aplasia affecting half of the arch and hemiaplasia to a unilateral or bilateral vertebral arch remnant and persistent posterior tubercle (Fig. 5.**54**) or complete aplasia (Fig. 5.**55**) (Huggare 1995).

Complete aplasia of the posterior arch may be accompanied by compensatory enlargement of the spinous process of the axis. Aplasia of the posterior arch may be associated with anterior atlantoaxial subluxation (Schulze et al. 1980) or with bilateral atlantoaxial lateral offset (Gehweiler et al. 1983) and can mimic a Jefferson fracture. Isolated ossicles may occur in the area of the unformed arch, representing a transitional form to aplasia of the entire posterior arch (Fig. 5.**56**).

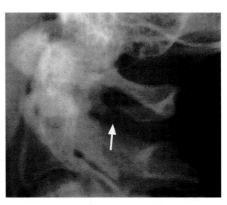

Fig. 5.**50**   Typical lateral cleft in the posterior arch of the atlas, located just behind the lateral mass (arrow). (From von Torklus and Gehle 1987.)

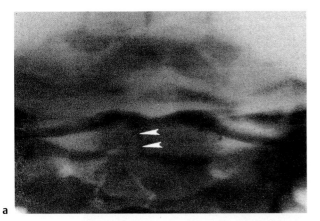

a

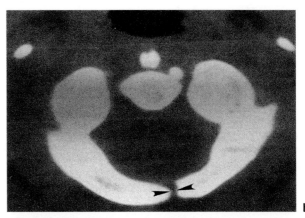

b

Fig. 5.**51 a, b**   Cleft in the posterior arch of the atlas.
a The cleft mimics a fracture of the axis in the transoral view (arrowheads).

b CT appearance of a posterior arch cleft (arrowheads). (From Smoker 1994.)

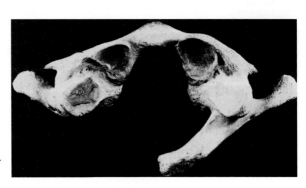

Fig. 5.**52**   Partial aplasia (hemiaplasia) of the posterior arch of ▷ the atlas in a specimen.

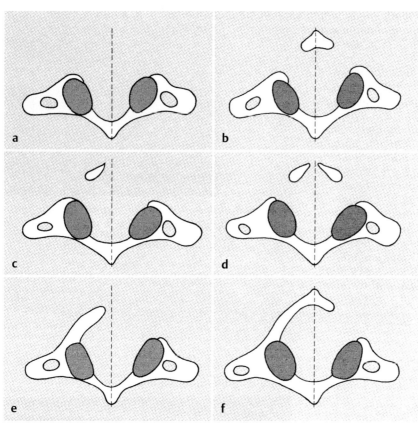

Fig. 5.**53 a–f**   Various types of partial or complete aplasia of the posterior arch of the atlas (after von Torklus).
a Total aplasia.
b Persistent posterior tubercle.
c Unilateral paramedian arch remnant.
d Bilateral arch remnant with cleft.
e Hemiaplasia.
f Partial aplasia affecting one half of the arch.

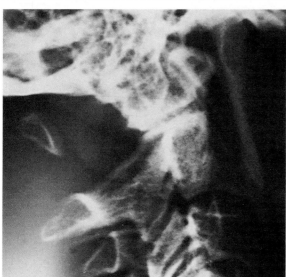

a

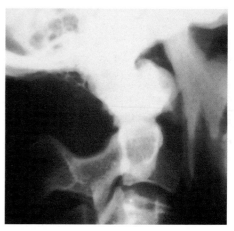

Fig. 5.**55**   Total aplasia of the posterior arch.

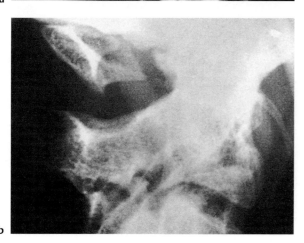

b

◁ Fig. 5.**54 a, b**   Partial aplasia of the posterior arch of the atlas in the lateral projection.
a   Bilateral hemiaplasia of the posterior arch with a persistent posterior tubercle.
b   Partial bilateral hemiaplasia of the posterior arch with a persistent posterior tubercle and adjacent arch rudiments.

Anterior Arch

Clefts in the anterior arch of the atlas are much less common than in the posterior arch and are nearly always accompanied by posterior arch anomalies (Desgrez et al. 1965, Stolze 1969, von Torklus and Gehle 1987, Chambers and Gaskill 1992, Haakonsen et al. 1995). The term "**bipartite atlas**" or "**split atlas**" refers to clefts in both arches (Fig. 5.**57**) (Wackenheim 1974, Lemaire et al. 1982, Chapman et al. 1991).

A split atlas has also been observed in connection with Klippel–Feil syndrome (Wolf and Klein 1997). Clefts in the anterior arch of the atlas are narrow (Geipel 1955, Chambers and Gaskill 1992). Occasionally, defects in both arches may be associated with instability of the atlas (Gamble and Rinsky 1985, von Torklus and Gehle 1987).

When an anterior arch cleft is present, the arch appears thickened and the anterior atlantodental joint space is difficult to define (Walker and Beggs 1995). The cortical boundary of the anterior arch may appear duplicated or indistinct. The cleft can be clearly visualized on CT scans. MRI may create the impression of a **pseudotumor** at the site of the cleft (Smoker 1994) (Fig. 5.**57**).

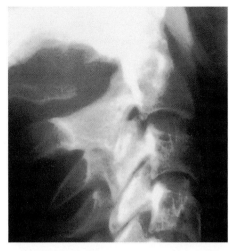

Fig. 5.**56**   Transitional form to total aplasia: an isolated ossicle in the area of the unformed atlas arch.

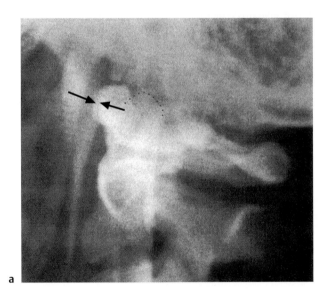

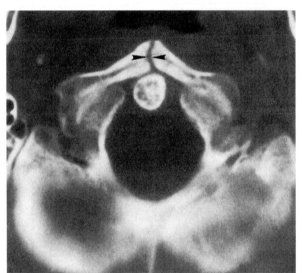

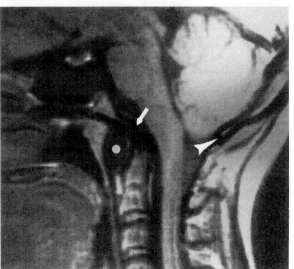

Fig. 5.**57 a–c**   Split atlas.
a Lateral radiograph shows a thickened anterior arch with a double outline (arrows). The atlantodental joint space cannot be identified. The anterior arch is slightly higher than the apex of the dens (dotted line). A cleft in the posterior arch is also present.
b CT appearance of the cleft in the anterior arch (arrowheads).
c Sagittal T1-weighted MRI shows an absence of fat marrow in the anterior arch of the atlas (white spot) with thickening of the arch. The cortical boundary of the posterior arch is not visualized in the midsagittal plane. The basion (arrow) and opisthion (arrowhead) can be clearly identified. (From Smoker 1994.)

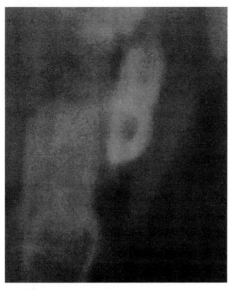

Fig. 5.**58** Duplication of the anterior arch of the atlas in a midsagittal tomogram. The duplicated arches are separated from each other by cortical bone.

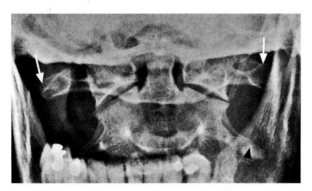

Fig. 5.**59** Laterally projecting transverse processes of the atlas (arrows) and axis (arrowhead).

Partial and **complete aplasias** of the anterior arch are very rare (Geipel 1955, Gentaz and Grellet 1969, Chapman et al. 1991). **Duplication** of the anterior arch has also been described (Fischer 1973), with only the lower part of the duplicated arch articulating with the dens. The two arches are separated from each other at the midline by cortical boundaries, and their cortical and cancellous bone are continuous with the lateral masses on each side. The upper arch projects above the apex of the dens and is below the anterior border of the clivus (Figs. 5.**58**, 5.**100**).

Transverse Processes

The transverse processes of the atlas normally exceed all the other cervical vertebrae in width (Fig. 5.**59**).

Clefts or defects in the transverse process of the atlas have occasionally been observed in both the anterior and posterior roots of the process. In other cases the process may be completely detached from the vertebra (Bock 1968). There have been rare reports describing **absence of the transverse foramen** (Vasudeva and Kumar 1995) and **pneumatization of the atlas** (Scialpi et al. 1994).

There may be bony bars on the atlas that partially or completely enclose the vertebral artery. The **lateral ponticulus** arises from the lateral border of the lateral mass and forms a bony arch over the transverse process for the artery (Fig. 5.**60**).

In most cases the lateral ponticulus is incomplete. It is poorly visualized on routine AP and lateral radiographs because it is projected obliquely in both planes. It is present in about 3% of the population (Törö and Szepe 1942, Mitchell 1998).

The **posterior ponticulus** is more common, with an incidence of approximately 13% (von Torklus and Gehle 1987). Known also as the **Kimmerle variant**, this bony projection arises from the posterior surface of the lateral mass of the atlas and forms a complete or partial bridge extending over the vertebral artery groove of the posterior arch (Figs. 5.**61**, 5.**62**).

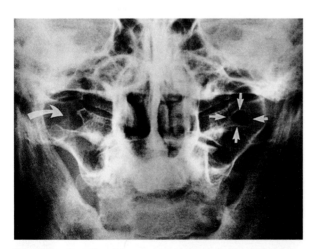

Fig. 5.**60** Complete lateral ponticulus on the left side of the atlas (arrow), incomplete lateral ponticulus on the right side (curved arrow).

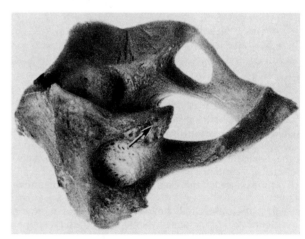

Fig. 5.**61** Posterior ponticulus of the atlas (Kimmerle variant, arcuate foramen) in an anatomic specimen. The ponticulus is complete on one side and rudimentary on the other.

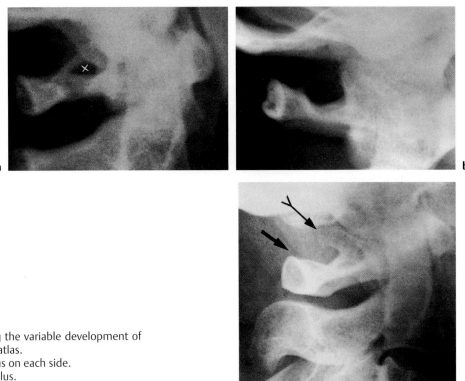

Fig. 5.**62 a–c**   Cases illustrating the variable development of the posterior ponticulus of the atlas.
a Complete posterior ponticulus on each side.
b Incomplete posterior ponticulus.
c Incomplete posterior ponticulus (arrow) with a stout, superiorly directed, hook-shaped anterior extension (double arrow).

When fully developed, the posterior ponticulus forms an **arcuate foramen** that transmits the vertebral artery, its accompanying veins, and the suboccipital nerve. It has been suggested that a connection may exist between a narrow arcuate foramen and cervical migraine (von Torklus and Gehle 1987).

Various theories have been proposed on the **origin of the ponticuli**. One theory holds that the lateral and posterior ponticuli are derived from embryonic tissue of the dorsal proatlas arch or the transverse process of the proatlas. Another theory suggests that the ponticuli arise from the upper half of the atlas segment and result from the ossification of ligaments that pass over the vertebral artery.

The **epitransverse process** is a peg-shaped bony prominence that arises from the transverse process of the atlas and whose apex is directed upward toward the occipital bone. The process usually shows a laterally convex curvature (Fig. 5.**63**). It can also occur as a separate bone that articulates with the transverse process of the atlas (Fig. 5.**64**).

The epitransverse process is distinguished from the **paracondylar process**, a peg-shaped bony prominence that arises by a broad base from the occipital bone next to the occipital condyle. It extends toward, and may articulate with, the lateral end of the transverse process of the atlas (Fig. 5.**65**).

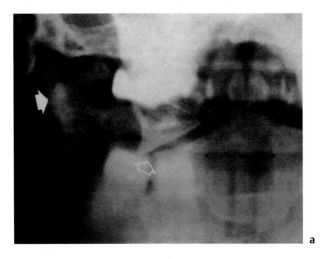

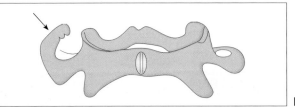

Fig. 5.**63 a, b**   Epitransverse process of the atlas.
a Epitransverse process (solid arrow) articulating with the skull base. Note the lateral displacement of the atlas to the right side (open arrow), indicating the pathological effect of the process on the function of C1. (From von Torklus and Gehle 1987.)
b Schematic drawing of an epitransverse process (arrow) (after von Torklus and Gehle).

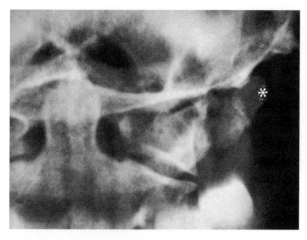

Fig. 5.**64** Isolated epitransverse process (asterisk) in the AP projection. (From von Torklus and Gehle 1987.)

The epitransverse and paracondylar processes may occur on one or both sides and may coexist. A bony process that is connected both to the occipital condyle and to the transverse process of the atlas is called a **paracondylar mass** (Fig. 5.**66**). The **infratransverse process** is a peg-shaped bony protuberance extending downward from the transverse process of the atlas to the transverse process of the axis (Figs. 5.**67**, 5.**68**).

Developmentally, the epitransverse process and paracondylar process are derived from portions of the transverse process of the proatlas, which is located between the occipital bone and the transverse process of the atlas during embryonic development. Incomplete regression results in varying degrees of persistence of the paracondylar and epitransverse processes (Fig. 5.**69**).

Variants of these anomalies in which a fixed or articular connection exists between the occiput and atlas are of clinical importance. This connection can limit the range of head motion and lead to atlantoaxial instability with torticollis and chronic head and neck pain. Ossification anomalies between the occiput and atlas show an association with other developmental abnormalities of the craniovertebral junction. Paracondylar and epitransverse processes require differentiation from a well-developed styloid process that is projected radiographically over the lateral transverse process of the atlas (Fig. 5.**70**).

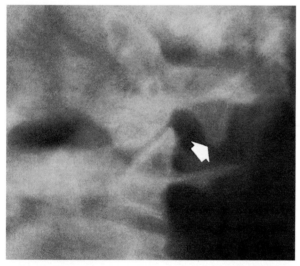

a

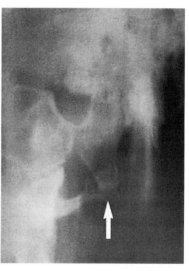

b

Fig. 5.**65a, b** Paracondylar process.
a AP tomogram shows a broad-based free-ending paracondylar process (arrow). (From von Torklus and Gehle 1987.)

b This paracondylar process has a jointlike connection with the transverse process of the atlas (arrow).

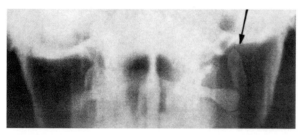

Fig. 5.**66** Paracondylar mass (arrow) linking the occipital condyle to the transverse process of C1. (From von Torklus and Gehle 1987.)

Fig. 5.**67** Tomogram shows supratransverse and infratrans- ▷ verse processes on the right side of the atlas, with assimilation of the atlas on the left side (arrowheads).

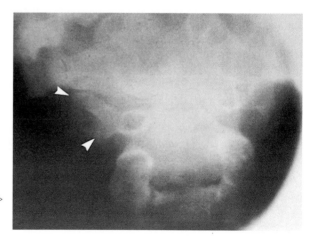

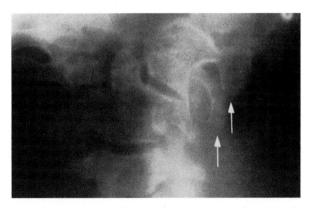

Fig. 5.**68** Tomogram shows infratransverse and paracondylar processes on the left side of the atlas (arrows), accompanied by assimilation of the atlas.

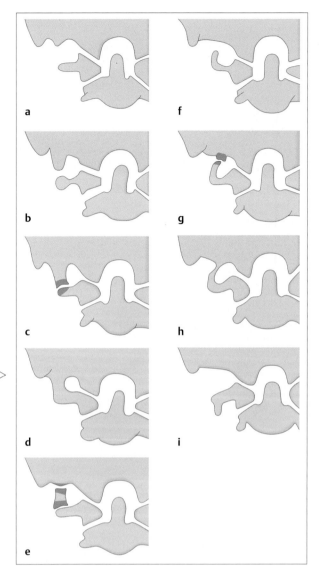

Fig. 5.**69 a–i** Varying prominence and interrelationships of ▷ the paracondylar and epitransverse processes. (From von Torklus and Gehle 1987.)
a Paracondylar tubercle.
b Freely terminating paracondylar process.
c Paracondylar process with an articular connection to the transverse process of the atlas.
d Paracondylar process fused to the transverse process of the atlas.
e Paracondylar mass linking the occiput to the transverse process of the atlas.
f Freely terminating epitransverse process.
g Epitransverse process articulating with the occiput.
h Epitransverse process fused to the occiput.
i Infratransverse process.

Fig. 5.**70** The styloid process is superimposed on the transverse processes of the atlas in the frontal tomogram, simulating an epitransverse process.

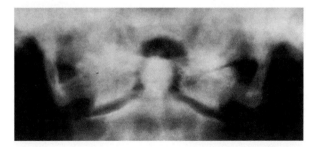

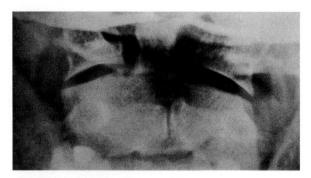

Fig. 5.**71**   Spina bifida of the axis, with displacement of the atlas toward the left side.

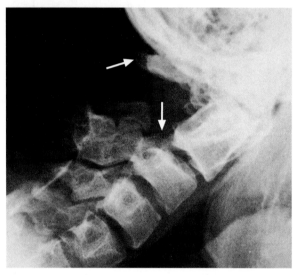

Fig. 5.**72**   Congenital defects in the arch of the axis and the posterior tubercle of the atlas (arrows). Suspected partial assimilation of the posterior arch rudiment.

Anomalies of the Axis

Vertebral Arch

Spina bifida of the axis is frequently combined with a cleft in the posterior arch of the atlas (Kirschbichler 1972) (Fig. 5.**71**).

Few reports have been published on **spondylolysis** of the axis (Kirschbichler 1972, Hanson et al. 1990, Jeanneret and Magerl 1990). Clefts and defects in the pedicle can lead to significant displacements of the vertebral bodies, but the anomaly may also be asymptomatic (Fig. 5.**72**).

> In children and adults, the spinolaminar line of the axis may appear posterior to that of C1 and C3. This finding is a normal variant and should not be interpreted as subluxation (Kattan 1977).

True **joint formation** has been observed between the spinous processes of the atlas and axis (Fig. 5.**47**). Figure 5.**73** illustrates an abnormal C2 spinous process.

Transverse Processes

Only a few variants and anomalies of the C2 transverse process have been described. The transverse process may be extremely long (Fig. 5.**59**), or it may feature an accessory process or a persistent apophysis (Fig. 5.**74**).

Vertebral Body

The ossicle at the apex of the dens, interpreted as the body of the proatlas (see During Growth), may persist as the **ossiculum terminale of Bergmann** (Figs. 5.**27**, 5.**28**, 5.**75**). Often, however, this variant cannot be reliably distinguished from other types of bone formation at the apex of the dens.

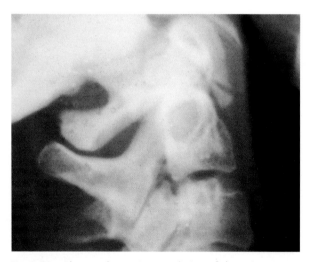

Fig. 5.**73**   Abnormal superior angulation of the spinous process of C2. An accessory ossicle is visible below the anterior arch of the atlas.

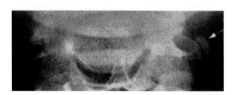

Fig. 5.**74**   Persistent apophysis of the C2 transverse process.

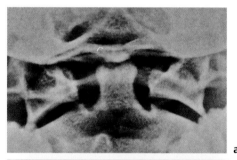

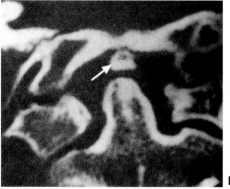

Fig. 5.**75 a, b**   Persistent ossiculum terminale.
a AP projection.
b Persistent ossiculum terminale in coronal CT. (From Smoker 1994.)

The **os odontoideum** is an independent bony element that appears above the axis on radiographs, generally taking the place of the normal dens (Juhl and Kjaergard 1983) (Fig. 5.76).

Von Torklus and Gehle (1987) dispute the common belief that the os odontoideum is an isolated ossification center of the dens that has failed to unite with the vertebral body. Rather, they characterize it as a hypoplasia of the dens that is accompanied by a separate os odontoideum. It is assumed that the os odontoideum results from an error in the development of the ossiculum terminale with irregular segmentation of the apex of the dens. Thus, the os odontoideum is equivalent developmentally to the ossiculum terminale of Bergman. The degree of **dens hypoplasia** in the presence of an os odontoideum is highly variable and ranges from complete absence (Fig. 5.76) to the presence of a dens stump (Fig. 5.77) or a short dens (Fig. 5.78).

The os odontoideum may be very small and visible only on sectional images. Large specimens may reach the size of a normal dens (Fig. 5.76). Besides its size, the os odontoideum is also variable in its position, i.e., it may be orthotopic or dystopic. An **orthotopic os odontoideum** occupies the position of the normal dens (Fig. 5.76) while a **dystopic os odontoideum** borders on the clivus (Fig. 5.79).

Fusion of the anterior arch of the atlas to the dens (Olbrantz and Bohrer 1984) and to the os odontoideum (Fig. 5.79) has been described. When an os odontoideum is present, the posterior arch of the atlas is often hypoplastic while the anterior arch is usually well developed. The causes of an **acquired os odontoideum** include inflammatory destruction of the dens during childhood. In this case the ossiculum terminale may continue to develop and even become hypertrophic. The term **os odontoideum verum** is used when the complete subdental synchondrosis persists into adulthood, isolating the dens and its base (McClellan et al. 1992) (Fig. 5.80).

The clinical importance of the os odontoideum lies in its ability to cause atlantoaxial instability, resulting in lateral or anteroposterior atlantoaxial displacement (Figs. 5.79, 5.81).

> With a dystopic os odontoideum, atlantoaxial displacement may already be present in the neutral position or may be detectable only by function studies.

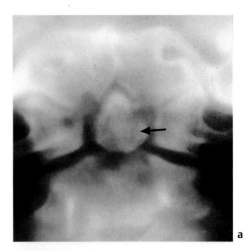

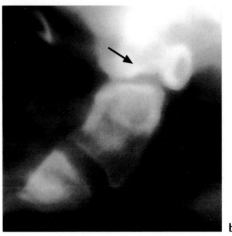

Fig. 5.**76 a, b**   Large os odontoideum in an orthotopic position (arrow). Note the elliptical shape and rounded edges. Marked hypoplasia of the dens.
a   Frontal tomogram.
b   Lateral tomogram.

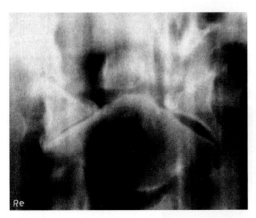

Fig. 5.**77**   Os odontoideum. Note the hypoplasia of the dens, which appears stublike.

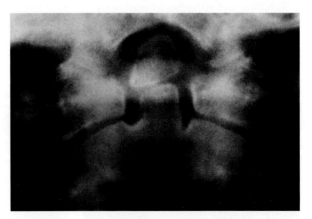

Fig. 5.**78**   Large os odontoideum atop a shortened dens in an AP tomogram. (From von Torklus and Gehle 1987.)

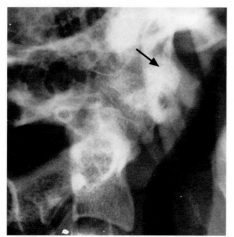
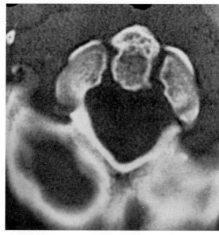

Fig. 5.**79a, b**   Dystopic os odontoideum fused to the anterior arch of the atlas.
a Lateral flexion view. The os odontoideum is above the anterior arch of the axis (arrow). Atlantoaxial displacement occurs when the neck is flexed, with widening of the atlantoaxial distance.
b CT demonstrates fusion of the os odontoideum to the anterior arch of the atlas.

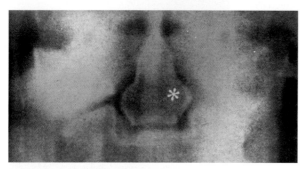

Fig. 5.**80**   Os odontoideum verum in an AP tomogram. The dens and its base (asterisk) are isolated by a persistent subdental synchondrosis. (From von Torklus and Gehle 1987.)

In cases of chronic instability with progressive anterior dislocation, there is a risk of injury to the medulla oblongata. A **dens fracture** (see Fig. 5.**105**) or **dens nonunion** differ from an os odontoideum in that the base of the fragment shows some degree of constriction and does not have the rounded or elliptical shape of an os odontoideum. Also, with an os odontoideum the gutterlike depressions that normally flank the dens are generally absent or less distinct (Fig. 5.**76**).

A **bicornuate dens** is one in which normal fusion of the bipartite apex has failed to occur, presumably due to persistence of the embryonic notochord. The result of this is an apex with two knobs in adulthood.

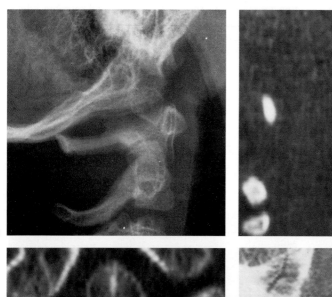
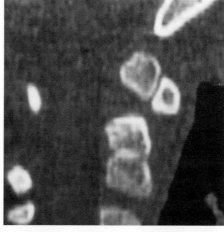
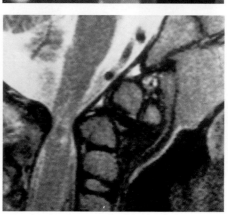

Fig. 5.**81**   Orthotopic os odontoideum. Anterior atlantoaxial subluxation with spinal stenosis and cervical myelopathy. The patient presented clinically with quadriparesis.
a Lateral radiograph.
b Sagittal multiplanar CT reconstruction.
c Coronal multiplanar CT reconstruction.
d Sagittal T2-weighted MRI of cervical myelopathy in the area of the foramen magnum.

Dysplasias of the dens mainly occur in association with assimilation of the atlas and abnormalities of atlantoaxial segmentation. Examples of dens dysplasia are shown in Fig. 5.**82**.

Dens hypoplasia refers to a shortened dens that does not reach the upper border of the anterior arch of the atlas (Fig. 5.**77**). A dens less than 11.9 mm long is classified as hypoplastic in both males and females (McManners 1983). The criteria for diagnosing **dens aplasia** are as follows:

- A dens or dens stump cannot be identified.
- There is no os odontoideum.
- The theoretical base of the dens is situated at an abnormally low level.

Dolichodens refers to an elongated dens whose apex extends more than 4 mm above the upper border of the anterior arch of the atlas (Fig. 5.**83**). In this anomaly, material from the centrum of the proatlas contributes to the formation of the dens apex. If the apex extends past the Chamberlain line, basilar invagination is present. If it touches the McRae line, a foramen magnum syndrome can result (Wackenheim 1974, Yanai and Tsuji 1985).

Dens hyperlordosis means that the angulation of the dens exceeds the normal slight dorsal angulation or curvature of 168° ± 8° (Fig. 5.**84**) (Decking and Ter Steege 1975). Known also as "**dens recurvatus**," this anomaly leads to a very high position of the atlas, which can restrict atlas motion and eventually lead to transverse ligament incompetence. Angular hyperlordosis of the dens may be mistaken for an old dens fracture (Fig. 5.**106**).

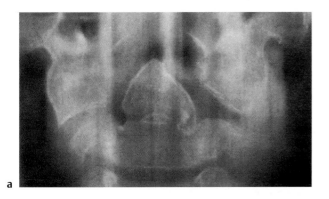

a

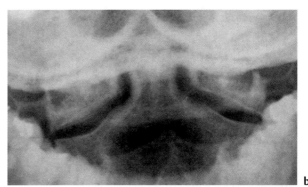

b

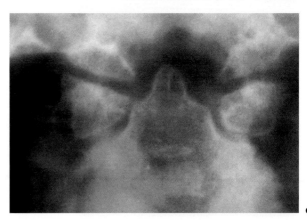

c

Fig. 5.**82 a–c**   Dysplasias of the dens. (From von Torklus and Gehle 1987.)
a Dysplastic dens with partial assimilation of the atlas in an AP tomogram.
b Broad base of the dens merges smoothly with the lateral articular facet on each side.
c Steplike dysplasia of the dens in an 11-year-old girl.

Fig. 5.**83 a, b**   Elongated dens (dolichodens). The dens projects 10 mm above the atlas. (From von Torklus and Gehle 1987.)
a Frontal tomogram.
b Lateral tomogram.

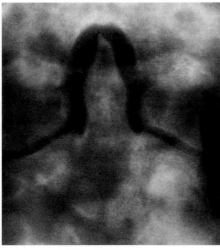

a

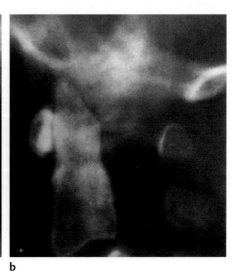

b

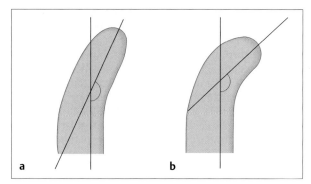

Fig. 5.**84 a, b** Determination of dens curvature.
a Normal angle (168° ± 8°).
b Angular hyperlordosis of the dens.

Lateral tilting of the dens is very rare. More than 5° of angulation is very suspicious for an acute or older fracture (Monu et al. 1987).

A **persistent synchondrosis** between the body and axis of the dens can also be difficult to distinguish from post-traumatic changes (Figs. 5.**38**, 5.**106**). **Scalloping** of the inferior end plate of the axis may indicate a failure of regression of the **notochord** (Fig. 5.**149**). Usually these changes are found in the mid- and lower thoracic spine and in the lumbar spine. They are uncommon in the axis and cervical spine.

Vertebral Assimilations

Assimilation of the upper cervical vertebrae with each another and with the occiput are important anomalies of the craniovertebral region (see Skull, Skull Base, and Occiput). Several forms of dysplasia may be encountered in the region of the craniovertebral junction:

- **Occipital dysplasia** confined to the occipital bone
- **Occipitocervical dysplasia** affecting the occipital bone and the first two cervical vertebrae
- **Suboccipital dysplasia** confined to the cervical vertebrae

These combined anomalies reflect the ontogenic relationships that exist between the first two cervical vertebrae and the fused occipital segments (see above). Here we shall limit our attention to the basic features of the latter two forms of dysplasia. A more detailed review can be found in the monograph by von Torklus and Gehle (1987).

Assimilations of the Atlas

Along with basilar invagination, assimilation of the atlas is among the most common craniovertebral junction abnormalities. It has a reported incidence of 0.25–0.4%. While assimilation of the atlas may be clinically asymptomatic, generally it is one of the most serious anomalies of the craniocervical region (McRae and Barnum 1953, Schmidt 1964, Schmidt and Fischer 1964, Chandraraj and Briggs 1992, Iwata et al. 1998, Jeanneret and Magerl 1990). It is accompanied by very severe degrees of occipital dysplasia (McRae 1953) and is very often associated with variants and dysplasias of the atlas and axis. Assimilation of the atlas is formally classified under the heading of occipital dysplasias (Schmidt and Fischer 1960).

> **Types of atlas assimilation** (Chandraraj and Briggs 1992)
> ➤ Complete assimilation of the atlas
> ➤ Partial assimilation of the atlas

Complete assimilation of the atlas is present when the atlas is completely occipitalized and cannot be identified as a separate structure (Fig. 5.**85**). **Partial assimilation** denotes a partial fusion of the atlas to the skull base (atlanto-occipital synostosis, Fig. 5.**86**).

◁ Fig. 5.**85 a–c** Complete assimilation of the atlas.
a Lateral projection. The posterior arch of the atlas is barely discernible (arrow).
b Frontal tomogram shows complete fusion of the occipital condyles with the lateral masses of the atlas.
c Lateral tomogram shows faint evidence of the anterior arch of the atlas interior to the clivus (arrows).

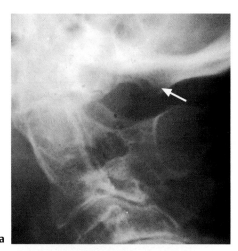

a

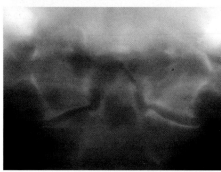

b

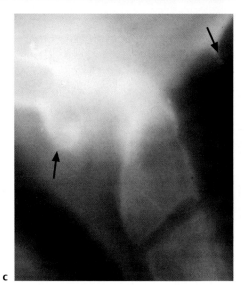

c

In the majority of cases, assimilation of the atlas does not occur in isolation but is combined with other anomalies, e.g.:

- Basilar invagination
- Various forms of occipital vertebra
- Fusion of adjacent vertebral bodies (block vertebrae)

A strong correlation exists between assimilation of the atlas and posterior arch defects. Assimilation of the atlas also has a high association with narrowing and deformity of the foramen magnum. With higher grades of atlas assimilation ranging to atlas aplasia, the dens assumes an increasingly high position with secondary narrowing of the foramen magnum (Ingelmark 1947, McRae and Barnum 1953, Iwata et al. 1998).

The morphology of atlas assimilation varies according to the degree and location of the anomaly. A unilateral or asymmetrical assimilation may be associated with bony torticollis, which is usually accompanied by craniofacial asymmetry. In most cases a synostosis exists between the anterior rim of the foramen magnum and the anterior arch of the atlas or between the lateral mass and the occipital condyles. Clinical symptoms are most likely to occur when these anomalies are combined with basilar invagination. An accompanying condylar reduction causes a high position of the dens. When this is combined with atlanto-occipital assimilation, progressive atlantoaxial subluxation can result (Iwata et al. 1998).

Atlantoaxial fusions differ from synostoses elsewhere in the spinal column due to the absence of an intervertebral space between C1 and C2 (Fig. 5.**87**). Atlantoaxial fusions are very rare (McRae and Barnum 1953, Soholm and Ingvardsen 1990, Gupta et al. 1993), disregarding fusions in Klippel–Feil syndrome and other complex differentiation anomalies (e.g., Goldenhar syndrome). Typically the fusion produces a new composite structure, the "atlas-axis," in which the anterior arch of the atlas is absent. Additionally, the dens is hypoplastic or aplastic (von Torklus and Gehle 1987) (Fig. 5.**88**).

Besides complete fusion, varying degrees of partial atlantoaxial fusion may occur, especially between the dens of the axis and the anterior arch of the atlas (Geipel 1955, Wackenheim and Dirheimer 1974). Unilateral assimilation of the atlas and axis represents a rare differentiation anomaly (Fig. 5.**89**).

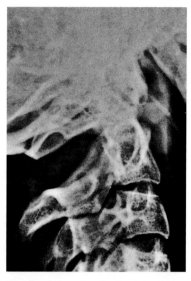

Fig. 5.**86**   Partial assimilation of the atlas. In the lateral projection, the anterior and posterior arch of the atlas are still partially delineated from the skull base.

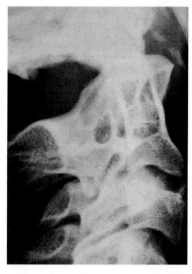

Fig. 5.**87**   Fusion of the atlas and axis. The anterior arch of the atlas can still be identified.

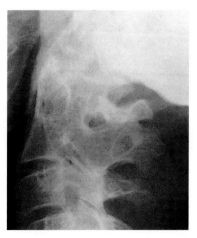

Fig. 5.**88**   Assimilation of the atlas and axis. The atlas lacks an anterior arch. (From von Torklus and Gehle 1987.)

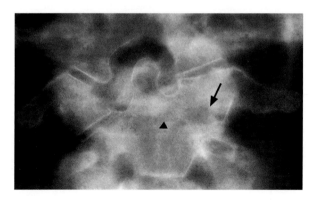

Fig. 5.**89**   Unilateral atlantoaxial fusion (arrow). The dens is fused to the lateral mass on one side (arrowhead). (From von Torklus and Gehle 1987.)

Unilateral irregular segmentation of the atlas and axis may occur alone or in conjunction with atlas assimilation. Either cranial portions of the axis are fused to the lateral mass on one side, or caudal portions of the lateral mass are fused to cranial portions of the axis. The joints between the vertebral bodies are not obliterated but are asymmetrically shifted upward or downward by one-half segment. As a result, joints that normally correspond are at different levels,

and joint mechanics are impaired. The displaced joint always shows a horizontal orientation (Fig. 5.**90**).

Irregular atlantoaxial segmentation is often associated with dysplasia of the dens (von Torklus and Gehle 1987). The irregular segmentation has been attributed to disturbances of notochordal development in early embryonic life. Figures 5.**91** and 5.**92** show various patterns of assimilation that can occur at the craniovertebral junction.

Other Accessory Ossicles

Accessory ossicles in the region of the foramen magnum, dens base, and lateral masses (Fig. 5.**93**) are usually not visible on standard radiographs. Sectional imaging views (conventional tomography, CT) are necessary for accurate localization.

Any isolated skeletal elements located between the dens apex, anterior arch of the atlas, and anterior border of the clivus, between the dens and lateral mass, or between the transverse process of the atlas and the lateral part of the occipital bone or immediate suboccipital area (Figs. 5.**21**, 5.**94**) may result from incomplete regression of the hypochordal bar.

The likelihood of this assumption is higher in younger patients and in patients who have no degenerative changes in the craniovertebral joints (Fig. 5.**93**). Frequently, however, these accessory ossicles cannot be accurately classified. Any connection with manifestations of an occipital vertebra (remnant of the hypochordal bar) is very unlikely unless a posterior ossicle is found in the region of the skull base (Fig. 5.**95**).

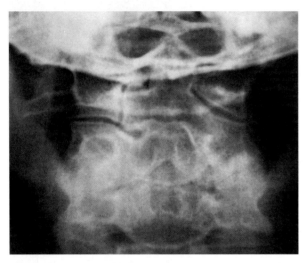

Fig. 5.**90**   Irregular atlantoaxial segmentation with dysplasia of the dens. The dens articulates with the lateral masses on both sides. Note the offset of the atlantoaxial articular surfaces and the horizontal position of the right articular surface. (From von Torklus and Gehle 1987.)

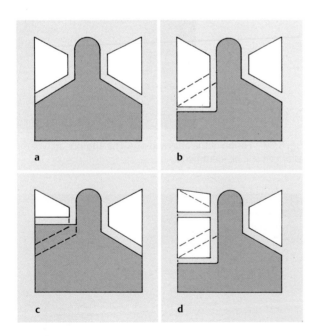

Fig. 5.**91 a–d**   Possible patterns of atlantoaxial assimilation (after Schmidt and Fischer).

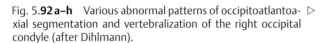

Fig. 5.**92 a–h**   Various abnormal patterns of occipitoatlantoa- ▷ xial segmentation and vertebralization of the right occipital condyle (after Dihlmann).

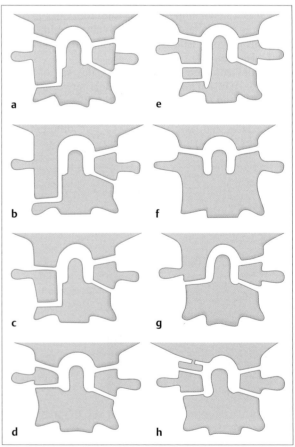

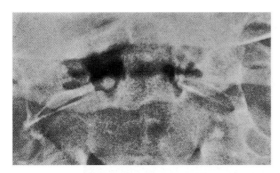

Fig. 5.**93**   A small, rounded ossicle is projected over the right dentolateral groove in a patient with degenerative arthritis of the right atlantoaxial joint.

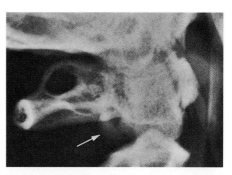

Fig. 5.**94**   Small, isolated bony element located behind and below the lateral mass. Note posterior ponticulus.

A **tertiary condyle** is usually located in the midline and articulates with the apex of the dens (Fig. 5.**96**). It may also show a more lateral location.

The different variations of the ossiculum terminale are included among the manifestations of an occipital vertebra (q.v.). Isolated ossicles below the anterior arch of the atlas as well as small anterosuperior bony elements are viewed as remnants of the hypochordal bar (Fig. 5.**97**).

The **os suboccipitale** (of Kerckring) represents an un-fused remnant of the neural arch of the proatlas (Fig. 5.**98**).

Accessory ossicles usually have no clinical relevance and should be differentiated from acquired calcifications and ossifications (see discussion below).

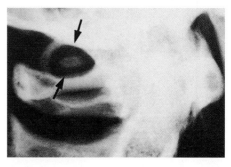

Fig. 5.**95**   Isolated bony element in the projection of a posterior ponticulus (arrows).

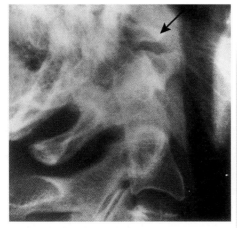

a

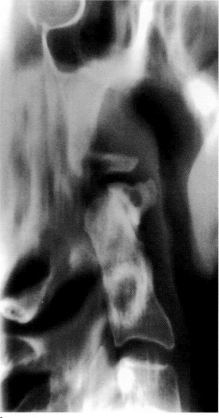

b

Fig. 5.**96 a, b**   Tertiary condyle (arrow).
a Lateral projection.
b Lateral tomogram.
Note the atlantodental osteoarthritis with joint space narrowing, subchondral sclerosis, and cystic changes in the anterior arch of the atlas (observation by Gläser, Aalen).

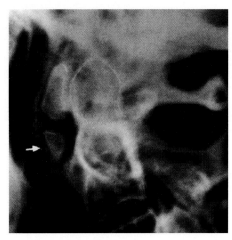

Fig. 5.**97** Anteroinferior ossicle (arrow) below the anterior arch of the atlas. This element is derived from the hypochordal bar. (From von Torklus and Gehle 1987.)

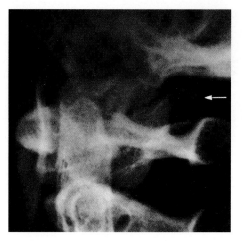

Fig. 5.**98** Os suboccipitale (of Kerckring) appears as a small ossicle below the posterior rim of the foramen magnum (arrow). (From von Torklus and Gehle 1987.)

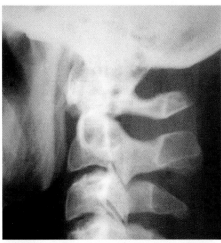

a

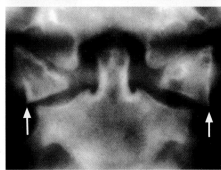

b

Fig. 5.**99a, b** Jefferson fracture.
a In the lateral view, the upper cervical spine appears normal.
b In the frontal tomogram, both lateral masses are displaced laterally. The articular facets of C1 overhang those of C2 (arrows).

 ## Fracture, Subluxation, or Dislocation?

In evaluating bony injuries of the atlas and axis, it is important to consider the many normal variants, anomalies, and imaging artifacts that can occur in order to avoid a misdiagnosis. If plain film findings are equivocal, CT or MRI should be employed.

This section deals with the principal fractures, subluxations, and dislocations of the upper cervical vertebrae and sources of diagnostic errors. A more detailed discussion of upper cervical traumatology can be found in standard reference works (e.g., Rogers 1992).

Fractures

An axial blow to the cranial vault can produce a **burst fracture** of the **atlas**, with fractures occurring through both the anterior and posterior arches on one or both sides (**Jefferson fracture**). The force drives down the occipital condyles into the articular facets and lateral masses of C1. Usually the lateral mass is broken into a medial fragment, which remains attached to the transverse ligament, and a lateral fragment that overhangs the lateral border of C2 (Figs. 5.**99**, 5.**100**).

A **posterior arch fracture** of the **atlas** (Figs. 5.**100**, 5.**101**), combined with a tear of the transverse ligament, leads to radiographically detectable instability with widening of the atlantodental joint space (Levine 1983).

A unilateral posterior arch fracture of C1 can occur if the traumatizing force ceases after one side has been fractured. An isolated, nondisplaced fracture of the **anterior tubercle** has been described in patients with multiple injuries sustained in motor vehicle accidents (Roush and Salciccioli 1982, Wiens et al. 1993).

Posterior arch fractures can be quite difficult to diagnose on plain films if the fragments are not displaced, especially when one considers the limited options for positioning patients who have sustained a serious injury (Hadley et al. 1985).

Superimposed **air in the auricle of the ear** or a **tilted lateral projection** can simulate a fracture of C1 (Fig. 5.**23**). A **paramedian cleft** in the posterior arch of C1, occurring as a normal variant, can also be misinterpreted as a fracture (Fig. 5.**50**). **Clefts** in the anterior and posterior arches can create the impression of a Jefferson fracture due to lateral displacement of the lateral masses. In children, ossification of the lateral masses may precede that of the body of C2, causing an apparent lateral displacement of the masses in relation to C2 and mimicking a C1 fracture (**pseudo-Jefferson fracture**). Aplasia of the C1 posterior arch may be associated with a bilateral atlantoaxial lateral offset (Gehweiler et al. 1983) and can mimic a Jefferson fracture.

Upper cervical fractures can be detected on **CT scans** with extremely high confidence (Woodring and Lee 1992). The ability to generate 3-D reconstructions also permits detailed visualization of the injury and the detection of rotational malalignment (Zinreich 1990).

A typical bony injury of C2 is the **hangman fracture**, a bilateral fracture of the vertebral arch (traumatic spondylolisthesis of the pars interarticularis) (Effendi et al. 1981, Mollan and Wyatt 1984, Saternus and Paul 1984) (Fig. 5.**102**).

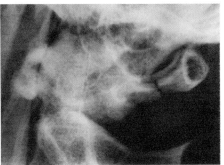
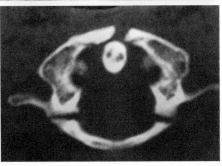

Fig. 5.**100 a, b** Jefferson fracture.
a Conspicuous fracture of the posterior arch of the atlas in the lateral projection. Note the double outline of the anterior arch as evidence of the fracture.
b Axial CT demonstrates a bilateral fracture of the posterior arch of the atlas and a midline fracture of the anterior arch.

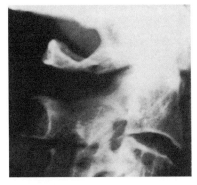

Fig. 5.**101** Lateral view of a posterior arch fracture of the atlas.

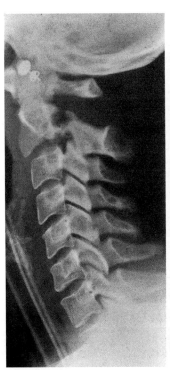
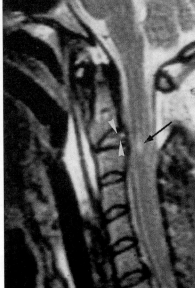

a   b

Fig. 5.**102 a, b** Traumatic spondylolysis of C2 (hangman fracture). Unstable type II fracture.
a Lateral view shows a bilateral fracture of the C2 vertebral arch with more than 15° angulation of the axis relative to C3.

b T2-weighted sagittal MRI shows a rupture of the intervertebral disk (arrowheads) and circumscribed edema (arrow) of the cervical cord, signifying a contusion. (From Buitrago-Tellez et al. 1997.)

Displacement of the fragments and slippage of C2 over C3 can lead to rupture of the C2/C3 intervertebral disk (Fig. 5.**102**). Traumatic spondylolisthesis following a motor vehicle accident was described in a five-month-old infant (Finnegan and McDonald 1982). Effendi et al. (1981) distinguished three different types of hangman fracture based on displacement and intervertebral dislocation (Fig. 5.**103**).

> **Effendi classification of the hangman fracture:**
> ➤ *Type I:* Fracture line runs through the posterior part of the C2 vertebral body or through the vertebral arch with no angulation or displacement.
> ➤ *Type II:* C2 is displaced more than 3 mm anteriorly relative to C3 or shows more than 15° of angulation.
> ➤ *Type III:* Type II fracture plus unilateral or bilateral dislocation of the C2/C3 apophyseal joints.

The injury is classified as stable if the intervertebral disk between C2 and C3 is intact. The intervertebral disk is always ruptured in type II and III fractures, and so these injuries are classified as unstable (Fig. 5.**102**). Isolated fractures of the body of C2 and transverse fractures are very rare

(Maki 1985). Usually a **hangman fracture** can easily be diagnosed on plain films. However, the rare **spondylolysis** of C2 can mimic a hangman fracture (Fig. 5.**72**).

CT can be helpful in diagnosing nondisplaced type I fractures (Baumgarten et al. 1985, Gerlock and Mirfakhraee 1983). **MRI** is necessary to exclude spinal injuries in type II and III fractures and to check for herniated disk tissue (Fig. 5.**102**).

Fractures of the dens have been classified into stable and unstable types by Anderson and d'Alonzo (1974) (Fig. 5.**104**).

> **Anderson-d'Alonzo classification of dens fractures:**
> ➤ *Type I:* Oblique fracture through the upper part of the dens (stable fracture type)
> ➤ *Type II:* Fracture line at the junction of the dens and vertebral body (unstable fracture type) (Fig. 5.**105**)
> ➤ *Type III:* Fracture line runs through the vertebral body, detaching the dens (stable fracture type)

Fractures of the dens have been described in infants and children (Savader et al. 1985) but occur predominantly in older individuals as a result of motor vehicle injuries and

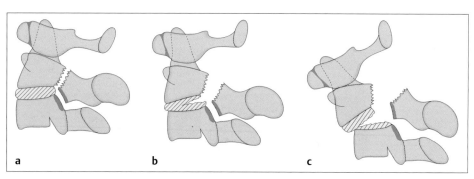

Fig. 5.**103 a–c**   Effendi classification of traumatic spondylolysis of C2 (hangman fracture).
a Type I: nondisplaced fracture of the C2 vertebral arch with an intact intervertebral disk between C2 and C3.
b Type II: more than 15° of anterior or posterior angulation between C2 and C3 and/or more than 3 mm of displacement of C2 relative to C3, with rupture of the intervertebral disk. The apophyseal joints articulate normally.
c Type III: same as type II but with dislocation of C2/C3 apophyseal joints. As in type II, the C2/C3 intervertebral disk is ruptured.

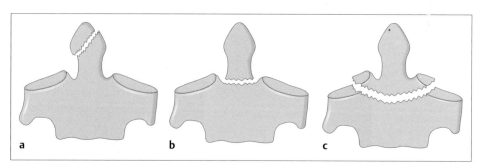

Fig. 5.**104 a–c**   Anderson–d'Alonzo classification of dens fractures.
a Type I: oblique fracture through the dens without involvement of the base. Stable fracture type.
b Type II: transverse fracture at the base of the dens without involvement of the vertebral body. The most common fracture type, unstable.
c Type III: oblique fracture at the base of the dens extending into the vertebral body. The second most common fracture type, stable.

Fig. 5.**105 a, b** Basal fracture of the dens. Note the sharp, angular fracture margins, which distinguish the fracture from an os odontoideum.
a Lateral projection.
b Sagittal CT reconstruction.

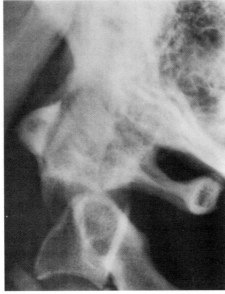

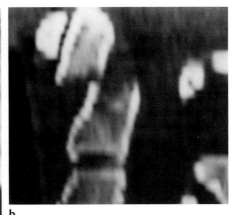

falls (Pepin et al. 1985). Fractures of the dens can show varying degrees of displacement.

Dens fractures are seen most clearly on **open-mouth** or **lateral radiographs**. Widening of the prevertebral soft-tissue shadow to more than 7 mm provides an indirect sign of a dens fracture. Nondisplaced horizontal fractures of the dens may be missed on axial **CT** and even in sagittal reconstructions. If a fracture is still suspected in such cases, a lateral **conventional tomogram** can establish the diagnosis (Pathria and Petersilge 1991).

Potential sources of diagnostic error include a **persistent synchondrosis remnant** at the base of the dens, which may be accompanied by anterior notching of the dens. This finding may be misinterpreted as a basal dens fracture (Fig. 5.**38**). **Mach effect**, as illustrated by the posterior arch of C1 superimposed on the body of the dens (Figs. 5.**34**, 5.**35**) and the interdental space of the maxillary incisors projected onto the dens (Fig. 5.**36**), can also produce **pseudofracture lines** leading to diagnostic error. If the normal variants are unknown, a **bifid dens** (bicornuate dens) can also cause errors of interpretation. **Clefts** in the anterior and posterior arch of C1 can mimic fractures of the dens (Haakonsen and Gudmundsen 1995) (Fig. 5.**49**). **Dens recurvatus** (Fig. 5.**84**) requires differentiation from an old consolidated dens fracture (Fig. 5.**106**).

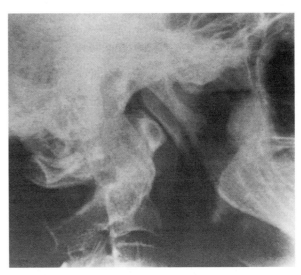

Fig. 5.**106** This fractured dens has healed in a position of marked anterior displacement relative to the body of the axis.

The development of a **nonunion** is mainly a complication of type II fractures of the dens. The presence of more than 6 mm of displacement is associated with an increased incidence of nonunions (Hadley et al. 1985). Type II and type III fractures have a considerably better prognosis (Hadley et al. 1985), but even these types can progress to nonunion (Clark and White 1985). It should be possible, however, to distinguish an **os odontoideum** from a nonunited dens fracture by applying the criteria noted above (Figs. 5.**76**, 5.**105**). Another potential complication of a bony atlantoaxial injury is secondary basilar invagination, which can lead to skull-base and facial asymmetries in growing patients (Schmidt and Fischer 1964).

The question of displaced bone fragments and their differentiation from **accessory ossicles** can be resolved by knowing the typical sites of occurrence and morphological features of adjuvant ossicles (see above). A **persistent apophysis** of the **transverse process of C2** (Fig. 5.**74**) requires differentiation from the rare fracture of the transverse process.

Subluxations and Dislocations

The range of motion of the cervical spine is generally greater in children than in adults, with the maximum between 11 and 14 years of age (Markuske 1981). Flexion-extension of the neck in these children is often associated with a marked displacement of C2 relative to C3 in the sagittal plane and with a less pronounced shifting of the C3 vertebral body relative to C4 (Markuske 1981). This disproportionately high mobility during flexion, known as "**pseudodislocation**," disappears by approximately 10 years of age (Fig. 5.**107**).

 Unlike a stepoff due to trauma, pseudodislocation is not observed in the neutral position.

The incidence of pseudodislocation in children is reported at 24% (Cattell and Filtzer 1965). It has even been noted in 40% of children under 8 years of age. The amount of the displacement is 2 mm on average and may be as much as 3 mm. A greater amount of pseudodislocation between C2 and C3 during flexion is known as **hypermobility syndrome**. Often this is associated with passive hyperextensibility of the joints. The posterior border of C2 undergoes a displacement of 3 mm or more through flexion/extension in approximately 50% of all children under 7 years of age (Cattell and Filtzer 1965).

On extension of the neck, the anterior arch of C1 may override the apex of the dens by more than two-thirds of its width in children up to 8 years of age (Cattell and Filtzer 1965) (Fig. 5.**108**). **Atlantoaxial pseudosubluxation** is manifested by a slightly increased atlantodental distance, which measures approximately 4 mm during flexion (Fig. 5.**107**), the predental space often acquiring a V shape (Bohrer et al. 1985). The angle of the V-shaped space in the normal population is 5.57° ± 4.13° (up to 22°) and 9.27° ± 5.06° in flexion (Monu et al. 1987).

Normal values for the predental distance (Hinck 1960, von Torklus and Gehle 1987)
➤ In women: 1.238 mm (0.0074 × age in years) ± 0.90 mm
➤ In men: 2.052 mm (0.0192 × age in years) ± 1.00 mm
➤ In 3- to 10-year-old children: 2.8 mm ± 0.5 mm. A value of 4 mm was observed in only 1 of 120 children (Markuske 1981)

Earlier we noted the relationship between aplasia of the C1 posterior arch and anterior atlantoaxial subluxation, and a bilateral atlantoaxial offset simulating a Jefferson fracture (Schulze 1980, Gehweiler et al. 1983). Clefts and defects in the pedicles can also lead to considerable displacement of the vertebral bodies (Fig. 5.**72**).

Atlanto-occipital dislocation is a very rare event (Fig. 5.**109**) (Kaufman et al. 1982, Grobovschek and Scheibelbrandner 1983).

Dislocations and subluxations of C1 that occur in association with a dens fracture are classified as **transdental dislocations**. An isolated dislocation of C1, called a **transligamentous dislocation**, is usually fatal. **Functional views** of the cervical spine are essential for detecting subtle anterior subluxation of C1.

The differential diagnosis should include anterior displacement of C1 as a result of rheumatoid disease (Fig. 5.**113**). **Anterior displacement of the atlas** in children is difficult to distinguish from **pseudodislocation** but is most likely present if the width of the atlantoaxial space is more than 4 mm. **Lateral displacement of the atlas** is a rare condition that can be diagnosed on cervical function views by noting a lateral offset when the head is tilted to the side (Fielding 1978, Kratzer et al. 1985).

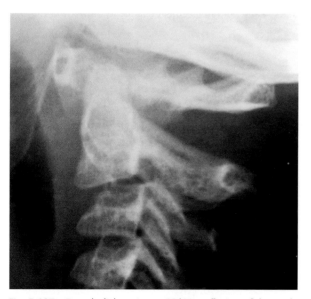

Fig. 5.**107** Pseudodislocation at C2/C3 on flexion of the neck. Note the increased atlantodental distance.

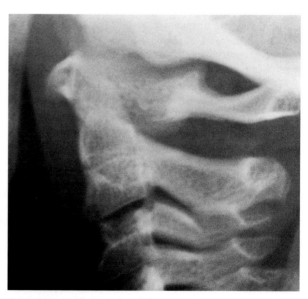

Fig. 5.**108** High position of the anterior arch of the atlas on extension of the neck.

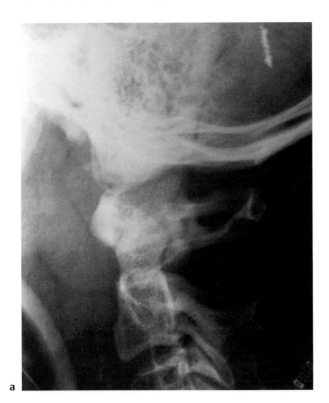

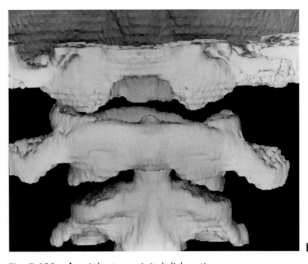

Fig. 5.**109a, b**   Atlanto-occipital dislocation.
a In the lateral view, there appears to be no contact between the occipital condyles and the articular facets of the atlas. The C1 vertebra is slanted, and the atlanto-occipital distance is increased. There is also evidence of atlantoaxial subluxation.
b Three-dimensional CT reconstruction confirms atlanto-occipital distraction and dislocation with widening of the atlanto-occipital joint space on the left side. Additionally there is atlantoaxial subluxation with distraction of the atlantoaxial joints.

Atlantoaxial rotatory subluxation, known also as **rotatory fixation**, may occur spontaneously or as a result of trauma. Clinically, the patient shows limited motion of the cervical vertebrae and in extreme cases may have a persistent torticollis.

With **rotatory subluxation of the axis**, C2 occupies a typical, fixed rotated position in relation to C1 (Fig. 5.**110**). The spinous process of C2 is shifted from the midline in the AP view while the C1 lateral masses appear symmetrical. In the lateral view, a lateral articular facet of C2 may define the anterior contour of the vertebra.

With **rotatory subluxation of the atlas**, the lateral masses of C1 are positioned asymmetrically in the AP projection (Fig. 5.**111**). In the lateral projection, the C1 lateral masses are not correctly superimposed and may jut out anteriorly and posteriorly. **CT** permits an accurate analysis of rotatory subluxations involving C1 and C2 (Jones 1984, Baumgarten et al. 1985).

Atlantoaxial displacement, possibly combined with rotatory fixation (El-Khoury et al. 1985), can occur in association with various congenital systemic diseases:

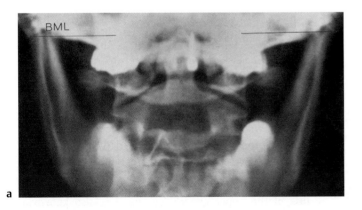

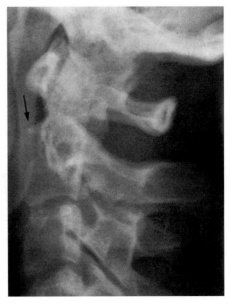

Fig. 5.**110a, b**   Spontaneous rotatory subluxation of the axis. (From von Torklus and Gehle 1987.)
a In the AP open-mouth view, the atlas appears symmetrical while the spinous process of the axis deviates 1 cm to the right from the midline. The bimastoid line (BML) is horizontal.
b In the lateral view, the right lateral articular facet of the axis defines the anterior contour of the vertebra as a result of the subluxation. The C2/C3 articular processes are not aligned.

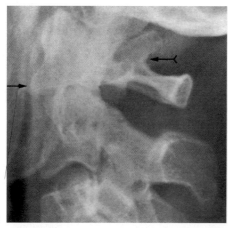 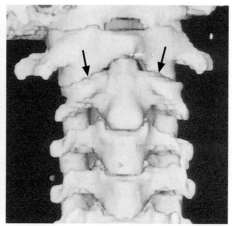

Fig. 5.**111 a, b**   Rotatory subluxation of the atlas.
a In the lateral view, one lateral mass of C1 overhangs the C2 lateral articular facet anteriorly (arrow) and the other posteriorly (double arrow). (From von Torklus and Gehle 1987.)

b Three-dimensional CT reconstruction of C1 rotatory subluxation in a different patient shows bilateral offset of the atlantoaxial joint surfaces (arrows). (From Buitrago-Tellez et al. 1997.)

- Down syndrome (Hvidarsson et al. 1982, Grobovschek and Strohecker 1985, Pueschel et al. 1984, Menezes and Ryken 1992, Trumble et al. 1994, Uno et al. 1996)
- Mucopolysaccharidosis type I (Hurler syndrome) (Thomas et al. 1985) and type IV (Morquio syndrome) (Pouliqueu et al. 1982)
- Larssen syndrome (Le Marec et al. 1994)
- Neurofibromatosis (Aprile et al. 1984)
- Spastic torticollis (Ryken and Menezes 1993)

In extreme cases the displacement can lead to compression of the cervical cord (Haaland et al. 1984).

In patients with **muscular torticollis** (see Midcervical Spine), which may result from congenital dysplasia of the sternocleidomastoid muscle, posttraumatic soft-tissue contractures and scars, or may develop suddenly due to an unknown cause, the axis on the affected side often remains lower and has a smaller articular surface. In these cases the dens is shifted and curved toward the convex side. Asymmetry and displacement of C1 are usually a result or accompanying feature of the condition. Most cases present with a transient or fixed **atlantoaxial rotatory subluxation**, which is best demonstrated by CT (Fig. 5.**111**) (Kratzer et al. 1985, Ono et al. 1985).

Atlantoaxial displacements also occur in **Grisel syndrome** (nasopharyngeal torticollis) (Grisel 1930). This condition mainly affects children and adolescents and occasionally young adults. Onset is related to a nasopharyngeal infection, tonsillitis, otitis media or otitis externa. Presumably, the pathogenesis is based on transient contractures of the suboccipital and paravertebral muscles caused by the venous or lymphogenous spread of an inflammatory process. Radiographs may show anterior displacement of C1 with or without rotatory subluxation. Typically there is widening of the prevertebral soft-tissue shadow consistent with an inflammatory process (Wetzel and La Rocca 1989, Mathern and Batzdorf 1989).

 Necrosis?

Avascular or aseptic **osteonecrosis** of the **dens** is a rare pathological process that has been discussed only sporadically in the literature (Freiberger et al. 1965, Dove and Yau 1982). It is assumed that the necrosis results from a fracture of the dens.

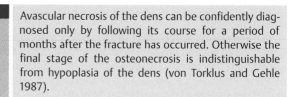

> Avascular necrosis of the dens can be confidently diagnosed only by following its course for a period of months after the fracture has occurred. Otherwise the final stage of the osteonecrosis is indistinguishable from hypoplasia of the dens (von Torklus and Gehle 1987).

Avascular necrosis of the dens has also been reported in patients treated for scoliosis by means of halo-pelvic distraction (Tredwell and O'Brien 1975). According to von Torklus and Gehle (1987), this reproducible dens necrosis confirms the essential role of the ligaments in the blood supply of the dens (Schiff and Parke 1973, Althoff and Goldie 1977). To the best of our knowledge, no reports have been published on **osteonecrosis** of the atlas.

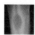 **Inflammation?**

Bacterial spondylitis may be caused by hematogenous spread or direct inoculation (Leach et al. 1967, Zigler et al. 1987). Block vertebrae and vertebral destruction can occur as sequelae to previous infections. **Tuberculous spondylitis** of the upper cervical vertebrae is also known as **malum suboccipitale**. Comprising some 2% of all cases of tuberculous spondylitis, this disease is a rare but important form of tuberculosis (Weaver and Lifeso 1984, Morvan et al. 1984, Dowd et al. 1986, Lifeso 1987, Corea and Tamimi 1987, Levin et al. 1992). The clinical symptoms are pain, dysphagia, and neurological deficits that may include tetraplegia. Progression of the disease is associated with bone erosions and increasing destruction of the affected joints, atlanto-occipital subluxation, and the development of pre-vertebral and intraspinal abscesses (Fig. 5.**112**). Similar changes can also be seen in **fungal infections**.

The following rheumatoid diseases can lead to changes in the cervical spine:

- **Rheumatoid arthritis**
- **Ankylosing spondylitis**
- Occasionally, other **seronegative spondyloarthropathies** (psoriasis, Reiter syndrome)

Rheumatoid arthritis is the leading cause of subluxations and malalignments in the occipitoatlantoaxial region. Cervical spine involvement is present in approximately 60–80% of rheumatoid arthritis patients (Bland 1974, Park et al. 1979). The changes include inflammatory destructive changes in the craniovertebral and apophyseal joints and intervertebral disk spaces and acro-osteolysis of the dens and spinous processes (see Midcervical and Lower Cervical Spine).

The following typical changes are observed in the occipitoatlantoaxial region:

- Arthritis of the atlanto-occipital and atlantoaxial joints
- Various forms of subluxation:
  - Anterior atlantoaxial subluxation
  - Vertical subluxation (cranial settling)
  - Lateral and posterior subluxation

Reportedly, these subluxations are present in 40–85% of patients with rheumatoid arthritis (Bland 1990).

Anterior atlantoaxial subluxation is a common finding in rheumatoid arthritis and may be detectable even in the early stage of the disease (Haaland et al. 1984, Halla et al. 1989). It reportedly occurs in 20–25% of rheumatoid arthritis patients (Mathews 1969). The normal atlantodental distance of 2 mm is increased in these cases to 4–10 mm (Fig. 5.**113**).

The pathogenesis of anterior atlantoaxial subluxation is related to laxity of the transverse ligament caused by inflammatory changes between the dens and transverse ligament. If the atlantodental distance is widened to more than 8 mm, laxity of the alar ligaments is also assumed (Werne 1959). **Posterior atlantoaxial subluxation** has also been reported in patients with rheumatoid arthritis (Redlund-Johnell 1984a). The extent of the inflammatory granulation tissue (pannus) and its relationship to the cervical cord are best evaluated with MRI (Fig. 5.**113**).

Vertical subluxation of the dens (pseudobasilar invagination, cranial settling) can also be observed in rheumatoid arthritis. It is caused by a decreased height of the lateral masses and occipital condyles and can become life-threatening. Vertical subluxation has been observed in 5–22% of patients with rheumatoid arthritis (El-Khoury et al. 1980, Weissman et al. 1982, Redlund-Johnell 1984b). MRI permits an early and comprehensive diagnosis that includes the effects of the subluxation on the spinal cord (Fig. 5.**113**).

Lateral subluxation of the atlantoaxial joints occurs in approximately 10–20% of rheumatoid arthritis patients and is generally associated with anterior atlantoaxial subluxation (Jackson 1983).

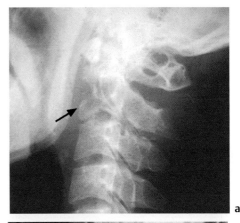
a

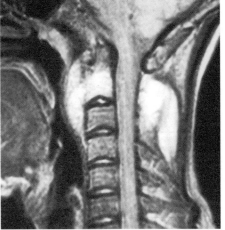
b

Fig. 5.**112 a, b** Tuberculous spondylitis of the axis (malum suboccipitale).
a Lateral radiograph shows osteolytic destruction of the C2 vertebral body (arrow).
b T1-weighted MRI after intravenous contrast administration demonstrates involvement of the C2 vertebral body and extensive perivertebral abscess formation on the anterior and posterior sides. There is no sign of abscess extension into the spinal canal (observation by D. Resnick, San Diego).

Arthritis of the atlanto-occipital joints is characterized by:

- Narrowing of the joint spaces
- Subchondral sclerosis and erosions of the articular surfaces in the atlanto-occipital and lateral atlantoaxial joints

The course of rheumatoid arthritis may be marked by **inflammatory erosions** of the **dens**, **dens atrophy**, and in extreme cases by almost complete destruction of the dens (Rosenberg et al. 1978) (Fig. 5.**114**). Pathological fractures of the dens (Storms et al. 1980) and atlas (Sandelin et al. 1985) have also been described. Rheumatoid arthritis and especially **juvenile rheumatoid arthritis** (Fried 1983) can lead to bony fusion of the craniovertebral joints with ankylosis of the occipitoatlantoaxial junction.

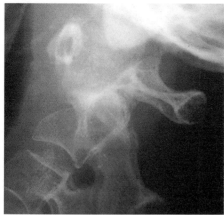

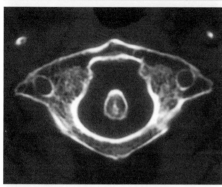

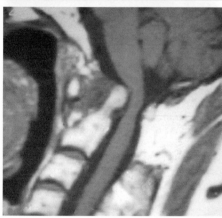

Fig. 5.**113 a–c**   Atlantoaxial displacement in rheumatoid arthritis.
a Lateral radiograph shows marked widening of the atlantodental distance due to posterior displacement of the dens.
b CT demonstrates the marked posterior displacement of the dens.
c Cord compression is evident on T1-weighted sagittal MRI. Note the pannus tissue between the anterior arch of the atlas and the dens.

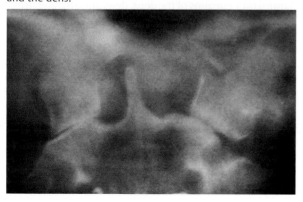

Ankylosing spondylitis usually spares the occipitoatlantoaxial joints, and **occipitoatlantoaxial fusion** is rare. The development of secondary **block vertebrae** is preceded by arthritis of the affected joints. The incidence of **atlantoaxial subluxation** is only about 2% (Sharp and Purser 1961, Schwägerle et al. 1981). **Psoriatic arthritis** and, less commonly, **Reiter syndrome** can also lead to occipitoatlantoaxial abnormalities with erosion of the dens and atlantoaxial subluxation. Bone proliferation at the apex of the dens may be found in all seronegative spondylarthropathies.

 Tumor?

Tumors and tumorlike lesions are relatively rare in the upper cervical spine (Fig. 5.**115**).

Chordomas and **aneurysmal bone cysts** show a predilection for this region (Hastings et al. 1968, von Torklus and Gehle 1987).

Chordomas arise from remnants of the primitive notochord and most commonly occur at the upper and lower ends of the spinal column. Approximately 15% of all chordomas affect the **upper cervical spine**, with other cases involving the spheno-occipital and sacrococcygeal regions. As a rule, chordoma is a locally aggressive and destructive tumor with an extensive extraosseous component; pure intraosseous forms are very rare (Darby et al. 1999). Advanced tumors can metastasize by the hematogenous route (Sundaresan et al. 1979). Chordomas show no sex predilection and occur in persons from 30 to 60 years of age (Mindell 1981). Radiographs show vertebral body **destruction** and a soft-tissue mass. Adjacent vertebral bodies may be involved. **Calcifications** are found in approximately 30% of cases. Affected vertebral bodies may also exhibit heavy sclerosis (ivory vertebra) (de Bruine and Kroon 1988). MRI defines the intraspinal extent of the tumor (Le Pointe et al. 1991). The radiographic features of chordoma are illustrated in the sections on the midcervical spine and sacrum (Figs. 5.**195**, 5.**439**).

Aneurysmal bone cysts typically affect the **posterior spinal elements**, especially the vertebral arches and spinous processes (Fig. 5.**190**). The vertebral body may also be affected, however. Radiographs typically show a circumscribed **cystic expansion** of the bone with obliteration and rarefaction of the cancellous trabeculae. The lesion is usually enclosed by a thin shell of bone. Differentiation from a large osteoblastoma may be difficult (Fig. 5.**116**) (Dias and Frost 1973, Capanna et al. 1985, Caro et al. 1991).

◁ Fig. 5.**114**   AP tomogram reveals pronounced erosions and mutilation of the dens in rheumatoid arthritis. (From von Torklus and Gehle 1987.)

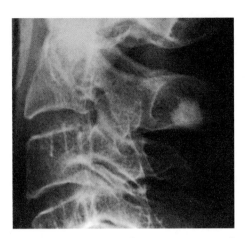

Fig. 5.**115**   Osteoma in the spinous process of C2.

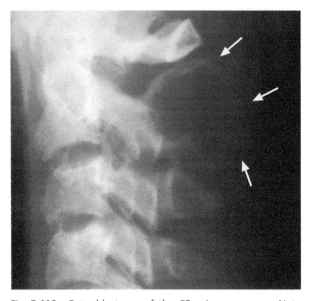

Fig. 5.**116**   Osteoblastoma of the C2 spinous process. Note the expansion of the spinous process and the thin bony shell enclosing the tumor (arrows) (observation by D. Resnick, San Diego).

A few reports have been published on the features of **osteoblastoma** (Gelberman and Olson 1974), **osteoid osteoma** (Jones 1987), **osteochondroma** (Wu and Guise 1978), and **juxtacortical chondroma** (Calderone et al. 1982).

Metastases from **breast, thyroid, prostatic, bronchial, and renal carcinoma** are frequently found in the atlas and axis of patients with skeletal metastases (Fig. 5.**117**). CT and MRI and extremely helpful in making a diagnosis and evaluating spinal stability.

Tumorlike changes can result from various disorders of the vertebral bodies. For example, a cleft in the anterior arch of C1 may appear as a "**pseudotumor**" on MRI (Fig. 5.**57**). The upper cervical spine may be involved by **fibrous dysplasia** or **Paget disease** (Figs. 5.**208**, 5.**363**, 5.**444**), and this can raise problems of differential diagnosis (Brown et al. 1971, Resnik and Liniger 1984). Marked **elongation** and **ectasia** of the **vertebral artery** can sometimes produce **lateral indentations** in the posterior margin and intervertebral foramen of C2, which may be mistaken for an expansile tumor. Typically this is observed at the C2/C3 level (Fig. 5.**118**).

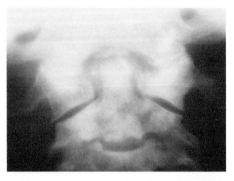

Fig. 5.**117**   Osteoblastic metastases in the atlas and axis from prostatic carcinoma.

 ## Other Changes?

Degenerative osteoarthritis produces the same changes in the craniovertebral and atlantoaxial joints as in other joints: joint space narrowing, sclerosis of the articular surfaces, marginal osteophytes, and calcification or ossifications in the capsule and ligaments.

Degenerative osteoarthritis of the **atlanto-occipital joints** is difficult to diagnose, because often these joints are not visualized on radiographs of the skull and cervical spine. Evaluation is also hampered by the notchlike changes in the medial border of the superior articular facets of C1 (Fig. 5.**24**). Degenerative osteoarthritis can also be difficult to diagnose in the **atlantoaxial joints** (Fig. 5.**119**), for even the normal articular margins of C1 can resemble osteophytic spurs (Figs. 5.**29**, 5.**36**, 5.**39**) (Halla and Hardin 1987).

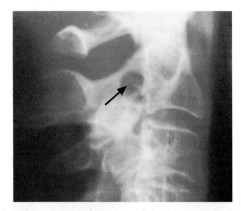

Fig. 5.**118**   Sharply marginated erosion of the intervertebral foramen (arrows) caused by elongation of the vertebral artery.

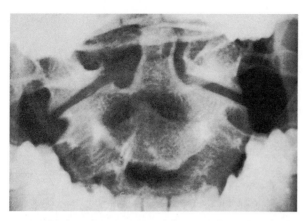

Fig. 5.**119** Degenerative osteoarthritis of the right atlanto-axial joint. Note the asymmetric positions of the C2 articular surfaces and the oblique position of the dens.

Degenerative osteoarthritis of the **atlantodental joint** is manifested by narrowing of the predental joint space in the lateral projection and by marginal osteophytes on the upper articular surface of the C1 anterior arch and, less commonly, on the apex of the dens (Fig. 5.**120**) (Fischer and Schmidt 1969).

Osteophytes on the superior margin of the C1 anterior arch or on the apex of the dens create a "**crowned dens**" configuration in the **AP projection** (Skaane and Klott 1981) and may be confused with calcification of the dens ligaments, which also may be caused by calcium pyrophosphate dihydrate crystal deposition in pseudogout (Dirheimer et al. 1983) (Fig. 5.**121**).

In contrast to the rare occurrence of degenerative osteoarthritis in the other craniovertebral joints, its prevalence in the anterior atlantoaxial joint is comparable to that of spondylosis deformans in the lower and midcervical spine (Olsson 1942, Aufdermaur 1960).

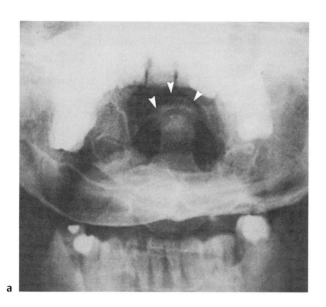

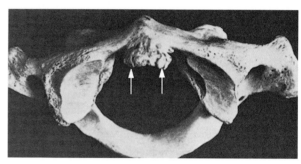

Fig. 5.**120 a, b** Osteoarthritis of the atlantodental joint.
a Peridental ossification ("crowned dens") in the AP projection.
b Specimen (different case) shows the structure corresponding to the crowned dens over the anterior arch of the atlas.

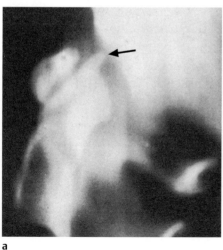

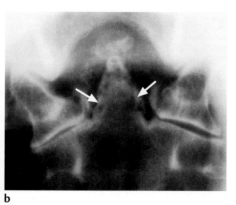

Fig. 5.**121 a, b** Calcified peridental ligaments.
a Radiographic appearance of a calcified dens apical ligament (arrow).
b Calcifications and ossifications of the alar ligaments (arrows), apical ligament, and calcifications in the apical bursa above the apex of the dens (arrowhead). Atlantoaxial osteoarthritis is also present (observation by W. Grochtmann, Gütersloh).

The shortened distance between the spinous processes of C1 and C2 can lead to **frictional sclerosis (Baastrup's phenomenon)** like that occurring elsewhere in the spine (Fig. 5.**122**, compare with Fig. 5.**47**).

Differentiation from **calcifications and ossifications** of the capsule and ligaments in the occipitoatlantoaxial region and from osteophytic reactions can be difficult (Prescher 1990). Bony projections on the upper and lower margins of the C1 anterior arch may represent ossification of the **anterior atlanto-occipital membrane**, a detached **osteophyte**, **accessory ossicles**, or **calcifying tendinitis** of the longus colli muscle (Newmark et al. 1986, Gamroth 1991) (Figs. 5.**123**–5.**127**).

Prevertebral calcifications are known to occur in **hypervitaminosis A** (Pennes et al. 1984). **Ossification** of the **transverse ligament** may be an early manifestation of ossification of the posterior longitudinal ligament (OPLL) but can also result from calcium pyrophosphate dihydrate crystal deposition in pseudogout (Wackenheim 1978, Dirheimer et al. 1983) (Fig. 5.**128**).

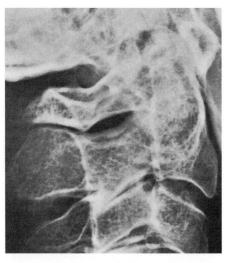

Fig. 5.**122** Baastrup's phenomenon between the spinous processes of the atlas and axis in a patient with a powerfully developed C2 spinous process.

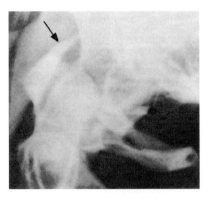

Fig. 5.**123** Bony prong extending upward from the anterior arch of the atlas to the skull base (arrow).

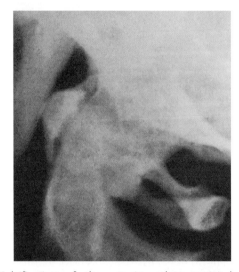

Fig. 5.**124** Calcification of the anterior atlanto-occipital membrane.

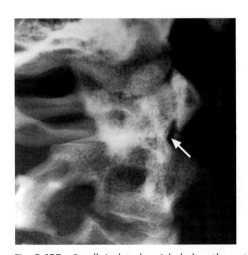

Fig. 5.**125** Small, isolated ossicle below the anterior arch of the atlas (arrow). An osteophytic outgrowth is visible on the upper margin of the anterior arch. A history of whiplash injury raised the possibility of an isolated fracture of the C1 anterior tubercle, but the same feature was visible on previous radiographs.

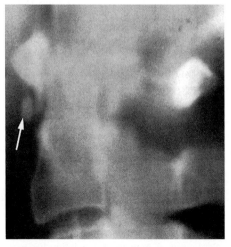

Fig. 5.**126** Ossicle below the anterior arch of the atlas.

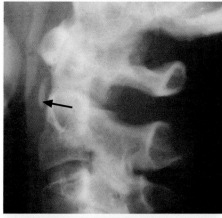

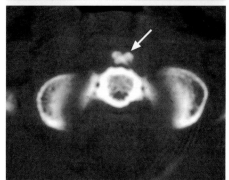

a

b

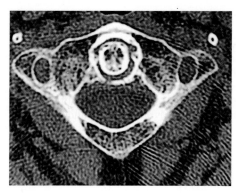

Fig. 5.**128**   Calcification of the transverse ligament on axial CT. The cause is unknown.

◁ Fig. 5.**127 a, b**   Calcifying tendinitis of the longus colli muscle. The images show an oblong calcified structure located just anterior to the axis (arrow).
a Lateral radiograph.
b Axial CT.

References

Althoff, B., J. I. F. Goldie: The arterial supply of the odontoid process of the axis. Acta orthop. scand. 48 (1977) 622

Anderson, L. D., R. T. d'Alonzo: Fractures of the odontoid process of the axis. J. Bone Jt Surg. 56-A (1974) 1663

Aprile, P. D. G. Krajewska, T. Parniola, M. Trizio, F. Federico, A. Carella: Congenital dislocation of dens of the axis in a crase neurofibromatosis. Neuroradiology 12 (1984) 405

Aufdermaur, M.: Die Spondylosis cervicalis. Hippokrates, Stuttgart 1960

Baumgarten, N., W. Mouradian, D. Boger, R. Watkins: Computed axial tomography in C1–C2 trauma. Spine 10 (1985) 187

Bland, J. H.: Rheumatoid arthritis of the cervical spine. J. Rheumatol. 1 (1974) 319

Bland, J. H.: Rheumatoid subluxation of the cervical spine. J. Rheumatol. 17 (1990) 134

Bock, H.: Querfortsatzfehlbildung am Atlas. Fortschr. Röntgenstr. 109 (1968) 111

Bohrer, S. P., J. A. Brody: More than just lip service. Skelet. Radiol. 21 (1992) 305

Bohrer, S. P., A. Klein, W. Martin III: „V" shaped predens space. Skelet. Radiol. 14 (1985) 11

Brown, H. P., H. LaRocca, J. K. Wickstrom: Paget's disease of the atlas and axis. J. Bone Jt Surg. 53-A (1971) 1441

de Bruine, F. T., H. M. Kroon: Spinal chordoma: radiologic features in 14 cases. Amer. J. Roentgenol. 150 (1988) 861

Buitrago-Téllez, C. H., S. J. Ferstel, M. Langer: Spine. In Heller, M., A. Fink: Radiology of Trauma. Springer, Berlin 1997 (pp. 59–94)

Calderone, A., A. Naimark, A. L. Schiffer: Juxtacortical chondroma of C2. Case report 196. Skelet. Radiol. 8 (1982) 160

Capanna, R., U. Albisinni, P. Picci et al.: Aneurysmal bone cyst of the spine. J. Bone Jt Surg. 67-A (1985) 527

Caro, P. A., G. A. Mandell, R. P. Stanton: Aneurysmal bone cyst of the spine in children. MRI imaging at 0,5 tesla. Pediat. Radiol. 21 (1991) 114

Cattell, H. S., D. L. Filtzer: Pseudosubluxation and other normal variations in the cervical spine in children. J. Bone Jt Surg. 47-A (1965) 1295

Chambers, A. A., M. F. Gaskill: Midline anterior atlas clefts: CT findings. J. Comput. assist. Tomogr. 16 (1992) 868

Chandraraj, S., C. A. Briggs: Failure of somite differentiation at the cranio-vertebral region as a cause of occipitalization of the atlas. Spine 17 (1992) 1249

Chapman, S., J. H. Goldin, R. G. Hendel, A. D. Hockley, M. C. Wake, P. Weale: The median cleft face syndrome with associated cleft mandible, bifid odontoid peg and agenesis of the anterior arch of atlas. Brit. J. oral max.-fac. Surg. 29 (1991) 279

Clark, Ch. R., A. A. White: Fractures of the dens. J. Bone Jt. Surg. 67-A (1985) 1340

Corea, J. R., T. M. Tamimi: Tuberculosis of the arch of the atlas. Case report. Spine 12 (1987) 608

Cramer, A.: Funktionelle Merkmale von Störungen der Wirbelsäulenstatik. In: Die Wirbelsäule in Forschung und Praxis, Bd. 5. Hippokrates, Stuttgart 1958 (S. 20)

Darby, A. J., V. N. Cassar-Pullicino, I. W. McCall, D. C. Jaffray: Vertebral intra-osseous chordoma or giant notochordal rest. Skelet. Radiol. 28 (1999) 342

Decking, D., W. Ter Steege: Röntgenologische Parameter der Halswirbelsäule im seitlichen Strahlengang. Hippokrates, Stuttgart 1975

Desgrez, H., R. Gentaz, J. P. Chevrel: Animalies congénitales des arcs de l'atlas. J. Radiol. Électrol. 46 (1965) 819

Dias, L. D. S., H. M. Frost: Osteoblastoma of the spine. A review and report of eight new cases. Clin. Orthop. 91 (1973) 141

Dihlmann, W.: Gelenke, Wirbelverbindungen. Thieme, Stuttgart 1987

Dirheimer, Y., C. Bonsimon, D. Christman, C. Wackenheim: Syndesmo-odontoid joint and calciumphyrophosphate dihydrate deposition disease (CPPD). Neuroradiol. 25 (1983) 319

Dolan, K. D.: Cervico-basilar relationships. Radiol. Clin. N. Amer. 15 (1977) 155

Dove, J., A. C. M. C. Yau: Avascular necrosis of the dens. A follow-up study. Spine 7 (1982) 408

Dowd, CH. F., D. J. Sartoris, P. Haghighi, D. Resnick: Tuberculous spondylitis resulting in atlantoaxial dislocation. Case report 344. Skelt. Radiol. 15 (1986) 65

Dvorak, J., M. Panjabi, M. Gerber, W. Wichmann: CT-functional diagnostics of the rotatory instability of upper cervical spine. Part 1. An experimental study on cadavers. Spine 12 (1987a) 197

Dvorak, J., J. Hayek, R. Zehnder: CT-functional diagnostics of the rotatory instability of the upper cervical spine. Part 2. An evaluation on healthy adults and patients with suspected instability. Spine 12 (1987b) 726

Effendi, B., D. Roy, B. Cornish, R. G. Dussault, C. A. Laurin: Fractures of the ring of the axis. A classification based on the analysis of 131 cases. J. Bone Jt Surg. 63 (1981) 319

El-Khoury, G. Y., M. H. Wener, A. H. Menezes et al.: Cranial settling in rheumatoid arthritis. Radiology 137 (1980) 637

El-Khoury, G. Y., C. R. Clark, R. R. Wroble: Fixed atlantoaxial rotary deformity with bilateral facet dislocation. Skelet. radiol. 13 (1985) 217

Ellis, J. H., W. Martel, J. H. Lillie, A. M. Aisen: Magnetic resonance imaging of the normal craniovertebral junction. Spine 16 (1991) 105

Endler, F., K. Fochem, U. H. Weil: Orthopädische Röntgendiagnostik. Thieme, Stuttgart 1984 (S. 4.6–4.12)

Fielding, J. W.: Atlantoaxial rotary deformities: Symposium on the upper cervical spine. Orthop. clin. N. Amer. 9 (1978) 955

Finnegan, M. A., H. Mc Donald: Hangman's fracture in an infant. Canad. med. Ass. J. 127 (1982) 1001

Fischer, E.: Doppelter vorderer Atlasbogen. Fortschr. Röntgenstr. 118 (1973) 228

Fischer, E., H. Schmidt: Die degenerativen Veränderungen des vorderen atlantodentalen Gelenks. Fortschr. Röntgenstr. 111 (1969) 552

Freiberger, R. H., P. D. Wilson, J. A. Nicholas: Acquired absence of the odontoid process. J. Bone Jt Surg. 47-A (1965) 1231

Fried, J. A.: The cervical spine in juvenile rheumatoid arthritis. Clin. Orthopaed. 170 (1983) 102

Gamble, J. G., L. A. Rinsky: Combined occipitoatlantoaxial hypermobility with anterior and posterior arch defects of the atlas. In Pierre-Robin syndrome. J. pediat. Orthop. 5 (1985) 475

Gamroth, A.: Tendinitis calcarea acuta of the musculus longus colli. Fortschr. Röntgenstr. 155 (1991) 189

Gehweiler, J. A., R. H. Daffner, S. L. Robert: Malformations of the atlas vertebra simulating the Jefferson fracture. Amer. J. Neuroradiol. 4 (1983) 187

Geipel, P.: Zur Kenntnis der Spaltbildung des Atlas und Epistropheus, Teil IV. Zbl. Path. 94 (1955) 19

Gelberman, R. H., C. O. Olson: Benign osteoblastoma of the atlas. A case report. J. Bone Jt Surg. 56-A (1974) 808

Gentaz, R., J. Grellet: Les aplasies de l'arc antérieur de l'atlas. A propos d'un cas d'aplasie partielle. Ann. radiol. 12 (1969) 681

Gerlock, A. J. jr., M. Mirfakhraee: Computed tomography and Hangman's fracture. South Med. J. 76 (1983) 727

Grisel, P.: Enucléation die l'atlas et toricolis nasopharyngien. Presse méd. 38 (1930) 50

Grobovschek, M., W. Scheibelbrandner: Atlantooccipital dislocation. Neuroradiology 25 (1983) 173

Grobovschek, M., J. Strohecker: Congenital atlantoaxial subluxation in Down's syndrome. Neuroradiology 27 (1985) 186

Gupta, S., R. V. Phadke, V. K. Jain: C1-C2 block vertebra with fusion of anterior arch of atlas and the odontoid. Aust. Radiol. 37 (1993) 95

Haakonsen, M., T. E. Gudmundsen, O. Histol: Midline anterior and posterior atlas clefts may simulate a Jefferson fracture. A report of 2 cases. Acta orthop. scand. 66 (1995) 369

Haaland, K., H. A. Aadland, T. K. Haavik, F. M. Vallersness: Atlantoaxial subluxation in rheumatoid arthritis. Scand. J. Rheumatol. 13 (1984) 319

Hadley, M. N., C. Browner, V. K. H. Sonntag: Axis fractures: a comprehensive review of management and treatment in 107 cases. Neurosurgery 17 (1985) 281

Halla, J. T., J. G. Hardin Jr.: Atlantoaxial (C1–C2) facet joint osteoarthritis: A distinctive clinical syndrome. Arthr. and Rheum. 30 (1987) 577

Halla, J. T., J. G. Hardin, J. Vitek et al.: Involvement of the cervical spine in rheumatoid arthritis. Arthr. and Rheum. 32 (1989) 652

Hanson, E. C., J. E. Shook, G. J. Wiesseman, V. E. Wood: Congenital pedicle defects of the axis vertebra. Report of a case. Spine 15 (1990) 236

Hastings, D. E., I. Macnab, V. Lawson: Neoplasm of the atlas and axis. Canad. J. Surg. 11 (1968) 290

Hinck, V. C., C. E. Hopkins: Measurement of the atlanto-dental interval in the adult. Amer. J. Roentgenol. 84 (1960) 945

Huggare, J.: Congenital absence of the atlas posterior arch. A case report. Brit. J. Orthodont. 22 (1995) 71

Huggare, J., S. Kylämarkula: Morphology of the first cervical vertebra in children with enlarged adenoids. Eurp. J. Orthodont. 7 (1985) 93

Hvidarsson, St., G. Magram, H. Singer: Symptomatic atlantoaxial dislocation in Down syndrome. Pediatrics 69 (1982) 568

Ingelmark, B. E.: Über das kraniovertebrale Grenzgebiet beim Menschen. Acta anat., Suppl. 6 (1947)

Iwata, A., M. Murata, N. Nukina, I. Kanazawa: Foramen magnum syndrome caused by atlanto-occipital assimilation. J. neurol. Sci. 154 (1998) 229

Jackson, H.: Atlanto-axial subluxation. Radiology 148 (1983) 864

Jeanneret, B., F. Magerl: Congenital fusion C0–C2 associated with spondylolysis of C2. J. Spinal Dis. 3 (1990) 413

Jirout, J.: Studien der Dynamik der Halswirbelsäule an der frontalen und horizontalen Ebene. Fortschr. Röntgenstr. 106 (1967) 236

Jirout, J.: Die Rolle des Axis bei Seitenneigung der Halswirbelsäule und die „latente Skoliose". Fortschr. Röntgenstr. 109 (1968) 74

Jones, D. A.: Osteoid osteoma of the atlas. J Bone Jt Surg. 69-B (1987) 149

Jones, R. N.: Rotary dislocation of both atlantoaxial joints. J. Bone Jt Surg. 66-B (1984) 6

Juhl, M., K. Kjaergard Seerup: Os odontoideum. Acta orthop. scand. 54 (1983) 113

Kamieth, H.: Röntgenbefunde von normalen Bewegungen in den Kopfgelenken. Hippokrates, Stuttgart 1983

Kamieth, H.: Röntgenfunktionsdiagnostik der Halswirbelsäule. Hippokrates, Stuttgart 1986

Kattan, K. R.: Backward „displacement" of the spinolaminal line at C2: a normal variation. Amer. J. Roentgenol. 129 (1977) 289

Kaufman, R. A., J. S. Dunbar, J. A. Botsford, R. L. McLaurin: traumatic longitudinal atlantooccipital distraction injuries in children. Amer. J. Neuroradiol. 3 (1982) 415

Kirschbichler, Th.: Die paarig angelegten Processus odontoidei epistrophei – Eine seltene Fehlbildung im kraniozervikalen Übergangsbereich. Fortschr. Röntgenstr. 117 (1972) 654

Kratzer, M., P. M. Karpf, M. Reiser: Zur Differentialdiagnose des kindlichen Schiefhalses: Die fixierte atlantoaxiale Rotationsluxation. Fortschr. Med. 101 (1985) 160

Leach, R. E., H. Goldstein, D. Younger: Osteomyelitis of the odontoid process. J. Bone Jt Surg. 49-A (1967) 369

Lemaire, J. P., J. F. Couaillier, P. Grammont, P. Machet: Atlas bipartites. Rev. Chir. Orthopéd. 68 (1982) 471

Le Marec, B., M. Chapuis, C. Treguier, S. Odent, H. Bracq: A case of Larsen syndrome with severe cervical malformations. Gen. Couns 5 (1994) 179

Le Pointe, H. D., P. Brugieres, X. Chevalier et al.: Imagerie des chordomes du rachis mobile. J. Neuroradiol. 18 (1991) 267

Levin, M. F., A. D. Vellet, P. L. Munk et al.: Tuberculosis of the odontoid bone: a rare but treatable cause of quadriplegia. J. Canad. Ass. Radiol. 43 (1992) 199

Levine, A. M.: Avulsion of the transverse ligament associated with a fracture of the atlas. Orthoped. 6 (1983) 1467

Lewit, K., L. Krausová: Messungen von Vor- und Rückbeuge in den Kopfgelenken. Fortschr. Röntgenstr. 99 (1963) 538

Lewit, K., L. Krausová: Mechanismus und Bewegungsausmaß der Seitneigung in den Kopfgelenken. Fortschr. Röntgenstr. 101 (1964) 194

Lifeso, R.: Atlanto-axial tuberculosis in adults. J. Bone Jt Surg. 69-B (1987) 183

Maki, N. J.: Transverse fracture through the body of the axis. Spine 10 (1985) 857

Markuske, H.: Besonderheiten im Röntgenbild der kindlichen Halswirbelsäule. Pädiat. und Grenzgeb. 20 (1981) 175

Mathern, G. W., U. Batzdorf: Grisel's syndrome. Cervical spine clinical, pathologic, and neurologic manifestations. Clin. Orthop. 244 (1989) 131

Mathews, J. A.: Atlanto-axial subluxation in rheumatoid arthritis. Ann. rheum. Dis. 28 (1969) 260

McClellan, R., T. el Gammal, S. Willing, T. Lott, G. Odell: Persistent infantile odontoid process: a variant of abnormal atlantoaxial segmentation. Amer. J. Roentgenol. 158 (1992) 1305

McManners, T.: Odontoid hypoplasia. Brit. J. Radiol. 56 (1983) 907

McRae, D. L.: Bony abnormalities in the region of the foramen magnum; correlation of the anatomic and neuroligic findings. Acta radiol. 40 (1953) 335

McRae, D. L., A. S. Barnum: Occipitalisation of the atlas. Amer. J. Roentgenol. 70 (1953) 23

Menezes, A. H.: Craniovertebral junction anomalies: diagnosis and management. Semin. pediat. Neurol. 4 (1997) 209

Menezes, A. H., T. V. Ryken: Craniovertebral abnormalities in Down's syndrome. Pediat. Neurosurg. 18 (1992) 24

Mindell, E. R.: Chordoma. J. Bone Jt Surg. 63-A (1981) 501

Mitchell, J.: The incidence of the lateral bridge of the atlas vertebra. J. Anat. 193 (1998) 283

Mollan, R. A. B., P. C. H. Wyatt: Hangman's fracture. Injury 14 (1984) 265

Morvan, G., N. Martini; C. Massare, H. Nahum: La tuberculose du rachis cervical. SO.F.C.O.T. Réunion ann., nov. 1983, Suppl. II. Rev. Chir. Orthop. (1984) 76

Muller, F., R. O'Rahilly: Occipitocervical segmentation in staged human embryos. J. Anat. 185 (1994) 251

Newmark III, H., D. Blackford, D. Roberts et al.: Computed tomography of acute cervical spine tendinitis. J. comput. Tomogr. 10 (1986) 373

Ogden, J. A.: Radiology of postnatal skeletal development. XI. The first cervical vertebra. Skelet. radiol. 12 (1984) 212

Ogden, J. A.: XII. The second cervical vertebra. Skelet. radiol. 12 (1984) 169

Olbrantz, K. St. P. Bohrer: Fusion of the anterior arch of the atlas and dens. Skelet. Radiol. 12 (1984) 21

Olsson, O.: Arthrosis deformans des vorderen Zahngelenkes. Fortschr. Röntgenstr. 66 (1942) 233

Ono, K., K. Yonenobu, F. Takeshi, K. Okada: Atlantoaxial rotatory fixation. Spine 10 (1985) 602

Park, W. M., M. O'Neill, I. W. McCall: The radiology of rheumatoid involvement of the cervical spine. Skelet. Radiol. 4 (1979) 1

Pathria, M. N., C. A. Petersilge: Spinal trauma. Radiol. Clin. N. Amer. 29 (1991) 847

Pennes, D. R., C. N. Ellis, K. C. Madison et al.: Skeletal hyperostoses secondary to 13-cis-retinoic acid. Amer. J. Roentgenol. 141 (1984) 979

Penning, L., J. T. Wilmink: Rotation of the cervical spine. A CT study in normal subjects. Spine 12 (1986) 732

Pepin, J. W., R. B. Bourne, R. J. Hawkins: Odontoid fractures, with special reference to the elderly patient. Clin. Orthop. Relat. Res. 193 (1985) 178

Phan, N., C. Marras, R. Midha, D. Rowed: Cervical myelopathy caused by hypoplasia of the atlas: two case reports and review of the literature. Neurosurgery 43 (1998) 629

Pouliqueu, J. C., G. F. Pennecot, J. Beneux, F. Chadoutaud, P. Lacert, G. Duval-Beaupere: Charnière crabiorachidienne et maladie de Morquio. Chir. Pédiat. 23 (1982) 247

Prescher, A.: The differential diagnosis of isolated ossicles in the region of the dens axis. Gegenbaurs morphol Jb., Abt. 1 136 (1990) 139

Prescher, A.: The craniocervical junction in man, the osseous variations, their significance and differential diagnosis. Anat. Anz. 179 (1997) 1

Pueschel, S. M., J. B. Herndon, M. M. Gelch, K. E. Seft, F. H. Scola, M. J. Goldberg: Symptomatic atlantoaxial subluxation in persons with Down syndrome. J. pediat. Orthop. 4 (1984) 682

Redlund-Johnell, I.: Posterior antlantoaxial dislocation in rheumatoid arthritis. Scand. J. Rheumatol. 13 (1984) 337

Redlund-Johnell, I.: vertical dislocation of the C1 and C2 vertebra in rheumatoid arthritis. Acta radiol. diagn. 25 (1984) 133

Resnik, C. S., J. R. Liniger: Monostotic fibrous dysplasia of the cervical spine: Case report. Radiology 151 (1984) 49

Rogers, L. F.: Radiology of Skeletal Trauma, 2nd ed. Churchill Livingstone, New York 1992

Rosenberg, F., R. Bataille, J. Sany et al.: Lyse de l'odontode au cours de la polyarthrite rhumatode. Rev. Rhum. 45 (1978) 249

Roush, R. D., G. G. Salciccioli: Fracture of the anterior tubercle of the atlas. J. Bone Jt Surg. 64-A (1982) 626

Ryken, T., A. H. Menezes: Nonrheumatoid cranial settling. Spine 18 (1993) 2525

Sandelin, J., S. Santavirta, F. Laasonen, P. Slätis: Spontaneous fracture of atlas of cervical spine affected by rheumatoid arthritis. Scand. J. Rheumatol. 14 (1985) 167

Saternus, K.-S., E. Paul: Hangman's fracture bei ventral-flexierter Traktion. Z. Rechtsmed. 93 (1984) 301

Savader, S. J., C. Martinez, F. R. Murtogh: Odontoid fracture in a 9-month-old infant. Surg. Neurol. 24 (1985) 529

Schiff, D. C. M., W. W. Parke: The arterial supply of odontoid process. J. Bone Jt Surg. 55-A (1973) 1450

Schmidt, H.: Über die Beweglichkeit in den Kopfgelenken bei basilarer Impression. Bericht über die 44. Tagung der Deutschen Röntgengesellschaft vom 24.–28.4.1963. Thieme, Stuttgart 1964 (S. 62–64)

Schmidt, H., E. Fischer: Die okzipitale Dysplasie. Thieme, Stuttgart 1960

Schmidt, H., E. Fischer: Zur röntgenologischen Differentialdiagnose von knöchernen Fehlbildungen am Schädel-Hals-Übergang. Radiol. clin. 33 (1964) 223

Schulze, P. J., R. Buurman: Absence of the posterior arch of the atlas. Amer. J. Roentgenol. 134 (1980) 178

Schwägerle, W., M. Sunder-Plassmann, H. Pröll, O. Scherak: Halswirbelsäule bei Morbus Bechterew und Polyarthritis. Z. Orthop. 119 (1981) 637

Schweitzer, M. E., J. Hodler, V. Cervilla, D. Resnick: Craniovertebral junction: normal anatomy with MR correlation. Amer. J. Roentgenol. 158 (1992) 1087

Scialpi, M., F. Boccuzzi, T. Magli, C. Scapati: Pneumatizzazione atlo-occipitale: dimostrazione mediante tomografia computerizzata. Radiol. med. 87 (1994) 880

Sharma, S., S. Gupta, A. K. Kalla, S. Khanna, I. P. Singh, F. Vogel: Computer-tomographic (CT) studies and anthropological measurements in patients with atlanto-occipital fusion. Anthropol. Anz. 49 (1991) 325

Sharp, J., D. W. Purser: Spontaneous atlanto-axial dislocation in ankylosing spondylitis and rheumatoid arthritis. Ann. rheum. Dis. 20 (1961) 47

Skaane, P., K.-J. Klott: Die peridentale Aureole (crowned odontoid process) bei der vorderen Atlantodentalarthrose. Fortschr. Röntgenstr. 134 (1981) 62

Smoker, W. R.: Craniovertebral junction: normal anatomy, craniometry, and congenital anomalies. Radiographics 14 (1994) 255

Soholm, S., O. Ingvardsen: Congenital atlantoaxial block vertebra. A case report. Fortschr. Röntgenstr. 153 (1990) 351

Stolze, Th.: Spalten des vorderen und hinteren Atlasbogens, seltene, für den Atlas typische Veränderungen. Radiologe 9 (1969) 304

Storms, G. E. M. G., M. W. M. Kruijsen, H. J. Van Beusekom et al.: Pathological fracture of the odontoid process in rheumatoid arthritis. Neth. J. Med. 23 (1980) 120

Sundaresan, N., J. H. Galicich, F. C. H. Chu et al.: Spinal chordomas. J. Neurosurg. 50 (1979) 312

Tänzer, A.: Durch Spalt im vorderen Bogen des Atlas vorgetäuschte Fraktur des Dens epistrophei. Fortschr. Röntgenstr. 86 (1957) 138

Thomas, S. L., M. H. Childress, B. Quinton: Hypoplasia of the odontoid with atlantoaxial subluxation in Hurler syndrome. Pediat. Radiol. 15 (1985) 353

Törö, J., L. Szepe: Untersuchungen über die Frage der Atlasassimilation und Manifestation des Atlas. Z. Anat. Entw. Gesch. 111 (1942) 186

von Torklus, D., W. Gehle: Die obere Halswirbelsäule, 3. Aufl. Thieme, Stuttgart 1987

Tredwell, S. J., J. P. O'Brien: Avascular necrosis of the proximal end of the dens—a complication of halo-pelvic distraction. J. Bone Jt Surg. 57-A (1975) 332

Trumble, E. R., J. S. Myseros, W. R. Smoker, J. D. Ward, J. J. Mickell: Atlantooccipital subluxation in a neonate with Down's syndrome. Case report and review of the literature. Pediat. Neurosurg. 21 (1994) 55

Uno, K., O. Kataoka, R. Shiba: Occipitoatlantal and occipitoaxial hypermobility in Down syndrome. Spine 21 (1996) 1430

Vasudeva, N., R. Kumar: Absence of foramen transversarium in the human atlas vertebra: a case report. Acta anat. 152 (1995) 230

Viehweger, A.: Die Darstellung des medialen Randes der kranialen Gelenkfläche des Atlas auf den Übersichtsaufnahmen der HWS in v. d. Strahlengang. Fortschr. Röntgenstr. 84 (1956) 492

Wackenheim, A.: Roentgen Diagnosis of the Craniovertebral Region. Springer, Berlin 1974

Wackenheim, A.: Ossification du ligament transverse. J. Radiol. Eléctrol. 59 (1978) 413

Wackenheim, A., Y. Dirheimer: La fusion congenitale de l'arc anterieure de l'atlas avec la dente de l'axis. Radiologie 58 (1974) 525

Wackenheim, A., E. Babin, M. S. D. Thiébaut, F. Lopez: Une nouvelle épreuve fonctionelle pour l'exploration de la dynamique cervico-occipitale. Concours méd. 91 (1969) 7130

Walker, J., I. Beggs: Bipartite atlas and hypertrophy of its anterior arch. A case report. Acta radiol. 36 (1995) 152

Weaver, P., R. M. Lifeso: The radiological diagnosis of tuberculosis of the adult spine. Skelet. radiol. 12 (1984) 178

Weissman, B. N. W.: Atlantoaxial subluxation (comment to Jackson's letter to the editor). Radiology 148 (1983) 866

Weissman, B. N. W., P. Aliabadi, M. Weinfeld, W. Thomas, J. Sosman: Prognostic features of atlantoaxial subluxation in rheumatoid arthritis patients. Radiology 144 (1982) 745

Werne, S.: The possibilities of movement in the craniovertebral joints. Acta orthop. scand. 28 (1959) 165

Wetzel, F. T., H. La Rocca: Grisel's syndrome. A review. Clin. Orthop. 240 (1989) 141

Wiens, J., J. Freyschmidt, A. Kasperczyk: Isolierte horizontale Fraktur des vorderen Atlasbogens. Fortschr. Röntgenstr. 159 (1993) 566

Wolf, R. F., J. P. Klein: Complete bipartition of the atlas in the Klippel-Feil syndrome. A radiologically illustrated case report. Surg. radiol. Anat 19 (1997) 339

Woodring, J. H., C. Lee: The role and limitations of computed tomographic scanning in the evaluation of cervical trauma. Trauma 33 (1992) 698

Wu, K. K., E. R. Guise: Osteochondroma of the atlas: a case report. Clin. Orthop. 136 (1978) 160

Yamashita, K., Y. Aoki, K. Hiroshima: Myelopathy due to hypoplasia of the atlas. A case report. Clin. Orthop. 338 (1997) 90

Yanai, Y., R. Tsuji, S. Ohmori, S. Kuberta, Ch. Nagashima: Foramen magnum syndrome caused by a dolichoodontoid process. Surg. Neurol. 24 (1985) 95

Zigler, J. E., H. H. Bohlman, R. A. Robinson et al.: Pyogenic osteomyelitis of the occiput, the atlas, and the axis. J. Bone Jt Surg. 69-A (1987) 1069

Zinreich, S. J., H. Wang, F. Abdo, R. N. Bryan: 3-D CT improves accuracy of spinal trauma studies. Diagn. Imag. 12 (1990) 102

Midcervical and Lower Cervical Spine

Normal Findings

 ### During Growth

The embryonic development of the cervical vertebral bodies was discussed in the general introduction to this chapter. The C3–C7 vertebrae each have three ossification centers. Additionally, the C7 vertebra usually has separate centers for the costal processes.

The **AP projection** in a **newborn** demonstrates three ossification centers in each of the subaxial cervical vertebrae, as in the rest of the spinal column (Fig. 5.**129**). One center is located in the vertebral body and one in each hemi-arch. The center for the vertebral body is separated from the arch centers laterally by neurocentral synchondroses (see p. 562). During the first year of life, ossification of the vertebral arch progresses until the halves finally unite. Before the bony union of the arch is completed, the multiple unfused arches may create the impression of a generalized spina bifida (Fig. 5.**130**).

Fusion of the neurocentral synchondrosis (epiphysis of the vertebral arch, Fig. 5.**131**) is completed by the seventh year of life (Table 5.**1**). The lateral portion of the vertebral arch and the pars interarticularis ossifies before the appendages of the vertebral arch. The development of the

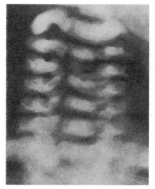
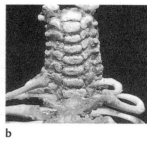

a

b

Fig. 5.**129 a, b**   Cervical spine of a newborn.
a AP projection with the head rotated to the left.
b Anatomic specimen of a neonatal cervical spine (Museum of Man, San Diego).

vertebral body ossification centers and marginal ridges was described earlier (see introductory section on the spinal column). Generally the marginal ridges begin to ossify in about the 10th year of life. By about the 12th year they form a closed bony ring, which fuses with the vertebral body between the 14th and 24th year of life. The vertebral

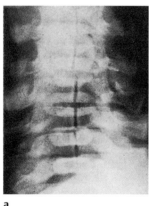
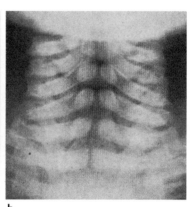

a   b

Fig. 5.**130 a, b**   Cervical spine and cervicothoracic junction in the AP projection.
a In a newborn.
b In a 6-month-old child.

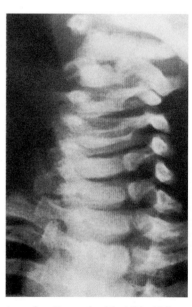

Fig. 5.**131**   Cervical spine of a 6-month-old child. Oblique projection demonstrates the neurocentral synchondroses.

bodies typically appear wedge-shaped in children (Fig. 5.**132**).

The ossified marginal ridges of the cervical vertebrae, or bony ring apophyses, generally appear as small, flat disks anteriorly and as punctate calcifications of the end plates posteriorly. The anterior steplike notches in the cervical vertebral bodies are generally much less pronounced than in the thoracic and lumbar vertebrae (Figs. 5.**133**, 5.**134**; compare with Figs. 5.**214** and 5.**215**).

A distinctive feature of the lower cervical spine in adolescents is that **apophyses** are visible on the **transverse processes** with greater regularity than in other regions (Fig. 5.**134**).

Fig. 5.**132 a–d** Radiographic appearance of the cervical vertebral bodies at different ages.
a 6 years.
b 9 years.
c 14 years.
d 16 years.
Note the elliptical and wedge-shaped vertebral bodies. Marginal ridge formation starts at 9 years of age.

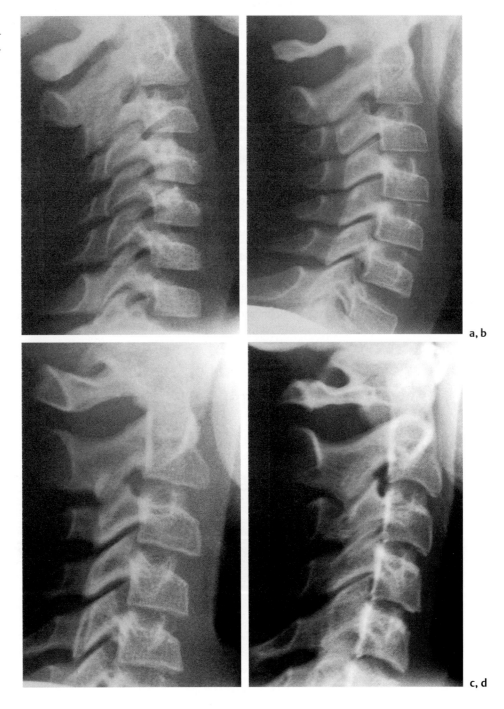

a, b

c, d

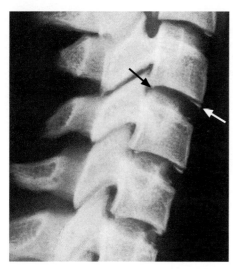

Fig. 5.**133** Ossification of the marginal ridge anteriorly (white arrow) and posteriorly (black arrow) in the cervical spine.

 ## In Adulthood

The C3 through C7 vertebral bodies are very similar to one another in appearance but show characteristic differences from the thoracic and lumbar vertebrae (Fig. 5.**135**).

The vertebral bodies are small compared with the vertebral arches and have an almost rectangular cross section. The lateral borders of the superior surface of the vertebral bodies are raised into a prominent lip (the uncinate process), contrasting with the rounded lateral borders of the inferior surface (Figs. 5.**134**, 5.**135**). This reciprocal arrangement of the upper and lower surfaces gives rise to the **uncovertebral joints** (of Luschka), which are peculiar to the cervical spine. Developmentally, the uncinate processes are derived from the neural arch and unite with the vertebral body only after the neurocentral synchondrosis has disappeared. They are still poorly developed in newborns and small children and do not become promi-

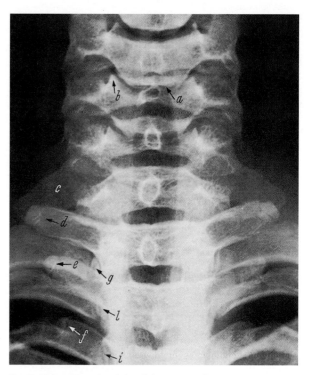

Fig. 5.**134** AP projection of the cervicothoracic junction in a 12-year-old girl.
a   Marginal ridges on the vertebral bodies
b   Uncinate process
c   Large transverse process of C7
d–f   Apophyses on the transverse process of T1–T3
g–l   Costovertebral joint spaces

nent until the ninth or tenth year. The uncovertebral joints are not true joints but result from the secondary, probably functional clefting of the intervertebral disk (Rauber and Kopsch 1998). With aging, they assume an increasingly important load-bearing function as the intervertebral disks lose their resiliency.

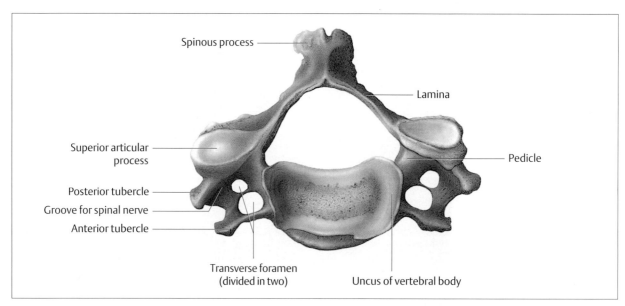

Fig. 5.**135** Superior view of the fifth cervical vertebra, showing how a bony septum can divide the transverse foramen into two parts. (From Rauber and Kopsch, 1998.)

The **pedicles** of the cervical vertebrae are short and run obliquely and posterolaterally at about a 45° angle. As a result, the intervertebral foramina open anterolaterally at an angle of approximately 30–55°. The articular processes overlie one another in a pillarlike arrangement and have almost flat articular surfaces angled 45° to the horizontal plane in an anterosuperior-to-posteroinferior direction (Fig. 5.**135**). The **transverse processes** of the cervical vertebrae are located in front of the articular processes. All are pierced by transverse foramina, through which the vertebral arteries ascend to the skull. The transverse foramina may be divided into two parts by a **bony septum** (Fig. 5.**135**), the smaller, posterior accessory foramen transmitting a vein and a vertebral nerve branch (Rauber and Kopsch 1998). Each of the transverse processes has an anterior and a posterior root, which terminate respectively in an anterior and a posterior tubercle. The anterior root corresponds to the rib rudiment of the cervical vertebra (see Fig. 5.**3**). The anterior tubercle of C6 is often raised into a protuberance called the **carotid tubercle**. Each of the transverse processes from C3 downward bears a **groove for the spinal nerve** (Fig. 5.**135**).

The **spinous processes** become longer and sturdier from above downward and, except for C7, have a bifid tip. The spinous processes can vary considerably in size (Fig. 5.**136**).

The spinous process of C7 is exceptionally long and is directed almost horizontally (**vertebra prominens**). Because of the relatively high intervertebral disk spaces in the cervical spine and the narrow thoracic disks, the normal disk space between the C7 and T1 vertebral bodies appears relatively thin.

The **AP projection** usually gives a satisfactory view of the vertebral bodies, disk spaces, lateral masses, and spinous processes (Fig. 5.**134**). The pedicles, apophyseal joints, vertebral arches, and transverse processes cannot be adequately evaluated in this projection. Given the physiological lordosis of the cervical spine and the rhomboid shape of the cervical vertebral bodies, the AP projection does not give an orthograde view of the upper and lower end plates of the vertebral bodies, making it difficult or impossible to evaluate the end plates and disk spaces, especially at the midcervical and lower cervical levels. The **uncinate processes** appear as characteristic spurlike projections at the lateral borders of the upper vertebral body end plates (Fig. 5.**134**).

The pedicles of the cervical vertebrae are poorly visualized because of their obliquity. The lateral contour of the cervical spine is formed on each side by the superimposed superior and inferior articular processes and is slightly undulated. The **transverse processes** are superimposed on the articular processes and, except for the elongated transverse processes of C7, are not delineated (Fig. 5.**137**).

The **pillar view**, an AP projection with the tube angled 35–40° downward, is useful for obtaining an orthograde view of the intervertebral disk spaces (Smith et al. 1975). The **spinous processes** generally appear as inverted V-shaped figures arranged vertically along the midline of the cervical spine. As mentioned, the spinous processes are usually split into two equal-size tubercles except on C1 and C7 (Fig. 5.**137**).

In evaluating the AP radiograph of the cervical spine, it should be noted that the lateral boundaries of the apophyseal joints and the spinous processes should be

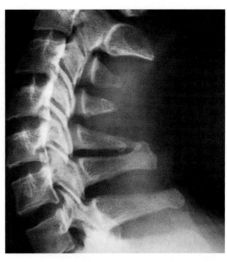

Fig. 5.**136** Variability in the size of the spinous processes in the cervical spine. The spinous processes of C3 and C4 are dwarfed by the very prominent spinous processes of C6 and C7.

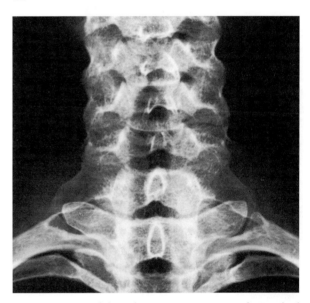

Fig. 5.**137** Large bilateral transverse processes of C7 with rib stubs.

vertically aligned with no offsets or discontinuities. The intervertebral disk spaces should be of uniform width, and the upper and lower end plates of adjacent vertebral bodies should be parallel.

Air in the **rima glottidis** may appear in the AP projection as a slitlike lucency projected onto a cervical vertebra (usually C4) and can simulate a gap in the bone (Fig. 5.**138**).

Similarly, air in the **piriform recess** can mimic an osteolytic area, and the lucent band of the **trachea** may be misidentified as the vertebral canal. Calcifications of the **thyroid cartilage** are also projected at the level of the C4 vertebral body on each side of the midline and can mimic accessory bone elements (Fig. 5.**139**).

The **lateral radiograph** is considerably better than the AP view for demonstrating the vertebral bodies, intervertebral disk spaces, lateral masses, apophyseal joints, spinal canal, and spinous processes.

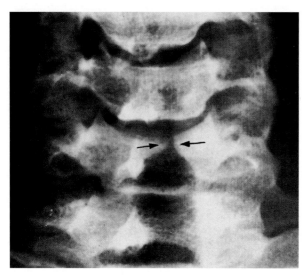

Fig. 5.**138** The rima glottis (arrows) can mimic a cleft in the vertebral arch.

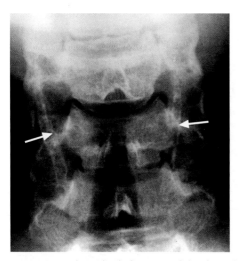

Fig. 5.**139** Bilateral calcifications of the thyroid cartilage (arrows) simulating accessory bone elements.

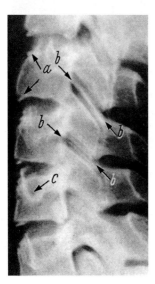

Fig. 5.**140** Mid-cervical spine in the lateral projection.
a Marginal ridges.
b Joint spaces.
c Groove between the tubercles of the transverse process (for the spinal nerve).

The cervical spine shows a **mild physiological lordosis** with maximum curvature at the level of the fourth disk space. The lordosis may be accentuated in the supine position. In about 20% of the population, the cervical spine shows no lordosis in the upright position or even shows a slight degree of kyphosis when the head is in the neutral position (Green et al. 1981).

The **spinal canal** is bounded anteriorly by the posterior cortical margins of the vertebral bodies and posteriorly by the spinolaminar line (Fig. 5.**142**). Lines drawn along these structures should be smooth and harmonious. The spinal canal is triangular in cross section, the transverse diameter being approximately twice the sagittal diameter (Wolf et al. 1956, Penning 1965).

As a general rule of thumb, the sagittal width of the spinal canal approximately equals the sagittal diameter of the corresponding cervical vertebral body.

The spinal canal in children is relatively wider than in adults and may show a funnel-shaped expansion inferiorly (Yousefzadeh et al. 1982). The **shape of the cervical vertebral bodies** resembles a rectangle or rhomboid, usually with a concave end plate inferiorly and a flat end plate superiorly. The upper end plate may be slightly shorter than the lower end plate (Fried 1966). Because of this, the superior corners of the vertebral bodies are blunter than the sharp anteroinferior corners, which may resemble osteophytes. The cervical vertebral bodies can vary considerably in size.

The height of the **intervertebral disk spaces** increases from above downward. The disk spaces appear slightly wedge-shaped, being somewhat higher anteriorly than posteriorly.

The **lateral masses** and **apophyseal joints** are projected behind the vertebral bodies in the lateral view. The **apophyseal joint spaces** are directed obliquely in the anterosuperior-to-posteroinferior direction. On an accurate lateral projection, the joint spaces on each side are precisely superimposed. With a slightly off-lateral projection, the joint spaces exhibit double contours (Fig. 5.**140**). With a somewhat more oblique projection, the joint spaces can mimic a vertebral arch fracture.

The **apophyseal joint spaces** in the C2/C3 segment are usually difficult to visualize because of their anteriorly convergent position (Fig. 5.**141**). This may be mistaken for ankylosis.

The posterior contour of the articular surface of the C5-C7 superior articular processes often shows shallow indentations (Fig. 5.**142**) that can simulate a fracture. They results from a change in the orientation of the articular surfaces at the cervicothoracic junction (Kattan and Joyce Pais 1982 a, b).

In the lateral projection, the **transverse processes** with their anterior and posterior tubercles for muscle attachments are projected over the corresponding vertebral bodies (unlike the rest of the spine, they are adjacent to the vertebral bodies and not behind them). Consequently the **groove for the spinal nerve** is projected onto the vertebral body and can mimic an **osteolytic area** rimmed by sclerosis (Figs. 5.**140**, 5.**142**).

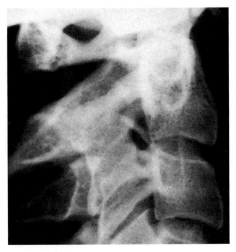

Fig. 5.**141** Apparent ankylosis of the C2 and C3 vertebrae. The superior and inferior articular processes are superimposed, obscuring the apophyseal joint space.

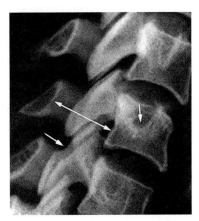

Fig. 5.**142** Sagittal diameter of the spinal canal (double arrow). Note the concavity behind the posterior margin of the inferior articular process (longer arrow) and the groove between the anterior and posterior tubercles projected onto the vertebral body in the lateral view (short arrow).

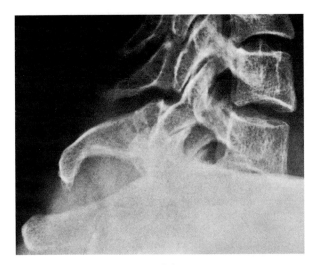

Fig. 5.**143** Caudal deviation of the C7 spinous process.

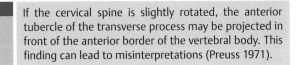

If the cervical spine is slightly rotated, the anterior tubercle of the transverse process may be projected in front of the anterior border of the vertebral body. This finding can lead to misinterpretations (Preuss 1971).

The **spinous processes** become longer in the craniocaudal direction, and generally they are completely visible on lateral radiographs. Significant downward **angulation of the spinous processes** can occur, as in the case of C7 (Fig. 5.**143**).

Oblique views of the spinal canal are useful for demonstrating the intervertebral foramina, the pedicles, the uncinate processes, and the apophyseal joints. A **45° oblique view** gives an orthograde projection of the intervertebral foramina on the examined side. The foramina of the lower cervical vertebrae are seen more clearly on **55° oblique views** (Marcelis et al. 1993). An approximately 70° oblique projection gives a nonsuperimposed view of the apophyseal joint spaces on each side (Abel 1982). The intervertebral foramina are bounded above and below by the inferior

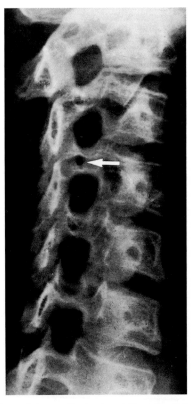

Fig. 5.**144** Oblique view of the cervical spine defines the full extent of the intervertebral foramina. The arrow indicates a foramen in the groove for the spinal nerve.

and superior vertebral notches of the adjacent vertebrae, in front by the uncinate process and posterolateral borders of the vertebral bodies, and behind by the articular processes. Generally a satisfactory view of the foramina and the apophyseal joints cannot be obtained on just one projection. The C2/C3 intervertebral foramen is circular and is usually larger than the other, more elliptical foramina (Fig. 5.**144**). The **groove for the spinal nerve** may resemble a foramen in the oblique projection.

Table 5.**2**   Total passive range of motion (in degrees) of the cervical spine Values are mean and standard deviation (from Dvorak et al. 1992)

Age (years)	Flexion-extension		Lateral bending		Rotation	
	Males	**Females**	**Males**	**Females**	**Males**	**Females**
20–29	152.7 ± 20.0	149.3 ± 11.7	101.1 ± 13.3	100.0 ± 8.6	183.8 ± 11.8	182.4 ± 10.0
30–39	141.1 ± 11.4	155.9 ± 23.1	94.7 ± 10.0	106.3 ± 18.1	175.1 ± 9.9	186.0 ± 10.4
40–49	131.1 ± 18.5	139.8 ± 13.0	83.7 ± 13.9	88.2 ± 16.1	157.4 ± 19.5	168.2 ± 13.6
50–59	136.3 ± 15.7	126.9 ± 14.8	88.3 ± 29.1	76.1 ± 10.2	166.2 ± 14.1	151.9 ± 15.9
Over 60	116.3 ± 18.7	133.2 ± 7.6	74.2 ± 14.3	79.6 ± 18.0	145.6 ± 13.1	154.2 ± 14.6

The **cervicothoracic junction** is very difficult to visualize on radiographs because of the numerous superimposed structures in the lateral and AP projections. The delineation of this region can be improved by using the **swimmer's projection** and other special views (McCall et al. 1973, Scher and Vambeck 1977, Boger and Ralls 1981). If findings are equivocal, the cervicothoracic junction should be evaluated by **CT** or **MRI** (LaMasters and Dorwart 1985, Acheson et al. 1987, Manaster and Osborn 1987, Pathria and Petersilge 1991). **Conventional tomography** should be used only in highly selected cases (Anderson et al. 1982).

Normal Range of Motion

Cervical spinal motion is evaluated in flexion-extension, rotation, and lateral bending (Kamieth 1986). The total range of spinal motion declines with aging, particularly during the fourth and fifth decades (Dvorak et al. 1992) (Table 5.**2**).

Flexion and Extension

The vertebral bodies normally shift 1–2 mm anteriorly and posteriorly during flexion-extension of the spine, producing a "stepladder" effect. This phenomenon is most pronounced at the C2/C3 level in children up to 10 years old during flexion of the cervical spine ("pseudodislocation") (Gaizler 1971) (Fig. 5.**107**). The juvenile spine shows the greatest mobility in flexion-extension at the C4/C5 level.

The **Penning method** has proved useful for determining the range of motion of individual spinal segments (Penning 1960, 1965, 1968, 1978, Dvorak et al. 1988) (Fig. 5.**145**). Different values have been found for the active and passive ranges of motion, with passive tests showing somewhat greater total and segmental ranges (Dvorak et al. 1992) (Table 5.**3**). Muhle et al. (1998 a) found comparable results for segmental motion in flexion and extension using **MRI**. Flexion in each or at least three levels is considered normal (Bohrer et al. 1990) (See also "Subluxations and Dislocations").

Fig. 5.**145**   Penning method of cervical motion analysis (Penning 1978). The extension film is superimposed on the flexion film with the C7 vertebral body and spinous process exactly matching, and a line is drawn along the right edge of the upper film. This process is repeated for all the cervical vertebral bodies, yielding angles for the segmental mobility of the different segments.

Table 5.**3**   Active and passive ranges of segmental flexion-extension (in degrees) in the cervical spine (from Muhle 1998 a)

Segment	Penning (1960) (active)	Dvorak et al. (1988) (active)	Dvorak et al. (1988) (passive)
C2–C3	12.5	10 ± 5	12 ± 5
C3–C4	18	15 ± 8	17 ± 7
C4–C5	20	19 ± 6	21 ± 7
C5–C6	21.5	20 ± 7	23 ± 7
C6–C7	15.5	19 ± 6	21 ± 8

Lateral Bending

Lateral bending of the spine is normally associated with rotation of the vertebral bodies, shifting of the spinous processes toward the convex side of the bend, and approximation of the vertebral bodies on the concave side. The rotation of the cervical spine is difficult to analyze on conventional radiographs because it occurs in the transverse plane (Werne 1959).

Rotation

CT is the best imaging modality for analyzing rotation (Penning and Wilmink 1986, Dvorak et al. 1987 a, b). Aside from the atlantoaxial joint, the midcervical spinal segments (C3–C6) undergo an average rotation of 6.5–6.9°. The average ranges of rotation in the segments C2/C3, C6/C7, and C7/T1 are 3.0°, 5.4°, and 2.1°, respectively (Penning and Wilmink 1986).

 ## Pathological Finding?

Normal Variant or Anomaly?

Variants

The anterior and posterior margins of the **vertebral bodies** are occasionally sites of **persistent epiphyseal centers**. They appear as isolated punctate or disk-shaped ossification centers, usually located on the anterior vertebral end plate and generally fitting into a small corresponding defect in the corner of the vertebral body (Figs. 5.**133**, 5.**146**).

If these changes first appear in adulthood, they probably represent calcification of the anulus fibrosus (Kerns et al. 1968). It is unclear whether the persistent epiphyseal centers are related to accessory ossicles at the anterior vertebral margins, which are found in approximately 3% of persons between the ages of 40 and 60 who do not have degenerative disk disease (Teichert 1956). Other isolated ossicles may be found in the area of the uncovertebral joints. They may appear temporarily during growth but are also seen in later life (Figs. 5.**146**, 5.**147**). Presumably they represent persistent epiphyseal centers. Occasional asymmetrical development of the uncinate processes (Fig. 5.**148**) can be attributed to the absence of an epiphyseal center on one side.

The normal **wedge shape** of the juvenile **cervical vertebral bodies** may persist into adulthood in some vertebrae (see During Growth above) and should not be mistaken for a compression fracture (see Fractures below).

Persistence of the **notochord** is manifested on radiographs by corresponding indentations in the posterior third of adjacent vertebral end plates (Fig. 5.**149**).

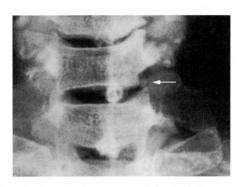

Fig. 5.**146**   Persistent ossification center of the C7 left uncinate process.

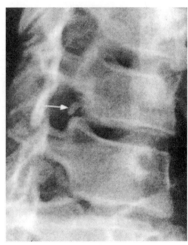

Fig. 5.**147**   Persistent ossification center of a right uncinate process.

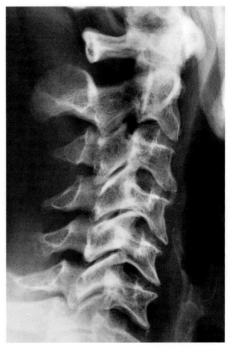

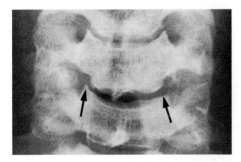

Fig. 5.**148**   Asymmetrical development of the C6 uncinate processes.

Fig. 5.**149**   Persistence of the notochord appears as conspicuous indentations in the posterior third of the lower end plates of C2–C7.   ▷

Persistent apophyses of the transverse processes mainly occur as variants in the region of the cervicothoracic junction (Figs. 5.**134**, 5.**150**). They require differentiation from traumatic changes. An **isolated transverse process of T1** has also been described (Reinhardt 1958). Foci of **isolated ossification** directly overlying the articulation of the first rib with the transverse process are fairly common and are classified as etiologically obscure accessory bones.

The **transverse processes** may feature enlarged or **elongated anterior tubercles**, which are most common in the lower cervical vertebrae (Lapoyowker 1960). Like **enlarged posterior tubercles**, they can apparently lead to a cervical syndrome. The tubercles on adjacent vertebrae may be elongated to form jointlike articulating surfaces. Several cases of this have been described at the C5/C6 level (Fig. 5.**151**) (Wendtland 1966, Op den Orth 1969, Applbaum et al. 1983).

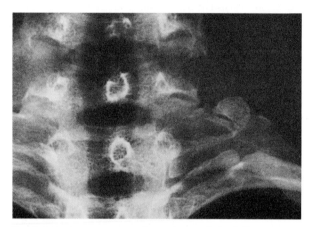

Fig. 5.**150** Persistent apical apophysis of the left transverse process of T1.

Accessory processes can also create jointlike connections between the transverse processes of the upper thoracic vertebrae (Fig. 5.**152**), resembling the accessory processes found in the upper cervical spine (Figs. 5.**63**–5.**69**). Elongated, riblike anterior tubercles of C2–C7 coexisting with an elongated transverse process of C2 (Pickern 1953) may be genetically related to the infratransverse and epitransverse processes of C1, the infratransverse process of C2, and the paracondylar process of the occipital bone, or they may be analogous to cervical ribs.

Cervical ribs and **elongation of the C7 transverse process** are among the most common variants that are encountered at the cervicothoracic junction (Fig. 5.**137**).

Cervical ribs most frequently arise from C7 and may be unilateral or bilateral. They have a synostotic or articular connection with the transverse process and are variable in shape. They reportedly occur in approximately 6% of the population (Wanke 1937). In more subtle forms the cervical rib is usually fused to its transverse process and does not project beyond it. In the most pronounced forms, the cervical rib resembles a true rib in size and shape and joins with the sternum. Intermediate forms may have a free end or may be connected to the first thoracic rib by a fibrous cord (Fig. 5.**153**).

Cervical ribs have also been described in the skeleton of fetuses with **Ullrich–Turner syndrome** (Kjaer and Fischer-Hansen 1997).

According to Kühne (1936), cervical ribs represent a **cranial variant** of the cervicothoracic junction in which C7, and occasionally C6, is transformed into a thoracic vertebra, featuring a closed transverse foramen and rib projections. In the **caudal variant** of the cervicothoracic junction, T1 assumes some of the features of a cervical vertebra, i.e., it gives rise to a slender, steeply placed first pair of ribs and its transverse processes are shortened. Occasionally a closed transverse foramen is found in the transverse processes of T1.

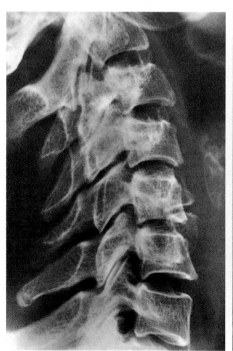
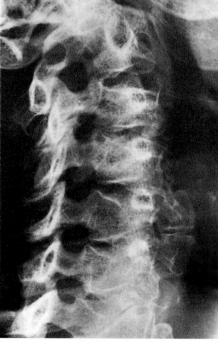

Fig. 5.**151 a, b** Jointlike connection between the elongated anterior tubercles of the C5 and C6 transverse processes.
a Lateral projection.
b Oblique projection.

a

b

Transitional vertebrae are a common finding at the cervicothoracic junction. Cranial variants are seen with much greater frequency than caudal variants. Very rarely, eight cervical vertebrae may be found in conjunction with a normal number of thoracic vertebrae. Skeletal variants at the cervicothoracic junction are also associated with variants in the nerves and blood vessels of that region. When a cervical rib is present, the subclavian artery passes over the cervical rib and not over the first thoracic rib. The vertebral artery in this situation enters the transverse foramen at the C5 level instead of the usual C6 level. The clinical manifestations of a cervical rib may resemble those of a scalenus syndrome:

- Arm pain
- Paresthesia
- Palsy
- Peripheral circulatory impairment

The **facets** of the **apophyseal joints** at C2/C3 may show congenital asymmetries of morphology and orientation (Overton and Grossmann 1952). Deviation of the joint axis from that of the other vertebral bodies, with an increased anterior inclination, was discussed above under Normal Findings (Fig. 5.**141**).

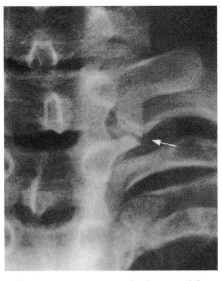

Fig. 5.**152**   A peglike bony process extends downward from the medial part of the left transverse process of T1, forming a jointlike connection with a corresponding stubby process arising from T2. The interface between the processes shows degenerative changes.

Fig. 5.**153 a, b**   Examples of cervical ribs.
a Bilateral cervical ribs.
b Right-sided cervical rib that articulates with the first rib (arrow).

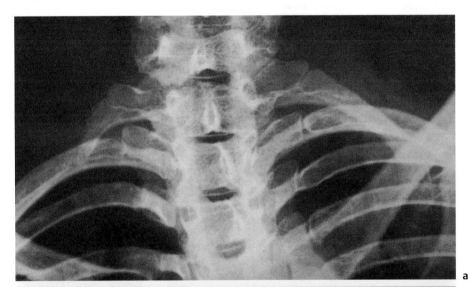

a

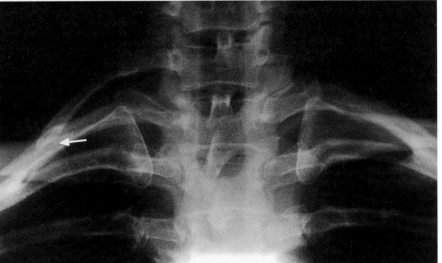

b

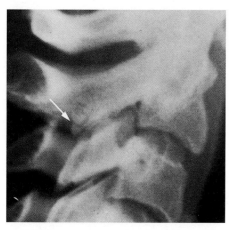

Fig. 5.**154**   Small epiphysis on the inferior articular process of C2.

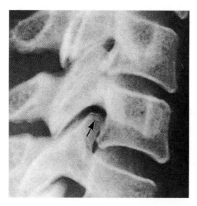

Fig. 5.**155**   Persistent epiphysis on the superior articular process in a 36-year-old woman.

Small ossicles, representing **persistent epiphyses**, are occasionally found at the tips of the articular processes (Figs. 5.**154**–5.**156**). Figure 5.**157** shows one such epiphysis located at the tip of the inferior articular process.

Occasionally a bony peg is seen projecting upward from an articular process (Fig. 5.**158**), or the tip of a superior articular process may show dysplastic thickening (Fig. 5.**159**).

Not all bony structures that are projected into the intervertebral foramina on lateral and oblique views can be accurately identified without sectional imaging procedures (Figs. 5.**160**, 5.**161**). Some may represent the articular processes of the apophyseal joints or the ends of a bifid spinous process. These findings are most common in the upper cervical spine, and most do not cause clinical complaints. Occasionally, though, the changes involve the lower cervical vertebral bodies in a clinically symptomatic patient (Fig. 5.**162**).

The **spinous processes** show considerable variability in their prominence and angulation (Figs. 5.**136**, 5.**143**).

> The unusual cranial or caudal angulation of a spinous process may cause apparent dorsal gaping in the affected segment, simulating an injury of the posterior ligaments.

Several authors have described unusual **unilateral hyperplasia** involving the C5–C7 spinous processes (Reinhardt 1956, Seibert-Deiker 1975). The **duplication** of a spinous process has also been described (Dahmen 1967). Sometimes a hypertrophic spinous process can extend far enough to produce a jointlike connection with the spinous process below it (Seibert-Deiker 1975). Figure 5.**163** shows a spike-shaped outgrowth projecting downward from the enlarged spinous process of C3.

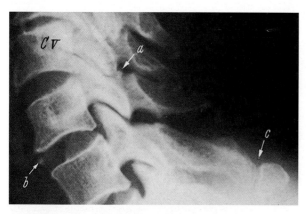

Fig. 5.**156**   Lateral projection of the cervical spine from C5 to C7.
a Accessory bone below the inferior articular process of C5.
b Calcific deposits in the anterior longitudinal ligament at the level of the C6/C7 disk space.
c Isolated ossicle on the C7 spinous process. Possible persistent apophysis.

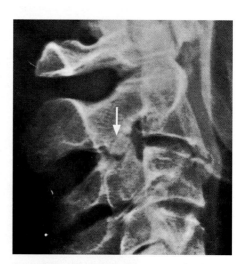

Fig. 5.**157**   Persistent, degeneratively altered apophysis of an articular process (arrow). The degenerative changes in the disk space at that level are associated with an osteophytic "buttress reaction" anteriorly (observation by Fellmann, Leukerbad).

Fig. 5.**158** Bilateral bone pegs projecting upward from the C3 articular processes (observation by Wendtland, Marl).

Fig. 5.**159** Stocky, dysplastic superior articular process (arrow).

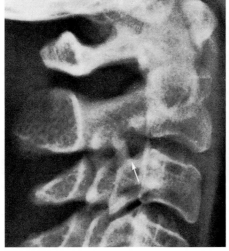

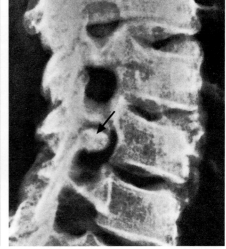

Fig. 5.**158**

Fig. 5.**159**

Fig. 5.**160** Narrow, horizontal bone spur projected into the intervertebral foramen at C2/C3.

Fig. 5.**161** Bone structure projected into the intervertebral foramen (arrow) on an oblique spinal view.

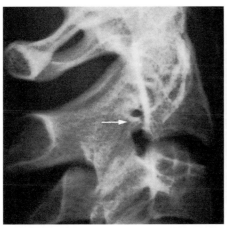

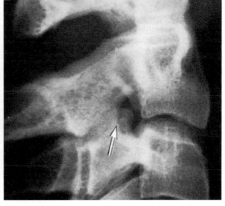

Fig. 5.**160**

Fig. 5.**161**

Fig. 5.**162** Bone spur projecting downward into the C5/C6 intervertebral foramen in a 23-year-old woman with neuralgic pain in the right arm (observation by Wendtland, Marl).

Fig. 5.**163** An unusually long C3 spinous process extends to the C5 level, arching over the hypoplastic C4 spinous process. The C2 spinous process is overgrown and has a downward-projecting tip.

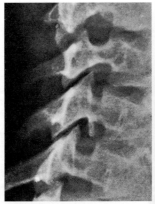

Fig. 5.**162**

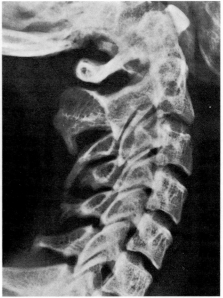

Fig. 5.**163**

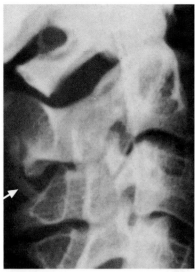

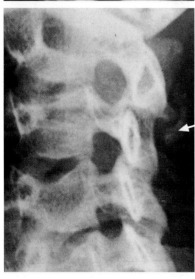

Fig. 5.**164a, b**   Isolated bone spurs (arrows) projecting into the soft tissues adjacent to the spinous processes.

Isolated bony bars are occasionally found around the spinous processes of the upper cervical spine (Fig. 5.**164**). Figure 5.**165** shows a bonelike structure between the C6 and C7 spinous processes that resembles an isolated bony process.

An isolated bony element found near the apex of a spinous process may represent the **persistent apophysis** of a spinous process or an **accessory ossification center** (Fig. 5.**156**).

Anomalies and Deformities

The **fusion** of **vertebral bodies** may involve two or more adjacent vertebrae. The developmental cause is a failure of segmentation of the primitive vertebral body. Synostosis in **block vertebrae** may be partial or complete. The fusion may additionally affect the vertebral arches, articular processes, and spinous processes, confirming its dysontogenic cause (Figs. 5.**166**, 5.**167**).

The fusion of vertebrae is often extensive and is particularly common in the cervical region. Only about 13% of all block vertebrae are congenital (Brown et al. 1964). **Acquired block vertebrae** may be caused by inflammatory disease (see below) or may occur in fetal alcohol syndrome (Tredwell et al. 1982).

The blocking most commonly involves the **C2–C3 area** (Fig. 5.**167**). Block vertebrae are often associated with a rudimentary disk, which appears as a narrow space with sclerotic margins. Most **congenital block vertebrae** additionally show a slight hourglass-shaped constriction. The sagittal diameter of block vertebrae is usually decreased relative to the normal adjacent vertebral bodies, and their total height is usually less than the sum of the corresponding normal segments. Congenital block vertebrae cause little or no positional change in the affected spinal segment. It may be difficult to distinguish congenital block vertebrae from acquired blocking in juvenile rheumatoid arthritis (Figs. 5.**166**, 5.**171**, 5.**172**, 5.**304**, 5.**346**, 5.**398**).

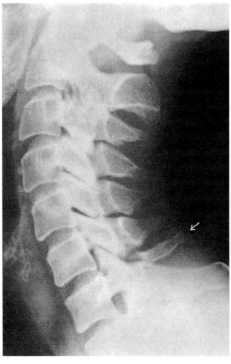

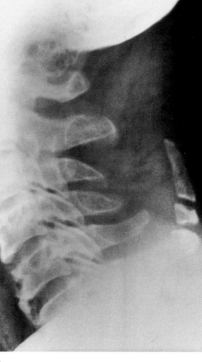

Fig. 5.**165a, b**   Accessory bone formation in the area of the spinous processes.
a An isolated, spinous process-like structure has formed between the spinous processes of C6 and C7 (observation by Köhler).
b A segmented bony structure projects upward from the C6 vertebra (observation by Witkops, Montabaur).

Fig. 5.**166** Congenital blocking of C3 and C4 with complete fusion of the vertebral body, neural arch, and spinous processes. Note the constricted contour and decreased sagittal diameter of the block vertebra.

Fig. 5.**167** Blocking of C2/C3 with partial synostosis of the spinous processes.

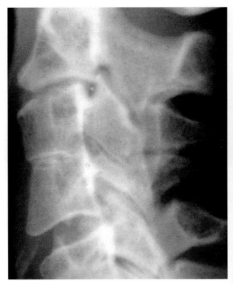

Fig. 5.**166**

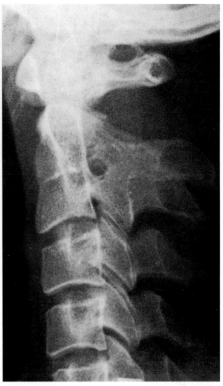

Fig. 5.**167**

Platyspondyly—flat and wedged vertebrae—may occasionally be observed in the cervical spine in patients with osteochondrodysplasias. It is far more common in the thoracic and lumbar spine. Congenital flat and wedged cervical vertebrae also occur as isolated anomalies. While congenital wedging is associated with hemivertebral shortening, a posttraumatic wedged vertebra usually shows some degree of elongation.

Hypoplasia of a vertebra is marked by a decrease in its sagittal and vertical dimensions. Acquired **vertebra plana** is discussed on p. 633. A **tall vertebra** whose vertical diameter is greater than its AP diameter is most commonly seen at the C3 and C7 levels. It is often found in association with dysostoses or may follow compensatory overgrowth adjacent to a vertebra that has become flattened as a result of disease.

Among the **lateral arch dysplasias**, underdevelopment of the pars interarticularis represents the mildest degree of developmental anomaly (Fig. 5.**168**).

Isolated cases of unilateral and bilateral **vertebral arch clefts** have been described at the C5–C7 levels, often combined with median posterior arch defects (Fig. 5.**169**) (Gaizler and Gaizler 1963, Holland and Stolle 1970, Azouz et al. 1974, Beck 1982, Forsberg et al. 1990, Kan and Matsubayashi 1995).

Clefts of the spinous processes are relatively common in the first thoracic vertebra (Fig. 5.**170**).

Horizontal clefts of the spinous process have also been observed at that level. Their pathogenesis is poorly understood (Heeren 1943, Schmitt and Rücker 1979). Larger defects may additionally involve the transverse and articular processes. This anomaly can lead to **spondylolisthesis**, which is rare in the cervical spine (Lissner 1956, Czákány and Almós 1959, Schwartz et al. 1982, Edwards et al. 1991, Black et al. 1991).

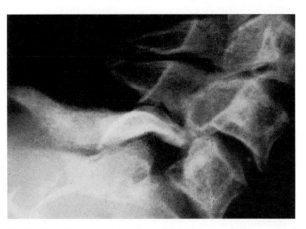

Fig. 5.**168** Pronounced unilateral hypoplasia of the vertebral arch and apophyseal joint of C6.

Diastematomyelia is a rare developmental anomaly that usually involves the conus medullaris and thoracic cord and is extremely rare in the cervical cord (Anand et al. 1985). Radiographs may occasionally demonstrate an ossified septum (Levine et al. 1985), but otherwise **MRI** is the diagnostic modality of choice (Prasad et al. 1995, Jäger et al. 1997).

Spinal canal stenosis can have various causes:
- Acquired diseases (see below)
- Spondylolisthesis
- Klippel–Feil syndrome (Bony and Denaro 1982, Prusick et al. 1985) (see below)
- C2/C3 fusion (de Graaf 1982)
- Achondroplasia (Morgan and Young 1980)
- Other skeletal dysplasias (Wackenheim 1985)

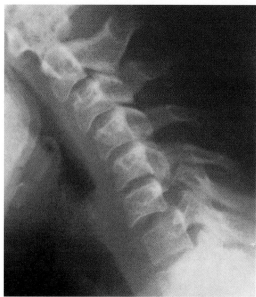

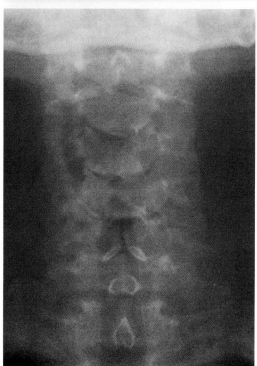

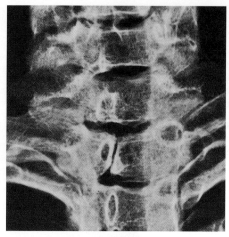

Fig. 5.**170**   Midline cleft of the T1 spinous process. The cervical vertebrae in the imaged segment are rotated to the left.

Fig. 5.**169a, b**   True spondylolysis with spondylolisthesis and clefting of the C6 spinous process. (From Beck 1982.)
a Lateral projection demonstrates a cleft in the C6 neural arch with spondylolisthesis during flexion.
b AP projection shows a midline cleft in the C6 spinous process.

These findings are best demonstrated by CT and MRI (Rodiek 1983).

Klippel–Feil syndrome is a complex developmental anomaly that was first described by Klippel and Feil in 1912 and referred to the cervical and upper thoracic spine (Klippel and Feil 1912, Sicard and Lemoyez 1923). Its cardinal feature in the cervical spine is the fusion of multiple cervical vertebrae including the vertebral bodies and arches (Fig. 5.**171**). The total number of cervical vertebrae may be diminished.

Klippel–Feil syndrome may be accompanied by atlanto-occipital dysplasia or by Sprengel's deformity (see chapter on the shoulder, p. 261) with cervical ribs and os omovertebrale (Fig. 5.**172**, see also Fig. 5.**205**) or congenital scoliosis, kyphosis (Winter et al. 1984) and spinal stenosis (Bony and Denaro 1982, Prusick et al. 1985).

Besides the partial or complete fusion of cervical vertebral bodies and a numerical reduction, clefts may be present in the vertebral bodies and arches (Wolf and Klein 1997). Hemivertebrae and wedged vertebrae may also be present in the syndrome (Figs. 5.**171**, 5.**173**).

The clinical manifestations of Klippel–Feil syndrome include a short neck and low nuchal hairline. Often there are concomitant developmental anomalies and malformations of the nervous system accompanied by paralysis, sensory disturbances, and contractures.

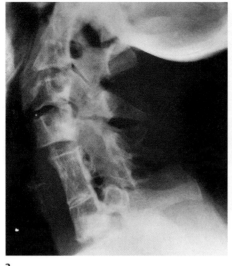

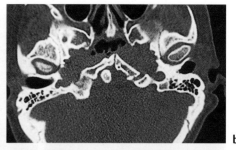

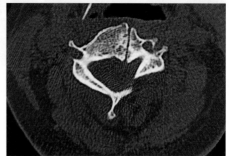

a

Fig. 5.**171 a–d**   Complex anomalies in Klippel–Feil syndrome. Only six cervical vertebral bodies are present. There is partial occipitalization of C1, which has a cleft in its anterior arch. Complete blocking of C5 and C6 accompanied by partial ankylosis of C7. Clefts are also present in the C4 vertebral body and the T1 neural arch.
a Lateral projection.
b–d Axial CT scans at the level of C1 (**b**), C4 (**c**), and T1 (**d**). Note the dysplastic C2 spinous process and the decreased sagittal diameter of the block vertebrae (observation by Möller, Lilienthal).

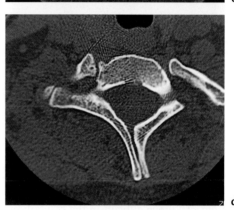

d

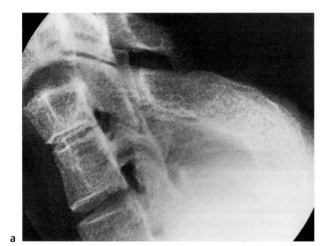

a

Fig. 5.**172 a, b**   Os omovertebrale.
a Klippel–Feil syndrome with block vertebrae and development of an unusually pronounced os omovertebrale (observation by Reichel, Wiesbaden).
b Sprengel deformity with an elevated scapula and an os omovertebrale that articulates with the medial border of the scapula.

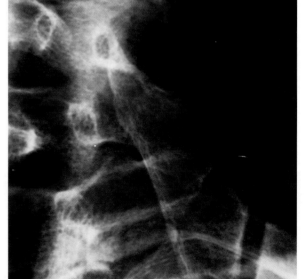

b

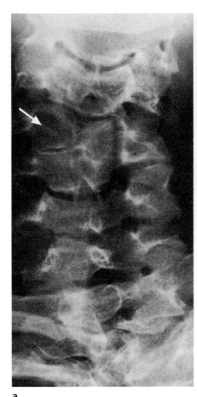

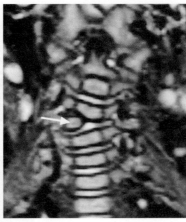

Fig. 5.**173 a, b**   Cervical hemivertebrae.
a Lateral hemivertebra at C4 (arrow).
b MRI appearance of a lateral hemivertebra at C4 (arrow).

 Fracture, Subluxation, or Dislocation?

The diagnosis of fractures, subluxations, and even dislocations can prove difficult in the cervical region. Reference was made earlier to the different radiographic projections and the information they can provide. While we recognize the definite value of **routine radiographs** and **special views** in acute diagnosis, we again emphasize that **CT** (including two- and three-dimensional reconstructions) and **MRI** are absolutely essential for scrutinizing details, investigating equivocal findings, and planning surgical procedures (Fig. 5.**174**) (Acheson et al. 1987, Goldberg et al. 1988, Pathria and Petersilge 1991, Fishman et al. 1991, Harris and Yeakley 1992, Mirvis and Wolf 1992). The limited sensitivity of conventional radiographs compared with conventional tomography and CT is known (Streitwieser et al. 1983, Acheson et al. 1987), but it should be noted that fine fracture lines, especially when horizontal, may be difficult to detect even with CT.

Fractures

The thickness of the **prevertebral soft-tissue shadow** can provide indirect evidence for the presence of a fracture. If the soft-tissue shadow in front of C3 and the superior border of C4 is thickened to more than 5–7 mm and the prevertebral soft tissues at the C6 and C7 level are widened to more than 20 mm, a fracture should be suspected (Rogers 1992). Displacement of the prevertebral fat stripe in front of the anterior longitudinal ligament can provide another indirect sign (Whalen and Woodruff 1970).

Axial trauma to the spine can produce **burst fractures** and **split fractures** of the cervical vertebral bodies, most commonly affecting C5 and C6 (Fig. 5.**174**).

Compression fractures of the cervical vertebral bodies in adults can be difficult to distinguish from a physiological decrease in the **height of C4 and C5** occurring as a normal variant.

 A fracture should be suspected if the anterior height of a vertebral body is 3 mm less than its posterior height.

A knowledge of the ossification centers and timing of ossification is of key importance in evaluating the **pediatric cervical spine** (Figs. 5.**129**–5.**132**). The **ossification centers** of the marginal ridges of the vertebral body end plates should not be mistaken for avulsed bone fragments (Fig. 5.**133**). The normal slight **anterior wedging** of the **juvenile vertebral body** (Fig. 5.**132**) requires differentiation from **compression fractures**, but this can be very difficult in practice. **Vertebra plana** may also be mistaken for a compression fracture (Figs. 5.**191**, 5.**312**).

With their typical location and arrangement, **persistent notochord remnants** should not be mistaken for old depressed fractures of the vertebral body end plates (Fig. 5.**149**). Finally, **degenerative arthritis of the uncovertebral joints** in the lateral projection can **mimic a horizontal fracture** of the vertebral body (Goldberg et al. 1982) (Fig. 5.**198**).

A special type of burst fracture caused by **hyperflexion** is the **teardrop fracture**, in which a triangular or rectangular fragment (the "teardrop") is broken from the anteriorly compressed vertebral body (Fig. 5.**175**). The vertebral body itself may be driven posteriorly into the spinal canal (Schneider and Kahn 1956). Anterior osteophytes may become detached through the same mechanism.

Fig. 5.**174a–d** Hyperflexion trauma.
a Burst fracture of C4 with evidence of a teardrop fragment (arrow). The apophyseal joints of C4 are not cleanly projected over one another, suggesting that the posterior arch has been fractured. Compression fracture of C6 with anterior wedging (arrowhead).
b CT demonstrates a vertical fracture of C4 with a right-sided fracture of the vertebral arch.
c View of the C4 vertical fracture in a three-dimensional CT reconstruction.
d T2-weighted sagittal MRI shows edematous changes in the C4 and C6 vertebral bodies and in the posterior soft tissues as evidence of the acute trauma and hyperflexion injury.

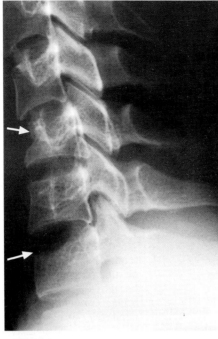
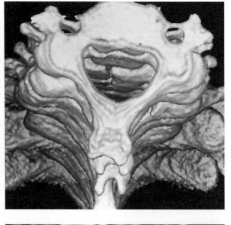
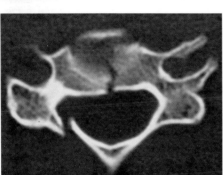
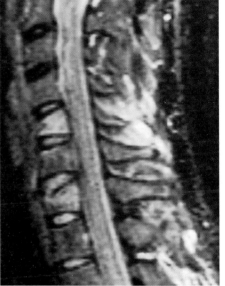

a

b

c

d

Widening of the interspinous distance as well as subluxations and dislocations of the apophyseal joints are signs of hyperflexion injury to the posterior ligaments (Fig. 5.**175**). It should be noted, however, that unusual cranial or caudal angulation of spinous processes can mimic posterior gaping (**pseudogaping**), especially at C3/C4. Given the variability of the spinous processes, the spacing of the spinous processes should be assessed at the level of the spinolaminar line.

The fracture line associated with a **vertical split fracture** is usually visible only in the AP projection. Air in the larynx (Figs. 5.**138**, 5.**174**) or **congenital clefts** in the neural arch can mimic this type of fracture. The typical sclerotic margins of congenital arch defects serve to distinguish them from vertical fractures, however (Fig. 5.**170**).

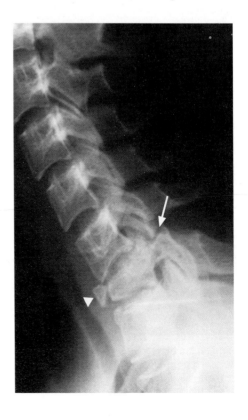

Fig. 5.**175** Teardrop fracture of the C7 vertebral body. Plain ▷ film shows concomitant dislocation of the C6/C7 apophyseal joints (arrows) with a characteristic anterior edge fragment (arrowhead) caused by compression of the C7 vertebral body. Gaping of the C6 and C7 spinous processes signify disruption of the posterior ligaments.

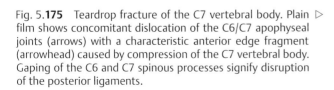

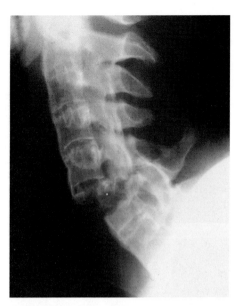

Fig. 5.**176**   Fracture of the lower cervical spine caused by hyperextension trauma in a patient with ankylosing spondylitis (observation by D. Resnick, San Diego).

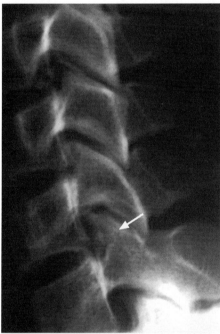

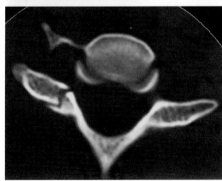

Fig. 5.**177 a, b**   Fracture of the superior articular process.
a Lateral projection demonstrates the very thin fracture line (arrow).
b CT confirms the finding.

Hyperextension fractures present the following radiographic signs:

- Widened disk spaces
- Spinous process fractures
- Vacuum phenomena
- Fractures of the vertebral arches and apophyseal joints (Gehweiler et al. 1980, Edeiken-Monroe et al. 1986)

It is also important to consider that **ankylosing spondylitis** makes the cervical spine more susceptible to fractures (Broom and Raycroft 1988, Amamilo 1989). These fractures are caused by hyperextension of the cervical spine, especially in the lower segments (Fig. 5.**176**).

Special attention should be given to fractures occurring in proximity to the **uncovertebral and apophyseal joints**. Often these injuries are difficult to diagnose and require special investigation by **CT** (Yetkin et al. 1985) (Fig. 5.**177**). **Accessory ossicles** of the **uncinate processes** (Figs. 5.**146**, 5.**147**) and persistent epiphyses of the inferior or superior articular process of the apophyseal joints can be difficult to distinguish from fractures (Figs. 5.**154**, 5.**155**). **Congenital clefts** of the vertebral arch and its appendages can be readily distinguished from fractures at those sites by their typical appearance and sclerotic borders (Figs. 5.**169**, 5.**170**).

> With a slightly oblique lateral projection of the cervical spine, the apophyseal joint spaces may project onto the vertebral arch and simulate a fracture.

An **indentation** that often occurs as a normal variant in the **superior articular surfaces** of the lower cervical apophyseal joints, especially at C7, can be difficult to distinguish from an injury (Figs. 5.**142**, 5.**177**).

Avulsion fractures of the lower spinous processes are usually caused by muscular traction due to repetitive overuse (Figs. 5.**178**, 5.**179**). This injury, known also as **clay shoveler's fracture**, predominantly affects the C6 and C7 spinous processes but can also affect T1 and T2 (Cancelmo 1972). The pull of the attached muscles tends to displace the fragment inferiorly, distracting the fracture line and predisposing to nonunion (Fig. 5.**180**).

The fracture is easy to diagnose on lateral radiographs (Fig. 5.**178**). In the **AP projection**, simultaneous visualization of the avulsed spinous process and the avulsion site can produce a characteristic "**double spinous process**" sign (Fig. 5.**179**). The **juvenile form** of this injury is an avulsion fracture of the spinous apophysis, known also as **Schmitt disease** (Schmitt and Wisser 1951, Cancelmo 1972). The juvenile avulsion fracture may heal with bony consolidation but may also proceed to nonunion (Fig. 5.**156**). It is important to differentiate the fracture from **spinous epiphyses** and persistent epiphyses. **Accessory bone elements** in the area of the spinous processes (Figs. 5.**164**, 5.**165**) and **calcifications** of the **nuchal ligament** (Fig. 5.**203**) are other potential sources of confusion.

Chronic overuse injury to the spinous processes may appear as a roughening of the spinous tip with a concave bony defect on the undersurface of the spinous process (Schmitt and Wisser 1951, Schmitt and Rücker 1979).

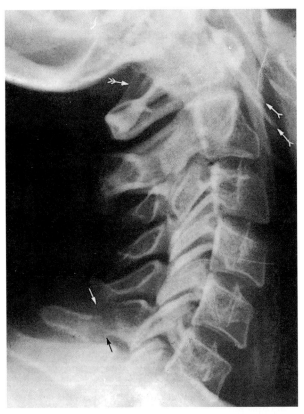

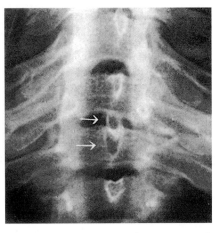

Fig. 5.**179**   "Double spinous process" sign of a spinous avulsion fracture. The narrow-rimmed upper ellipse is the base of the fractured spinous process, and the broader-rimmed lower ellipse is the detached apical fragment, which is displaced inferiorly.

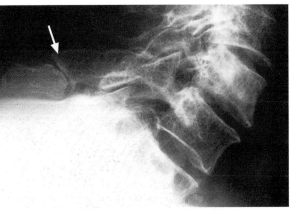

Fig. 5.**178**   Fracture of the C6 spinous process (arrow). The styloid process of the temporal bone is visible on each side (arrow). A posterior ponticulus of C1 is also defined (double arrow).

Fig. 5.**180**   Old, nonunited clay shoveler's fracture of C7 ▷ (arrow).

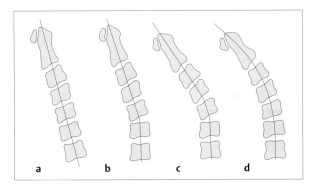

Subluxations and Dislocations

Whiplash injuries are two-phase injuries caused by sudden acceleration–deceleration forces. Phase one is marked by an S-shaped cervical curve with flexion in the upper segments and hyperextension in the lower segments. In phase two, all of the cervical segments are extended while the neck is maximally hyperextended (Panjabi et al. 1998). This produces injuries of varying magnitude ranging from mild pain, malalignments, and reversible subluxations to dislocations and fracture-dislocations (Grifka et al. 1998).

Loss of the **normal lordotic position** of the cervical spine and possibly its reversal to kyphosis following a **whiplash injury** may be attributable to reflex muscle splinting but may also fall within the range of normal variation. **Pseudodislocation** at the C2/C3 level in children should also be kept in mind as a normal variant (see Fig. 5.**107**).

In whiplash injuries, functional views in the flexion and extension are done to detect injuries to the interrelated disk, apophyseal joint capsule, and posterior stabilizing ligaments.

Soft-tissue injuries may be manifested on **functional views** as **isolated rotation** or **fixed limitation of motion** in individual spinal segments, possibly combined with the displacement of vertebrae (Ross 1964a, b). A **decrease** or **increase in interspinous distances** suggests injury to the posterior stabilizing ligaments, but only after variants of the spinous processes have been excluded.

On the **functional views** of the cervical spine in flexion-extension, the detection of zero flexion or flexion in just one segment implies significant soft-tissue injury (muscle, ligaments), while flexion in two adjacent segments suggests limitation of motion and minor soft-tissue injuries (Bohrer et al. 1990) (Fig. 5.**181**).

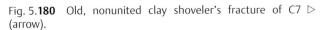

Fig. 5.**181**   Flexion patterns observed in 150 patients (Bohrer et al. 1990). **a** No angle. **b** One angle. **a** and **b** are abnormal and may indicate significant soft tissue injuries. **c** Two flexion angles. Indicates less than full flexion without significant injury, corresponding to mild soft tissue injuries. **d** Three or more angles represent normal flexion pattern.

Cervical flexion occurring in more than three segments is considered a normal finding (Bohrer et al. 1990).

Criteria for the instability of a cervical spinal segment (Cintron et al. 1981, Scher 1982, Rogers 1992)
➤ A horizontal shift of more than 3 mm or an angulation of more than 11° between two adjacent vertebral bodies
➤ Unilateral disk space narrowing
➤ Widening of the precervical soft-tissue space
➤ Widening of the interspinous distance (see Variants above)
➤ Widening of a disk space in the lateral projection

Rotatory subluxation refers to the fixation of two adjacent cervical vertebrae in an abnormally rotated position and may be spontaneous or posttraumatic. It most commonly affects the craniovertebral joints.

Subluxations and **dislocations** below C2 are almost invariably caused by trauma. Subluxations, in which the articular processes are still in broad contact with each other, are distinguished from dislocations, in which the tips of the articular processes may still touch (Fig. 5.**182**) or may be separated by a gap (Fig. 5.**175**).

A **unilateral dislocation** leads to vertebral rotation with a corresponding lateral shift of the spinous process in the AP projection. A **bilateral dislocation** of the apophyseal joints leads to flexion deformity of the cervical spine.

 ## Necrosis?

Osteonecrosis of the vertebral bodies is discussed in the section on the thoracic spine, as **Kümmel–Verneuil disease** and **steroid necrosis** are unusual in the cervical spine. **Vertebra plana** (Calvé disease), once considered a form of aseptic necrosis, is further discussed in the section on tumors.

 ## Inflammation?

Bacterial spondylitis and **spondylodiscitis** are rare in the cervical spine compared with other spinal regions except the sacrum (Garcia and Grantham 1960, Cahill et al. 1991). Most patients are in the fifth or sixth decade, but older persons may also be affected. Generally the infection is manifested in the vertebral body. Osteomyelitis of the vertebral arch and its appendages is rare (Peris et al. 1992). Specific causes of spondylitis and spondylodiscitis include the following:

● Complications of diagnostic endoscopy (Barr et al. 1988)
● Intubation (Lloyd and Johnson 1980)
● Dental extractions (Pinckney et al. 1980)

Tuberculous spondylitis and **spondylodiscitis** are relatively rare in the cervical spine. Multiple vertebral bodies are affected in typical cases (Wurtz et al. 1993). A case involving complete **synostosis** of the cervical spine following tuberculous spondylitis has been described (Lukoscheck and Niethard 1995).

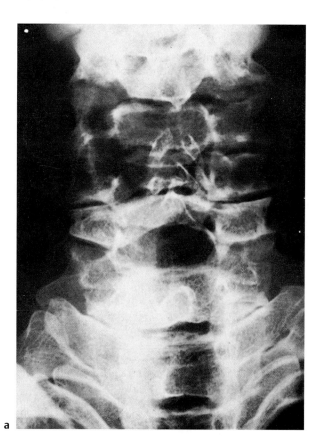

a

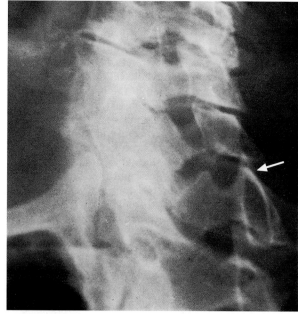

b

Fig. 5.**182a, b**   Apophyseal joint dislocation between C5 and C6.
a The dislocation is difficult to detect on the AP radiograph.
b The dislocated apophyseal joint is clearly visible in the oblique view (arrow). Note the offset in the row of intervertebral foramina.

Rare involvement of the spine by **actinomycosis** is typically manifested in the cervical spine (Crank et al. 1982). Spondylitis in the setting of **syphilis** predominantly affects the cervical spine (Sgalitzer 1941, 1960).

Gouty osteoarthropathy rarely involves the cervical spine but can lead to erosions of the dens and vertebral end plates, disk space narrowing, and vertebral malalignment, displaying features that may resemble intervertebral osteochondrosis and spondylodiscitis (Aaron 1984, Das 1988). Involvement of the cervical spine by **sternocosto-clavicular hyperostosis** ("pustulotic arthro-osteitis") with vertebral sclerosis and bandlike ossification at the anterior border of the vertebrae and disks has been described (Resnick 1985).

Rheumatoid arthritis and the **seronegative spondylar-thropathies** (ankylosing spondylitis, psoriasis, Reiter syndrome) have many radiographic features in common. They affect synovial joints, synchondroses, symphyses, tendon and ligament attachments, and bone. Nevertheless, they differ in their sites of involvement and the extent of the changes.

Rheumatoid arthritis has an affinity for the cervical spine (Fig. 5.**183**). Characteristic findings include:

- Osteoporosis
- Narrowing and erosion of the apophyseal joint spaces
- Mild sclerosis

The disk spaces are narrowed, and the vertebral end plates show irregularities and sclerosis. Bony ankylosis may occur. Osteophytes are not present in typical cases.

Sharp tapering of the **spinous processes** is among the typical features of cervical rheumatoid arthritis and can range to osteolysis, especially in the spinous processes of the lower cervical spine (Fig. 5.**183**) (Schilling et al. 1963). Inflammation of the ligamentous attachments and adjacent bursa has been cited as the possible cause (Bywaters 1982). This feature should be distinguished from **chronic overuse injuries** of the lower cervical spinous processes, which are characterized by roughening of the spinous tips

and concave bony defects on the undersurface of the spinous process (Schmitt and Wisser 1951, Schmitt and Rücker 1979).

Subluxations of cervical vertebrae in rheumatoid arthritis usually occur only after a prolonged course of illness. They lead to typical stepladder displacements of the cervical vertebrae as evidence of segmental instability (Redlund-Johnell 1984) (Fig. 5.**184**).

Figure 5.**185** illustrates typical radiographic changes in the cervical spine that may be observed in rheumatoid arthritis.

Spondylarthropathy in patients on **chronic hemodialysis** can lead to vertebral subluxations that mimic the features of rheumatoid arthritis (Orzincolo et al. 1990).

Juvenile rheumatoid arthritis typically involves the cervical spine. Besides subluxations, which primarily affect the atlantoaxial joint, the changes correspond to those of rheumatoid arthritis. The upper and middle segments of the cervical spine are especially prone to rheumatoid changes and eventual **ankylosis** (Fig. 5.**186**). Exclusive involvement of the lower cervical spine is unusual. In pronounced cases, the ligamenta flava may ossify and there may be partial **fusion of the vertebral bodies**. The features of juvenile rheumatoid arthritis are often unmistakable because of the severe effects on the growth and development of the intervertebral disks, vertebral bodies, neural arches, and spinous processes. The intervertebral foramina may appear enlarged (Dihlmann and Friedmann 1977). **Klippel–Feil syndrome** can mimic juvenile rheumatoid arthritis but is consistently associated with synostosis of the spinous processes and the scapula may be elevated. An os omovertebrale is occasionally present (Figs. 5.**171**, 5.**172**).

Ankylosing spondylitis is typically manifested first in the sacroiliac joint region and, over time, spreads upward to involve the cervical spine (Fig. 5.**187**). Involvement of the cervical spine appears to be somewhat more common in women (Resnick et al. 1976, Spencer et al. 1979, Maldonado-Cocco et al. 1985).

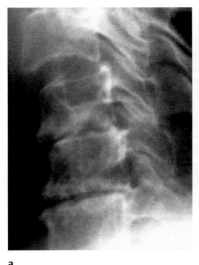
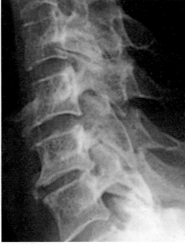
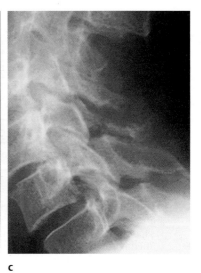

a   b   c

Fig. 5.**183 a–c**   Rheumatoid arthritis of the cervical spine.
a Narrowing of the disk spaces with erosion and sclerosis of the vertebral end plates. The vertebral bodies show a mild degree of subluxation.

b Apophyseal joint involvement with joint space narrowing and subchondral sclerosis.
c Erosions and destructive changes in the spinous processes.

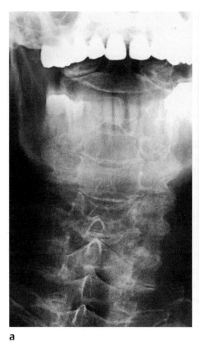
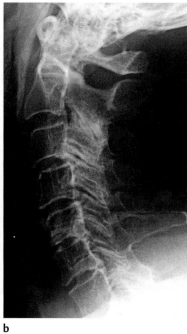

a

b

Fig. 5.**184a, b**   Rheumatoid arthritis of the cervical spine. Instability is manifested by the left convex bowing of the neck and mild subluxation of the vertebral bodies.
a AP projection.
b Lateral projection. Note the "stepladder" alignment of the vertebral bodies and the sclerosis of the apophyseal joints.

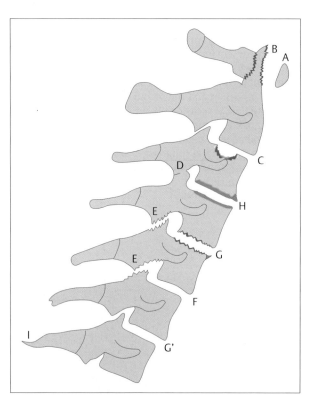

Fig. 5.**185**   Synopsis of the cervical spinal changes that may be found in adult rheumatoid arthritis (after Dihlmann).

A	Anterior displacement of C1
B	Erosion of the dens
C	Rheumatoid spondylodiscitis
D	Bony ankylosis of the apophyseal joints
E	Erosive arthritis of the apophyseal joints with pseudo-slippage (pseudospondylolisthesis)
F	Rheumatoid discitis or chondrosis
G, G′	Early stage of rheumatoid spondylodiscitis with disk narrowing and ill-defined vertebral end plates
H	Typical intervertebral osteochondrosis
I	Osteolysis of the spinous process

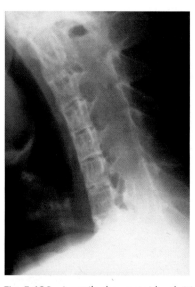

Fig. 5.**186**   Juvenile rheumatoid arthritis with extensive ankyloses of the cervical spine. Note the small sagittal diameter of the vertebral bodies as a sign of impaired growth (observation by D. Resnick, San Diego).

Fig. 5.**187 a, b**   Ankylosing spondylitis of
the cervical spine.
a Narrowing of the disk spaces with erosions of the vertebral end plates.
b Late stage with bony ankylosis of the apophyseal joints. Evidence of syndesmophytes.

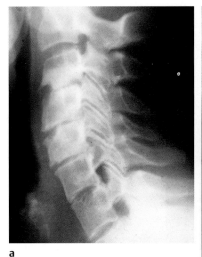

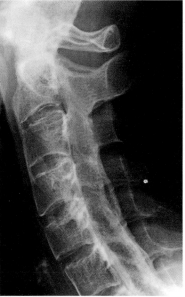

a

b

Complete **ankylosis** of the C2–C7 **apophyseal joints** is a classic feature of ankylosing spondylitis. In contrast to juvenile rheumatoid arthritis, there is no narrowing of the vertebral bodies or intervertebral disk spaces.

Ossification of the posterior longitudinal ligament has been described in patients with ankylosing spondylitis (Olivieri et al. 1988). While **atlantoaxial subluxation** is occasionally found in ankylosing spondylitis, subluxations below C2 are very rare and are more characteristic of rheumatoid arthritis. As in rheumatoid arthritis and psoriatic arthritis, ankylosing spondylitis is associated with **erosion** and **sclerosis** of the **vertebral end plates**, similar to that in spondylodiscitis. The **spinous processes** may be **eroded** in ankylosing spondylitis, as they may be in rheumatoid ar-

thritis (Bywaters 1982). Erosion of the spinous processes may also be a feature of psoriasis and Reiter syndrome. Reference was made earlier to the frequency of **fractures** in ankylosing spondylitis (Broom and Raycroft 1988).

The spinal changes in **psoriasis** and **Reiter syndrome** are almost identical, but involvement of the cervical spine is more common in psoriasis (Killebrew et al. 1973) (Fig. 5.**188**). Both diseases can be difficult to distinguish from ankylosing spondylitis, but **ankylosis** of the apophyseal joints is **less common**. Marked **paravertebral ossification** is occasionally observed (Killebrew et al. 1973; Moilanen et al. 1984). **Instability** of the cervical spine is very rare except at the atlantoaxial level.

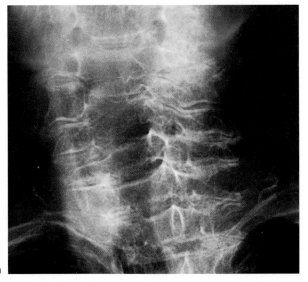

a

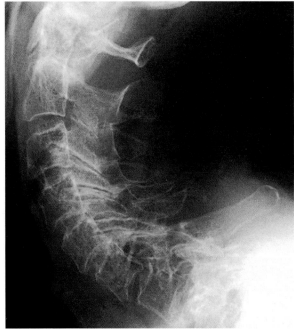

b

Fig. 5.**188 a–c**   Psoriatic arthritis of the cervical spine, characterized by apophyseal joint space narrowing and sclerosis with irregularities of the vertebral end plates.
a AP projection.
b Lateral projection. Note the hyperlordosis of the cervical spine.

Fig. 5.**188 c** ▷

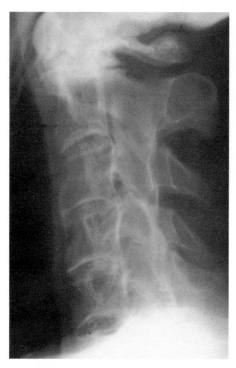

Fig. 5.**188c**   Late stage of the disease with bony ankylosis of the apophyseal joints.

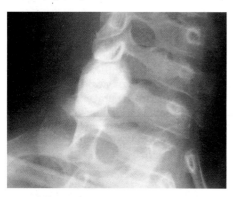

Fig. 5.**189**   Osteoblastoma of the C6 vertebral arch. Radiograph shows expansion and sclerosis of the pars interarticularis (observation by D. Resnick, San Diego).

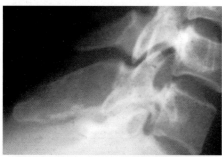

a

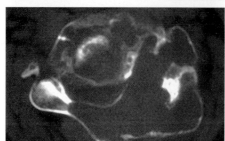

b

 Tumor?

Levine et al. (1992) analyzed 41 cases of **benign tumors** of the cervical spine in a recent study. They found the following tumors in descending order of frequency:

- Osteoid osteoma
- Osteoblastoma
- Aneurysmal bone cyst
- Eosinophilic granuloma
- Giant cell tumor
- Osteochondroma
- Hemangioma

The most commonly affected vertebrae were C2 and C4. Osteoid osteomas and osteoblastomas were usually located in the vertebral arches and apophyseal joints while giant cell tumors, aneurysmal bone cysts, and eosinophilic granulomas occurred predominantly in the vertebral bodies. Although most tumors of the cervical spine are visible on plain films, the complex anatomy of that region calls for sectional imaging procedures, which can also narrow the differential diagnosis. Superimposed structures can produce false positive findings on radiographs. For example, air in the piriform recess can mimic an osteolytic lesion in the AP projection while the groove for the spinal nerve can mimic osteolysis in the lateral projection (Figs. 5.**140**, 5.**142**).

Osteoid Osteoma

Osteoid osteomas most commonly involve the vertebral arches and their appendages, especially the pedicles and apophyseal joints (Fielding et al. 1977). The cardinal sign on plain films is **osteosclerosis**. Tomography or CT is usually necessary to detect the radiolucent **nidus** (Fig. 5.**362**).

Osteoblastoma

Osteoblastoma also arises predominantly from the posterior spinal elements. Usually it is associated with well-defined osteolytic bone expansion and may show partial or complete sclerosis (Fig. 5.**189**) (Dias and Frost 1973).

Aneurysmal Bone Cyst

An aneurysmal bone cyst can be difficult to distinguish from other lesions (Fig. 5.**190**) (Dahlin and McLeod 1982). Approximately 14% of all aneurysmal bone cysts involve the spine. Both the vertebral bodies and posterior elements may be affected. When the lesion is located in the spinous process or transverse process in a child or adolescent, the correct diagnosis can usually be made, but it may be difficult to distinguish the lesion from osteoblastoma. Expansion of the pedicle or lamina may be less pronounced, making diagnosis more difficult. The radiographic signs of an aneurysmal bone cyst are least specific in the vertebral body.

◁ Fig. 5.**190a, b**   Aneurysmal bone cyst of the vertebral arch (observation by D. Resnick, San Diego).
a Aneurysmal bone cyst of the spinous process with a pathological fracture (lateral radiograph).
b Lesion extending in the vertebral arch and transverse process (CT).

Giant Cell Tumor

Giant cell tumors affect the axial skeleton in 7% of cases. The cervical spine is the third most common site of occurrence after the sacrum and thoracic spine (Sanjay et al. 1993). The tumor is usually located in the vertebral body, making it easier to distinguish from an aneurysmal bone cyst or osteoblastoma.

Eosinophilic Granuloma

Eosinophilic granuloma is the most common form of Langerhans-cell histiocytosis (histiocytosis X), accounting for 70% of cases. The typical spinal manifestation is **vertebra plana**, which is found mainly in children (Fig. 5.**191**) (Berning and Freyschmidt 1985, Robert et al. 1987).

Eosinophilic granuloma can also lead to vertebral body expansion with osteolytic changes affecting both the vertebral body and the posterior spinal elements (Baber et al. 1987, Johnson et al. 1993).

Osteochondroma

Spinal involvement by osteochondroma is rare (Fig. 5.**192**). The tumor can cause narrowing of the spinal canal (Fielding and Ratzan 1973, Esposito et al. 1985).

Hemangioma

Hemangiomas most commonly affect the vertebral bodies of the thoracic spine (Fig. 5.**359**) but also occur in the cervical spine and may spread to the vertebral arches or involve them primarily (Laredo et al. 1986).

Neurinoma

Figure 5.**193** shows the classic enlargement of an intervertebral foramen caused by a spinal neurinoma.

Fibrous Dysplasia

Involvement of the cervical spine by fibrous dysplasia was mentioned earlier (Fig. 5.**194**).

Chordoma

Chordoma was discussed in the section on C1 and axis (Fig. 5.**195**).

Additional spinal tumors are described in the section on the lumbar spine.

Metastases

Cervical metastases occur with some frequency during the systemic spread of malignant tumors (Rao et al. 1992), but metastases to the thoracic and lumbar spine are more common.

Erosions

An erosion in the intervertebral foramen caused by **elongation of the vertebral artery** appears as a sharply demarcated impression in the vertebral body and requires differentiation from an expansile tumor. The erosion is typically located at the C2/C3 level but has also been described at C4/C5 (Fig. 5.**118**) (Roy-Camille and Thibierge 1982, Dory 1985).

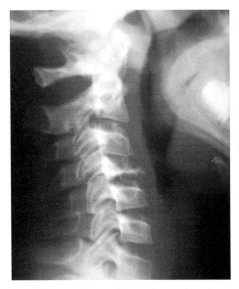

Fig. 5.**191**   Eosinophilic granuloma of C4 with vertebra plana.

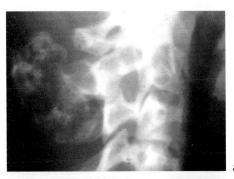

a

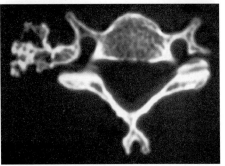

b

Fig. 5.**192a, b**   Osteochondroma of the upper cervical spine arising from the C2 transverse process.
a Lateral projection.
b CT (observation by D. Resnick, San Diego).

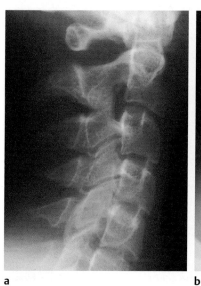 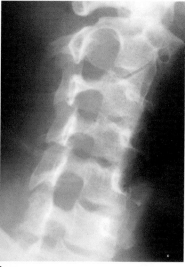

a   b

Fig. 5.**193 a, b** Typical enlargement of the intervertebral foramina by multiple neurinomas in neurofibromatosis.
a Lateral projection.
b Oblique projection.

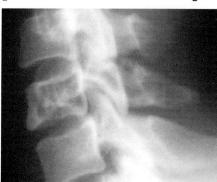

a

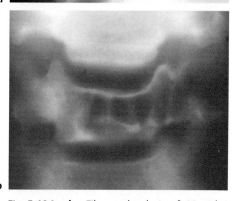

b

Fig. 5.**194 a, b** Fibrous dysplasia of C6 with involvement of the vertebral body and spinous process.
a Lateral projection.
b Frontal tomogram.

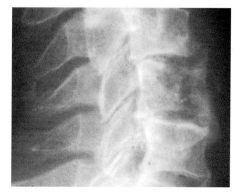

Fig. 5.**195** Osteolytic destruction of the C5 vertebral body by a chordoma.

 ## Other Changes?

Degenerative Changes

Degenerative changes in the cervical spine are a common finding after age 40 and increase with aging. Multiple segments of the lower cervical spine are usually affected, especially C5/C6 and C6/C7 (Lestini and Wiesel 1989). This pertains to **intervertebral osteochondrosis**, **spondylarthrosis**, and **uncovertebral arthrosis**. Each of the degenerative conditions can lead to narrowing of the intervertebral foramina, most commonly at C3/C4, C4/C5, and C5/C6. A 45° oblique projection is necessary for an accurate evaluation of the intervertebral foramina.

Degenerative changes correlate poorly with clinical manifestations in older patients and somewhat better in younger patients (McRae 1960, Friedenberg and Miller 1963). Additional procedures should be used for treatment planning, especially MRI and functional examinations in various degrees of flexion, extension, and rotation (Muhle et al. 1998 b, c, Muhle et al. 1999).

This section deals with the most important degenerative changes that may be encountered in the cervical spine. Standard reference works may be consulted for more detailed information (Dihlmann 1987, Resnick 1995, Freyschmidt 1997).

Intervertebral chondrosis is associated with dehydration of the nucleus pulposus, disk space narrowing, and tears in the anulus fibrosus, all of which can lead to a **vacuum phenomenon**, mostly occurring in the lumbar spine, and occasionally also in the cervical spine (Bohrer and Chen 1988). The vacuum phenomenon was noted on CT scans in approximately 30% of patients with cervical disk disease, especially in the marginal region of the disks (Isu et al. 1983).

With loss of intervertebral disk height and loss of the pressure- and shock-absorbing function of the disk, subchondral changes develop in the vertebral body end plates leading to **intervertebral osteochondrosis**. This condition is manifested by sclerosis of the end plates and the formation of **marginal spondylophytes**. Breaks can develop in the end plates, allowing disk material to protrude into the vertebral body (**Schmorl's nodes**). These changes affect the entire spine but are most pronounced in the lower cervical and lumbar regions. Finally, there may be **erosive changes**

Table 5.**4**   Differential diagnosis of intervertebral disk narrowing and sclerosis of the vertebral end plates (after Resnick et al.)

Disease	Mechanism	Roentgen signs
Intervertebral osteochondrosis	Degeneration of the nucleus pulposus and cartilage end plate Schmorl nodes	Disk space narrowing Vacuum phenomenon Well-defined sclerotic end plates
Infection	Osteomyelitis Discitis	Disk space narrowing Ill-defined sclerotic end plates Soft-tissue swelling
Trauma	Intervertebral disk injury Degeneration Intraosseous cartilage prolapse	Disk space narrowing Well-defined sclerotic end plates Fractures Soft-tissue swelling
Neuropathic osteoarthropathy	Loss of proprioception Repetitive trauma	Disk space narrowing Pronounced sclerosis Spondylophyte formation Fragmentation Malalignment
Rheumatoid arthritis	Apophyseal joint instability with excessive loads Effects of inflammatory tissue on neighboring joints	Disk space narrowing Sclerotic end plates with sharp or ill-defined margins Subluxation Apophyseal joint changes
Calcium pyrophosphate dihydrate crystal deposition (pseudogout)	Crystal deposition in the cartilaginous end plate and intervertebral disk with degeneration	Disk space narrowing Calcifications Sclerotic end plates with sharp or ill-defined margins Fragmentation Subluxation
Alkaptonuria	Crystal deposition in the cartilaginous end plate and intervertebral disk with degeneration	Disk space narrowing Vacuum phenomenon Well-defined end plates Calcifications

in the vertebral body end plates and synostoses may be observed.

The differential diagnosis includes various other diseases that can cause loss of intervertebral disk height and similar changes in the vertebral body end plates (Table 5.**4**).

Intervertebral osteochondrosis may also be associated with **hemispheric spondylosclerosis**, but this is more common in the lumbar spine (Fig. 5.**373**). The differential diagnosis of sclerotic vertebral changes is covered in the section on the lumbar spine.

Spondylosis deformans, which may or may not be associated with disk space narrowing, is characterized by the development of **submarginal spondylophytes** (Resnick 1985). Pathophysiologically, it is thought that tears of the anulus fibrosus at its attachment to the vertebral body, along with slight anterior and anterolateral displacements of the disk, exert tensile forces on the outer fibers of the anulus fibrosus, causing traction osteophytes to develop several millimeters below the marginal ridge. As its base broadens, the spondylophyte is able to reach the edge of the vertebra. Initially it grows straight laterally and anteriorly before turning upward or downward below the anterior longitudinal ligament. Spondylophytes that extend posteriorly from the posterior vertebral margin are relatively rare, in contrast to the more common lateral and anterior spondylophytes. Severe spondylosis deformans can narrow the intervertebral foramen and cause neurological complaints or osteophyte-induced dysphagia (Fig. 5.**196**).

An isolated **accessory bone** can form in the anterior longitudinal ligament as a result of metaplastic bone formation with or without spondylosis deformans (Teichert 1956). An underlying **osteoblastic diathesis** can lead to the formation of **hyperostotic spondylophytes** that give the anterior surface of the cervical spine a "sugar-coated" appearance (Fig. 5.**197**) (see also DISH, Thoracic Spine).

When segmental resiliency has been lost as a result of disk wear, the uncovertebral joint connections are subject to greater stresses leading to uncovertebral arthrosis or **uncovertebral spondylosis**. This condition is marked by broadening, increased density, deformity, and posterolateral elongation of the uncinate processes, affecting the segments C3–C7 (Fig. 5.**198**).

With severe uncovertebral arthrosis, lateral radiographs of the lower cervical spine may show a cleftlike lucent line projected over the vertebral body (Fig. 5.**198**) resulting from a Mach effect (Dihlmann and Dörr 1970) or the uncovertebral joint line projected over the vertebral body (Goldberg et al. 1982). This can simulate a fracture line (**pseudofracture**). Intraosseous vacuum phenomena and pneumatoceles may occur (Fig. 5.**199**).

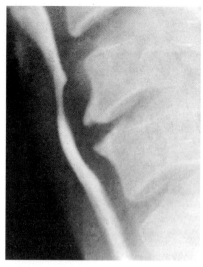

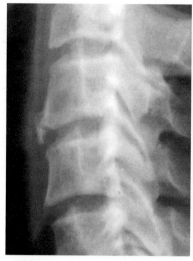

a

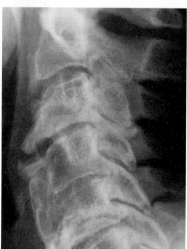

c

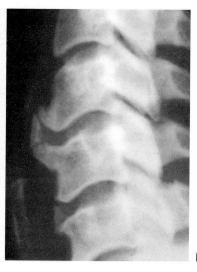

b

Fig. 5.**196** Deviation of the esophagus at the level of anterior osteophytes in C5/C6 intervertebral osteochondrosis. The patient presented clinically with dysphagia.

Fig. 5.**197 a–c** Various degrees of calcification and ossification of the anterior longitudinal ligament.
a Circumscribed metablastic calcification in the anterior longitudinal ligament.
b Accessory bone formation with marginal osteophytes.
c Severe degenerative changes, hyperostotic spondylophytes, and extensive flowing bone outgrowths anterior to the vertebral bodies (DISH syndrome).

The radiographic features of osteoarthritis of the apophyseal joints, or **spondylarthrosis deformans**, are basically the same as in other joints of the body: joint space narrowing, increased density of the subchondral cancellous bone, and marginal osteophytes (Figs. 5.**338**, 5.**376**, 5.**377**). The additional stresses imposed by intervertebral disk narrowing and loss of the shock-absorbing function of the disk promote the development of spondylarthrosis deformans. Osteophytic outgrowths on the articular processes and uncovertebral joints can lead to **narrowing** of the **intervertebral foramina** with radicular symptoms and may also cause **vertebral artery compression** with impairment of blood flow (Elies 1984).

Intervertebral osteochondrosis and **spondylarthrosis** predispose to segmental instabilities with **retrolisthesis** or **pseudospondylolisthesis** (Daburge 1984) (Fig. 5.**200**). Other subaxial **subluxations** can result from **rheumatoid arthritis** and spinal **trauma**.

Stenosis of the **cervical spinal canal** can result from a combination of spondylosis deformans, uncovertebral arthrosis, spondylarthrosis, and ossification of the posterior longitudinal ligament and may be aggravated by pseudo-spondylolisthesis or retrolisthesis secondary to degenerative changes.

Scheuermann disease can affect the cervical vertebrae, producing characteristic changes such as flat and wedged vertebrae, but it is more common in the thoracic and lumbar spine (q.v.). Significant scoliosis of the cervical spine can occasionally lead to frictional sclerosis of the transverse processes between C7 and T1 (Fig. 5.**201**).

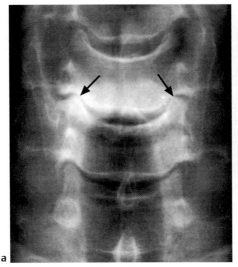
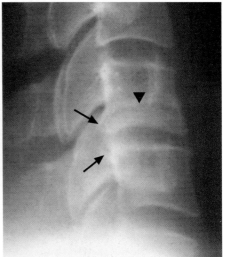

Fig. 5.**198 a–c**   Uncovertebral osteoarthritis.
a AP projection shows elongation of the uncinate processes and increased sclerosis of the uncovertebral joints (arrows).
b Lateral projection shows uncovertebral spondylosis (arrow) and a pseudofracture caused by uncovertebral osteoarthritis (arrowhead).
c The intervertebral foramen has been narrowed by uncovertebral spondylosis (arrow).

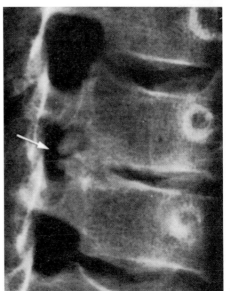

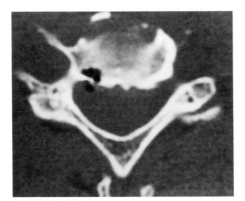

Fig. 5.**199**   Pneumatocele caused by a vacuum effect in uncovertebral osteochondrosis.

Fig. 5.**200**   Retrospondylolisthesis in a patient with interver- ▷
tebral osteochondrosis.

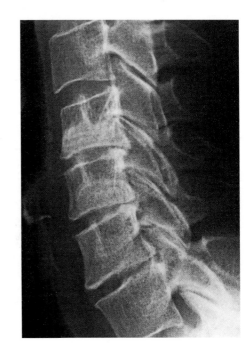

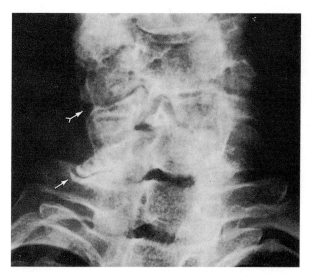

Fig. 5.**201**   Left convex scoliosis of the lower cervical spine with a sclerosis-rimmed pressure erosion and pseudoarticulation between the transverse processes of C7 and T1 (arrow). Calcified laryngeal cartilage (double arrow).

Calcification and Ossification

Ossification of the posterior longitudinal ligament (OPLL) was first described by Tsukimoto (1960) and has an increased incidence in the Japanese population (Op den Orth 1975, Terayama 1989). The disease predominantly affects men in the fifth to seventh decades of life and may be asymptomatic, although encroachment on the spinal canal can produce neurological symptoms (Fig. 5.**202**).

The ossification occurs just posterior to the vertebral bodies, usually at the C3–C5 level. It may extend contiguously over several vertebral bodies or may show a segmental distribution. OPLL can occur in the thoracic or lumbar spine, most commonly affecting T4–T7 and L1–L2. The precise cause of the disease is unknown but is apparently related to diffuse idiopathic skeletal hyperostosis (Resnick et al. 1978, Tsuyama 1984). Simultaneous ossification of the ligamenta flava may occur. OPLL has a characteristic appearance on MR images (Widder 1989, Yamashita et al. 1990).

Calcification of the nuchal ligament has a metaplastic cause and may be found all along the **supraspinous ligament**, especially at the level of the C6 and C7 spinous processes (Fig. 5.**203**). Ossification and bone formation between the spinous processes was discussed under Variants (Figs. 5.**164**, 5.**165**). These calcifications require differentiation from old spinous process fractures and bony avulsions (Figs. 5.**178**–5.**180**) and from ossification of the interspinous ligament (Fig. 5.**204**).

Paraosseous soft-tissue calcifications and ossifications can occur in **myositis ossificans traumatica, postopera-**

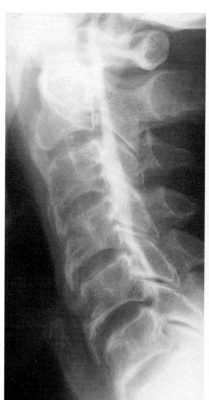

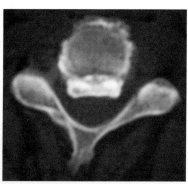

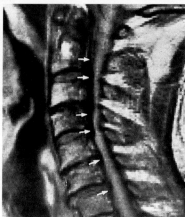

Fig. 5.**202 a–c**   Ossification of the posterior longitudinal ligament.
a Retrovertebral calcifications and ossifications from C2 to C5 in the lateral projection.
b CT appearance of OPLL (**a** and **b** courtesy of D. Resnick, San Diego).
c Retrovertebral signal voids from C2 to C4 with pronounced atrophy of the cervical cord (different case).

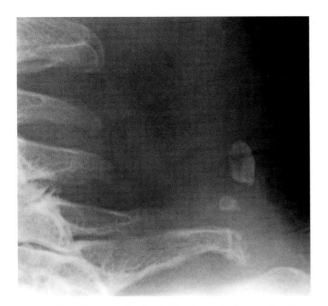

Fig. 5.**203**   Circumscribed calcification of the nuchal ligament.

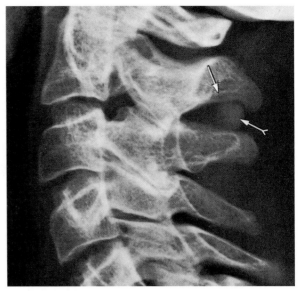

Fig. 5.**204**   Round, hazelnut-size bone between the C2 and C3 spinous processes (arrows).

tively (Fig. 5.**205**), or in the rare **myositis ossificans progressiva** (Fig. 5. **206**) (Arcq 1970, Thickman et al. 1982).

Melorheostosis is characterized by the formation of bony outgrowths that resemble melted wax flowing down a candle (Fig. 5.**207**). Typical streaky sclerotic changes are also found in **Paget disease** of the spine (Fig. 5.**208**).

Diffuse calcifications of the **intervertebral disk** can result from systemic diseases that include the following:

- Alkaptonuria
- Hemochromatosis
- Hyperparathyroidism
- Poliomyelitis
- Acromegaly
- Amyloidosis
- Calcium pyrophosphate dihydrate crystal deposition (pseudogout) (Weinberger and Myers 1978).

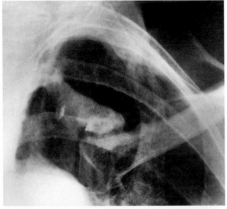

a

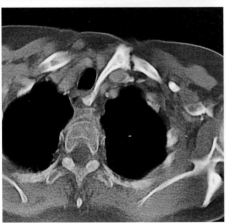

b

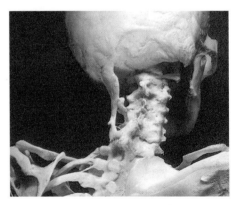

Fig. 5.**206**   Myositis ossificans progressiva with bone formation in the paravertebral muscles along the back of the neck (Museum of Man, San Diego).

◁ Fig. 5.**205 a, b**   Postoperative heterotopic mediastinal bone formation at a former drain site following esophageal resection.
a AP projection. The heterotopic bone formation looks like a skeletal variant (compare with os omovertebrale).
b CT clearly demonstrates heterotopic bone formation at the surgical access site.

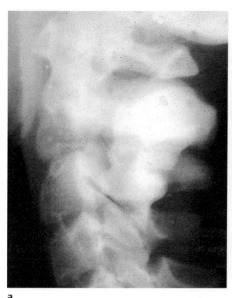
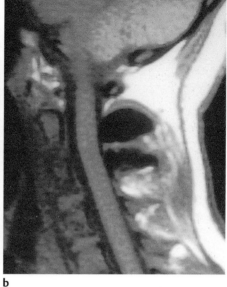

Fig. 5.**207 a, b**   Melorheostosis of the upper cervical spine with flowing ossifications on the C2 and C3 vertebral arches.
a Lateral projection.
b Sagittal T1-weighted MRI demonstrates signal voids within the solid ossifications (observation by D. Resnick, San Diego).

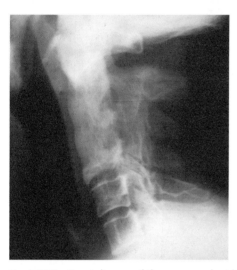

Fig. 5.**208**   Paget disease of the upper and midcervical spine (observation by D. Resnick, San Diego).

Isolated disk calcifications in adults occur as a result of **degenerative processes** and may be located in the anulus fibrosus, nucleus pulposus, and cartilaginous end plates of the vertebral bodies. **Calcifying discitis** has been described as a special form of disk calcification in children and adolescents (Kristensen et al. 1984, Girodias et al. 1991). It occurs predominantly in the cervical spine but is also observed in the thoracic and lumbar spine (Figs. 5.**209**, 5.**210**). The cause of the sudden disk calcifications is unknown but is presumably based on an inflammatory or traumatic etiology (Mainzler 1973, Kristensen et al. 1984).

Approximately 75% of affected children experience clinical complaints in the form of pain, limited motion, and torticollis. Temperature elevation and leukocytosis have been reported.

Radiographs demonstrate single or multiple, flat or elliptical **calcifications** of the **nucleus pulposus**. Rupture of the calcium deposits into the vertebral bodies, intervertebral foramina, spinal canal, or surrounding soft tissues has been observed (Mainzler 1973, Girodias et al. 1991) and can lead to neurological complaints and dysphagia.

The disease has a good overall prognosis. Generally the calcifications regress over a period of weeks or months, but they may also persist (Fig. 5.**211**).

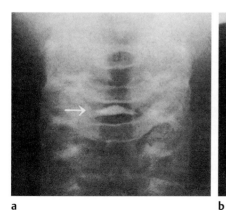
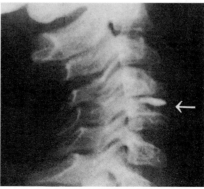

Fig. 5.**209 a, b**   Calcifying discitis of the cervical spine in a child. The dense calcification creates the impression of a vertebra plana (arrow).
a AP projection.
b Lateral projection.

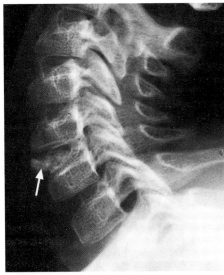

a

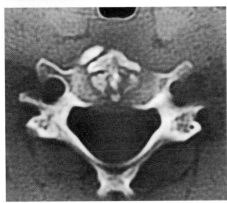

b

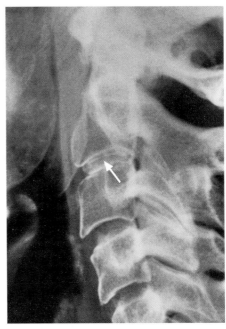

Fig. 5.**211** Complete calcification or ossification of the C2/C3 intervertebral disk (arrow) (observation by Hildebrand, Bad Wildungen).

◁ Fig. 5.**210a, b**   Calcifying discitis at C5/C6.
a Calcifications in the C5/C6 disk space (arrow).
b Calcifications on axial CT.

References

Aaron, S. L., J. D. R. Miller, J. S. Percy: Tophaceous gout in the cervical spine. J. Rheumatol. 11 (1984) 862

Abel, M.S.: The exaggerated supine oblique view of the cervical spine. Skelet. Radiol. 8 (1982) 213

Acheson, M. B., R. R. Livingston, M. L. Richardson et al.: High-resolution CT scanning in the evaluation of cervical spine fractures: Comparison with plain film examinations. Amer. J. Roentgenol. 148 (1987) 1179

Amamilo, S. C.: Fractures of the cervical spine in patients with ankylosing spondylitis. Orthop. Rev. 18 (1989) 339

Anand, A. K., E. Kuchner, R. James: Cervical Diastematomyelia: Uncommon presentation of a rare congenital disorder. Comput. Radiol. 9 (1985) 45–49

Anderson, L. D., B. L. Smith, J. DeTorre et al.: The role of polytomography in the diagnosis and treatment of cervical spine injuries. Clin. Orthop. 165 (1982) 64

Applbaum, G., P. Gerard, D. Bryk: Elongation of the anterior tubercle of a cervical vertebral transverse process: An unusual variant. Skelet. Radiol. 10 (1983) 265–267

Arcq, M.: Ungewöhnliche Lokalisation einer Myositis ossificans traumatica an der Halswirbelsäule. Z. Orthop. 108 (1970) 176–183

Azouz, E. M., J. D. Chan, R. Wee: Spondylosis of the cervical vertebrae. Report of three cases, with a review of the English and French literature. Radiology 111 (1974) 315–318

Baber, W. W., Y. Numaguchi, J. M. Nadell et al.: Eosinophilic granuloma of the cervical spine without vertebrae plana. J. comput Tomogr 11 (1987) 346

Barr, R. J., D. G. Hannon, I. V. Adair et al.: Cervical osteomyelitis after rigid oesophagoscopy: brief report. J. Bone Jt Surg. 70-B (1988) 147

Beck, G.: Ein Fall von echter Spondylolisthesis im Halsteil. Fortschr. Röntgenstr. 136 (1982) 93

Berning, W., J. Freyschmidt: Zur Klinik und Radiologie der Histiozytose X am Skelett – eine retrospektive Studie an 18 Patienten. Röntgenblätter 38 (1985) 400

Black, K. S., M. T. Gorey, B. Seideman et al.: Congenital spondylolisthesis of the 6th cervical vertebra: CT findings. J. Comput. assist. Tomogr. 15 (1991) 335

Boger, D., P. W. Ralls: New traction device for radiography of the lower cervical spine. Amer. J. Roentgenol. 137 (1981) 1202

Bohrer, S. P., Y. M. Chen: Cervical spine annulus vacuum. Skelet. Radiol. 17 (1988) 324

Bohrer, S. P., Y. M. Chen, D. G. Sayers: Cervical spine flexion patterns. Skelet. Radiol. 19 (1990) 521

Bony, M., V. Denaro: The cervical stenosis syndrome with a review of 83 patients treated by operation. Int. Orthop. 6 (1982) 185–195

Broom, M. J., J. F. Raycroft: Complications of fractures of the cervical spine in ankylosing spondylitis. Spine 13 (1988) 763

Brown, M. W., A. W. Templeton, F. J. Hodges III: The incidence of acquired and congenital fusions in the cervical spine. Amer. J. Roentgenol. 92 (1964) 1255

Bywaters, E. G. L.: Rheumatoid and other diseases of the cervical interspinous bursae and changes in the spinous processes. Ann. Rheum. Dis. 41 (1982) 360

Cahill, D. W., L. C. Love, G. R. Rechtine: Pyogenic osteomyelitis of the spine in the elderly. J. Neurosurg. 74 (1991) 878

Cancelmo, J. J. Jr.: Clay shoveler's fracture: a helpful diagnostic sign. Amer. J. Roentgenol. 115 (1972) 540

Cintron, Elsie A., L. A. Gilula, W. A. Murphy, J. A. Gehweiler: The widened disc space: A sign of cervical hyperextension injury. Radiology 141 (1981) 639–644

Crank, R. N., M. Sundaram, J. B. Shields: Cervical actinomycosis with spinal involvement. Case Report 197. Skelet. Radiol. 8 (1982) 164–167

Csákány, G., S. Almós: Echte Spondylolisthese der Halswirbelsäule. Fortschr. Röntgenstr. 91 (1959) 277–280

Daburge, A.: Instabilité dur rachis cervical par arthrose. Rev. Chir. Orthop. 70 (1984) 397–399

Dahlin, D. C., R. A. McLeod: Aneurysmal bone cyst and other non-neoplastic conditions. Skelet. Radiol. 8 (1982) 243

Dahmen, G.: Über die Doppelanlage eines Dornfortsatzes. Z. Orthop. 102 (1967) 621–622

Das De, A.: Intervertebral disc involvement in gout: brief report. J. Bone Jt Surg. 70-B (1988) 671

Dias, L. D. S., H. M. Frost: Osteoblastoma of the spine. A review and report of eight new cases. Clin. Orthop. 91 (1973) 141

Dihlmann, W., W. M. Dörr: Der zervikale Pseudospalt nach D. Schoen bei der Spondylosis uncovertebralis. Spezielle, weniger beachtete Röntgenbefunde am Stütz- und Gleitgewebe. Fortschr. Röntgenstr. 113 (1970) 522–527

Dihlmann, W.: Gelenke, Wirbelverbindungen. Thieme, Stuttgart 1987

Dihlmann, W., G. Friedmann: Die Röntgenkriterien der juvenil-rheumatischen Zervikalsynostose im Erwachsenenalter. Fortschr. Röntgenstr. 126 (1977) 536–541

Dory, M. A.: CT-Demonstration of cervical vertebral erosion by tortuous vertebral artery. Amer. J. Neuroradiol. 6 (1985) 641–642

Dvorak, J., M. Panjabi, M. Gerber, W. Wichmann: CT-functional diagnostics of the rotatory instability of upper cervical spine. Part 1. An experimental study on cadavers. Spine 12 (1987 a) 197

Dvorak, J., J. Hayek, R. Zehnder: CT-functional diagnostics of the rotatory instability of the upper cervical spine. Part 2. An evaluation on healthy adults and patients with suspected instability. Spine 12 (1987 b) 726

Dvorak, J., J. A. Antinnes, M. Panjabi, D. Loustalot, M. Bonomo: Age and gender related normal motion of the cervical spine. Spine 17, Suppl. (1992) 393

Dvorak, J., D. Froehlich, L. Penning, H. Baumgartner, M. M. Panjabi: Functional radiographic diagnosis of the cervical spine: flexion/extension. Spine 13 (1988) 748

Edeiken-Monroe, Beth, L., K. Wagner, J. H. Harris jr.: Hyperextension dislocation of the cervical spine. Amer. J. Neuroradiol. 7 (1986) 135–140

Edwards, M. G., D. Wesolowski, M. T. Benson et al.: Computed tomography of congenital spondylolisthesis of the sixth cervical vertebra. Clin. Imag. 15 (1991) 191

Elies, W.: HWS-bedingte Hör- und Gleichgewichtsstörungen. HNO 32 (1984) 485–493

Esposito, P. W., A. H. Crawford, C. Vogler: Solitary osteochondroma occurring on the transverse process of the lumbar spine. A case report. Spine 10 (1985) 398

Fielding, J. W., H. A. Keim, R. J. Hawkins et al.: Osteoid osteoma of the cervical spine. Clin. Orthop. 128 (1977) 163

Fielding, J. W., S. Ratzan: Osteochondroma of the cervical spine. J. Bone Jt Surg. 55-A (1973) 640

Fishman, E. K., D. Magid, D. R. Ney et al.: Three-dimensional imaging. Radiology 181 (1991) 321

Forsberg, D. A., S. Martinez, J. B. Vogler III et al.: Cervical spondylolysis: Imaging findings in 12 patients. Amer. J. Roentgenol. 154 (1990) 751

Freyschmidt, J.: Skeletterkrankungen. Klinisch-radiologische Diagnose und Differentialdiagnose. Springer, Berlin 1997

Fried, K.: Die zervikale juvenile Osteochondrose (Scheuermannsche Krankheit). Fortschr. Röntgenstr. 105 (1966) 69–77

Friedenberg, Z. B., W. T. Miller: Degenerative disc disease of the cervical spine. J. Bone Jt Surg. 45-A (1963) 1171

Gaizler, Gy.: Das Treppenphänomen an der Halswirbelsäule. Fortschr. Röntgenstr. 114 (1971) 317–322

Gaizler sen. Gy., Gy. Gaizler jun: Fehlen einer Bogenwurzel an der Halswirbelsäule. Fortschr. Röntgenstr. 99 (1963) 421–423

Garcia, A. Jr., S. A. Grantham: Haematogenous pyogenic vertebral osteomyelitis. J. Bone Jt Surg. 42-A (1960) 429

Gehweiler, J. A., R. L. Osborne, R. S. Becker: The Radiology of Vertebral Trauma. Saunders, Philadelphia 1980

Girodias, J.-B., E. M. Azouz, D. Marton: Intervertebral disc space calcification. A report of 51 children with a review of the literature. Pediat. Radiol. 21 (1991) 541

Goldberg, R. P., H. S. Vine, B. A. Sacks et al.: The cervical split: a pseudofracture. Skelet. Radiol. 7 (1982) 267

Goldberg, A. L., W. E. Rothfus, Z. L. Deeb et al.: The impact of magnetic resonance on the diagnostic evaluation of acute cervico-thoracic spinal trauma. Skelet. Radiol. 17 (1988) 89

de Graaf, R.: Congenital blockvertebrac C2–C3 in patients with cervical myelopathy. Acta Neurochir. 61 (1982) 111–162

Green, J. D., T. S. Harle, J. H. Harris: Anterior subluxation of the cervical spine: hyperflexion sprain. Amer. J. Neuroradiol. 2 (1981) 243

Grifka, J., A. Hedtmann, H. G. Pape, H. Witte, H. F. Bär: Beschleunigungsverletzung der Halswirbelsäule. Orthopäde 27 (1998) 802

Guldberg, R. P., H. S. Vine, B. A. Sacks, H. P. Ellison: The cervical split: A pseudofracture. Skelet. Radiol. 7 (1982) 267–272

Harris, J. H. Jr., J. W. Yeakley: Hyperextension-dislocation of the cervical spine: ligament injuries demonstrated by magnetic resonance imaging. J. Bone Jt Surg. 74-B (1992) 567

Heeren, I. G.: Horizontale Spaltbildung im Wirbelkörperdornfortsatz. Röntgenpraxis 15 (1943) 18

Holland, C., W. Stolle: Fehlbildungen der Wirbelbogenreihe. Fortschr. Röntgenstr. 112 (1970) 120–121

Isu, T., K. Miyasaka, Y. Iwasaki, T. Ito, M. Tsuru, H. Takei, S. Abe: Computed tomographic findings of vacuum phenomenon in cervical intervertebral discs. Surg. Neurol. 19 (1983) 528–531

Jäger, H. J., A. Schmitz-Stolbrink, K. D. Mathias: Cervical diastematomyelia and syringohydromyelia in a myelomeningocele patient. Europ. Radiol. 7 (1997) 477

Johnson, S., T. Klostermeier, A. Weinstein: Case report 768. Skelet. Radiol. 22 (1993) 1993

Kann, S., T. Matsubayashi: Symptomatic cervical spondylolysis. Neuroradiology 37 (1995) 559

Kamieth, H.: Röntgenfunktionsdiagnostik der Halswirbelsäule. Hippokrates, Stuttgart 1986

Kattan, K. R., M. Joyce Pais: Some borderlands of the cervical spine. Part I: The normal (and nearly normal) that may appear pathologic. Skelet. Radiol. 8 (1982 a) 1–6

Kattan, K. R., M. Joyce Pais: Some borderlands of the cervical spine. Part II: The subtile and the hidden abnormal. Skelet. Radiol. 8 (1982 b) 7–12

Kerns, S., T. L. Pope Jr., E. E. de Lange, R. E. Fechner, T. E. Keats, C. Cimmino: Annulus fibrosus calcification in the cervical spine: radiologic-pathologic correlation. Skelet. Radiol 15 (1986) 605

Killebrew, K., R. H. Gold, S. D. Sholkoff: Psoriatic spondylitis. Radiology 108 (1973) 9

Kjaer, I., B. Fischer-Hansen: Cervical ribs in fetuses with Ullrich-Turner syndrome [see comments]. Amer. J. med. Genet. 71 (1997) 219

Klippel, M., A. Feil: Anomalie de la colonne vertébrale par absence des vertèbres cervicales, cage thoracique remontant jusqu'á la du crâne. Bull. mém. Soc. Anat. (Paris) 87 (1912) 185–188

Kristensen, S., A. Juul, K. Larsen, Vivian Bertelsen: Cervical intervertebral disc classification in childhood. Arch. Oto-Rhino-Laryngol. 240 (1984) 239–242

Kühne, K.: Die Vererbung der Variationen der menschlichen Wirbelsäule. Z. Morph. Anthropol. 35 (1936) 1

LaMasters, D. L., R. H. Dorwart: High-Resolution, cross-sectional computed tomography of the normal spine. Orthop. Clin. N. Amer. 16 (1985) 359–379

Lapayowker, M. S.: An unusual variant of cervical spine. Amer. J. Roentgenol. 83 (1960) 656–659

Laredo, J.-D., D. Reizine, M. Bard et al.: Vertebral hemangiomas: radiologic evaluation. Radiology 161 (1986) 183

Lestini, W. F., S. W. Wiesel: The pathogenesis of cervical spondylosis. Clin. Orthop. 239 (1989) 69

Levine, A. M., S. Boriani, M. Donati, M. Campanacci: Benign tumors of the cervical spine. Spine 17 (1992) 399

Levine, R. S., G. K. Geremia, Th. W. McNeill: CT demonstration of cervical diastematomyelia. J. Comput. Assist. Tomogr. 9 (1985) 592–594

Lissner, J.: Spondylolisthese der Halwirbelsäule. Fortschr. Röntgenstr. 84 (1956) 626–628

Lloyd, T. V., J. C. Johnson: Infectious cervical spondylitis following traumatic endotracheal intubation. Spine 5 (1980) 478

Lukoschek, M., F. U. Niethard: Komplette Synostosierung der Halswirbelsäule im jugendlichen Alter. Ein bisher unveröffentlichtes Krankheitsbild. Z. Orthop. 133 (1995) 120

Mainzer, F.: Herniation of the nucleus pulposus. A rare complication of intervertebral-disc calcification in children. Radiology 107 (1973) 167–170

Maldonado-Cocco, J. A., S. Babini, O. Garcia-Morteo: Clinical features of ankylosing spondylitis in women and men and its relationship with age of onset. J. Rheumatol. 12 (1985) 179

Manaster, B. J., A. G. Osborn: CT patterns of facet fracture dislocations in the thoracolumbar region. Amer. J. Roentgenol. 148 (1987) 335

Marcelis, S., F. C. Seragani, J. A. M. Taylor et al.: Reevaluation of oblique radiography of the cervical spine: Comparison of 45 degree and 55 degree anteroposterior oblique projections. Radiology 253 (1993) 188

McCall, I., W. Park, T. McSweeney: The radiological demonstration of acute lower cervical injury. Clin. Radiol. 24 (1973) 235

McRae, D. L.: The significance of abnormalities of the cervical spine. Amer. J. Roentgenol. 84 (1960) 3

Mirvis, S. E., A. L. Wolf: MRI of acute cervical spine trauma. Appl. Radiol. 12 (1992) 15

Moilanen, A., U. Yli-Kerrtula, A. Vilppula: Cervical spine involvements in Reiter's syndrome. Fortschr. Röntgenstr 141 (1984) 84

Monu, J., S. P. Bohrer, G. Howard: Some upper cervical spine norms. Spine 12 (1987) 515

Morgan, D. F., R. F. Young: Spinal neurological complications of achondroplasia. J. Neurosurg. 52 (1980) 463

Muhle, C., J. Wiskirchen, D. Weinert, A. Falliner, F. Wesner, G. Brinkmann: Biomechanical aspects of the subarachnoid space and cervical cord inhealthy individuals examined with kinematic magnetic resonance imaging. Spine 23 (1998a) 556

Muhle, C., L. Bischoff, D. Weiner, V. Lindner, A. Falliner, C. Maier: Exacerbated pain in cervical radiculopathy at axial rotation, flexion, extension, and coupled motions of the cervical spine. Invest. Radiol. 33 (1998b) 279

Muhle, C., J. Metzner, D. Weinert, A. Falliner, G. Brinkmann, M. H. Mehdorn: Classification system based on kinematic MR imaging in cervical spondylitic myelopathy. Amer. J. Roentgenol. 19 (1998c) 1763

Muhle, C., J. Metzner, D. Weinert, R. Schön, E. Rautenberg, A. Falliner: Kinematic MR imaging in surgical management of cervical disc disease, spondylosis and spondylotic myelopathy. Acta radiol. 40 (1999) 146

Olivieri, I., D. Trippi, G. Gemignani et al.: Ossification of the posterior longitudinal ligament in ankylosing spondylitis. Arthr. and Rheum. 31 (1988) 452

Op den Orth, J. O.: Seltene, miteinander artikulierende Knochenfortsätze an den unteren zervikalen Wirbeln. Fortschr. Röntgenstr. 111 (1969) 684–687

Op den Orth, J. O.: Verkalkung bzw. Verknöcherung des Lig. longitudinale posterius der Halswirbelsäule. Fortschr. Röntgenstr. 122 (1975) 442–687

Orzincolo, C., P. L. Bedani, P. N. Scutellari et al.: Destructive spondyloarthropathy and radiographic follow-up in hemodialysis patients. Skelet. Radiol. 19 (1990) 483

Overton, L. M., J. W. Grossmann: Anatomical variations in the articulation between the second and third vertebrae. J. Bone Jt Surg. 34-A (1952) 155–161

Panjabi, M. M., J. Cholewicki, K. Nibu, J. N. Grauer, L. B. Babat, J. Dvorak: Biomechanik ds Beschleunigungstrauma. Orthopäde 27 (1998) 813

Pathria, M. N., C. A. Petersilge: Spinal trauma. Radiol. Clin. N. Amer. 29 (1991) 847

Penning, L.: Functional Pathology of the Cervical Spine. Radiographic Studies of Function and Dysfunction in Congenital Disorders, Cervical Spondyloses and Injuries. Excerpta Medica, Amsterdam 1968 (p. 41)

Penning, L.: Functioneel Roentgenonderzoek Bij Degenerative en Traumatische Afwijkingen der Laag-Cervicale Bewegingsegmenten (Thesis). The Netherlands, University of Groningen 1960

Penning, L., J. T. Wilmink: Rotation of the cervical spine. A CT study in normal subjects. Spine 12 (1986) 732

Penning, L.: Normal movements of the cervical spine. Amer. J. Roentgenol. 130 (1978) 317–326

Penning, L.: The Cervical Spine. Excerpta Medica, Amsterdam 1965

Peris, P., M. A. Brancs, J. Gratacs et al.: Septic arthritis of spinal apophyseal joint. Report of two cases and review of the literature. Spine 17 (1992) 1514

Pickern, F.: Verlängerte Proc. costotransversarii am 2. HWK. Fortschr. Röntgenstr. 79 (1953) 777

Pinckney, L. E., G. Currarino, C. L. Highgenboten: Osteomyelitis of the cervical spine following dental extraction. Radiology 135 (1980) 335

Prasad, V. S., R. L. Sengar, B. P. Sahu, D. Immaneni D.: Diastematomyelia in adults. Modern imaging and operative treatment. Clin. Imag. 19 (1995) 270

Preuss, H. J.: Ergänzende Bemerkungen zu „seltenen, miteinander artikulierenden Knochenfortsätzen an den zervikalen Wirbeln". Fortschr. Röntgenstr. 114 (1974) 323–327

Prusick, V. C., L. C. Samberg, D. P. Wesolowski: Klippel-Feil Syndrome associated with spinal stenosis. J. Bone Jt Surg. 67-A (1985) 161–164

Rao, S., K. Badani, D. Orth, T. Schildhauer, M. Borges: Metastatic malignancy of the cervical spine. Spine 17 (1992) 407

Rauber/Kopsch: Bewegungsapparat, Bd. 1. Hrsg. von Tillmann, B., G. Töndury. In Rauber/Kopsch. Anatomie des Menschen. Lehrbuch und Atlas, 2. Aufl. Hrsg. Leonhardt, H., B. Tillmann, G. Töndury, K. Zilles. Thieme, Stuttgart 1998

Redlund-Johnell, Inga: Subaxial caudal dislocation of the cervical spine in rheumatoid arthritis. Neuroradiology 26 (1984) 407–410

Reinhard, K.: Isolierter Querfortsatz am ersten Brustwirbel. Fortschr. Röntgenstr. 88 (1958) 624

Reinhardt, K.: Eine ungewöhnliche Anomalie an den Dornfortsätzen des 5., 6. und 7. Halswirbels. Fortschr. Röntgenstr. 85 (1956) 253–255

Resnick, Ch. S.: Cervical spine involvement in sternoclavicular hyperostosis. Spine 10 (1985) 846–848

Resnick, D.: Degenerative diseases of the vertebral column. Radiology 156 (1985) 3

Resnick, D.: Diagnosis of Bone and Joint Disorders, 3rd ed. Saunders, Philadelphia 1995.

Resnick, D., I. L. Dwosh, T. G. Goergen et al.: Clinical and radiographic abnormalities in ankylosing spondylitis: a comparison of men and women. Radiology 119 (1976) 293

Resnick, D., J. Guerra, Ch. A. Robinson, V. C. Vint: Association of diffuse idiopathic skeletal hyperostosis (DISH) and calcification and ossification of the posterior longitudinal ligament. Amer. J. Roentgenol. 131 (1978) 1049–1053

Robert, H., J. Dubousset, L. Miladi: Histiocytosis X in the juvenile spine. Spine 12 (1987) 167

Rodiek, S. O.: Computertomographische Untersuchungen bei zervikaler spinaler Stenose. Fortschr. Röntgenstr. 139 (1983) 383–389

Rogers, L. F.: Radiology of Skeletal Trauma. Churchill Livingston, New York 1992

Ross, E.: Die Varianten des Verschiebungsphänomens an der Halswirbelsäule. Fortschr. Röntgenstr. 100 (1964a) 242–253

Ross, E.: Verschiebungsphänomen und Wirbelblockierung an der Hals- und Lendenwirbelsäule. Fortschr. Röntgenstr. 100 (1964b) 367–382

Roy-Camille, R., M. Thibierge, J. Metzger: Exploration d'une lacune de l'axis chez une patiente cervicalgique. Nouv. Presse Med. 11 (1982) 453–454

Sanjay, B. K. S., F. H. Sim, K. K. Unni et al.: Giant-cell tumours of the spine. J. Bone Jt Surg. 75-B (1993) 148

Scher, A., V. Vambeck: An approach to the radiological examination of the cervicodorsal junction following injury. Clin. Radiol. 28 (1977) 243

Scher, A. T.: Radiographic indicators of traumatic cervical spine instability. S. Afr. med. J. 62 (1982) 562–565

Schilling, F., M. Schacherl, A. Bopp, A. Gampp, J. P. Haas: Veränderungen der Halswirbelsäule (Spondylitis cervicalis) bei der chronischen Polyarthritis und bei der Spondylitis ankylopoetica. Radiologe 3 (1963) 484

Schmitt, H. G., P. Wisser: Die Schipperkrankheit beim Jugendlichen. Langenbecks Arch. klin. Chir. 268 (1951) 333

Schmitt, W. G. H., H. C. Rücker: Langzeitbeobachtungen an der jugendlichen Meta- und Apophyse des Dornfortsatzes des 1. Brustwirbels (Schmittsche Krankheit). Fortschr. Röntgenstr. 131 (1979) 623

Schneider, R. C., E. A. Kahn: Chronic neurological sequelae of acute trauma to the spine and spinal cord. Part I. The significance of the acute flexion or „tear drop" fracture dislocation of the cervical spine. J. Bone Jt Surg. 38 (1956) 985–997

Schwartz, A. M., R. J. Wechsler, M. D. Landy, St. M. Wetzner, Susan A. Goldstein: Posterior arch defects of the cervical spine. Skelet. Radiol. 8 (1982) 135–139

Seibert-Deikert, F. M.: Über eine halbseitige Dornfortsatzhyperplasie des 5. Halswirbels, verbunden mit einer persistierenden Apophyse des 7. Halswirbels. Fortschr. Röntgenstr. 122 (1975) 366–377

Sgalitzer, M.: Roentgenographic diagnosis of vertebral syphilis. Radiology 37 (1941) 75–78

Sgalitzer, M.: Zur Röntgendiagnostik der destruktiven Wirbelsäulensyphilis. Wien. klin. Wschr. 72 (1960) 714–719

Sicard, J. A., J. Lermoyez: II. Formes frustes, évolutive, familiale du syndrome de Klippel-Feil. Rev. neurol. 39 (1923) 71

Smith, G. R., M. S. Abel, L. Cone: Visualization of the posterolateral elements of the upper cervical vertebrae in the anteroposterior projection. Radiology 115 (1975) 219

Spencer, D. G., W. M. Park, H. M. Dick, S. N. Papazoglu, W. Watson Buchanan: Radiological manifestations in 200 patients with ankylosing spondylitis. Correlations with clinical features and HLA B27. J. Rheumat. 6 (1979) 305–315

Streitwieser, D. R., R. Knopp, L. R. Wales et al.: Accuracy of standard radiographic views in detecting cervical spine fractures. Ann. Emerg. Med. 12 (1983) 538

Teichert, G.: Schaltknochen der Zwischenwirbelscheiben und Spondylosis deformans. Fortschr. Röntgenstr. 84 (1956) 457–462

Terayama, K.: Genetic studies on ossification of the posterior longitudinal ligament of the spine. Spine 14 (1989) 1184

Thickman, D., A. Bonakdar-Pour, M. Clancy, J. van Orden, H. Steel: Fibrodysplasia ossificans progressiva. Amer. J. Roentgenol. 139 (1982) 935

Tredwell, St. J., D. F. Smith, P. J. MacLeod, Betty J. Wood: Cervical spine anomalies in fetal alcohol syndrome. Spine 7 (1982) 331–334

Tsukimoto, H.: An autopsy report of syndrome of compression of spinal cord owing to ossification within spinal canal of cervical spine. Arch. jap. Chir 29 (1960) 1003

Tsuyama, N.: Ossification of the posterior longitudinal ligament of the spine. Clin. Orthop. 184 (1984) 71

Wackenheim, A.: Chirolumbar dysostosis and constitutional narrowness of the cervical spinal canal. Skelet. Radiol. 14 (1985) 47–52

Wanke, R.: Scalenussyndrom und Hals-Brust-Übergangswirbel. Langenbecks Arch. klin. Chir. 189 (1937) 512

Weinberger, A., A. R. Myers: Intervertebral disc calcification in adults: a review. Semin. Arthr. Rheum. 8 (1978) 1978

Wendtland, K.: Halsrippen am 5. und 6. Halswirbelkörper. Fortschr. Röntgenstr. 105 (1966) 121–122

Werne, S.: The possibilities of movement in the craniovertebral joints. Acta orthop. scand. 28 (1959) 165–173

Whalen, J. P., C. L. Woodruff: The cervical prevertebral fat stripe. A new aid in evaluating the cervical prevertebral soft tissue space. Amer. J. Roentgenol. 109 (1970) 445–451

Widder, D. J.: MR imaging of ossification of the posterior longitudinal ligament. Amer. J. Roentgenol. 153 (1989) 194

Winter, R. B., J. H. Moe, J. E. Lonstein: The incidence of Klippel-Feil syndrome in patients with congenital scoliosis and kyphosis. Spine 9 (1984) 363–366

Wolf, B. S., M. Khilmani, L. Malis: The sagittal diameter of the bony cervical spinal and its significance in cervical spondylosis. Mt. Sinai J. Med. (NY) 23 (1956) 283

Wolf, R. F., J. P. Klein: Complete bipartition of the atlas in the Klippel-Feil syndrome. A radiologically illustrated case report. Surg. radiol. Anat. 19 (1997) 339

Wurtz, R., Z. Quader, D. Simon et al.: Cervical tuberculous vertebral osteomyelitis: case report and discussion of the literature. Clin. infect. Dis. 16 (1993) 806

Yamashita, Y., M. Takahashi, Y. Matsuno et al.: Spinal cord compression due to ossification of ligaments: MR imaging. Radiology 175 (1990) 843

Yetkin, Z., Anne G. Osborne, D. S. Gallis, V. M. Haughton: Uncovertebral and facet joint dislocation in cervical articular pillar fractures. CT Evaluation. Amer. J. Neuroradiol. 6 (1985) 633–637

Yousefzadeh, D. K., G. Y. El-Khoury, W. L. Smith: Normal sagittal diameter and variation in the pediatric cervical spine. Radiology 144 (1982) 319–325

Thoracic Spine

Normal Findings

During Growth

The embryological development of the thoracic vertebral bodies was reviewed in the introductory section. As noted in the section on the cervical spine, the ossification centers of the vertebral arches remain unfused during the **first year of life** (Figs. 5.**129**–5.**131**, 5.**212**).

The ossification centers in the vertebral bodies have reached the anterior and posterior surfaces of the vertebral bodies by the time the child is born. As in the cervical spine, the neurocentral synchondroses (the epiphyses of the vertebral arch) remain visible until at least the third year of life (Figs. 5.**131**, 5.**264**, 5.**265**).

The vertebral bodies are initially egg-shaped in the newborn. As remnants of the intersegmental clefts in the embryonic spine, notches are present in the anterior and posterior margins of the vertebral bodies. They appear on radiographs as bandlike transverse lucencies at the center of the vertebral bodies and often remain visible after the first year of life (Fig. 5.**213**). They represent nutrient canals ("Hahn clefts") through which arterial and venous vascular bundles enter and exit the vertebra (Figs. 5.**213**, 5.**217**).

By the first and second years of life, the vertebral bodies gradually develop a rectangular shape with rounded edges. On lateral radiographs, the ringlike **cartilaginous marginal ridge** of the end plates produces a steplike indentation at the corners of the vertebral body (Fig. 5.**214**).

Between the 10th and 12th years, **ossification centers** develop in the cartilaginous marginal ridges, appearing triangular or disk-shaped on lateral radiographs (Fig. 5.**215**).

The ossified apophyseal ring may appear on AP and lateral radiographs as a continuous linear density along the vertebral body end plates (Fig. 5.**216**). The opposing surface of the vertebral body is lined by radial ridges that reinforce the attachment of the apophyseal ring. The ossified ridges fuse with the rest of the vertebral body by the 24th year.

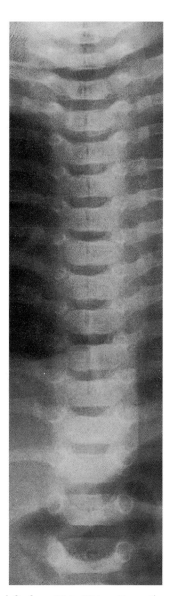

Fig. 5.**212**   Vertebral arch clefts from T1 to T9 in a 6-month-old boy.

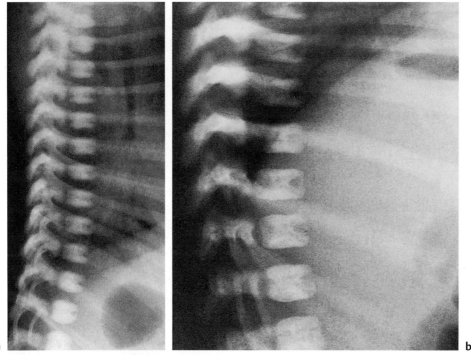

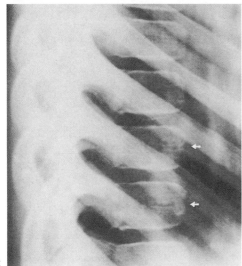

Fig. 5.**213 a–c**   Special features of pediatric thoracic vertebral bodies.

a Vertebral bodies in a 3-month-old infant are egg-shaped with the narrow end forward.

b Vertebral bodies of a 3-month-old infant show distinct notches in their anterior and posterior margins where vessels enter and leave the vertebrae.

c Anterior nutrient canals (arrows) are a normal finding in children.

Fig. 5.**214a, b**   Ossification of thoracic vertebral bodies at different ages.
a Five years: steps at the anterior corners of the thoracic vertebrae.
b Seven years: steps at the anterior corners of the lumbar vertebrae. Note the beveled anteroinferior corner of T11.

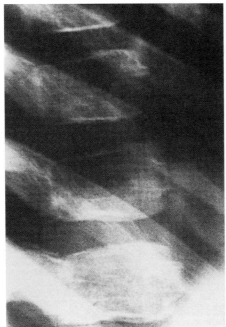

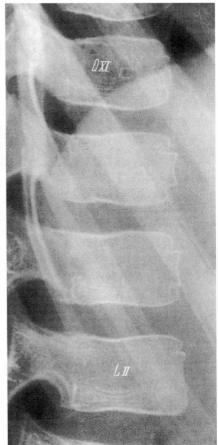

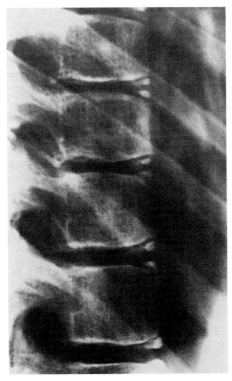

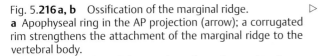

Fig. 5.**215**   Triangular or disk-shaped ossification centers in the marginal ridge cartilage form steplike features in the anterior corners of the vertebral bodies.

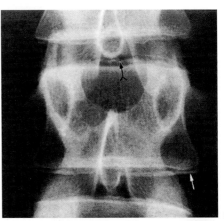

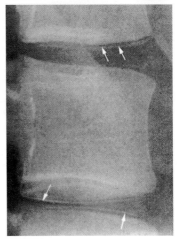

Fig. 5.**216a, b**   Ossification of the marginal ridge.   ▷
a Apophyseal ring in the AP projection (arrow); a corrugated rim strengthens the attachment of the marginal ridge to the vertebral body.
b Partial ossification of the apophyseal ring (arrows) in the lateral projection.

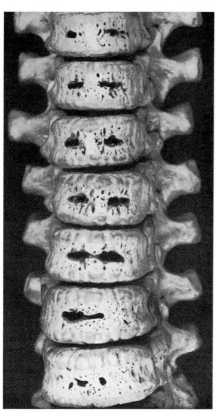

 In Adulthood

The thoracic vertebrae gradually increase in size from above downward and are connected by intervertebral disks approximately 5 mm in height. The vertebral bodies have roughly equal sagittal and transverse dimensions (Fig. 5.**218**) and, like the intervertebral disk spaces, show a slight degree of anterior wedging.

The **physiological wedging** of the thoracic vertebrae is most pronounced at the T8 and T11–T12 levels (Lauridsen et al. 1984). The anterior height of the thoracic vertebral body is 1–2 mm less than its posterior height (Maiman and Pintar 1992). This height discrepancy may be as much as 20% in normal individuals (Lauridsen et al. 1984). The anterior, posterior, and lateral surfaces of the vertebral bodies are slightly concave. The concavity is greatest on the posterior aspect where blood vessels enter the vertebral body (Fig. 5.**219**).

◁ Fig. 5.**217**   Nutrient canals (Hahn clefts) in the juvenile spine. Note the corrugation of the vertebral body margins.

Fig. 5.**218 a, b**   Anatomy of a thoracic vertebra. (From Rauber and Kopsch 1998.)
a Lateral aspect. The arrows indicate the superior and inferior vertebral notches.
b Superior aspect.
▽

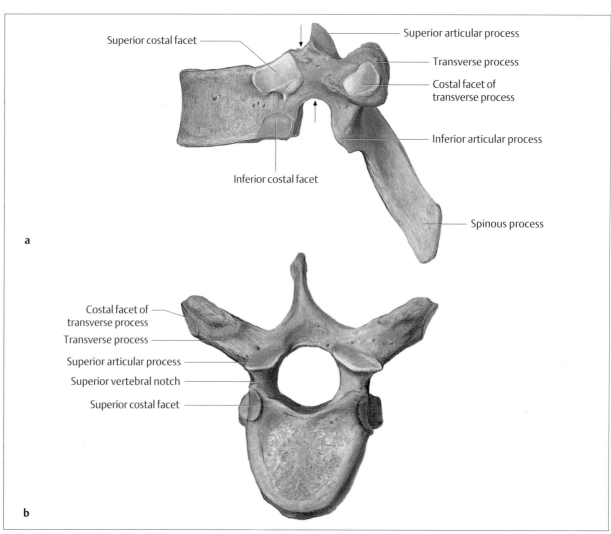

Superior costal facet

Superior articular process

Transverse process

Costal facet of transverse process

Inferior articular process

Inferior costal facet

Spinous process

a

Costal facet of transverse process

Transverse process

Superior articular process

Superior vertebral notch

Superior costal facet

b

The pedicles extend almost straight back from the vertebral body. The intervertebral foramina are elliptical in shape and open laterally. The articular facets, and thus the joint spaces, are oriented almost on the frontal plane. The transverse processes are posterior to the articular processes and bear costal facets from T1 through T10. The spinous processes are nearly horizontal in the upper thoracic spine, while in the midthoracic spine they slant backward and downward and overlap like the shingles on a roof. The spinous processes in the lower thoracic spine are again directed more horizontally and are shorter than those at higher levels.

The T1 vertebra resembles C7 in its high lateral margins and very long spinous process. The T12 vertebra, by contrast, resembles a lumbar vertebra in the placement of its articular processes and the shape of its vertebral foramen.

The ribs articulate with the thoracic vertebrae close to the pedicles (costovertebral joints) and, except for the 11th and 12th ribs, also articulate with the transverse processes (costotransverse joints). The heads of the ribs (except for the 1st, 11th, and 12th) each articulate with two vertebrae and the intervertebral disk between them. This pattern of articulations may or may not hold for the 10th rib.

In the **AP projection**, the vertebral bodies and disk spaces are clearly defined in the mid- and lower thoracic spine but are less well defined in the upper thoracic spine due to its kyphotic curvature. The pedicles are seen in an "end-on" projection, appearing as round or elliptical structures. The distance between the medial contours of the pedicles, the **interpedicular distance**, equals the width of the spinal canal. This width increases in the craniocaudal direction (Hinck et al. 1966).

> As a rule of thumb, the interpedicular distance should approximately equal the sum of the widths of both pedicles (Wackenheim 1985).

The **transverse processes** and **costotransverse joints** are generally well defined despite their superimposed position on radiographs. An **AP radiograph** of T9–T10 gives a clear projection of the costotransverse joints. If the more cranial segments are not defined with sufficient clarity, the central ray aimed at T6 can be angled 39–40° cephalad to provide a better view (Hohmann and Gasteiger 1970). The posterior elements, especially the laminae and articular processes, are difficult to analyze in the AP view, which gives an almost end-on projection of the **spinous processes** of T1, T11, and T12. The tips of the spinous processes of the remaining vertebrae are projected over the underlying vertebral bodies. Often the spinous processes are directed obliquely and deviate from the midline.

In the **lateral projection**, it can be difficult to define and evaluate the cervicothoracic junction. The upper three or four thoracic vertebrae are superimposed by the shoulder girdle. The thoracic vertebral bodies and disk spaces show a slight anterior wedging that contributes to the physiological kyphosis of the thoracic spine. The anterior and posterior margins of the vertebral bodies show a slight concavity that is most distinct posteriorly (Fig. 5.**219**). These features are remnants of the Hahn clefts, where blood vessels enter or leave the posterior aspect of the vertebral body (Fig. 5.**219**). CT can define the venous channels that run through the vertebral body. With their sclerotic edges and typical bifurcation patterns, there should be no danger of mistaking these lucencies for a frac-

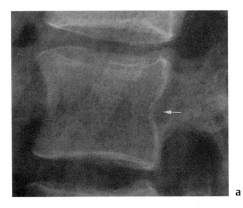

a

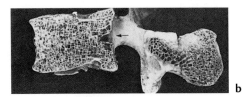

b

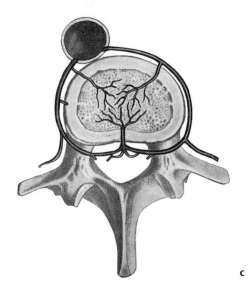

c

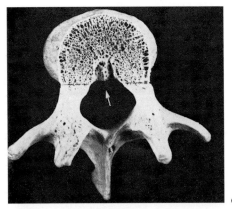

d

Fig. 5.**219 a–d** Vascular entry and exit sites in the vertebral bodies.
a Site of vascular entry at the posterior vertebral margin, lateral projection.
b Site of vascular entry at the posterior vertebral margin, sagittal section of a specimen.
c Diagram showing the vascular supply of a vertebral body.
d Site of vascular entry at the posterior vertebral margin, cross section through a specimen.

ture (Fig. 5.**219**). For the most part, the pedicles and intervertebral foramina are clearly defined despite the superimposed ribs. The facet joints are slanted in an anterosuperior-to-posteroinferior direction, forming an angle of 20–25° with the longitudinal axis of the thoracic spine. Because the articular facets are almost in the frontal plane, as noted above, the joint spaces are usually well defined.

> When obscured by superimposed ribs and lung, the facet joints can be defined more clearly by rotating the spine slightly. The posterior portions of the vertebral arch cannot be evaluated in the lateral projection, and the spinous processes are usually difficult to define. As a result, the sagittal diameter of the thoracic spinal canal cannot be reliably determined.

The jugular notch of the sternal manubrium superimposed on an upper thoracic vertebra in the **AP projection** can mimic a vertebral compression fracture (Fig. 5.**220**). The absence of a spinous process on the apparently compressed vertebra helps to identify the artifact. A similar phenomenon can be produced by superimposition of the manubriosternal synchondrosis, simulating a horizontal cleft in an upper thoracic vertebra (Fig. 2.**221**).

In the **lateral projection** the glenoid cavity can mimic a wedged vertebra (Fig. 5.**222**) (Schmitt 1938). The **scapular angle** can often produce irregular summation effects at the level of the T7 vertebral body (Fig. 5.**223**).

The vertebral end plates that border the nucleus pulposus may develop depressions surrounded by fine, curvilinear, sclerotic densities (Fig. 5.**224**). Schmorl nodes may develop in this area.

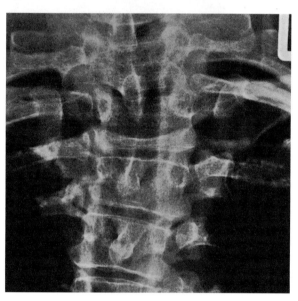

Fig. 5.**220**   The superimposed upper border of the manubrium sterni mimics a compression fracture of the T2 vertebral body.

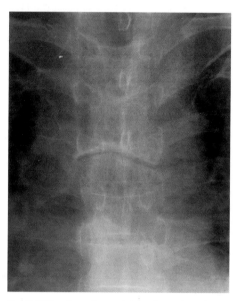

Fig. 5.**221**   Superimposition of synchondrosis manubriosternalis and an upper thoracic vertebra simulating horizontal vertebral cleft.

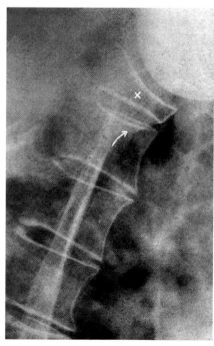

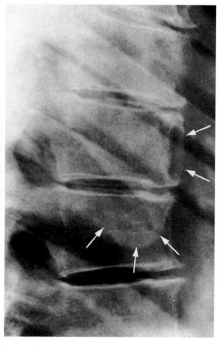

Fig. 5.**222**

Fig. 5.**223**

Fig. 5.**222**   The superimposed glenoid and scapular border (arrow) mimic a wedged thoracic vertebra (×) (observation by Schmitt, Worms).

Fig. 5.**223**   The interior angle of the scapula is superimposed over the T7 vertebral body, and its medial border is projected anterior to the T6 vertebral body.

Rudimentary ribs on the T12 vertebra may be missed in the lateral projection, causing an error in the numbering of the thoracic vertebral bodies.

Posture and Range of Motion

In the embryo, the spine follows a simple kyphotic curve that is almost completely straight at birth. In children 8 to 16 years of age, thoracic kyphosis is least pronounced in the 10th through 12th years and increases with growth, showing a somewhat different pattern in girls and boys (Willner and Johnson 1983).

In girls, a correlation exists between body height and the frequency of scoliosis and kyphosis. The incidence of both deformities is significantly higher in taller girls (Skogland et al. 1985).

In 80% of adults, radiographs of the cervicothoracic junction show a mild degree of left convex scoliosis that is most pronounced at the T3 and T5 levels.

Textbooks and manuals of orthopedics and radiology may be consulted for details on techniques for measuring scoliosis, kyphosis, and lordosis (Schinz 1986, Hellinger 1955). The most commonly used methods are reviewed in Figs. 5.**225**–5.**229**.

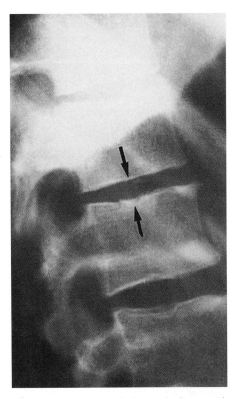

Fig. 5.**224** Pressure-bearing zones of the end plates with sclerotic changes (arrows).

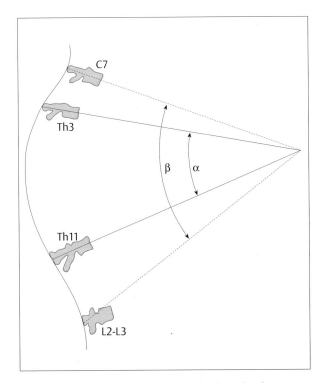

Fig. 5.**225** Measurement of thoracic kyphosis by the Neugebauer method (after Hellinger).
α T3/T11 kyphosis angle (normal = 25°)
β C7/L2–L3 kyphosis angle (normal = 40°)

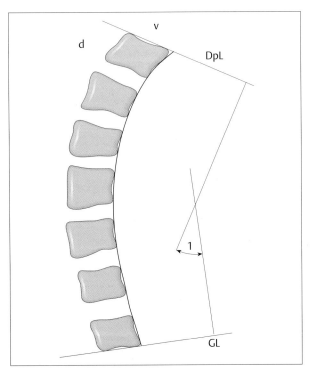

Fig. 5.**226** Measurement of thoracic kyphosis (after Hellinger). Normal angle = 20–40°.
1   Kyphosis angle
d   Dorsal
Dpl Line through upper end plate
GL   Line through lower end plate
v   Ventral

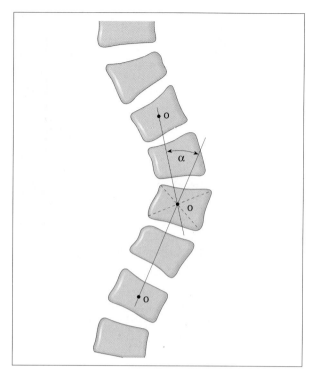

Fig. 5.**227**   Measurement of scoliosis by the Ferguson method (after Hellinger).

o   Center of vertebral body
Lines   Lines connecting the vertebral body centers
– – –   Diagonals inside the vertebral body
α   Ferguson angle

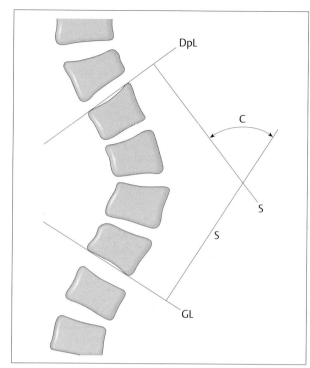

Fig. 5.**228**   Measurement of scoliosis by the Cobb method (after Hellinger).
C   Cobb angle
DpL Line through upper end plate
GL   Line through lower end plate
S   Perpendicular

The Cobb method is simpler than the Ferguson measurement but is less accurate (Neugebauer 1972). The Ferguson method is preferred in children, because the still-cartilaginous end plates can be difficult to define on radiographs.

The **range of motion** of the thoracic spine in flexion, extension, rotation, and sidebending is small in relation to its length. **Functional views** of the thoracic spine are important only in the treatment of scoliosis. Sidebending views give information on the ability of the spine to compensate for the deformity. The same applies to backbending views of the thoracic spine, which can be used to evaluate extension of the kyphotic spine. White and Panjabi (1978) may be consulted for more detailed information on the mobility of specific segments.

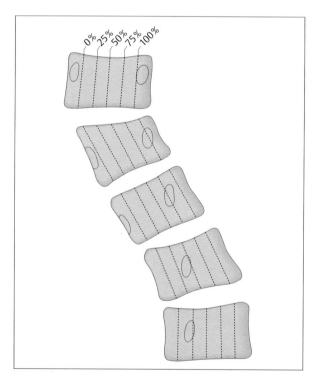

Fig. 5.**229**   Determination of vertebral rotation by the method of Nash and Moe. This method evaluates the relationship of the pedicle shadows to the percentage zones.

Pathological Finding?

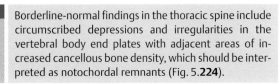

Normal Variant or Anomaly?

Variants

> Borderline-normal findings in the thoracic spine include circumscribed depressions and irregularities in the vertebral body end plates with adjacent areas of increased cancellous bone density, which should be interpreted as notochordal remnants (Fig. 5.**224**).

The normally elliptical pedicles in the lower thoracic spine occasionally show a reniform outline with a slight flattening or concavity on the medial side. This **thinning of the pedicles** at the thoracolumbar junction is found in approximately 7% of the population (Benzian et al. 1971). The interpedicular distance remains constant due to an absence of appositional bone growth on the inner surface of the vertebral arches after childhood. The interpedicular distance is slightly greater in men than in women (Fischer 1970).

> When thinned pedicles are noted in the presence of a normal interpedicular distance, it should not be assumed that an intraspinal mass is present.

Accessory diarthrosis is the term applied to extremely rare supernumerary vertebral articulations in the thoracolumbar region located at the level of L1. They result from anomalous development of the mamillary process (Figs. 5.**263** and 5.**291**) (Ricci 1964).

In patients with a cranial or caudal shift of vertebral segmentation at the thoracolumbar junction, the ribs of the two lowest thoracic vertebrae may be underdeveloped or there may be accessory rudimentary ribs on the first lumbar vertebra. These variants may show an asymmetrical arrangement (Fig. 5.**230**).

Because of the frequent accompanying shift in other regional boundaries of the spinal column in these cases, the only way to assign a precise number to transitional vertebrae in the thoracolumbar region in questionable cases is to radiograph the spine up to the cranial level and count downward from C1. Possible variants are shown schematically in Fig. 5.**231**.

Caudal shifts have been found in association with several other anomalies:

- Esophageal atresia with or without tracheoesophageal fistulae (Stevenson 1972, Hodson and Shaw 1973)
- Anal atresia
- Hirschsprung disease (Melham and Fahl 1985)

Conversely, associated spinal anomalies were found in nearly 40% of 94 patients with anal atresia (Denton 1982). Most of these anomalies involved the sacrococcygeal region but some involved the thoracic spine, including one case found to have 14 pairs of ribs.

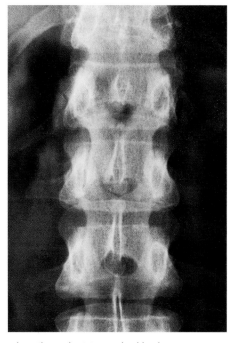

Fig. 5.**230** Lumbar rib on the L1 vertebral body.

Anomalies and Deformities

In **newborns**, it is more common to find a morphological anomaly in the form of a mild **wedge-shaped deformity at the thoracolumbar junction**, usually at L1 or L2 (Fig. 5.**232**).

This developmental deficiency, which usually has a favorable prognosis, is thought to result from mechanical stresses acting at the vertex of the flexed embryo. It is especially pronounced in certain congenital systemic diseases, where a postnatal disturbance of enchondral growth can make the deformity more severe (Swoboda 1950, Seyss 1951, 1968, Swischuk 1970).

> **Typical vertebral body anomalies**
> ➤ Vertebral body clefts
> ➤ Vertebral body defects
> ➤ Synostosis of two or more vertebrae

Vertebral body clefts (somatic clefts) can occur in the sagittal or coronal plane. A **complete sagittal cleft** is very rare and usually is not compatible with life. **Partial sagittal clefts** most commonly affect the anterior and posterior aspects of the vertebral body. They presumably result from a notochord anomaly during early embryonic development. A **persistent notochord** separates the halves of the vertebral body from each other, in which case the anterior or posterior cleft communicates with a persistent chordal canal (Diethelm 1974).

The typical **butterfly vertebra** is visible on AP radiographs (Figs. 5.**233**, 5.**234**). The hemivertebrae narrow toward the unfused center, resembling two cones that have been placed apex to apex (Fig. 5. **235**).

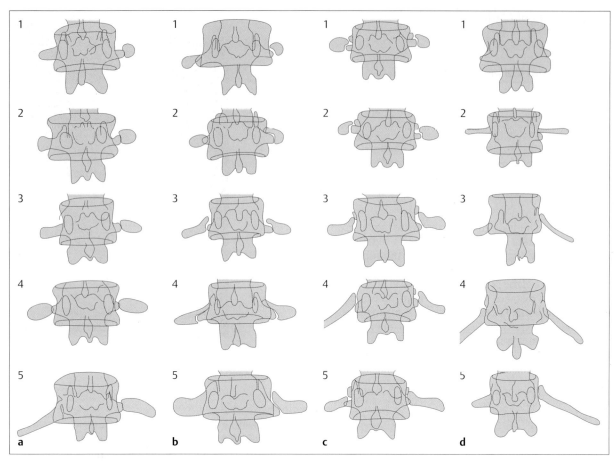

Fig. 5.**231 a–d**   Variable appearance of lumbar ribs (after Schertlein).

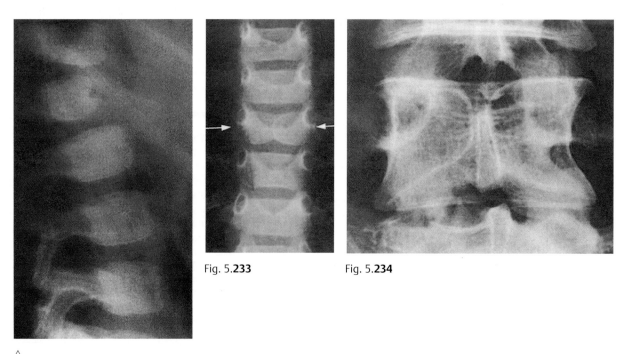

△
Fig. 5.**232**   Wedge-shaped deformity
of the L1 vertebral body in a small
child with associated kyphosis.

Fig. 5.**233**   Butterfly vertebra in a one-year-old child (arrows).

Fig. 5.**234**   Butterfly vertebra in a 23-year-old man.

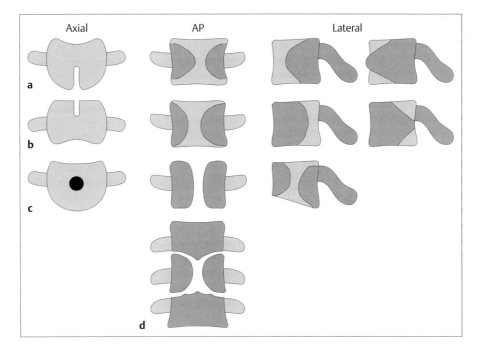

Fig. 5.**235 a–d**   Radiographic projections of various vertebral body anomalies.
a Sagittal cleft with an anterior defect = butterfly vertebra.
b Sagittal cleft with a posterior defect. Butterfly vertebra with a dorsal cleft.
c Persistent chordal canal.
d Butterfly vertebra with scalloping of the adjacent vertebrae.

The lateral borders of the butterfly vertebra may extend past the sides of the adjacent vertebrae. Adaptive changes may be evident in the adjacent vertebrae, as the opposing end plates adapt their shape to the deformity of the dysplastic vertebra (van den Bos et al. 1984).

A **persistent chordal canal** is based on a failure of normal notochord regression with the formation of fibrocartilage in its place, producing features very similar to the partial sagittal vertebral clefts described above (Diethelm 1974).

Coronal clefts in the vertebral bodies are extremely rare. They are detectable on lateral radiographs and CT scans (Brocher 1980). Coronal cleft vertebrae are often wedge-shaped with corresponding kyphotic deformity. Differentiation is required from traumatic deformities and osteolytic lesions of the vertebral body.

Two main types of **vertebral body defects** are recognized:

- Vertebral body aplasia
- Partial vertebral body defects

Vertebral body aplasia, in which the chondral and/or ossification centers of the vertebral body are absent (asoma), is extremely rare (Rathke 1977).

Partial vertebral body defects are fairly common and present as posterior, anterior, or lateral hemivertebrae. To avoid confusion with acquired wedging, developmental anomalies of this kind should be referred to as **hemivertebrae** rather than wedged vertebra. **Hemisoma** (half of a vertebral body with a complete vertebral arch) is distinguished from **hemispondylus** (half of a vertebral body with half of an arch) (Fig. 5.**236**).

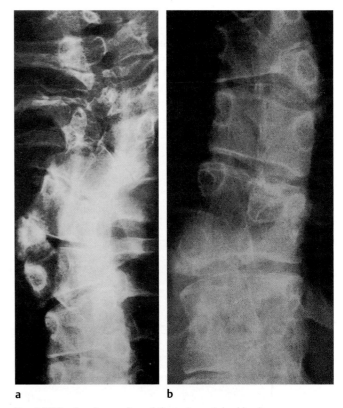

Fig. 5.**236 a, b**   Anomalies of thoracic vertebral bodies.
a Butterfly deformity of several upper thoracic vertebrae with a T7 hemivertebra (displaced toward the right side).
b Fused T9 hemivertebra on the left side, fused T12 hemivertebra on the right side.

In other cases one or more quadrants may be missing from the vertebral body, resulting in a one-quarter or three-quarter vertebra. The pathogenesis of hemivertebrae may be based on a **hemimetameric segmentation anomaly** that occurs during the precartilaginous stage. In this anomaly the primitive vertebral halves skip a segment and fuse in an incorrect order, often resulting in the irregular blocking of vertebrae (Fig. 5.**237**).

The definitive form of the anomaly cannot be evaluated until skeletal growth is complete. Vertebral rudiments may still appear rectangular during childhood but later may assume a wedge shape in response to physiological loading (Brocher 1936). While **lateral hemivertebrae** result in scoliosis, **posterior hemivertebrae** lead to kyphotic deformity. Anterior hemivertebrae with a defect in the posterior vertebral body are much less common.

Angular kyphosis secondary to a posterior wedged vertebra requires **differentiation** from an inflammatory (tuberculous) process, osteolytic skeletal metastases, posttraumatic vertebral wedging, and spondyloepiphyseal dysplasias. Posterior hemivertebrae are characteristically shortened in the sagittal dimension.

Lateral hemivertebrae are among the most common spinal anomalies and may be single or multiple. They occur predominantly in the thoracic and lumbar spine. The lateral hemivertebra always has a rib anlage, which is frequently hypoplastic and fused to adjacent ribs. Usually the hemivertebra also possesses a hemiarch, recognized by the elliptical outline of its pedicle (Fig. 5.**238**).

All hemivertebrae may show a partial or complete synostosis with adjacent vertebral bodies (Fig. 5.**236b**). Frequently the height of adjacent vertebral bodies is increased to compensate for the faulty statics.

Fusions of adjacent vertebrae (**block vertebrae**) were discussed in the section on the mid- and lower cervical spine. The blocking may be complete, with small but intact intervertebral foramina, or various types of partial blocking may occur:

Types of partial blocking
➤ Fusion of the anterior or posterior third of the vertebral body
➤ Fusion of the entire vertebral body
➤ Fusion limited to the posterior and central portions of the neural arch

Block vertebrae may coexist with other anomalies. The more pronounced the blocking, the higher its correlation with other abnormalities. Meanwhile, more severe anomalies have a higher association with block vertebrae and vertebral synostoses (Fig. 5.**239**) (Diethelm 1974).

According to Reeder (1993), segmentation anomalies of the vertebral bodies are commonly encountered in the following malformations and syndromes:

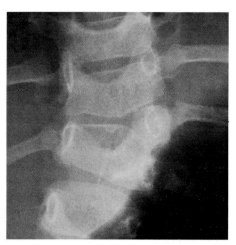

Fig. 5.**238** T11 hemivertebra. The vertebral arch and rib are present on the left side.

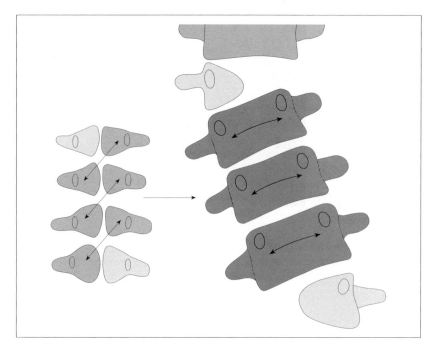

Fig. 5.**237** Pathogenesis of a hemimetameric segmentation anomaly, in which the primitive vertebral halves skip one segment and fuse together in the incorrect order. This leaves one lateral, wedge-shaped hemivertebra above and below the anomalously fused segments (after Dihlmann).

- Chondrodysplasia punctata (Conradi disease)
- Diastematomyelia
- Klippel–Feil syndrome
- Myelomeningocele

Progressive, noninfectious anterior vertebral fusion is considered a special form of vertebral blocking. It usually affects multiple vertebrae in the region of the thoracolumbar junction and is based on the fusion of the anterior thirds of the vertebral bodies. In newborns it produces kyphosis with anterior loss of intervertebral disk height and leads to progressive kyphotic blocking that may span up to five vertebral bodies (Knutsson 1949). It is probably caused by a congenital dysplasia of the affected intervertebral disks (Christensen et al. 1973) (Fig. 5.**240**). Another potential cause is thalidomide embryopathy (Smith et al. 1986).

Fig. 5.**239** Multiple spinal anomalies in a 19-year-old woman. ▷
AP projection of the thoracic spine shows underdevelopment of the first rib on each side, a T4 hemivertebra on the right side, blocking of T5 and T6, deformities at T7 and T8, and a butterfly vertebra at T9.

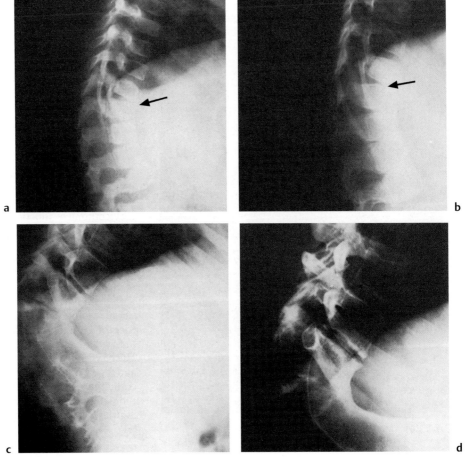

Fig. 5.**240 a–d** Progressive noninfectious vertebral fusion (arrows). (From Christensen et al. 1973.)
a November 1951.
b February 1951.
c November 1964.
d February 1973.

Vertebral arch clefts, especially in the last two thoracic vertebrae, are usually vertical midline clefts (Fig. 5.**241**) but may also involve the pars interarticularis (Probst 1957, Tomsick et al. 1974). They can cause mild, nonspecific pain or may be clinically asymptomatic and are occasionally detected in abdominal CT examinations. **Aplasia** of the **spinous processes** in the lower thoracic spine has also been described (Schulze and Gulbin 1965).

Diastematomyelia was described briefly in the section on cervical anomalies. This congenital longitudinal diastasis of the spinal cord may be associated with other vertebral anomalies, particularly neural arch clefts as well as myelodysplasias and vertebral body abnormalities (Goldberg et al. 1984). It most commonly occurs in the lumbar spine (Mathieu et al. 1982, Marchini et al. 1983, Han Jong et al. 1985) and is discussed under that heading. The same applies to dysrhaphism, clefts and other anomalies of the vertebral arch, and anomalies of the arch processes.

Spondylocostal dysplasia is a severe dysplasia of the thoracic spine that is analogous to the Klippel–Feil anomaly of the cervical spine. The changes often extend to the upper lumbar spine and include multiple anomalies of the vertebral bodies and arches and numerous rib anomalies with shortening and deformity of the thorax. The disease may occur in isolation or in the setting of malformation syndromes (Kozlowski 1984). Numerous **systemic skeletal malformations** lead to a variety of spinal deformities that commonly affect the thoracic vertebral bodies. All grades of dysplasia may be encountered ranging from early forms of elliptical vertebrae to **flat vertebrae**. The interested reader can find more information in the *Atlas of Con-*

stitutional Disorders by Spranger et al. (1974). The paper by Kozlowski (1974) on platyspondyly in childhood may also be of interest.

Fracture, Subluxation, or Dislocation?

The discussion of spinal injuries in this section applies equally to the lumbar spine including the thoracolumbar junction, because the mechanisms of injury and fracture patterns are very similar and follow the same AO classification scheme (Magerl et al. 1994). A comprehensive review of all forms of vertebral trauma and associated injuries would exceed the scope of this book. Details can be found in textbooks and monographs (e.g., Rogers 1992).

The thoracolumbar junction is affected by trauma more frequently than any other spinal region. Fractures of the thoracic spine are rare, aside from compression fractures secondary to osteoporosis. Only about 30% of all thoracic vertebral fractures occur above T10 (Maiman and Pintar 1992). Because the thoracic spine is integrated into the thoracic cage and has relatively limited mobility, large forces are necessary to fracture the thoracic vertebral bodies. This fact, plus the relatively small width of the spinal canal, account for the relatively high incidence of neurological complications that are associated with fractures of the thoracic spine (El-Khoury and Whitten 1993).

The radiographic evaluation of thoracic spinal injuries is challenging, especially at the cervicothoracic junction, because of the numerous superimposed structures in the **lateral projection**. The value of the **swimmer's view** was mentioned in the section on the cervical spine. The **AP projection**, then, is of primary value in the analysis of this region. It should be noted that the jugular notch of the sternal manubrium can simulate a compression fracture in the AP projection when it is superimposed over an upper thoracic vertebra (Fig. 5.**220**). The absence of a spinous process on the apparent compressed vertebra helps to identify the artifact in these cases. In the lateral view, diagnostic errors can result from an orthograde projection of the glenoid cavity of the shoulder, which resembles a wedged vertebra (Fig. 5.**222**) (Schmitt 1938). Additionally, the scapular angle can produce misleading summation effects at the level of the T7 vertebral body (Fig. 5.**223**).

CT is the best modality for diagnosing unstable spinal injuries and detecting involvement of the middle and posterior columns. Small compression wedge fractures do not require further CT evaluation, but scans should be obtained if the fracture has caused more than a 50% decrease in vertebral body height. Streak artifacts in the area of the cervicothoracic junction can limit CT evaluation of the spine (Pathria and Petersilge 1991). CT also has limitations in the diagnosis of transverse fractures (Chance fractures) and the detection of posterior element disruptions in flexion-distraction injuries (Taylor and Eggli 1988). Two-dimensional reformatted images are recommended for evaluating these kinds of injury. The value of three-dimensional reconstructions is controversial (Zinreich et al. 1990, Saeed et al. 1994). It is clear, however, that 3-D images have major value in detecting rotational malalignment to distinguish type C fractures in the AO classification from type A and type B injuries. **MRI** is useful for the diagnosis of spinal cord injuries, ruptures of the anterior and posterior longitudinal ligaments (Kliewer et al. 1993), intervertebral disk injuries, and radiographically occult bony lesions (Fig. 5.**174**).

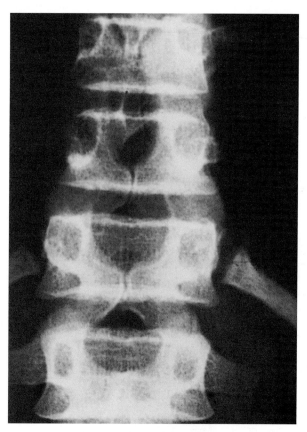

Fig. 5.**241** Median neural arch clefts at T11 and T12.

Of the many systems that have been devised for classifying injuries of the thoracic and lumbar spine, those of Denis (1983), Ferguson and Allen (1984), and McAfee et al. (1983) are the most widely used. These classification systems are based on the **three-column model**:

- The anterior column consists of the anterior longitudinal ligament, the anterior two-thirds of the vertebral body, and the anterior portion of the anulus fibrosus.
- The middle column consists of the posterior third of the vertebral body and anulus fibrosus and of the posterior longitudinal ligament.
- The posterior column contains the vertebral arch including the articular processes, apophyseal joint capsule, and the supra- and interspinous ligaments.

The middle column is critical for spinal stability. Isolated injuries of the anterior or posterior column are inherently stable, whereas the concomitant involvement of an element in the middle column leads to instability.

The **AO classification** of thoracolumbar spinal injuries is based on the mechanism of the injury, common morphological features, and prognostic aspects and also on the two-column biomechanical model of the spine developed by Whitesides et al. (1977) (Magerl 1994). Three main fracture types are distinguished in the ASIF classification:

- Vertebral body compression injuries (type A)
- Distraction injuries (type B)
- Rotational injuries (type C) (Fig. 5.**242**)

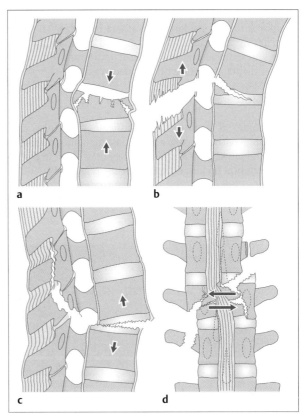

Fig. 5.**242 a–d**   AO classification of fractures of the thoracic and lumbar spine (after Magerl).
a Type A: compression fractures.
b Type B: distraction injury with posterior disruption.
c Type B: distraction injury with anterior disruption.
d Type C: rotatory injury.

AO classification of fractures of the thoracic and lumbar spine

➤ *Type A:* Vertebral body compression
  – *A1:* impacted fracture (end plate depression)
  – *A2:* coronal split fracture
  – *A3:* incomplete burst fracture
➤ *Type B:* Injury of the anterior and posterior elements with distraction
  – *B1:* flexion–distraction (posterior disruption through the joints)
  – *B2:* posterior disruption through the vertebral arch
  – *B3:* hyperextension–shear injury (anterior disruption through the intervertebral disk)
➤ *Type C:* Injury of the anterior and posterior vertebral elements with rotation
  – *C1:* type A with rotation
  – *C2:* type B with rotation
  – *C3:* rotation-shear injury

Vertebral body compression injuries (type A) are caused by axial compression and are often combined with flexion, resulting in a compression wedge fracture, for example. Minor wedge fractures of the thoracic spine may be difficult to distinguish from mild physiological wedging of a thoracic vertebra (see In Adulthood). When axial trauma is inflicted in the neutral position, the primary effect is a concave depression of the vertebral end plate (usually upper) combined with a decrease in intervertebral disk height. A greater traumatizing force can drive the disk into the vertebral body, causing it to split apart (burst fracture). If the axial loading is combined with flexion, a "teardrop fragment" may be broken from the anterior margin of the vertebral body (see Midcervical and Lower Cervical Spine, Fig. 5.**175**).

Injuries of the anterior and posterior elements with distraction (type B) most commonly affect the thoracolumbar junction. Whiplash injuries are caused by flexion and distraction forces that can damage the posterior ligaments (inter- and supraspinous ligaments), disrupt the apophyseal joints and neural arches, and even disrupt the posterior vertebral margin or intervertebral disks. A horizontal fracture of the neural arch and vertebral body caused by this mechanism is called a **Chance fracture** after the author who first described it (Fig. 5.**243**) (Chance 1948, Rogers 1971, Dehner 1971).

This type of injury usually occurs at the level of the L1–L2 vertebral bodies in adults but tends to affect the midthoracic spine in children (Rogers 1971, Taylor and Eggli 1988). **Hyperextension-shear injuries** seldom affect the thoracolumbar region of the spine. These injuries involve a transverse rupture of the intervertebral disk with variable posterior extension and may include fractures of the pars interarticularis and articular processes. Severe cases are marked by anteroposterior displacement or fracture-dislocation and neurological involvement.

Injuries of the anterior and posterior elements with rotation (type C) cause the most serious damage. They occur in conjunction with depressed fractures, split fractures, burst fractures, and flexion and hyperextension injuries. It can be difficult to appreciate the rotatory component on plain radiographs and CT scans. Three-dimensional reconstructions are advantageous in these cases

(Saeed et al. 1994). Distraction injuries with a rotatory component are considered extremely unstable. They are consistently associated with unilateral or bilateral fractures and dislocations of the facet joints and lateral or sagittal displacements with encroachment on the spinal canal (Manaster and Osborn 1987). Rotational shear fractures (C3) represent the highest grade of unstable spinal injuries.

Pathological fractures are insufficiency fractures that occur when pathologically altered bone becomes unable to withstand physiological stresses. They may occur in one or more vertebral bodies at the same time (Fig. 5.**244**).

Reeder (1993) lists the following **frequent causes** for the **pathological fracture of a single vertebral body:**

- Eosinophilic granuloma (histiocytosis X)
- Hemangioma
- Hyperparathyroidism
- Brown tumor
- Lymphoma
- Leukemia
- Metastases
- Multiple myeloma
- Plasmacytoma
- Osteomyelitis
- Osteoporosis
- Paget disease
- Steroid therapy
- Cushing syndrome

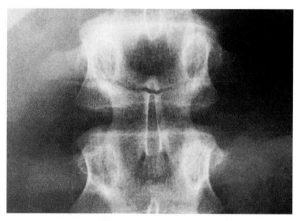

a

Fig. 5.**243 a, b** Chance fracture.
a Flexion-distraction fracture of L1.
b Corresponding injury with pedicular involvement in a lateral tomogram (different case).

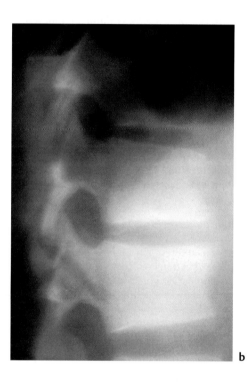

b

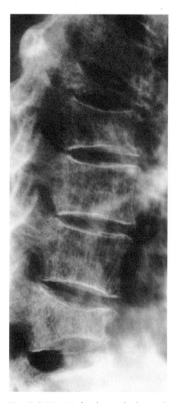

Fig. 5.**244** Multiple pathological vertebral fractures in a patient with multiple myeloma.

Less frequent causes include:

- Amyloidosis
- Primary benign and malignant spinal tumors
- Osteomalacia
- Sarcoidosis
- Scheuermann disease
- Kümmell–Verneuil disease

The following are the most likely causes of **pathological fractures in multiple vertebral bodies** (Reeder 1993):

- Primary and secondary hyperparathyroidism
- Metastases
- Multiple myeloma
- Neuropathy (e.g., diabetic, syphilitic)
- Osteomalacia
- Osteomyelitis
- Osteoporosis
- Scheuermann disease
- Sickle cell anemia and other anemias
- Steroid therapy
- Cushing disease

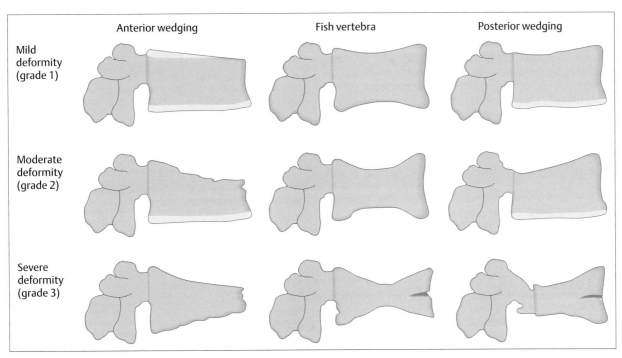

	Anterior wedging	Fish vertebra	Posterior wedging
Mild deformity (grade 1)			
Moderate deformity (grade 2)			
Severe deformity (grade 3)			

Fig. 5.**245** Semiquantitative method of grading vertebral body deformities (after Genant et al.).

Grade 1 Decrease in height $< 20\%$
Grade 2 Decrease in height 20–40%
Grade 3 Decrease in height $> 40\%$

Less frequent causes include:

- Amyloidosis
- Gaucher disease
- Non-Hodgkin lymphoma
- Leukemias
- Paget disease
- Rheumatoid arthritis

Osteoporotic fractures of varying degree are common incidental findings in evaluations of the thoracic spine (Melton et al. 1989). Whereas **wedged vertebrae** develop in the thoracic spine, **fish vertebrae** tend to occur in the lumbar spine. The degree of vertebral body deformity can be graded on a semiquantitative scale as mild ($< 20\%$), moderate (20–40%), or severe ($> 40\%$) (Genant et al. 1993) (Fig. 5.**245**) or determined quantitatively by vertebral morphometry (Black et al. 1995).

It is common to find increased kyphosis, which can occasionally lead to **age-related blocking** and, through pressure necrosis of the anterior disk, to a **senile kyphotic block vertebra** (Fig. 5.**246**).

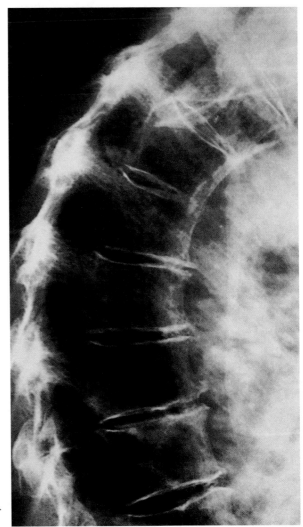

Fig. 5.**246** Senile kyphotic partial block vertebrae at the ▷ midthoracic level.

Often it is very difficult to distinguish osteoporotic collapse from pathological fractures due to neoplasia. Radiographs usually do not reveal tumor-associated destruction of bony trabeculae because they are obscured by compressed bone substance. Fractures in bone weakened by osteoporosis or osteomalacia are less common in the upper thoracic spine, however. A paravertebral soft-tissue mass also suggests a neoplastic process, although it may have an inflammatory cause.

A **special form** of pathological fracture occurs in **ankylosing spondylitis** (Thorngren et al. 1981), whose traumatic complications usually involve the cervical region and occasionally the thoracic and lumbar spine (see Midcervical and Lower Cervical Spine, Fig. 5.**176**). **Vertebra plana** and its etiology were discussed in the section on the subaxial cervical spine (Fig. 5.**191**), and the statements made there are also valid for the other vertebrae.

 ## Necrosis?

Kümmell–Verneuil Disease

First described by Kümmell in 1891, Kümmell–Verneuil disease refers to the delayed posttraumatic collapse of a vertebral body (Brower and Downey 1981). Initially the disease was attributed to traumatic, vasomotor, and neurological causes (Brower and Downey 1981). Today it is generally agreed that the pathogenesis is based on osteonecrosis of the vertebral body (Maldague et al. 1979, Brower and Downey 1981, Malghem et al. 1993). It is thought that a traumatic event leads to an **ischemic episode** that results in **osteonecrosis** and delayed ischemic collapse of the affected vertebral body (Maldague et al. 1978).

It is common in these cases to find a vacuum phenomenon at the center of the vertebral body or along the end plates, which is most pronounced when traction is placed on the spine. Intervertebral gas collections, principally nitrogen, can be clearly demonstrated by **CT** (Malghem et al. 1993). On **MRI**, the intravertebral vacuum cleft shows a high T2-weighted signal intensity suggestive of fluid within the cleft (Naul et al. 1989, Malghem et al. 1993). The horizontal zone of high signal intensity within the vertebral body is considered to be specific for osteonecrosis.

In children, it is important to exclude **eosinophilic granuloma** as the cause of a collapsed vertebral body.

It should be added that the intravertebral vacuum phenomenon is found almost exclusively in association with **nonneoplastic** lesions of the vertebral bodies (Resnick et al. 1981, Malghem et al. 1993).

Steroid-Induced Osteonecrosis

Necrosis of the vertebral bodies can also occur as a complication of corticosteroid therapy (Maldague et al. 1978, 1979). As in Kümmell–Verneuil disease, intravertebral vacuum phenomena can be found as evidence of osteonecrosis (Maldague et al. 1978, 1979, Lemaire et al. 1983, Modena et al. 1985) (Fig. 5.**247**).

Scheuermann Disease

Scheuermann disease (adolescent kyphosis) is discussed below under Other Changes.

 ## Inflammation?

The thoracic spine is the second most common site of involvement by **bacterial infections** (spondylitis, spondylodiscitis) after the lumbar spine (Garcia and Grantham 1960). Hence these infections are discussed under Lumbar Spine. This also applies to **tuberculous spondylitis**, which most commonly affects the L1 vertebral body (Hodgson 1975). The sections on the cervical spine and especially the lumbar spine should be consulted for general information on spinal inflammatory diseases.

In children it is important to differentiate progressive noninfectious anterior vertebral fusion from infectious fusions (see Anomalies and Deformities, Fig. 5.**240**) (Knutsson 1949, Christensen et al. 1973, Smith et al. 1986).

Involvement of the thoracic spine by **rheumatoid arthritis** is known to occur (Heywood and Meyers 1986, Redlund-Johnell and Larsson 1993) but, in contrast to ankylosing spondylitis, psoriatic arthritis, and Reiter syndrome, it is rare. Rheumatoid arthritis of the thoracic spine is manifested by disk space narrowing and subchondral end plate irregularities with erosions and sclerosis. Similar changes take place in the intervertebral and costovertebral joints.

Ankylosing spondylitis generally starts in the sacroiliac joint area and often produces early changes at the lumbosacral and thoracolumbar junctions. From there it spreads cephalad with passage of time. Isolated involvement of the thoracic spine with no sacroiliac joint changes is unusual (Cheatum 1976). Early changes in the thoracic spine are more difficult to detect than the typical accompanying lesions of the sacroiliac joints (Mau et al. 1990). Ankylosing spondylitis of the thoracic spine produces changes at the discovertebral junctions, the intervertebral and costovertebral joints, and the attachments of the posterior ligaments (Figs. 5.**248**, 5.**249**).

A special feature in the thoracic spine is **involvement of the costotransverse joints**. These changes are difficult to detect on plain films. Sectional imaging studies show typical inflammatory erosions of the subchondral bone, sclerotic changes, and sites of partial or complete **ankylosis**. When ankylosis is present, it is common to find associated thickening and sclerosis of the adjacent ribs (Huang et al. 1993). Because these capsular and ligamen-

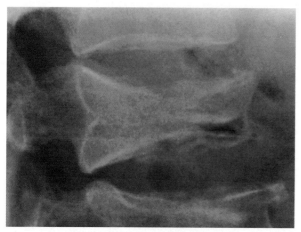

Fig. 5.**247** Intervertebral vacuum phenomenon.

tous ossifications can also occur in degenerative arthritis, the presence of syndesmophytes should be a criterion for the diagnosis of ankylosing spondylitis (Fig. 5.**249**). Less common manifestations are erosions of the articular surfaces, generally starting at T1–T2 and T10–T12. A typical clinical feature of ankylosing spondylitis is a potentially severe **thoracic kyphosis**, but this signifies a late stage of the disease.

Psoriatic arthritis, **Reiter syndrome**, and **enteropathic spondylarthropathie**s are discussed in the section on the lumbar spine.

 ## Tumor?

Bone tumors and tumorlike lesions of the spine are discussed in the section on the lumbar spine. Tumors are not known to have a special affinity for the thoracic spine except for hemangiomas, and statements made about the lumbar spine apply with equal validity to the thoracic spine.

 ## Other Changes?

Common characteristics of diseases of the thoracic and lumbar spine are discussed in the section on the lumbar spine. Here we shall focus on a few findings that are typical of the thoracic spine.

Degenerative diseases of the thoracic spine are less important than in the cervical and lumbar regions. **Intervertebral osteochondrosis** predominantly affects the midthoracic spine, while **spondylosis deformans** tends to affect the mid- and lower thoracic spine. **Costotransverse and costovertebral osteoarthritis** occur as features of degenerative thoracic spine disease more commonly in women than in men and predominantly affect the two lowest pairs of ribs. One should be careful when interpreting osteophytic changes in the costotransverse and costovertebral joints, because they may simply represent **calcified attachments of the radiate ligaments** of the heads of the first through seventh ribs. Nevertheless, osteoarthritis of the costovertebral joints can lead to complete ankylosis between the ribs and vertebral bodies. This finding often correlates with **hyperostosis** of the **heads of the ribs** and the articulating **transverse process** and represents a form of **perivertebral hyperostosis** (Fischer and Stecher 1972, Macones et al. 1989). It is thought to result from abnormal stress, as it is most commonly found in men and heavy laborers and predominantly affects the right side (Macones et al. 1989). Similar **bilateral hyperostosis** occurs in various spinal diseases such as:

- Ankylosing spondylitis
- Psoriatic spondylitis
- DISH (Huang et al. 1993)

Differentiation from osteoblastic metastases and other sclerotic bone changes can be difficult (Fig. 5.**250**).

Diffuse idiopathic skeletal hyperostosis (DISH) (Resnick et al. 1975, Resnick and Niwayama 1976), known also as **spondylosis hyperostotica** (Ott 1973) and **ankylosing hyperostosis** or **Forestier disease** (Forestier and Ròtes-Queról 1950, Forestier et al. 1969, Forestier and Lagier 1971), is a skeletal disorder that predominates in men over 50 years of age (Forestier and Lagier 1971, Harris et al. 1974, Resnick et al. 1975, Resnick and Niwayama 1976). Patho-

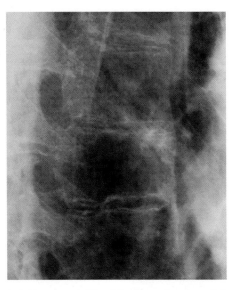

Fig. 5.**248**   Ankylosing spondylitis of the thoracic spine: disk space narrowing, syndesmophytes, and partial ankylosis.

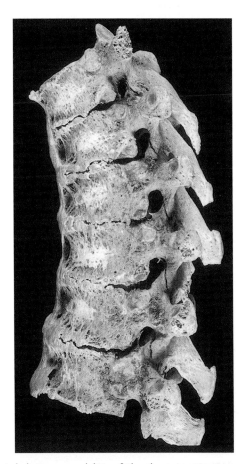

Fig. 5.**249**   Ankylosing spondylitis of the thoracic spine in a specimen. Note the ankylosis of the vertebral bodies and costotransverse joints and the ossification of the anterior longitudinal ligament.

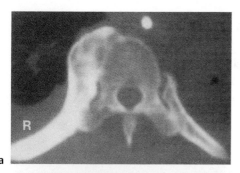

a

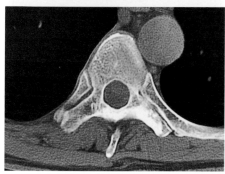

b

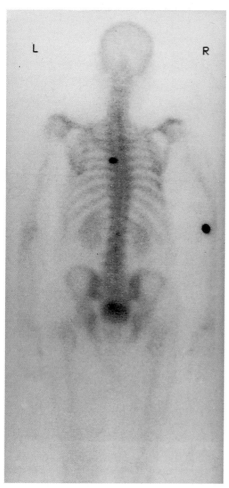

c

Fig. 5.**250a–c**   Sclerotic changes in the proximal ribs and vertebral arches.
a Stress-induced hyperostosis of the rib and transverse process. (From Macones 1989.)
b Osteosclerosis of the vertebral arch and transverse process due to a single osteoblastic metastasis from prostatic carcinoma. Note the absence of sclerosis in the proximal rib.
c Bone scan corresponding to **b**.

logically, it involves **calcification and ossification of the anterior longitudinal ligament** accompanied by **spondylosis deformans** and **fibro-ostosis** at the sites of attachment of the anterior longitudinal ligament to the vertebral bodies. The precise cause of the disease is unknown, but it may relate to disturbances of glucose metabolism (Julkunen 1971, Littlejohn and Smythe 1981) and an increased prevalence of the HLA-B8 antigen (Rosenthal et al. 1977).

> **Criteria for the diagnosis of spinal involvement by DISH**
> ➤ *Flowing ossification and calcification* along the anterolateral aspect of at least four contiguous vertebral bodies, with or without bony excrescences at the intervening discovertebral junctions
> ➤ The relative preservation of *intervertebral disk height* and the absence of pronounced signs of degenerative disk disease, including vacuum phenomena and vertebral body marginal sclerosis
> ➤ The *absence of apophyseal jointbony ankylosis* and *sacroiliac joint changes* such as erosion and sclerosis

DISH-related **vertebral body changes** are most commonly found in the thoracic spine (Fig. 5.**251**), especially between T7 and T11.

Flowing calcification and ossification appear along the anterior and lateral aspects of contiguous vertebral bodies. The frequent undulating contours result from heavy bone deposition at the level of the disk space in the presence of spondylophytes (Fig. 5.**252**).

The deposited bone ranges from a few millimeters to 20 mm in thickness and is often heavier on the right side, presumably because the pulsations of the descending aorta inhibit ossification on the left side. Ossification along the posterior aspect of the vertebral bodies is rare. **Ossification of the posterior longitudinal ligament (OPLL)**, which apparently is related to DISH, was described in the section on the mid- and lower cervical spine (Fig. 5.**253**).

Scheuermann disease (adolescent kyphosis) is among the physeal osteochondroses and affects the spine. The **osteochondroses** have several features in common:

- Predilection for the immature skeleton
- Involvement of an epiphysis, apophysis, or equivalent bones
- Fragmentation
- Collapse and sclerosis on radiographs, often followed by a reconstitution of bony contours (Resnick 1995)

The older view that these features were caused by osteonecrosis has been disproved. Scheuermann disease has a reported incidence of 4–8% (Wassman 1951). The changes usually appear between 13 and 17 years of age and are very rare before age 10. As the degree of thoracic kyphosis increases between the ages of 12 and 16, the incidence of Scheuermann disease also rises (Skogland et al. 1985). **Scheuermann disease** is characterized by **increased kyphosis** of the spine, which usually affects the thoracic spine (75%) but may also involve the thoracolumbar junction (20–25%) and rarely the lumbar spine (up to 5%) (Lamb 1954, Fried 1966). The kyphotic curve is usually round and infrequently angular. While kyphotic deformity is not invariably present, it can lead to a **fatigue fracture of a spinous process** (**Müller sign**). Scoliosis is often found in addition to the thoracic kyphosis (Deacon et al. 1985).

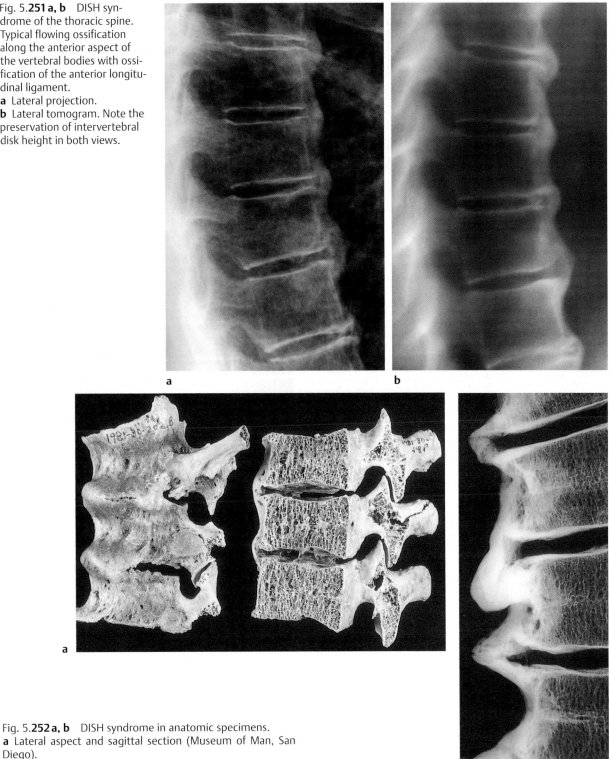

Fig. 5.**251 a, b** DISH syndrome of the thoracic spine. Typical flowing ossification along the anterior aspect of the vertebral bodies with ossification of the anterior longitudinal ligament.
a Lateral projection.
b Lateral tomogram. Note the preservation of intervertebral disk height in both views.

Fig. 5.**252 a, b** DISH syndrome in anatomic specimens.
a Lateral aspect and sagittal section (Museum of Man, San Diego).
b DISH syndrome in a lateral specimen radiograph.

Early signs consist of anterior disk space narrowing and anterior convexity of the vertebral bodies with slight anterior wedging (Figs. 5.**254**, 5.**255**).

The vertebral body ceases to grow in height, and its anteroposterior diameter increases (**Knutsson's sign**) (Knutsson 1948). As the disease progresses, the **contours of the upper and lower surfaces of the vertebral bodies** become undulant, irregular, and sclerotic but sharply defined (Fig. 5.**256**). Intradiscal **vacuum phenomena** are occasionally observed.

The **marginal ridges** appear irregular and crumbly, especially in the anterior pressure-bearing zone of the kyphotic curve, and may be absent. In this case the anterior corners of the vertebral bodies acquire a stepped or beveled appearance (Figs. 5.**255**, 5.**256**). In the **late stage**, the vertebral deformities along with degenerative sequelae and any osteophytic deposits are still visible on the anterior aspects of the vertebrae (Fig. 5.**257**).

Schmorl nodes (cartilaginous nodes), caused by the extrusion of disk material into the vertebral body through

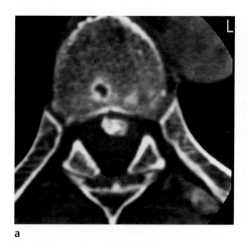 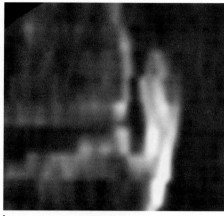

Fig. 5.**253 a, b** Ossification of the posterior longitudinal ligament (OPLL) (observation by Weber, Damme).
a Axial CT.
b Sagittal reconstruction.

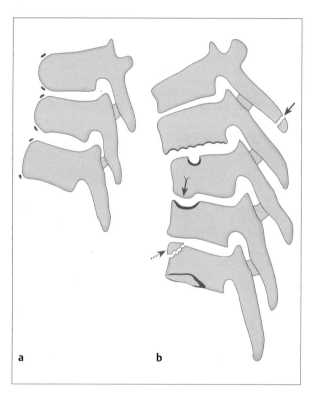 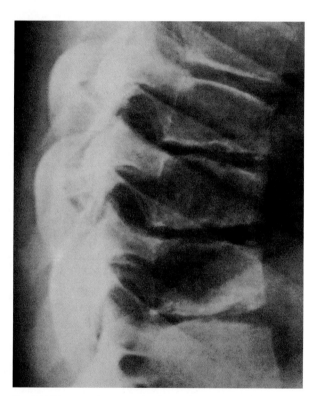

Fig. 5.**254 a, b** Radiographic features of Scheuermann disease (after Dihlmann).
a Early radiographic signs consist of anterior disk space narrowing, anterior vertebral body convexity (barrel-shaped vertebra), and mild vertebral wedging.
b Examples of typical radioraphic signs: sharp and irregular vertebral contours, anterior vertebral wedging, anterior disk space narrowing, increased AP vertebral diameters, Schmorl nodes with dense margins (typically in the anterior third of the vertebral body), retromarginal disk prolapse with a corner fracture (dotted arrow), fatigue fracture of the spinous process due to pathological kyphosis (Müller sign) (arrow), and the Edgren–Vaino sign (double arrow).

Fig. 5.**255** Anterior vertebral wedging in Scheuermann disease.

Fig. 5.**256** Scheuermann disease of the thoracic spine. Irregular vertebral end plates and anterior wedging (arrowheads). Edgren–Vaino sign (arrow).

Fig. 5.**257 a, b** Late stage of Scheuermann disease is characterized by pronounced kyphosis, irregular and sclerotic vertebral contours, relatively long and low vertebral bodies, and significant degenerative reactions.

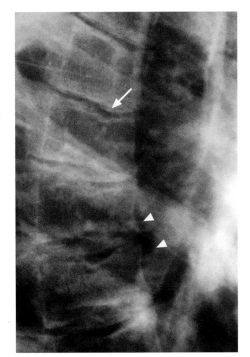

Fig. 5.**256**

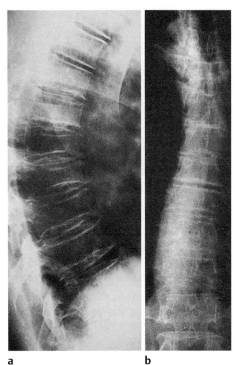

a   b

Fig. 5.**257**

breaks in the end plate, are observed in 50% of patients with Scheuermann disease, making them a cardinal feature of the disease. The nodes are rimmed by sclerosis within the cancellous bone of the vertebral body (Figs. 5.**254**, 5.**258**).

Due to the reduction in disk volume, the disk space diminishes in height. Cartilaginous nodes located near the anterior or posterior edge may break through the wall of the vertebral body, causing the detachment of a corner including the ring apophysis. In this situation the nucleus pulposus may prolapse beneath the anterior longitudinal ligament or toward the intervertebral foramen or spinal canal, producing neurological symptoms (von Meyenburg 1946). The detached ring apophysis can continue to

develop in isolation, producing a **limbus vertebra** (Fig. 5.**254**). With a large Schmorl node, the opposing end plate may show a circumscribed, exostosis-like bony outgrowth: the **Edgren–Vaino sign** (Figs. 5.**254**, 5.**256**, 5.**259**, 5.**386**).

There are reports that the vertebral bodies of one or more thoracic or thoracolumbar segments may become fused anteriorly (Bischofsberger 1949–1951, Butler 1971).

Sickle cell anemia is associated with a vertebral deformity that resembles osteoporotic fish vertebrae (Reynolds 1966), but instead of biconcave deformity there is a **saucer-shaped depression** in the central portion of the end plates with an apparent thickening of the depressed bone (Fig. 5.**260**).

Fig. 5.**258 a, b** Schmorl nodes.
a Lateral projection.
b Radiograph of a specimen.

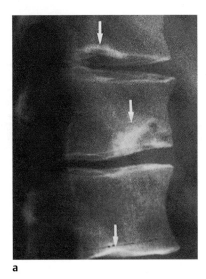

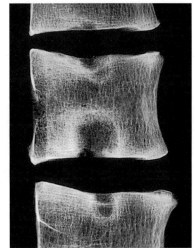

a   b

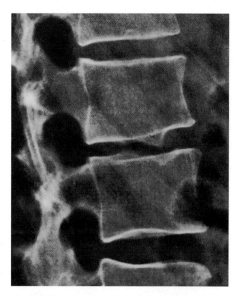

Fig. 5.**259** Bony outgrowth from the anterior lower end plate of T12. The opposing depression in the upper end plate of L1 has the appearance of a Schmorl node.

As described in the section on the cervical spine, a **calcifying discitis** can develop in children and lead to the posterior extrusion of disk material (Schapira et al. 1988) (Fig. 5.**261**). In adult patients as well, disk herniations at the thoracic level have been described in association with disk calcifications (Williams 1954).

Aortic ectasia or an **aneurysm** of the descending aorta can produce **erosive changes in the left anterior contours of the vertebral bodies** (Boldt and Bücheler 1971).

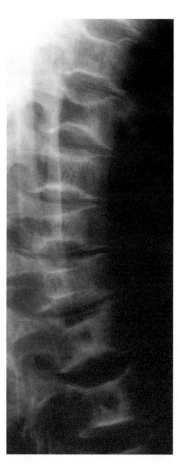

Fig. 5.**260** Sickle cell anemia. Typical saucer-shaped depressions are visible in the upper and lower end plates.

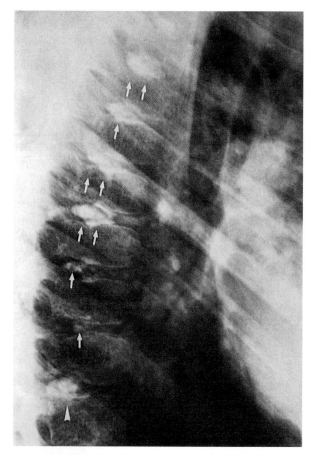

Fig. 5.**261** Multiple calcifications of the nucleus pulposus in thoracic intervertebral disks.

References

Benzian, S. R., F. Mainzer, C. A. Gooding: Pediculate thinning, a normal variant at the thoracolumbar junction. Brit. J. Radiol. 44 (1971) 936

Bischofsberger, C.: Partielle Synostosen von Wirbelkörpern als besonderes Endbild der juvenilen Kyphose. Arch. orthop. Unfall-Chir. 44 (1949–51) 73–85

Black, D. M., L. Palermo, M. C. Nevitt, H. K. Genant, R. Epstein, R. San Valentin et al.: Comparison of methods for defining prevalent vertebral deformities: the study of osteoporotic fractures. J. Bone Mineral Res. 10 (1995) 890

Boldt, I., E. Bücheler: Ein luisches thorakolumbales Aortenaneurysma mit Wirbelkörperarrosion. Fortschr. Röntgenstr. 114 (1971) 846

Bos, van den, R. W., G. J. Vielvoye, J. G. Blickman: Vertebral anomalies in monozygotic twins. Diagn. Imag. clin. 53 (1984) 259–261

Brocher, J. E. W., H.-G. Willert: Differentialdiagnose der Wirbelsäulenerkrankungen, 6. Aufl. Thieme, Stuttgart 1980

Brocher, J. E. W.: Unvollständige Blockwirbelbildung in der oberen Brustwirbelsäule. Röntgenpraxis 8 (1936) 440–447

Brower, A. C., E. Downey Jr.: Kummell disease: report of a case with serial radiographs. Radiology 141 (1981) 363

Butler, R. W.: Spontaneous anterior fusion of vertebral bodies. J. Bone Jt Surg. 53-B (1971) 230

Chance, G. Q.: Note on a type of flexion fracture of the spine. Brit. J. Radiol. 21 (1948) 452

Cheatum, D. E.: "Ankylosing spondylitis" without sacroiliitis in a woman without the HLA B27 antigen. J. Rheumatol. 3 (1976) 420

Christensen, E. R., Anna L. Jensen, E. M. Schalimtzek: Non-infectious vertebral fusion. Abstract from the 10th Meeting of the European Society of Pediatric Radiology. Birmingham, April 10–13, 1973

Deacon, P., C. R. Berkin, R. A. Dickson: Combined idiopathic kyphosis and scoliosis. An analysis of the lateral spinal curvatures associated with Scheuermann's disease. J. Bone Jt Surg. 67-B (1985) 189

Dehner, J. R.: Seabelt injuries of the spine and abdomen. Amer. J. Roentgenol. 111 (1971) 833

Denis, F.: The three column spine and its significance in the classification of acute thoracolumbar spinal injuries. Spine 8 (1983) 817

Denton, J. R.: The association of congenital spinal anomalies with imperforate anus. Clin. Orthop. 162 (1982) 91

Diethelm, L.: Fehlbildungen des Corpus vertebrae. In: Röntgendiagnostik der Wirbelsäule, Teil 1, red. v. L. Diethelm. In Diethelm, L., F. Heuck, O. Olsson, K. Ranniger, F. Strnad, H. Vieten, A. Zuppinger: Handbuch der Medizinischen Radiologie, Bd. VI. Springer, Berlin 1974 (S. 190–263)

El-Khoury, G. Y., C. G. Whitten: Trauma of the upper thoracic spine. Anatomy, biomechanics, and unique imaging features. Amer. J. Roentgenol. 160 (1993) 95

Ferguson, R. L., B. L. Allen Jr.: A mechanistic classification of thoracolumbar spine fractures. Clin. Orthop. 189 (1984) 77

Fischer, E.: Interpedunkularabstände und das Verhältnis des Interpedunkularabstandes zur Wirbelbreite an der Brust- und Lendenwirbelsäule. Z. Orthop. 107 (1970) 624

Fischer, E., W. Stecher: Die Hyperostose der Rippenköpfchen, ein Teilbild der perivertebralen Hyperostose. Fortschr. Röntgenstr. 117 (1972) 336–342

Forestier, J., R. Lagier: Ankylosing hyperostosis of the spine. Clin. Orthop. 74 (1971) 65

Forestier, J., J. Rotès-Quérol: Hyperostose ankylante vertébrale sénile. Rev. Rhum. 17 (1950) 525–534

Forestier, J., R. Lagier, A. Certony: Le concept d'hyperostose vertébrale ankylosante. Approche anatomoradiologique. Rev. Rhum. 36 (1969) 655–661

Fried, K.: Die zervikale juvenile Osteochondrose (Scheuermannsche Krankheit). Fortschr. Röntgenstr. 105 (1966) 69

Garcia, A. Jr., S. A. Grantham: Haematogenous pyogenic vertebral osteomyelitis. J. Bone Jt Surg. 42-A (1960) 429

Genant, H. K., C. Y. Wu, C. van Kuijk, M. C. Nevitt: Vertebral fracture assessment using a semiquantitative technique. J. Bone Mineral Res. 8 (1993) 1137

Goldberg, Caroline, G. Fenelon, N. S. Blake, F. Dowling, B. F. Regan: Diastematomyelia: A critical review of the natural history and treatment. Spine 9 (1984) 367–372

Han, Jong S., Jane E. Benson, B. Kaufman, H. Rekate, R. J. Alfidi, H. H. Bohlman, B. Kaufman: Demonstration of diastematomyelia and associated abnormalities with MR Imaging. Amer. J. Neuroradiol. 6 (1985) 215–219

Harris, J., A. R. Carter, E. N. Glick et al.: Ankylosing hyperostosis. I. Clinical and radiological features. Ann. rheum. Dis. 33 (1974) 210

Hellinger, J.: Meßmethoden in der Skelettradiologie. Thieme, Stuttgart 1995.

Heywood, A. W. B., O. L. Meyers: Rheumatoid arthritis of the thoracic and lumbar spine. J. Bone Jt Surg. 68-B (1986) 362

Hinck, V. C., W. M. Clark jr., C. E. Hopkins: Normal interpedunculate distances (minimum and maximum) in children and adults. Amer. J. Roentgenol. 97 (1966) 141–153

Hodgson, A. R.: Infectious disease of the spine. In Rothman, R. H., F. A. Simeone: The Spine. Saunders, Philadelphia 1975 (p. 567)

Hodson, C. J., D. G. Shaw: Congenital atresia of the esophagus and thirteen pairs of ribs. Pediat. Radiol. 1 (1973) 248

Hohmann, D., W. Gasteiger: Röntgendiagnostik der Kostotransversalgelenke. Fortschr. Röntgenstr. 112 (1970) 783–789

Huang, G.-S., Y.-H. Park, J. A. M. Taylor et al.: Hyperostosis of ribs: association with vertebral ossification. J. Rheumatol. 20 (1993) 2073

Julkunen, H., O. P. Heinonen, K. Pyorrala: Hyperostosis of the spine in an adult population, its relationship to hyperglycemia and obesity. Ann. rheum. Dis. 30 (1971) 605

Kliewer, M. A., L. Gray, J. Paver, W. D. Richardson, J. B. Vogler, J. H. McElhaney et al.: Acute spinal ligament disruption: MR imaging with anatomic correlation. Magn. Reson. Imag. 3 (1993) 855

Knutsson, F.: Observations of the growth of the vertebra body on Scheuermann's disease. Acta radiol. 30 (1948) 97–104

Knutsson, F.: Fusion of vertebrae following noninfectious disturbance in the zone of growth. Acta Radiol. 32 (1949) 404–411

Kozlowski, K.: Platyspondylie in childhood. Pediat. Radiol. 2 (1974) 81–88

Kozlowski, K.: Spondylo-costal-dysplasia. A further report-review of 14 cases. Fortschr. Röntgenstr. 140 (1984) 204–209

Lamb, D. W.: Localised osteochondritis of the lumbar spine. J. Bone Jt Surg. 36-B (1954) 591

Lauridsen, K. N., A. De Carvalho, A. H. Andersen: Degree of vertebral wedging of the dorso-lumbar spine. Acta radiol. 25 (1984) 29

Lemaire, M., M. Alealay, G. Touchard, J. Payen, A. Desplats, B. Malapart et al.: Ostéonécrose vertébrale. Sem. Hôp. Paris 59 (1983) 296

Littlejohn, G. O., H. A. Smythe: Marked hyperinsulinemia after glucose challenge in patients with diffuse idiopathic skeletal hyperostosis. J. Rheumatol. 8 (1981) 965

Macones, A. J. Jr., M. S. Fisher, J. L. Locke: Stress-related rib and vertebral changes. Radiology 170 (1989) 117

Magerl, F., M. Aebi, S. D. Gertzbein, J. Harms, S. Nazarin: A comprehensive classification of thoracic and lumbar injuries. Europ. Spine J. 3 (1994) 184

Maiman, D. J., F. A. Pintar: Anatomy and clinical biomechanics of the thoracic spine. Clin. Neurosurg. 38 (1992) 296

Maldague, B. E., H. M. Noel, J. J. Malghem: The intravertebral vacuum cleft: a sign of ischemic vertebral collapse. Radiology 129 (1978) 23

Maldague, B. E., J. Malghem, J. P. Huaux et al.: Ischemic collapse of the vertebral body: myth or reality. J. belge Radiol. 62 (1979) 61

Malghem, J., B. Maldague, M. Labaisse: Intravertebral vacuum cleft: changes in content after supine positioning. Radiology 187 (1993) 483

Manaster, B. J., A. G. Osborn: CT patterns of facet fracture dislocations in the thoracolumbar region. Amer. J. Roentgenol. 148 (1987) 335

Marchini, C., F. Schiavi, M. Leonardi, C. Cecotto: Diastematomyelia in an adult. Ital. J. Neurol. Sci. 2 (1983) 211–214

Mathieu, J.-P., M. Decarie, J. Dube, D. Marton: La diastématomyelie. Chir. Pédiat. 23 (1982) 29–35

Mau, W., H. Zeidler, R. Mau, A. Majewski, J. Freyschmidt, W. Stangel et al.: Evaluation of early diagnostic criteria for ankylosing spondylitis in a 10 year follow-up. Z. Rheumatol. 49 (1990) 82

v. Meyenburg, H.: Über „Abtrennung" der hinteren Wirbelkörperkante als Ursache von Ischias. Radiol. clin. (Basel) 15 (1946) 215–223

McAfee, P. C., H. A. Yuan, B. E. Fredrickson et al.: The value of computed tomography in thoracolumbar fractures: an analysis of one hundred consecutive cases and a new classification. J. Bone Jt Surg. 65-A (1983) 461

Melhem, R. E., M. Fahl: Fifteen dorsal vertebras and rib pairs in two siblings. Pediat. Radiol. 15 (1985) 61

Melton, L. J., S. H. Kann, M. A. Frye et al.: Epidemiology of vertebral fractures in women. Amer. J. Epidemiol. 129 (1989) 1000

Modena, V., I. Maiocco, C. Bosio, A. Bianchi, P. G. De Fillippe, V. Daneo: Intervertebral vacuum cleft: notes on five cases. Clin. exp. Rheumatol. 3 (1985) 23

Naul, L. G., G. Peet, W. B. Maupin: Avascular necrosis of the vertebral body: MR imaging. Radiology 172 (1989) 219

Neugebauer, H.: Cobb oder Ferguson. Eine Analyse der beiden gebräuchlichsten Röntgenmeßmethoden von Skoliosen. Z. Orthop. 110 (1972) 342

Ott, V. R.: Über die Spondylosis hyperostotica. Schweiz. med. Wschr. 83 (1953) 790

Pathria, M. N., C. A. Petersilge: Spinal trauma. Radiol. Clin. N. Amer. 29 (1991) 847

Probst, J.: Interartikulärspaltbildung am Brustwirbel und ihre Darstellung im Röntgenbild. Fortschr. Röntgenstr. 86 (1957) 762–766

Rathke, F. W.: Über Wirbelkörperaplasie. Fortschr. Röntgenstr. 127 (1977) 248–254

Redlund-Johnell, I., E.-M. Larsson: Subluxation of the upper thoracic spine in rheumatoid arthritis. Skelet. Radiol. 22 (1993) 105

Reeder, M. M.: Reeder and Felson's. Gamuts in Bone, Joint and Spine Radiology. Springer, Berlin 1993

Resnick, D.: Diagnosis of Bone and Joint Disorders, 3rd ed. Saunders, Philadelphia 1995

Resnick, D., G. Niwayama: Radiographic and pathologic features of spinal involvement in diffuse idiopathic skeletal hyperostosis (DISH). Radiology 119 (1976) 559

Resnick, D., S. R. Shaul, J. M. Robins: Diffuse idiopathic skeletal hyperostosis (DISH): Forestier's disease with extraspinal manifestations. Radiology 115 (1975) 513

Resnick, D., G. Niwayama, J. Guerra Jr. et al.: Spinal vacuum phenomena: anatomical study and review. Radiology 139 (1981) 341

Reynolds, J.: A re-evaluation of the "fish vertebra" sign in sickle cell hemoglobinopathy. Amer. J. Roentgenol. 97 (1966) 693

Ricci, A.: Anomalie dei tuberoli mamillari delle vertebre lombari: processo stiloideo e diatrosi accessorie. Riv. Radiol. 4 (1964) 697

Rogers, L. F.: The roentgenographic appearance of transverse or Chance fractures of the spine: the seat belt fracture. Amer. J. Roentgenol. 111 (1971) 844

Rogers, L. F.: Radiology of Skeletal Trauma. Churchill Livingston, New York 1992

Rosenthal, M., I. Bahous, W. Muller: Increased frequency of HLA B8 in hyperostotic spondylitis. J. Rheumatol. 4, Suppl 3 (1977) 94

Saeed, M., C. H. Buitrago-Téllez, F. J. Ferstl, S. Boos, B. Wimmer, M. Langer: Three-dimensional CT in the diagnosis of spinal trauma: comparison with plain film and two-dimensional CT examinations. Europ. Radiol. 4 (1994) 161

Schapira, D., D. Goldsher, M. Nahir, Y. Scharf: Calcified thoracic disc with herniation of the nucleus pulposus in a child. Postgrad. med. J. 64 (1988) 160

Schmitt, H.: Vorgetäuschter Keilwirbel. Röntgenpraxis 10 (1938) 609

Schulze, R., P. Gulbin: Über das Fehlen der Dornfortsätze an der Brust-/Lendenwirbelgrenze. Fortschr. Röntgenstr. 103 (1965) 627

Seyss, R.: Zur Röntgenologie der kindlichen Wirbelsäule. Fortschr. Röntgenstr. 74 (1951) 434

Seyss, R.: Zur Deutung der Genese des Angelhakenwirbels. Kinderärztl. Prax. 36 (1968) 85

Skogland, L. B., H. Stehen, O. Trygstad: Spinal deformities in tall girls. Acta orthop. scand. 56 (1985) 155

Smith, J. R. G., I. R. Martin, D. G. Shaw, R. O. Robinson: Progressive non-infectious anterior vertebral fusion. Skelet. Radiol. 15 (1986) 599–604

Spranger, J., L. O. Langer, H.-R. Wiedemann: Bone Dysplasias: An Atlas of Constitutional Disorders of Skeletal Development. Saunders, Philadelphia 1974

Stevenson, R. E.: Extra vertebrae associated with esophageal atresias and tracheoesophageal fistulas. J. Pediat. 81 (1972) 1123

Swischuk, L. E.: The beaked, notched, or hooked vertebra. Its significance in infants and young children Radiology 95 (1970) 661

Swoboda, W.: Dorsolumbale Kyphose als unbekanntes Skelettzeichen beim angeborenen Myxödem. Fortschr. Röntgenstr. 73 (1950) 740

Taylor, G. A., K. D. Eggli: Lap-belt injuries of the lumbar spine in children: a pitfall in CT diagnosis. Amer. J. Roentgenol. 150 (1988) 1355

Thorngren, K.-G., E. Liedberg, P. Aspelin: Fractures of the thoracic and lumbar spine in ankylosing spondylitis. Arch. orthop. trauma. Surg. 98 (1981) 101

Tomsick, T. A., M. E. Lebowith, C. Campbell: The congenital absence of pedicle in the thoracic spine. Report of two cases. Radiology 111 (1974) 587–589

Wackenheim, A.: Analyse structuraliste de l'image radiologique. Radiologie. J. Cepur 5 (1985) 873–878

Wassman, K.: Kyphosis juvenilis Scheuermann—an occupational disorder. Acta orthop. scand. 21 (1951) 65

White, A. A., M. M. Panjabi: Clinical Biomechanics of the Spine. Lippincott-Raven, Philadelphia 1978

Whitesides, T. E. jr.: Traumatic kyphosis of the thoracolumbar spine. Clin. Orthop. 128 (1977) 78

Williams, R.: Complete protrusion of a calcified nucleus pulposus in the thoracic spine. Report of a case. J. Bone Jt Surg. 36-B (1954) 597

Willner, S., B. Johnson: Thoracic kyphosis and lumbar lordosis during the growth period in children. Acta pediat. scand. 72 (1983) 873–878

Zinreich, S. J., H. Wang, F. Abdo, N. Bryan: 3-D CT improves accuracy of spinal trauma studies. Diagn. Imag. Int. 4 (1990) 24

Lumbar Spine

Normal Findings

The five lumbar vertebrae are particularly massive, due to the greater mechanical stresses that act upon the lumbar region (Fig. 5.**262**).

The shape of the lumbar vertebrae depends on gender and especially on the degree of lumbar lordosis (Cheng et al. 1998). The **pedicles** are short and, with the exception of L5, are directed straight backward. The articular facets of the **apophyseal joints**, unlike those of the cervical and

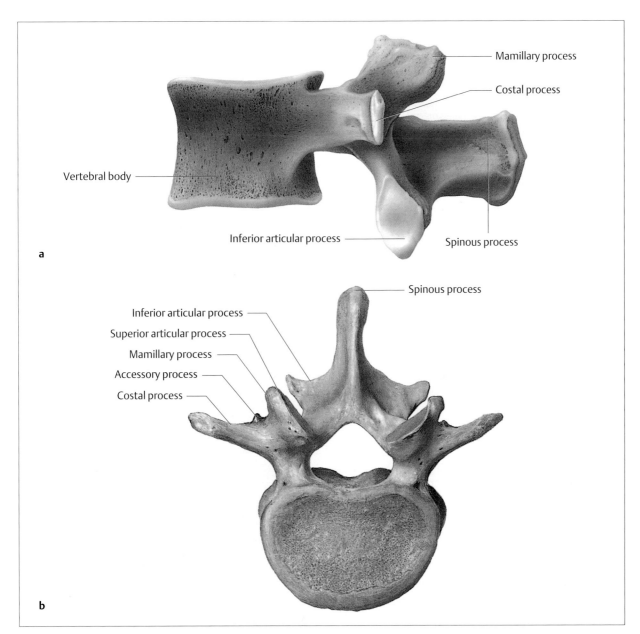

Fig. 5.**262 a, b**   Anatomy of a lumbar vertebra. (From Rauber and Kopsch 1998.)

a Lateral aspect.
b Superior aspect.

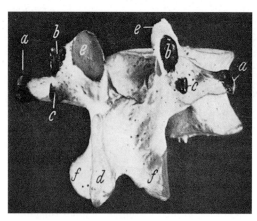

Fig. 5.**263**   Posterior oblique view of a lumbar vertebra with accessory ossification centers.
a   Apophysis of costal process
b   Mamillary process
c   Accessory or styloid process
d   Spinous process
e   Superior articular process
f   Inferior articular process

thoracic vertebrae, are curved. The superior **articular processes** bear concave articular facets that face posteromedially, while the inferior articular processes have convex facets that face anterolaterally. The **costal processes** correspond to fused, rudimentary ribs. The anlages of the transverse processes are represented by the **accessory processes** (Fig. 5.263).

The **fifth lumbar vertebra** has several distinctive features:

- It is usually taller anteriorly than posteriorly.
- The pedicles are directed posterolaterally.
- The articular facets are often asymmetrical and have a more frontal orientation.

During Growth

Lateral radiographs in infants demonstrate a typical pattern of unfused neurocentral synchondroses along the lumbar spine (compare with Thoracic Spine) (Figs. 5.264, 5.265).

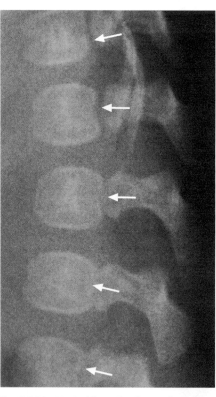

Fig. 5.**264**   Typical lateral radiograph of a 2-month-old infant demonstrates open neurocentral synchondroses (arrows).

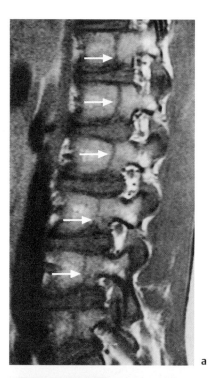

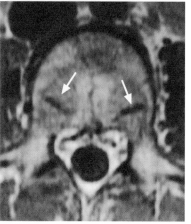

Fig. 5.**265a, b**   Remnants of the neurocentral synchondrosis ▷ in an 11-year-old child.
a The remnants of the neurocentral synchondrosis appear as vertical bands of low signal intensity (arrows) on sagittal T1-weighted MRI.
b Corresponding features on axial MRI show a typical location and alignment (arrows) (observation by Winterstein, Buchholz).

In **children**, the corners of the marginal ridges often form spurlike anterior projections at approximately 8 years of age (Fig. 5.**214**). Differentiation of **lumbar ribs** (see above) from the **apophyses** of the **costal processes** can be difficult in adolescents (Figs. 5.**266**, 5.**270**).

The **apophyses** of the **spinous processes** appear on lateral radiographs as very thin crescents (Fig. 5.**267**), and may be visible due to overpenetration.

 ## In Adulthood

In the **AP projection**, the upper and especially the lower lumbar vertebrae appear distorted due to the physiological lordosis of the lumbar spine. The **vertebral bodies** appear box-shaped with slightly concave sidewalls. The intervertebral disk spaces are clearly defined. The fourth lumbar vertebra is at the level of the iliac crests. The fifth lumbar vertebra appears foreshortened because of the physiological lordosis and is poorly delineated on most films. With aging, the vertebral bodies in both sexes normally become broader at the equator, especially in the lower third of the thoracic and lumbar spine (Erdheim 1931).

The **pedicles** of L1 through L4 appear as elliptical lucencies. The posterior portions of the lumbar **vertebral arches** are clearly portrayed in the AP projection. The **articular processes** and **laminae** form characteristic butterfly figures that enclose the **interlaminar window**. This feature can mimic lucencies within the vertebral body. In the AP view the anteroinferior corners of the L5 vertebral body may be projected over the interlaminar window and resemble calcified ligaments (Fig. 5.**268**).

The spinous processes are projected over the vertebral body and the intervertebral disk space. Because of their obliquity, the **apophyseal joint spaces** appear only sporadically as lucencies between the vertical lines of the articular processes and may appear to cut the pedicles vertically in half.

The **costal processes** arise at the level of the pedicles and are directed laterally. They are usually longest at L3, and they may angle slightly upward at L4. If the superior articular process or a costal process is projected onto the pedicle, it can appear to have a double outline. The portions of the vertebral body not covered by the vertebral arch then have the appearance of rounded defects (Fig. 5.**269**). The psoas muscle outlines superimposed over the costal processes can mimic a fracture (Fig. 5.**270**).

The **width of the spinal canal** is measured by the interpedicular distance in the AP projection. By 5 years of age the interpedicular distance increases by approximately 2 mm, and by age 15 it increases by an additional millimeter (Larsen 1981), with no further increase thereafter (Fischer and Giere 1970). Sex differences are minimal (1–2 mm more in males than females). The average spinal canal width in adults is 22–24 mm at the level of the first four lumbar vertebrae and approximately 25 mm at the L5 level. Interpedicular distances that remain constant or even decrease caudally are evidence for a narrow spinal canal. The sagittal diameter is somewhat smaller on average and decreases from above downward. The width of the vertebra, unlike its length and height, does not correlate

Fig. 5.**269** Projection-related lucencies at the inferior corners of the vertebral body (double arrow). Styloid process (arrow). ▷

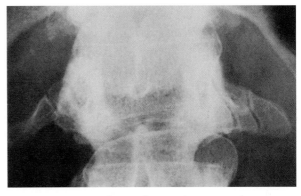

Fig. 5.**266** L1 vertebra with articulating costal processes. Two articulations are visible on the left side.

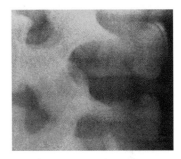

Fig. 5.**267** Spinous apophyses in an 18-year-old.

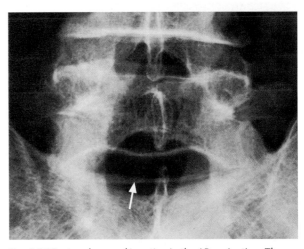

Fig. 5.**268** Lumbosacral junction in the AP projection. The anteroinferior margin of L5 is projected into the "interlaminar window" (arrow) and might be confused with calcified ligaments.

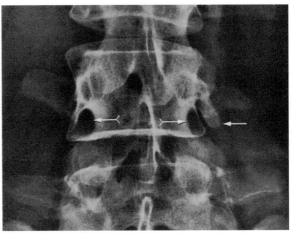

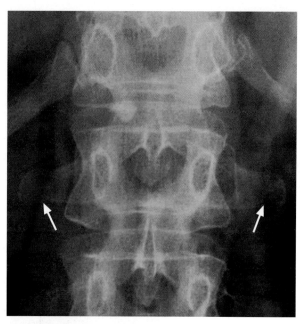

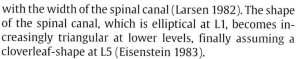

Fig. 5.**270**   Pseudofracture of the L1 costal processes caused by the superimposed psoas muscle outlines (arrows). A small vertebral body osteoma at L1 is noted as an incidental finding.

with the width of the spinal canal (Larsen 1982). The shape of the spinal canal, which is elliptical at L1, becomes increasingly triangular at lower levels, finally assuming a cloverleaf-shape at L5 (Eisenstein 1983).

The **lateral projection** gives an excellent general view of the lumbar vertebral bodies and intervertebral disk spaces. The **spinous processes**, **vertebral arches**, and **intervertebral foramina** are also well visualized. The **vertebral bodies** display an approximately rectangular shape except for L5, whose body is up to 6 mm taller anteriorly than posteriorly (posterior wedging). The vertebral body end plates and posterior border are flat or slightly concave (Fig. 5.**271**). The radiographic morphometry of vertebral bodies is based on determination of the lumbar vertebral index (Fig. 5.**272**). Corresponding values have been published in the literature (Cheng et al. 1998).

The intervertebral disk spaces normally increase in height from L1/L2 to L4/L5. Their height then remains constant or diminishes from L4/L5 to L5/S1. In one series, however, this typical "disk height sequence" was found in just 35% of men and 55% of women (Biggemann et al. 1997). An abrupt, discontinuous change in disk space height is most likely to signify a pathological process (Fig. 5.**273**).

A decrease in intervertebral disk height of the pre-sacral segment in itself should not be interpreted as degenerative change but as a tendency toward lumbosacral assimilation (Wichtl 1940, Dihlmann 1987).

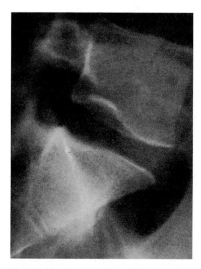

Fig. 5.**271**   Depression of the L5 lower end plate with flattening of the opposing upper surface of the first sacral vertebra.

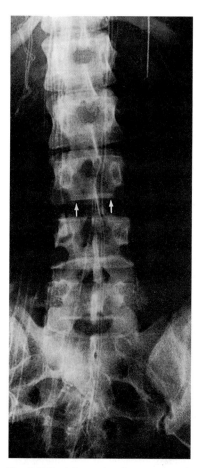

Fig. 5.**273**   Distraction fracture at L3/L4.

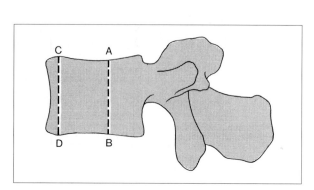

Fig. 5.**272**   Lumbar vertebral index (*AB/CD*) of Barnett–Nordin.

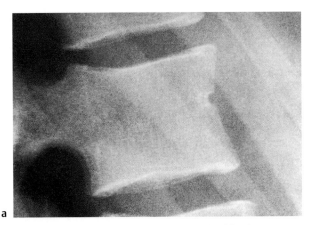

a

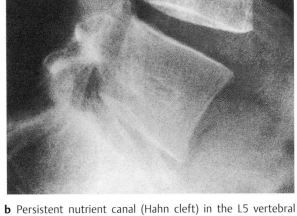

b

Fig. 5.**274 a, b** Vascular features in vertebral bodies.
a Vascular foramen in the anterior border of the L1 vertebral body.

b Persistent nutrient canal (Hahn cleft) in the L5 vertebral body.

The anterior and posterior margins of the vertebral bodies normally lie along uniformly curved lines. This line may be interrupted at the base of the sacrum (S1). A congenitally short sacral base creates a steplike discontinuity in the posterior contour line with an apparent backward slippage of L5 upon S1, known as **pseudoretrolisthesis** (see Fig. 5.**378**). Unlike a true spondyloretrolisthesis, there is no offset in the anterior contour line and a normal distance is measured between the tip of the S1 articular process and the pedicle of L5.

The **posterior surfaces of the vertebral bodies** sometimes show discontinuities or funnel-shaped pits that represent the sites of entry of basivertebral veins (see under Thoracic Spine, Fig. 5.**219**). Remnants of the **Hahn cleft** may also be found in the anterior margin of the vertebral body and within its substance (Fig. 5.**274**).

Occasionally, a **bone-in-bone appearance** may be produced by **growth recovery lines** (transverse lines, stress lines, Park and Harries lines), which indicate intermittent bone growth (Fig. 5.**275**) (Garn et al. 1968). They do not occur after growth has ceased and have been observed in healthy and in sick persons, both in adults and in children. They have been reported in association with heavy metal poisoning.

The **intervertebral foramina** appear as ear-shaped lucencies, becoming smaller and narrower at lower levels, especially at L5/S1. The intervertebral joints, transverse processes, and laminae are superimposed in the lateral projection. The **transverse processes** appear as elliptical densities projected over the vertebral arches. The **apophyseal joint spaces** are visible only at L5/S1, if at all.

The overlap of the L4 vertebral body and ilium in the lateral view can produce a **Mach effect** that resembles a transverse cleft (Fig. 5.**276**). The **epiphyseal ring** of the lumbar vertebra in children and adolescents may appear as a fine line within the intervertebral space in a slightly oblique projection (Fig. 5.**216**).

When the costal processes are superimposed over the vertebral arch, they can sometimes cause an **apparent spondylolysis (pseudospondylolysis)**, especially at the L2 and L3 levels (El-Khoury et al. 1981) (Fig. 5.**277**). Unlike true spondylolysis, pseudospondylolysis presents with sharply defined margins of the cleft and is located in the pars interarticularis at a higher lumbar level than a true cleft (Fig. 5.**320**).

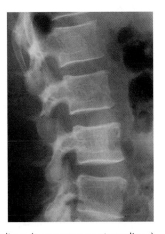

Fig. 5.**275** Growth recovery lines (transverse or stress lines) in multiple lumbar vertebrae, creating a bone-in-bone appearance.

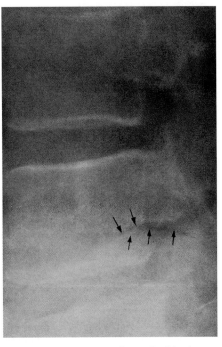

Fig. 5.**276** The superimposed ilium and vertebral body create a Mach band effect that mimics a horizontal cleft in the vertebral body (arrows).

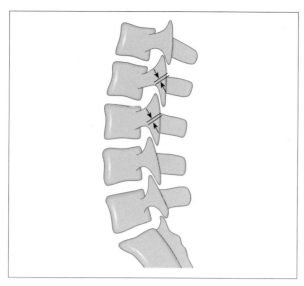

Fig. 5.**277**   Pseudospondylolysis of L2 and L3 (arrows) caused by the costal processes superimposed over the vertebral arch (after Dihlmann).

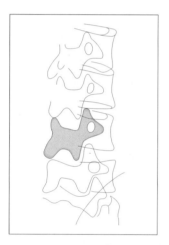

Fig. 5.**278**   "Scotty dog" sign of Lachapèle in an oblique view of the lumbar spine.

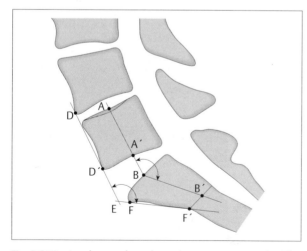

Fig. 5.**279**   Lumbosacral angle and promontory angle. The lumbosacral angle is formed by the central axes of the L5 and S1 vertebral bodies. The promontory angle is formed by anterior tangents to the L5 and S1 vertebral bodies (after Hellinger).

Oblique views of the lumbar spine at a **45° angle** are useful for demonstrating the vertebral arches and apophyseal joints. The appearance of the vertebral arches and facet joints on oblique radiographs is best described by the **scotty dog sign of Lachapel** (Fig. 5.279) (Brown and Evans 1973).

Oblique films of the lumbar spine, unlike oblique cervical films, usually do not afford a clear view of the intervertebral foramina. Nonsuperimposed views of the lumbosacral junction can be obtained with **CT** (Dorwart and Genant 1983) and **MRI**.

Normal Posture and Range of Motion

Various methods can be used to evaluate the **position** of the vertebrae at the **lumbosacral junction** in the lateral view. The **lumbosacral angle** between the central axes of the L5 and S1 vertebral bodies has a reported average value of 143°. The **promontory angle**, formed by the anterior tangents to L5 and S1, is approximately 14° less than the lumbosacral angle (Fig. 5.279).

Other angle measurements can be found in references on skeletal radiology (Hellinger 1995). Several simple geometric constructions can be used to detect abnormalities of vertebral position (Fig. 5.280).

A decreased lumbosacral angle is referred to as **acute sacrum** (sacrum acutum) and can lead to instability. A greater proportion of the body weight is then transmitted to L5, increasing the tendency for this vertebra to slip forward on the sacrum. With an **arched sacrum** (sacrum arcuatum), the lumbosacral angle is decreased and the lum-

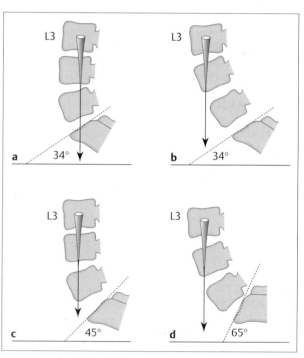

Fig. 5.**280 a–d**   Lumbosacral angle of Ferguson. With a stable lumbosacral alignment, the weight-bearing axis (perpendicular line from the center of L3) should pass through the anterior part of the sacrum.
a Good alignment with a normal lumbosacral angle of 34°.
b Increased lumbar lordosis with a normal lumbosacral angle.
c Increased lumbosacral angle with a normal degree of lordosis.
d Increased lumbosacral angle with increased lordosis.

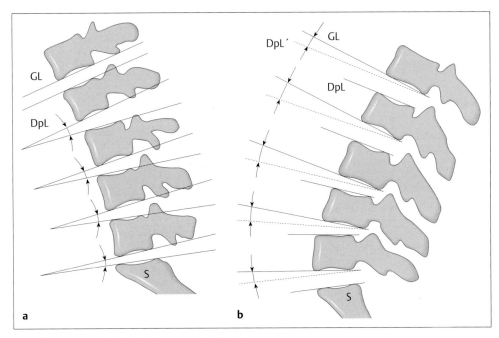

Fig. 5.**281 a, b** Measurement of flexion-extension in the lumbar spine. Normally the intervertebral spaces wedge open toward the convex side. Normal values for the ranges of intersegmental motion: L1/L2 = 11°; L2/L3 = 12°; L3/L4 = 18°; L4/L5 = 24°; L5/S1 = 18° (after Hellinger).
a Flexion.

b Extension.
DpL   Tangents to upper vertebral end plates
DpL′   Lines parallel to upper vertebral end plate tangents
GL   Tangents to lower vertebral end plates
S   Sacrum

bosacral junction is less angular and more curved. Both conditions lead to a marked forward and downward inclination of the sacral base (see Fig. 5.**424**).

Normal values for **functional examinations** of the lumbar spine in flexion, extension, and lateral bending can be found in the literature (Figs. 5.**281**, 5.**282**) (Dvorak et al. 1991 a, b).

Methods for measuring spinal curvature in the coronal and sagittal planes and vertebral body rotation are presented in the section on the thoracic spine (Figs. 5.**22**–5.**26**).

▌ *Pathological Finding?*

 Normal Variant or Anomaly?

Variants

Persistent **vertebral body apophyses** (unfused marginal ridges) are most commonly found at the posteroinferior corners of the lumbar vertebrae (Fig. 5.**283**). **Beveled corners** are also occasionally found at this location.

> Remnants of the **Hahn cleft**, which may appear as notches in the anterior or posterior margins of vertebral bodies or as transverse lucent lines with sclerotic edges within the vertebral body, fall within the range of normal findings (Fig. 5.**274**).

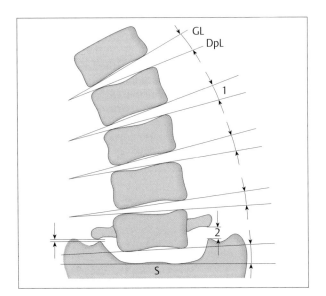

Fig. 5.**282** Lateral bending of the lumbar spine. The range is measured to detect limitations of lumbar sidebending. Lines drawn tangent to the upper and lower end plates normally open toward the convex side. Generally the L5/S1 segment shows the smallest range of motion. The normal total range of lateral bending is 40°, i.e., 20° toward the right side and 20° toward the left (after Hellinger).
DpL Tangents to upper vertebral end plates
GL Tangents to lower vertebral end plates
1   Frontal intersegmental angle
2   Distance from L5 transverse process to sacrum

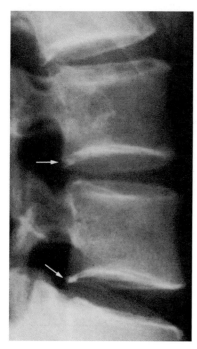

Fig. 5.**283**   Persistent posterior apo-physeal centers in the lumbar vertebrae of a 24-year-old man.

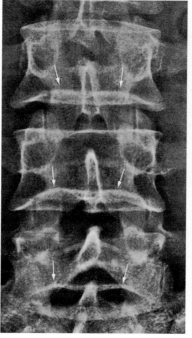

a

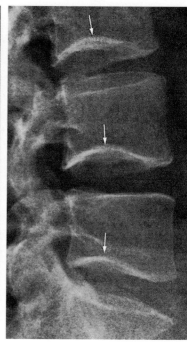

b

Fig. 5.**284 a, b**   Cupid's bow contour of the lower lumbar vertebral bodies. Typical broad-based concavities are visible in the lower vertebral end plates (arrows) (observation by Kohlbach, Witzenhausen).
a AP projection.
b Lateral projection.

Morphological variants of the vertebral bodies include bi-concave upper and lower end plates, with a corresponding biconvex configuration of the intervening disk spaces. **Concavity of the lower end plates** of the L3–L5 vertebral bodies is a relatively common finding and has been called the **Cupid's bow** (Dietz and Christensen 1976, Firooznia et al. 1983, Chan et al. 1997). Typical broad-based indentations are visible in both planes (Fig. 5.**284**) and may produce an **"owl's eyes"** configuration on axial CT scans (Ramirez et al. 1984).

The AP projection shows symmetrical, parasagittal concavities of the vertebral end plates. In the lateral view, these concavities are located in the posterior portion of the lower end plate. The cause of the Cupid's bow contour is unknown. It is found with greater frequency in tall individuals, especially men (Tsuji et al. 1986). It appears to be unrelated to osteopenia or mechanical stresses on the spine (Chan et al. 1997).

> The posterior scalloping of vertebral bodies can occur as a normal variant and is not necessarily pathological (Mitchell et al. 1967).

Large **notches in the anterior and posterior vertebral margins** may be found in bone marrow hyperplasias such as thalassemia major (Cooley anemia) and in Gaucher disease and other myelopathies (Mandell and Kricoun 1979). Tortuous venous collaterals from the ascending lumbar vein in **portal hypertension** can also produce deep notches in the lumbar vertebral bodies, probably by the transmission of aortic pulsations (Kam and Funston 1980).

Bony bridges of variable size may extend between the **costal processes** of adjacent lumbar vertebrae (Figs. 5.**285**–5.**287**). Occasionally these bridges establish a jointlike connection with the costal processes of adjacent vertebrae. Phenotypically, these changes resemble similar bony bridges in the cervical spine such as the epitransverse and infratransverse processes of C1. A congenital etiology is likely, therefore, but has not yet been proved (Meves 1939, de Cuveland 1956, Rettig 1959, Schmitz-Dräger 1959, Vielberg 1970). At the same time, **posttraumatic new bone formation** after costal process fractures can lead to similar bony extensions as a result of myositis ossificans.

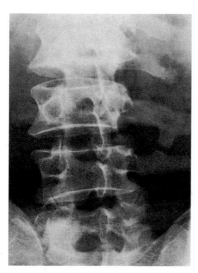

Fig. 5.**285**   Bony process on the long costal process of L3 forms a jointlike connection with the costal process of L4 (observation by Kremser, Altona).

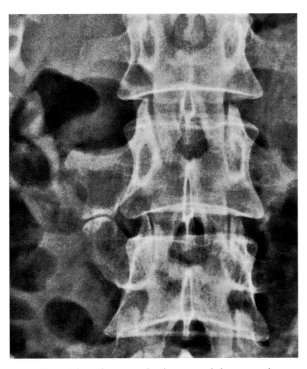

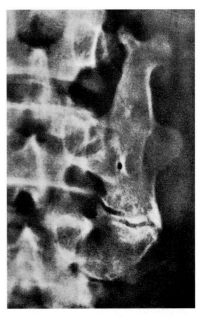

Fig. 5.**287** Powerful bony bridge between the costal processes of L2 and L4 has a jointlike connection with L3/L4 (observation by Wirth, Zug).

Fig. 5.**286** A broad osseous bridge extends between the costal processes of the L3 and L4 vertebrae, establishing a jointlike connection.

The following findings point to a **congenital etiology:**

- The broad connection of the transverse processes resembles a synostosis or articular connection more than a bony bar.
- Bilateral changes.
- Additional anomalies of the articular processes or other arch elements.
- Additional vertebral body anomalies such as block vertebrae and sagittal clefts.
- No angular or steplike deformities in the transverse processes that might indicate a fracture.

The findings below are more consistent with a **traumatic etiology:**

- Initial changes detected on serial examinations.
- Unilateral or isolated finding.
- Deformity, thickening, or angulation of the costal processes.
- The affected costal process is still clearly demarcated.
- No additional anomalies of the vertebral bodies or neural arches.
- Associated costal and/or pelvic fractures.

An accessory **riblike process** (Portmann 1961) between the transverse processes of L4 and L5 is probably analogous to the description of a heterotopic rib in the pelvis (see also Pelvis, Sacrum, and Coccyx). Figure 5.**288** illustrates a **bony bar** between the **articular and transverse processes**.

Vertical foramina at the base of the transverse processes are called **costotransverse foramina**. They are usually 2–3 mm in diameter, have cortical boundaries, and transmit veins (Fig. 5.**289**) (Beers et al. 1984).

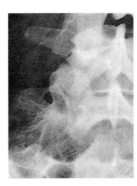

Fig. 5.**288** Bony bridge spanning the costal and articular processes of L5.

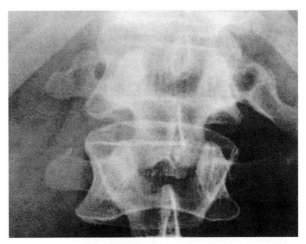

Fig. 5.**289** Costotransverse foramina in the costal processes of L1 (observation by Wendtland, Marl).

Scrutiny of the vertebral arches may show **intervertebral bony bars** (Fig. 5.**290**) that resemble **ossification of the ligamentum flavum** (Voss 1972).

The **mamillary process** is a rudimentary process arising from the superior articular process of the lumbar vertebrae. An exceptionally long mamillary process can be identified on radiographs (Fig. 5.**291**).

The **accessory process** runs obliquely downward below the mamillary process and is visible on radiographs when at least 3–5 mm long. It is then termed the **styloid process** (Figs. 5.**263**, 5.**269**, 5.**292**) (Ricci 1964).

This process has been observed with a frequency of 7.9% and occurs mainly in the lower lumbar spine (Verbiest 1955). One case was described in which the process formed a pseudarthrosis with a broad pedestal on the next lower lumbar transverse process (Fig. 5.**290**) (Kiefer and Emmrich 1964). The length of the styloid process may depend on the pull of the medial intertransverse muscles of the lumbar spine.

Exostosis-like bony processes have been described on the pedicles, laminae, and articular processes (Figs. 5.**293**, 5.**294**), and less common **cartilaginous exostoses** have been observed on the pars interarticularis (von Torklus and Braband 1963). These outgrowths may be associated with neurological complaints.

Foraminal spur is the term applied to a small bone spur that projects downward from the pedicle (behind the nerve root), occurs on one or both sides, and is located at the attachment of the ligamentum flavum (Helms and Sims 1986).

The potential for **persistence** of the **apophyses of articular processes** was noted in the previous sections on the cervical and thoracic spine (see Fig. 5.**8**). These persistent apophyses may be found on the inferior and superior articular processes and are variable in their size and shape (Fig. 5.**295**). They occur predominantly in males (Boisot et al. 1962). Their occasional association with other anomalies (spondylolysis, median neural arch cleft) may suggest a dysplastic etiology (Fig. 5.**296**). **Supernumerary ossicles** located medial to a site of spondylolysis have been described (Oppenheimer 1942, Mathias and Lössl 1975), and CT studies have confirmed their nontraumatic etiology (Raymond and Dumas 1983, Pech and Haughton 1985).

The **tip** of the **inferior articular process** may be notched (Figs. 5.**297**, 5.**298**). **Longitudinal clefts** in the inferior articular process have been reported (Oppenheimer 1941). The case of a symmetrical **duplicated superior articular process** of L4 has been described (Mathias and Lössl 1975). The occurrence of **accessory ribs** in the lower lumbar spine was noted in the section on variants at the thoracolumbar junction (Fig. 5.**231**). They are particularly common in

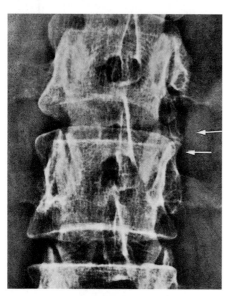

Fig. 5.**290** Small osseous bridge forms a jointlike connection between the vertebral arches (arrows).

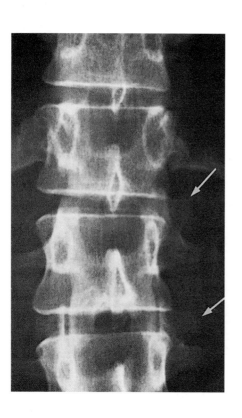

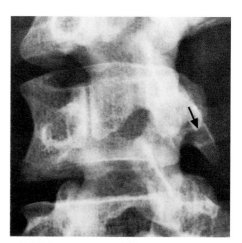

Fig. 5.**291** Long mamillary processes on the left side of the L1 and L2 vertebrae (observation by Holthusen, Hamburg).

◁ Fig. 5.**292** Styloid process of a lumbar vertebra.

Fig. 5.**293 a–d** Exostoses of the vertebral arch.

a–c Exostoses projecting medially toward the spinal canal from the vertebral arch (arrows).

d Exostosis-like outgrowth from the L3 superior articular process appears to articulate with the slightly arched transverse process of L2 (observation by Ribbing).

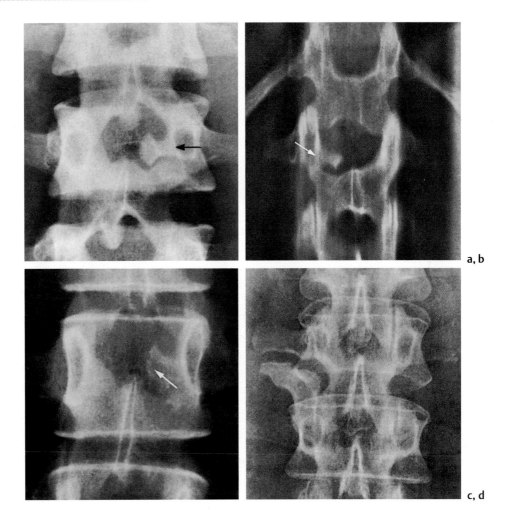

a, b

c, d

patients who also have sacral dysplasia (Bohutová et al. 1980).

The **lumbosacral junction** is subject to numerous variants (Brocher 1958). With **sacralization**, the boundary between the lumbar and sacral regions is shifted upward by one segment (cranial variant). The vertebra located at the L5 level is assimilated into the sacrum. With **lumbarization**, S1 is present as a separate lumbar vertebral body (caudal variant). Sacralization is approximately four times more common than lumbarization (Hasner et al. 1953). The assimilation process chiefly affects the transverse processes but also involves the articular processes, vertebral arches, and vertebral bodies. The assimilation may be unilateral (Fig. 5.**299**) or bilateral (Fig. 5.**300**). If it is unclear whether a vertebra has been sacralized or lumbarized, it is described as a **transitional vertebra**.

Junctional anomalies can range from an **assimilation tendency** with stout transverse processes directed toward the sacrum to a complete **synostosis**. Mixed forms in which one half of a vertebra is sacralized and the other appears lumbarized are called **asymmetric transitional vertebrae** and may be connected to the lateral mass of the sacrum by a hyperplastic transverse process. These connections may be fibrous or articular, with articular cartilage and a joint capsule.

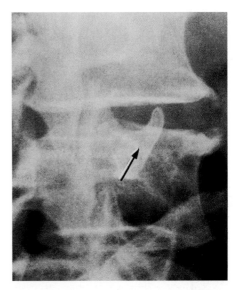

Fig. 5.**294** Exostosis projecting upward from the pedicle of L4 (arrow).

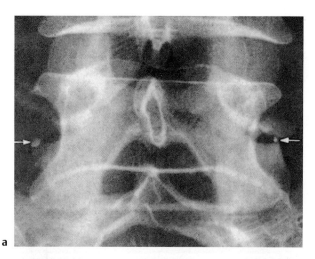

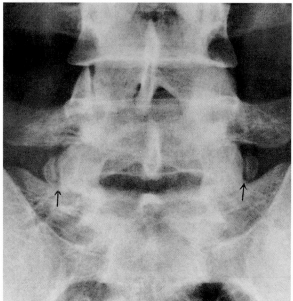

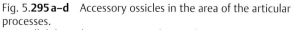

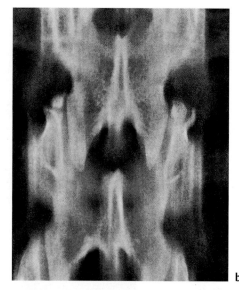

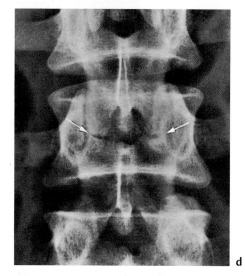

Fig. 5.295 a–d Accessory ossicles in the area of the articular processes.
a Small, bilateral accessory ossicles on the superior articular processes (arrows).
b Large accessory ossicles on the superior articular processes of L3 (observation by Hoeffkan, Cologne).

c Large accessory ossicles on the superior articular processes at the lumbosacral junction (arrows).
d Fairly large accessory ossicles at the tips of the inferior articular processes (arrows), with a symmetrical transverse cleft.

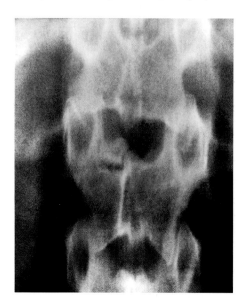

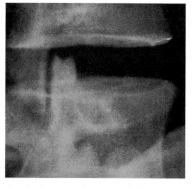

Fig. 5.**297**   Notched tip of the L5 superior articular process.

◁ Fig. 5.**296**   Vertebral arch dysplasia with spondylolysis and an isolated bony element on the L1 vertebral body (observation by Kretzschmar, Rheine).

The possible variants are too numerous to be described in detail. Consequently, the illustrations of radiographic findings and anatomic specimens represent only a selection (Figs. 5.**299**–5.**302**).

The accessory joints of partial or asymmetrical transitional vertebrae are subject to degenerative processes (Fig. 5.**301**).

The clinical significance of lumbosacral transitional vertebrae is controversial. They are a predisposing factor for the development of degenerative disk disease and may be a cause of low back pain (Fig. 5.**303**) (Jonsson et al. 1989). This particularly applies to asymmetric transitional vertebrae.

> Complete sacralization with a rigid bony connection has no clinical significance.

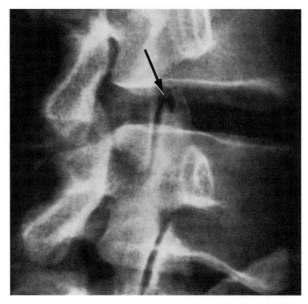

Fig. 5.**298**   Bifid superior articular process of L4 on the left side.

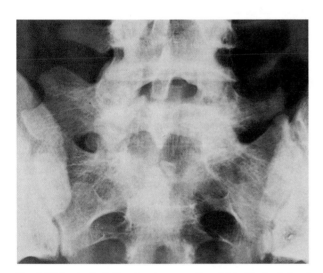

Fig. 5.**299**   Assimilation tendency on the right side (unilateral transitional vertebra).

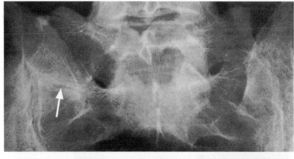

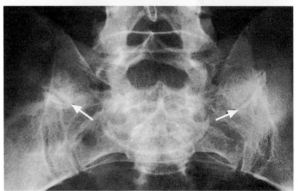

Fig. 5.**301 a, b**   Bilateral transitional vertebrae.
a With nearthrosis and frictional sclerosis on the right side (arrow).
b Bilateral nearthrosis and frictional sclerosis (arrows).

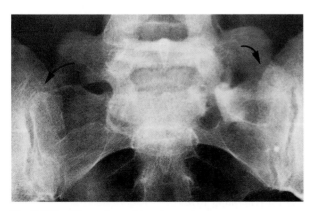

Fig. 5.**300**   Bilateral transitional vertebra.

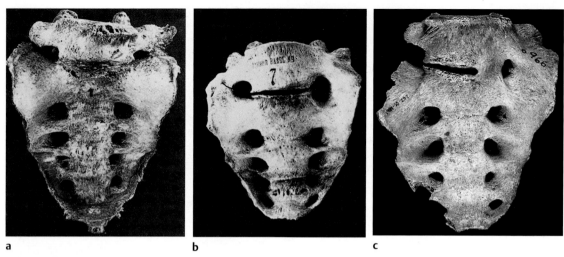

a   b   c

Fig. 5.**302 a–c** Sacral specimens illustrating variants of the lumbosacral junction.
a Partial asymmetric sacralization.

b Partial lumbalization.
c Asymmetric transitional vertebra with partial sacralization.

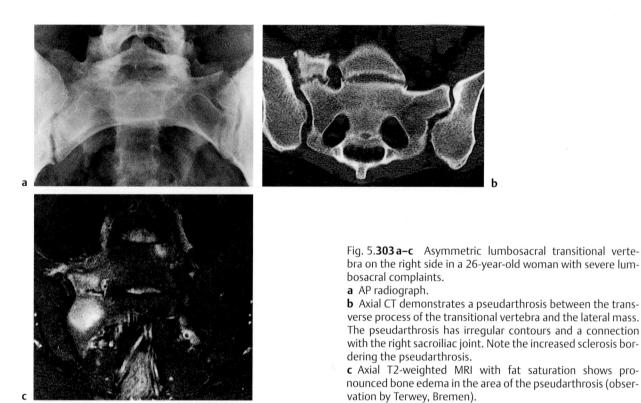

a   b

c

Fig. 5.**303 a–c** Asymmetric lumbosacral transitional vertebra on the right side in a 26-year-old woman with severe lumbosacral complaints.
a AP radiograph.
b Axial CT demonstrates a pseudarthrosis between the transverse process of the transitional vertebra and the lateral mass. The pseudarthrosis has irregular contours and a connection with the right sacroiliac joint. Note the increased sclerosis bordering the pseudarthrosis.
c Axial T2-weighted MRI with fat saturation shows pronounced bone edema in the area of the pseudarthrosis (observation by Terwey, Bremen).

Anomalies and Deformities

Vertebral body anomalies include synostoses, vertebral body defects, and vertebral body clefts (somatic clefts). Block vertebrae (Fig. 5.**304**), vertebral body defects (Fig. 5.**305**), and sagittal vertebral body clefts (Fig. 5.**306**) were discussed in detail in the section on the thoracic spine.

Coronal cleft vertebrae are very rare and occur predominantly in the lumbar spine (Brocher and Willert 1980). A connecting element is present between the ossification centers, probably consisting of an intervertebral

disklike structure and based on persistence of the perichordal septum (Fig. 5.**307**). These transient clefts are found in newborns, frequently combined with additional anomalies. In approximately 50% of cases, multiple vertebrae are affected. The clefts are usually located in the posterior third of the vertebral body at the site of the notochord, increasing the anteroposterior diameter of the vertebral body by the width of the cleft. The cleft itself contains hyaline cartilage, which generally ossifies within 2–4 months (Diethelm 1974).

Former coronal vertebral body clefts can be recognized in later life by lengthening of the vertebral body and indentations in the vertebral end plates at the site of the fused cleft. Vertebrae with coronal clefts often show concomitant wedging with associated angular kyphosis. These anomalies are mainly of differential diagnostic interest and should be distinguished from other traumatic deformities and osteolytic vertebral body processes.

According to Reeder (1993), coronal cleft vertebrae occur as normal variants in the lower thoracic and upper lumbar spine of normal children, especially preterm boys, occurring also in chondrodysplasia punctata (Conradi disease), Kniest dysplasia, and metatropic dysplasia.

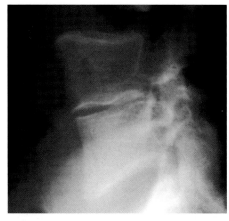

Fig. 5.**304**   Incomplete blocking of the L4 and L5 vertebrae.

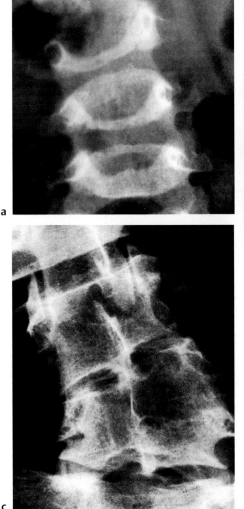

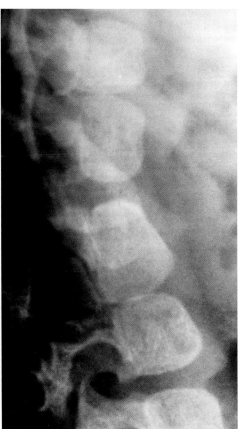

Fig. 5.**305 a–c**   Hemivertebrae in the lumbar spine.
a Right-sided L2 hemivertebra in the AP projection.
b Lateral projection of the same case.
c L5 hemivertebra fused on the left side, with resultant scoliosis.

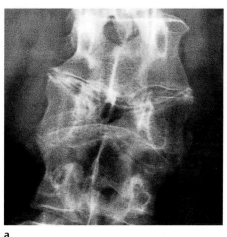
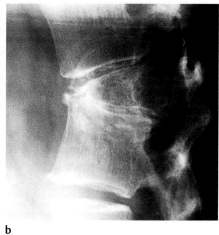

Fig. 5.**306 a, b**   Butterfly vertebra in the lumbar spine.
a AP projection.
b Lateral projection.

a   b

The causes of coronal vertebral body clefts include a **persistent chordal canal**, in which physiological notochord regression fails to occur and fibrocartilage develops in its place (Fig. 5.**235**). **Notochordal remnants** in the vertebral bodies appear as vertical lucent bands rimmed by sclerosis (Krause 1940).

General **underdevelopment of the lower lumbar spine** (Fig. 5.**308**) may be associated with underdevelopment of the sacrum. This may represent a *forme frustre* of lumbar or lumbosacral agenesis (Carlo et al. 1982). The focal or unilateral hypoplasia of vertebral bodies can result from radiotherapy applied before the patient has reached skeletal maturity (Fig. 5.**309**).

The vertebral bodies in **Down syndrome** are taller and narrower than normal with a concave anterior margin (Janovec 1972). **Tall vertebrae** are also seen in **hypotonic infants** and **Rubella syndrome** and occasionally in Marfan syndrome, arachnodactyly, and spondylocostal dysplasia (Reeder 1993).

Finally, a regional **compensatory vertebral body height increase** can occur in pathological processes that have caused decreased vertebral height in adjacent or other spinal regions, such as tuberculosis, kyphosis, and scoliosis. Height changes in vertebral bodies, including localized changes, are also seen when the causal disease process is active before the patient has attained his or her full body height (Fig. 5.**310**).

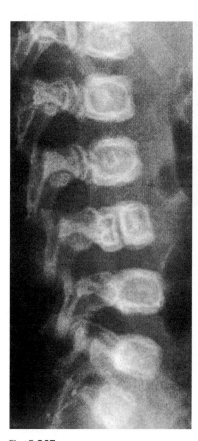
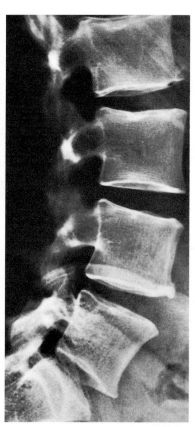

Fig. 5.**307**   Coronal vertebral cleft (observation by Swoboda).

Fig. 5.**308**   Dysplasia of the L5 vertebra, which is underdeveloped inferiorly.

Fig. 5.**307**   Fig. 5.**308**

Posterior scalloping of the vertebral bodies (Frey-schmidt 1997) may occur as a normal variant, especially at L4 and L5, but is more commonly found in association with achondroplasia (Fig. 5.**341**), an intraspinal mass, neuro-fibromatosis, acromegaly, constitutional disorders, or cal-cification of the posterior longitudinal ligament (Lagemann 1972, Reeder 1993). **Biconvex lumbar verte-brae** have been observed in several adults from the same family (Fig. 5.**311**).

Classification of vertebral arch anomalies after Brocher and Willert (1980)

➤ Vertebral arch anomalies that are associated with anomalies of the spinal cord or cauda equina and corre-sponding neurological abnormalities
➤ Vertebral arch anomalies that involve only the bony arch

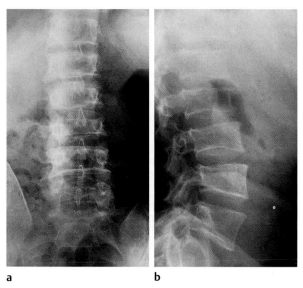

a   b

Fig. 5.**309** Left unilateral hypoplasia of L1–L6 after radio-therapy for a Wilms tumor in childhood.

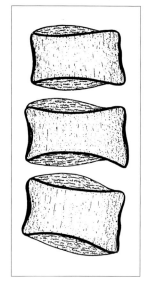

Fig. 5.**311** Biconvex lumbar vertebrae occurring as a family trait (observation by Lasserre).

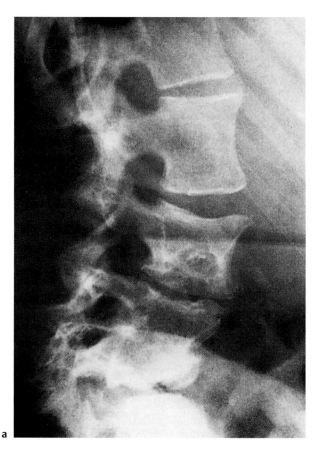

a

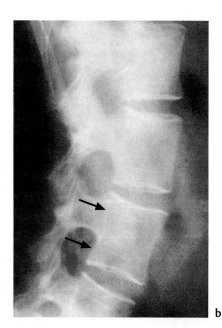

b

Fig. 5.**310 a, b** Compensatory increases in vertebral body height.
a Compensatory height increase in the L3 vertebral body. The patient had a history of spondylitis/spondylodiscitis at L4/L5 in early childhood.
b Compensatory height increase in all the lumbar vertebral bodies. Note the streaklike densities at the original growth boundaries (arrows).

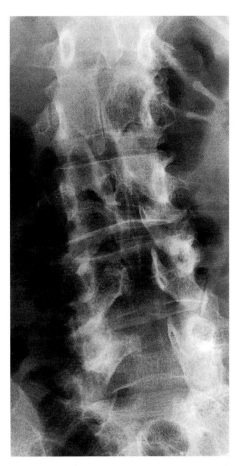

Fig. 5.**312**   Spina bifida with vertebral arch defects from L2 to L5.

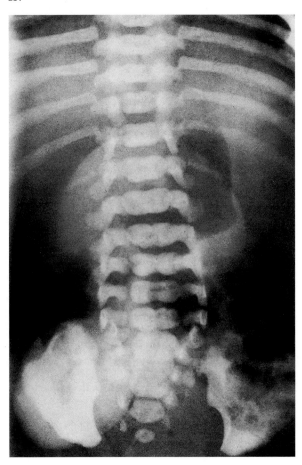

Fig. 5.**313**   Meningocele.

The first group, characterized by neurological abnormalities, falls under the heading of **dysraphism**. It includes the following:

- **Rachischisis** (araphia)
- **Spina bifida** (e.g., with myelocele or meningocele)
- **Diplomyelia**
- **Diastematomyelia**

The second group (without neurological abnormalities) includes the following:

- Median and lateral **arch clefts**
- **Arch dysplasias**
- **Anomalies of the arch processes**

The spectrum of **dysraphic abnormalities** ranges from simple clefts in spinous processes to extensive arch defects (Fig. 5.**312**) and the most severe form, spina bifida aperta.

With a **meningocele** or **myelomeningocele**, the AP radiograph shows a fusiform expansion of the spinal canal with widening of the interpedicular distance. Absence of the spinous processes and posterior arch elements is characteristic (Fig. 5.**313**). The spinous processes and arch elements are also absent in the lateral view. **MRI** has a critical role in the diagnosis and management of dysraphic anomalies (Altman and Altman 1987).

Diplomyelia, in which the spinal cord is partially or completely divided in two by a longitudinal fissure, is not associated with specific changes in the spinal column. **Diastematomyelia** occurs in approximately 15% of patients with congenital scoliosis and is twice as common in girls as in boys. In this anomaly the spinal cord is split into halves by a sagittal septum, which may be partly ossified, within the vertebral canal (Banniza von Bazan 1984) (Fig. 5.**314**). Diastematomyelia may be associated with other developmental anomalies such as:

- Congenital scoliosis
- Rib anomalies
- Elevated scapula
- Myelomeningocele

Clinical symptoms usually first appear in the growing child when the septum hampers the physiological ascent of the conus medullaris in the lumbar region, but occasionally symptoms do not appear until adulthood (Maroun et al. 1982). AP radiographs may demonstrate **fusion of the vertebral arches**, **vertebral arch defects**, and fusiform **widening of the spinal canal** with an increased interpedicular distance (Banniza von Bazan 1984). Lateral radiographs may show **posterior scalloping of the vertebral bodies**. The anomaly is frequently associated with scoliosis, but the spine may appear completely normal. Ossified septa can occasionally be seen on conventional radiographs and are defined more clearly by **CT** (Arredondo et al. 1980). But **MRI** is the modality of choice for evaluating the spinal canal and its abnormalities (Fig. 5.**314**) (Prasad et al. 1995).

> **Median arch clefts** in L5 and S1 have an incidence of approximately 20% and fall within the range of borderline-normal findings (Figs. 5.**315**, 5.**316**).

Median arch clefts (spinous clefts) generally have no clinical importance and can be classified as a type of vertebral arch dysplasia. Concomitant defects in the spinal cord and/or its membranes (myelomeningoceles) are extremely

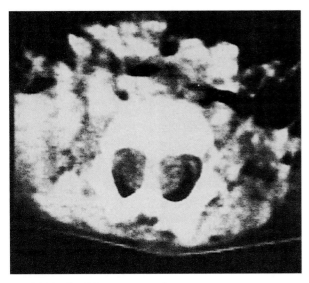

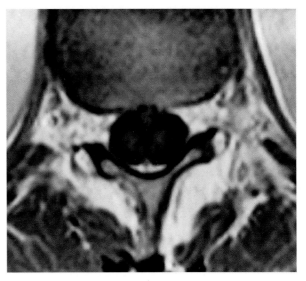

Fig. 5.**314a, b**   Diastematomyelia.
a Bony septum in axial CT.

b Axial T1-weighted MRI demonstrates the two parts of the spinal cord (different case).

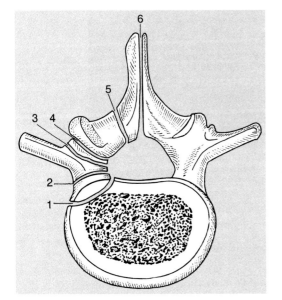

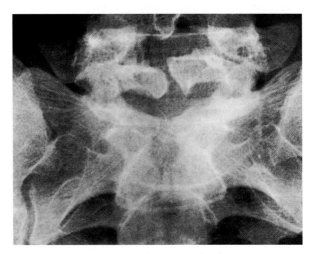

Fig. 5.**316**   Median arch clefts of L5 and S1.

Fig. 5.**315**   Clefts in the vertebral arch.
1, 2   Retrosomatic clefts
3, 4   Clefts in the pars interarticularis
5   Retroisthmic cleft
6   Median (spinous) cleft

rare. The term "spina bifida" should be used only if the cleft is combined with neurological abnormalities, and "spina bifida occulta" if there is no protrusion of cord or meninges through the bony defect.

The median arch defect may lie on an oblique plane, producing an asymmetry in the lateral view that can mimic duplication of the spinous process (Fig. 5.**317**). The spinous process may be completely absent or may be vestigial, consisting of a separately developed apical ossification center (see under variants and anomalies of C1). The affected vertebral arch may be hypoplastic or may show compensatory extension across the midline.

Lateral arch clefts may be retrosomatic, may involve the pars interarticularis (spondylolysis), or may involve the lamina (retroisthmic).

Retrosomatic clefts are very rare and occasionally bilateral and have been observed from T12 to L5 (Fig. 5.**318**) (Olsson 1948, Johansen et al. 1983, Niethard and Pfeil 1985). Fatigue fractures (Niethard and Pfeil 1985) and persistence of the neurocentral synchondrosis (Olsson 1948) have been suggested as causes. To date, however, no case of a persistent neurocentral synchondrosis has been described, and besides, the synchondrosis is located at a more anterior site in the vertebral body (Fig. 5.**265**). Aplastic and hypoplastic pedicles (Bardsley and Hanelin 1971, Morin and Palacios 1974), which may show circumscribed notching, presumably represent a special subtype of retrosomatic clefts (Fig. 5.**319**).

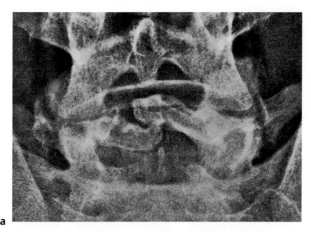
a

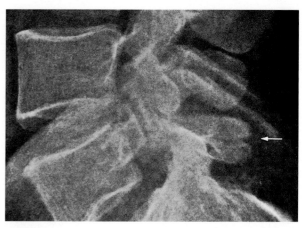
b

Fig. 5.**317 a, b**   Incomplete closure of the L5 vertebral arch.
a The halves of the vertebral arch are overlapped in the AP projection.

b Apparent duplication of the spinous process in the lateral projection (arrow).

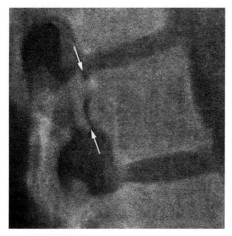

Fig. 5.**318**   Retrosomatic cleft of L2 (arrows).

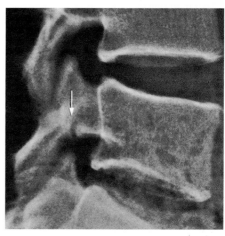

Fig. 5.**319**   Small notch at the base of the pars interarticularis.

Retroisthmic clefts, located in the lamina just behind the inferior articular process, are even rarer than retrosomatic clefts (Seegelken and Schulte 1972, Seegelken and Keller 1974). The more than coincidental association of these clefts with a median arch cleft suggests a dysplastic etiology.

The **most common site of occurrence** of neural arch clefts is the **pars interarticularis** (isthmus). A pars cleft is known also as **spondylolysis** (Figs. 5.**315**, 5.**320**). Its incidence is approximately 4–5 % (Wiltse 1962, Abel 1985, Hensinger 1989) and is three times higher in the white population than in people of color. A genetic predisposition has been confirmed. Vertebral arch defects were detected in 34 % of Alaskan Eskimos, the most common defect being a pars cleft in the fifth lumbar vertebra (Stewart 1953).

The principal sites of occurrence are the arches of L4 and L5. Spondylolysis is rare above L2. Usually only bilateral spondylolysis causes complaints, which are very rare with unilateral defects (Libson et al. 1982). Clefts may be present in multiple, usually adjacent vertebrae. Two or rarely three vertebrae are usually affected in these cases.

To date there have been no reports of finding spondylolysis in a fetus or newborn, and it is rarely detected prior to the fifth year. By the seventh year, however, the incidence corresponds to that in adults (Wiltse et al. 1975, Hensinger 1989). Almost all pars defects have developed by 18 years of age.

The potential **causes** of **spondylolysis** are diverse:

● Congenital anomaly (Hensinger 1989)
● Trauma (Kaiser et al. 1972)
● Stress fracture sustained during skeletal growth
● Secondary form due to destruction of the pars interarticularis (by tumor, inflammatory disease, or trauma), Paget disease, neurogenic spondylarthropathy, osteomalacia, or osteogenesis imperfecta

Wiltse et al. (1976) have classified lumbar spondylolysis and spondylolisthesis into five types:

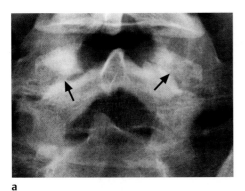

a

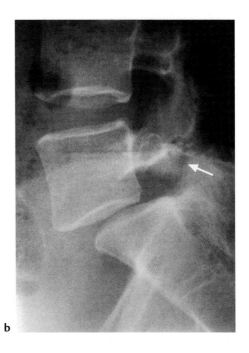

b

Fig. 5.**320 a, b** Bilateral spondylolysis of L5 with spondylolisthesis.
a Typical appearance of the clefts in the AP projection (arrows).
b Spondylolysis (arrow) and spondylolisthesis in the lateral projection.

Classification of lumbar spondylolysis and spondylolisthesis after Wiltse et al.
➤ *Type 1:* Congenital dysplasia of the upper sacrum or the L5 vertebral arch.
➤ *Type 2:* A defect in the pars interarticularis, which may be caused by:
 – 2 a: a fatigue fracture
 – 2 b: dysplasia and elongation of an intact pars interarticularis, or
 – 2 c: an acute fracture of the pars interarticularis
➤ *Type 3:* Degenerative, resulting from intersegmental instability
➤ *Type 4:* Traumatic, caused by fractures of the vertebral arch outside the pars
➤ *Type 5:* Pathological, due to local or generalized bone disease

The most common types of spondylolysis are 2 a, 2 b, and 3. Type 2 b lesions may progress to type 2 a.

It should be assumed that a fatigue fracture is present in the following circumstances:

● Histological examination of the bony gap reveals fibrous connective tissue interspersed with osteochondral tissue (Zippel and Runge 1976).
● The spondylolysis is first diagnosed after surgical spinal fusion (Brunet and Wiley 1984).
● The spondylolysis occurs in a high-performance athlete whose actions include sudden movements into a position of hyperlordosis (Schwerdtner and Schobert 1973, Luther and Legal 1975).
● Therapeutic immobilization cures the spondylolysis.

The following features distinguish spondylolysis from other types of fatigue fracture:

● It develops at an early age, shows a genetic predisposition, and is rarely associated with periosteal callus formation (Ciullo and Jackson 1985).

● It develops after minor trauma, and the stress-related damage in the pars interarticularis persists as spondylolysis (Wiltse et al. 1975).

The arch segments outside the pars interarticularis may also be affected by fatigue fractures, but this is very rare. Stress fractures of the retroisthmic arch and pedicles have been described (Abel 1985). Fatigue fractures of the inferior articular processes have also been detected by CT following laminectomy and facetectomy (Rothmann et al. 1985).

Spondylolysis can often be detected **radiographically** in the AP and lateral projections. In the **AP projection**, the spondylolysis defect runs laterally downward (Fig. 5.**320**), contrasting with the more medially downward course of the apophyseal joint line (Amato et al. 1984). The best views are obtained by angling the x-ray tube 30° cephalad (Amato et al. 1984). Compensatory enlargement and sclerosis of the contralateral vertebral arch are occasionally found (Fig. 5.**321**). Spondylolysis is usually well visualized in the **lateral projection**. The defect runs in a posterior-superior to anterior-inferior direction through the pars interarticularis (Figs. 5.**320**, 5.**321**).

Secondary signs of spondylolysis and spondylolisthesis include more than a 20% loss of posterior vertebral body height compared with the anterior margin, especially when the L5 vertebral body is affected (Hensinger 1989). Occasionally the vertebra shows a trapezoidal configuration or hypoplasia (Fig. 5.**322**). Anteroposterior shortening of the vertebral body can mimic spondylolisthesis if only the posterior vertebral contours are evaluated. The normal alignment of the anterior vertebral margins serves to distinguish this condition from true spondylolisthesis.

The **oblique projection** can define the full extent of the pars interarticularis and the pars defect (Figs. 5.**323**, 5.**324**). Oblique **tomograms** can clarify findings that are difficult to evaluate on the summation image (Fig. 5.**325**). Interpretation is facilitated by referral to the **scotty dog sign of Lachapèle** (Lachapèle 1939) (Fig. 5.**278**).

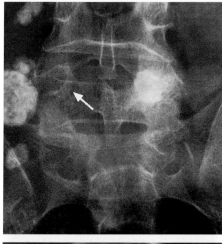

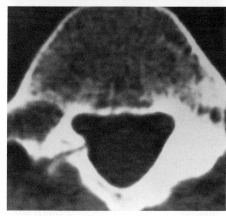

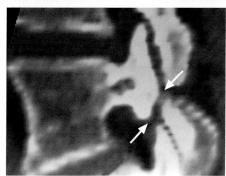

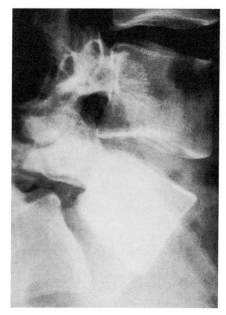

Fig. 5.**322**   Anterior displacement of an underdeveloped L5 relative to S1 and L4.

◁ Fig. 5.**321 a–c**   Compensatory pedicular hypertrophy in response to unilateral spondylolysis.
a Left-sided sclerosis of the vertebral arch with right-sided spondylolysis of L5 (arrow) (observation by Westermann, Hannover).
b Axial CT scan in a different case shows marked sclerosis and hypertrophy of the contralateral vertebral arch due to spondylolysis on the right side (observation by Breunsbach, Cologne).
c Spondylolysis in the sagittal reformatted image (arrows) (observation by Breunsbach, Cologne).

A cleft in the pars interarticularis appears as a "collar" on the dog, while a retroisthmic cleft appears as a band around the dog's abdomen (Fig. 5.**326**). **Dysplasia** of the pars causes the neck of the dog to appear longer and thinner (Fig. 5.**327**). Reference was made earlier to **pseudospondylolysis** caused by superimposing the costal processes over the vertebral arches at the L2 and L3 levels (Fig. 5.**277**).

CT examinations, especially using high resolution and multiplanar reformations (Fig. 5.**321**), provide a valuable addition to imaging options (Rothmann and Glenn 1984, Langston and Gavant 1985, Teplick et al. 1986). **Radionuclide scanning** and particularly single-photon emission computed tomography (**SPECT**) can reliably detect fatigue fractures of the pars interarticularis (Fig. 5.**323**) (Pennell et

al. 1985, Bellah et al. 1991). Increased tracer uptake may correlate with pain symptoms and signify an early, radiographically occult stage of spondylolysis, whereas longstanding spondylolysis may be negative on radionuclide scans (Pennell et al. 1985, Kollier et al. 1985, Bellah et al. 1991). In summary, bone scans are more sensitive than conventional radiographs, and SPECT is more sensitive and specific than bone scans. On the other hand, bone scans and SPECT are less specific for spondylolysis than conventional radiography and CT (Harvey et al. 1998).

MRI can demonstrate the pars defect, bone edema, as well as narrowing of the intervertebral foramen and spinal canal as a result of spondylolisthesis (Grenier et al. 1989). The signal intensity changes of the bone marrow in the pedicles, however, are not specific for spondylolysis, but

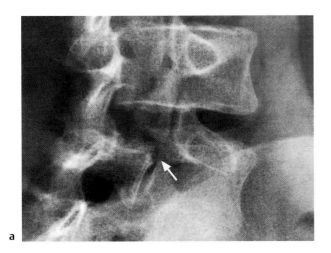

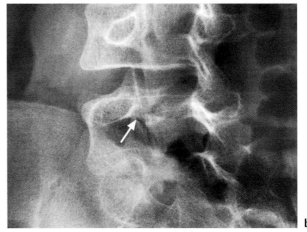

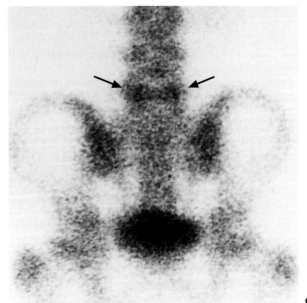

Fig. 5.**323 a–c**   Spondylolysis and interarticular dysplasia in the oblique projection.
a Complete spondylolysis of L5 on the left side (arrow).
b Marked interarticular dysplasia of L5 on the right side (arrow).
c Bilateral areas of increased uptake in a bone scan (arrows).

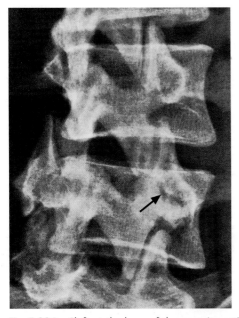

Fig. 5.**324**   Cleft at the base of the superior articular process (arrow) with probable degenerative deformity in a 25-year-old man (observation by Wendtland, Marl).

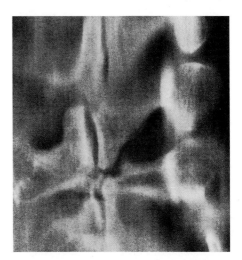

Fig. 5.**325**   Spondylolysis with a double pars fracture in an oblique tomogram.

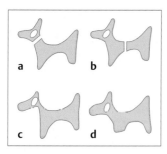

Fig. 5.**326a–d** Spondylolysis and dysplasia of the vertebral arch. Schematic diagram (after Dihlmann).
a Typical spondylolysis due to a pars defect.
b Retroisthmic cleft.
c Dysplasia of the pars and hypoplasia of the superior articular process.
d Aplasia of the inferior articular process.

are more frequently encountered in spondylarthrosis deformans (Morrison et al. 2000).

Spondylolysis can lead to **spondylolisthesis**, or anterior vertebral slippage (Fig. 5.**328**). For this slippage to occur, degenerative changes must be present in the associated intervertebral disk and there must be laxness of the posterior ligaments and loss of tonus in the anterior muscles.

Generally the slippage starts before 20 years of age and is completed in adulthood. The two lower lumbar vertebrae are most commonly affected, particularly L5, which is involved in approximately 80–90% of all cases.

Pseudospondylolisthesis and **spondyloretrolisthesis** (retroposition, reverse spondylolisthesis) are discussed in the section on degenerative changes in the lumbar spine.

In the strict sense of the term, spondylolisthesis is actually a pseudospondylolisthesis in that the break in the pars interarticularis allows only the vertebral body to slip for-

ward and not the entire vertebra. Meanwhile, pseudospondylolisthesis is actually a spondylolisthesis in the strict sense as it denotes slippage of the entire vertebra, including its appendages, rather than a portion of it (Fig. 5.**329**).

Spondylolisthesis of the L5 vertebra is characterized in the **AP projection** by the appearance of the "inverted Napoleon hat" sign (Fig. 5.**330**).

In the **lateral projection**, the degree of spondylolisthesis and pseudospondylolisthesis can be evaluated quantitatively by the method of Sim (1973) or semiquantitatively by the method of Meyerding (1932) (Figs. 5.**331**, 5.**332**). Wiltse and Winter (1983) may be consulted for a review of the various methods of measurement.

The mobility of the displaced vertebra can be measured on **functional views** taken in flexion and extension (Penning and Blickman 1980, Dvorak et al. 1991 a, b). Hypermobility of the displaced vertebra, and especially unstable gliding, lead to segmental instability with a "drawer phenomenon" (Fig. 5.**333**).

Dysplasia of the vertebral arch has the following radiographic features:

- Thin laminae (Fig. 5.**334**)
- Elongation of the arch
- Elongation of the pars interarticularis with narrowing or angulation
- Hypoplasia of the articular processes
- Abnormal orientation of the apophyseal joints

Arch dysplasias are hereditary and are probably a significant factor in the pathogenesis of vertebral slippage. **Asymmetries of joint space position** are included among the congenital anomalies. They may occur in one segment (Fig. 5.**335**) or may involve several segments with various joint space orientations (Fig. 5.**336**) and can lead to gaping of the joint space with clinical complaints (Fig. 5.**337**).

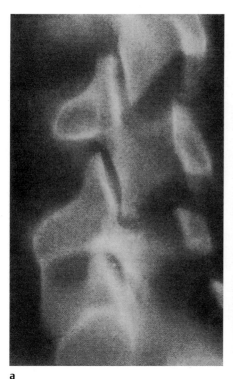

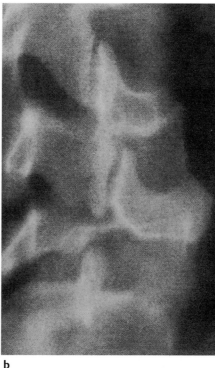

Fig. 5.**327a, b** Dysplasia of the articular process (observation by Brocher, Genf).
a Well-developed but sclerotic pars interarticularis on the right side.
b Hypoplastic L5 inferior articular process with a narrow pars.

a

b

Fig. 5.**328 a–c** Spondylolisthesis.
a Mild degree of spondylolisthesis (grade I).
b Grade III spondylolisthesis.
c Spondyloptosis.

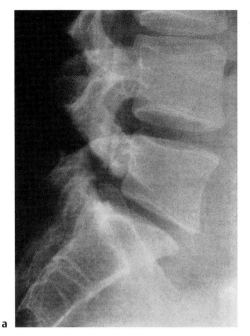

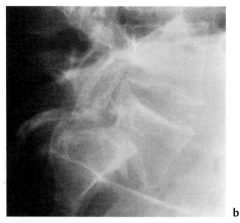

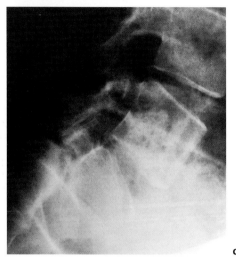

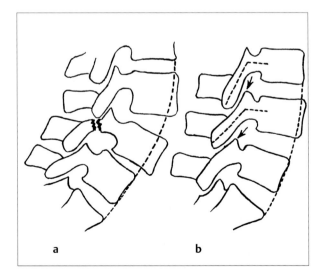

Fig. 5.**329 a, b** Spondylolisthesis and pseudospondylolisthesis.
a Spondylolisthesis.
b Pseudospondylolisthesis. Note the increased inclination of the articular surfaces and the increased angle of the vertebral arch (dashed line).

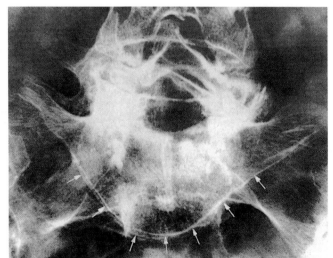

Fig. 5.**330** "Inverted Napoleon hat" sign of spondylolisthesis of L5 on an AP radiograph.

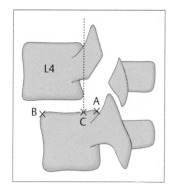

◁ Fig. 5.**331**   Roentgenometry of spondylolisthesis and pseudospondylolisthesis by the method of Sim. The ratio (*AC/AB*) × 100 % gives the slippage of the affected vertebra in percent (after Dihlmann).

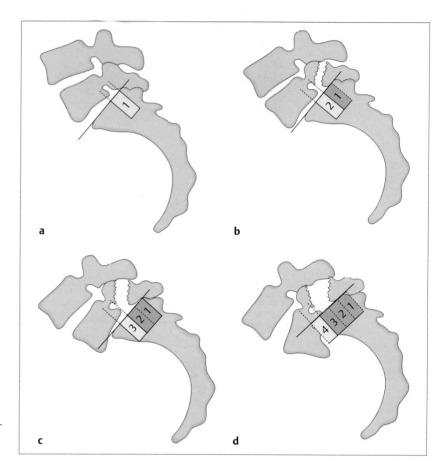

Fig. 5.**332 a–d**   Meyerding classification of spondylolisthesis and pseudospondylolisthesis.

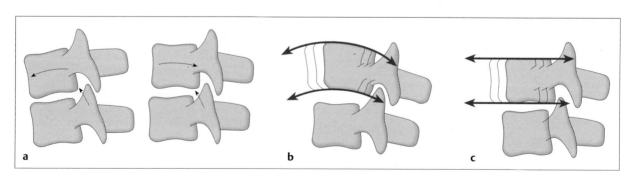

Fig. 5.**333 a–c**   Flexion-extension functional views for the evaluation of segmental instability (after Dihlmann).
a No segmental instability (hypomobility, immobility).

b Moderate segmental instability (hypermobility).
c Severe segmental instability (vertebral slippage, "drawer phenomenon").

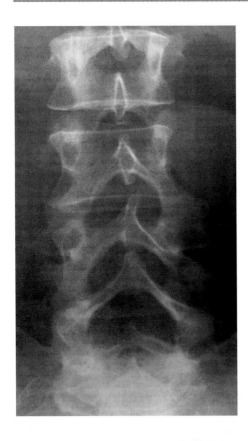

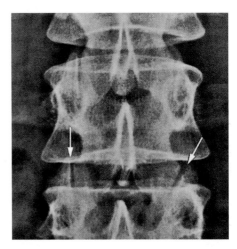

Fig. 5.**335**   Axial malalignment of the apophyseal joint on the left side (arrows). This abnormality is frequently missed on AP radiographs.

◁ Fig. 5.**334**   Dysplasia of the L4 and L5 vertebral arches with laminar hypoplasia (from Schinz 1986).

Fig. 5.**336**   Axial malalignment (dashed lines) of two apophyseal joints of the lower lumbar spine.

Fig. 5.**337**   Gaping apophyseal joint (arrow).

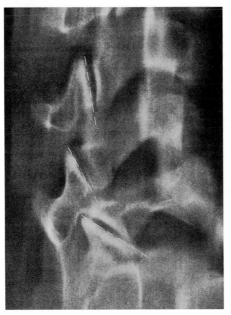

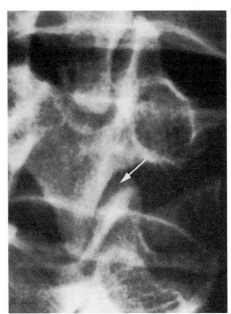

Fig. 5.**336**

Fig. 5.**337**

Aplasia, **hypoplasia**, and **dysplasia** of the **articular processes** in the lumbosacral region are particularly common findings in transitional vertebrae (Fig. 5.**338**) (Ruckensteiner 1939). The underdevelopment of an articular process can incite a sclerotic reaction in the underlying pars region.

Aplasia of the articular processes is extremely rare (Fig. 5.**339**). These changes are demonstrated much better by CT than plain films (Arcomano and Karas 1982, Boeck et al. 1982, Yousefzadeh et al. 1982, Wortzmann and Steinhardt 1984). Males predominate (61%), and the aplasia

tends to occur on the left side (Stelling 1981). Pain usually brings the condition to light. These anomalies have also been observed in children (Yousefzadeh et al. 1982) and may be combined with other anomalies (Wortzmann and Steinhardt 1984). They can lead to instability and degenerative changes, and unilateral aplasia can lead to scoliosis (Ruckensteiner 1939, Wigh 1981).

A constitutionally **narrow lumbar canal** in adults means that the interpedicular distance is less than 13 mm wide. A sagittal diameter of less than 10 mm on CT scans provides a useful cutoff point for diagnosing spinal steno-

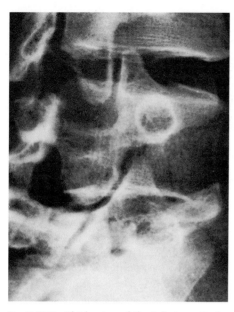

Fig. 5.**338**   Thickening of the inferior articular process of L4. Spondylarthrosis deformans at L5/S1.

sis. It should be considered that, with aging, it becomes increasingly difficult to distinguish primary congenital narrowing from acquired narrowing, which is usually due to degenerative disease (Fig. 5.**340**) (Lassale et al. 1983).

A narrow lumbar canal is a common feature of **certain skeletal dysplasias**, most notably:

- Achondroplasia (Fig. 5.**341**)
- Hypochondroplasia
- Pseudoachondroplasia
- Acromegaly
- Dystrophic dysplasia
- Klippel–Feil syndrome

A narrow lumbar canal may also be found in Paget disease (Weisz 1983, Reeder 1993).

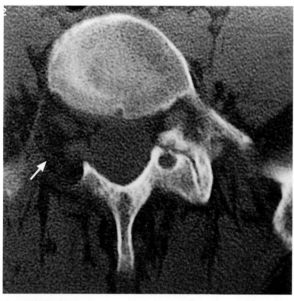

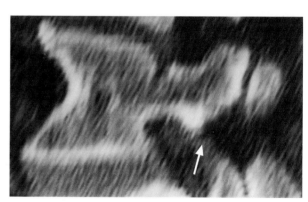

Fig. 5.**339a, b**   Aplasia of the inferior articular process.
a Absence of the inferior articular process on axial CT (arrow). Degeneration of the contralateral apophyseal joint with cyst formation.

b Aplasia of the inferior articular process in a sagittal reformatted image (arrow) (observation by Weidner, Osnabrück).

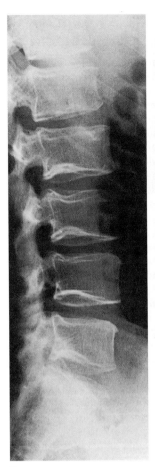
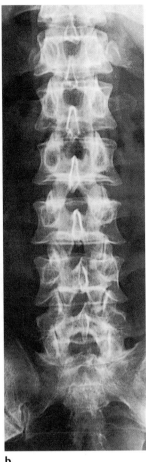

a   b

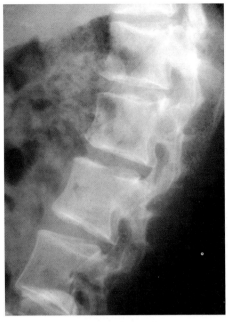

Fig. 5.**341**   Achondroplasia with a narrow spinal canal. There is marked posterior scalloping of the vertebral bodies.

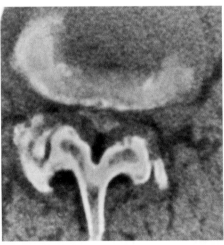

c

Fig. 5.**340 a–c**   Narrow lumbar canal in a 38-year-old man.
a, b Biplane radiographs of the lumbar spine demonstrate round pedicles, narrow interlaminar windows in the AP view, and a small sagittal diameter in the lateral view. All of these signs suggest a narrow spinal canal.
c CT appearance of significant spinal stenosis. Note the hypertrophy of the articular processes and ligamenta flava and the marked compression of the dural sac.

Fracture, Subluxation, or Dislocation?

Traumatic changes in the lumbar spine are basically the same as those affecting the thoracic spine and thoracolumbar junction. Fractures in these regions have a common classification system and are discussed in the section on the thoracic spine.

Isolated **transverse process fractures** caused by paraspinous muscle traction or direct trauma are associated with lateral and especially upward displacement of the lateral fragments. Multiple fractures are common. The psoas margin superimposed on the transverse process can mimic this type of fracture, which should not be confused with the apophysis of a transverse process (Figs. 5.**266,** 5.**270**). **Persistent apophyses** differ from avulsed fragments in that they have intact cortical margins and are usually located further laterally. **Fractures of the L5 costal processes** may signify posterior **instability of the pelvic ring** in trauma patients (Reis and Keret 1985). It should be added that myositis ossificans following costal process fractures can cause secondary bony bridges to form between the transverse processes, and these can simulate a congenital variant (Figs. 5.**285**–5.**287**). A "limbus vertebra" can mimic **traumatically avulsed bone fragments** from vertebral bodies (Figs. 5.**384**–5.**386**). **Fatigue fractures of the vertebral arch** are discussed under spondylolysis in the section on anomalies and deformities.

Necrosis?

Necrotic changes in vertebrae (Kümmell–Verneuil disease, steroid-induced necrosis) were discussed in the section on the thoracic spine. **Acute intervertebral disk narrowing** combined with a "nibbled" appearance of adjacent vertebral contours and increased calcium deposition in vertebral areas bordering the disk may be observed following surgical sympathectomy. It has been attributed to a segmental chondromalacia of the disk brought on by a sudden disruption of the arterial blood supply (Güssel 1949).

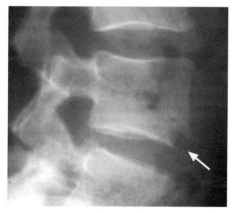

Fig. 5.**342** Anterior spondylitis in tuberculous spondylitis, marked by erosion of the anteroinferior corner of the vertebral body (arrow).

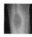 ## Inflammation?

Bacterial spondylodiscitis most commonly affects the lumbar spine, followed by the thoracic and cervical spine and the sacrum (Garcia and Grantham 1960, Cahill et al. 1991). It occurs predominantly in the fifth and sixth decades but may also affect children and the elderly. Generally the infection is manifested within the vertebral body and less commonly in the vertebral arch and its appendages (Peris et al. 1992). Besides the usual hematogenous route, bacteria can reach the site by direct inoculation through an open spinal injury, surgical wound (Nielsen et al. 1990), or needle tract (Buetti and Ldi 1958, Hadden and Swanson 1982). The spread of adjacent soft-tissue infections to the spine can also occur (Gordon 1977). Defects in the vertebral surfaces and intervertebral disks and sclerosis of the T9–L4 vertebrae have been described following **lumbar sympathetic blockade** and interpreted as subacute postinfectious sequelae.

A **hematogenous infection** is usually manifested in the anterior subchondral region of the vertebral body. From there it may spread upward or downward to the adjacent intervertebral disk or anteriorly below the anterior longitudinal ligament. The infection may also track upward and downward below the ligament, causing numerous erosions in the anterior and lateral surfaces of multiple vertebrae. This is found mainly in **tuberculosis** and is known as **superficial anterior tuberculous spondylitis** (Wiesmayr 1952, Brocher 1953) (Fig. 5.**342**).

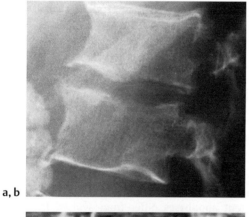
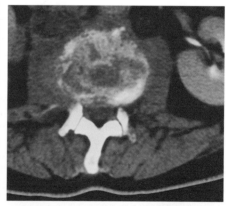

a, b

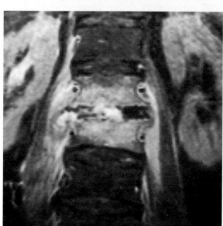
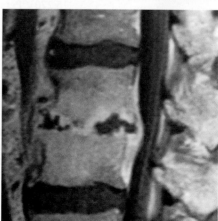

c, d

Fig. 5.**343 a–d** Spondylodiscitis.
a Plain film shows narrowing of the L2/L3 disk space with unsharpness of the adjacent vertebral end plates.
b Erosions of the discovertebral junctions on axial CT.
c Coronal MRI (STIR sequence) shows edematous changes in the affected vertebral bodies, the intervertebral disk, and the psoas muscles with abscess formation on the right side.
d T1-weighted sagittal MRI after contrast administration defines the intraspinal extent of the inflammation and shows narrowing of the spinal canal.

With **spondylitis** of acute onset, isolated paravertebral periosteal reactions may occur (Schmitt 1949). The infection spreads from the infected disks (discitis) to the adjacent vertebral body. Disk space narrowing may be an early sign of **infectious spondylodiscitis**. Destructive changes in the adjacent vertebral end plates are initially subtle but progress over time. Even the slightest **loss of disk height** and circumscribed **thinning** of the adjacent **end plates** may be the radiological signs of an infection (Figs. 5.**343**, 5.**344**).

The destruction of two adjacent vertebral bodies and the intervening disk is typical of an infectious etiology (Fig. 5.**345**). Approximately two-thirds of all cases of spondylodiscitis involve the disk space and adjacent vertebral bodies. It is less common to find involvement of multiple segments or of a single vertebral body or disk (Malawski 1977).

Differentiation is required from **tumor-associated destruction**, which almost never causes loss of disk height even when two adjacent vertebrae are affected. Problems can also arise in differentiating spondylodiscitis from **erosive osteochondrosis** (Fig. 5.**371**).

Reparative processes eventually lead to **vertebral body sclerosis** adjacent to the end plates (Griffiths and Jones 1971). Possible late sequelae include the development of diffuse vertebral body sclerosis (**ivory vertebra**) and **block vertebrae** (Fig. 5.**437**), which may be accompanied by angular deformity of the spine. Unlike the more harmonious forms and structures of congenital block vertebrae (Figs. 5.**166 a**, 5.**304**), acquired block vertebrae are usually

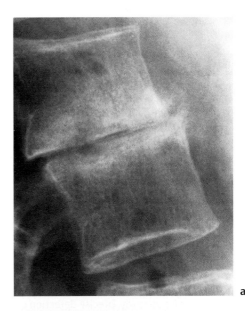
a

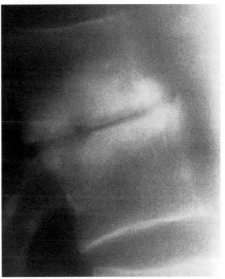
b

Fig. 5.**344 a, b** Advanced spondylodiscitis, characterized by disk space narrowing and erosions of the discovertebral junctions. Marked subchondral sclerosis is present in the form of hemispheric spondylosclerosis.
a Lateral radiograph.
b Lateral tomogram.

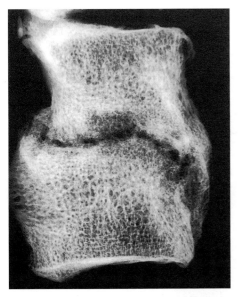

Fig. 5.**345** Specimen illustrating the late sequelae of spondylodiscitis (specimen courtesy of D. Resnick, San Diego).

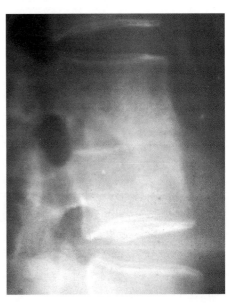

Fig. 5.**346** Postinfectious block vertebrae. In contrast to congenital block vertebrae, there is no waistlike constriction of the vertebral bodies.

associated with irregularities of shape, structure, and contour.

This **basic pattern** of spondylitis applies to all types of inflammation (Frottier et al. 1983):

- **Tuberculosis** (Gorse et al. 1983)
- **Nonspecific osteomyelitis**, which is associated with monosymptomatic discitis, especially in children (Eggert 1970, Galil et al. 1983)
- **Salmonellosis** (Lé 1982)
- Spinal **brucellosis** (Bang disease), which has become a rarity (Mohan et al. 1990)

Gouty osteoarthropathy may be associated with erosions of the vertebral bodies and posterior elements (Lagier and MacGee 1983), and this can create the impression of an infection or intervertebral osteochondrosis (Jajic 1982, Stepàn et al. 1983, Das 1988).

Information on the differential diagnosis of the various forms of spondylodiscitis can be found in textbooks and manuals (Schinz 1986, Resnick 1995, Freyschmidt 1997).

CT permits the early, precise detection of bone destruction and involvement of the paravertebral soft tissues (Fig. 5.**343**) (Hermann et al. 1983, Raininko et al. 1985). **MRI** is superior to CT for analyzing the paravertebral soft tissues, detecting intervertebral disk involvement, and detecting the spread of inflammation into the spinal canal (Fig. 5.**343**) (Kramer et al. 1990, Sharif 1992).

Changes in the lumbar spine due to **rheumatoid arthritis** are rare, as in the thoracic spine, and are discussed under that heading (Heywood and Meyers 1986).

The lumbar spine is a common site of involvement by **seronegative spondylarthropathies** (ankylosing spondylitis, Reiter disease, psoriatic arthritis, enteropathic spondylarthropathy). **Ankylosing spondylitis** generally occurs between 15 and 35 years of age with a male preponderance. In classic cases the disease starts in the sacroiliac joints and later spreads to the thoracolumbar and lumbosacral junction (Kinsella et al. 1966). In long-standing cases, the disease eventually affects the midlumbar and upper thoracic spine and less commonly the cervical spine. Involvement of the spine without sacroiliac joint involvement is unusual (Gran et al. 1985).

Ankylosing spondylitis presents **radiographically** with changes in the discovertebral junction, apophyseal joints, costovertebral joints, and posterior ligaments. In the **vertebral bodies**, subdiscal and marginal destruction lead to a focal contour defect at the anterior corner and occasionally the posterior corner of the vertebral body known as a **Romanus lesion** or **marginal spondylitis** (Fig. 5.**347**) (Romanus and Ydén 1952). These changes are most commonly found in L3–L5. The corner defect is usually surrounded by a rim of reactive sclerosis, which may occur in the absence of a defect, producing a "**shiny corner**" sign (Fig. 5.**348**) (Dihlmann 1966). Marginal spondylitis is seen in approximately 10% of all patients with ankylosing spondylitis, so it is relatively rare. Destructive foci in the vertebral body end plates are termed **Andersson lesions** (Andersson 1937).

A **round** or **barrel-shaped vertebra** results from the enlargement of anterior corner defects, thereby rounding off the anterior surface of the vertebral body (Dihlmann 1966). A **square vertebra** can result from anterior spondylitis when the concave anterior surface of the vertebral body becomes straightened as a result of productive bone-forming processes or cortical bone loss (Fig. 5.**349**). The **differential diagnosis** of squared vertebrae includes Paget disease and, less commonly, psoriatic arthritis, Reiter syndrome, and rheumatoid arthritis.

CT has demonstrated deep **erosions** in the **vertebral arches** and **spinous processes** of patients with long-standing **ankylosing spondylitis** (Grossman et al. 1983).

A characteristic feature of ankylosing spondylitis is the formation of **syndesmophytes**, which appear initially at the thoracolumbar junction, particularly on the anterior and lateral aspects, in approximately 60% of cases (Figs. 5.**350**, 5.**351**, 5.**353**–5.**355**). They result from ossification of the outer layers of the anulus fibrosus and in advanced cases may additionally involve the anterior longitudinal ligament and the entire intervertebral disk (Figs. 5.**350**, 5.**351**) (Dihlmann 1987). Syndesmophytes appear as thin, vertical radiodensities along the spine (Figs. 5.**354**, 5.**403**).

Other spinal changes of ankylosing spondylitis are seen in the **apophyseal** and **costovertebral joints**, which show erosive and sclerotic changes and may eventually ankylose (Dihlmann 1987). **Ossification** of the **apophyseal joints**

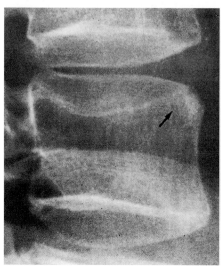
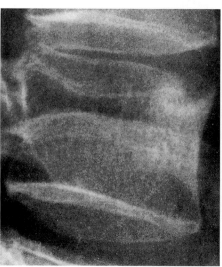

Fig. 5.**347 a, b**   Romanus lesion (anterior spondylitis).
a Destruction and sclerosis of the anterior vertebral margin.
b Film four years later shows persistence of sclerosis with partial filling-in of the concavity (arrow).

a   b

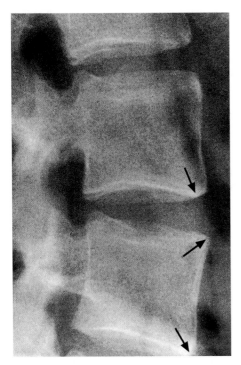

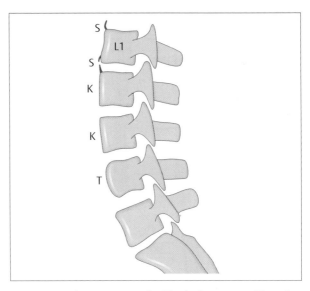

Fig. 5.**349** Changes in vertebral body shape caused by anky-
losing spondylitis (after Dihlmann).
K   Square vertebrae
S   Syndesmophytes
T   Barrel-shaped vertebra

Fig. 5.**348** Anterior spondylitis with sclerosis of the anterior
corners of the vertebral bodies ("shiny corners," arrows).

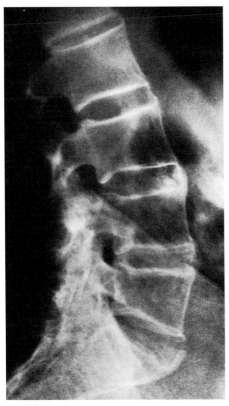

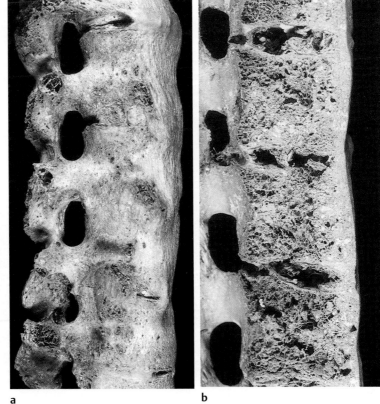

a   b

Fig. 5.**350** Lateral view of the lumbar spine
in ankylosing spondylitis demonstrates ossification of the anterior longitudinal ligament.

Fig. 5.**351 a, b** Ankylosing spondylitis in a specimen.
a Ankylosis of the lumbar spine due to ossification of the anterior longitudinal
ligament and anulus fibrosus.
b Sagittal cross section of the specimen (Museum of Man, San Diego).

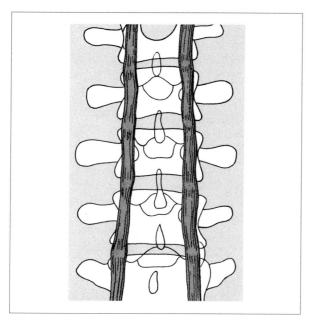

Fig. 5.**352** Ankylosing spondylitis. No syndesmophytes, but extensive ossification of the apophyseal joints and ligamentum flavum (after Dihlmann).

and **ligamenta flava** creates paired vertical radiodense lines called a **double trolley track** (Figs. 5.352, 5.353). A **triple trolley track** is produced by ossification of the interspinous and supraspinous ligaments (Fig. 5.354).

Mixed osteophytes occur when syndesmophytes develop at sites where there are preexisting degenerative spondylophytes (Fig. 5.403) (Dihlmann 1987). In its advanced stage, **ankylosing spondylitis** produces a "bamboo spine" contour with undulant bony outgrowths at the level of the disk spaces (Fig. 5.355).

Psoriatic arthritis is characterized by **paravertebral ossification (parasyndesmophytes)** involving the thoracic and upper lumbar spine (Figs. 5.356, 5.403). Sundaram and Patton (1975) observed this pattern of ossification in 62% of patients with psoriatic arthritis and normal sacroiliac joints and in 81% of patients who also had normal-appearing joints of the hands and feet. The calcifications were typically directed parallel to the lateral surfaces of the vertebral bodies and the intervertebral disk spaces (Fig. 5.356).

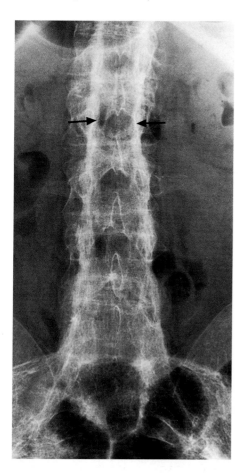

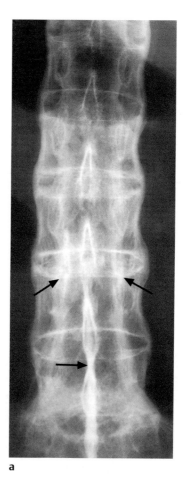

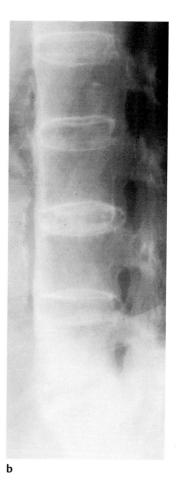

a

b

△
Fig. 5.**353** Ankylosing spondylitis of the lumbar spine. Ankylosis of the apophyseal joints has produced a double trolley-track sign (arrows). There is concomitant ankylosis of the sacroiliac joints.

Fig. 5.**354a, b** Ankylosing spondylitis of lumbar spine. Ankylosis of the apophyseal joints (arrows) and ossification of the interspinous and supraspinous ligaments (arrowheads) have produced a triple trolley-track sign. The anulus fibrosus and anterior longitudinal ligament are also ossified.
a AP projection.
b Lateral projection.

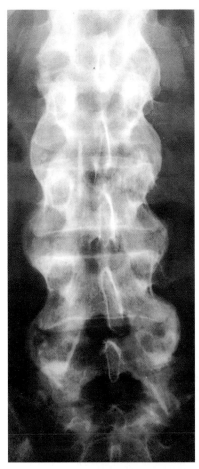

Films occasionally show extensive **paravertebral ossifications** that fuse with the adjacent structures of the axial skeleton. Sometimes they resemble the syndesmophytes of ankylosing spondylitis, but generally they are distinguished by their larger size, their typical unilateral or asymmetrical pattern of occurrence, and their slightly greater distance from the spine. There may also be **osteitis** of the vertebral bodies and apophyseal joint involvement with **arthritis** and **ankylosis**, although this is less common than in ankylosing spondylitis.

Involvement of the spine in **Reiter syndrome** is less common than in ankylosing spondylitis and psoriatic arthritis. As in psoriatic arthritis, the early stage of Reiter syndrome is marked by **paravertebral ossification** along

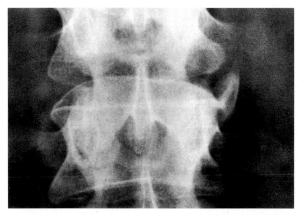

Fig. 5.**355** Bamboo spine in the late stage of ankylosing spondylitis.

Fig. 5.**356** Typical parasyndesmophyte in psoriatic arthritis.

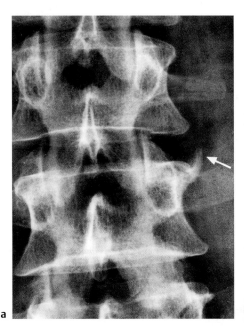

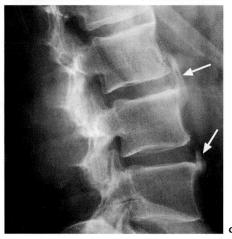

Fig. 5.**357 a–c** Parasyndesmophytes in Reiter disease (arrows).
a Small parasyndesmophyte.
b Large ossified parasyndesmophyte.
c Parasyndesmophytes in the lateral projection.

the lower three thoracic vertebrae and upper three lumbar vertebrae in up to 35% of patients (Sundaram and Patton 1975). The radiographic appearance resembles that of psoriatic arthritis and may be an early manifestation of the disease that precedes changes in the peripheral joints (Fig. 5.**357**).

Apophyseal joint changes may also be present in Reiter syndrome. Syndesmophytes can develop in Reiter syndrome and in psoriatic arthritis, eventually producing a "bamboo spine" contour as in ankylosing spondylitis and preventing any further differentiation of the diseases.

Enteropathic spondylarthropathies occur in association with Crohn disease, ulcerative colitis, and Whipple disease (McEwen et al. 1971, Moll et al. 1974, Dekker-Saeys et al. 1978). The changes closely resemble those of ankylosing spondylitis.

 ## Tumor?

A comprehensive discussion of tumors and tumorlike lesions of the spine is beyond our scope and can be found in standard reference works on the subject (Freyschmidt 1986, Campaniaci 1990, Resnick 1995, Freyschmidt 1998). Here we shall briefly review the most important spinal tumors and their sites of predilection, to the extent that this information has not been covered in previous sections.

Generally a spinal tumor is suspected on the basis of increased or decreased radiographic density, which may be focal or diffuse. Contour changes in the form of a reduced volume (destruction, collapse) or increased size are also suspicious for neoplasia. Thus, the differential diagnosis of the various patterns has special significance in the spine.

The **most frequent causes of focal vertebral body sclerosis** are as follows (Reeder 1993):

- Bone islands
- Compression fractures or consolidating fractures
- Osteoblastic metastases
- Spondylarthrosis
- Intervertebral osteochondrosis

Hemispheric spondylosclerosis in particular can mimic an osteosclerotic spinal tumor (Figs. 5.**344**, 5.**373**).

The following diseases and conditions are **less frequent** causes of focal sclerosis (Reeder 1993):

- Osteoma
- Histiocytosis X
- Lymphoma
- Osteoblastoma
- Osteoid osteoma
- Chronic osteomyelitis
- Sarcoidosis
- Sarcoma (especially osteosarcoma)
- Tuberous sclerosis
- Sclerotic vertebral arch (see below)

Homogeneous or **nonhomogeneous osteosclerosis** of one or more vertebral bodies in an older patient is strongly suspicious for metastasis. Prostatic carcinoma is the leading source in males, but metastases can also arise from lymphoma, plasmacytoma, and chordoma (see below). **Osteopoikilosis** can produce multiple bone islands that resemble osteoblastic metastases (Lagier et al. 1984). The same applies to certain manifestations of melorheostosis (Fig. 5.**207**) (Garver et al. 1982).

The **dense sclerosis of one or more vertebral bodies (ivory vertebrae)** may be caused by osteosclerotic metastases, especially from prostatic carcinoma. They can also result from any of the following conditions:

- Paget disease
- Myelosclerosis
- Lymphoma
- Fluorosis
- Osteopetrosis
- Rarely, chordoma, osteosarcoma or plasmacytoma (Fig. 5.**358**)

These changes require differentiation from:

- The typical appearance of vertebral hemangioma (Fig. 5.**359**)
- Rugger jersey spine due to renal osteodystrophy (Fig. 5.**360**)
- Osteosclerotic changes in the various stages of osteopetrosis (Fig. 5.**361**)

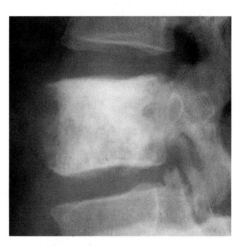

Fig. 5.**358** Vertebral plasmacytoma, associated with dense sclerosis of the vertebral body.

Fig. 5.**359 a–c** Hemangioma of a lumbar vertebra. The lesion involves both the vertebral body and the neural arch.
a AP projection.
b Lateral projection.
c Typical CT appearance.

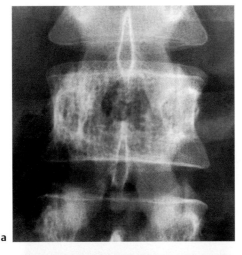
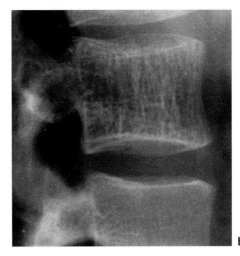
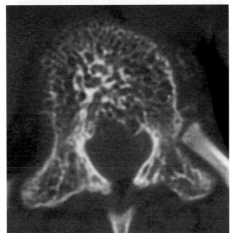

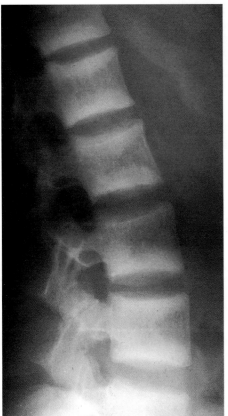

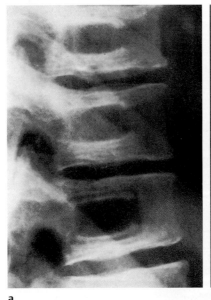
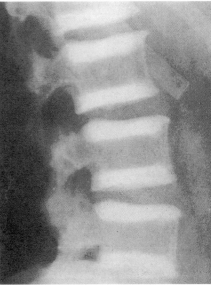

Fig. 5.**361 a, b** Osteopetrosis (Albers–Schönberg disease).
a Initial stage is marked by dense vertebral end plates with a laminated appearance.
b Late stage shows typical zones of increased density near the end plates (sandwich vertebrae).

◁ Fig. 5.**360** Involvement of the lumbar spine by renal osteodystrophy ("rugger jersey" spine).

The **sclerosis** of a **vertebral arch** may have **congenital causes:** hypoplasia or aplasia of the pedicle or articular process (Fig. 5.**339**), spina bifida occulta, or apophyseal joint asymmetry. Other causes are unilateral **spondylolysis** with contralateral reactive sclerosis due to increased stresses (Fig. 5.**321**), **tumors** (osteoma, osteoid osteoma, osteoblastoma, osteoblastic metastases, lymphoma, myeloma, Ewing sarcoma, osteosarcoma) (Figs. 5.**189**, 5.**362**, 5.**368**), **tumorlike changes** (Paget disease, fibrous dysplasia, sarcoidosis, tuberous sclerosis), **infections**, **surgical procedures** (laminectomy), or no detectable cause (**idiopathic**) (Yochum et al. 1990).

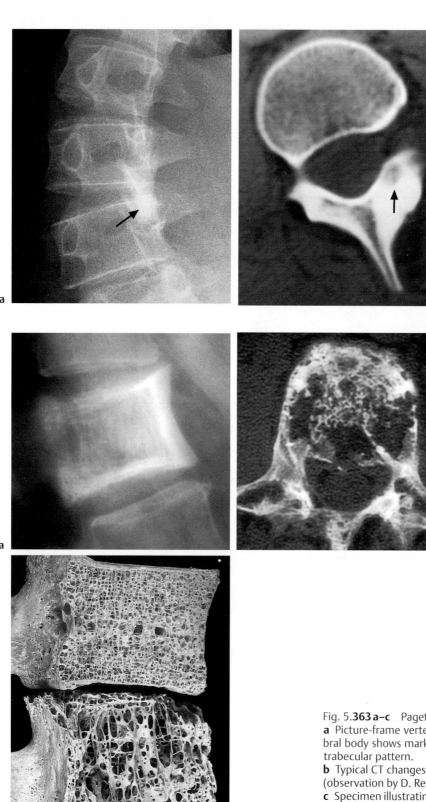

Fig. 5.**362 a, b**   Osteoid osteoma of the lumbar spine.
a Right convex torsional scoliosis of the lumbar spine, secondary to an osteoid osteoma in the left superior articular process of L3 (arrow).
b CT demonstrates the nidus and increased sclerosis (arrow).

Fig. 5.**363 a–c**   Paget disease.
a Picture-frame vertebra in the lateral projection. The vertebral body shows marked cortical thickening with a coarsened trabecular pattern.
b Typical CT changes with involvement of the entire vertebra (observation by D. Resnick, San Diego).
c Specimen illustrating Paget disease. Note the coarse trabeculations compared with a normal vertebra (Museum of Man, San Diego).

Cortical thickening of vertebral bodies occurs with **osteosclerosis** and especially with **Paget disease** (Fig. 5.**363**). A very **thin cortex** (as if drawn with a pencil) is a typical finding in all forms of **osteopenia** (Fig. 5.**365**).

The **coarse trabecular pattern** seen in **Paget disease** differs from the finer and more uniform trabecular condensation observed in **fluorosis** (Fig. 5.**364**). There is generalized involvement of all cancellous bone areas in fluorosis (Fig. 5.**364**), contrasting with the predominantly monotopic or oligotopic distribution of Paget disease.

The differential diagnosis of increased **vertical trabeculation** in one or more vertebral bodies should include the following:

- Paget disease (Fig. 5.**362**)
- Osteoporosis (Fig. 5.**365**)
- Hemangioma (Fig. 5.**359**)
- Primary anemia
- Less common diseases such as:
  – Lymphoma
  – Leukemia
  – Diffuse metastasis
  – Multiple myeloma (Fig. 5.**366**)

Overlying bowel gas can mimic the appearance of **osteolytic areas** in bone. In the AP projection, the interlaminar window or other **projection-related effects** can create the impression of increased density (Fig. 5.**268**). Osteolytic metastases in the vertebral arch can cause **destruction of the pedicle**, which is most clearly demonstrated in the AP projection (**Elsberg–Dyke sign**, Fig. 5.**367**).

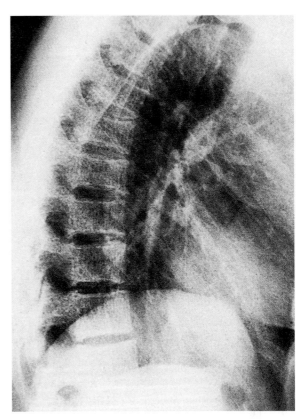

Fig. 5.**364**   Fluorosis of the spine. Radiograph shows a finely striated pattern of sclerosis of the thoracic and lumbar vertebrae.

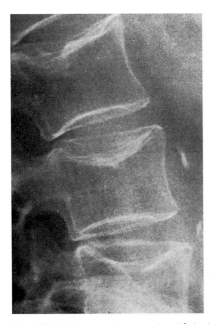

Fig. 5.**365**   Severe osteoporosis with incipient fish vertebrae caused by central collapse. Cortical thinning is pronounced.

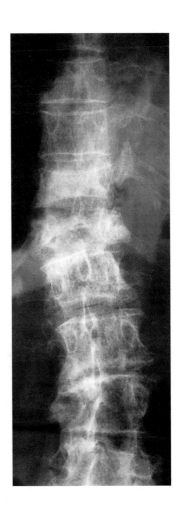

Fig. 5.**366**   Multiple myeloma. Diffuse, finely striated sclerosis of all vertebral bodies with a pathological fracture of T12.   ▷

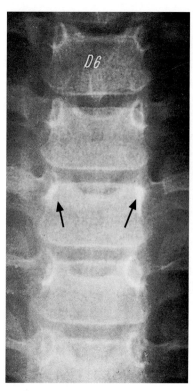

Fig. 5.**367**   Destruction of both T8 pedicles by a tumor (Elsberg–Dyke sign).

Small osteolytic lesions of the vertebral bodies no larger than 15 mm in size are very difficult to detect on **plain films**. This is accomplished better with **conventional tomography** (Schröder et al. 1968) or **CT**, which can detect lesions as small as 2–3 mm (Haller 1990a, b). **MRI** is better suited for diagnosing vertebral metastases and is superior to CT and bone scans, especially for evaluating paraosseous extension and infiltration of the spinal canal (Smoker et al. 1987, Frank et al. 1990, Kattapuram et al. 1990, Algra et al. 1991).

Loss of vertebral body height occurs when the load-bearing capacity of the cancellous trabeculae has been compromised as a result of **bone destruction** or **osteopenia** (Andresen et al. 1999). Pathological fractures of vertebral bodies due to metastasis require differentiation from compression fractures due to osteoporosis, osteomalacia, or multiple myeloma. **Pathological fractures of the upper thoracic spine** are likely to have a malignant cause, since osteoporosis and osteomalacia are less common in that region. Vertebra plana in children is a typical feature of **eosinophilic granuloma** (Fig. 5.**191**) (Whitehouse and Griffiths 1976, Weinstein et al. 1984).

The detection of an intravertebral **vacuum phenomenon** suggests an ischemic cause (Kümmell–Verneuil disease, Fig. 5.**247**) and largely excludes a malignant process. **Intervertebral disk height** is generally **preserved** in the presence of **malignant vertebral body collapse**, whereas it is typically **reduced** in **spondylodiscitis**.

The **enlargement** of vertebral bodies in their transverse and sagittal dimensions is found in **acromegaly** among other diseases (Erdheim 1931, Lang and Bessler 1961, Erbe et al. 1975). Films show periosteal productive bone changes, especially on the anterior and lateral aspects of the vertebral bodies, while the proliferation of marginal

ridge segments increases the posterior convexity of the vertebra (**scalloping**). Another typical feature of this disease is an increase in intervertebral disk height caused by the proliferation of discal tissue. **Scheuermann disease** is among the conditions that can lead to an increase in the sagittal diameter of vertebral bodies (see section on the thoracic spine). Expansion of vertebral contours can also occur with **giant cell tumors**, **aneurysmal bone cysts**, and **fibrous dysplasia** (Figs. 5.**190**, 5.**194**).

Earlier reference was made to the ability of **aortic aneurysms** to produce **concavities and contour defects** in the anterior and left lateral surfaces of a vertebra (see section on the thoracic spine). The differential diagnosis of posterior vertebral scalloping was discussed under Normal Variant or Anomaly.

Enostosis

Enostosis (bone island, osteoma) of the spine most commonly affects the thoracic and lumbar vertebrae (Broderick et al. 1978). Enostomas appear as insular densities with relatively sharp margins (Figs. 5.**115**, 5.**270**, 5.**368**) (Broderick et al. 1978). These benign lesions require differentiation from osteosclerotic metastases.

Osteoid Osteoma, Osteoblastoma

Osteoid osteomas of the spine are most commonly found in the lumbar and cervical spine (Francis et al. 1980). They usually occur in the posterior portions of the vertebra and can lead to diffuse **sclerosis** (Fig. 5.**189**). **Osteoid osteoma** and **osteoblastoma** of the thoracic and lumbar spine often lead to scoliosis of the affected segment (Dias and Frost 1973, Griffin 1978, Adelwahab et al. 1986). Typically the lesion is located at the apex of the concavity (Fig. 5.**362**). Any otherwise unexplained **painful scoliosis** in adolescence should raise suspicion of an osteoid osteoma and prompt further radiological investigation. Generally the **nidus** is easier to detect with **CT** than radiographs (Stojanovič et al. 1982, Gamba et al. 1984). Osteoid osteoma and osteoblastoma show intense tracer uptake on bone scans (Onimus et al. 1985, Pettine and Klassen 1986). **MRI** is very sensitive in detecting bone edema (Azouz 1994) but is less specific because of its relatively poor ability to visualize the nidus (Assoun et al. 1994). The difficulty of diagnosing osteoid osteoma is reflected in the fact that often more than one year passes from the painful onset of the disease to a definitive diagnosis (Mau 1982).

Osteosarcoma

Osteosarcomas, usually of the conventional type, very rarely affect the spine. They tend to occur in vertebral bodies, where they produce a focal or diffuse sclerosis (ivory vertebra). Involvement of the vertebral arch can be difficult to distinguish from osteoid osteoma (Shives et al. 1986).

Fig. 5.**368 a–d**   Osteomas of the vertebral bodies.
a Large osteoma of L1 in the AP projection.
b Lateral projection. Same case as in **a**.
c Small osteoma.
d Small osteoma appears as an exostosis-like outgrowth from the right side of the vertebral body.

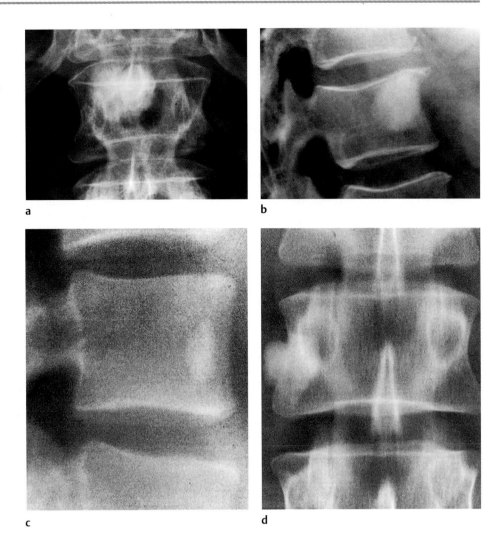

a

b

c

d

Cartilage-Forming Tumors

Benign cartilage-forming tumors are rare in the spine. The occurrence of **enchondromas** and **chondroblastomas** has been described (Buraczewski et al. 1957, Hoeffel et al. 1987, Morard et al. 1993). Approximately 2% of all **osteochondromas** occur in the vertebral bodies, most commonly involving the posterior elements of the lumbar and cervical vertebrae (Fig. 5.**192**) (von Torklus and Braband 1963, Fielding and Ratzan 1973, Marchand et al. 1986). Only about 7% of **chondrosarcomas** are found in the vertebral bodies (Shives et al. 1989).

Giant Cell Tumors

Giant cell tumors involve the axial skeleton in approximately 7% of all cases, affecting the sacrum, thoracic spine, cervical spine, and lumbar spine in descending order of frequency (Fig. 5.**440**) (Dahlin 1977, Schwimer et al. 1981, Sanjay et al. 1993). In the vertebrae they affect the vertebral body more often than the posterior elements. This distinguishes them from aneurysmal bone cyst and osteoblastoma, which tend to affect the posterior elements (Figs. 5.**189**, 5.**190**).

Aneurysmal Bone Cyst

Aneurysmal bone cysts (Lifeso and Younge 1985) are relatively common in the spine and are discussed more fully in the section on the cervical spine (Fig. 5.**190**). They are frequently expansile and can spread past the boundaries of the vertebral body into the disk, adjacent vertebra, or spinal canal.

Fibrous Dysplasia

Fibrous dysplasia of vertebrae is very rare and may be associated with an increase in vertebral body size. It is characterized by a soap-bubble structure with severe vertebral body deformity and intact contours (Fig. 5.**194**) (Nyúl-Toth and Joós 1974).

Hemangioma

Hemangioma is the most common of the vascular tumors. It occurs predominantly in the thoracic spine but may also affect the cervical and lumbar spine. Most hemangiomas are located in the vertebral bodies (Sherman and Wilner 1961, Laredo et al. 1986). They show a characteristic spoked-wheel pattern with coarsened, vertically oriented trabeculae (Fig. 5.**359**). Extension into the surrounding soft tissues or spinal canal can mimic a malignant tumor. **MRI** typically shows increased signal intensity in T2-weighted spin-echo sequences. Hemangiomas may show a high or low signal intensity on T1-weighted images. They enhance intensely after intravenous contrast administration (Ross et al. 1987, Laredo et al. 1990).

Chordoma

Chordomas occur predominantly in the sacrococcygeal region and upper cervical spine and are discussed more fully under those headings (Figs. 5.**195**, 5.**439**). Involvement of the lumbar and thoracic spine has been observed (Meyer et al. 1984, de Bruine and Kroon 1988, Darby et al. 1999). Radiographically, they can resemble skeletal metastases, chondrosarcoma, giant cell tumor, skeletal lymphoma, infection, and plasmacytoma.

Ewing Sarcoma

Ewing sarcoma affects the spine in 6% of all cases (Whitehouse and Griffiths 1976, Weinstein et al. 1984). Usually this tumor leads to osteolysis and eventual vertebral body collapse. Vertebral sclerosis is occasionally observed.

Eosinophilic Granuloma

Eosinophilic granuloma most commonly affects the thoracic and lumbar spine, but cervical involvement can occur (Fig. 5.**191**). **Vertebra plana** (Calve disease) is a more common finding in children than adults.

Multiple Myeloma

The axial skeleton is a site of predilection for multiple myeloma, which produces a honeycomb pattern of osteolytic lesions of fairly uniform size, particularly in the vertebral bodies (Freyschmidt 1986). The posterior vertebral elements are less commonly affected, which can help distinguish multiple myeloma from multiple osteolytic metastases (Jacobson et al. 1958b). Diffuse sclerotic bone changes are also occasionally seen with this tumor (Hall and Gore 1988) (Fig. 5.**366**).

Plasmacytoma

Plasmacytoma (solitary myeloma) occurs predominantly in the thoracic and lumbar spine and may present as a cystic, expansile lesion with thickened trabeculae or as a purely osteosclerotic or osteolytic lesion (Maurer 1958, Krull et al. 1972, Spiro et al. 1988). Plasmacytoma may be concealed within a diffusely sclerotic vertebral body (ivory vertebra) (Roberts et al. 1974). Plasmacytoma should be considered in every middle-aged patient with a solitary osteolytic lesion in a vertebral body, possibly accompanied by a pathological fracture, or with a process spreading into the spinal canal and/or adjacent vertebral body. **POEMS syndrome** (polyneuropathy, organomegaly, endocrinopathy, M-protein, skin changes) is a type of plasma cell dyscrasia that is associated with sclerosing plasmacytomas of the spine and pelvis (Resnick et al. 1981a, Resnick et al. 1984, Aggarwal et al. 1990).

Lymphomas

Skeletal involvement by **non-Hodgkin lymphoma** and **Hodgkin lymphoma** most commonly affects the spine and other bones that contribute to hematopoiesis. Radiographically, these tumors may be purely osteolytic, purely sclerotic (ivory vertebra), or may show a mixed pattern of osteolytic and sclerotic features (Gaudin et al. 1992, Farrés 1993).

Lymphomas can be difficult to distinguish from metastases and Paget disease (see differential diagnosis of ivory vertebrae) (Fig. 5.**363**).

Others

It is very rare to encounter **simple bone cysts** in the spine (Matsumoto et al. 1990). Other rare entities at this location are **lipoma, lymphangioma, lymphangiomatosis** (Oppermann et al. 1979), **cystic hemangiomatosis** (Fig. 5.**369**) (Reid et al. 1989), and **malignant fibrous histiocytoma** (Huvos et al. 1985).

Solitary neurofibromas and **neurinomas (schwannomas)** can also occur in the lumbar and thoracic spine. Their typical radiographic features are described in the section on the cervical spine (Fig. 5.**193**).

Metastases

The spine is the most common location for **skeletal metastases**. This is due in part to the high content of hematopoietic bone marrow (Galasko 1981). Metastases are most frequent in the lumbar spine, followed by the thoracic spine and cervical spine. They arise in the vertebral body more often than in the neural arch, although arch involvement is more common with skeletal metastases than with multiple myeloma (Harrington 1986). **Osteolytic metastases** most commonly originate from cancers of the thyroid, kidney, adrenal, gastrointestinal tract, and uterus. On CT, intravertebral disk herniation may be suspicious for an osteolytic metastasis (Fig. 5.**383**). **Mixed-form metastases** occur mainly with bronchial, breast, cervical and ovarian cancers, while purely **osteoblastic metastases** are seen mainly with prostatic carcinoma. The most common primary tumors that metastasize to the spine are bronchial, breast and prostatic carcinoma.

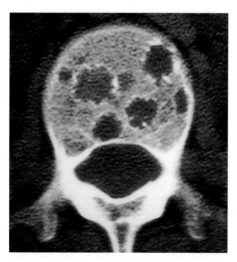

Fig. 5.**369** CT appearance of cystic hemangiomatosis of a vertebral body (observation by D. Resnick, San Diego).

Other Changes?

Degenerative changes in the lumbar vertebrae are quite common and predominantly affect L4–S1, with relatively frequent concomitant involvement of the L3/L4 segment (Miller et al. 1988). The basic forms of degenerative spinal changes—chondrosis, intervertebral osteochondrosis, spondylosis deformans, and spondylarthrosis deformans—are described in the chapters on the cervical and thoracic spine.

The relationship between radiographic changes and back pain is controversial (Torgerson and Dotter 1976, Witt et al. 1984, Collee et al. 1990). It appears, however, that a connection does exist between intervertebral osteochondrosis and pain, whereas no such link has yet been established for spondylosis deformans or spondylarthrosis deformans.

Intervertebral Osteochondrosis

Intervertebral osteochondrosis in its **generalized form** can affect the entire lumbar spine (Fig. 5.**370**). Similar changes combined with disk calcifications can occur in the setting of alkaptonuria (**ochronosis**) (Fig. 5.**392**) (Sakkas et al. 1987).

The **erosive form** of intervertebral osteochondrosis, which is associated with sclerosis, erosions, and focal end plate defects caused by Schmorl node formation, can be difficult to distinguish from spondylodiscitis (Fig. 5.**371**) (Lagier et al. 1979, Lagier and MacGee 1979). **MRI** is helpful in making this differentiation, however. Stäbler et al. (1998) found that spondylodiscitis was associated with significantly greater edema in the adjacent vertebral bodies. Meanwhile, the discovertebral junctions in erosive osteochondrosis were almost always clearly delineated and of low signal intensity, while these findings were not seen in spondylodiscitis. Another criterion for erosive osteochondrosis is the typically low signal intensity of the intervertebral disks in T2-weighted and STIR images, contrasting with the generally high signal intensity found in spondylodiscitis. Contrast enhancement of the affected intervertebral disks was present in both diseases and was not a useful differentiating criterion (Stäbler et al. 1998).

Intervertebral osteochondrosis is characterized on **MRI** by a decreased signal intensity in the intervertebral disks on T2-weighted images. It is associated with typical signal intensity changes in the vertebral body marrow adjacent to the end plates, which Modic et al. (1988 a, b) classified into three types (Fig. 5.**372**).

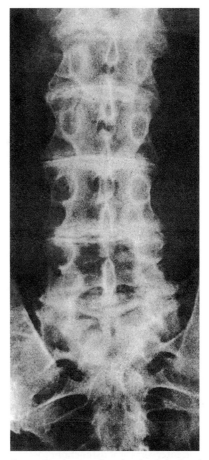

Fig. 5.**370** Generalized osteochondrosis of the lumbar intervertebral disks.

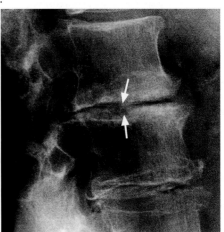

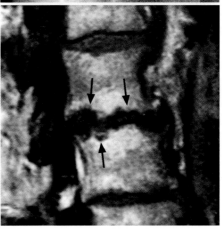

Fig. 5.**371 a, b** Erosive osteochondrosis. ▷
a Lateral radiograph shows erosions of the vertebral end plates (arrows) with increased sclerosis, disk space narrowing, and vacuum phenomenon.
b Sagittal T1-weighted MRI reveals marked erosive changes (arrows).

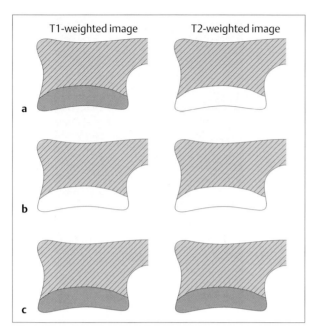

T1-weighted image   T2-weighted image

a

b

c

Fig. 5.**372 a–c** Signal intensity changes in vertebral body marrow in intervertebral osteochondrosis (after Modic).
a Type 1: edema of the vertebral body.
b Type 2: fatty degeneration of the vertebral body.
c Type 3: vertebral body sclerosis.

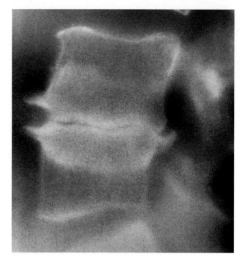

Fig. 5.**373** Hemispheric spondylosclerosis in a patient with intervertebral osteochondrosis. Lateral tomogram.

Typical signal intensity changes in the vertebral body narrow in intervertebral osteochondrosis (after Modic et al.)

➤ *Type 1:* Decreased signal intensity on T1-weighted images and increased signal intensity on T2-weighted images. Enhancement occurs after intravenous contrast administration. The changes are attributed to increased vascularization of the vertebral marrow.

➤ *Type 2:* Increased signal intensity on T1-weighted images and isointense or increased signal intensity on T2-weighted images. These changes relate to the conversion of hematopoietic marrow to yellow marrow.

➤ *Type 3:* Decreased signal intensity on T1- and T2-weighted images due to sclerosis of the vertebral body.

Hemispheric Spondylosclerosis (Dihlmann Syndrome)

Hemispheric spondylosclerosis, known also as **Dihlmann syndrome**, refers to a broad, hemispherical area of sclerosis that affects the cancellous bone overlying the intervertebral disk. It most commonly affects the two lower lumbar vertebrae but can also occur at L3, the thoracolumbar junction, and the midcervical spine (Fig. 5.**368**) (Dihlmann 1981, 1987).

Hemispheric spondylosclerosis is a painful, reversible process that is more common in women than men. In almost 90% of cases it is associated with loss of height in the adjacent intervertebral disk, and anterior osteophyte formation occurs in 80% of cases. Two-thirds of cases also show sclerosis of the vertebral body adjacent to the disk. Associated erosions of the lower end plate are a characteristic accompanying feature. Hemispheric spondylosclerosis occurs mainly in degenerative diseases but is also observed in inflammatory diseases (e.g., ankylosing spondylitis, tuberculosis) (Fig. 5.**344**).

Vacuum Phenomenon

The **vacuum phenomenon** in intervertebral osteochondrosis is caused by the formation of fissures within the nucleus pulposus (Fig. 5.**374**) (Knutsson 1942, Kröker 1949/1950, Resnick et al. 1981). The clefts contain either fluid (MRI: low T1-weighted signal intensity, high T2-weighted signal intensity) or gas (vacuum phenomenon, MRI: low T1- and T2-weighted signal intensity) (Schiebler et al. 1991, Schweitzer and El-Noueam 1998).

Traction on the lumbar spine improves radiographic detection by generating negative pressures. Small gas collections over the anterosuperior corner of the vertebra in the area of the anulus fibrosus are interpreted as an early sign of disk damage (Fig. 5.**375**) and are most commonly found after trauma to the cervical spine (Bohrer 1986).

Spondylarthrosis deformans

As in intervertebral osteochondrosis, CT scans of **spondylarthrosis deformans** may show intra-articular gas collections (vacuum phenomenon) (Lefkowitz and Quencer 1982). Spondylarthrosis deformans can contribute to the development of **spinal stenosis** when combined with intervertebral disk protrusion, hypertrophy and subluxation of the facet joints (pseudo- or degenerative spondylolisthesis), synovial cyst formation (Fig. 5.**376**), enlargement of the laminae, and hyperplasia or ossification of the ligamenta flava (Plötz and Benini 1998). The L4/L5 and L5/S1 segments are most commonly affected (Fig. 5.**340**).

The CT cutoff values for spinal stenosis are a sagittal diameter of 11.5 mm, an interpedicular distance of 16 mm, and a cross-sectional area of 1.45 cm^2 (Fig. 5.**340**) (Ullrich et al. 1980, Lee et al. 1988). The normal width of the lumbar root canals is approximately 5 ± 0.7 mm at L4, 4.6 ± 0.75 mm at L5, and 4.8 ± 0.9 mm at S1 (Lassale et al. 1984).

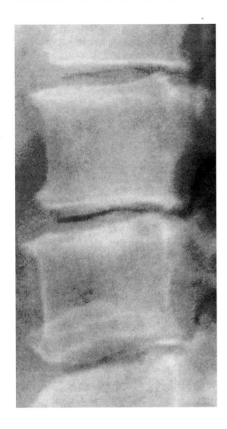

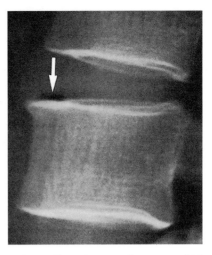

Fig. 5.**375** Air crescent over the anterosuperior corner of L4 (arrow), which disappears with inclination. This finding suggests early disk pathology.

◁ Fig. 5.**374** Gas collections in various intervertebral disks in intervertebral osteochondrosis.

A reduction in the sagittal diameter of the lateral recess (anterior to the superior articular process and posterior to the vertebral body) to less than 3 mm is definitely pathological, and 3–5 mm represents borderline stenosis of the lateral recess (Mikhael et al. 1981).

Finally, spondylarthrosis can lead to narrowing of the intervertebral foramina (Osborne et al. 1984).

On **MRI**, pedicular bone marrow changes can be frequently seen: type 1—low signal intensity on T1-weighted spin-echo MRI and high signal intensity on fast T2-weighted spin-echo MRI, corresponding to fibrovascular changes (4%); type 2—high signal intensity on T1 and fast T2-weighted spin-echo MR images, corresponding to fatty degeneration (Morisson et al. 2000).

Pseudospondylolisthesis, Spondyloretrolisthesis

Spondylarthrosis deformans may be associated with pseudospondylolisthesis and spondyloretrolisthesis (degenerative spondylolisthesis) (Plötz and Benini 1998).

Pseudospondylolisthesis is usually a result of spondylarthrosis but may also occur after inflammatory destruction of the articular processes, as may occur in rheumatoid arthritis. Pseudospondylolisthesis refers to the anterior slippage of an entire vertebra without spondylolysis, usually due to flatness or subluxation of the facet joints (Fig. 5.**377**).

Elongation of the pars interarticularis and other dysplasias can be demonstrated in pseudospondylolisthesis, preferably by sectional imaging (Fig. 5.**327**, 5.**336**, 5.**338**). Pseudospondylolisthesis usually does not develop before

Fig. 5.**376 a, b** Synovial cyst of the apophyseal joint in spondylarthrosis.
a Axial CT demonstrates a small gas collection in the synovial cyst (arrow).
b T2-weighted sagittal MRI (observation by Dieckob, Bielefeld).

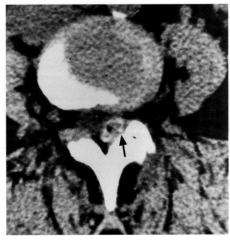

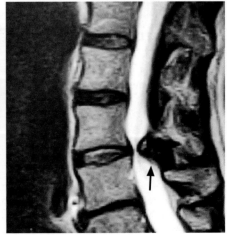

a

b

40 years of age. The L4/L5 segment is most commonly affected.

Spondyloretrolisthesis most commonly results from chondrosis and narrowing of the underlying intervertebral disk. It usually affects the L5 vertebra but may also be seen in the upper lumbar, thoracic, and cervical spine, where inflammatory processes can also play a causal role (Gillespie 1951).

To diagnose spondyloretrolisthesis, it is necessary to scrutinize the posterior corners of the vertebrae. A steplike discontinuity is found at the level of the displaced segment, and a decreased distance is measured between the tip of the S1 articular process and the L5 vertebral arch

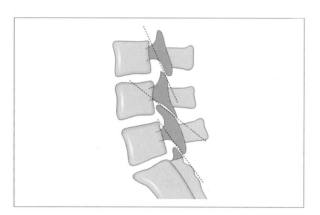

Fig. 5.**377**   Pseudospondylolisthesis of L4 in spondylarthrosis and obliquity of the articular processes in the corresponding segment (compare tangent slopes) (after Dihlmann).

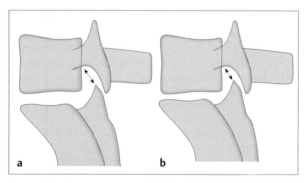

Fig. 5.**378 a, b**   Pseudoretrolisthesis and spondyloretrolisthesis (after Dihlmann).
a Pseudoretrolisthesis of L5: the S1 end plate is smaller than L5, and the distance between the tip of the S1 articular process and the L5 vertebral arch (arrow) is not decreased.
b Spondyloretrolisthesis of L5: the L5 end plate approximately equals S1, and the tip of the S1 articular process is abnormally close to the L5 vertebral arch (arrow).

(Fig. 5.**378**). The approximation of both vertebrae can occur only if the articular surfaces of the corresponding articular processes also move in relation to each other. Because the articular surfaces are slanted, the L5 vertebra must slip backward slightly in order to move closer to S1 (Dihlmann 1987).

In **pseudoretrolisthesis**, the upper end plate of S1 has an unusually short sagittal diameter in relation to the lower end plate of L5, creating the appearance of posterior slippage. This can be determined by measuring the opposing end plates of L5 and S1 (Fig. 5.**378**).

Schmorl Nodes

Degeneration of the nucleus pulposus and vertebral end plate in intervertebral osteochondrosis can allow the intraosseous herniation of disk material, producing a Schmorl node. In a recent study, an association with a straight or fractured vertebral end plates was found and the authors noted an association with abnormalities of the discovertebral junction, but not with advanced degenerative disk disease (Pfirrmann and Resnick 2001). Schmorl nodes can also occur in other conditions such as Scheuermann disease, trauma, infection, and metabolic disorders (Resnick and Niwayama 1978). Scheuermann disease is less common in the lumbar spine, but lumbar involvement is generally associated with more severe clinical symptoms (Lings and Mikkelsen 1982) and with very prominent Schmorl nodes, usually located in the region of the thoracolumbar junction (Figs. 5.**379**, 5.**380**).

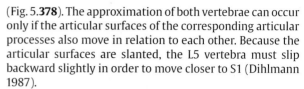

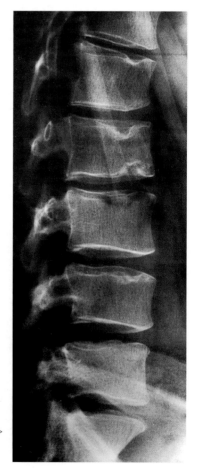

Fig. 5.**379**   Scheuermann disease of the lumbar spine with ▷ conspicuous Schmorl nodes. Note the irregularities at the discovertebral junctions and the wedging of L1.

Schmorl nodes are more common in males and tend to affect the lower end plate of a vertebral body. Almost all Schmorl nodes are found in the lower thoracic spine and the thoracolumbar junction, especially between T7 and L2. About two-thirds of Schmorl nodes are located in the posterior part of the vertebral end plate, one-third in the middle part, and only rarely in the anterior part (Pfirrmann and Resnick 2001). A recent study found evidence that a relationship exists between clinical complaints and the vascularization, size and marrow edema of Schmorl nodes (Stäbler et al. 1997). Leibner and Floman (1998) described the rare case of large **communicating Schmorl nodes** of the upper and lower end plates forming a vertical channel through the affected vertebral body (Figs. 5.**381**, 5.**382**). This may result from a congenital weakness, a persistent notochord, or a traumatic event. Occasionally, massive intravertebral disk herniations are ovserved, which may simulate an osteolytic process (Fig. 5.**383**).

The **limbus vertebra** is a **special form** of Schmorl node that can occur in intervertebral osteochondrosis and other diseases. It develops when disk tissue prolapses through a relative weak point at the periphery of the vertebra, i.e., between the ring apophysis and vertebral body or through vascular foramina. When the material reaches the outer surface of the vertebral body, it creates an **isolated corner fragment** (limbus vertebra) (Figs. 5.**384**, 5.**385**).

Most corner fragments are located anteriorly, but some are lateral or posterior (von Meyenburg 1946, Keller 1974, Techekapusch 1981). The isolation may develop during the stage of marginal ridge formation in adolescence, or it may occur in adults as a result of repetitive microtrauma or excessive loading (Micheli 1985). It is very rarely caused by a single injury (usually posterior) (Laredo et al. 1986, Kolin and Kol 1989, Banerian et al. 1990, Epstein and Epstein 1991). A **posterior corner fragment** may be associated with neurological complaints (von Meyenburg 1946, Goldman et al. 1990) and is a characteristic finding in CT and MRI (Kolin and Kol 1989, Banerian et al. 1990).

Isolated corner fragments detected incidentally after trauma can easily lead to misinterpretation, especially when confined to a single vertebra (Fig. 5.**386**). Finding a smooth, deep concavity with broad sclerotic margins in the cancellous bone with an isolated anterior vertebral corner is so typical that the traumatic detachment of the anterior corner (normal structure and contour, jagged fracture margins) may not even be considered in the differential diagnosis.

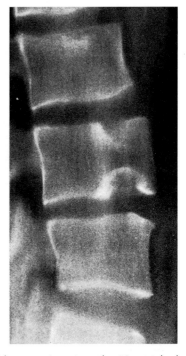

Fig. 5.**380** Anterior disk protrusions into the L3 vertebral body from its upper and lower end plates, with slight elongation of the vertebra.

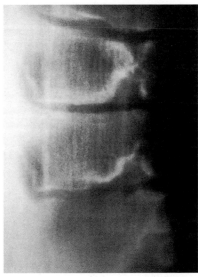

Fig. 5.**381** Deep intravertebral disk herniations appear to communicate within the vertebral body. Isolation of the anterior corners is presumed.

Fig. 5.**382a, b** Deep, communicating Schmorl nodes in the upper and lower end plates of a vertebral body. (From Leibner 1998.)
a Axial CT.
b Coronal reformation demonstrates the communicating tract.

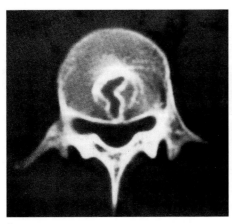

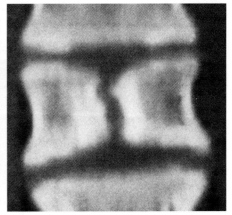

a   b

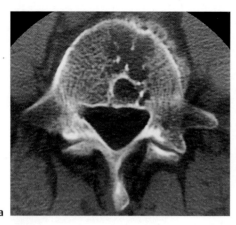 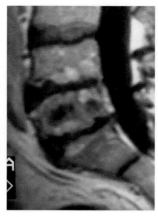

Fig. 5.**383**   Intravertebral disk herniation simulating osteolytic metastasis.
a Transaxial CT.
b Sagittal T1-weighted MRI.

a   b

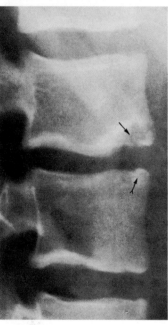 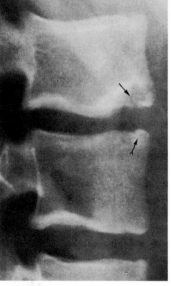 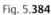

Fig. 5.**384**

Fig. 5.**385**

Fig. 5.**384**   Marked anterior corner separations at opposing sites on the L1 and L2 vertebral bodies with Schmorl nodes.

Fig. 5.**385**   Anterosuperior corner separations of L3 and L4 (Limbus vertebrae).

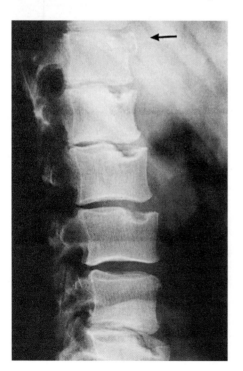

Narrowing of the Interspinous Distance, Basstrup Syndrome

A marked reduction of intervertebral disk height in the setting of intervertebral osteochondrosis or lumbar hyperlordosis can lead to narrowing of the interspinous distance, particularly in the midlumbar spine. This can allow contact between the spinous processes, leading to reactive new bone and cartilage formation. The touching surfaces of the spinous processes can undergo wear and sclerosis with associated pain—a condition known as **Baastrup syndrome (interspinous osteoarthritis, kissing spines)** after the author who first described it (Fig. 5.**387**) (Baastrup 1933, Babin 1980, Sartoris et al. 1985).

Loss of intervertebral disk height can also lead to **frictional sclerosis** between the superior articular processes and the inferior border of the overlying vertebral arch (Fig. 5.**388**).

◁ Fig. 5.**386**   Upper end plates show anterior Schmorl nodes throughout the lumbar spine, with a corner separation at T12 (arrow). This was detected incidentally after a riding accident and was not caused by trauma. Note the slight downward bulging of the T12 and L1 lower end plates below the site of the upper end plate disruption (Edgren–Vaino sign).

Fig. 5.**387 a, b**   Baastrup syndrome (arrows) of the lumbar spine.
a Marked interspinous osteoarthritis is apparent in the lateral projection.
b AP projection.

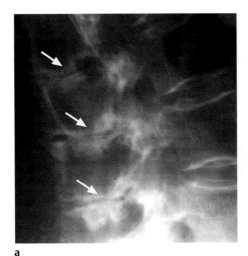

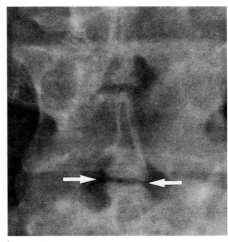

a

b

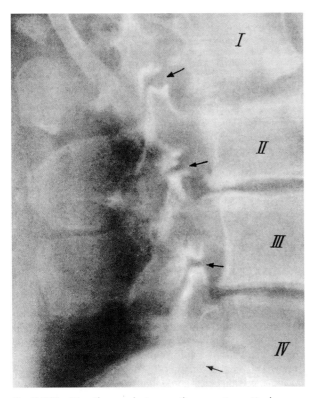

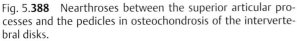

Fig. 5.**388**   Nearthroses between the superior articular processes and the pedicles in osteochondrosis of the intervertebral disks.

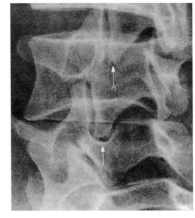

Fig. 5.**389**   The articular processes of L4 and L5 are displaced downward and upward with concave dysplasia (arrow) of the L5 pars (swayback syndrome). Note the bifid tip of the L3 inferior articular process (double arrow).

A typical deformity occurs when the superior articular process of a lumbar vertebra is displaced upward while the inferior articular process of the next higher vertebra is displaced downward (Fig. 5.**389**). The inferior articular process of the upper vertebra becomes engaged in a depression in the dysplastic pars interarticularis of the lower vertebra. Known as **swayback syndrome**, this can occur in lumbar hyperlordosis with Baastrup-type contact between the spinous processes (Jacobson et al. 1958 a).

Hyperostotic Spondylosis, DISH Syndrome

Hyperostotic spondylosis or DISH syndrome is almost as common in the lumbar spine as in the thoracic spine and has already been discussed under that heading (Figs. 5.**251**, 5.**252**). The L1–L3 vertebral bodies are predominantly affected (Fig. 5.**390**).

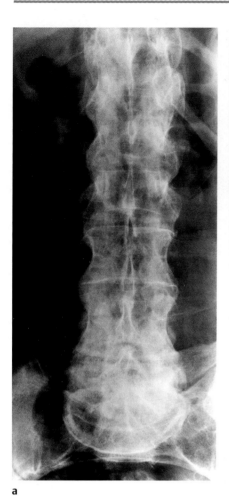

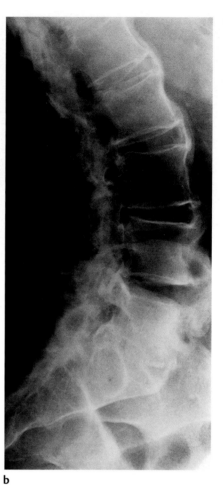

a   b

Fig. 5.**390 a, b**   DISH syndrome of the lumbar spine.
a AP projection.
b Lateral projection.

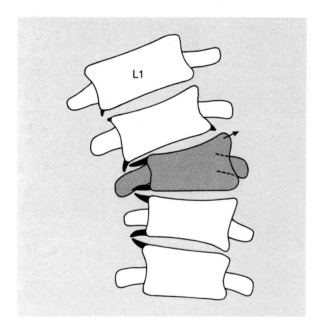

Fig. 5.**391**   Rotational slippage of L3 (arrow) in left convex lumbar scoliosis. Buttressing osteophytes (black) form predominantly on the concave side of the scoliosis (after Dihlmann).

Posture

Scoliosis of the lumbar spine may develop de novo with aging or may progress from a preexisting curve (Robin et al. 1982). Scoliotic deformity of the lumbar spine predisposes to degenerative changes, which in turn can aggravate the postural deformity. Intervertebral osteochondrosis and other degenerative changes of the lumbar spine do not in themselves lead to scoliosis.

The lateral displacement of vertebrae, or **rotatory slippage**, is a painful complication of lumbar scoliosis. The ligaments on the tense opposite side give way, allowing the vertebra to slip toward the side of the convexity and also rotate. This is accompanied by degenerative changes on the concave side of the curve (Fig. 5.**391**). Rotatory slippage can occur only if there is a change in the shape and position of the degenerative articular processes.

In extreme cases, degenerative diseases of the lumbar spine can lead to a loss of physiological lordosis and even to a kyphotic deformity (Takemitsu et al. 1988).

Calcification and Ossification

Calcification of intervertebral disks is noted in approximately 6% of all abdominal radiographs (Cohen and Abraham 1973, Weinberger and Myers 1978). Disk calcifications can also occur in many systemic diseases, e.g.:

- Hemochromatosis
- Calcium pyrophosphate dihydrate crystal deposition (CPPD)
- Hyperparathyroidism
- Poliomyelitis
- Acromegaly
- Amyloidosis
- Alkaptonuria

When **ochronosis** develops during the course of alkaptonuria (Fig. 5.**392**), the late stage is characterized by extensive bandlike calcifications in the thoracic and lumbar intervertebral disks accompanied by degenerative changes. The concomitant presence of osteopenic vertebral bodies creates a "stuffed waffle" configuration. In **chondrodystrophia calcificans** (stippled epiphyses), multiple small punctate calcifications are found in the intervertebral disks.

Disk calcifications can also occur after surgical **spinal fusion** and **ankylosis** in patients with rheumatic and seronegative spondylarthropathies. Disk calcification in **children (calcifying discitis)** was discussed in the section on the cervical spine. A less common and less symptomatic form of calcifying discitis can also occur in the lumbar and thoracic spine (Girodias et al. 1991).

In **adults**, degenerative disk calcifications are ten times more common in the anulus fibrosus than in the nucleus pulposus (Schorr and Adler 1954), occurring at a typical site in the posterior third of the disk space (Figs. 5.**393**, 5.**394**). Most of the calcifications are composed of hydroxyapatite.

Calcifications of the **nucleus pulposus** may be single or multiple and can occur in several regions at the same time (Fig. 5.**395**). Calcifications can also occur in the anterior portions of the intervertebral disks (Fig. 5.**396**). With symmetrical calcifications located under the posterior base of a lumbar vertebra near the chordal region, the cause of the calcifications may be based on a developmental abnormality (Figs. 5.**397**, 5.**398**) (Dihlmann 1964).

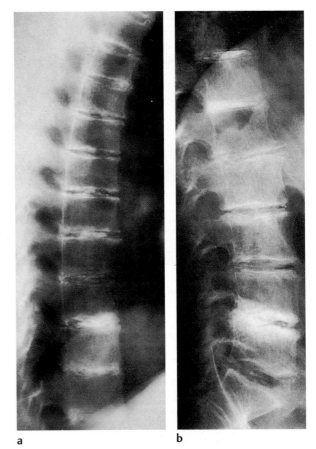

a   b

Fig. 5.**392 a, b**   Ochronosis in alkaptonuria. Bandlike calcifications are visible in the intervertebral disks (observation by Hillenbrand-Eckard, Augsburg).
a Thoracic spine.
b Lumbar spine.

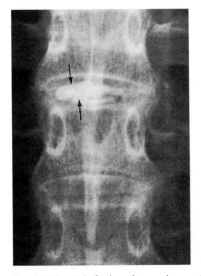

Fig. 5.**393**   Calcified nucleus pulposus (arrows).

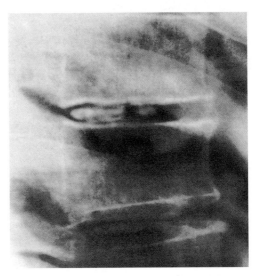

Fig. 5.**394**   Calcifications in the nucleus pulposus.

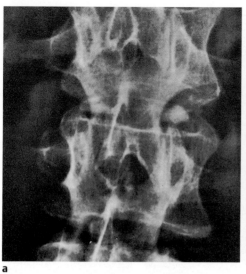
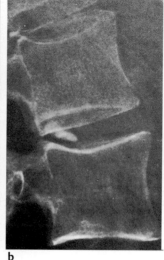
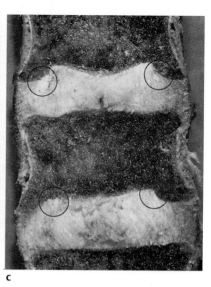

a   b   c

Fig. 5.**395 a–c**   Calcifications of intervertebral disks (observation by Teichert, Hamburg).

a, b Large, bilateral calcium deposits in the posterior L1/L2 disk space of a 53-year-old woman. AP and lateral projections.
c Calcium deposits (circles) in an anatomic section.

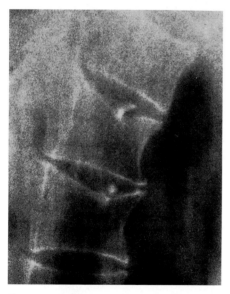

Fig. 5.**396**   Older, nontraumatic collapse of the upper end plate with disk calcification.

Calcifications of the intervertebral disk can appear as signal voids on **MRI** or may show increased signal intensity on T1-weighted images (Major et al. 1993, Bangert et al. 1995). Disk calcifications may prolapse in any direction and produce clinical symptoms (Smith 1976, Williams 1954).

Calcifications of the **anulus fibrosus** are difficult to distinguish from calcifications of the posterior longitudinal ligament (Figs. 5.**399**–5.**401**). Extensive calcium deposits and **bone formation** in the fibrous ring and **ossification of the entire intervertebral disk** can occur in children (Silverman 1954), especially when combined with congenital anomalies (Sonnabend et al. 1982), but are also found in adults (Figs. 5.**209**, 5.**211**, 5.**402**). **Gouty osteoarthropathy** can lead to the ossification of vertebral ligaments and tendons as well as calcification and hyperostosis (Jajic 1982, Stepán et al. 1983). Other typical calcifications and ossifications in the area of the intervertebral disks are shown schematically in Fig. 5.**403**.

Ossification of the **posterior longitudinal ligament (OPLL)** is very rare in the lumbar spine and is covered more fully in the section on the cervical spine (Tsuyama 1984, Hiramatsu and Nobechi 1971). One observation describes concomitant posterior scalloping of the vertebral bodies (Lagemann 1972).

Ossification of the **iliolumbar ligament** can occasionally lead to clinical complaints (Fig. 5.**404**) (Simon 1930, Broudeur et al. 1982). The precise cause of the ossification is unknown but may relate to instability due to rotatory lumbar scoliosis, injuries, or idiopathic skeletal hyperostosis (DISH).

Diffuse **paravertebral soft-tissue calcifications** can result from a hematoma in the psoas region (Fig. 5.**405**). They may also occur in paraplegia or occasionally in the setting of progressive myositis ossificans (Fig. 5.**406**) and are often referable to intimal calcifications of the abdominal aorta and major pelvic arteries (Fig. 5.**407**).

Fig. 5.**397 a, b**   Calcific foci in the posterior part of the lumbar disk in a patient with conspicuously tall lumbar vertebral bodies (dysplasia?) (observation by Weil-Lechner).
a AP projection (arrows).
b Lateral projection (arrows).

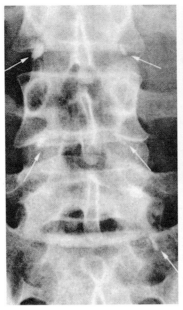 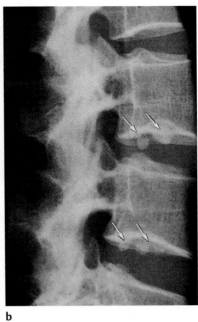

a   b

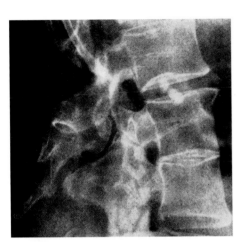

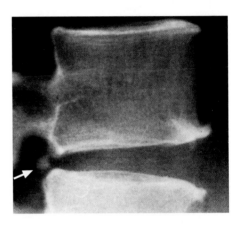

Fig. 5.**398**   Calcific foci in the posterior part of the intervertebral disk. Note the tall lumbar vertebral bodies and incomplete block vertebrae. Dysplasia of the lumbar spine is present in this region.

Fig. 5.**399**   Calcium deposit just behind the posterior vertebral corners at the level of the intervertebral disk space (arrow).

Fig. 5.**400**   Calcification behind the level of the posterior corners of L3 and L4 (arrow).

Fig. 5.**401**   Small calcium shadows at the posterior border of the lumbar intervertebral disks.

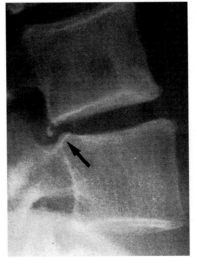 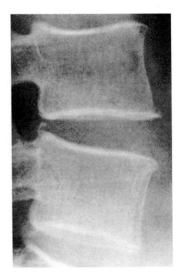

Fig. 5.**400**   Fig. 5.**401**

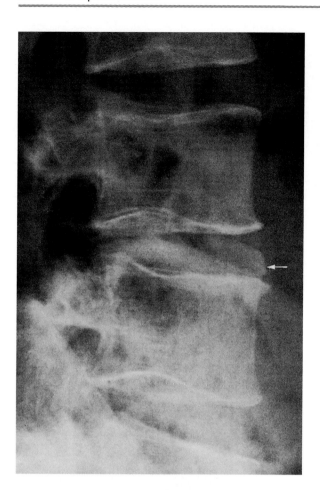

Fig. 5.**402** Extensive disk calcifications in a man with generalized meniscal calcification (arrow).

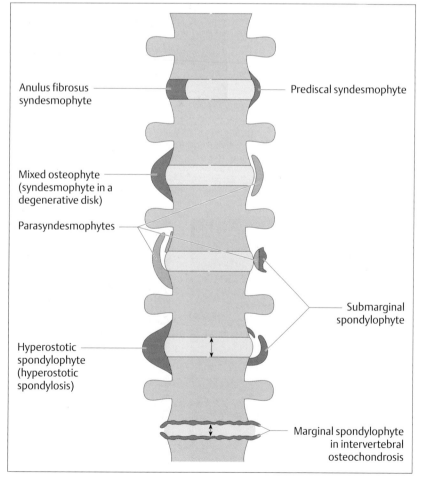

Anulus fibrosus
syndesmophyte

Prediscal syndesmophyte

Mixed osteophyte
(syndesmophyte in a
degenerative disk)

Parasyndesmophytes

Submarginal
spondylophyte

Hyperostotic
spondylophyte
(hyperostotic
spondylosis)

Marginal spondylophyte
in intervertebral
osteochondrosis

Fig. 5.**403** Differential diagnosis of vertebral osteophytes. The submarginal spondylophytes of spondylosis deformans and the hyperostotic spondylophytes of hyperostotic spondylosis are generally associated with a disk space of normal height. Marginal spondylophytes in intervertebral osteochondrosis are associated with disk space narrowing (after Dihlmann).

Fig. 5.**404** Unusually heavy ossification of the ilio-lumbar ligament on both sides. Scoliosis of the lower lumbar spine.

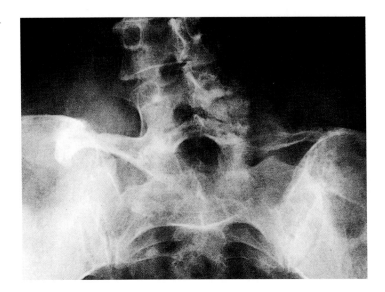

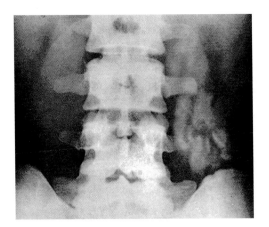

Fig. 5.**405** Calcified hematoma in the psoas region.

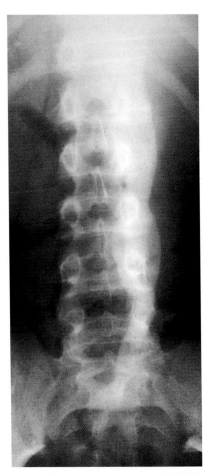

Fig. 5.**406** Extensive ossification along the left side of the lumbar spine in progressive myositis ossificans (observation by D. Resnick, San Diego).

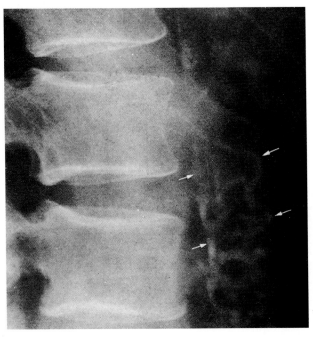

◁ Fig. 5.**407** Intimal calcifications of the abdominal aorta (arrows).

References

Abel, M. S.: Jogger's fracture and other stress fractures of the lumbo-sacral spine. Skelet. Radiol. 13 (1985) 221

Abdelwahab, I. F., V. H. Frankel, M. J. Klein: Aggressive osteoblastoma of the third lumbar vertebra. Skelet. Radiol. 15 (1986) 164–169

Aggarwal, S., R. K. Goulatia, A. Sood et al.: POEMS syndrome: a rare variety of plasma cell dyscrasia. Amer. J. Roentgenol. 155 (1990) 339

Algra, P. R., J. L. Bloem, H. Tissing et al.: Detection of vertebral metastases: comparison between MR imaging and bone scintigraphy. Radiographics 11 (1991) 219

Altman, N. R., D. H. Altman: MR imaging of spinal dysraphism. Amer. J. Neuroradiol. 8 (1987) 533

Amato, M., W. G. Totty, L. A. Gilula: A. Spondylolysis of the lumbar spine: demonstration of defects and laminal fragmentation. Radiology 153 (1984) 627

Andersson, O.: Röntgenbilder vid spondylarthritis ankylopoetica. Nord. Med. Tidskr. 14 (1937) 200

Andresen, R., M. A. Haidekker, S. Radmer, D. Banzer: CT determination of bone mineral density and structural investigations on the axial skeleton for estimating the osteoporosis-related fracture risk by means of a risk score. Brit. J. Radiol. 72 (1999) 569

Arcomano, J. P., S. Karas: Congenital absence of the lumbosacral articular processes. Skelet. Radiol. 8 (1982) 133

Arredondo, F., V. M. Haughton, D. C. Hemmy et al.: The computed tomographic appearance of the spinal cord in diastematomyelia. Radiology 13 (1980) 685

Assoun, J., G. Richardi, J.-J. Railhac et al.: Osteoid osteoma: MR imaging versus CT. Radiology 191 (1994) 217

Azouz, E. M.: Bone marrow edema in osteoid osteoma. Skelet. Radiol. 23 (1994) 53

Baastrup, C. J.: Processus spinosi vertebrae lumbales und einige zwischen diesen liegende Gelenkbildungen mit pathologischen Prozessen in dieser Region. Fortschr. Röntgenstr. 48 (1933) 430

Babin, E.: Radiology of the Narrow Lumbar Canal. Radiologic Signs and Surgery. In Wackenheim, A., E. Babin: The Narrow Lumbar Canal. Springer, New York 1980 (p. 4–10)

Banerian, K. G., A.-M. Wang, L. C. Samberg, et al.: Association of vertebral end plate fracture with pediatric lumbar intervertebral disk herniation: value of CT and MR imaging. Radiology 177 (1990) 763

Bangert, B. A., M. T. Modic, J. S. Ross, N. A. Obuchowski, J. Perl, P. M. Ruggieri et al.: Hyperintense disks on T1-weighted MR images: correlation with calcification. Radiology 195 (1995) 437

Banniza von Bazan, U.: Diasthematomyelie. In: Junghanns H. Die Wirbelsäule in Forschung und Praxis. Bd. XCIX. Hippokrates, Stuttgart 1984

Bardsley, J. L., L. G. Hanelin: The unilateral hypoplastic lumbar pedicle. Radiology 101 (1971) 315

Beers, G. J., A. P. Carter, W. F. McNary: Vertical foramina in the lumbosacral region: CT appearances. Amer. J. Neuroradiol. 5 (1984) 617

Bellah, R. D., D. A. Summerville, S. T. Treves et al.: Low-back pain in adolescent athletes: detection of stress injury to the pars interarticularis with SPECT. Radiology 180 (1991) 509

Biggemann, M., W. Frobin, P. Brinckmann: Physiologisches Muster lumbaler Bandscheibenhöhen. Fortschr. Röntgenstr. 167 (1997) 11

Boeck, M., E. de Smedt, R. Potvliefe: Computed tomography in the evaluation of a congenital absent lumbar pedical. Skelet. Radiol. 8 (1982) 197

Bohrer, S. P.: The annulus vacuum sign. Skelet. Radiol. 15 (1986) 233

Bohutová, J., J. Kalár, J. Vitovec, L. Whyánek: Accessory caudal axial and pelvic ribs. Fortschr. Röntgenstr. 133 (1980) 641

Boisot, J., C. Lagarde, C. Laurens: Apophyse articulaire accessoire des vertébres lombaires. J. Radiol. Électrol 43 (1962) 470

Brocher, J. E. W.: Die Wirbelsäulentuberkulose. Thieme, Stuttgart 1953

Brocher, J. E. W.: Die Wirbelverschiebung in der Lendengegend, 3. Aufl. Thieme, Stuttgart 1958

Brocher, J. E. W., H.-G. Willert: Differentialdiagnose der Wirbelsäulenerkrankungen, 6. Aufl. Thieme, Stuttgart 1980

Broderick, T. W., D. Resnick, T. G. Goergen, N. Alazraki: Enostosis of the spine. Spine 3 (1978) 167–170

Broudeur, P., C. H. Larroque, R. Passeron et al.: The iliolumbar syndrome. Rev. Rhum. 50 (1982) 393

Brown, R. C., E. T. Evans: What causes the "eye in the Scotty dog" in the oblique projection of the lumbar spine? Amer. J. Roentgenol. 116 (1973) 435

de Bruine, F. T., H. M. Kroon: Spinal chordoma: Radiologic features in 14 cases. Amer. J. Roentgenol. 150 (1988) 861

Brunet, J. A., J. J. Wiley: Acquired spondylolysis after spinal fusion. J. Bone J Surg. 66-B (1984) 720

Buetti, V. C., H. Ldi: Spondylitis nach Paravertebralanästhesie. Helv. chir. Acta 25 (1958) 261

Buraczewski, J., J. Lysakowska, W. Rudowski: Chondroblastoma (Codman's tumour) of the thoracic spine. J. Bone Jt Surg. 39-B (1957) 705

Cahill, D. W., L. C. Love, G. R. Rechtine: Pyogenic osteomyelitis of the spine in the elderly. J. Neurosurg. 74 (1991) 878

Campanacci, M.: Bone and Soft Tissue Tumors. Springer, Berlin 1990

Carlo, W. A., R. Kliegman, M. S. Dixon, B. D. Fletcher, A. A. Fanaroff: Vertebral agenesis. Amer. J. Dis. Child. 136 (1982) 533–537

Chan, K. K., D. J. Sartoris, P. Haghighi, P. Sledge, E. Barrett-Connor, D. T. Trudell et al.: Cupid's bow contour of the vertebral body: evaluation of pathogenesis with bone densitometry and imaging-histopathologic correlation. Radiology 202 (1997) 253

Cheng, X. G., Y. Sun, S. Boonen, P. H. F. Nicholson, P. Brys, J. Dequeker, D. Felsenberg: Measurements of vertebral shape by radiographic morphometry: sex differences and relationships with vertebral level an lumbar lordosis. Skelet. Radiol. 27 (1998) 380

Ciullo, J., W. Jackson: Pars interarticularis stress reaction, spondylolysis, and spondylolisthesis in gymnasts. Clin. Sports Med. 4 (1985) 95

Cohen, J. A., E. Abraham: The calcified intervertebral disc. J. med. Soc. N. J. 70 (1973) 459

Collée, G., H. M. Kroon, B. A. C. Dijkmans et al.: Radiological findings in relation to clinical features in low back pain. J. orthop. Rheumatol. 3 (1990) 147

Cuveland, E., de: Über die Herkunft von Knochenbrüchen zwischen den Lenden-Wirbel-Querfortsätzen. Fortschr. Röntgenstr. 85 (1956) 93–95

Dahlin, D.C.: Giant-cell tumor of vertebrae above the sacrum. A review of 31 cases. Cancer 39 (1977) 1350

Darby, A. J., V.N. Cassar-Pullicino, I. W. McCall, D. C. Jaffray: Vertebral intra-osseous chordoma or giant notochordal rest. Skelet. Radiol. 28 (1999) 342

Das De, A.: Intervertebral disc involvement in gout: Brief report. J. Bone Jt Surg. 70-B (1988) 671

Dehner, J. R.: Seabelt injuries of the spine and abdomen. Amer. J. Roentgenol. 111 (1971) 833

Dekker-Saeys, B. J., S. G. M. Meuwissen, E. M. Van Den Berg-Loonen et al.: Ankylosing spondylitis and inflammatory bowel disease. II. Prevalence of peripheral arthritis, sacroiliitis and ankylosing spondylitis in patients suffering from inflammatory bowel disease. Ann. rheum. Dis. 37 (1978) 33

Dias, L. D. S., H. M. Frost: Osteoblastoma of the spine. A review and report of eight new cases. Clin. Orthop. 91 (1973) 141

Diethelm, L.: Fehlbildungen des Corpus vertebrale. b.) Frontale Wirbelkörperspalten. In: Röntgendiagnostik der Wirbelsäule, Teil 1, red. v. L. Diethelm. In Diethelm, L., F. Heuck, O. Olsson, K. Ranninger, F. Strnad, H. Vieten, A. Zuppinger: Handbuch der Medizinischen Radiologie, Bd. VI. Springer, Berlin 1974 (S. 202–208)

Dietz, G. W., E. E. Christensen: Normal "Cupid's bow" contour of the lower lumbar. Vertebrae 121 (1976) 577–579

Dihlmann, W.: Kalkschatten im Zwischenwirbelraum. Fortschr. Röntgenstr. 101 (1964) 558

Dihlmann, W.: Die sog. Spondylitis anterior, Discitis und Spondylodiscitis bei Morbus Bechterew. Fortschr. Röntgenstr. 104 (1966) 699–718

Dihlmann, W.: Hemispherical spondylosclerosis—a polyetiologic syndrome. Skeletal Radiol. 7 (1981) 99–106

Dihlmann, W.: Die sogenannte Spondylitis anterior, Discitis und Spondylodiscitis bei Morbus Bechterew – Schlüssel zum Verständnis dieser Erkrankung. Fortschr. Röntgenstr. 104 (1966) 699

Dihlmann, W.: Gelenke, Wirbelverbindungen, 3. Aufl. Thieme, Stuttgart 1987

Dorwart, R. H., H. K. Genant: Anatomy of the lumbosacral spine. Radiol. Clin. N. Amer. 21 (1983) 201

Dvořák, J., M. M. Panjabi, D. G. Chang, R. Theiler, D. Grob: Functional radiographic diagnosis of the lumbar spine. Flexion-extension and lateral bending. Spine 16 (1991 a) 562

Dvořák, J., M. M. Panjabi, J. E. Novotny, D. G. Chang, D. Grob: Clinical valadidation of functional flexion-extension Roentgenograms of the lumbar spine. Spine 16 (1991 b) 943

Eggert, D.: Unspezifische Spondylitis im Kindesalter. Fortschr. Röntgenstr. 113 (1970) 697–703

Eisenstein, St.: Lumbar vertebral canal morphometry for computerized tomography in spinal stenosis. Spine 8 (1983) 187–191

El-Khoury, G. Y., D. K. Yousefzadeh, M. H. Kathol et al.: Pseudospondylolysis. Radiology 139 (1981) 71

Erbe, W., G. Stephan, H. Böttcher: Das Muster der Skelettveränderungen bei der Akromegalie. Fortschr. Röntgenstr. 122 (1975) 317–322

Erdheim: Über die Wirbelsäulenveränderungen der Akromegalie. Virchows Arch. path. Anat. 281 (1931) 197–296

Epstein, N. E., J. A. Epstein: Limbus lumbar vertebral fractures in 27 adolescents and adults. Spine 16 (1991) 962

Farrés, M. T., W. Dock, I. Augustin et al.: Radiologisches Erscheinungsbild des primären Knochenlymphoms. Fortschr. Röntgenstr. 158 (1993) 589

Fielding, J. W., S. Ratzan: Osteochondroma of the cervical spine. J. Bone Jt Surg. 55-A (1973) 640

Firooznia, H., Ira Tyler, Cornelia Golimbu, Mahvash Rafii: Computerized tomography of the Cupid's bow contour of the lumbar spine. Comput. Radiol. 7 (1983) 347–350

Fischer, E., W. Giere: Größenänderungen von Skelettabschnitten der Wirbelsäule und der unteren Extremität im Erwachsenenalter bei Männern und Frauen. 1. Mitteilung: Breitenänderung der normalen Brust- und Lendenwirbelsäule. Z. Orthop. 107 (1970) 620–624

Francis Jr., W. R. T. Einhorn, J. W. Fielding: Osteoid osteoma of the thoracic spine: report of a case. Clin. Orthop. 149 (1980) 175

Frank, J. A., A. Ling, N. J. Patronas et al.: Detection of malignant bone tumors: MR imaging vs scintigraphy. Amer. J. Roentgenol. 155 (1990) 1043

Freyschmidt, J.: Tumoren der Wirbelsäule und des Sakrums. In Schinz, H. R.: Radiologische Diagnostik, 7. Aufl. hrsg. von W. Frommhold, W. Dihlmann, H.-St. Stender, P. Thurn; Bd. V/2: Wirbelsäule – Rückenmark, hrsg. von W. Dihlmann, H.-St. Stender. Thieme, Stuttgart 1986 (S. 249–318)

Freyschmidt, J.: Tumoren der Wirbelsäule und des Sakrums. In Schinz, H. R.: Radiologische Diagnostik, 7. Aufl. Bd. V/2: Frommhold, W., W. Dihlmann, H.-S. Stender, P. Thurn: Wirbelsäule und Rückenmark. Thieme, Stuttgart 1986 (S. 249–318)

Freyschmidt, J.: Skeletterkrankungen. Klinisch-radiologische Diagnose und Differentialdiagnose. Springer, Berlin 1997

Freyschmidt, J., H. Ostertag, G. Jundt: Knochentumoren. Klinik, Radiologie, Pathologie. Springer, Berlin 1998

Frottier, J., J.-L. Vildé, F. Bricaire, C. Leport: Les spondylodiscites. Aspects actuels. Maladies infect. 33 (1983) 2413–2421

Galasko, C. S. B.: The anatomy and pathways of skeletal metasasis. In Weiss, L., H. A. Gilbert: Bone Metastasis. Hall, Boston 1981 (p. 49)

Galil, A., R. Gorodischer, J. Bar-Ziv, T. Hallel, Ch. Malkin, R. Garty: Intervertebral disc infection (Discitis) in childhood. Eur. J. Pediat. 139 (1982) 66–70

Gamba, J. L., S. Martinez, J. Apple et al.: Computed tomography of axial skeletal osteoid osteomas. Amer. J. Roentgenol. 142 (1984) 769

Garcia Jr., A., S. A. Grantham: Haematogenous pyogenic vertebral osteomyelitis. J. Bone Jt Surg. 42-A (1960) 429

Garn S. M., F. N. Silverman, K. P. Hertzog et al.: Lines and bands of increased density. Their implication to growth and development. Med. Radiogr. Photogr. 44 (1968) 58

Garver, P., D. Resnick, P. Haghighi, J. Guerra: Melorheostosis of the axial skeleton with associated fibrolipomatous lesions. Skeletal Radiol. 9 (1982) 41–44

Gaudin, P., R. Juvin, Y. Rozand et al.: Skeletal involvement as the initial disease manifestation of Hodgkin's disease: a review of 6 cases. J. Rheumatol. 19 (1992) 146

Gillespie, H. W.: Vertebral reposition (reversed spondylolithesis). Brit. J. Radiol. 24 (1951) 193

Girodias, J.-B., E. M. Azouz, D. Marton: Intervertebral disk space calcification. A report of 51 children with a review of the literature. Pediat. Radiol. 21 (1991) 541

Goldman, A. B., B. Ghelman, J. Doherty: Posterior limbus vertebrae: a cause of radiating back pain in adolescents and young adults. Skelet. Radiol. 19 (1990) 501

Gordon, E. J.: Infection of disc space secondary to fistula from pelvic abscess. Sth. med. J. 70 (1977) 114

Gorse, G. J., M. Joyce Paris, J. A. Kusske, th. C. Cesario: Tuberculous spondylitis. Medicine 62 (1983) 178–193

Gran, J. T., G. Husby, M. Hordvik: Spinal ankylosing spondylitis: A variant form of ankylosing spondylitis or a distinct disease entity? Ann. rheum. Dis. 44 (1985) 368

Grenier, N., H. Y. Kressel, M. L. Schiebler et al.: Isthmic spondylolysis of the lumbar spine: MR imaging at 1,5 T. Radiology 170 (1989) 489

Griffin, J. B.: Benign osteoblastoma of the thoracic spine. Case report with fifteen-year follow-up. J. Bone Jt Surg. 60-A (1978) 833

Griffiths, H. E. D., D. M. Jones: Pyogenic infection of the spine. A review of twenty-eight cases. J. Bone Jt Surg. 53-B (1971) 383

Grossman, H., R. Gray, E. L. St. Louis: CT of long-standing ankylosing spondylitis with cauda equina syndrome. Amer. J. Neuroradiol. 4 (1983) 1077–1080

Güssel, E.: Akute Osteochondrose der Wirbelsäule beim Erwachsenen. Fortschr. Röntgenstr. 71 (1949) 109–113

Hadden, W. A., A. J. G. Swanson: Spinal infection caused by acupuncture mimicking a prolapsed intervertebral disc. A case report. J. Bone Jt Surg. 64-A (1982) 624

Hahn, P. Y., J. J. Strobel, F. J. Hahn: Verification of lumbosacral segments on MR images: identification of transitional vertebrae (see comments). Radiology 182 (1992) 580

Hall, F. M., S. M. Gore: Osteosclerotic myeloma variants. Skelet. Radiol. 17 (1988) 101

Haller, J., M. P. Andre, D. Resnick, C. Miller, B. A. Howard, M. J. Mitchell: Detection of thoracolumbar vertebral body destruction with lateral spine radiography. Part I: Investigation in cadavers. Invest. Radiol. 25 (1990 a) 517

Haller, J., M. P. Andre, D. Resnick, C. Miller, B. A. Howard, M. J. Mitchell: Detection of thoracolumbar vertebral body destruction with lateral spine radiography. Part II: Clinical investigation with computed tomography. Invest. Radiol. 25 (1990 b) 523

Harrington, K. D.: Metastatic disease of the spine. J. Bone Jt Surg. 68-A (1986) 1110

Harvey, C. J., J. L. Richenberg, A. Saifuddin, R. L. Wolman: The radiological investigation of lumbar spondylolysis. Clin. Radiol. 53 (1998) 723

Hasner, E., H. H. Jacobsen, M. Schalimtzek, E. Snorrason: Lumbosacral transitional vertebrae: a clinical and roentgenologic study of 400 cases of low back pain. Acta radiol. 39 (1953) 225

Hellinger, J.: Meßmethoden in der Skelettradiologie. Thieme, Stuttgart 1995

Helms, C. A., R. Sims: Foraminal spurs: a normal variant in the lumbar spine. Radiology 160 (1986) 153–154

Hensinger, R. N.: Current concepts review: Spondylolysis and spondylolisthesis in children and adolescents. J. Bone Jt Surg. 71-A (1989) 1098

Hermann, G., D. S. Mendelson, B. A. Cohen, J. S. Train: Role of computed tomography in the diagnosis of infectious spondylitis. J. Comp. Assist. Tomogr. 7 (1983) 961–968

Heywood, A. W. B., O. L. Meyers: Rheumatoid arthritis of the thoracic and lumbar spine. J. Bone Jt Surg. 68-B (1986) 362

Hiramatsu, Y., T. Nobechi: Calcification of the posterior longitudinal ligament of the spine among Japanese. Radiology 100 (1971) 307–312

Hoeffel, J. C., F. Brasse, M. Schmitt et al.: About one case of vertebral chondroblastoma. Pediat. Radiol. 17 (1987) 392

Huvos, A. G., M. Heilweil, S. S. Bretsky: The pathology of malignant fibrous histiocytoma of bone. A study of 130 patients. Amer. J. surg. Pathol. 9 (1985) 853

Jacobson, H. G., M. E. Tausend, J. H. Shapiro, M. H. Poppel: The "sway back" syndrome. Amer. J. Roentgenol. 79 (1958 a) 677

Jacobson, H. G., M. H. Poppel, J. H. Shapiro et al.: The vertebral pedicle sign: a roentgen finding to differentiate metastatic carcinoma from multiple myeloma. Amer. J. Roentgenol. 80 (1958 b) 817

Jajic, I.: Gout in the spine and sacro-iliac joints: radiological manifestations. Skeletal Radiol. 8 (1982) 209–212

Janovec, M.: Diagnostik des Down-Syndroms mit Hilfe des Wirbelknochenindexes. Radiol. Diagn. (Berl.) 13 (1972) 129–139

Johansen, J. G., D. J. McCarty, V. M. Haughton: Retrosomatic Clefts: computed tomographic appearance. Radiology 148 (1983) 447

Jonsson, B., B. Stromqvist, N. Egund: Anomalous lumbosacral articulations and low-back pain. Evaluation and treatment. Spine 14 (1989) 831

Kaiser, E., F. Biedermann, R. Lehmann, D. Szdzny: Lumbosakrale Wirbelluxation mit konsekutiver Spondylolisthesis. Fortschr. Röntgenstr. 117 (1972) 223

Kam, J., M. R. Funston: Venous collaterals causing vertebral body notching. Brit. J. Radiol. 53 (1980) 491–493

Kattapuram, S. V., J. S. Khurana, J. A. Scott et al.: Negative scintigraphy with positive magnetic resonance imaging in bone metastases. Skelet. Radiol. 19 (1990) 113

Keller, R. H.: Traumatic displacement of the cartilaginous vertebral rim: a sign of intervertebral disc prolapse. Radiology 110 (1974) 21

Kiefer, H., J. Emmrich: Abnorm großer Processus styloides der Lendenwirbelsäule mit reaktiver Pseudarthrosebildung. Fortschr. Röntgenstr. 100 (1964) 280–281

Kinsella, T. D., F. R. MacDonald, L. G. Johnson: Ankylosing spondylitis: a late re-evaluation of 92 cases. J. Canad. med. Ass. 95 (1966) 1

Knutsson, F.: The vacuum phenomenon in the intervertebral discs. Acta radiol. 23 (1942) 173

Kolin, J., J. Kol: Posterior lumbar apophyseal ring fracture simulating a mass lesion in computed tomograms. Fortschr. Röntgenstr. 151 (1989) 114

Kollier, B. D., R. P. Johnson, G. F. Carrera et al.: Painful spondylolysis or spondylolisthesis studied by radiography and single-photon emission computed tomography. Radiology 154 (1985) 207

Kramer, J., M. Schratter, N. Pongracz et al.: Spondylitis: Erscheinungsbild und Verlaufsbeurteilung mittels Magnetresonanztomographie. Fortschr. Röntgenstr. 153 (1990) 131

Krause, G. R.: Persistence of the notochord. Amer. J. Roentgenol. 44 (1940) 719–725

Kröker, P.: Sichtbare Rißbildungen in den Bandscheiben der Wirbelsäule. Fortschr. Röntgenstr. 72 (1949/50) 1–20

Krull, P., H. Holsten, A. Seeberg et al.: Klinische und röntgenologische Besonderheiten des solitären Plasmozytoms. Fortschr. Röntgenstr. 117 (1972) 324

Lachapèle, A.-P.: Un moyen simple pour faciliter la lecture des radiographies vertébrales obliques de la région lumbo-sacrée. Bull. Mém. Soc. radiol. med. France (1939) 175

Lagemann, K.: Hintere Längsbandverkalkungen kombiniert mit Wirbelkörperexkavationen. Fortschr. Röntgenstr. 116 (1972) 834–835

Lagier, R., G. Guelpa, J.-C. Gerster: Lumbar erosive intervertebral osteochondrosis. Anatomico-radiological study of a case. Fortschr. Röntgenstr. 130 (1979) 204–209

Lagier, R., W. MacGee: Erosive intervertebral osteochondrosis in association with generalized osteoarthritis and chondrocalcinosis. Anatomicoradiological study of a case. Z. Rheumat. 38 (1979) 405–414

Lagier, R., W. MacGee: Spondylodiscal erosions due to gout: anatomicoradiological study of a case. Ann. rheum. Dis. 42 (1983) 350

Lagier, R., A. Mbakop, A. Bigler: Osteopoikilosis: a radiological and pathological study. Skelet. Radiol. 11 (1984) 161

Lang, E. K., W. T. Bessler: Roentgenologic features of acromegaly. Amer. J. Roentgenol. 86 (1961) 321

Langston, J. W., M. L. Gavant: Incomplete ring sign: a simple method for CT detection of spondylolysis. J. Comput. assist. Tomogr. 9 (1985) 728

Laredo, J.-D., M. Bard, J. Chretien, M.-F. Kahn: Lumbar posterior marginal intra-osseous cartilaginous node. Skelet. Radiol. 15 (1986) 201

Laredo, J.-D., D. Reizine, M. Bard et al.: Vertebral hemangiomas: Radiologic evaluation. Radiology 161 (1986) 183

Laredo, J.-D., E. Assouline, F. Gelbert et al.: Vertebral hemangiomas: fat content as a sign of aggressiveness. Radiology 177 (1990) 467

Larsen, J. L.: The lumbar spinal canal in children. Part II: The interpedicular distance and its relation to the sagittal diameter and transverse pedicular width. Europ. J. Radiol. 1 (1981) 312–321

Larsen, J. L.: The lumbar spinal canal in children. Part III: Development of the lumbar spinal canal in relation to the development of the lumbar vertebral bodies. Europ. J. Radiol. 2 (1982) 66–71

Lassale, B., M. Benoist, G. Morvan, C. Massare, A. Deburge, J. Cauchoix: Sténose du canal lombaire. Étude nosologique et séméiologique. Rev. Rhum. 50 (1983) 39–45

Lassale, B., G. Morvan, M. Gottin: Anatomy and radiological anatomy of the lumbar canals. Anat. Clin. 6 (1984) 195

Lé, Ch. T.: Salmonella vertebral osteomyelitis. Amer. J. Dis. Child. 136 (1982) 722–724

Lee, S. H., P. E. Coleman, F. J. Hahn: Magnetic resonance imaging of degenerative disc disease of the spine. Radiol. Clin. N. Amer. 26 (1988) 949

Lefkowitz, D. M., R. M. Quencer: Vacuum facet phenomenon: a computed tomographic sign of degenerative Spondylolisthesis. Radiology 144 (1982) 562

Leibner, E. D., Y. Floman: Tunneling Schmorl's nodes. Skelet. Radiol. 27 (1998) 225

Libson, E., R. A. Bloom, G. Dinari: Symptomatic and asymptomatic spondylolysis and spondylolisthesis in young adults. Int. Orthop. 6 (1982) 259

Lifeso, R., D. Younge: Aneurysmal bone cysts of the spine. Intern. Orthop. (SICOT) 8 (1985) 281–285

Lings, S., L. Mikkelsen: Scheuermann's disease with low localisation. Scand. J. Rehab. Med. 14 (1982) 77–79

Luther, R., H. Legal: Spondylolyse bei Leistungssport? Orthop. Prax. 11 (1975) 50

Mandell, G. A., M. E. Kricoun: Exaggerated anterior vertebral notching. Pediatr. Radiol. 31 (1979) 367–369

Maroun, F., J. C. Jacob, M. A. Mangan, M. Hardjasudarma: Adult diastematomyelia: a complex dysraphic state. Surg. Neurol. 18 (1982) 289–294

Major, N. M., C. A. Helms, H. K. Genant: Calcification demonstrated as high signal intensity on T1-weighted MR images of the disks of the lumbar spine. Radiology 189 (1993) 494

Malawski, S. K.: Pyogenic infection of the spine. Int. Orthop. (SICOT) 1 (1977) 125

Marchand, E. P., J.-G. Villemure, J. Rubin et al.: Solitary osteochondroma of the thoracic spine presenting as spinal cord compression. A case report. Spine 11 (1986) 1033

Mathias, K. D., H.-J. Lössl: Symmetrische Verdoppelung des Processus articularis superior des 4. LWK. Fortschr. Röntgenstr. 123 (1975) 277

Matsumoto, K., S. Fujii, T. Mochizuki et al.: Solitary bone cyst of a lumbar vertebra. A case report and review of literature. Spine 15 (1990) 605

Mau, H.: Das Osteoid-Osteom der Wirbelsäule. Z. Orthop. 120 (1982) 761–766

Maurer, H.-J.: Sklerotische Wirbelveränderungen bei einem Plasmozytom. Fortschr. Röntgenstr. 89 (1958) 114

McEwen, C., D. DiTata, C. Lingg et al.: Ankylosing spondylitis and spondylitis accompanying ulcerative colitis, regional enteritis, psoriasis and Reiter's disease. Arthr. and Rheum. 14 (1971) 291

Meves, F.: Angeborene Mißbildung der Lendenwirbelsäule. Röntgenpraxis 11 (1939) 628–630

Meyer, J. E., R. A. Lepke, K. K. Lindfors et al.: Chordomass: their CT appearance in the cervical thoracic and lumbar spine. Radiology 153 (1984) 693

v. Meyenburg, H.: Über Abtrennung der hinteren Wirbelkörperkante als Ursache von Ischias. Radiol. Clin. (Basel) 15 (146) 215–224

v. Meyenburg, H.: Die Abtrennung der hinteren Wirbelkante als Ursache von Ischias. Radiol. clin. 15 (1946) 217

Meyerding, H. W.: Spondylolisthesis. Surg. Gynecol. Obstet. 54 (1932) 371

Micheli, Lyle J.: Back injuries in gymnastics. Clin. Sports Med. 4 (1985) 85–93

Mikhael, M. A., I. Ciric, J. A. Tarkington et al.: Neuroradiological evaluation of lateral recess syndrome. Radiology 140 (1981) 97

Miller, J. A. A., C. Schmatz, A. B. Schultz: Lumbar disc degeneration: Correlation with age, sex, and spine level in 600 autopsy specimens. Spine 13 (1988) 173

Mitchell, G. E., H. Louri, A. Bernie: A. Various causes of scalloped vertebrae with notes of their pathogenesis. Radiology 89 (1967) 67

Modic, M. T., T. J. Masaryk, J. S. Ross et al.: Imaging of degenerative disk disease. Radiology 168 (1988 a) 177

Modic, M. T., P. M. Steinberg, J. S. Ross et al.: Degenerative disk disease: Assessment of changes in vertebral body marrow with MR imaging. Radiology 166 (1988 b) 193

Mohan, V., R. P. Gupta, T. Marklund et al.: Spinal brucellosis. Int. Orthop. (SICOT) 14 (1990) 63

Moll, J. M. H., I. Haslock, I. F. Macrae et al.: Associations between ankylosing spondylitis, psoriatic arthritis, Reiter's disease, the intestinal arthropathies, and Behçet's syndrome. Medicine 53 (1974) 343

Morard, M., N. de Tribolet, R. C. Janzer: Chondromas of the spine: report of two cases and review of the literature. Brit. J. Neurosurg. 7 (1993) 551

Morin, M. E., E. Palacios: The aplastic hypoplastic lumbar pedicle. Amer. J. Roentgenol. 122 (1974) 639

Morrison J. L., P. A. Kaplan, R. G. Dussault, M. W. Anderson: Pedicle marrow signal intensity changes in the lumbar spine: a manifestation of facet degenerative joint disease. Skeletal Radiol. 29 (2000) 703

Nielsen, V. A. H., E. Iversen, P. Ahlgren: Postoperative discitis. Radiology of progress and healing. Acta radiol. 31 (1990) 559

Niethard, F. U., J. Pfeil: Retrosomatische Spondylolyse des 5. Lendenwirbels mit Segmentationsstörung des zugehörigen Wirbelbogens. Z. Orthop. 123 (1985) 859

Nyúl-Toth, P., M. Joós: Über die Wirbelmanifestation der fibrösen Dysplasie. Fortschr. Röntgenstr. 120 (1974) 744–747

Olsson, O.: Über eine Spaltbildung in den Bogenwurzeln des 2. Lendenwirbels. Acta radiol. 30 (1948) 243

Onimus, M., J. M. Laurain, M. Guidet: L'ostéome ostéoide vertébral. Rev. Chir. Orthop. 71 (1985) 63–69

Oppenheimer, A.: Longitudinal fissures in the vertebral articular processes. J. Bone Jt Surg. 23-A (1941) 280

Oppenheimer, A.: Supernumerary ossicle at the isthmus of the neural arch. Radiology 39 (1942) 98

Oppermann, H. C., I. Greinacher, F. Ball et al.: Die Knochenlymphangiomatose im Kindesalter. Fortschr. Röntgenstr. 131 (1979) 60

Osborne, D. R., E. R. Heinz, D. Bullard et al.: Role of computed tomography in the radiological evaluation of painful radiculopathy after negative myelography: foraminal neural entrapment. Neurosurgery 14 (1984) 147

Pech, P., V. M. Haughton: CT appearance of unfused ossicles in the lumbar spine. Amer. J. Neuroradiol. 6 (1985) 629

Pennell, R. G., A. H. Maurer, A. Bonakdarpour: Stress injuries of the pars interarticularis: radiologic classification and indications for scintigraphy. Amer. J. Roentgenol. 145 (1985) 763

Penning, L., J. R. Blickman: Instability in lumbar spondylolisthesis: a radiologic study of several concepts. Amer. J. Roentgenol. 134 (1980) 293

Peris, P., M. A. Brancs, J. Gratacs et al.: Septic arthritis of spinal apophyseal joint. Report of two cases and review of the literature. Spine 17 (1992) 1514

Pettine, K. A., R. A. Klassen: Osteoid-osteoma and osteoblastoma of the spine. J. Bone Jt Surg. 68-A (1986) 354

Pfirrmann C. W. A., D. Resnick: Schmorl nodes of the thoracic and lumbar spine: radiographic-pathologic study of prevalence, characterization, and correlation with degenerative changes in 1,650 spinal levels in 100 cadavers. Radiology 219 (2001) 368

Plötz, G. M., A. Benini: Lumbar degenerative spondylolisthesis: review of 106 operated cases with degenerative anterior vertebral translation as the predominant aspect of spondylosis. Neurosurgery 8 (1998) 271

Portmann, J.: Ein zusätzlicher, rippenähnlicher Querfortsatz. Fortschr. Röntgenstr. 95 (1961) 856–857

Prasad, V. S., R. L. Sengar, B. P. Sahu, D. Immaneni: Diastematomyelia in adults. Modern imaging and operative treatment. Clin. Imag. 19 (1995) 270

Raininko, R. K., A. J. Aho, M. O. Laine: Computed tomography in spondylitis. CT versus other radiographic methods. Acta orthop. scand. 56 (1985) 372

Ramirez jr., H., J. E. Navarro, W. F. Bennett: "Cupid's bow" contour of the lumbar vertebral endplates detected by computed tomography. J. Comp. Assist. Tomogr. 8 (1984) 121–123

Raymond, J., J.-M. Dumas: Anomalous ossicle of the articular process: arthrography and facet block. Amer. J. Roentgenol. 141 (1983) 1233

Reeder, M. M.: Reeder and Felson's. Gamuts in Bone, Joint and Spine Radiology. Springer, Berlin 1993

Reid, A. B., I. L. Reid, G. Johnson et al.: Familial diffuse cystic angiomatosis of bone. Clin. Orthop. 238 (1989) 211

Reis, N. D., D. Keret: Fracture of the tranverse process of the fifth lumbar vertebra. Injury 16 (1985) 421

Resnick, D., P. Haghighi, J. Guerra: Bone sclerosis and proliferation in a man with multisystem disease. Invest. Radiol. 19 (1984) 1–6

Resnick, D.: Diagnosis of Bone and Joint Disorders, 3rd ed. Saunders, Philadelphia 1995

Resnick, D., G. Niwayama: Intervertebral disc herniations: cartilaginous (Schmorl's) nodes. Radiology 126 (1978) 57

Resnick, D., G. D. Greenway, P. A. Bardwick et al.: Plasma-cell dyscrasia with polyneuropathy, organomegaly, endocrinopathy, M-protein, and skin changes: The POEMS syndrome. Radiology 140 (1981 a) 17

Resnick, D., G. Niwayama, J. Guerra et al.: Spinal vacuum phenomena: anatomical study and review. Radiology 139 (1981 b) 341

Rettig, H.: Patho-Physiologie angeborener Fehlbildungen der Lendenwirbelsäule. Beilage Z. Orthop. 91 (1959)

Reynolds, J.: A re-evaluation of the "fish-vertebra" sign in sickle cell hemoglobinopathy. Amer. J. Roentgenol. 97 (1966) 693

Ricci, A.: Anomalie die tuberoli mamillari delle vertebre lombari: Processo stiloideo e diartrosi accessorie. Riv. Radiol. 4 (1964) 697–702

Roberts, M., P. A. Rinaudo, J. Vilinskas et al.: Solitary sclerosing plasma-cell myeloma of the spine. Case report. J. Neurosurg. 40 (1974) 125

Robin, G. C., Y. Span, R. Steinberg et al.: Scoliosis in the elderly. A follow-up study. Spine 7 (1982) 355

Romanus, R., S. Ydén: Destructing and ossifying spondylitic changes in rheumatoid ankylosing spondylitis (pelvospondylitis ossificans). Acta orthop. Scand. 22 (1952) 88–99

Ross, J. S., T. J. Masaryk, M. T. Modic et al.: Vertebral hemangiomas: MR imaging. Radiology 165 (1987) 165

Rothmann, S. L. G., W. V. Glenn jr.: CT multiplanar reconstruction in 253 cases of lumbar spondylolysis. Amer. J. Neuroradiol. 5 (1984) 81

Rothmann, S. L. G., W. V. Glenn jr., C. W. Kerber: Postoperative fractures of lumbar articular facets. Amer. J. Roentgenol. 143 (1985) 779

Ruckensteiner, E.: Beobachtungen bei Aplasie von Zwischengelenken der Wirbelsäule. Fortschr. Röntgenstr. 59 (1939) 334–339

Sakkas, L., B. Thomas, P. Smyrnis et al.: Low back pain and ochronosis. Int. Orthop. (SICOT) 11 (1987) 19

Sanjay, B. K. S., F. H. Sim, K. K. Unni et al.: Giant-cell tumours of the spine. J. Bone Jt Surg. 75-B (1993) 148

Sartoris, D. J., D. Resnick, R. Tyson, P. Haghighi: Age-related alterations in the vertebral spinosus processes and intervening tissues. Amer. J. Roentgenol. 145 (1985) 1025

Schiebler, M. L., N. Grenier, M. Fallon et al.: Normal and degenerated intervertebral disk: In vivo and in vitro MR imaging with histopathologic correlation. Amer. J. Roentgenol. 157 (1991) 93

Schmitt, G., H.: Periostreaktion als einziges anfängliches Zeichen einer alten Wirbelosteomyelitis. Fortschr. Röntgenstr. 71 (1949) 105–108

Schmitz-Dräger, H. G.: Angeborene Querfortsatzanomalien der Lendenwirbelsäule. Fortschr. Röntgenstr. 90 (1959) 611–614

Schorr, S., E. Adler: Calcified intervertebral disc in children and adults. Acta radiol. (Stockh.) 41 (1954) 498–504

Schröder, H., K. H. Rotte, H. J. Eichhorn: Über die Leistungsfähigkeit tomographischer Untersuchungen zum Nachweis von osteolytischen Wirbelkörpermetastasen. Fortschr. Röntgenstr. 108 (1968) 761–766

Schweitzer, M. E., K. I. El-Noueam: Vacuum disc: frequency of high signal intensity on T2-weighted MR images. Skelet. Radiol. 27 (1998) 83

Schwerdtner, H. P., H. Schobert: Die Spondylolyse im Hochleistungssport bei Geräteturnerinnen. Z. Orthop. 111 (1973) 934

Schwimer, S. R., L. W. Bassett, A. A. Mancuso et al.: Giant cell tumor of the cervicothoracic spine. Amer. J. Roentgenol. 136 (1981) 63

Seegelken, K., G. A. Schulte: Spaltbildungen des Wirbelbogens. Fortschr. Röntgenstr. 116 (1972) 473

Seegelken, K., H. Keller: Retroisthmische Spalte der Lendenwirbelsäule. Fortschr. Röntgenstr. 121 (1974) 659

Sharif, H. S.: Role of MR imaging in the management of spinal infections. Amer. J. Roentgenol. 158 (1992) 1333

Sherman, R. S., D. Wilner: The roentgen diagnosis of hemangioma of bone. Amer. J. Roentgenol. 86 (1961) 1146

Shives, T. C., D. C. Dahlin, F. H. Sim et al.: Osteosarcoma of the spine. J. Bone Jt Surg. 68-A (1986) 660

Shives, T. C., R. A. McLeod, K. K. Unni et al.: Chondrosarcoma of the spine. J. Bone Jt Surg. 71-A (1989) 1158

Silverman, F. N.: Calcification of the intervertebral disks in childhood. Radiology 62 (1954) 801–816

Sim, G. P. G.: Vertebral contour in spondylolisthesis. Brit. J. Radiol. 46 (1973) 250

Simon, W.: Die Verknöcherung des Ligamentum iliolumbale. Acta chir. scand. 67 (1930) 767

Smith, D. M.: Acute back pain associated with a calcified Schmorl's node. A case report. Clin. Orthop. 117 (1976) 193

Smoker, W. R. K., J. C. Godersky, R. K. Knutzon et al.: The role of MR imaging in evaluating metastatic spinal disease. Amer. J. Roentgenol. 149 (1987) 1241

Sonnabend, D. H., T. K. Taylor, G. K. Chapman. Intervertebral disk calcification syndromes in children. J. Bone Jt Surg. 64-B (1982) 25–31

Spiro, T.C., J. Freyschmidt, H. Schlomer: Zur Klinik und Radiologie des Plasmozytoms. Analyse von 116 Fällen. Fortschr. Röntgenstr. 148 (1988) 516

Stäbler, A., M. Bellan, M. Weiss, C. Gartner, J. Brossmann, M. Reiser: MR imaging of enhancing intraosseous disc herniation (Schmorl's nodes). Amer. J. Roentgenol. 168 (1997) 933

Stäbler, A., A. Baur, A. Krüger, M. Weiss, T. Helmberger, M. Reiser: Differentialdiagnose der erosiven Osteochondrose und bakteriellen Spondylitis in der Magnetresonanztomographie (MRT). Fortschr. Röntgenstr 168 (1998) 421

Stelling, C. B.: Anomalous attachment of the transverse process to the vertebral body: an accessory finding in congenital absence of a lumbar pedicle. Skelet. Radiol. 6 (1981) 47

Stepán, J., J. Kolár, A. Šusta, F. Čáp: Die Wirbelsäule und polytope Hyperostosen bei Gicht und Hyperurikämie. Radiologe 23 (1983) 371–374

Stewart T. D.: The age incidence of neural arch defects in Alaskan natives, considered from the standpoint of etiology. J. Bone Jt Surg. 35-A (1953) 937

Stojanovič, J., J. Papa, T. Bajraktarevic Čičin-Šain: Das computertomographische Bild eines Osteoidosteoms der Wirbelsäule. Fortschr. Röntgenstr. 137 (1982) 226–229

Sundaram, M., J. T. Patton: Paravertebral ossification in psoriasis and Reiter's disease. Brit. J. Radiol. 48 (1975) 628

Takemitsu, Y., Y. Harada, T. Iwahara et al.: Lumbar degenerative kyphosis. Clinical, radiological and epidemiological studies. Spine 13 (1988) 1317

Techekapuch, S.: Rupture of the lumbar cartilage plate into the spinal canal in an adolescent. J. Bone Jt Surg. 63-A (1981) 481

Teplick, G. J., P. A. Laffey, A. Berman et al.: Diagnosis and evaluation of spondylolisthesis and/or spondylolysis on axial CT. Amer. J. Neuroradiol. 7 (1986) 479

Torgerson, W. R., W. E. Dotter: Comparative roentgenographic study of the asymptomatic and symptomatic lumbar spine. J. Bone Jt Surg. 58-A (1976) 850

v. Torklus, D., H. Braband: Kartilaginäre Exostosen kleiner Wirbelgelenke im Lumbalbereich. Fortschr. Röntgenstr. 99 (1963) 682–684

Tsuji, H., T. Yoshioka, H. Sainoh: Developmental balloon disc of the lumbar spine in healthy subjects. Spine 10 (1986) 907

Tsuyama, N.: Ossification of the posterior longitudinal ligament of the spine. Clin. Orthop. 184 (1984) 71

Ullrich, C. G., E. F. Binet, M. G. Sanecki et al.: Quantitative assessment of the lumbar spinal canal by computed tomography. Radiology 134 (1980) 137

Verbiest, H.: Further experiences on the pathological influence of developmental narrowness of the bony lumbar vertebral canal. J. Bone Jt Surg. 37-B (1955) 576–583

Vielberg, H.: Beobachtung seltener Wirbelkörperanomalien an der Lendenwirbelsäule eines Erwachsenen. Fortschr. Röntgenstr. 113 (1970) 60–67

Voss, A.-C.: Die Verknöcherung des Lig. flavum. Fortschr. Röntgenstr. 117 (1972) 226–227

Weinberger, A., A. R. Myers: Intervertebral disc calcification in adults: a review. Semin. Arthr. Rheum. 8 (1978) 69

Weinstein, J. B., M. J. Siegel, R. C. Griffith: Spinal Ewing sarcoma: Misleading appearances. Skelet. Radiol. 11 (1984) 262

Weisz, G. W.: Lumbar spinal canal stenosis in Paget's disease. Spine 8 (1983) 192

Whitehouse, G. H., G. J. Griffiths: Roentgenologic aspects of spinal involvement by primary and metastatic Ewing's tumor. J. Canad. Ass. Radiol. 27 (1976) 290

Wichtl, O.: Über Erniedrigung der letzten Lendenbandscheibe und das Vorkommen lumbosacraler Übergangsbandscheiben. Fortschr. Röntgenstr. 62 (1940) 229

Wiesmayr, W.: Über die Spondylitis tuberculosa anterior. Wien. Med. Wschr. 102 (1952) 468–469

Wigh, R. E.: The transitional lumbosacral osseous complex. Skelet. Radiol. 8 (1981) 127

Williams, R.: Complete protrusion of a calcified nucleus pulposus in the thoracic spine. Report of a case. J. Bone Jt Surg. 36-B (1954) 597–600

Wiltse, L. L.: The etiology fo spondylolisthesis. J. Bone Jt Surg. 44-A (1962) 539

Wiltse, L. L., E. H. Widell Jr., D. W. Jackson: Fatigue fracture. The basic lesion in isthmic spondylolisthesis. J. Bone Jt Surg. 57-A (1975) 17

Wiltse, L. L., P. H. Newman, I. Macnab: Classification of spondylolysis and spondylolisthesis. Clin. Orthop. 117 (1976) 23

Wiltse, L. L., R. B. Winter: Terminology and measurement of spondylolisthesis. J. Bone Jt Surg. 65-A (1983) 768

Witt, I., A. Vestergaard, A. Rosenklitt: A comparative analysis of x-ray findings of the lumbar spine in patients with and without lumbar pain. Spine 9 (1984) 298

Wortzmann, G., M. Steinhardt: Congenitally absent lumbar pedicle: a reappraisal. Radiology 152 (1984) 713

Yochum, T. R., L. T. Sellers, D. A. Oppenheimer et al.: The sclerotic pedicle—how many causes are there? Skelet. Radiol. 19 (1990) 411

Yousefzadeh, D. K., G. Y. El-Khoury, A. R. Lupetin: Congenital aplastic-hypoplastic lumbar pedicle in infants and young children. Skelet. Radiol. 7 (1982) 259

Zippel, H., H. Runge: Pathologische Anatomie und Pathogenese von Spondylolyse und Spondylolisthese im Kindesalters. Z. Orthop. 114 (1976) 189

Sacrum and Coccyx

Normal Findings

 During Growth

The **sacrum** is composed of five originally separate vertebrae that fuse after birth to form one bone. Like the rest of the vertebrae, each sacral vertebra has a body, arch, transverse processes, and articular processes. The upper three sacral vertebrae have one ossification center in the body, two ossification centers in the vertebral arch, and a lateral ossification center for each costal element (Fig. 5.**408**). Separate ossification centers for the inferior articular process are occasionally present.

The lateral centers become visible on radiographs in the fifth or sixth month. During the first years of life they fuse with the main centers to form the **lateral mass** of the sacrum.

> This can create an apparent bifid malformation of the fetal sacrum on **sonography** after 20–25 weeks and should not be mistaken for a true anomaly (Kliewer et al. 1995).

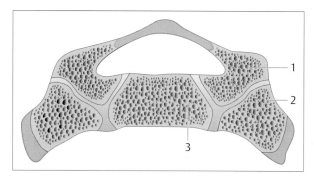

Fig. 5.**408** Cross-section through the first sacral vertebra of a one-year-old child. The five ossification centers are shown schematically (after Rauber and Kopsch).
1 Ossification center in the vertebral arch anlage
2 Ossification center in the costal anlage
3 Ossification center in the vertebral body anlage

In the full-term **newborn**, the vertebral bodies of S1–S5 and the vertebral arches of S1–S4 are already ossified (Figs. 5.**409**, 5.**410**). The upper three sacral segments appear as large, triangular bony structures located between the arch centers and the iliac wings. The lateral centers are

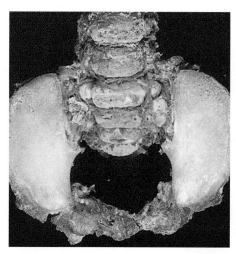

Fig. 5.**409** Specimen of a neonatal sacrum, anterior view (Museum of Man, San Diego).

Fig. 5.**410** Lateral radiograph of the sacrum in a 2-month-old ▷ infant.

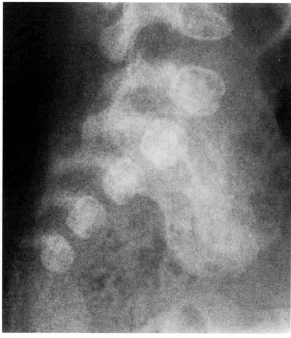

sometimes absent at S1, or the S1 centers may be the last to appear during this period.

The **intervertebral disk spaces** appear relatively high, and the disk between S1 and S2 resembles the last lumbar disk (Schwabe 1933). The last two sacral disks do not contain a nucleus pulposus (Lippert 1966).

Fusion of the individual sacral vertebrae to form the sacrum starts around the sixth year of life and continues into the fourth decade. Ossification proceeds from above downward, starting with the vertebral arches and spreading to the costal processes and finally to the spinous

processes and vertebral bodies. Fusion of the vertebral arches and costal processes is completed between 15 and 25 years of age (Fig. 5.**411**) (Rauber and Kopsch 1998).

Shell-like **epiphyses** typically appear in the lateral portion of the upper two sacral vertebrae between 11 and 20 years of age (Figs. 5.**412**, 5.**413**). Similar epiphyses are also occasionally seen at the inferior border of the sacrum (Fig. 5.**414**).

Ossification of the intervertebral disks begins in the two middle segments, followed by the fourth disk. The first disk is the last to ossify. Fusion of the first and second sacral

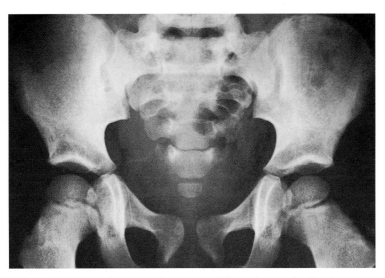

Fig. 5.**411**   Pelvis and sacrum of a 15-year-old boy. The vertebral arches are still unfused.

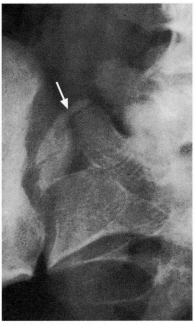

Fig. 5.**412**   Shell-like growth zone along the upper lateral border of the lateral mass of the sacrum (arrow) in a 13-year-old girl.

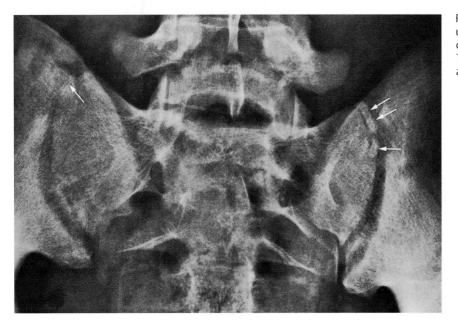

Fig. 5.**413**   Growth centers at the upper lateral border of the sacrum (arrow) in a 15-year-old boy. The wide sacroiliac joint spaces are normal for this age.

vertebrae may not occur until 20 to 30 years of age. The posterior longitudinal ligament also ossifies (Schwabe 1933). Thus, the fusion of the sacral vertebrae remains superficial until middle age, and sacral disk remnants may still be found even in old age (Fig. 5.**415**).

The **coccygeal vertebrae** vary in number from three to six. Four vertebrae are usually present. The rudimentary vertebrae of the coccyx ossify from a single center and usually do not have apophyseal centers. The first ossification center appears at 1–5 years of age, and the last ossification center appears at age 15–20 (Rauber and Kopsch 1998).

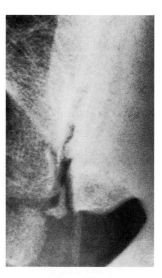

Fig. 5.**414**   Shell-like growth zone along the lower articular margin of the lateral mass in an 18-year-old male.

Fig. 5.**415**   Typical appearance of the sacrum and part of the coccyx, showing the arcuate lines of the anterior (pelvic) sacral foramina (arrowheads) and the intervertebral canals (arrows). Note the sacrocaudal transitional vertebra.

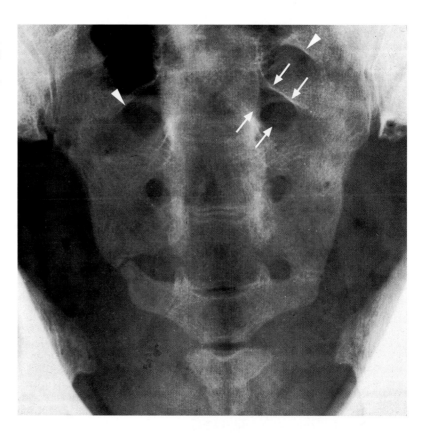

 In Adulthood

The **lateral mass** of the sacrum is formed by the fusion of the transverse processes and costal elements. The fused spinous processes of the sacral vertebrae form the **median sacral crest** (Fig. 5.**416**). The paired **lateral sacral crests** on the dorsal surface are formed by the fused accessory processes and are lateral to the sacral foramina. They can project far anteriorly in the lateral view (Fig. 5.**417**). The **intermediate sacral crest**, formed from remnants of the articular processes, runs parallel to the lateral crest and medial to the sacral foramina. The intermediate crests terminate inferiorly in the **sacral cornua**, which articulate with the coccygeal cornua.

The **sacral hiatus** is a gap in the posterior wall of the sacral canal resulting from an absence of fusion of the spinous processes of S5 and usually of S4. The upper border of the sacral hiatus is usually located between S4 and the first coccygeal vertebra, but it may occur at a higher level.

The **first coccygeal vertebra** is often fused to the sacrum in males. The **lower coccygeal vertebrae** are often fused together (Fig. 5.**418**) while the upper coccygeal vertebrae are loosely interconnected. It is very common to find an articular connection between the first and second coccygeal vertebrae (Fig. 5.**419**).

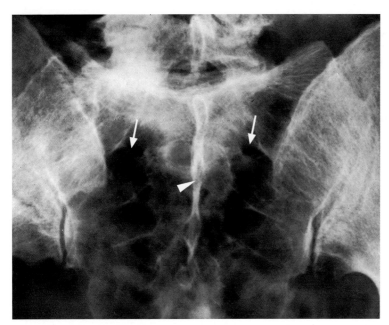

Fig. 5.**416**   Median sacral crest (arrowhead) and posterior sacral foramina (arrows).

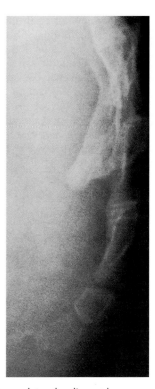

Fig. 5.**417**   Lateral sacral crest on a lateral radiograph.

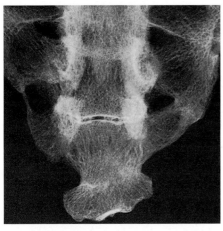

Fig. 5.**418**   Asymmetric synostosis of the last coccygeal vertebrae. Sacrocaudal transitional vertebra with sclerotic margins along the intervertebral junction.

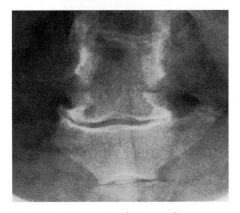

Fig. 5.**419**   Connection between the sacrum and coccyx. Sacrocaudal transitional vertebra with sclerotic margins and osteophytes along the intervertebral junctions.

The **intervertebral foramina** of the sacrum consist of short bony canals that open on the ventral and dorsal surface as the **anterior** and **posterior sacral foramina** (Figs. 5.**415**, 5.**416**). The foramina of the lower sacral vertebrae may be fully open or partially closed. Segments with open foramina are indistinguishable from **sacrocaudal transitional vertebrae** with articular-process-like structures (Figs. 5.**415**, 5.**418**, 5.**419**). A true joint or a cartilaginous attachment may exist between the sacral apex and the **coccyx**.

The sacrum is difficult to evaluate in the **AP projection** because its curvature and tilt toward the long axis of the body give it a considerably foreshortened appearance. A better projection of the sacrum can be obtained by angling the tube 15–25° cephalad. The vertebral canal is difficult to define in the sacrum due to the absence of true pedicles (Figs. 5.**415**, 5.**416**). As noted, the intervertebral foramina in the sacrum take the form of **intervertebral canals** that open anteriorly and posteriorly as the **anterior** and **posterior sacral foramina**. The outlines of the intervertebral canals are often visible as faint, slightly curved linear shadows (Figs. 5.**415**, 5.**416**). The anterior sacral foramina generally do not appear as ringlike structures in the standard **AP radiograph**. Usually only their superomedial border is visible as a curved line while their inferolateral border blends indistinctly with the pelvic surface of the sacrum. As a rule, only the fourth foramen is visualized without distortion. The **posterior sacral foramina** are smaller and are rarely visualized (Figs. 5.**415**, 5.**416**). In an orthograde view of the sacrum obtained by angling the tube cephalad, the anterior and posterior sacral foramina are superimposed. The posterior foramina are offset superiorly from the anterior foramina in the AP projection. The greater the sacral tilt relative to the film plane, the greater the degree of offset (Fig. 5.**416**).

Fig. 5.**420**   "Transverse clefts" in the sacrum: a projection artifact.

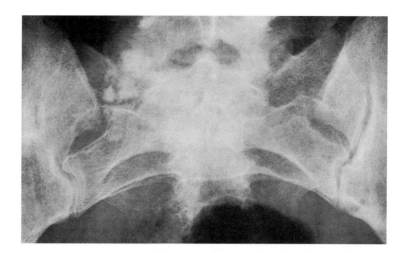

Transverse **cleftlike lucencies** in the lateral mass between the first and second sacral vertebrae are fairly common projection-related phenomena (Fig. 5.**420**). **Arched soft-tissue densities** may be superimposed over the sacrum on each side; they are caused by the gluteal soft tissues (Fig. 5.**421**).

The **lateral projection** mainly provides information on the shape of the sacrum. As in the AP view, the sacral canal is difficult to evaluate. Usually only the anterior wall is defined. Sites of fusion between the sacral vertebrae are marked by slight indentations or low prominences on the anterior contour of the sacrum. Rudimentary intervertebral disks are occasionally found.

> The sacral foramina may appear as lucent areas or "pseudocysts" in the lateral projection (the "foramen effect," Fig. 5.**422**). (Portmann 1962)

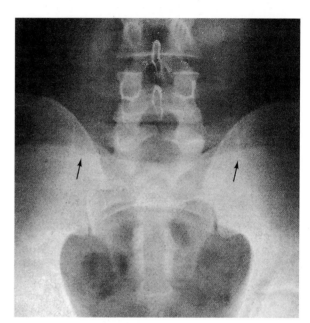

Fig. 5.**421**   Gluteal tissue folds can appear as curved soft-tissue shadows (arrows) projected over the sacrum and pelvis.

Fig. 5.**422 a, b**   Pseudocysts of the sacrum (observation by Fliegel, Basel).
a Typical lucent area in the lateral projection (arrow).
b Another example of sacral pseudocysts (arrows).

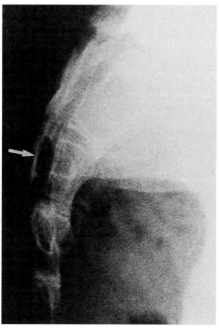

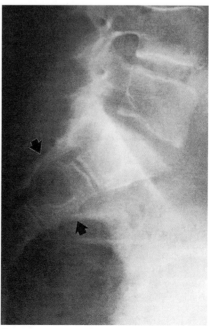

a

b

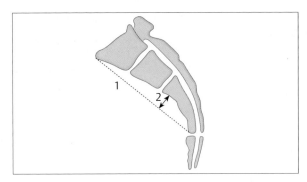

Fig. 5.**423**   Sacral index of Radlauer (after Hellinger). Sacral index = (2/1) × 100 %.
1   Ventral chord
2   Maximum depth of sacrum

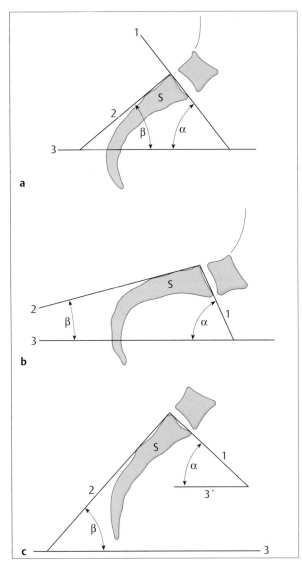

Fig. 5.**424 a–c**   Sacral base angle and sacral tilt (after Hellinger).
a Normal pelvis.
b Horizontal pelvis.
c Steep pelvis.
1   Tangent to upper end plate of S1
2   Tangent to dorsal surface of sacrum
3, 3′   Parallels to horizontal film baseline
α   Sacral base angle
β   Sacral tilt

Well-defined linear lucencies along the dorsal aspect of S1 and S2 have been found in 30 % of cases and have been interpreted as a normal finding (Kreyenbühl and Hessler 1973).

Normal Position and Posture

The curvature of the sacrum increases in the newborn from a more flattened shape in the fetus. The promontory angle is already present during the last two-thirds of fetal development. The promontory is formed by S2 in the fetus and newborn, later shifting to the upper border of the first sacral vertebra during puberty (Schoberth 1956). The anterior concavity of the sacrum shows very great individual variation in adults. The curvature of the sacrum can be stated in terms of the sacral index (Fig. 5.**423**) (Radlauer 1908, Hellinger 1995).

The sacral index changes in later life, suggesting that the sacrum acquires a deeper curvature with aging (Schoberth 1956). The degree of sacral curvature is hereditary. The angle of sacral tilt is measured as illustrated in Fig. 5.**424**.

Pathological Finding?

Variation or Anomaly?

Variants

The sacrococcygeal region shows considerable morphological diversity even when normally developed. This includes varying types of **angulation** in the frontal and sagittal planes (Figs. 5.**425**, 5.**426**) as well as **dysplasias** and partial **aplasias** (Figs. 5.**427**, 5.**432**). Generally these variations have no clinical importance, but they can be a source of misinterpretation in trauma cases. Atypical **angular deviation** of the sacrum may be indistinguishable from posttraumatic changes (Fig. 5.**428**).

Marked **displacements** can occur between S1 and S2 and between S2 and S3 **during growth**. In each case the upper vertebra always shifts anteriorly in relation to the next lower vertebra (Cacciarelli 1977).

Persistent ossification centers. Secondary ossification centers like those occurring in the upper and lower portions of the lateral mass (Figs. 5.**412**–5.**414**) may be a cause of accessory ossicles (Fig. 5.**429**).

Accessory ribs can occur at various sites in the sacropelvic region. They are usually connected to the sacrum, but a small number arise from the coccyx (Ireberger 1936, Cornwall and Ramsey 1957, Halloran 1960, Greenspan and Norman 1982, Dunaway et al. 1983). **Pelvic ribs** may be single or multiple (Van Derslice et al. 1992), and they are highly variable in their size, shape, and course. Jointlike discontinuities are occasionally present, giving rise to the term "**pelvic digit**" (Greenspan and Norman 1982). Pelvic ribs may have a direct bony attachment to the sacrum, or they may be connected by cartilage or ligaments to the pelvic wall (see the chapter on the pelvis). Differentiation is required from other calcifications and ossifications of the soft tissues and ligaments (Fig. 5.**443**).

Small, symmetrical **cystlike lucencies** in the **lateral mass** of the sacrum are incidental findings of uncertain etiology that have no clinical significance (Fig. 5.**430**).

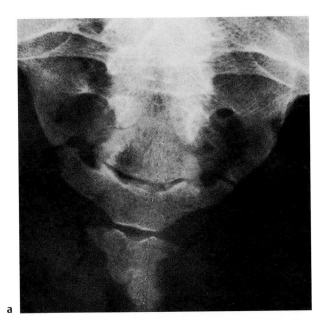

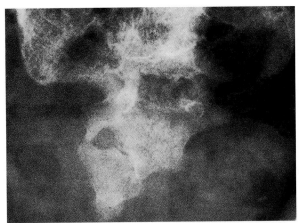

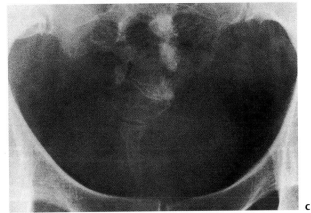

Fig. 5.**425 a–c** Variants of the sacrococcygeal region.
a Right convex bowing of the sacrococcygeal junction.
b The lowest coccygeal vertebra is deformed and deviated toward the right side.
c Right convex bowing of the coccyx.

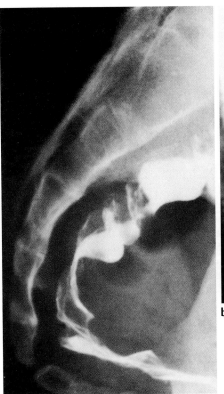

Fig. 5.**426 a–c** Morphological variants of the coccyx.
a Extremely long, angulated, horizontally directed coccyx in a patient who complained of pain on sitting.
b Anterior angulation of the coccyx on T1-weighted sagittal MRI.
c Posterior angulation of the coccyx on T1-weighted sagittal MRI.

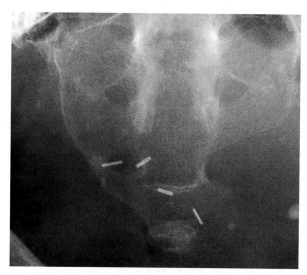

Fig. 5.**427**   Circumscribed defect in the left side of the sacrum due to incomplete formation of the lowest sacral foramen. The metallic clips are from previous lower abdominal surgery.

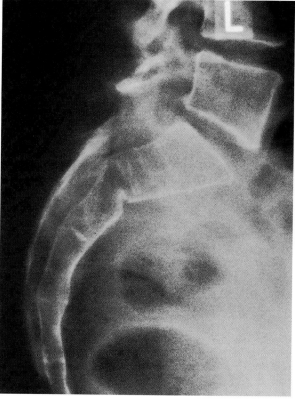

Fig. 5.**428**   Deep notch in the pelvic surface of the sacrum, ▷ located opposite a slight angular deformity on the dorsal side (observation by Etter, Lucerne). Old trauma? Anomaly?

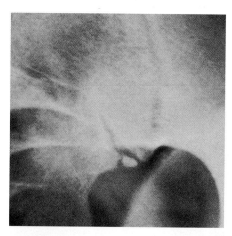

Fig. 5.**429**   Accessory bone (persistent ossification center?) below the sacroiliac joint.

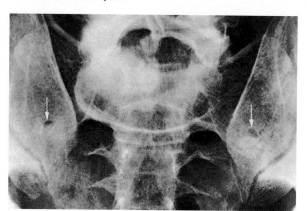

Fig. 5.**430**   Symmetrical cystlike lucencies in the sacral ala.

Cystic lucencies with sclerotic margins in the first sacral vertebra (**pseudocysts**) near the sacroiliac joints represent fossae in the posterior sacral wall, which are partially bounded by the S1 transverse processes (Fig. 5.**431**). All changes of this kind are typically located at a far lateral site in the sacral lateral mass.

Concavities in the anterior wall of the **sacral canal** can mimic sites of tumor destruction and have been described as common anatomic variants (Coutte and de Carvalho 1983).

The synostosis between individual sacral segments may be absent, resulting in **horizontal clefts** (Fig. 5.**432**). Failure of closure of the sacral foramina can lead to **sacral asymmetries**. These asymmetries are difficult to distinguish from **sacrocaudal transitional vertebrae**, which are connected to the lateral mass of the sacrum by transverse-process-like structures (Figs. 5.**415**, 5.**418**, 5.**419**).

Anomalies and Deformities

Vertebral Arch Defect:
Mild anomalies of the upper sacral vertebrae predominantly affect the spinous processes, where it is common to find a **medial arch defect** due to a failure of arch closure. The **arch of S1** is often rudimentary and sometimes develops only on one side. One root of the arch may be higher than the other (Figs. 5.**316**, 5.**317**, 5.**450**), and occasionally an isolated center for the apex of the spinous process may be interposed between them.

Fig. 5.**431 a–d**   Pseudocysts in the lateral mass of the sacrum. Regularly shaped lucent areas, mostly bordered by cortex, are visible in the lateral portions of the sacrum at the level of S1 (arrows).
a Summation image in the AP projection.
b Frontal tomogram.
c Deep fossa (×) in the lateral mass of an anatomic specimen.
d Oblique radiograph of the finding in **c** (arrows).

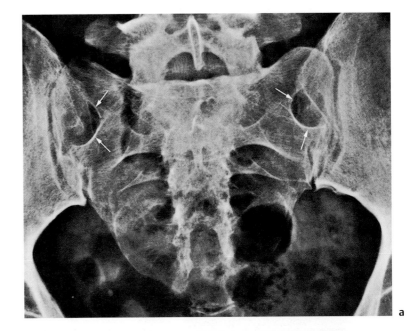

a

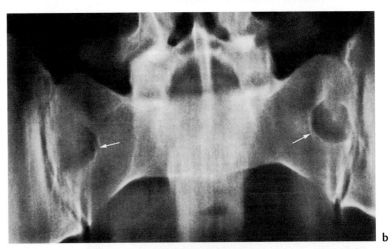

b

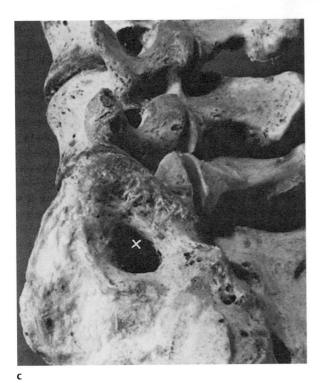

c

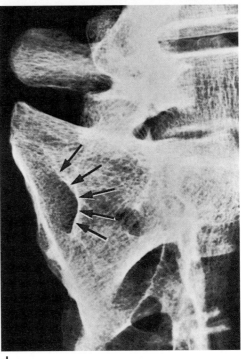

d

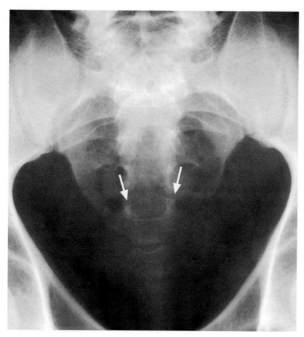

Fig. 5.**432** Horizontal cleft in the lower part of the sacrum (arrows).

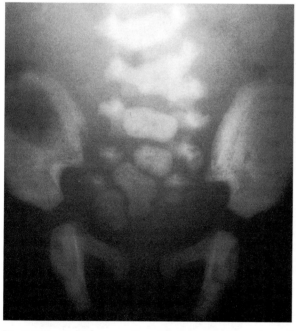

Fig. 5.**433** Multiple anomalies of the lower lumbar and sacral vertebrae (observation by D. Resnick, San Diego).

Hemivertebra:

The presence of a hemivertebra has been described at the S1 level (Heim and Marcovich 1995). The authors identified this anomaly as a very rare cause of backache in patients with no neurological abnormalities (Fig. 5.**433**).

There have also been sporadic reports of agenesis of an S1 pedicle (Sener 1997).

Sacrococcygeal Agenesis:

A severe anomaly is subtotal or total sacrococcygeal agenesis (**caudal regression syndrome**), which occurs with increased frequency in the children of diabetic mothers (Figs. 5.**434**, 5.**435**) (Stanley et al. 1979).

The sacrum and coccyx may be partially or completely absent (Nour et al. 1989). The iliac bones in these cases are fused at the midline and articulate with each other or with the lowest vertebral body. With partial sacral agenesis, the remaining sacral segments occupy a normal position between the iliac bones. Sacral agenesis combined with complete fusion of the lower extremities is termed "**mermaid syndrome**" (Guidera et al. 1991). Vertebral anomalies and scoliosis are consistently found above the sacrum, and occasionally the lumbar spine and lower thoracic spine are not formed (Guidera et al. 1991). A single case of focal lumbar agenesis with an intact sacrum has been described (Grace et al. 1971).

Sacrococcygeal agenesis is often part of a complex developmental abnormality (Weaver et al. 1986), which may be accompanied by:

- Urogenital tract anomalies
- Anomalies of the sacral and coccygeal plexus, occasionally with the formation of myelomeningoceles
- Gastrointestinal anomalies (Loder and Dayioglu 1990, Guidera et al. 1991, Estin and Cohen 1995)

Partial agenesis of the sacrum has been observed in association with an anterior sacral meningocele (Sumner et al. 1980). Accompanying congenital presacral teratomas have been reported (Hunt et al. 1977, O'Riordain et al. 1991). Contractures of the lower extremity and congenital hip dislocation are common associated features (Fig. 5.**435**).

MRI is of major importance in the diagnosis of complex anomalies (Nievelstein et al. 1994, Estin and Cohen 1995).

Dysraphic Anomalies: Dysraphic anomalies, covered in the section on the lumbar spine, can also affect the sacrum. If the vertebral arch defect involves all of the sacral segments and includes the sacral hiatus, a **total sacral hiatus** is said to be present (Fig. 5.**436**).

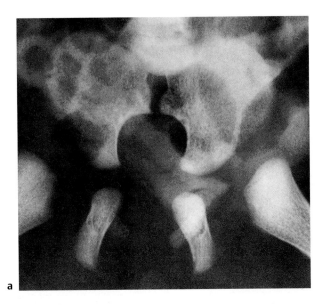

a

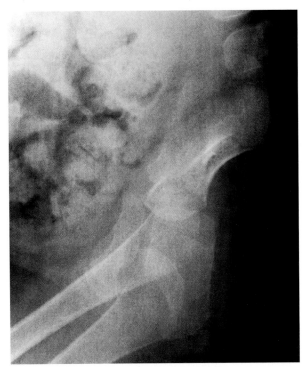

b

Fig. 5.**434a, b**   Sacral agenesis in a child.
a AP projection.
b Lateral projection.

 Fracture, Subluxation, or Dislocation?

Fractures

Isolated Fractures:
Isolated fractures of the sacrum and coccyx are caused by direct violence and are classified as stable injuries of the pelvic ring (type A3 in the AO classification). The majority are transverse fractures located below the sacroiliac joint space at the level of the third and fourth sacral segments (Fountain et al. 1977). Generally the caudal fragment is tilted anteriorly. **Transverse fractures** of S2 are considered extremely rare and reportedly account for just 2% of sacral injuries (Hadley and Carter 1985, Kerboul et al. 1985).

Isolated **oblique or vertical fractures** of the sacrum occur so rarely that their presence should warrant a thorough search for additional signs of a pelvic ring fracture. Sacral fractures are more common in association with complex injuries of the pelvic ring (types B and C in the AO classification, see chapter on the pelvis).

Denis et al. (1988) classified sacral fractures into three types based on the location of the fracture line: lateral to the sacral foramina in the lateral mass (type 1), through the sacral foramina (type 2), or through the sacral canal (type 3). The closer the fracture line is to the sacral canal, the greater the degree of neurological impairment.

Fractures of the **coccyx** occur more commonly in isolation than sacral fractures. They reportedly occur in 3–6% of pelvic fractures (Schild et al. 1981). Nondisplaced coccygeal fractures are difficult to diagnose (see Normal Variants).

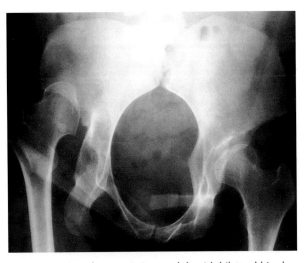

Fig. 5.**435**   Sacral agenesis in an adult with bilateral hip dysplasia and a dislocated right hip.

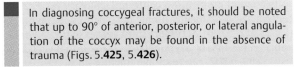

In diagnosing coccygeal fractures, it should be noted that up to 90° of anterior, posterior, or lateral angulation of the coccyx may be found in the absence of trauma (Figs. 5.**425**, 5.**426**).

Up to 30% of sacral and coccygeal fractures are missed on **standard AP radiographs** (Schild et al. 1981, Heller and Jend 1986, Rogers 1992). This is due to the apparent foreshortening of the sacrum in the AP projection and the presence of superimposed bowel structures. Most fractures appear only as slight discontinuities or irregularities in the margins of the sacral foramina (Fig. 5.**437**).

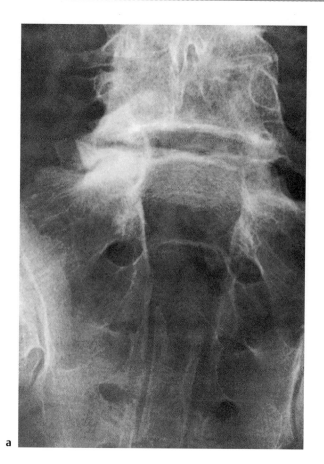

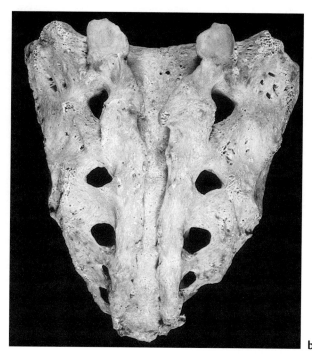

Fig. 5.**436a, b** Total sacral hiatus.
a AP radiograph.
b Posterior view of a specimen.

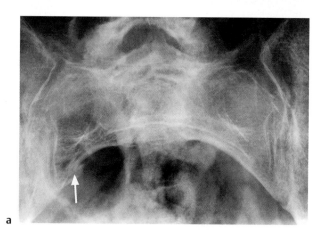

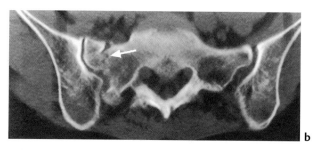

Fig. 5.**437a, b** Sacral fracture following a lateral compression injury of the pelvic ring.
a AP radiograph (arrow).
b Axial CT (arrow).

Persistent ossification centers. Secondary ossification centers can occasionally mimic detached bone fragments (Figs. 5.**412**–5.**414**). **Accessory joint spaces** in the sacroiliac joints (Fig. 5.**448**) or **asymmetrical transitional vertebrae** (Fig. 5.**299**–5.**302**) can resemble fracture lines.

The **lateral projection** can occasionally show contour irregularities in the anterior or posterior cortex and demonstrate dislocations.

CT is the simplest and most reliable study for evaluating the sacrum and the sacroiliac joints (Schild et al. 1981, Heller and Jend 1986, Rogers 1992). **MRI** is very sensitive in the detection of bone contusions and occult fractures (Brahme et al. 1990, Staatz et al. 1997).

Insufficiency Fractures:
Insufficiency fractures of the sacrum typically consist of vertically oriented fracture lines located close to one or both sacroiliac joints (Fig. 5.**438**). Horizontal fractures can also occur.

Sacral insufficiency fractures have been described in children (Grier et al. 1993, Martin et al. 1995), athletes (Czarnecki et al. 1988, Guttner et al. 1990, McFarland and Giangarra 1996, Eller et al. 1997), women with postmenopausal osteoporosis, patients with rheumatoid arthritis or corticosteroid medication (West et al. 1994), and in patients who have undergone radiation therapy (Renner 1990, Newhouse et al. 1992, Blomlie et al. 1993). The frac-

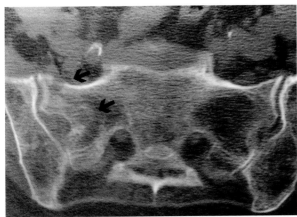
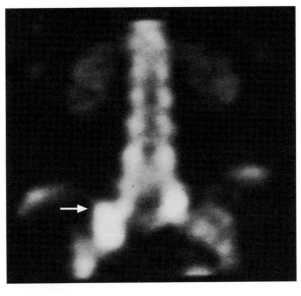

Fig. 5.**438 a, b** Insufficiency fracture of the sacrum.
a Cortical and cancellous discontinuities in the right lateral mass on axial CT (arrows).
b Increased tracer uptake in the right lateral mass (arrow).

tures are difficult to diagnose on **conventional radiographs** and occasionally are manifested by faint discontinuities in the arcuate line or increased sclerosis of the lateral mass. **Bone scans** show increased tracer uptake at the site of insufficiency fractures (Abe et al. 1992), which may show an H-shaped pattern (**Honda sign**). But **CT** and especially **MRI** are best for the detection of these fractures (Gacetta and Yandow 1984, Brahme et al. 1990, Lien et al. 1992, Staatz et al. 1997). There is debate as to whether the intraosseous vacuum phenomenon sometimes seen in sacral insufficiency fractures is useful as a differentiating feature from other disorders (Arafat and Davies 1994, Stäbler et al. 1995, Stäbler et al. 1996, Peh and Ooi 1997).

Dislocations

Dislocations of the **sacrum** occur in cases of complete, bilateral sacroiliac joint disruption and are discussed in the section on the sacroiliac joints.

With dislocations of the **coccyx**, the lower segment is usually displaced anteriorly and rarely is displaced posteriorly (Becker 1937). Dislocations of the coccyx can also occur as obstetric injuries.

 ## Necrosis?

To our knowledge, there have been no published reports on spontaneous avascular osteonecrosis of the sacrum. Meanwhile, relatively frequent reference has been made to the link between therapeutic irradiation and **radiation necrosis** of the sacrum (Rubin and Probhasawat 1961, Bragg et al. 1970, Holler et al. 1998). **Sickle cell anemia** is associated with erosive and sclerotic changes about the sacroiliac joints, presumably a result of ischemia (Kaklamanis 1984). In one study, avascular necrosis was identified as the cause of **coccygodynia** in 2 of 16 adult patients (Lourie and Young 1985).

 ## Inflammation?

Osteomyelitis of the sacrum and coccyx is very rare. It may be caused by the spread of pelvic abscess and fistula formation in patients with **Crohn disease** (Faerber et al. 1981, Schwartz et al. 1987). Involvement of the axial skeleton is known to occur in **drug addicts** but predominantly affects the sacroiliac joint.

 ## Tumor?

The diagnosis of tumors on **conventional radiographs** is limited by overlying bowel gas and stool, which can occasionally mimic areas of osteolysis. "**Pseudocysts**" of the sacrum mentioned previously (Figs. 5.**422**, 5.**431**) and occasional anterior protrusions of the sacral canal (Coutte and de Carvalho 1983) can lead to diagnostic errors in the lateral projection. This also applies to "pseudo-osteolytic lesions" in the AP projection (Fig. 5.**431**). The osteolytic phase of **Paget disease** in the sacrum can mimic a destructive malignant process.

Tumors of the axial skeleton were discussed fully in the sections on the cervical spine and especially the lumbar spine (see also Campanacci 1990, Resnick 1995, Freyschmidt 1998).

Below we shall consider only tumors that have special relevance to the sacrum and coccyx.

Chordomas

Derived from remnants of the notochord, chordomas affect the sacrococcygeal region in 50–60% of all cases (Rich et al. 1985). They are most prevalent in the **fifth and sixth decades of life**. Chordomas are three times more common in men than women.

Radiographs usually show nonspecific osteolysis. Marginal sclerosis is occasionally present, and intratumoral calcifications are seen in approximately 30–50% of cases (Fig. 5.**439**). Extensive paraosseous soft-tissue masses are often present.

Chordomas can be difficult to distinguish from chondrosarcoma. Differentiation from aneurysmal bone cysts, giant cell tumors (no calcifications), and metastases may

also be difficult. Osteolysis of the sacrum with an associated soft-tissue mass should suggest a chordoma in cases where there is no reason to suspect metastases.

Giant Cell Tumor

Giant cell tumors of the spinal column predominantly affect the sacrum (Sanjay et al. 1993), and transarticular extension of the tumor may be noted (Fig. 5.**440**).

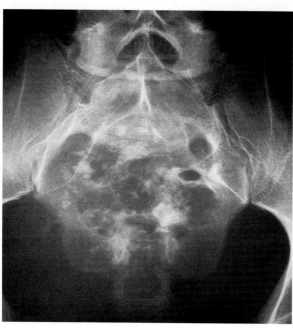
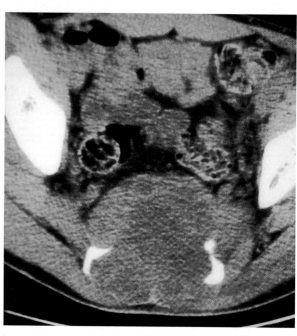

Fig. 5.**439 a, b**   Chordoma of the sacrum (observation by D. Resnick, San Diego).
a AP radiograph shows a large osteolytic lesion in the sacrum with flecks of calcification.

b Destruction of the sacrum with a large soft-tissue mass on axial CT.

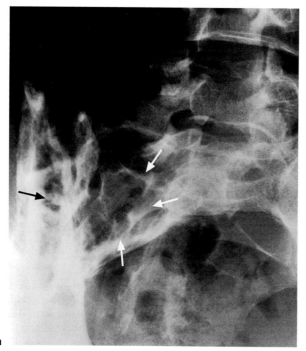
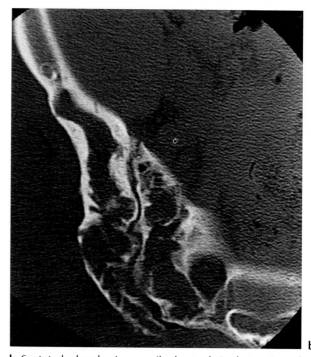

Fig. 5.**440 a, b**   Giant cell tumor of the sacrum.
a Osteolytic destruction of the sacrum in an AP radiograph (arrows).

b Septated, sharply circumscribed osteolytic destruction of the lateral mass of the sacrum with extension to the adjacent ilium on axial CT.

Solitary plasmacytoma may have a trabeculated or soap-bubble-like appearance on radiographs, resembling a giant cell tumor. Osteolytic lesions usually have sharply circumscribed margins.

Metastases

The sacrum is a common site of occurrence for skeletal metastases. Conventional radiographs show abnormalities only if extensive destruction has occurred. Destruction of the arcuate line is a particularly helpful diagnostic feature (Amorosa et al. 1985).

Tumors of Neurogenic Origin

The sacrum is a frequent site of occurrence of **neurogenic cysts** (Willinsky and Fazl 1985, Willinsky et al. 1988) and occasional solid tumors such as **neurofibromas** and **ependymomas** (Fig. 5.**441**).

Congenital Cysts, Teratomas

Congenital cysts and teratomas have been described in the sacrococcygeal region (Stojavinovič et al. 1982).

Glomus Tumors

There is controversy as to the occurrence of glomus tumors in the coccyx and their relationship to coccygodynia (Pambakian and Smith 1981, Albrecht 1990).

 ## Other Changes?

Calcifications and Ossifications

A small calcification is occasionally seen in the **intervertebral disk** between the last sacral and first coccygeal vertebrae (Fig. 5.**442**). It is a relatively common finding in children.

Calcifications and ossifications of the **sacrotuberal** and **sacrospinal ligaments** can occur in the setting of **DISH syndrome** and after **trauma** (Fig. 5.**443**). The ligament ossifications can resemble pelvic ribs and require differentiation from them.

Paget Disease

Sacral involvement by Paget disease is relatively common (Guyer et al. 1981) and presents mainly with osteolytic changes that can make diagnosis difficult (Fig. 5.**444**). In most cases, however, there is concomitant involvement of other pelvic regions.

Osteopoikilosis

Osteopoikilosis (osteopathia condensans disseminata) is an asymptomatic osteosclerotic dysplasia that is very rare (Jonasch 1955). It is marked by numerous small, homogeneous, well-circumscribed, rounded osteosclerotic areas that represent cortical bone islands and show no radiotracer uptake (Fig. 5.**445**).

Osteopoikilosis can be distinguished from osteoblastic **metastases**, **mastocytosis**, and **tuberous sclerosis** by the uniform size of the lesions, their symmetry, and the absence of radionuclide uptake.

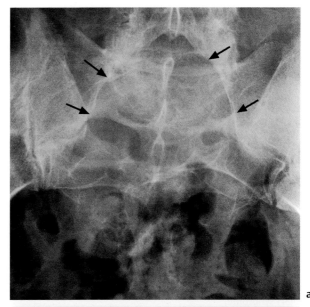
a

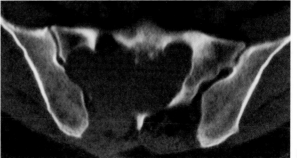
b

Fig. 5.**441 a, b** Neurofibroma of the sacrum.
a Large, smoothly marginated osteolytic defect in the sacrum (arrows) in the AP projection.
b Axial CT.

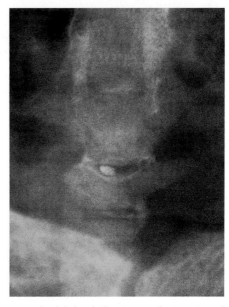

Fig. 5.**442** Intervertebral disk calcifications at the junction of the sacrum and coccyx.

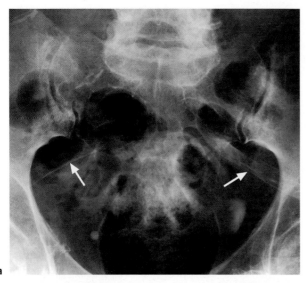

a

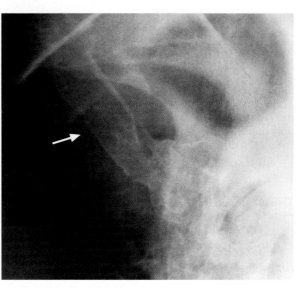

b

Fig. 5.**443 a, b** Ossified sacrospinal ligament in a patient with DISH syndrome.

a AP projection (arrows).
b Lateral projection (arrow).

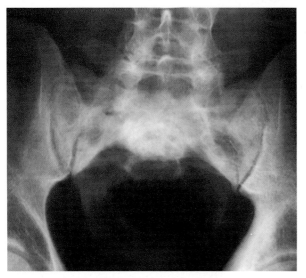

Fig. 5.**444** Paget disease of the sacrum. Typical changes are evident in the bony structure of the sacrum and the left hemipelvis.

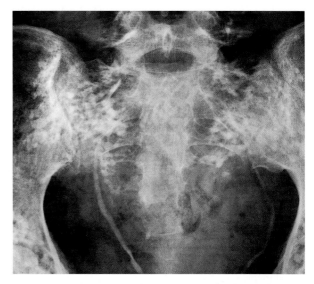

Fig. 5.**445** Involvement of the sacrum and pelvic skeleton by osteopoikilosis.

References

Abe, H., M. Nakamura, S. Takahashi, et al.: Radiation-induced insufficiency fractures of the pelvis: Evaluation with 99mTc-methylene diphosphonate scintigraphy. Amer. J. Roentgenol. 158 (1992) 599

Albrecht, S., I. Zbieranowski: Incidental glomus coccygeum. When a normal structure looks like a tumor. Amer. J. surg. Pathol 14 (1990) 922

Amorosa, Judith, K., St. Weintraub, L. F. Amorosa, J. N. Safer, M. Rafii: Sacral destruction foraminal lines revisited. Amer. J. Roentgenol. 145 (1985) 773–775

Arafat, Q. W., A. M. Davies: Sacral insufficiency fracture with intraosseous gas. Europ. J. Radiol. 18 (1994) 232

Bársony, T.: Zirkumskripte Aufhellungen im lateralen Anteil des Kreuzbeins. Kein pathologischer Befund. Brun's Beitr. Klein. Chir. 157 (1933) 359–363

Becker, F.: Traumatische Luxation des Steißbeins nach hinten durch Skiunfall. Beitrag zur Kenntnis der seltenen Formen der Steißbeinverletzungen. Zbl. Chir. 146 (1937) 2877–2880

Blomlie, V., H. H. Lien, T. Iversen et al.: Radiation-induced insufficiency fractures of the sacrum: Evaluation with MR imaging. Radiology 188 (1993) 241

Bragg, D. G., H. Shidnia, F. C. H. Chu et al.: The clinical and radiographic aspects of radiation osteitis. Radiology 97 (1970) 103

Brahme, S. K., V. Cervilla, V. Vint et al.: Magnetic resonance appearance of sacral insufficiency fractures. Skelet. Radiol. 19 (1990) 489

Cacciarelli, A. A.: Posterior widening of the S1–S2 interspace in children. A normal variant of sacral development. Amer. J. Roentgenol. 129 (1977) 305–309

Campanacci, M.: Bone and Soft Tissue Tumors. Springer, Berlin 1990

Cornwell, W. S., H. Ramsey: Unusual bilateral sacrococcygeal ossicles. Brit. J. Radiol. 68 (1957) 70–73

Coutte, A., A. de Carvalho: The cribriform fossa of the sacrum. A source of abusive interpretation of osteolysis. J. Radiol. 64 (1983) 437

Czarnecki, D. J., E. W. Till, J. L. Minikel: Unilateral sacral stress fracture in a runner. Amer. J. Roentgenol. 151 (1988) 1255

Denis, F., S. Davis, T. Comfort: Sacral fractures: an important problem. Retrospective analysis of 236 cases. Clin. Orthop. 227 (1988) 67

Dunaway, C. L., J. P. Williams, B. G. Brogdon: Sacral and coccygeal supernumerary ribs (pelvic ribs). Skeletal Radiol. 9 (1983) 212–214

Eller, D. J., D. S. Katz, A. G. Bergman, M. Fredericson, C. F. Beaulieu: Sacral stress fractures in long-distance runners. Clin. Sports Med 7 (1997) 222

Estin, D., A. R. Cohen: Caudal agenesis and associated caudal spinal cord malformations. Neurosurg. Clin. N. Amer. 6 (1995) 377

Faerber, E. N., J. C. Leonidas, L. L. Leape: Retroperitoneal iliac abscess with periostitis. Amer. J. Roentgenol. 136 (1981) 828

Fountain, S. S., R. D. Hamilton, R. M. Jameson: Transverse fractures of the sacrum. J. Bone Jt Surg. 59-A (1977) 486–489

Freyschmidt, J.: Tumoren der Wirbelsäule und des Sakrums. In Schinz: Radiologische Diagnostik, 7. Aufl. Bd. V/2: Wirbelsäule und Rückenmark. Thieme, Stuttgart 1986 (S. 249–318)

Freyschmidt, J., H. Ostertag, G. Jundt: Knochentumoren. Klinik, Radiologie, Pathologie. Springer, Berlin 1998

Gacetta, D. J., D. R. Yandow: Computed tomography of spontaneous osteoporotic sacral fractures. J. Comput. Assist. Tomogr. 8 (1984) 1190–1191

Grace, E., J. Drennan, D. Colver et al.: The 13 q-deletion syndrome. J. med. Genet. 8 (1971) 351

Greenspan, A., A. Norman: The "pelvic digit"—an unusual developmental anomaly. Skeletal Radiol. 9 (1982) 118–122

Grier, D., S. Wardell, J. Sarwack et al.: Fatigue fractures of the sacrum in children: two case reports and a review of the literature. Skelet. Radiol. 22 (1993) 515

Guidera, K. J., E. Raney, J. A. Ogden, M. Highhouse, M. Habal: Caudal regression: a review of seven cases, including the mermaid syndrome. J. pediat. Orthop. 11 (1991) 743

Guttner, B., J. Freyschmidt, P. Hohlweg-Majert: Stressfraktur des Os sacrum. Fortschr. Röntgenstr. 152 (1990) 236

Guyer, P. B., A. T. Chamberlain, D. M. Ackery et al.: The anatomic distribution of osteitis deformans. Clin. Orthop. 156 (1981) 141

Hadley, M. N., L. Ph. Carter: Sacral fracture with pseudomeningocele and cerebrospinal fluid fistula: Case report and review of the literature. Neurosurgery 16 (1985) 843–846

Halloran, W.: Sacral ribs. Quart. Bull. Northw. Med. Sch. 34 (1960) 304–309

Heim, M., C. Marcovich: A rare cause of low back pain. Amer. J. Orthop. 24 (1995) 273

Heller, M., H. H. Jend: Pelvic injuries. In Heller, M., H. H. Jend, H. K. Genant: Computed tomography of Trauma. Thieme, Stuttgart 1986 (pp. 89–102)

Hellinger, J.: Meßmethoden in der Skelettradiologie. Thieme, Stuttgart 1995

Holler, U., A. Petersein, W. Golder, S. Hoecht, T. Wiegel: Osteoradionekrose des Beckens versus knöcherne Metastasierung – eine schwierige Differentialdiagnose. Akt. Radiol 8 (1998) 196

Hunt, P. T., K. C. Davidson, K. W. Ashcraft et al.: Radiography of hereditary presacral teratoma. Radiology 122 (1977) 187

Ireberger: Rippenrudimente am Steißbein. Anat. Anz. (Jena) 86 (1936) 396

Jonasch, E.: 12 Fälle von Osteopoikilie. Fortschr. Röntgenstr. 82 (1955) 344

Kaklamanis, P.: Osteoarticular manifestations in sickle-cell disorders. Clin. Rheumatol. 3 (1984) 419

Kerboul, B., J. Le Saout, F. Chevalier, Ph. Meriot, B. Courtois: La fracture transversale de la deuxième vertèbre sacrée avec signes neurologiques. Neurochirurgie 31 (1985) 464–467

Kliewer, M. A., B. S. Hertzberg, P. George et al.: Fetal bifid sacrum artifact: normal developmental anatomy simulating malformation. Radiology 195 (1995) 673

Kreyenbühl, W., Ch. Hessler: A variation of the sacrum on the lateral view. Radiology 109 (1973) 49–52

Lien, H. H., V. Blomlie, K. Talle et al.: Radiation-induced fracture of the sacrum: findings on MR. Amer. J. Roentgenol. 159 (1992) 227

Lippert, H.: Anatomie der Wirbelsäule unter den Aspekten von Entwicklung und Funktion. Med. Klein. 61 (1966) 41–46

Loder, R. T., M. M. Dayioglu: Association of congenital vertebral malformations with bladder and cloacal exstrophy. J. pediat. Orthop. 10 (1990) 389

Lourie, J., St. Young: Avascular necrosis of the coccyx: a cause of coccygodynia? Brit. J. Clin. Pract. 16 (1985) 247–248

Martin, J., E. A. Brandser, M. J. Shin, J. A. Buckwalter: Fatigue fracture of the sacrum in a child. Canad. Ass. Radiol. J. 46 (1995) 468

McFarland, E. G., C. Giangarra: Sacral stress fractures in athletes. Clin. Orthop. 329 (1996) 240

Newhouse, K. E., G. Y. El-Khoury, J. A. Buckwalter: Occult sacral fractures in osteopenic patients. J. Bone Jt Surg. 74-A (1992) 227

Nievelstein, R. A., J. Valk, L. M. Smit, C. Vermeij-Keers: MR of the caudal regression syndrome: embryologic implications. Amer. J. Neuroradiol. 15 (1994) 1021

Nour, S., D. Kumar, J. A. Dickson: Anorectal malformations with sacral bony abnormalities. Arch. Dis. Childh. 64 (1989) 1618

O'Riordain, D. S., P. R. O'Connell, W. O. Kirwan: Hereditary sacral agenesis with presacral mass and anorectal stenosis: the Currarino triad. Brit. J. Surg. 78 (1991) 536

Pambakian, H., M. A. Smith: Glomus tumours of the coccygeal body associated with coccydynia. A preliminary report. J. Bone Jt Surg. 63-B (1981) 424

Peh, W. C., G. C. Ooi: Vacuum phenomena in the sacroiliac joints and in association with sacral insufficiency fractures. Incidence and significance. Spine 22 (1997) 2005

Portmann, J.: Der Forameneffekt am Kreuzbein. Fortschr. Röntgenstr. 96 (1962) 823–828

Radlauer, C.: Beiträge zur Anthropologie des Kreuzbeines. Gegenbaurs morph. Jb. 38 (1908) 322–447

Rauber/Kopsch: Bewegungsapparat, Bd. 1. In Rauber/Kopsch: Anatomie des Menschen. Lehrbuch und Atlas, 2. Aufl. Thieme, Stuttgart 1998

Renner, J. B.: Pelvic insufficiency fractures. Arthr. and Rheum. 33 (1990) 426

Resnick, D.: Diagnosis of Bone and Joint Disorders, 3rd ed. Saunders, Philadelphia 1995

Rich, T. A., A. Schiller, H. D. Suit et al.: Clinical and pathological review of 48 cases of chordoma. Cancer 56 (1985) 182

Rogers, L. F.: Radiology of Skeletal Trauma. Churchill Livingston, New York 1992

Rubin, P., D. Probhasawat: Characteristic bone lesions in post irradiated carcinoma of the cervix—metastases versus osteonecrosis. Radiology 76 (1961) 703

Sanjay, B. K. S., F. H. Sim, K. K. Unni et al.: Giant-cell tumours of the spine. J. Bone Jt Surg. 75-B (1993) 148

Schild, H., H. A. Müller, K. Klose, J. Ahlers, H. Nüwel: Anatomie, Röntgenologie und Klinik der Sakrumfrakturen. Fortschr. Röntgenstr. 134 (1981) 522–527

Schoberth, H.: Fehlstellungen des Kreuzbeins, röntgenologische und klinische Studien. Z. Orthop. 87 (1956) 216–218

Schwabe, R.: Untersuchungen über die Rückbildung der Bandscheiben im menschlichen Kreuzbein. Virchows Arch. path. Anat. 287 (1933) 651–713

Schwartz, C. M., T. C. Demos, J. M. Wehner: Osteomyelitis of the sacrum as the initial manifestation of Crohn's disease. Clin. Orthop. 222 (1987) 181

Sener, R. N.: Sacral pedicle agenesis. Comput. med. Imag. 21 (1997) 361

Staatz, G., G. Adam, M. Kilbinger, R. W. Günther: Osteoporotische Stressfrakturen des Os sacrum: MR-tomographische Befunde. Fortschr Röntgenstr 166 (1997) 307

Stäbler, A., R. Beck, R. Bartl, D. Schmidt, M. Reiser: Vacuum phenomena in insufficiency fractures of the sacrum. Skelet. Radiol. 24 (1995) 31

Stäbler, A., W. Steiner, P. Kohz, R. Bartl, H. Berger, M. Reiser: Time-dependent changes of insufficiency fractures of the sacrum: intraosseous vacuum phenomenon as an early sign. Europ. Radiol. 6 (1996) 655

Stanley, J. K., R. Owen, S. Koff: Congenital sacral anomalies. J. Bone Jt Surg. 61-B (1979) 401

Stojavinovič, J., J. Pappa, Š. Čičin-Šain, M. Agbaba, K. Čavka: Kongenitale Zysten und Teratome in der Sakrokokzygealgegend. Fortschr. Röntgenstr. 137 (1982) 560–563

Sumner, T. E., J. E. Crowe, C. R. Phelps II et al.: Occult anterior sacral meningocele. Amer. J. Dis. Child. 134 (1980) 385

Van Derslice, R., R. Gembala, P. P. Zekavat: Case report. Pelvic rib/digit. Spine 17 (1992) 1264

Weaver, D. D., C. L. Mapstone, P. Yu: The VATER association: Analysis of 46 patients. Amer. J. Dis. Child. 140 (1986) 225

West, S. G., J. L. Troutner, M. R. Baker, H. M. Place: Sacral insufficiency fractures in rheumatoid arthritis. Spine 19 (1994) 2117

Willinsky, R. A., M. Fazl: Computed tomography of a sacral perineural cyst. J. Comput. Tomogr. 9 (1985) 599–601

Willinsky, R. A., H. Grossman, P. W. Cooper et al.: The radiology of sacral cysts. J. Canad. Ass. Radiol. 39 (1988) 21

Normal Findings

During Growth

The pelvis develops from primordial connective tissue and forms a closed ring with residual blastema in the sacroiliac joints and pubic symphysis. While the symphysis becomes fibrocartilaginous after birth, the blastemic remnants at the site of sacroiliac joint spaces are not transformed into cartilage. This leaves a gap that later develops into a narrow joint cavity, forming a diarthrosis or rigid amphiarthrosis with articular cartilage, a synovial membrane, fibrous capsule, and reinforcing and auxiliary ligaments (Rauber and Kopsch 1998). The very firm capsule of the sacroiliac joint is strengthened on its ventral and dorsal sides by the sacroiliac ligaments (Fig. 5.**446**).

The ventral sacroiliac ligaments are considerably weaker than the dorsal ligaments. The synovial membrane blends posteriorly with the interosseous sacroiliac ligaments that span the retroauricular space. These ligaments are covered by the powerful dorsal sacroiliac ligaments (Fig. 5.**446**), which consist of long and short fiber tracts.

The sacroiliac joint is between the auricular surfaces of the ilium and sacrum. The articular surface of the sacrum in children is formed by the lateral parts of the first and second sacral vertebrae (Töndury 1958, Rauber and Kopsch 1998). The articular surface contours of the sacrum and ilium are almost identical, and in children they are generally subdivided into two main facets and a narrow anterior border.

In adolescents from 10 to 16 years of age, the iliac contours of the sacroiliac joint may be indistinct or absent on radiographs. Contour irregularities due to minor developmental errors in the iliac articular surfaces can produce one or two depressions along the upper or lower joint space called "**pseudoerosions**." The contours of the sacrum may appear serrated at growth zones.

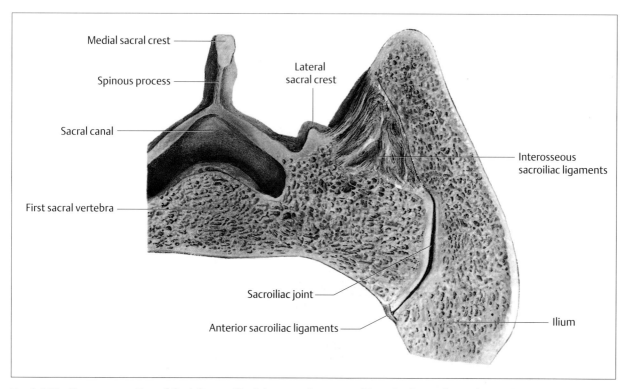

Fig. 5.**446**   Transverse section of the left sacroiliac joint, superior aspect. (From Rauber and Kopsch 1998.)

In Adulthood

After skeletal growth is completed, the sacroiliac joint space has a radiographic width of 3–5 mm. The cranial part of the third sacral vertebra is usually incorporated into the articular surface. The shape and size of the articular surfaces show individual variations and depend on the curvature of the spinal column. A small degree of spinal curvature in the sagittal plane is associated with an upright sacrum and a more vertical orientation of the articular surfaces, while greater degrees of sagittal spinal curvature are associated with greater angulation of the articular surfaces.

The articular cartilage on the auricular surface of the sacrum is about twice as thick as on that of the ilium. The auricular surfaces are slightly offset in relation to each other, creating an interlock that restricts movements. This is reinforced by irregularities in the articular surfaces, including elevations of several millimeters above the articular surface level. It is very common to find a large iliac prominence that fits a matching depression in the sacrum (Fig. 5.**447**) (Rauber and Kopsch 1998).

The **retroauricular space** is narrow in males and is the most reliable skeletal criterion for **sex determination** used by anthropologists and forensic pathologists. The broad base of the sacrum generally projects upward at the anterior sacroiliac joint margin in women and downward in men. A postauricular sulcus about 2 mm deep located between the iliac tuberosity and the posterior part of the auricular surface occurs mainly in women and is rare in men (Işcán and Derrick 1984).

Radiographic visualization of the sacroiliac joints is difficult to achieve on standard projections. Due to the varying angles and curvatures of the sacroiliac articular surfaces at different levels, it is rarely possible to define the entire joint space on one or both sides.

 A single projection is rarely sufficient for visualization of the sacroiliac joint space.

The **retroauricular space**, like the joint space, may be visualized in a fortuitous oblique projection that happens to be oriented correctly. But as a general rule, films centered on the sacroiliac joints in the supine position or especially in the lithotomy position, as well as AP and PA pelvic and lumbar spine films, are better than oblique views for defining the sacroiliac joints (Jaeger 1949, Dory and Francois 1978, Chevrot 1979, Dihlmann 1987). If additional information is needed, **CT** is preferred over conventional tomography (Carrera et al. 1981, Shirkhoda et al. 1984, Vogler 1984). **MRI** is advantageous for analyzing the articular cartilage and subchondral bone and is at least comparable to CT in diagnosing inflammatory conditions of the sacroiliac joints (Ahlström et al. 1990, Murphey et al. 1991, Docherty et al. 1992).

Functional views of the pelvic ring with weight-bearing on one leg are useful for detecting **pelvic ring laxity** by the position of the pubic bones at the symphysis. Spot films, fluoroscopy, and films using a compression tube (Kamieth 1956, 1958) are among the direct methods that can detect relative motion between the sacrum and ilium. A modified method is also available for diagnosing complete or incomplete pelvic rigidity (Dihlmann 1973).

▌ *Pathological Finding?*

Variation or Anomaly?

In addition to the sacroiliac joints, **accessory joint spaces** are present in 10–30% of the population (Fig. 5.**448**). They communicate with the true joint spaces and occur between the posterior superior iliac spine and lateral sacral crest at the level of the second sacral foramen or between the iliac and sacral tuberosities (Ehara et al. 1988). These accessory joint spaces are more common in whites than blacks, in men than women, and in older than younger individuals (Dihlmann 1978). They may be congenital true joints (diarthrosis) or, more typically, they may be fibrocartilaginous connections that develop after birth in response

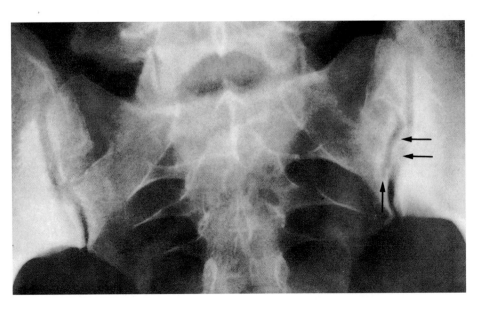

Fig. 5.**447** A prominence on the ilium (arrows) articulates with a notch in the sacrum (arrow) in the left sacroiliac joint.

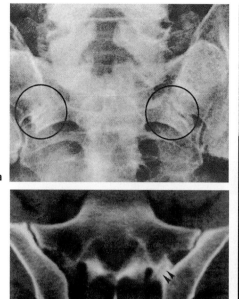

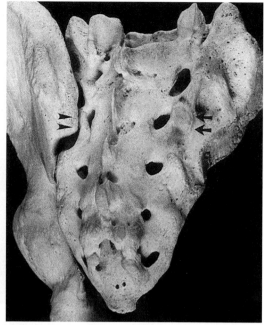

Fig. 5.**448 a–c** Accessory sacroiliac joints.
a Bilateral accessory articulation between the posterior superior iliac spine and the sacrum. A median arch defect at L5 and S1 is noted as an incidental finding.

b Accessory sacroiliac joints in a specimen, posterior aspect. The posterior superior iliac spine (arrowheads) articulates with the sacrum (arrows). (From Ehara et al. 1988.)
c Accessory sacroiliac joint (arrowheads). (From Ehara et al. 1988.)

to weight bearing (Ehara et al. 1988). A synostosis is sometimes found in accessory joint spaces (Dihlmann 1978).

A posterior **sacral protuberance** is occasionally present and is associated with a notchlike indentation in the iliac and sacral borders of the posteroinferior sacroiliac joint space (encoche sacrée) (Figs. 5.**447**, 5.**449**).

 A stepoff seen in this area should not be mistaken for a fracture.

A **bony bridge** across the lower part of the sacroiliac joint space has been classified as an **anomaly** (Dihlmann 1978).

Variants and anomalies of the joint space that go beyond the changes described above may be associated with or caused by deformities of the sacrum or ilium. Those that are within the scope of this book are discussed under the appropriate headings.

 ## Fracture, Subluxation, or Dislocation?

Injuries of the sacroiliac joints can occur in association with isolated sacral injuries and are more common in patients with pelvic ring injuries. Fractures of the ilium and sacrum may involve the sacroiliac joints (Rogers 1992) as a result of sagittal and lateral compression and shear mechanisms. Occasional stepoffs in the sacroiliac joint contours can mimic fracture lines (Figs. 5.**447**, 5.**449**).

In an **AP radiograph** of the pelvis, injuries to the sacroiliac joint may be manifested by widening of the sacroiliac joint space, displacement of the ilium, or asymmetry of the iliac wings (Fig. 5.**450**). Concomitant fractures of the L5

costal processes were mentioned previously as indirect signs of posterior instability.

CT is definitely superior to conventional radiographs in the detection of sacroiliac joint injuries (Heller and Jend 1986). Four types of injury can be defined on the basis of CT findings (Fig. 5.**451**):

CT classification of sacroiliac joint injuries

➤ *Type 1:* No bony or ligamentous injury. Vacuum phenomenon in the sacroiliac joint indicates that a stretch injury has occurred.

➤ *Type 2:* Rupture of the ventral sacroiliac ligaments with widening of the anterior joint space and a normal width of the posterior joint space.

➤ *Type 3:* Widening of the anterior and posterior sacroiliac joint space, signifying rupture of the ventral and dorsal sacroiliac ligaments.

➤ *Type 4:* Dislocation of the sacrum. Complete bilateral rupture of the ventral and dorsal sacroiliac ligaments, allowing anterior or posterior displacement of the sacrum.

Type 1 injuries are stable. Type 2 injuries are characterized by rotational instability and translational stability (type B injury in the AO classification of pelvic ring injuries). Type 3 and 4 injuries are characterized by rotational and translational instability (type C injury in the AO classification of pelvic ring injuries) (see chapter on the pelvis).

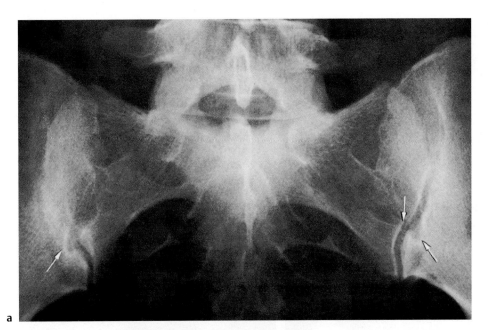

Fig. 5.**449a, b**   Stepoffs (encoche sacrée) in the sacroiliac joint lines.
a Bilateral notches in the sacroiliac joints (arrows).
b Pronounced notchlike step in the sacroiliac joint line.

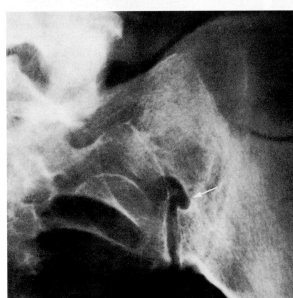

Necrosis?

Necrosis of the sacroiliac joint is discussed in the sections on the sacrum and ilium. **Sickle cell anemia** is associated with erosive and sclerotic changes in the sacroiliac joints, which presumably are caused by ischemia (Kaklamanis 1984, Sueoka et al. 1985).

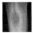
Inflammation?

Various diseases can mimic an inflammatory condition of the sacroiliac joints. They include the following:

- Erosive form of osteoarthritis
- Ochronosis
- Articular chondrocalcinosis
- Sacral osteochondrosis
- Hyperparathyroidism (Fig. 5.**458**)

Normal variants such as "**pseudoerosions**," which are distinguished from multiple inflammatory erosions by their isolated occurrence in the upper or lower joint margins, and **contour irregularities in the joint spaces of adolescents** 16–18 years of age can also lead to misinterpretations.

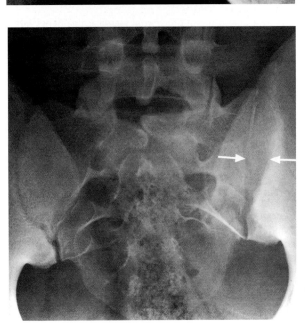

◁ Fig. 5.**450**   Traumatic disruption of the left sacroiliac joint with significant widening of the joint space (arrows). A median arch cleft in S1 is noted as an incidental finding.

Fig. 5.**451 a–d**   Classification of sacroiliac joint injuries (after Heller and Jend).
a Vacuum phenomenon due to a stretching injury.
b Rupture of the ventral sacroiliac ligaments with widening of the anterior joint space.
c Rupture of the ventral and dorsal sacroiliac ligaments with anterior and posterior joint space widening.
d Dislocation of the sacrum due to complete, bilateral rupture of the anterior and posterior ligaments.

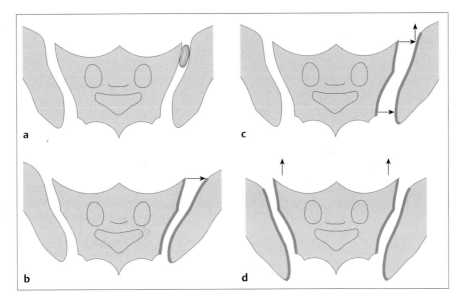

Sacroiliitis

Bacterial, nontuberculous forms of sacroiliitis can develop by the hematogenous route, by contiguous spread, by direct inoculation, or as a postoperative complication. They are particularly common in **drug abusers** (Guyot et al. 1987). Pelvic inflammatory processes have been known to spread to the sacroiliac joints by direct extension, and iatrogenic infections can result from surgery, injections, and percutaneous procedures.

Infections of the sacroiliac joint usually affect only one side and are rarely bilateral (Oka and Mottonen 1983), making it easier to distinguish them from other processes. Radiographic changes appear just 2–3 weeks after the onset of the disease and generally are most pronounced in the anteroinferior portion of the joint.

Cartilage destruction leads initially to joint space narrowing and blurring of the joint contours and subchondral cancellous bone structures. Marginal erosions can spread, causing destruction of the entire joint (Fig. 5.**452**). Reactive sclerosis is variable and depends on the causative organism. Treated cases may heal with partial or complete ankylosis of the sacroiliac joint (Haanpää et al. 1989).

Infantile Infectious Sacroiliitis:
Infantile infectious sacroiliitis takes a more acute course than in adults and may be mistaken clinically for the more common nonspecific coxitis. Radionuclide scans can detect changes just 4 days after the symptoms first appear (Sueoka et al. 1985).

Tuberculous Sacroiliitis:
Tuberculous sacroiliitis is the most common form of pelvic tuberculosis. Most cases are hematogenous (Richter et al. 1983, Pouchot et al. 1988), but some are caused by contigu-

Fig. 5.**452 a–c**   Bacterial sacroiliitis in a drug addict.
a Normal right sacroiliac joint.
b Affected left joint shows widening of the lower part of the synovial joint and erosive changes, which are most pronounced in the iliac articular surface.

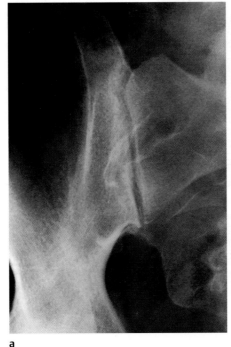

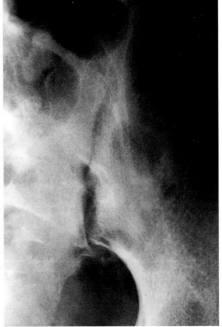

a

b

Fig. 5.**452 c** ▷

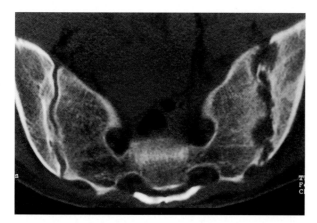

Fig. 5.**452 c** Appearance of the changes on axial CT.

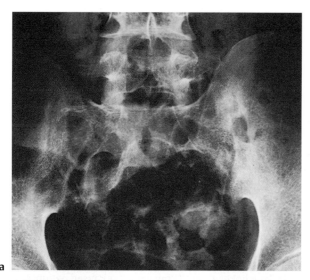

a

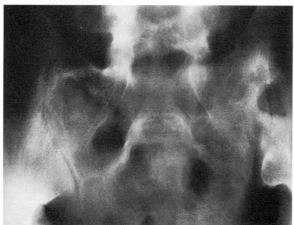

b

Fig. 5.**453 a, b** Tuberculous sacroiliitis.
a AP radiograph shows an inflammatory process of the left sacroiliac joint.
b Tomogram shows foci of advanced tuberculous destruction with reactive marginal sclerosis. The right sacroiliac joint also shows destructive changes.

ous spread from a gravitation abscess and affect both joints (Fig. 5. **453**).

Many cases are relatively asymptomatic initially, and it takes some time for clinical symptoms to appear. Because decalcification and bone destruction are delayed, radionuclide scans are often necessary for the early detection of sacroiliac joint involvement. Erosive changes with destruction and demineralization of the subchondral bone are delayed compared with a bacterial inflammation. Subchondral demineralization, together with marginal areas of bone destruction, cause apparent widening of the joint space, as in all forms of sacroiliitis. An early increase in cancellous bone density may signify a mixed infection or a functional adaptation of healthy bone areas. The impaction of atrophic bone areas can mimic osteosclerosis, however (Fig. 5.**453**). Predominantly productive sacroiliac tuberculosis can be detected earlier on radiographs because of the early destructive changes.

Brucellosis

Among the nontuberculous microorganisms, Gram-negative brucellae have a special affinity for the sacroiliac joints. Some 35–37% of patients with brucellosis have sacroiliac joint involvement, usually limited to one side. In some cases this is the only manifestation of the disease. Statistically, sacroiliitis is a somewhat less common manifestation than spondylitis but is more common than coxitis (Rotès-Queról 1963, Abeles and Mond 1989). Brucellosis is rare in children and adolescents, who occasionally show sacroiliac involvement (Neinstein and Goldenring 1983).

Other Infections

Drug addicts are susceptible to infection by rare causative organisms such as *Pseudomonas*, *Klebsiella*, *Serratia*, *Enterobacter*, streptococci, *Candida albicans*, and others (Guyot et al. 1987, Brancs et al. 1991).

Congenital and acquired **syphilis** can also involve the sacroiliac joints in rare cases.

Involvement of the sacroiliac joints can occur in the setting of **SAPHO syndrome** (Kahn and Chamot 1992). Unilateral involvement is more common.

Rheumatoid Arthritis

Sacroiliac joint involvement occurs only in advanced stages of rheumatoid arthritis (Resnick and Resnick 1985) and rarely leads to sclerosis. Sacroiliac joint involvement appears to be more common in women than in men (Sievers and Laine 1963). One or both joints may be affected, but asymmetrical involvement is the rule. Radiographs usually show only moderate joint space narrowing. Erosions principally affect the articular surface of the ilium. They are usually superficial, well circumscribed, and associated with minimal sclerosis. Ankylosis is rare and can be appreciated only on sectional images. Ossification of the sacroiliac ligaments is unusual. Involvement of the sacroiliac joints by **juvenile rheumatoid arthritis** has been described in 5–20% of cases (Martel et al. 1962, Bywaters and Ansell 1965).

Seronegative Spondylarthropathies

The seronegative spondylarthropathies (ankylosing spondylitis, psoriatic arthritis, Reiter syndrome, enteropathic spondylarthropathies) consistently affect the sacroiliac joints.

Ankylosing Spondylitis:

Sacroiliitis is a hallmark of ankylosing spondylitis. The process spreads initially from the sacroiliac joint to involve the thoracolumbar and lumbosacral junction (Kinsella et al. 1966). Spinal involvement preceding sacroiliac joint affection is seen in less than 1% of patients with ankylosing spondylitis (Dihlmann 1978).

The changes in the sacroiliac joint predominantly affect the iliac portion of the synovial joint and the ligaments.

The changes typically consist of periarticular osteoporosis, blurring of the articular surfaces, erosive changes, joint space widening, and marked sclerosis resulting from an aggressive, proliferating chondroid metaplasia at the chondro-osseous junction and in the subchondral bone (Dihlmann et al. 1977, Oliveri et al. 1990, Dihlmann 1991). As proliferative changes in the sacroiliac joint become more pronounced, **bony bridges** form across the joint space and may eventually cause complete ankylosis.

In contrast to other inflammatory sacroiliac joint diseases in which these features appear consecutively, the simultaneous triad of destruction, sclerosis, and ankylosis marks the "**variegated pattern**" that is virtually pathognomonic of ankylosing spondylitis (Figs. 5.**454**–5.**456**) (Dihlmann 1973, 1976, 1983). Further progression is marked by the appearance of **calcifications** and **ossifications** in the

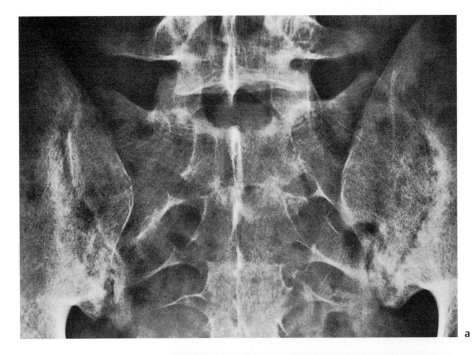

Fig. 5.**454a, b** Sacroiliitis in ankylosing spondylitis.
a Bilateral, variegated type of sacroiliitis on a survey radiograph.
b Variegated type of sacroiliitis on CT (different case).

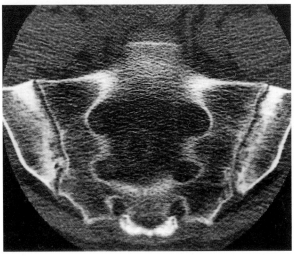

a

b

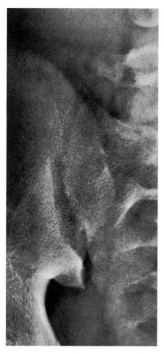

Fig. 5.**455**   Sacroiliitis in ankylosing spondylitis. Widening of the sacroiliac joint.

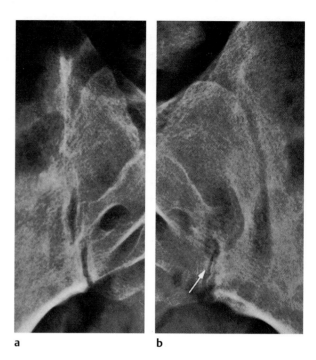

a   b

Fig. 5.**456a, b**   Ankylosing spondylitis.
a Fusion of the joint space, sclerotic bridging in the upper part of the joint.
b Osteolytic lesion projected over a joint contour.

Table 5.**5**   Involvement of the sacroiliac joints in various diseases (after Resnick 1995).

Disease	Bilateral, symmetrical	Bilateral, asymmetrical	Unilateral
Degenerative diseases	+	+	+
Osteitis condensans ilii	+	–	–
Ankylosing spondylitis	+	–	–
Inflammatory bowel disease	+	–	–
Psoriatic arthritis	+	+	+
Reiter disease	+	+	+
Infection	–	–	+
Rheumatoid arthritis	–	+	+
Gout	+	+	+
Calcium pyrophosphate dihydrate (CPPD) crystal deposition disease	+	+	+
Hyperparathyroidism	+	–	–

sacroiliac ligaments, which can result in complete fusion of the sacrum and ilium. Tomograms (Fig. 5.454) facilitate the diagnosis and follow-up (Dihlmann 1983, Dale and Vinje 1985).

The sacroiliac joint changes in ankylosing spondylitis are typically bilateral and symmetrical, but a unilateral onset is found in approximately 10% of patients (Dihlmann 1974a, 1976, 1991, Forrester 1990). The unilateral or bilateral occurrence of the changes and their possible asymmetry are of considerable value in the differential diagnosis of various diseases in this region (Table 5.5) (Resnick and
Resnick 1985).

There is no single imaging sign in the sacroiliac joint that is specific for ankylosing spondylitis. Even the "**variegated pattern**" is not pathognomonic, but it does narrow the differential diagnosis to a few diseases that can be clinically differentiated (psoriatic arthritis, Reiter syndrome, enteropathic spondylarthropathy) (Peterson and Silbiger 1967, Schilling 1969, Marcusson et al. 1983) (see below).

Psoriatic Arthritis:
Involvement of the sacroiliac joints occurs in 30–50% of patients with psoriatic arthritis (Killebrew et al. 1973, Harvie et al. 1976). Approximately 10–25% of all patients with psoriasis show sacroiliac joint involvement (Harvie et al. 1976, Moller and Vinge 1980). The radiographic signs resemble those of ankylosing spondylitis, but ankylosis is less common (Fig. 5.457). Articular involvement is usually bilateral and symmetrical, although an asymmetrical or

unilateral distribution may be seen (Table 5.**5**) (Peterson and Silbiger 1967, Jajič 1968, Schilling 1969, Killebrew et al. 1973, Resnick and Resnick 1985). As in ankylosing spondylitis, ossification of the sacroiliac ligaments may be observed.

Reiter Syndrome:

Reiter syndrome is frequently associated with sacroiliitis, which is found in 40–60% of cases following a protracted course (Weldon and Scalettar 1961, Peterson and Silbiger 1967, Schilling 1969). The radiographic signs resemble those of the spondylarthropathies described above. Intra-articular ankylosis is less common than in ankylosing spondylitis and the enteropathic spondylarthropathies. Most cases show bilateral changes, which may be symmetrical or asymmetrical (Fig. 5. **458**). Unilateral joint involvement can also occur. Intra-articular ankylosis is less common than in ankylosing spondylitis. The iliac and sacral tuberosities of the retroauricular space are occasionally involved in the disease process, appearing hazy and sclerotic (Martel et al. 1979).

Enteropathic Spondylarthropathies:

The enteropathic spondylarthropathies, which include Whipple disease (Canoso et al. 1978, Bussiere et al. 1980), Crohn disease (Moll et al. 1974, Mueller et al. 1974), and ulcerative colitis (McEwen et al. 1971, Moll et al. 1974), lead to changes in the sacroiliac joints that are indistinguishable from those of classic ankylosing spondylitis.

Bilharzial Arthropathy

Bilharzial arthropathy may involve the sacroiliac joints with a bilateral, asymmetrical distribution of erosive and sclerotic changes that can occasionally ankylose (Bassiouni and Kamel 1984).

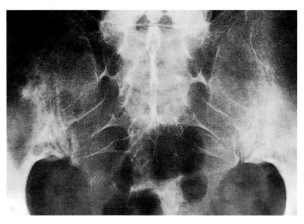

Fig. 5.**457**   Sacroiliitis in psoriatic arthritis. "Variegated" type of bilateral sacroiliitis.

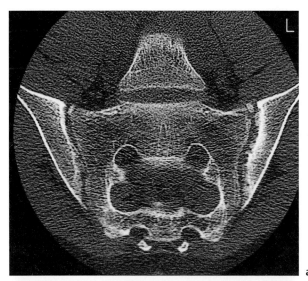

a

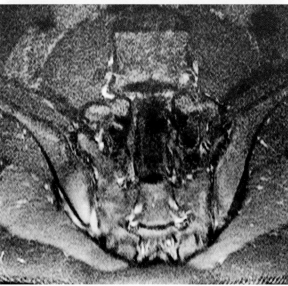

b

Fig. 5.**458 a, b**   Sacroiliitis in Reiter syndrome. Asymmetrical ▷ involvement of the sacroiliac joints with different degrees of activity.
a CT shows variegated changes on the left side with only minor changes on the right side.
b MRI (fat-saturated T2-weighted image) shows bone edema on the right side as evidence of a florid inflammation. The left side shows no edematous changes.

Other Changes?

Osteoarthritis

Osteoarthritis has the same manifestations in the sacroiliac joints as in other joints of the body:

- Joint space narrowing due to cartilage wear
- Sclerosis of the joint margins
- Subchondral cysts
- Osteophyte formation (Resnick and Resnick 1985)

Joint space narrowing is most evident in the lower part of the sacroiliac joint. Erosive changes are rarely found (Resnick et al. 1975).

Osteophytes are most often found along the upper and lower portions of the joint line but can occur at any level. They may produce circumscribed zones of increased density that require differentiation from osteoblastic metastases.

Osteophytes may bridge the joint space and cause **peri-articular ankylosis**, which should not be confused with the intra-articular ankylosis of ankylosing spondylitis. Partial or complete **fibrous ankylosis** of the sacroiliac joint is more frequent (Resnick et al. 1975, Resnick et al. 1977, Walker 1986). **Calcifications** and **ossifications** of the **ilio-lumbar ligament** and **sacroiliac ligaments** are also occasionally found.

Symmetrical sacroiliac osteoarthritis with joint space narrowing, erosions, sclerosis, and ankylosis can be difficult to distinguish from ankylosing spondylitis.

Osteoarthritis of the sacroiliac joints may be associated with a **vacuum phenomenon**, but this is not specific for osteoarthritis and can occur in articular chondrocalcinosis and other diseases (Shorter et al. 1984, Wendling et al. 1985). Intra-articular gas collections may occur in subchondral cysts (**pneumatoceles**), which are usually located in the ilium (Freyschmidt and Holland 1990, Wendt 1993).

Alkaptonuric ochronosis can produce unusually severe arthrotic changes. Detritus cysts can lead to osteolytic processes as well as reactive new bone formation with joint space consolidation, especially in the upper part of the joint. Marginal osteophytes appear as fine projections near the paraglenoid sulcus.

Articular Chondrocalcinosis

Articular chondrocalcinosis (pseudogout) can involve the cartilage of the sacroiliac joints (Martel et al. 1981) as well as the interosseous sacroiliac ligaments (Resnick and Pineda 1984). Findings consist of unilateral or bilateral subchondral erosions, sclerosis, and cyst formation that may be associated with joint space narrowing and bridging osteophytes (Martel et al. 1981, Littlejohn et al. 1982). As noted earlier, vacuum phenomena of the sacroiliac joints may occur in this disease.

Sacral Osteochondrosis

This disease is characterized by unilateral or bilateral destructive changes in the sacroiliac joints (Dihlmann 1974). Impaired apophyseal ossification of the lateral mass of the sacrum becomes apparent between 16 and 20 years of age. The affected apophysis appears dense and fragmented with indistinct margins while the contour of the ilium appears smooth (Dihlmann 1974).

Uric Arthropathy

Sacroiliac joint involvement by uric arthropathy leads to marginal erosions, subchondral sclerosis, and ankylosis, most commonly affecting both joints. The sacroiliac joints are affected with a reported frequency of approximately 17% (Alarcón-Segovia et al. 1973). Tophi are a characteristic feature of this disease (Malawista et al. 1965, Jajič 1982).

Hyperparathyroidism

As in gout, subchondral resorption in hyperparathyroidism (Dihlmann and Müller 1969, Dihlmann 1978) can lead to bilateral, symmetrical **pseudo-widening** of the sacroiliac joint space (Fig. 5.**459**).

The changes in hyperparathyroidism resemble those in ankylosing spondylitis but are distinguished from them by an absence of joint space narrowing and less pronounced articular surface irregularities (Hooge and Li 1981).

Connective Tissue Diseases

Rarely, the sacroiliac joints may be involved by connective tissue diseases (lupus erythematosus, polyarteritis nodosa, polymyositis, progressive scleroderma) (Dihlmann 1978).

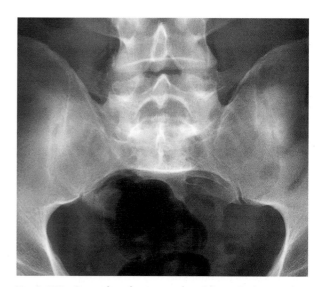

Fig. 5.**459** Secondary hyperparathyroidism. Both sacroiliac joints show areas of bone resorption with increased subchondral sclerosis.

Sickle Cell Anemia

Sickle cell anemia is marked by erosive and sclerotic changes in the sacroiliac joints, presumably due to ischemia (Schumacher et al. 1973, Kaklamanis 1984).

Ossification and Calcification

Ossifications of the **ventral sacroiliac ligaments** and **iliolumbar ligaments** (Fig. 5.**404**) are clearly demonstrated by radiographs, as are **capsuloligamentous ossifications** that are tangentially imaged below the arcuate line and appear as transverse osteophytes or bony bridges (Figs. 5.**460**, 5.**462**). Larger areas of ligament ossification can produce opacities that resemble those of hyperostosis triangularis of the ilium (see chapter on the pelvis).

Reparative bone formation in the sacroiliac capsule and ligaments is seen twice as often in men as women and can lead to bony fixation with **pelvic rigidity** (Figs. 4.**460**–5.**462**).

Multiple Hyperostosis

Multiple hyperostosis is a special form of ankylosing hyperostotic spondylarthropathies that also includes the sternocostal form (see section on the shoulder girdle, p. 261). Six cases have been described with involvement of the sacroiliac joints (all unilateral) and manubriosternal joints (Beranek et al. 1984).

Sacroiliac Joint Laxity

Abnormal laxity in both sacroiliac joints occasionally leads to an increased angle of pelvic tilt. Unilateral laxity leads to projection asymmetries in the pubic bones (Dihlmann 1978). Downward or forward slippage of the sacrum at both joints (with a corresponding displacement at the symphysis) is known as **sacrolisthesis**.

Diseases in Paraplegics

Paraplegics often develop periarticular osteoporosis and narrowing of the sacroiliac joints (Abel 1950). A few patients also develop intra-articular ankylosis that resembles ankylosing spondylitis.

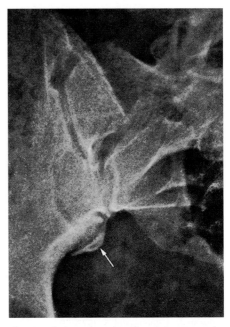

Fig. 5.**460**   Ossification below the sacroiliac joint near the subarcuate fossa (observation by Jacob, Chemnitz). Ossified ligament? Accessory bone?

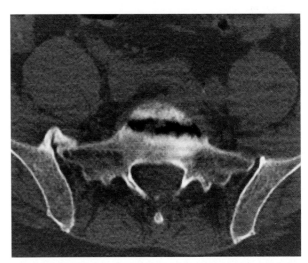

Fig. 5.**462**   Ossification of the anterior sacroiliac ligaments on axial CT section.

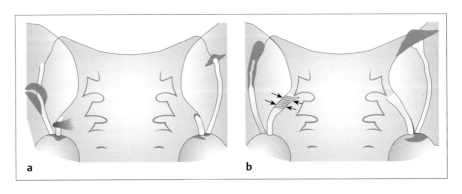

Fig. 5.**461 a, b**   Reparative ossification of the sacroiliac capsule and ligaments following overuse injury, gross trauma, and inflammatory disease (after Dihlmann).

References

Abel, M. S.: Sacroiliac joint changes in traumatic paraplegics. Radiology 55 (1950) 235

Abeles, M., C. B. Mond: Sacroiliitis and brucellosis. J. Rheumatol. 16 (1989) 136

Ahlström, H., N. Feltelius, R. Nyman et al.: Magnetic resonance imaging of sacroiliac joint inflammation. Arthr. and Rheum. 33 (1990) 1763

Alarcón-Segovia, D., J. A. Cetina, E. Diaz-Jouanen: Sacroiliac joints in primary gout. Amer. J. Roentgenol. 188 (1973) 438–443

Bassiouni, M., M. Kamel: Bilharzial arthropathy. Ann. rheum. Dis. 43 (1984) 806

Beranek, L., G. Kaplan, M. Benoist, J. P. Bouchon, A. Prost, J. P. Vassal, M. F. Kahn: Hyperostose multiple avec sacroilite unilatérale: Une nouvelle, spondylarthropathie. Presse Méd. (1984) 2001–2004

Brancs, M. A., P. Peris, J. M. Mir et al.: Septic arthritis in heroin addicts. Semin. Arthr. Rheum. 21 (1991) 81

Bussiere, J. L., J. L. Epifanie, B. Leblanc et al.: Maladie de Whipple et spondyloarthrite ankylosante. Rev. Rhum. 47 (1980) 577

Bywaters, E. G. L., B. M. Ansell: Sacroiliitis in juvenile chronic polyarthritis. Z. Rheumaforsch. 24 (1965) 122

Canoso, J. J., M. Saini, J. A. Hermos: Whipple's disease and ankylosing spondylitis: simultaneous occurrence in HLA-B27 positive male. J. Rheumatol. 5 (1978) 79

Carrera, G. F., W. D. Foley, F. Kozin et al.: CT of sacroiliitis. Amer. J. Roentgenol. 136 (1981) 41

Chevrot, A.: Incidence cranio-caudale oblique unilatérale de l'articulation sacro-iliaque. J. Radiol. 60 (1979) 143

Dale, K., O. Vinje: Radiography of the spine and sacroiliac joints in ankylosing spondylitis and psoriasis. Acta. Radiol. Diagn. 26 (1985) 145–159

Dihlmann, W.: Röntgendiagnostik der Sakroiliakalgelenke und ihrer nahen Umgebung, 2. Aufl. Thieme, Stuttgart 1978

Dihlmann, W.: Röntgen – Wer? Wie? Wann? Bd. III: Gelenke – Wirbelverbindungen. Thieme, Stuttgart 1973

Dihlmann, W.: Röntgendiagnostische Basisinformation: Das „bunte" Sacroiliacalbild. Akt. Rheumat. 1 (1976) 17

Dihlmann, W.: Kritik der Sacroiliitis-Stadieneinteilung („grading", „staging") bei Spondylitis ankylosans. Z. Rheumatol. 42 (1983) 49–57

Dihlmann, W., G. Müller: Iliakalveränderungen als Frühsymptome des Hyperparathyreoidismus. Beitrag zur Differentialdiagnose der Spondylitis ankylopoetica. Fortschr. Röntgenstr. 111 (1969) 558–565

Dihlmann, W., R. Lindenfelser, W. Selberg: Sakroiliakale Histomorphologie der ankylosierenden Spondylitis als Beitrag zur Therapie. Dtsch. Med. Wschr. 102 (1977) 129–132

Dihlmann, W.: Entwicklungsstörungen der Kreuz-Darmbein-Gelenke einschließlich der sogenannten Osteochondritis sacri. (Röntgendiagnostische Studien an den Kreuz-Darmbein-Gelenken VI). Fortschr. Röntgenstr. 101 (1974a) 285

Dihlmann, W.: Das „bunte Sakroiliakalbild" – das röntgenologische Frühkriterium der ankylosierenden Spondylitis. Fortschr. Röntgenstr. 121 (1974b) 564

Dihlmann, W.: Gelenke, Wirbelverbindungen. Thieme, Stuttgart 1987

Dihlmann, W.: Osteitis condensans ilii und sacroiliitis. J. Rheumatol. 18 (1991) 1430

Docherty, P., M. J. Mitchell, L. MacMillan et al.: Magnetic resonance imaging of sacroiliitis. J. Rheumatol. 19 (1992) 393

Dory, M. A., R. J. Francois: Craniocaudal axial view of the sacroiliac joint. Amer. J. Roentgenol. 130 (1978) 1125

Ehara, S., G. Y. El-Khoury, R. A. Bergman: The accessory sacroiliac joint: a common anatomic variant. Amer. J. Roentgenol. 150 (1988) 857

Forrester, D. M.: Imaging of the sacroiliac joints. Radiol. Clin. N. Amer. 28 (1990) 1055

Freyschmidt, J., B. Holland: Zum seltenen Phänomen intraossärer Gasansammlungen (sog. Pneumatozelen). Fortschr. Röntgenstr. 152 (1990) 6

Guyot, D. R., A. Manoli II, G. A. Kling: Pyogenic sacroiliitis in IV drug abusers. Amer. J. Roentgenol. 149 (1987) 1209

Haanpää, M., P. Hannonen, P. Kaira et al.: Clinical sequelae and sacroiliac joint changes by computed tomography after recovery from septic sacroiliitis. Clin. Rheumatol. 8 (1989) 197

Harvie, J. N., R. S. Lester, A. H. Little: Sacroiliitis in severe psoriasis. Amer. J. Roentgenol. 127 (1976) 579

Heller, M., H. H. Jend: Pelvic injuries. In Heller, M., H. H. Jend, H. K. Genant: Computed Tomography of Trauma. Thieme, Stuttgart 1986 (pp. 89–102)

Hooge, W. A., D. Li: CT of sacroiliac joints in secondary hyperparathyroidism. J. Canad. Ass. Radiol. 31 (1981) 42

Işcán, Y. M., Karen Derrick: Determination of sex from the sacroiliac joint: a visual assessment technique. Florida Scientist 47 (1984) 94–98

Jaeger, E.: Zur Aufnahmetechnik der Sacroiliacalgelenke. Fortschr. Röntgenstr. 71 (1949) 630

Jajič, I.: Gout in the spine and sacro-iliac joints. Radiological manifestations. Skelet. Radiol. 8 (1982) 209–212

Jajič, I.: Radiological changes in the sacroiliac joints and spine of patients with psoriatic arthritis and psoriasis. Ann. rheum. Dis. 27 (1968) 1

Kahn, M.-F., A.-M. Chamot: SAPHO syndrome. Rheum. Dis. Clin. N. Amer. 18 (1992) 225

Kaklamanis, P.: Osteoarticular manifestations in sickle-cell disorders. Clin. Rheumatol. 3 (1984) 419

Kamieth, H.: Röntgenologische Veränderungen an den Sakroiliakalgelenken bei der Beckenringlockerung. Fortschr. Röntgenstr. 84 (1956) 188–199

Kamieth, H.: Die Beckenringlockerung (BRL) – Aufnahmetechnik und Beurteilung. Hippokrates 29 (1958) 372–376

Killebrew, K., R. H. Gold, S. D. Sholkoff: Psoriatic spondylitis. Radiology 108 (1973) 9

Kinsella, T. D., F. R. MacDonald, L. G. Johnson: Ankylosing spondylitis: a late re-evaluation of 92 cases. J. Canad. med. Ass. 95 (1966) 1

Littlejohn, G. O., M. Baron, M. B. Urowitz: Sacroiliac joint abnormalities in calcium pyrophosphate crystal deposition disease. Rheumatol. Int. 1 (1982) 195

Malawista, S. E., J. E. Seegmiller, B. E. Hathaway, L. Sokoloff: Sacroiliac gout. J. Amer. med. Ass. 194 (1965) 954–961

Marcusson, J. A., H. Ström, N. Lindvall: Psoriasis, peripheral arthritis, sacroiliitis and juvenile chronic arthritis: a family study in relation to segregation of HLA Antigens. J. Rheumatol. 10 (1983) 619–623

Martel, W., J. F. Holt, J. T. Cassidy: Roentgenologic manifestations of juvenile rheumatoid arthritis. Amer. J. Roentgenol. 88 (1962) 400

Martel, W., E. M. Braunstein, G. Borlaza et al.: Radiologic features of Reiter's disease. Radiology 132 (1979) 1

Martel, W., D. K. McCarter, M. A. Solsky et al.: Further observations on the arthropathy of calcium pyrophosphate crystal deposition disease. Radiology 141 (1981) 1

McEwen, C., D. DiTata, C. Lingg et al.: Ankylosing spondylitis and spondylitis accompanying ulcerative colitis, regional enteritis, psoriasis and Reiter's disease. Arthr. and Rheum. 14 (1971) 291

Moll, J. M. H., I. Haslock, I. F. Macrae et al.: Associations between ankylosing spondylitis, psoriatic arthritis, Reiter's disease, the intestinal arthropathies, and Behçet's syndrome. Medicine 53 (1974) 343

Moller, P., O. Vinge: Arthropathy and sacro-iliitis in severe psoriasis. Scand. J. Rheumatol. 9 (1980) 113

Mueller, C. E., J. F. Seeger, W. Martel: Ankylosing spondylitis and regional enteritis. Radiology 112 (1974) 579

Murphey, M. D., L. H. Wetzel, J. M. Bramble et al.: Sacroiliitis: MR imaging findings. Radiology 180 (1991) 239

Neinstein, L. S., J. Goldenring: Brucella sacroiliitis. Clin. Pediat. 22 (1983) 645–648

Oka, M., T. Mottonen: Septic sacroiliitis. J. Rheumatol. 10 (1983) 475

Olivieri, I., G. Gemignani, G. Pasero: Ankylosing spondylitis with exuberant sclerosis in the sacroiliac joints, symphysis pubis and spine. J. Rheumatol. 17 (1990) 1515

Peterson jr., C. C., M. L. Silbinger: Reiter's syndrome and psoriatic arthritis. Their roentgen spectra and some interesting similarities. Amer. J. Roentgenol. 101 (1967) 860–871

Pouchot, J., P. Vinceneux, J. Barge et al.: Tuberculosis of the sacro-iliac joint: Clinical features, outcome, and evaluation of closed needle biopsy in 11 consecutive cases. Amer. J. Med. 84 (1988) 622

Rauber/Kopsch: Bewegungsapparat, Bd. 1. In: Rauber/Kopsch: Anatomie des Menschen. Lehrbuch und Atlas, 2. Aufl. Thieme, Stuttgart 1998

Resnik, C. S., D. Resnick: Radiology of disorders of the sacroiliac joints. J. Amer. med. Ass. 253 (1985) 2863–2866

Resnick, D., G. Niwayama, T. G. Goergen: Degenerative disease of the sacroiliac joint. Invest. Radiol. 10 (1975) 608

Resnick, D., G. Niwayama, T. G. Goergen: Comparison of radiographic abnormalities of the sacroiliac joint in degenerative disease and ankylosing spondylitis. Amer. J. Roentgenol. 128 (1977) 189

Resnick, D., C. Pineda: Vertebral involvement in calcium pyrophosphate dihydrate crystal deposition disease. Radiographic-pathologic correlation. Radiology 153 (1984) 55

Richter, R., W. Nubling, G. Kohler et al.: Die Tuberkulose der Iliosakralgelenke. Z. Orthop. 121 (1983) 564

Rogers, L. F.: Radiology of Skeletal Trauma. Churchill Livingston, New York 1992

Rotès-Querol, J.: Osteo-articular sites of Brucellosis. Ann. Rheumat. Dis. 22 (1963) 194–199

Schilling, F.: Differentialdiagnose der Spondylitis ankylopoetica, Spondylitis psoriatica, chronisches Reiter-Syndrom und Spondylosis hyperostotica. Therapiewoche 6 (1969) 249–256

Schumacher, H. R., R. Andrews, G. McLaughlin: Arthropathy in sickle-cell disease. Ann. Intern. Med. 78 (1973) 203–209

Shirkhoda, A., H. R. Brashear, M. E. Zelenek et al.: Sacral abnormalities—computed tomography versus conventional radiography. J. Comput. assist. Tomogr. 8 (1984) 41

Shorter, A. M., D. A. Burrows, W. P. Cockshott: Is the vacuum sign in the sacroiliac joint a useful radiological sign of chondrocalcinosis? Diagn. Imag. 53 (1984) 141

Sievers, K., V. Laine: The sacro-iliac joint in rheumatoid arthritis in adult females. Acta rheumatol. scand. 9 (1963) 222

Sueoka, B. L., J. F. Johnson, R. Enzenauer, J. S. Kolina: Infantile infectious sacroiliitis. Pediat. Radiol. 15 (1985) 403–405

Töndury, G.: Entwicklungsgeschichte und Fehlbildungen der Wirbelsäule. Hippokrates, Stuttgart 1958

Vogler, J. B. III, W. H. Brown, C. A. Helms, et al.: The normal sacroiliac joint: a CT study of asymptomatic patients. Radiology 151 (1984) 433

Walker, J. M.: Age-related differences in the human sacroiliac joint: a histological study; implications for therapy. J. Orthop. Sports Phys. Ther. 7 (1986) 325

Weldon, W. V., R. Scalettar: Roentgen changes in Reiter's syndrome. Amer. J. Roentgenol. 86 (1961) 344

Wendling, D., J. L. Magnet, M. Guidet, J. Strauss: Une image peu connue: Le phénomène du vide sacroiliaque. Rev. Rhum. 52 (1985) 109–113

Wendt, B.: Juxtaartikuläre Pneumatozele des Os illium. Fortschr. Röntgenstr. 158 (1993) 604

6 Pelvis

J. Freyschmidt

General Aspects

Normal Anatomy

Figure 6.**1** shows the normal anatomy of a male pelvis with the principal structures labeled.

The stability of the pelvis relies critically on ligamentous attachments, which are shown in drawings from anatomic specimens in Fig. 6.**2**.

A knowledge of these structures is important in the interpretation of ligament calcifications. The female pelvis has more broadly projecting iliac wings than the male pelvis, often with a broader sacrum and larger diameters of the pelvic inlet and outlet (Fig. 6.**3**).

> The true conjugate is the distance from the sacral promontory to the most prominent point on the dorsal surface of the symphysis. It normally measures 11 cm. The mean transverse diameter of the pelvis is 13 cm, and the mean oblique pelvic diameter is 12 cm.

The development of the **bony pelvis** from birth to 10 years is shown in Fig. 6.**63**.

Examination Technique

The basic radiograph of the pelvis is the AP view, which is supplemented as needed by alar and obturator views and the lateral sacral view.

The **inlet and outlet views** of Pennal are very helpful in trauma cases.

> **Pelvic inlet and outlet views of Pennal**
> ➤ *Inlet view:* The beam is directed from the head to the mid-pelvis at a 40° angle to detect anterior or posterior displacement of the pelvic ring.
> ➤ *Outlet view:* The beam is directed from the foot to the symphysis at a 40° angle to detect sacral fractures and craniocaudal displacements.

In addition to this static radiographs, **functional views** can be obtained if there is clinical suspicion of **pelvic instability or rigidity**. Pelvic instability can result from acute or chronic injury to the sacroiliac ligaments. It should be noted that the posterior pelvic ring is subject to much greater weight-bearing loads than the anterior pelvic ring (Fig. 6.**4**).

On the other hand, the bony and ligamentous structures of the anterior pelvic ring are considerably weaker and more susceptible to fractures, and yet fractures in that area cause fewer stability problems in the pelvic ring as a whole. The pubic symphysis is located at the end of a long lever arm extending from the sacroiliac joints. Because of this arrangement, small movements in the sacroiliac joints (with a fixed sacrum) are translated into larger excursions at the pubic symphysis.

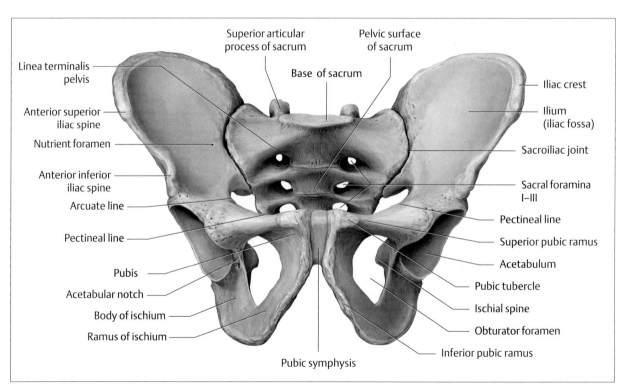

Fig. 6.**1**   Anatomic specimen of a male pelvis. (After Wolf-Heidegger 1961.)

If a sacroiliac joint becomes instable because of disease or injury, this instability will be transferred over time to the pubic symphysis, which is only weakly stabilized by ligaments.

It would exceed our scope to discuss the diverse etiology of sacroiliac joint instability and symphyseal instability and their manifestations. Pelvic rigidity is a result of reactive and/or reparative bone formation in the capsule and ligaments of the sacroiliac joints, completely eliminating any

degree of motion in these joints, which have only a minimum of physiological motion.

Functional views of the sacroiliac joints and pubic symphysis are obtained as follows.

- First an AP pelvic radiograph is obtained in the supine position.
- If asymmetries are noted that suggest pelvic instability or rigidity (Fig. 6.**5**), a second AP pelvic radiograph is taken in the standing position after 10 minutes of asymmetrical weight bearing (the patient walks around for 10 minutes while holding a 5-kg weight in one hand). If

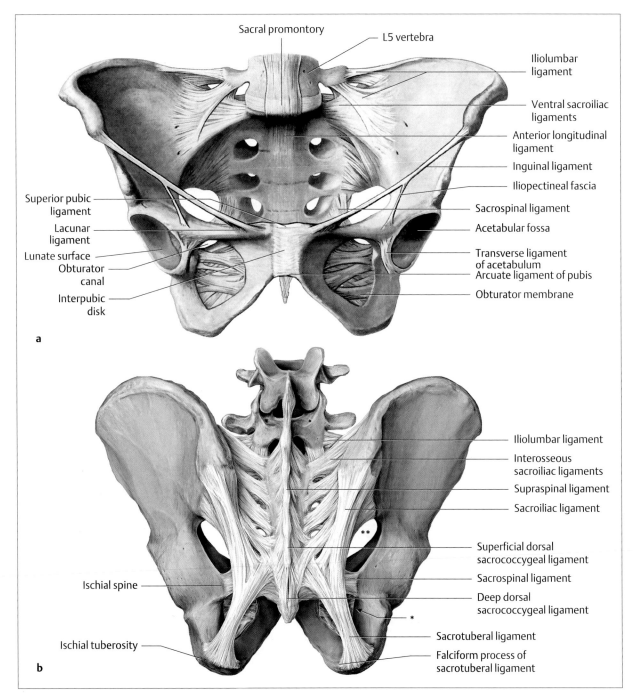

Fig. 6.**2a, b** Ligamentous attachments in a male pelvis. (After Wolf-Heidegger 1961.)
a Anterior aspect.
b Posterior aspect.

* Lesser ischial foramen
** Greater ischial foramen

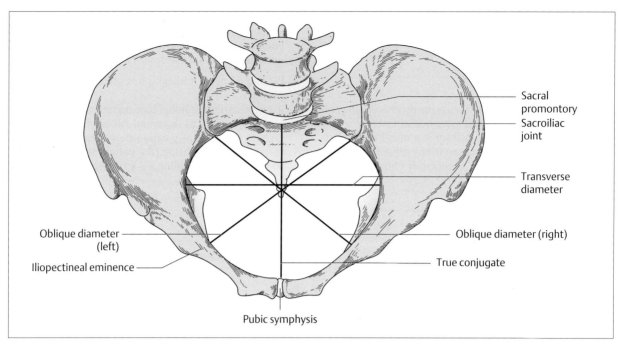

Fig. 6.**3**   Principal anatomic diameters of a female pelvis at the level of the pelvic inlet. (After Wolf-Heidegger 1961.)

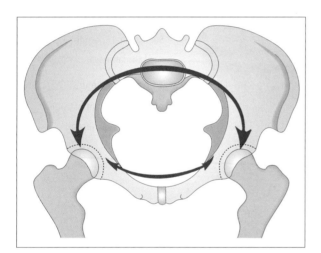

Fig. 6.**4**   Mechanical weight-bearing zones of the anterior and posterior pelvic ring (after Kane).

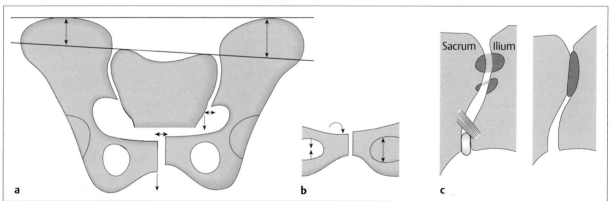

Fig. 6.**5 a–c**   Basic radiographic criteria for diagnosing pelvic instability (**a**, **b**) or pelvic rigidity (**c**) (after Dihlmann).
a Supine AP pelvic radiograph. When pelvic laxity is present, lines drawn tangent to the superior borders of the sacrum and iliac wings will diverge. Instability is also indicated by a stepoff between the ilium and sacrum on the arcuate line and by a gaping lower sacroiliac joint space or a stepoff at the upper and lower edges of the pubic symphysis, with symphyseal widening.

b Detail view of the pubic symphysis. Asymmetry of the obturator foramina and unequal heights of the opposing pubic rami may signify rotation on one side of the anterior pelvic ring.
c Diagram of the radiographic signs of ossification in the sacroiliac joint capsule and ligaments.

pelvic instability is present, the standing radiograph will show increased asymmetry compared with the static film.

- Additional spot films are taken of the pubic symphysis in one-legged stance to determine:
  - whether the pelvic instability is unilateral or bilateral;
  - whether there is any block (impaction) of the lax sacroiliac joint (no motion of the asymmetrical pubic rami when weight is shifted from leg to leg, but increased motion in the sacroiliac joint);
  - whether complete or incomplete pelvic rigidity is present (incomplete: slight motion of the pubic rami when weight is shifted from leg to leg despite ossifications in the sacroiliac joint capsule and ligaments).

CT examination is reserved for cases that cannot be resolved by conventional radiographs in multiple projections (all traumatic changes involving the posterior ilium and sacrum, all traumatic changes involving the hip, neoplastic changes, etc.).

MRI is used mainly in obstetric pelvimetry and for evaluating the hip and sacroiliac joints in children.

Trauma

Trauma to the pelvis will be discussed to the extent necessary for understanding and interpreting lucencies, densities, and asymmetries that occur as normal variants in the pelvic region.

Pelvic Injuries

The Tile classification of pelvic injuries is used at many institutions (Tile 1988). The classification is based on trauma mechanism, clinical stability, and radiographic criteria (Table 6.**1**).

- Type A (Fig. 6.**6**) consists of **peripheral pelvic fractures** that do not disrupt the continuity of the pelvic ring and thus do not compromise pelvic stability. Peripheral fractures of the iliac crest and wing, **coccygeal fractures**, and **transverse fractures of the lower sacrum** are a result of direct violence. **Avulsion fractures of the iliac spines**, especially during growth, are discussed more fully in the section on the ilium.
- Type B injuries cause rotational instability of the pelvis, but stability in the vertical direction is preserved. AP compression causes the external rotation of one or both hemipelves (open-book mechanism), often leading to symphyseal rupture. Lateral compression causes the internal rotation of one hemipelvis. Both mechanisms can lead to **anterior** as well as **posterior injuries of the pelvic ring** (Fig. 6.**7**). The posterior pelvic ring is never completely disrupted, because the open-book mechanism leaves the posterior sacroiliac ligament intact while lateral compression leaves the anterior sacroiliac ligament intact, stabilizing the posterior ring. The pelvis is unstable only in rotation.
- Type C injuries cause both rotational and vertical instability (translational instability). With a vertical shearing force, one hemipelvis is displaced upward. This can occur only if there is complete bony or ligamentous disruption of the anterior and posterior pelvic ring. **Sacroiliac joint fractures** and **sacral foraminal fractures** usually occur. A type C injury can also result from severe anteroposterior compression causing **complete**

Table 6.**1** Tile classification of pelvic injuries

Type	Description
Type A	Stable injuries
• A1	Peripheral pelvic fractures
• A2	Stable, minimally displaced anterior pelvic ring fractures
Type B	Rotational instability, vertical stability
• B1	AP compression: open-book injuries
• B2	Lateral compression: ipsilateral injury of the anterior and posterior pelvic ring
• B3	Lateral compression: contralateral injury of the anterior and posterior pelvic ring
Type C	Rotational and vertical instability
• C1	Injury with unilateral rotational and vertical instability
• C2	Injury with bilateral rotational and vertical instability
• C3	Pelvic ring fractures associated with an acetabular fracture

disruption of the posterior pelvic ring. It should be added that **pelvic ring fractures through the acetabulum** without vertical instability are also classified as type C injuries, as the acetabular fracture implies an unfavorable prognosis.

Ligamentous Injuries of the Sacroiliac Joint

Injuries of the sacroiliac ligaments can be accurately diagnosed with CT. The following criteria are used to grade the severity of the injury:

Criteria for grading ligamentous injuries
- ➤ *Grade I:* Symmetrical sacroiliac joints with no true pathological findings
- ➤ *Grade II:* Unilateral widening of the sacroiliac joint space due to rupture of the anterior ligaments
- ➤ *Grade III:* Marked unilateral widening of the sacroiliac joint space due to complete rupture of the sacroiliac ligament complex
- ➤ *Grade IV:* Marked widening of both sacroiliac joint spaces due to bilateral ligamentous injuries

---

As noted earlier, the comparison of normally symmetrical structures like the sacroiliac joints, the arcuate lines, the upper border of the pubic symphysis, and the obturator foramina is of practical importance in the diagnosis of pelvic ring fractures and instabilities. Discontinuities in the sacral foramina on plain radiographs are a useful indicator of sacral fractures.

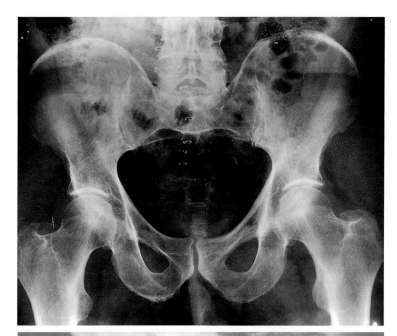

Fig. 6.**6**   Peripheral pelvic fractures (type A1 injuries in the Tile classification).
1   Avulsion fracture of the anterior superior iliac spine
2   Avulsion fracture of the anterior inferior iliac spine
3   Avulsion fracture of the ischial tuberosity
4   Isolated fracture of the inferior pubic ramus
5   Fracture of the iliac crest
6   Fracture of the iliac wing

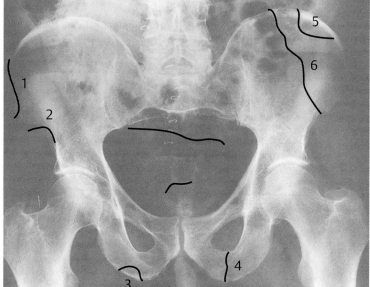

Osteonecrosis of the Acetabulum, Femoral Head, and Femoral Neck

These conditions are discussed in the section on the hip joint.

Ossification and Calcification of Soft-Tissue Structures

The diagram in Fig. 6.**8** illustrates various reparative and reactive ossifications that commonly occur in the sacroiliac joint capsule and ligaments and can be recognized on pelvic radiographs.

These ossifications can provide evidence of pelvic rigidity when corresponding clinical symptoms are present (see above).

Widespread **ossification of the pelvic ligaments** (Fig. 6.**2**) can occur as a normal variant or in the setting of fluorosis, DISH syndrome (diffuse idiopathic skeletal hyperostosis), or metaplastic ossification in seronegative spondylarthritides (e.g., ankylosing spondylitis). Their classification therefore depends on possible associated findings such as:

Fig. 6.**7**   Typical pelvic ring fractures.
1   Transiliac fracture
2   Transiliac or transacral sacroiliac joint
    fracture
3   Central sacral fracture
4   Transforaminal sacral fracture
5   Transalar sacral fracture
6   Sacroiliac joint separation
7   Transacetabular fracture
8   Transsymphyseal fracture
9   Transpubic fractures

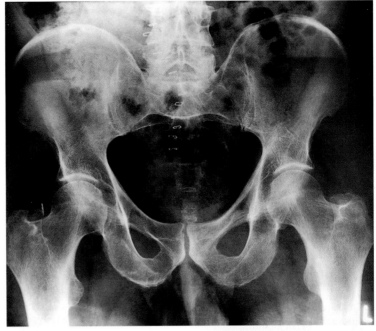

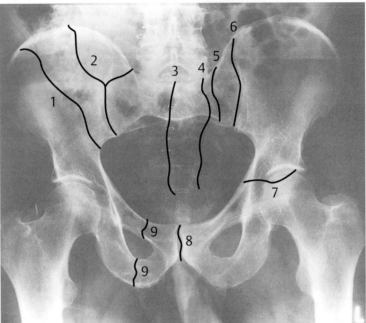

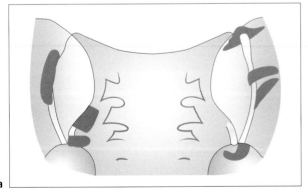

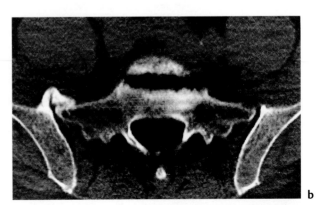

a

Fig. 6.**8 a, b**   Ossifications in the sacroiliac capsule and ligaments.

a Typical ossifications in the capsule and ligaments of the sacroiliac joints. They may indicate pelvic rigidity (see also Fig. 6.**5**).

b CT scan through the upper part of the sacroiliac joints shows heavy ossification of the anterosuperior portion of the right joint capsule and ligaments.

b

- Increased bone density (in fluorosis)
- Variegated type of sacroiliitis
- Signs of fibro-ostosis or fibro-osteitis in the iliac spines, ischia, and greater trochanters
- Calcifications in the hip joint capsule, etc.

Ossifications are most commonly observed in the sacrospinal, sacrotuberal and iliolumbar ligaments (Figs. 6.9–6.11, 6.19 a).

Ossification of the sacrotuberal ligament can be differentiated from an unusually long dystrophic calcification due to thrombotic occlusion of the femoral and external iliac vein when, for the latter, the lower part of the calcification extends past the ischial tuberosity (Fig. 6.12). Ossification of the pectineal ligament is rare and has been the subject of several publications (Fig. 6.13).

Productive and rarifying changes in the **fibro-osseous junctional region** of the pelvis are discussed more fully in the appropriate sections.

"**Pelvic digit**" is a rare anomaly consisting a solid, fingerlike ossification that contains a jointlike structure. Digits with two articulations have been described in the literature. A pelvic digit is most often found adjacent to the ilium (Fig. 6.14) or ischium.

Granieri and Bacarini (1996) describe the radiographic features of five new cases in which the digits resemble carpal bones, metacarpals or phalanges, sometimes in a rudimentary form. The authors do not speculate on the possible origin of these peculiar structures, and we are unable to offer any insights ourselves. Pelvic digits require differentiation from a heterotopic **lumbar rib**, which is usually distinguished by a well-defined cortex, normal-appearing trabecular bone, and sometimes by structures such as a costal head, neck, and tubercle (Sullivan and Cornwell 1974, Pais et al. 1978).

The differential diagnosis of pelvic digits also includes myositis ossificans and pelvic avulsion fractures. These conditions are symptomatic, however, whereas pelvic digits are always detected incidentally.

The overlapping abdominal creases in obese patients can lead to misinterpretation due to the shadows from the soft tissues themselves (differential diagnosis: enlarged uterus, full bladder, etc.) and also from air trapped in the creases (lucent line mimicking a fracture) or foreign material such as skin ointment (Fig. 6.15).

Dystrophic calcifications, rather than true ossifications, usually originate from the pelvic organs (Fig. 6.16).

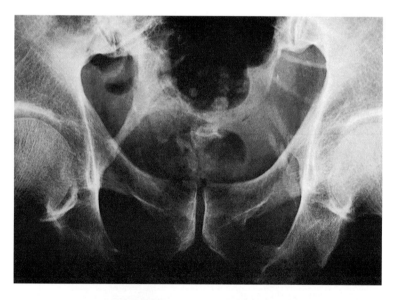

Fig. 6.**9** Ossification of both sacrospinal ligaments and the sacrotuberal ligament on the left side.

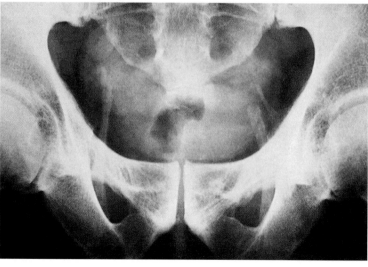

Fig. 6.**10** Ossification of both sacrotuberal ligaments and the sacrospinal ligament on the left side.

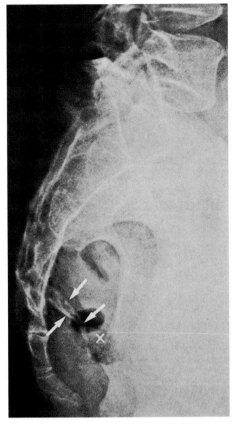

Fig. 6.**11**   Ossification of the sacrospinal ligament (arrows) in a profile view of the sacrum.
×   Ischial tuberosity

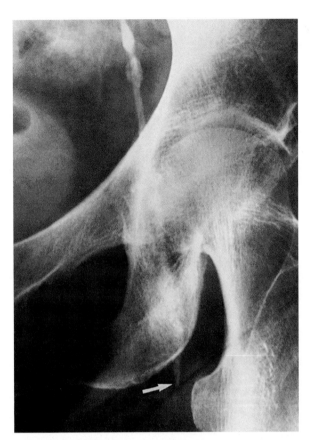

Fig. 6.**12**   Calcification in a venous trunk.

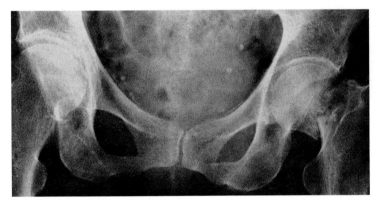

Fig. 6.**13**   Calcification of the pectineal ligament (from Sartor 1972). Note the fine linear densities above the horizontal pubic rami, running from the pecten of the pubis to the symphysis.

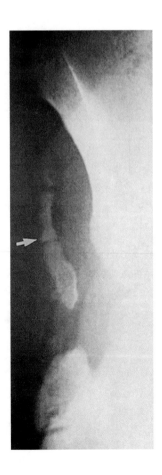

Fig. 6.**14**   "Pelvic digit" (arrow).

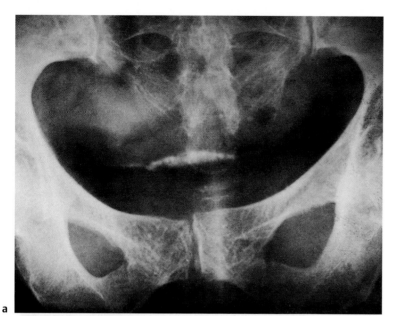

a

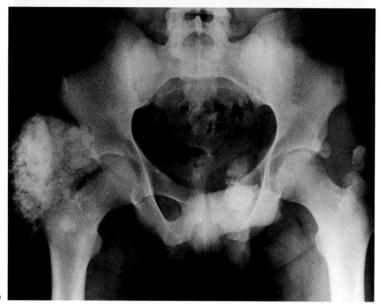

b

Fig. 6.**15 a, b**   Calcifications.
a Ointment in an abdominal crease appears as a transverse density projected over the lower sacrum.
b Extensive interstitial calcinosis in a chronic hemodialysis patient with an overdose of vitamin D replacement. Other prominent interstitial calcifications are present in the shoulder girdle region, hands, etc.

Fig. 6.**16**   Diagram of possible intrapelvic soft-tissue calcifications.
1 Calcified lymph node
2 Calcified fallopian tubes
3 Calcified spermatic cords
4 Phleboliths
5 Prostatic calcifications
6 Metallic injection residues in the gluteal muscle
7 Ovarian calcification
8 Aortic and pelvic arterial wall calcifications
9 Calcified postinjection abscess
10 Rudimentary tooth in an ovarian teratoma

Anomalies and Deformities

Anomalies and deformities are often manifested in the pelvis, and pelvic imaging should be included in the diagnostic workup of complex malformation syndromes. The principal development abnormalities of the pelvis are illustrated in Fig. 6.**17**.

Congenital syndromes that are associated with pelvic anomalies are listed in Table 6.**2** (Kozlowski and Beighton 1984).

A typical pelvic deformity in **neurofibromatosis** is shown in Fig. 6.**18**.

Structural Changes

A general **decrease in bone density** with increased radiolucency, especially in the iliac wings, pubis, and femoral necks, is a feature of advanced **osteoporosis** and **osteomalacia**. Osteomalacia is also associated with typical pseudofractures (so called Looser zones) in the pubis and iliac wings (oblique, following vascular channels, Fig. 6.**18d**), in the femoral necks, and below the lesser trochanters. Also, the bone structure often appears blurred as if rubbed with an eraser (ground-glass phenomenon). **Hyperparathyroidism** may show increased bone density in its early stages, while advanced cases show a fine honeycomb transformation of the bone structure.

A **generalized increase** in body density with "white" iliac wings and "white" symphyseal bones and hips may be seen in various conditions that include:

- Marble bone disease (combined with tree-ring densities in the iliac wings, Fig. 6.**18c**)
- Endosteal hyperostosis
- Osteomyelosclerosis syndrome
- Fluorosis

Table 6.**2** Congenital syndromes that are associated with pelvic anomalies (Kozlowski and Beighton 1984)

Common	Less common
• Achondroplasia: small trident acetabulum with short ilia, a narrow sacrum, small or slitlike ischial notches, squared-off iliac wings, and flat acetabular roofs • Mucopolysaccharidosis: flaring iliac wings, steep acetabular roofs, narrow pelvic inlet, coxa valga • Trisomy 21 syndrome: flaring, hypoplastic iliac wings, flat acetabular roofs, ischial tapering	• Achondrogenesis: failure of ossification of the sacrum, pubis, and ischium; flattened acetabula • Asphyxiating thoracic dysplasia (Jeune syndrome): flaring iliac wings, trident pelvis • Campomelic dysplasia: narrow pelvis with poor ossification • Caudal hypoplasia or aplasia: narrow pelvis with absent or hypoplastic sacrum • Chondrodysplasia punctata (Conradi–Hünermann disease): trapezoidal ilium • Chondroectodermal dysplasia (Ellis–van Creveld syndrome): trident pelvis • Cleidocranial dysplasia: broad pubic symphysis • Cockayne syndrome: small, square pelvis • Diastrophic dysplasia: short, thick ilia • Hypochondroplasia: small pelvis • Kniest dysplasia: broad iliac wings with hypoplasia of lower ilium; broad, short femoral necks with coxa vara • Marfan syndrome: vertical ilia, broad pelvis

→

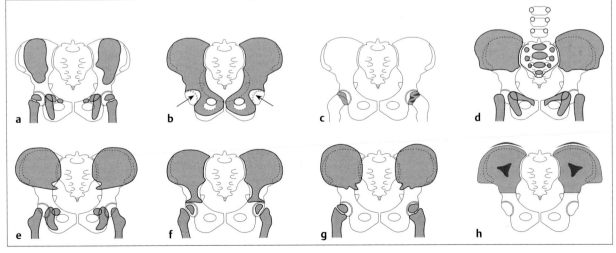

Fig. 6.**17a–h** Development abnormalities of the pelvis.
a Cleidocranial dysplasia
b Osteogenesis imperfecta
c Hypothyroidism
d Achondroplasia
e Mucopolysaccharidosis type 4 (Morquio)
f Dysostosis multiplex (mucopolysaccharidosis 1 and other mucopolysaccharidoses and mucolipidoses)
g Chondroectodermal dysplasia (Ellis–van Creveld syndrome)
h Nail–patella syndrome (osteoonychodysostosis)

Table 6.**2**   (Continue)

Common	Less common
	• Metaphyseal chondrodysplasia: abnormal acetabula
	• Metatrophic dysplasia: short ilia and small or slit-like ischial notches
	• Nail-patella syndrome: iliac horns
	• Osteodysplastia (Melnick – Needles syndrome): narrow pelvis with flaring iliac wings, shallow acetabula, and sharply tapered ischia
	• Osteogenesis imperfecta: protrusio acetabuli
	• Osteopetrosis: alternating bands of increased density in the iliac wings
	• Rubinstein – Taybi syndrome: flaring iliac wings
	• Spondyloepiphyseal dysplasia: square ilia, delayed ossification of the pubis and femoral heads
	• Thanatophoric dysplasia: square ilia with small sacrosciatic notches, trident pelvis
	• Trisomy 18 syndrome: small "antimongoloid" pelvis with vertical ilia, steep acetabular roofs
	• Tuberous sclerosis: patchy hyperdensities

Numerous small foci of increased density, showing a predilection for the articular regions of the pelvis (sacroiliac joints and hips), are typical of **osteopoikilosis** (Fig. 6.**19 a, b**). These lesions should not be confused with fine disseminated osteosclerotic metastases. Radionuclide bone scans in osteopoikilosis are normal, and the changes are detected incidentally. Figure 6.**19** illustrates the patterns of small, circumscribed densities that are seen in various disorders.

A coarse trabecular pattern and cortical thickening in the upper and posterior portions of the iliac wings as well as enlargement of the pubis and ischium are generally a result of **Paget disease**, which can involve large areas of the pelvis in advanced cases (Fig. 6.**19 d**). We need not explore the differential diagnosis of solitary and multiple osteolytic and osteosclerotic changes in this chapter. The occurrence of these changes as normal variants and the potential for confusing them with true pathological structures are discussed under the appropriate headings.

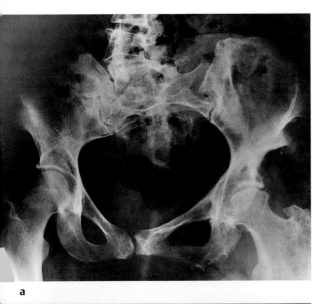

a

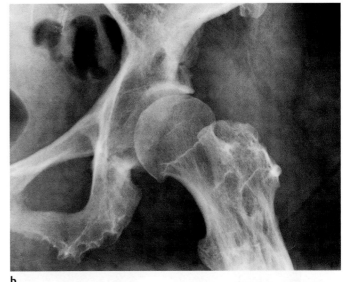

b

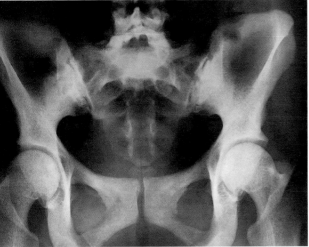

c

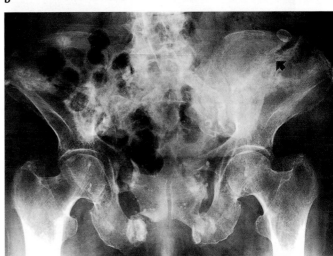

d

Fig. 6.**18 a–d**   Changes in pelvic shape and structure.
a, b Pelvic deformity in a 33-year-old woman with neurofibromatosis. Vertebral wedging is apparent in the lower lumbar spine and sacrum. The left hemipelvis shows severe dysplasia with tubercle-like foci of new bone formation on the ischium and in the area of the anterior inferior iliac spine (spiny pelvic contours). The left hip is dysplastic, and there is significant thickening of the left intertrochanteric region.
c Typical appearance of marble bone disease (osteopetrosis, Albers–Schönberg disease) with a uniform increase in the density of all imaged bone regions. This case does not show the otherwise typically alternating bands of increased and de-

creased density paralleling the iliac crest. The differential diagnosis should include osteomyelosclerosis, but this disease shows a more coarsely porous pattern of increased density.
d Severe osteomalacia with posterior and anterior pelvic ring instability. Looser zones (pseudofractures) are seen throughout the pubis. Also, there is an unusual fracture area running across the left iliac wing, following the course of larger blood vessels in that area. Similar incipient changes are visible on the right side. The changes regressed quickly in response to vitamin D replacement, with bony consolidation of the Looser zones.

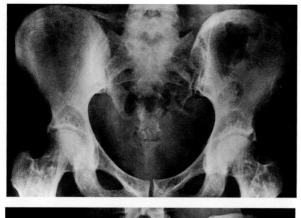

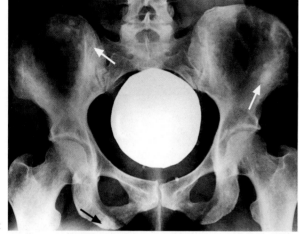

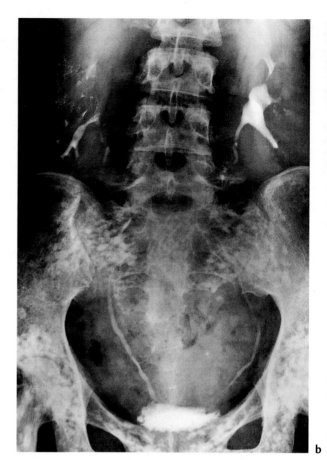

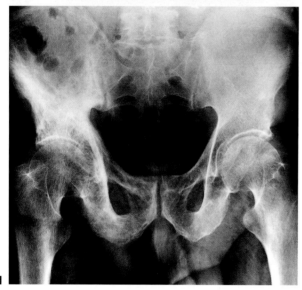

Fig. 6.**19 a–f** Differential diagnosis of spotty sclerosis and coarsened trabecular pattern of the pelvic bones.

a, b Different degrees of osteopoikilosis (spotted bones). Note also the ossification of the right iliolumbar ligament in film **a**.

c Circumscribed cancellous bone densities up to 1 cm in size reflect a patchy distribution of bone marrow necrosis in a patient who underwent chemotherapy (corticosteroids, cytostatics). Initially the foci were positive on bone scans, but their uptake faded during subsequent years. The arrows indicate selected foci or clusters of foci.

d Typical radiographic appearance of Paget disease, with a coarsened trabecular pattern in the lower right iliac wing, acetabulum, and right ischium and pubis.

Abb. 6.**19e, f**   Follow-up of small osteomas detected incidentally in the ilium. An osteoma is visible on the left side in film **e**, while the right side is unremarkable. In film **f**, taken 16 years later, the osteoma on the left side has become considerably larger, and a small osteoma is now visible on the right side (*). Note the small, footlike attachments of the large tumor in **f**, which are typical of osteoma. Larger osteomas usually show only little tracer uptake on bone scans, contrasting with the intense uptake that occurs in osteoplastic metastases.

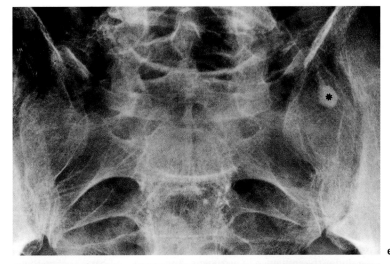

e

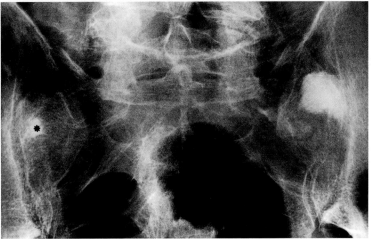

f

References

Adam, Ph., Y. Alberge, S. Castellano et al.: Pelvimetry by digital radiography. Clin. Radiol. 36 (1985) 327

Bettenhäuser, K.: Versprengte Lendenrippe. Fortschr. Röntgenstr. 100 (1964) 784

Bohutová, J., J. Kolár, J. Vitovec et al.: Accessory caudal axial and pelvic ribs. Fortschr. Röntgenstr. 133 (1980) 641

Dalinka, M. K., P. Arger, B. Coleman: CT in pelvic trauma. Orthop. Clin. N. Amer. 16 (1985) 471

Dihlmann, W.: Gelenke – Wirbelverbindungen, 2. Aufl. Thieme, Stuttgart 1982

Freyschmidt, J.: Skeletterkrankungen, 2. Aufl. Springer, Berlin 1997

Granieri, G. F., L. Bacarini: The pelvic digit: five new examples of an unusual anomaly. Skelet. Radiol. 25 (1996) 723

Greenspan, A., A. Norman: The "pelvic digit" – an unusual developmental anomaly. Skelet. Radiol. 9 (1982) 118

Hamilton, S.: Pelvic digit. Brit. J. Radiol. 58 (1985) 1010

Kaufmann, H. J.: Röntgenbefunde am kindlichen Becken bei Skelettaffektionen und chromosomalen Aberrationen. Thieme, Stuttgart 1964

Kempmann, G.: Verkalkte Beckenvenenthrombose und Stauungsossifikation am Unterschenkel – seltene Spätfolge der chronisch-venösen Insuffizienz. Fortschr. Röntgenstr. 127 (1977) 74

Kozlowski, K., P. Beighton: Gamut index of skeletal dysplasias. Springer, Berlin 1984 (S. 56–57)

Müller-Färber, J., K. H. Müller: Instabile Beckenringverletzungen. Unfallheilkunde 87 (1984) 441

Pais, M. J., A. Levine, S. O. Pais: Coccygeal ribs: development and appearance in two cases. Amer. J. Roentgenol. 131 (1978) 164

Sartor, K.: Symmetrische Verkalkung der Arcus iliopectinei. Fortschr. Röntgenstr. 116 (1972) 120

Sullivan, D., W. S. Cornwell: Pelvic rib: report of a case. Radiology 110 (1974) 355

Tile, M.: Pelvic ring fractures: should they be fixed? J. Bone Jt Surg. 70-A (1988) 1

Torode, I., D. Zieg: Pelvic fractures in children. J. pediat. Orthop. 5 (1985) 76

Wolf-Heidegger, G.: Atlas der systematischen Anatomie des Menschen, Bd. I., 2. Aufl. Karger, Basel 1961

Pelvis, Specific Section

Ilium

Normal Findings

During Growth

The ossification center for the ilium appears in the 9-week-old fetus. At birth, the ilium is already well developed with streaklike densities radiating from the center toward the periphery. A male type of ilium is initially present in both sexes and in females is later transformed into the female type under the influence of estrogens. **Apophyses** appear along the iliac crest (Figs. 6.**20**, 6.**46 f, g**) and anterior superior iliac spine between 12 and 15 years of age (Fig. 6.**20**). Their appearance in females is closely linked to the menarche. The apophysis of the iliac crest may ossify from multiple centers.

The apophyseal line may have a rippled appearance, similar to the apophyseal rings of the vertebral bodies (Fig. 6.**21**). Fusion of the iliac apophysis occurs between 21 and 25 years of age. According to Risser (1964), fusion of the iliac apophysis coincides with the cessation of longitudinal bone growth. Since the risk of scoliosis progression is thought to decrease with the cessation of longitudinal body growth, ossification processes in the iliac crest are a

helpful guide in determining the need for early surgical intervention. Many orthopedists still recommend the radiographic assessment of iliac crest maturation, particularly since radiographs of the left hand alone are inadequate for assessing skeletal maturity. They base this recommendation on the fact that the trunk, and thus the spinal column, continue to grow after the extremities have completed their growth. It is essential to obtain an AP projection of the iliac apophysis, since on a PA projection the apophysis is superimposed over the ilium and is difficult to evaluate (Izumi 1995). Other authors, such as Little and Sussman (1994), have found that the Risser sign (Fig. 6.22) is a less accurate indicator of skeletal maturity than chronological age and feel that it should not be used as a substitute for hand radiographs in determining skeletal age. The Risser sign, they maintain, is no better than chronological age as a criterion for predicting the progression of scoliosis.

Many orthopedists also use the "openness" of the triradiate (y-)cartilages as a factor in calculating skeletal maturity for timing posterior arthrodesis (e.g., Sanders et al. 1995). If the triradiate cartilages are still open at the time of posterior spinal fusion, there is greater risk of a "crankshaft phenomenon" (torsional deformity due to continued anterior spinal growth) than if the cartilages are closed. This led Roberto et al. (1997) to recommend a combined anterior and posterior fusion for these cases.

The **anterior inferior iliac spine** has its own apophyseal ossification center (Fig. 6.23) that appears on radiographs at about 13–15 years of age and fuses with the ilium at

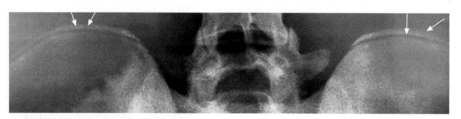

Fig. 6.**20**   Symmetrical arrangement of iliac apophyses in a 17-year-old male.

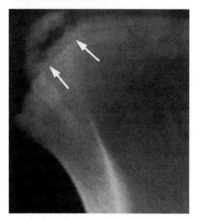

Fig. 6.**21**   Rippling of the iliac crest apophysis (arrows).

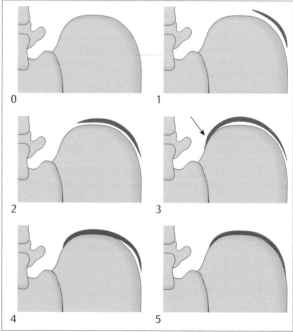

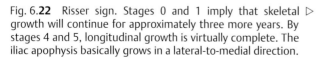

Fig. 6.**22**   Risser sign. Stages 0 and 1 imply that skeletal ▷ growth will continue for approximately three more years. By stages 4 and 5, longitudinal growth is virtually complete. The iliac apophysis basically grows in a lateral-to-medial direction.

about 16–18 years. This iliac spine is of some importance in traumatology, since a very powerful contraction of the inferior rectus muscle can avulse it from the ilium regardless of whether the apophyseal plate is open or closed (Figs. 6.**29**, 6.**30**).

A Y-shaped lucency with sharp, sclerotic margins located at the center of the iliac wing is a well-developed

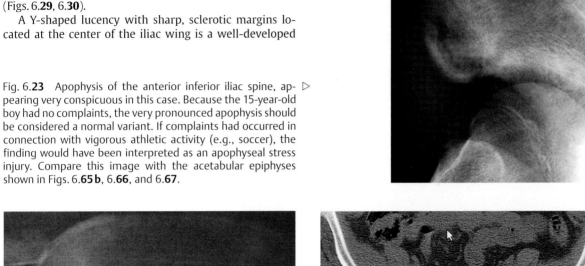

Fig. 6.**23** Apophysis of the anterior inferior iliac spine, appearing very conspicuous in this case. Because the 15-year-old boy had no complaints, the very pronounced apophysis should be considered a normal variant. If complaints had occurred in connection with vigorous athletic activity (e.g., soccer), the finding would have been interpreted as an apophyseal stress injury. Compare this image with the acetabular epiphyses shown in Figs. 6.**65 b**, 6.**66**, and 6.**67**. ▷

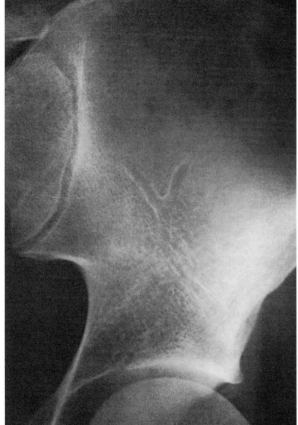

a

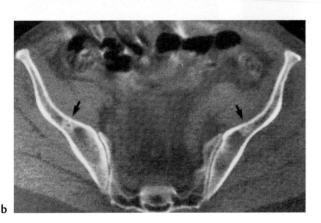

b

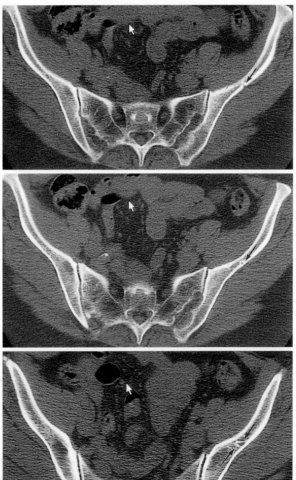

c

d

e

Fig. 6.**24 a–e**
a, b Nutrient canals.
a Typical Y-shaped nutrient canal at the center of the ilium.
b Nutrient canals cut transversely by a CT scan on both sides of the ilium, mimicking structural abnormalities in the cancellous bone (tumor? chronic trauma?).
c–e CT sections through a nutrient canal in the left ilium (black arrows in the ilium; the white arrow in the abdominal soft tissues has no importance).

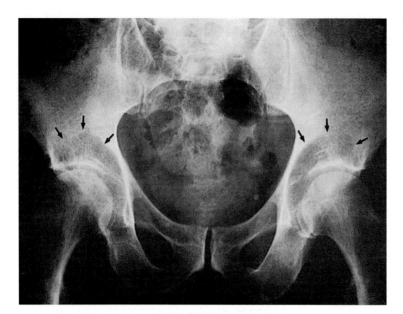

Fig. 6.**25**   The crescent-shaped lucencies over each acetabular roof are a completely normal phenomenon caused by a relative paucity of cancellous bone and an increased proportion of fatty marrow.

nutrient canal (Fig. 6.**24**). This feature is most commonly seen during the growth period but can also be observed in diseases with abnormally increased remodeling (e.g. in hyperparathyroidism), with consecutive augmentation of blood flow. These normal nutrient canals also create a point of least resistance for insufficiency fractures in cases where the bone has been structurally weakened due to osteomalacia or other disease (Fig. 6.**18d**). Nutrient canals in the ilium are easily mistaken for fracture lines on CT scans (Fig. 6.**24b-e**) (Richardson et al. 1985).

> Crescent-shaped lucencies above the acetabula can be confusing for the novice (Fig. 6.**25**). They are normal areas that contain a relative paucity of cancellous bone and a relatively large amount of marrow fat.

Pathological Finding?

Normal Variant or Anomaly?

The iliac wings show relatively little variation in their radiographic morphology. Irregularities on the iliac crests and spines in adults result from bony proliferation at sites of tendon attachment and usually have no pathological significance (p. 787).

A **spiny contour of the iliac crest** is found in Dyggve–Melchior–Clausen syndrome (also short, broad iliac wings), in parastremmatic dysplasia (with small iliac wings), in Smith–McCaught syndrome, and in neurofibromatosis (Fig. 6.**18a, b**).

"**Iliac horns**" are pathognomonic for nail-patella syndrome (osteo-onychodysostosis; Fig. 6.**26**). They are sym-

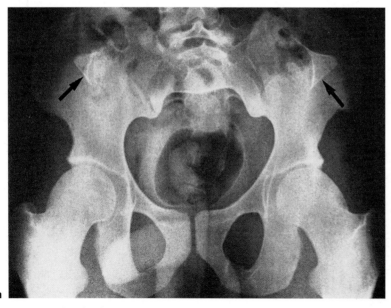

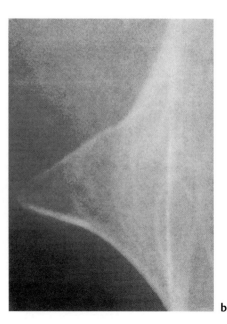

a   b

Fig. 6.**26a, b**   Iliac horns (arrows).
a AP projection.
b Tangential view.

metrically arranged, pyramid-shaped bony prominences that arise from the posterior iliac surface 2–3 fingerwidths from the center of the sacroiliac joints and may be up to 4 cm high. The horns are palpable on physical examination.

Hypoplasia of the iliac wings with a narrow pelvis may be found in Turner syndrome and other chromosomal abnormalities. A trapezoidal ilium is characteristic of Conradi–Hünermann disease (chondrodysplasia punctata), and a square ilium is seen in Cockayne syndrome, spondyloepiphyseal dysplasia, and thanatophoric dysplasia. A short ilium with a small or slitlike sacrosciatic notch is found in metatropic dysplasia (see also Table 6.**2**).

The **paraglenoid sulcus** is subject to marked variations in width and depth (Fig. 6.**27**). It is a notch or groove located in the ilium just lateral to the inferior end of the sacroiliac joint. When located on the sacral side of the sacroiliac joint, it is called the **preauricular notch**. The paraglenoid sulcus is considered to be a normal variant. It is located at the attachment of the anterior sacroiliac ligament and is analogous to the deep ligamentous groove in the clavicle at the attachment of the costoclavicular ligament (p. 307). Contrary to earlier claims, the notch is not a canal for the internal iliac artery. Since it is virtually absent in males and is particularly deep in females, the paraglenoid sulcus is useful for sex determination in forensic tests and anthropological studies (Houghton 1974, Dee 1981, Schemmer et al. 1995). The latter authors published a particularly worthwhile study on the origin and prevalence of the paraglenoid sulcus.

An important observation is that the sulcus or groove is not a primary structure but is caused by stress-induced bone resorption at the insertion of the anterior sacroiliac ligament.

Schemmer et al. (1995) found a definite relationship to parturition in 70 adult women, with deep grooves occurring only in multiparous women. The hormone-induced laxity of the sacroiliac joints during pregnancy apparently leads to greater stresses on the sacroiliac ligaments. These authors also found an association with hyperostosis triangularis ilii (osteitis condensans ilii) (Fig. 6.**34**, p. 785) and with increased lumbosacral lordosis.

The paraglenoid sulci may be misinterpreted as areas of bone destruction, especially on CT scans and especially when the sulci are asymmetrical or are cut only partially by the scan (Fig. 6.**27 b, c**).

Fracture?

Like the ischial tuberosity, the **anterior superior and anterior inferior iliac spines** are sites of predilection for avulsion fractures, especially when they are still apophyseal (Metzmaker and Pappas 1980, Fernback and Wilkinson 1981, Khouri et al. 1985, Sundar and Carty 1994, Brandser et al. 1995, Rossi et al. 2001). Most of these fractures are caused by a sudden, powerful contraction of the muscles attached to the spines (Table 6.**3**). A smaller percentage can result from chronic repetitive traction in the absence of acute trauma (comparable to a stress fracture).

Adolescents whose spines have not yet fused to the ilium are predominantly affected. Table 6.**3** lists the types of athletic activities that are most often associated with apophyseal avulsion fractures. In our experience, a missed

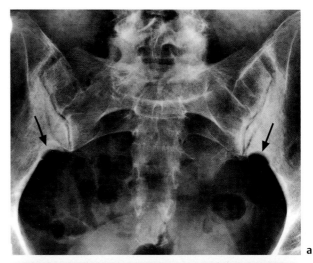

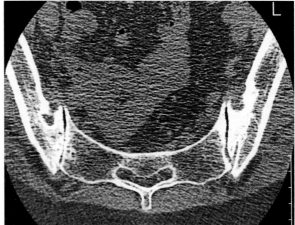

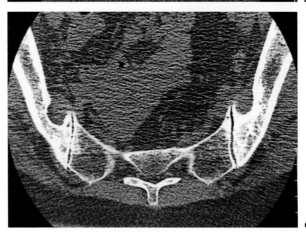

Fig. 6.**27 a–c**   Very deep paraglenoid sulci (arrows).
a AP radiograph.
b, c   CT scans in a multiparous woman.

kick at a soccer ball is the most common mechanism leading to avulsion of the anterior inferior iliac spine (Figs. 6.**28**–6.**30**).

Avulsion injuries of the anterior and lower pelvis have a broad spectrum of radiographic features. In most cases the AP projection or an extra oblique projection will clearly demonstrate a fresh avulsion fracture (Fig. 6.**29**).

  Differentiation between an avulsion fracture and an irregularly ossified apophysis is required.

Table 6.**3** Avulsion fractures in adolescence. Sites of occurrence, anatomy, and predisposing sports activities (after Sundar and Carty)

Location	Attached muscles	Types of sport leading to avulsion fractures
Anterior superior iliac spine	Sartorius, tensor fasciae latae	Running while playing soccer, sprinting
Anterior inferior iliac spine	Rectus femoris	Kicking a soccer ball, sprinting
Ischial tuberosity	Adductor magnus, quadratus femoris, semimembrano-sus, semitendino-sus, biceps femo-ris (long head)	Gymnastics (especially splits), sprinting, soccer (running, kicking), rugby (running, kicking)

This can be accomplished relatively easily by comparison with the opposite side. Of course, if the apophysis in children is not yet ossified, trauma cannot be detected radiographically in the acute stage (although CT or MRI may show an abnormal, tumorlike soft-tissue mass). Follow-up radiographs are needed to detect metaplastic ossification. A chronic avulsion fracture is more difficult to diagnose (resembling the findings in Fig. 6.**23**), particularly if

early hematoma- or edema-related ossification occurs around the fragment in an adolescent patient, in extreme cases producing a kind of myositis ossificans. This type of finding is easily confused with osteosarcoma. Chronic trauma to the apophyses can also produce inflammatory-like changes with blurring of the apophyseal region. A careful history is essential, and the patient should be questioned about any sports activities that may have caused sudden pain in the affected apophyseal area, exertional pain relating to chronic trauma, and so on.

 MR images can be very confusing, as they can demonstrate even slight edematous changes that are easily mistaken for inflammation or tumor.

Most avulsion fractures will heal completely with 20–30 days' immobilization. A protracted course with persistent pain and disability, often lasting for years, has been known to occur in nonimmobilized cases.

So-called **Looser transformation zones** (pseudofractures, insufficiency fractures) in the ilium typically occur in the area of nutrient canals (Figs. 6.**18 d**, 6.**31**). The most frequent cause is osteomalacia, which is not uncommon in older women (Fig. 6.**18 d**). The vessels in the iliac wings (see above) apparently contribute to the pathogenesis of Looser zones, also referred to as pseudofractures or insufficiency fractures. The pulsations in these vessels appear to play a role (Griffin 1982).

Insufficiency (stress) are most common in the supra-acetabular area of overweight women who have osteo-

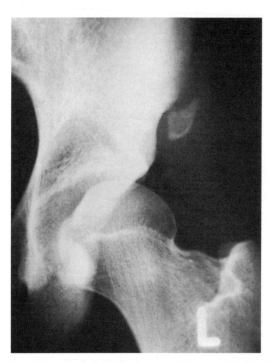

Fig. 6.**28** Acute avulsion fracture of the anterior inferior iliac spine. Postinjury radiograph of a 16-year-old girl who tripped and fell onto her left hip while playing ball. There was immediate swelling over the anterior inferior iliac spine and tenderness to pressure.

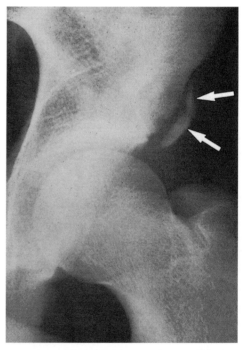

Fig. 6.**29** Avulsion of the anterior inferior iliac spine (arrows). Not a persistent apophysis.

Fig. 6.**30 a–d**   Follow-up of a typical avulsion fracture of the anterior inferior iliac spine in a 17-year-old boy.

a Radiograph taken two weeks after the patient felt acute right-sided groin pain while playing soccer (he kicked at the ball but missed it). The shell-like fragment is displaced laterally and inferiorly and is surrounded by metaplastic ossification.

b Approximately three months later, the foci of ossification appear more solid.

c CT appearance of **b**.

d MRI concurrent with **b** and **c** shows a hyperintense feature representing the bony fragment and heterotopic ossification with fatty marrow tissue. The MRI findings were misinterpreted as a tumor. After three months abstinence from sports, the fracture was fully consolidated along with the heterotopic ossifications, and the patient was free of complaints.

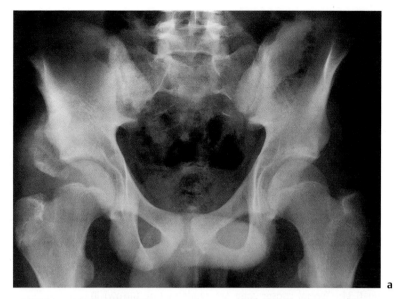

a

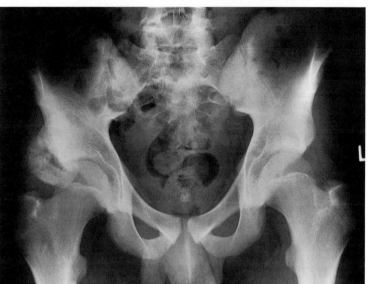

b

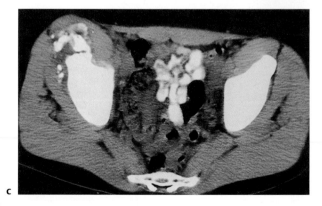

c

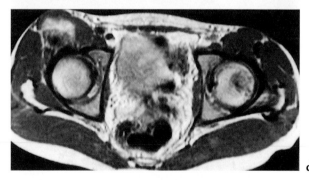

d

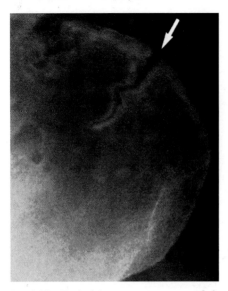

Fig. 6.**31** Typical Looser zone or pseudofracture (arrow) in osteomalacia. The same was found on the contralateral side.

porosis. They appear as a more or less dense sclerotic zone on radiographs and show intense tracer uptake on bone scans (Fig. 6.**32**).

Insufficiency (stress) fractures can also result from steroid therapy and radiotherapy, and they can occur in rheumatoid arthritis (Cooper et al. 1985).

> In their initial stage, Looser zones and other stress fractures represent true transitional states between normal and pathological. Nutrient canals in the ilium should not be mistaken for fresh traumatic fractures (Fig. 6.**24**).

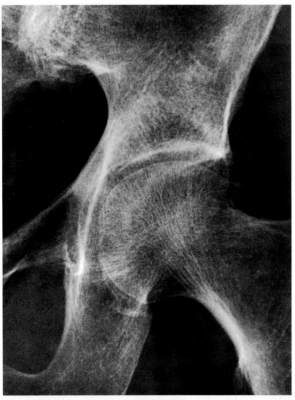

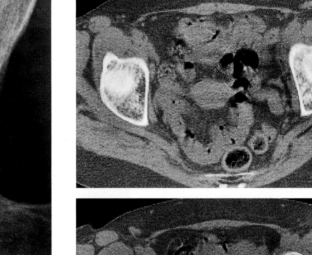

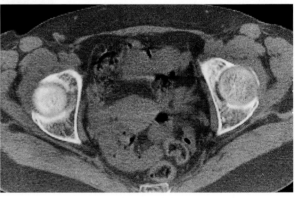

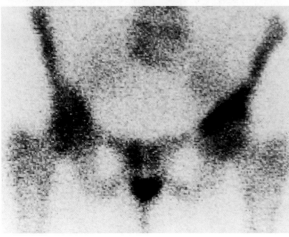

Fig. 6.**32a–d** Typical supra-acetabular stress fracture (insufficiency fracture) in an elderly woman with osteoporosis.
a AP radiograph does not suggest a definite diagnosis other than osteoporosis.
b Since the patient had severe pain in the left hip area, a bone scan was obtained, showing massive tracer uptake in and above the acetabular region.
c, d CT scans show patchy sclerotic foci in the left medial and anterior acetabular region. The scans do not show the structural abnormalities just above the acetabulum.

Necrosis?

It is rare for necrosis to affect large portions of the iliac wings. More common but more difficult to evaluate are circumscribed osteonecrotic lesions affecting the marrow spaces of the ilium following treatment with cytostatic drugs or steroids, for example, or in patients with chronic recurring pancreatitis. These lesions appear as circumscribed zones of reactive sclerosis (Fig. 6.**19c**).

Radiation-induced structural changes in the dorsal areas of the iliac bones—adjacent to the sacroiliac joints—are often difficult to detect on plain films and better visualized in CT images. In advanced stages they can lead to insufficiency fractures.

 ## Inflammation?

Basically any form of osteomyelitis and osteitis can occur in the pelvis. Generally, though, the findings are not difficult to distinguish from a possible normal variant.

Circumscribed, rounded, asymmetrical sclerotic lesions up to 1.5 cm in diameter are usually osteomas (see Fig. 6.**19e, f**). More streaklike, unilateral sclerotic areas may be a sign of **melorheostosis** (Fig. 6.**33**).

A triangular area of sclerosis on the iliac aspect of the sacroiliac joint, known traditionally as "**osteitis condensans ilii**," was given the more appropriate term **hyperostosis triangularis ilii** by Dihlmann (1976). The older term is misleading in that 50% of cases also have an area of sacral sclerosis, whose shape is highly variable. Much like the paraglenoid sulcus, hyperostosis triangularis ilii occurs predominantly in women 30–50 years of age, or during and after the childbearing years. The process may be unilateral or bilateral and is more common in parous than nonparous women. Pathoanatomically, hyperostosis triangularis ilii is based on a purely reactive increase in cancellous bone density due to a localized increase in mechanical stresses. This is evidenced in part by the fact that the hyperostosis can regress spontaneously. Its tendency to accompany osteoarthritis also suggests that it is a stress-related condition. Dihlmann also made the following discovery on the pathogenesis of hyperostosis triangularis ilii. In CT scans or macerated transverse sections of the ilium in normal sacroiliac joints, he noted a small, triangular area of sclerosis at the anteroinferior articular border of the ilium that was not visible on AP radiographs. In its three-dimensional geometry, this sclerotic zone is shaped like a pyramid with its apex pointing upward. Its location marks the pressure center of the sacroiliac joint when the individual is standing on both legs. Now if the pressure across the sacroiliac joint increases, due for example to increased pelvic laxity in pregnancy or a loss of shock-absorbing articular cartilage due to osteoarthritis, the increased stresses will incite reactive new bone formation around the inferior bony angle of the ilium, eventually producing the triangular sclerosis that is the hallmark of hyperostosis triangularis ilii. This condition should not be confused with the sclerosis that accompanies the "variegated" type of sacroiliitis (q.v.). Problems of differential diagnosis, especially with regard to the adjacent sacroiliac joint, are best resolved by CT (Fig. 6.**35**).

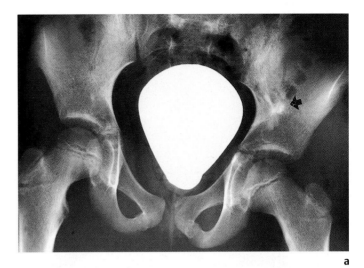

a

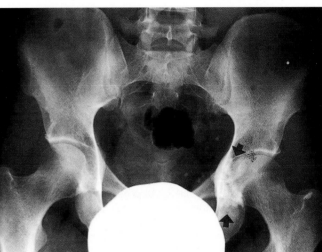

b

Fig. 6.**33 a, b**   Foci of cancellous bone sclerosis (arrows) in the pelvis of patients with melorheostosis. In both cases the pelvic foci were just the tip of the iceberg, as other ossifications were found in the bones and soft tissues of the left lower extremity.

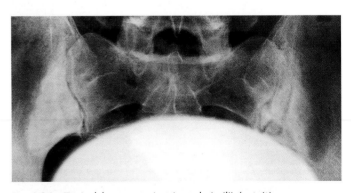

Fig. 6.**34**   Typical hyperostosis triangularis ilii (osteitis condensans ilii), affecting both sides but predominantly affecting the right ilium of a 46-year-old multipara. (Case courtesy of Professor V. Niehaus, Norden.)

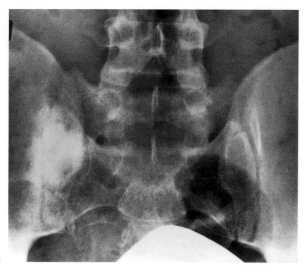

a

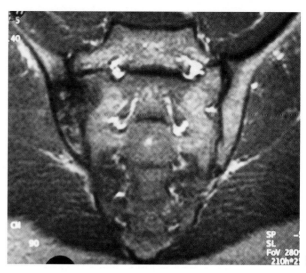

b

Fig. 6.**35 a, b**   Differential diagnosis of hyperostosis triangularis ilii. The extensive sclerosis in the posterior right ilium is caused by an Ewing sarcoma in a young man. The tumor has already spread to the sacrum (postcontrast MRI in panel **b**), and

additional MR images confirmed soft-tissue infiltration. The epicenter of the sclerosis is not located in the inferior angle of the ilium, as would be the case in hyperostosis triangularis ilii. (Case courtesy of Professor Dr. D. Hahn, Wurzburg.)

It is uncertain whether hyperostosis triangularis ilii has pathological significance in all cases or whether it should be classified as a normal variant in patients who are asymptomatic. This particularly applies to multiparous women, in whom the condition is often detected incidentally and definitely represents a physiological adaptation process.

Coarsened trabecular structures in the ilium of asymptomatic patients older than 50 years are pathognomonic for **Paget disease** (Fig. 6.**36**).

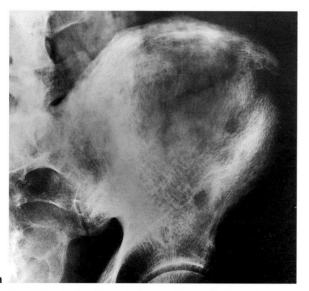

a

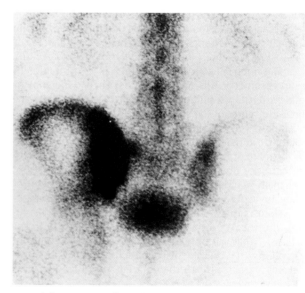

b

Fig. 6.**36 a, b**   In this typical case of Paget disease, coarsened trabecular pattern and cortical thickening are observed throughout the left ilium in an elderly man. The pattern is so

typical that it is virtually pathognomonic. In the corresponding bone scan in **b**, the most intense uptake occurs medially where the increased remodeling is still the most active.

Tumor?

Osteomas and melorheostosis are discussed under "Inflammation". The pelvis is a flat bone, making it a site of predilection for tumors that have an affinity for regions that contain red bone marrow, most notably:

- Skeletal metastases
- Plasmacytoma
- Malignant non-Hodgkin lymphoma of bone

Rapidly progressive bone destruction in the pelvis, like that caused by Ewing sarcoma, often incites a circumscribed osteonecrosis that appears as irregular "white" bone on radiographs (Fig. 6.**35**).

> Except for normally rarefied trabecular areas above the acetabula, effects due to overlying bowel gas, and "physiological" hyperostosis triangularis ilii, there are no anatomic structures in the pelvis or normal variants that can mimic pathological bone destruction or osteosclerosis.

Several works have been published in recent years on **subchondral synovial cysts of the sacroiliac joint** (Fig. 6.**37**) (e.g., Weinberg 1982, Graf and Freyschmidt 1988).

Of course, these lesions can be detected only by sectional imaging procedures and are often discovered incidentally. When asymptomatic, they can still be considered an extreme normal variant in some cases. Nothing definite is known about their pathogenesis, but it is conceivable, for example, that small cracks in the subchondral plate could allow synovial structures, especially synovial fluid, to enter the subchondral area and cause circumscribed bone resorption. The cracks would not always be visible on radiographs. We have seen many such cases in recent years, including some in which intra-articular air (vacuum phenomenon) entered the subarticular cavities. This always occurs when traction produces a regional negative pressure causing nitrogen to exit the blood and collect in a gaseous form. Another term for these air-filled cavities is **intraosseous pneumatocysts** (Ramirez et al. 1984, Hall and Turkel 1989, Freyschmidt and Holland 1990).

Other Changes?

As noted in the section on normal variants, hyperostotic spicules on the iliac crests and spines reflect a productive fibroostosis (enthesiopathy) occurring at the sites of attachment of the capsule and ligaments (Fig. 6.**38**).

They have real diagnostic significance only in connection with inflammatory joint conditions that are associated with destructive and proliferative changes—particularly diseases from the group of seronegative spondylarthritides.

Fig. 6.**37 a–d** Pseudotumors in the ilium.
a Subchondral synovial cyst or intraosseous ganglion in the right ilium below the sacroiliac joint. Intra-articular air, generated by a vacuum phenomenon, has entered the subchondral cavity. Water-equivalent attenuation values may also be found in such osteolytic areas.

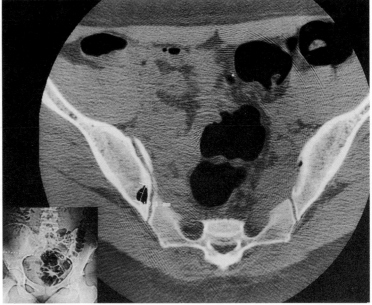

a

Fig. 6.**37 a–d** ▷

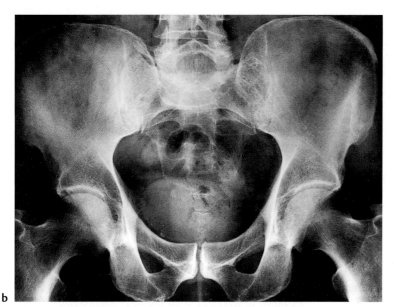

Fig. 6.**37 b–d**   This longstanding lesion in the posterior left ilium has undergone fatty transformation. AP radiograph in **b** shows a rarefication of the bony structures in the posterior left ilium. Paget disease? The CT scan in **c** clearly shows fat within the lesion, raising the possibility of a fatty cyst, fibrous dysplasia, or lipoma. The lesion was detected incidentally, so biopsy was omitted. The CT scan in **d**, acquired at a lower level than **c**, shows a coarsened trabecular pattern that was interpreted as a response to the altered mechanical stresses caused by the lesion. (Case courtesy of Dr. Kammerer, Weiden.)

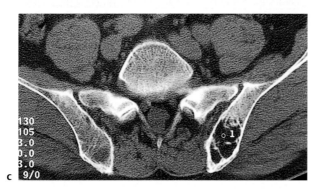

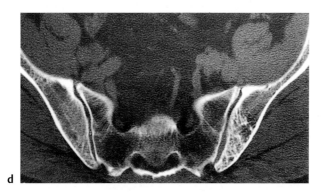

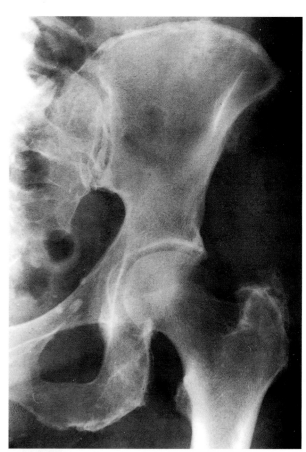

Fig. 6.**38**   Productive fibro-ostosis in an asymptomatic elderly man with a long history of diabetes mellitus. The film shows conspicuous areas of new bone formation in the iliac crest, anterior superior iliac spine, ischium, and around the greater trochanter. The spinal column displays classic features of DISH syndrome.

References

Brandser, E. A., G. Y. El-Khoury, M. H. Kathol et al.: Hamstring injuries: radiographic, conventional tomographic, CT, and MR imaging characteristics. Radiology 197 (1995) 257

Cooper, K. L., J. W. Beabout, R. A. McLeod: Supraacetabular insufficiency fractures. Radiology 157 (1985) 15

Dee, P. M.: The preauricular sulcus. Radiology 140 (1981) 354

Dihlmann, W.: Die Hyperostosis triangularis ilii – das sakroiliakale knöcherne Streß-Phänomen. 2. Teil (Inzidenz, Prognose, Pathogenese, Ätiologie, Tracerstudium, Differentialdiagnose). Fortschr. Röntgenstr. 124 (1976) 154

Dihlmann, W.: Gelenke – Wirbelverbindungen, 2. Aufl. Thieme, Stuttgart 1982

Exner, G. U., L. Kaufmann, A. Schreiber: Beziehungen zwischen der Entwicklung der Beckenkammapophysen („Rissersches Zeichen") und der Handskelettentwicklung bei Mädchen mit Skoliose. Z. Orthop. 123 (1985) 910

Fernback, S. K., H. R. Wilkinson: Avulsion injuries of pelvis and proximal femur. Am. J. Roentgenol. 17 (1981) 581

Freyschmidt, J., B. Holland: Zum seltenen Phänomen intraossärer Gasansammlungen (sog. Pneumatozelen). Fortschr. Röntgenstr. 152 (1990) 6

Graf, I., J. Freyschmidt: Die subchonrale Synovialzyste (intraossäres Ganglion). Fortschr. Röntgenstr. 148 (1988) 398

Griffin jr., C. N.: Symmetrical ilial pseudofractures: a complication of chronic renal failure. Skelet. Radiol. 8 (1982) 295

Hall, F. M., D. Turkel: Case report 526. Intraosseous pneumocyst of the ilium. Skelet. Radiol. 18 (1989) 127

Houghton, P.: The relationship of the pre-auricular groove of the ilium to pregnancy. Amer. J. phys. Anthropol. 41 (1974) 381

Izumi, J: The accuracy of Risser staging. Spine 20 (1995) 1868

Khouri, M. B., D. R. Kirks, S. Martinez et al.: Bilateral avulsion fractures of the anterior superior iliac spines in sprinters. Skeletal Radiol. 13 (1985) 65

Lester, P.D., W. H. McAlister: Congenital iliac anomaly with sciatic palsy. Radiology 96 (1970) 397

Little, D. G, M. D. Sussman: The Risser sign: a critical analysis. J. pediat. Orthop. 14 (1994) 569

Lombardo, St. J., A. C. Retting, R. K. Kerlan: Radiographic abnormalities of the iliac apophysis in adolescent athletes. J. Bone Jt Surg. 65-A (1983) 443

McAlister, W. H., M. J. Siegel, G. D. Shackelford: A congenital iliac anomaly often associated with sacral lipoma and ipsilateral lower extremity weakness. Skelet. Radiol. 3 (1978) 161

Metzmaker, J. N., A. M. Tappas: Avulsion fractures of the pelvis. Orthop. Trans. 4 (1980) 52

Peter, E., W. Dihlmann: Symmetrische Loosersche Umbauzonen (Milkman-Syndrom) neben den Kreuzdarmbeingelenken im Ilium. Fortschr. Röntgenstr. 100 (1964) 540

Ramirez jr., H., E. S. Blatt, H. F. Cable et al.: Intraosseous pneumatocysts of the ilium. Radiology 150 (1984) 503

Richardson, M. L., M. A. Montana: Nutrient canals of the ilium: a normal variant simulating disease on computed tomography. Skelet. Radiol. 14 (1985) 117

Risser, J. C.: Scoliosis past and present. J. Bone Jt Surg. 46-A (1964) 167

Roberto, R. F., J. E. Lonstein, R. B. Winter: Curve progression in Risser stage 0 or 1 patients after posterior spinal fusion for idiopathic scoliosis. J. pediat. Orthop. 17 (1997) 718

Rossi, F., S. Dragoni: Acute avulsion fractures of the pelvis in adolescent competitive athletes: prevalence, location and sports distribution of 203 cases collected. Skeletal Radiol. 30 (2001) 127

Sanders, J. O., J. A. Herring, R. H. Browne: Posterior arthrodesis and instrumentation in the immature (Risser-grade-O) spine in idiopathic scoliosis. J. Bone Jt Surg. 77-A (1995) 39

Schemmer, D., Ph. G. White, L. Friedman: Radiology of the paraglenoid sulcus. Skelet. Radiol. 24 (1995) 205

Sundar, M., H. Carty: Avulsion fractures of the pelvis in children: a report of 32 fractures and their outcome. Skeletal Radiol. 23 (1994) 85

Trede, H.: Symmetrische Umbauzonen (Looser-Milkman) in den Beckenschaufeln. Fortschr. Röntgenstr. 110 (1969) 279

Weinberg, S.: Intraosseous ganglion of the ilium. Skelet. Radiol. 9 (1982) 61

Pubis, Pubic Symphysis, and Ischium

Normal Findings

During Growth

The first ossification center of the pubis appears in the superior ramus, adjacent to the obturator foramen, during the 5th or 6th month of fetal development. At birth the ossification center usually encompasses the anterior border of the foramen.

The development of the ischial ossification centers parallels that in the pubis. At birth the acetabular part of the ischium, the ischial spine, and the ischial ramus and tuberosity are not yet ossified. The junction between the ischium and pubis, the **ischiopubic synchondrosis**, is of variable width (Fig. 6.**63**) and fuses over an extended period from the 4th to the 8th year of life. This timetable is somewhat uncertain because it is based on conventional radiographic studies. The bone ends that meet at the synchondrosis are generally oblique and are superimposed in the standard AP projection, so that the space between them cannot be seen (Fig. 6.**46b**).

 The synchondrosis between the pubis and ischium may appear markedly expanded (Figs. 6.**39**, 6.**46** on the left side) and mimic a pathological process (see below).

It is normal for the contours of the pubic symphysis to have a rippled appearance at about 10 years of age (Fig. 6.**39**).

During growth, isolated epiphyseal and apophyseal **ossification centers** appear about the pubic symphysis, appearing either on one side or symmetrically on both sides (Figs. 6.**40**–6.**42**).

Fine **apophyseal centers** normally appear along the lateral **ischial border,** coinciding with the appearance of centers along the iliac wing (Fig. 6.**40b**). Occasionally, a concomitant apophyseal center can be seen at the ischial tuberosity in the lateral view (Fig. 6.**40c**). Additional small, separate centers may also be visible on the ischial spine.

Like all apophyseal and epiphyseal centers, those of the pubis and ischium may persist beyond the growth period.

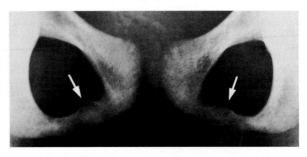

Fig. 6.**39** Ischiopubic synchondrosis (arrows) in a 12-year-old girl. The somewhat bulky shape of the synchondrosis is normal and should not be mistaken for necrosis or tumor (Fig. 6.**46**). Note also the rippled appearance of the symphyseal contours.

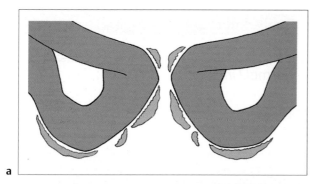

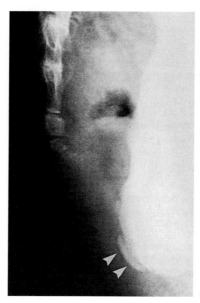

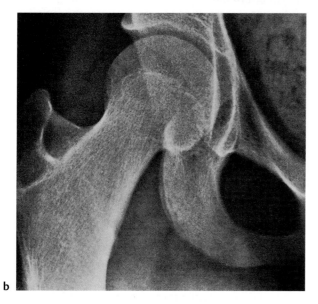

Fig. 6.**40 a–c**   Development of the ossification centers about the ischium and pubis.
a Symphyseal centers about the pubis and ischium.
b Thin apophyseal stripe along the ischium of a 13-year-old girl.
c Apophyseal centers near the ischial tuberosity (arrowheads).

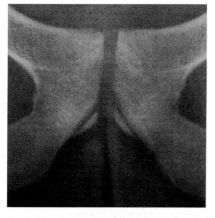

Fig. 6.**41**   Symmetrical apophyses located just below the ischia and adjacent to the pubic symphysis.

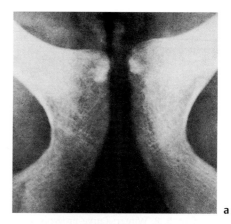

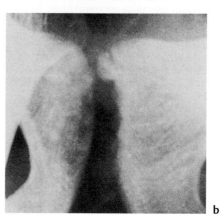

Fig. 6.**42 a, b**   Symmetrical ossification centers at the superior edge of the symphysis.   ▷
a Symmetrical projection.
b Oblique projection.

In Adulthood

Radiographs in adults will occasionally show an oblique linear or bandlike lucency, sometimes rimmed by sclerosis, located in the superior pubic ramus lateral to the tubercle. It may represent a fine groove or nutrient canal (Fig. 6.**43**).

The pubic symphysis rarely appears as a uniform space with straight, vertical edges. Usually the contours show some degree of undulation, curvature, or obliquity (Fig. 6.**43**). The space that contains fibrous and cartilaginous structures (see below) is rarely more than 5–6 mm in width.

> Small height disparities or stepoffs in the tangent to both horizontal pubic rami should not be considered pathological, especially in multiparous women.

The apposing bone ends of the pubis are covered by cartilage. Between them is a symphyseal cavity in which vacuum phenomena can occur (Fig. 6.**44**).

The pubic symphysis is spanned superiorly by the pubic ligament, which is firmly adherent to the fibrocartilaginous plate in the symphysis and extends laterally to the pubic tubercle. The symphysis is spanned inferiorly by the arcuate pubic ligament.

Pathological Finding?

 Normal Variant or Anomaly?

Reference was made above to the apophyseal structures that may be seen about the pubic symphysis. They may also occur in the form of comma-shaped ossifications at the inferior border of the body of the pubis, especially in young adults 25–27 years of age. They have no pathological significance (Fig. 6.**45**).

Fusiform expansion of the **ischiopubic synchondrosis**, even when unilateral, is a normal variant and should not be interpreted as a tumor, inflammation, or old fracture, especially when detected incidentally (Fig. 6.**46**).

An isolated ossification center may also occur within the synchondrosis.

Radiographs will occasionally show **multicentric bony elements** in the **lateral portions of the ischium**, located between the tuberosity and the acetabular part of the bone, in asymptomatic adolescents. These elements are congruent with corresponding "defects" in the adjacent portions of the ischium. They represent an extreme variant of apophyseal ossification and are not osteonecrotic lesions, especially when asymptomatic. They may be caused by increased mechanical stresses, but this is unclear (Fig. 6.**46i**). Besides the absence of clinical complaints, the bilaterality of the findings does not support a diagnosis of apophyseal necrosis. Another extreme variant of ischial apophyseal ossification is illustrated in Fig. 6.**56c–e**. In this case, delayed ossification of the many small centers mimics osteolytic lesions of the ischia.

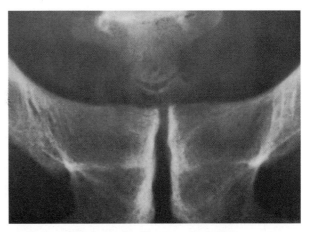

Fig. 6.**43** Oblique, groovelike structural changes passing through both superior pubic rami in a 47-year-old man.

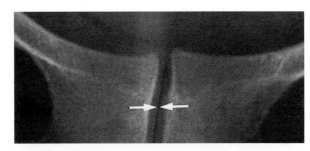

Fig. 6.**44** Vacuum cleft sign (vacuum phenomenon) in the pubic symphysis of a male (arrows). The finding is not pathological and is not even a normal variant.

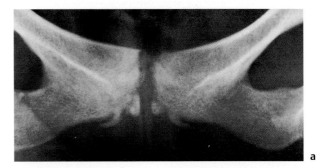

a

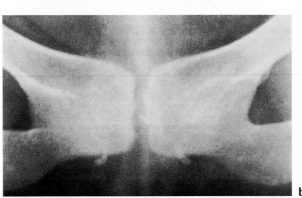

b

Fig. 6.**45a, b** Pubic symphysis.
a Symphysis with "comma-shaped ossifications" and inferior symphyseal centers in a 17-year-old girl.
b Symphysis with bilateral comma-shaped ossifications.

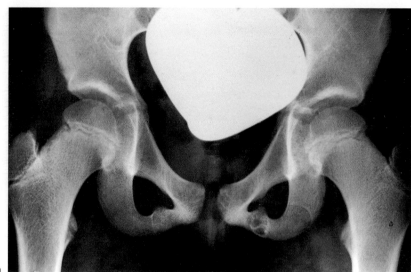

a

Fig. 6.46

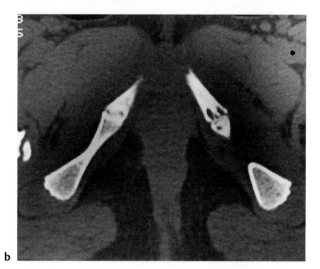

b

Fig. 6.**46 a–i**   Changes in the ischiopubic synchondrosis. Normal variants and pathological findings in the pubic and ischial region.
a–g Long-term follow-up of a tumor-simulating lesion in the left ischiopubic synchondrosis. When images **a–d** were taken, the 9-year-old boy complained of hip discomfort not inconsistent with "growing pains." The radiograph shows an "osteolytic process" involving the left ischiopubic synchondrosis. The synchondrosis on the right side is incompletely closed (see CT section in **b**) but has a fusiform shape. The CT scans show a hole-shaped defect on the left side (**b–d**), raising the possibility of a chondroma, other bone tumor, or an inflammatory process. Because the boy's complaints most likely are not referable to the finding, we regard it as a normal but extreme variant in the ossification of the ischiopubic synchondrosis, although we feel that osteonecrosis of the ischiopubic synchondrosis (van Neck disease) should still be considered as a possible diagnosis. The boy underwent no further studies or treatment. Six years later (**e**) the synchondrosis is still expanded but solid, and the patient is free of complaints. Two years after that (**f**), there is very little evidence of the original finding at the left ischiopubic junction. The final radiograph (**g**, taken four years after **f**) is essentially normal. The series of pelvic radiographs clearly document the appearance and fusion of the apophyses of the ischium and iliac crest.

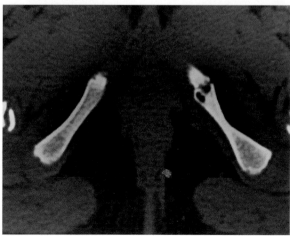

c

d

Fig. 6.**46 e–g**

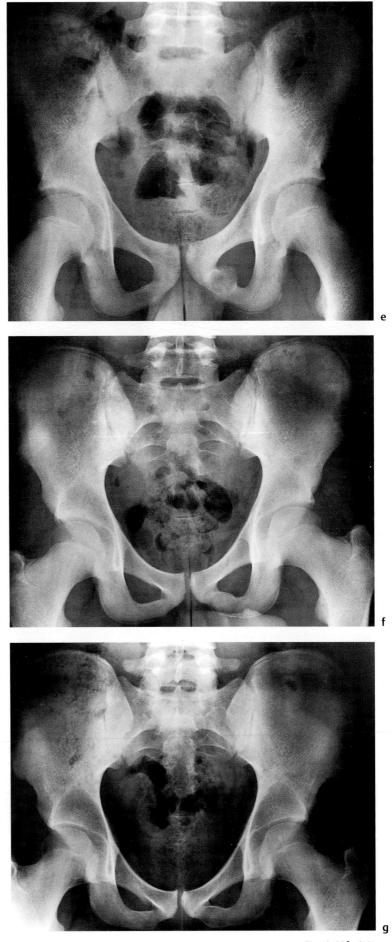

e

f

g

Fig. 6.**46 h–i** ▷

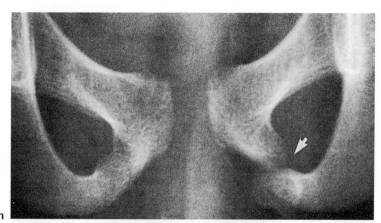

h

Fig. 6.**46 h, i**
h Broad gaping of the ischiopubic synchondrosis (arrow) and marked symphyseal separation following trauma.
i Irregular "bony outgrowths" along the lateral borders of both ischia, very likely an extreme variant (in an asymptomatic patient) due to the persistence of multiple apophyseal centers (arrows).

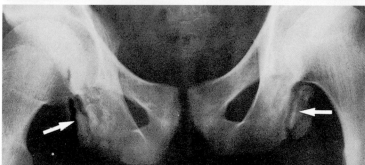

i

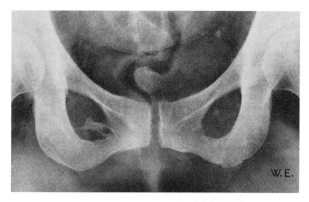

Fig. 6.**47** Unilateral bony process in the right inferior pubic angle: a normal variant in an asymptomatic patient.

Various **bony processes** of different origins may project toward the **obturator foramen** from the ischium. The rarest of these variants is illustrated in Fig. 6.**47**.

These processes most likely represent variable ossifications at the numerous ligamentous attachments that make up the obturator membrane. They also occur physiologically on the lateral border of the obturator foramen. The inferior surface of the superior pubic ramus may bear more or less pronounced tubercle-like bony protuberances that point toward the obturator foramen (Fig. 6.**48**).

Normally the processes are symmetrical on both sides but may appear asymmetrical in a nonorthograde projection. Tubercle-like prominences may form at the attachments of the gracilis muscles. Apparently these "**gracilis tubercles**" develop during growth and are not a result of productive fibro-ostosis. In any case, they are too solid to be fibro-ostotic (Fig. 6.**49**).

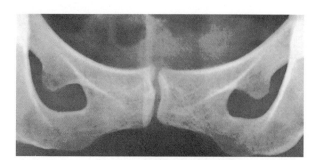

Fig. 6.**48** Symmetrical, exostosis-like protuberances jutting into the obturator foramina from the superior pubic rami. A normal variant.

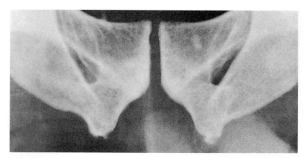

Fig. 6.**49** "Gracilis exostoses" are simply prominent, nonpathological sites of attachment for the gracilis muscles.

Sometimes it is difficult to draw a dividing line between atypical pubic configurations that are normal variants (Fig. 6.**50**) and true malformations and deformities. Often this distinction can be made only within the context of associated changes.

Mild unilateral hypoplasias of the pubis and ischium may be found in patients with hip dysplasia, muscular paralysis, etc. during skeletal growth and can lead to symphyseal laxity. A difficult situation arises when a failure of ossification of large portions of the pubis and other anomalies of the bony pelvis are detected purely by chance in an otherwise healthy young patient (Fig. 6.**51**).

Delayed or defective ossification of the pubis occurs in the congenital syndromes listed in Table 6.**4**.

A failure of pubic ossification, especially in the form of hypoplasia or aplasia, is often associated with other anomalies:

- Exstrophy of the bladder
- Epispadias or hypospadias
- Anal atresia
- Anomalies of the abdominal and pelvic muscles

Another pathological condition is **congenital fusion** of the pubic symphysis combined with **bilateral sacroiliac fusion**.

Table 6.**4** Congenital syndromes that are associated with delayed or defective ossification of the pubis (after Reeder)

Common	Rare
• Chondrodystrophy	• Achondrogenesis
• Cleidocranial dysplasia	• Camptomelic dysplasia
• Ehlers–Danlos syndrome	• Chondrodysplasia punctata (Conradi–Hünermann disease)
• Prune belly syndrome (Eagle–Barrett syndrome)	
• Congenital spondyloepiphyseal dysplasia	• Chromosome 4 p syndrome (Wolf syndrome)
	• Cryptophthalmos syndrome
	• Dyggve–Melchior–Clausen syndrome
	• Focal dermal hypoplasia (Goltz syndrome)
	• Severe hypophosphatasia
	• Larsson syndrome
	• Sjögren–Larsson syndrome
	• Taybi–Linder syndrome
	• Trisomy 9 p+ syndrome

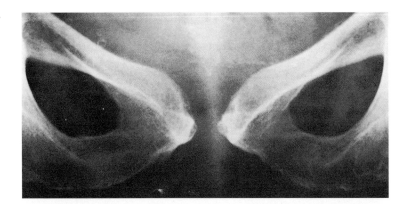

Fig. 6.**50** Symphyseal widening in an asymptomatic multipara.

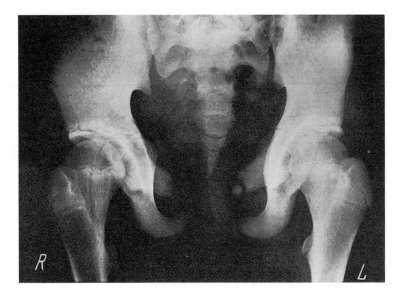

Fig. 6.**51** Absence of the symphysis in a 12-year-old girl. Complaints occurred only after the patient engaged in sports activities. (Case courtesy of Kremser, Altona.)

Fracture, Subluxation, or Dislocation?

Persistent open ischiopubic synchondroses should not be mistaken for fractures. In contrast to fractures, the contours of the still-open synchondroses usually show some degree of tapering. Also, there are no stepoffs like those seen with fractures (Fig. 6.**46h**).

Fracture-mimicking lucent lines about the ischiopubic synchondroses are occasionally caused by air trapped in the skin folds of the groin (Fig. 6.**52**).

Symphyseal ruptures are extremely difficult to diagnose in children as long as the pubic bones are not yet completely ossified. In the case shown in Fig. 6.**46h**, however, there can be no doubt about the abnormal gapping of the symphysis as there is a concomitant rupture of the ischiopubic synchondrosis on the left side.

A symphyseal rupture generally creates a more or less pronounced stepoff in the tangent to the superior pubic contours. Thus, if the symphysis gapes by more than 5–6 mm and there is a stepoff in its superior contour, it is appropriate to obtain functional views as described on p. 764.

Calcifications in the symphyseal cartilage may be a suggestive sign of a previous symphyseal rupture.

The apophyses of the ischium are subject to **traumatic apophysiolysis**, usually caused by a sudden, rapid leg movement or less commonly by chronic stress. Painful cases with increased separation of the apophysis from the parent bone are observed in sprinters, hurdlers, long jumpers, high jumpers, and pole vaulters. Further details on avulsion fractures of the ischial tuberosity during growth can be found in Table 6.**3**.

To a degree, the pubis is a site of predilection for the development of so-called **Looser transformation zones** (insufficiency or pseudo fractures) (Figs. 6.**18d**, 6.**53**). Apparently this is due to the relatively high mechanical stresses, and especially tensile stresses, that the numerous attached muscles (rectus abdominis, pectineus, adductor longus and brevis, etc.) exert on the pubis in relation to the strength of the thin bone.

Looser zones occur predominantly in the weakest parts of the horizontal pubic rami and at the junction between the pubis and ischium, i.e., the ischiopubic synchondrosis. In many cases, only radionuclide scans can detect the early structural changes that will culminate in Looser zones.

Stress fractures (fatigue type) (Fig. 6.**54**) occur at locations that follow the patterns of mechanical stresses on the pubis. In our experience, they have a tendency to occur in the acetabular part of the pubis (Fig. 6.**54**). Resnick and Guerra (1980) describe stress fractures of the inferior pubic ramus following hip operations.

Insufficiency (stress) fractures of the pubis like those occurring in osteoporosis are described by de Smet and Neff (1985).

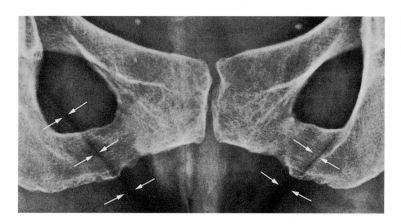

Fig. 6.**52**   Inguinal skin folds in a 45-year-old woman appear as bilateral lucent lines in the pubis, mimicking fracture lines (arrows).

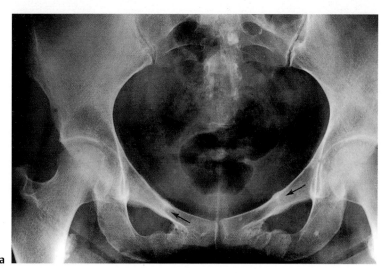

Fig. 6.**53a, b**   Looser zones (pseudofractures or insufficiency type of stress fractures) in the pubis.
a In a woman with osteomalacia. Looser zones are visible in the horizontal pubic rami and at the ischiopubic junctions, the latter showing an expanded configuration (arrows).

a

Fig. 6.53 b Bone scan from a different patient with osteomalacia due to resorption disturbances. The multiple hot spots in the pubis and ischium show a similar distribution to the case in panel **a**. An insufficiency fracture is also noted in the left femoral neck and, as is typically the case, bone resorption in the region of the right lesser trochanter and somewhat deeper in the medial femoral cortex.

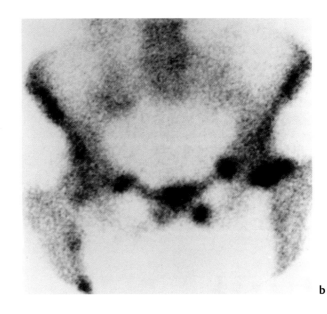

b

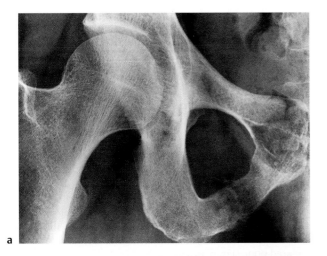

a

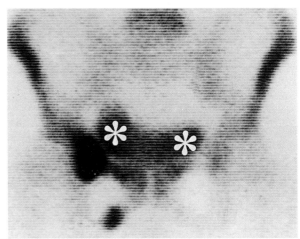

b

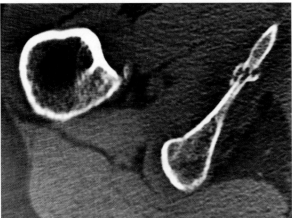

c

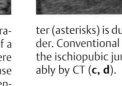

d

Fig. 6.54 a–d Stress fractures in the right horizontal pubic ramus near the acetabulum and at the ischiopubic junction of a young woman who jogged 10–15 km daily. She had severe pain on weight bearing. Bone scan shows areas of very intense uptake at both fracture sites. The increased uptake at the center (asterisks) is due to tracer accumulation in the urinary bladder. Conventional radiograph shows only the stress fracture at the ischiopubic junction. Both fractures are defined unmistakably by CT (**c, d**).

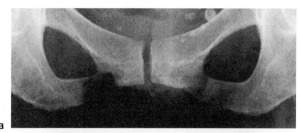

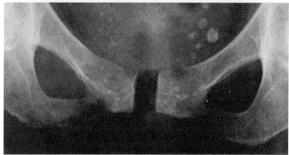

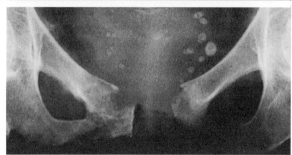

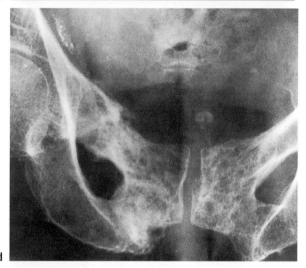

Fig. 6.**55 a–d**   Osteoradionecrosis of the pubis following radiotherapy for a gynecological tumor.
a–c Follow-ups: (**a**) 30 May 1975, (**b**) 1 September 1975, (**c**) 23 July 1976.
d Classic appearance of osteoradionecrosis with spongy rarefaction of bone structures, fragmentation, etc.

 ## Necrosis?

Osteonecrotic changes in the pubis mainly require differentiation from the many apophyseal centers that can occur about the pubis. Posttraumatic necrosis of the pubis was described by Luschnitz et al. (1967). It is unclear whether the radiographic changes that are among the features of **gracilis syndrome** also represent true osteonecrotic changes or result from a strongly rarefying fibro-ostosis. The following changes are seen in the lower portion of the pubic symphysis (Fig. 6.**61 b, c**):

● Irregular lucent areas, some with sclerotic borders
● Comma-shaped calcifications (necrotic bone?)
● Asymmetry of the symphysis
● Blurring of the pubic border on the opposite side
● Ossifications at pubic ligament attachments (Fig. 6.**61 b**) (see also Other Changes)

At one time it was more common to encounter **osteoradionecrosis** of the pubis than it is today, particularly after the radiotherapy of gynecological tumors.

The hallmarks of osteoradionecrosis are as follows:

● Increasing radiolucency
● Gradual fragmentation
● Disruption of the pubic symphysis (Fig. 6.**55 a–c**)

Advanced stages are unmistakable on radiographs and pose no problems of differential diagnosis (Fig. 6.**55 d**), whereas early stages often elude radiographic detection.

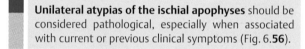

Unilateral atypias of the ischial apophyses should be considered pathological, especially when associated with current or previous clinical symptoms (Fig. 6.**56**).

These apophyseal disturbances are probably preceded by transient osteonecrosis in the growth region, as in many other necrotic conditions seen in adolescents. Interposed reparative tissue hinders apposition of the apophysis, which may remain isolated and more or less fragmented or may fuse with the parent bone via structures that are initially fibrous and later ossify. If the apophysis has sufficient growth potential, it may also enlarge to form a separate, isolated bone (Fig. 6.**56 b**).

The case in Fig. 6.**56 c–e** shows that atypical but nonpathological ossifications of the ischial apophyses can mimic "osteolytic lesions" in the ischia.

Ischiopubic osteochondrosis (van Neck disease) is basically a type of osteonecrosis or at least a growth disturbance that has a necrotic component (Fig. 6.**46 a–g**). It occurs predominantly in children 9–12 years of age. It is characterized by fusiform expansion of the ischiopubic synchondrosis, which shows marked structural irregularities and often has an isolated central "ossicle" which may correspond to a necrotic element. Diagnosis is extremely difficult, since marked expansion of the synchondrosis can occur as a normal finding (Fig. 6.**39**). Severe pain localized to the area of the synchondrosis is more suggestive of a pathological condition, as is a history of strenuous physical activity in children. Finally, a positive radionuclide bone scan can help to confirm the diagnosis.

Fig. 6.**56a–e**   Abnormalities of the ischial apophyses.
a Thickened bony contours of the ischium in a 21-year-old man. This finding is attributable to heavy mechanical stresses, which probably caused partial avulsion of the apophysis with heterotopic bone formation due to small hemorrhages.
b Older apophyseal avulsion in a 25-year-old man, which was followed by "autonomous enlargement" of the avulsed apophysis.

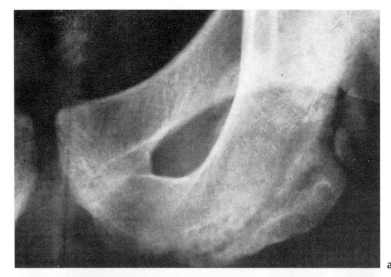

a

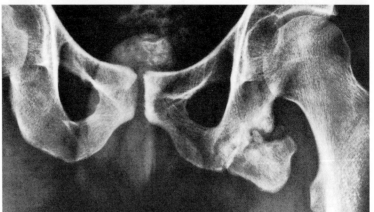

b

Fig. 6.**56c–e** ▷

 Inflammation?

Osteomyelitis can basically occur in any bone, including the pubis and ischium, although the latter bones are rarely affected. Our scope here is limited to **osteitis pubis**, which can occur after childbirth, after gynecological and urological operations, and in drug abusers (Gorricho et al. 1985). Patients present clinically with circumscribed pain, and a firm, painful mass can often be felt over the pubic symphysis. Abscess formation results in a fluctuant mass, but this is very rare and occurs only in cases of osteitis pubis that have an obvious bacterial etiology. Most cases run a slowly progressive course, and very often a causative organism cannot be detected in biopsy samples by conventional bacteriological methods because the patient has been taking antibiotics for a predominantly nonosseous inflammatory condition (cystitis, pyelonephritis, etc.). This led some authors to believe that most cases of pubic osteitis were nonspecific and abacterial, but today we must be very careful in interpreting these assessments. Based on our own experience in consultant cases and a great many percutaneous biopsies followed by more sensitive microbiological test methods (e.g., PCR), it appears that, at least in a large percentage of patients, osteitis pubis is indeed based on a bacterial infection.

Figure 6.**57** shows the progression of osteitis pubis following a transvaginal hysterectomy. The first radiograph shows only a slight blurring of the left symphyseal margin—an inherently borderline finding that must be considered pathological due to complaints of local pain on weight bearing. Eight weeks later, the symphysis has widened due to ligament destruction and shows the typical features of an inflammatory process (subchondral sclerosis, ragged bone margins, etc.). Eighteen months later, marked reparative changes have appeared and the only apparent abnormalities are those of osteoarthritis.

Osteitis pubis requires differentiation from nonspecific "**symphysitis**" (Fig. 6.**58**) in patients with a seronegative spondylarthritis. The process is the same as that occurring in the manubriosternal synchondrosis, for example (p. 335).

A final condition that can cause pubic inflammatory changes is **Paget disease**, which leads to a coarsened trabecular pattern and thickening of the cortex with a progressive increase in density and volume (Fig. 6.**19d**). Early changes are not visible on conventional radiographs and are detectable only on bone scans, appearing as large areas of abnormally increased uptake.

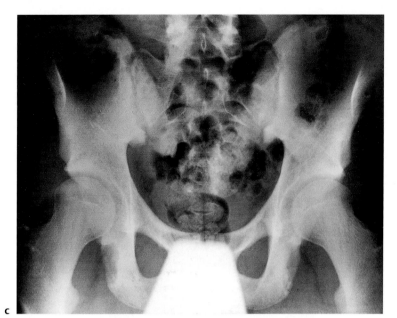

c

Fig. 6.**56 c–e**   Atypical, bilateral apophyseal ossification of the ischium of an athletically active young man 16 years of age. The patient was asymptomatic, and the finding was noted incidentally. The "osteolytic lesions" in both ischia (enlarged view of the right side in **d**) prompted a bone scan, which shows slightly increased uptake in the growth centers but no definite abnormalities. The left side of the AP radiograph (**c**) and the right side of the enlarged view (**d**) show many small apophyseal centers. The multiplicity of centers probably led to a delay in ossification.

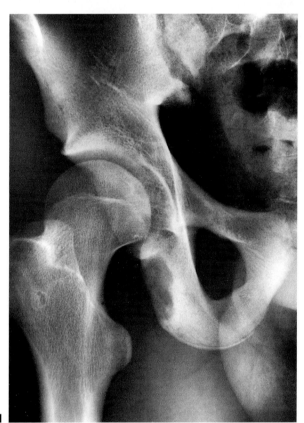

d

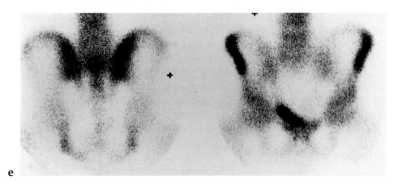

e

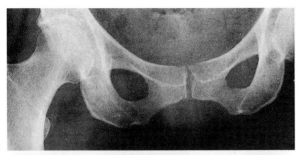
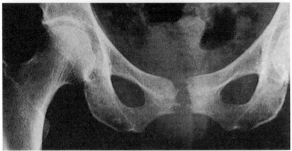
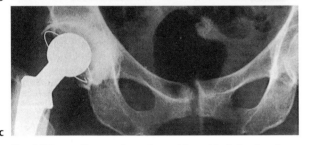

Fig. 6.**57 a–c** Progression of osteitis pubis following transvaginal hysterectomy.
a 13 June 1973.
b 8 August 1973.
c 12 February 1975.

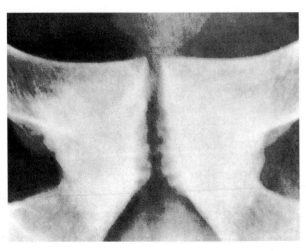

Fig. 6.**58** Symphyseal irregularities in ankylosing spondylitis.

Tumor?

Destruction of the pubis and ischium is most often caused by **metastases**. Destruction by **primary bone tumors** is very rare. Malignant lymphomas with involvement of the pubis have also been described. **Osteochondromas** of the pubis are most common in hereditary osteochondromatosis, and larger lesions are usually malignant (truncal location). Very expansile lesions with eggshell-like periosteal ossification are suspicious for an **aneurysmal bone cyst**. Approximately 3% of all aneurysmal bone cysts occur in the pubis and ischium. We will not further discuss bone destruction in the pubis by tumors, as this does not create any borderline findings with a normal pubis or with variants. **Pseudotumor-like prominences** about the ischiopubic synchondrosis can occasionally mimic a neoplasm (Fig. 6.**46 a–g**).

Figure 6.**59** illustrates the unusual case of a **giant osteoma** or **melorheostosis**. Of course, this case is definitely pathological and is not a borderline finding; but in keeping with the tradition of this book, it is presented as a special finding. The patient, a young woman, underwent radiographic examination for somewhat vague complaints in both gluteal regions. The radiological finding was incidental, therefore. A bone scan was obtained to differentiate it from a chronic inflammatory process (in the past, the finding would have been classified as osteitis condensans ischii) and from osteosarcoma. The bone scan was completely normal. This established that the lesion did not require biopsy and was an incidental finding, presumably a large osteoma or melorheostosis. Several year later the patient developed pain in her left hip with remarkable loss of motion. CT sections revealed dense bandlike fibrotic structures around the hip joint and a round calcification adjacent to the lesser trochanter, that—retrospectively—was visible on the plain film. This pattern allowed the definitive diagnosis of melorheostosis of bone with soft tissue involvement.

Other Changes?

Degenerative changes in the pubic symphysis are not unusual in older individuals, especially women who have borne several children (Fig. 6.**60**).

The finding in Fig. 6.**61 a** definitely falls within the borderline range between normal/normal variant and pathological. The patient is a 25-year-old professional soccer player with occasional pain in the symphyseal area. The radiograph shows narrowing of the symphysis, possibly due to a latent, protracted chondronecrosis, along with fine resorptive changes that are most evident on the medial aspect of the pubis on the left side, just below the symphysis. Both tubercles are slightly prominent, and there is subtle evidence of ligamentous ossification on the right side. If sports activities are continued, the present condition could develop into a **gracilis syndrome** (p. 798). Figure 6.**61 b, c** illustrates the classic gracilis syndrome in professional soccer players. In principle, the resorptive contour changes and surrounding (reactive) sclerosis correspond to a marked rarefying fibro-ostosis, probably combined with osteochondronecrosis (see Necrosis above).

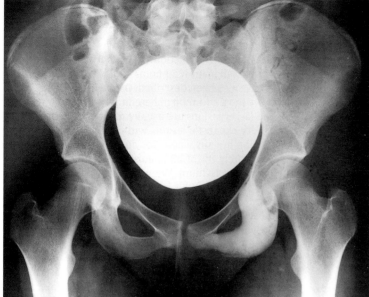

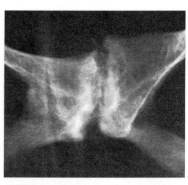

Fig. 6.**60** Chronic pelvic ring laxity with symphyseal displacement and reactive sclerosis in a 61-year-old woman.

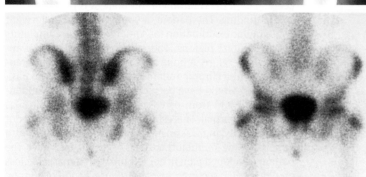

Fig. 6.**59 a, b** Giant osteoma or melorheostosis in the left ischium? Bone scans were normal (see text for a detailed case description). Note the small ossification adjacent to the lesser trochanter.

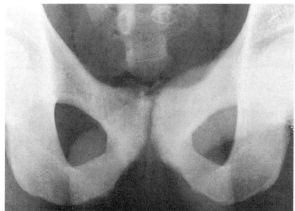

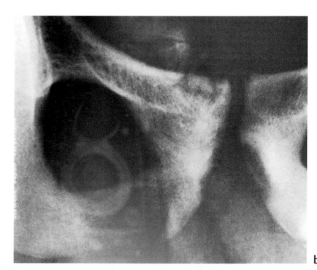

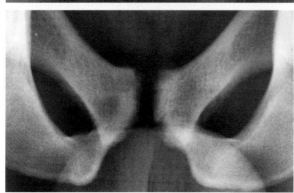

Fig. 6.**61 a–c** Regressive symphyseal changes in professional soccer players.
a Symphyseal narrowing and resorptive changes at the inferior border of the symphysis (see also text pp. 798, 801).
b Severe resorptive changes surrounded by reactive sclerosis. Comma-shaped calcification in a long, deep resorption lacuna on the left side.
c The patient presented clinically with highly acute tenderness over the symphysis. Radiograph shows slight symphyseal widening, frayed contours, and traces of "gracilis tubercles" (see p. 794).

Soft-tissue calcifications adjacent to the ischium may well result from a calcific bursitis (Fig. 6.**62**).

Differentiation is required from old apophyseal necrosis, myositis ossificans, and from dystrophic calcifications in a neoplastic process.

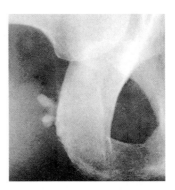

Fig. 6.**62** Bursal calcification over the ischial tuberosity. Not apophyseal necrosis.

References

de Smet, A. A., J. R. Neff: Pubic and sacral insufficiency fractures: clinical course and radiologic findings. AJR 145 (1985) 601

Dihlmann, W.: Seltene Beckenveränderungen bei der Spondylitis ankylopoetica (Morbus Bechterew). Fortschr. Röntgenstr. 97 (1962) 109

Fischer, P.: Verknöcherung am Ramus inferior pubis. Fortschr. Röntgenstr. 87 (1957) 667

Gonik, B., A. Stringer: Postpartum osteitis pubis. J. S. C. med. Ass. 78 (1985) 213

Gorricho, P., F. J. Busnea, A. Guerrero et al.: Osteomyelitis del pubis. Rev. clin. esp. 176 (1985) 138

Hillger, H., H. Schwenkenbecher: Verkalkung im Symphysenknorpel nach Symphysenruptur. Fortschr. Röntgenstr. 85 (1956) 113

Junge, H., F. Heuck: Die Osteopathia ischiopubica (gleichzeitig ein Beitrag zur normalen Entwicklung der Scham-Sitzbeinbegrenzung im Wachstumsalter). Fortschr. Röntgenstr. 78 (1953) 656

Luschnitz, E., J. Riedeberger, B. Bauchspiess: Das röntgenologische Bild der Osteonecrosis pubica posttraumatica. Fortschr. Röntgenstr. 107 (1967) 113

Maurer, H. J.: Ungewöhnliche Form eines Tuberculum obturatum anterius. Fortschr. Röntgenstr. 83 (1955) 889

Meurman, K. O. A., S. Elfving: Stress fracture in soldiers. A multifocal bone disorder. Radiology 134 (1980) 483

van Neck, M.: Ostéochondrite du pubis. Arch. franco-belg. chir. 27 (1924) 238

Nehrkorn, O.: Ungewöhnliche Apophysenentwicklungsstörung des linken Sitzbeines. Fortschr. Röntgenstr. 101 (1964) 100

Noakes, T. D., J. A. Smith, G. Lindenberg et al.: Pelvic stress fractures in long distance runners. Amer. J. Sports Med. 13 (1985) 120

Resnick, D., J. Guerra jr.: Stress fractures of the inferior pubic ramus following hips surgery. Radiology 137 (1980) 335

Rispoli, P.: Schambeinsyndrom bei Fußballspielern. Z. Orthop. 99 (1964) 87

Sandomenico, C., O. Tamburrini: Bilateral accessory ossification center of ischiopubic synchondrosis in a female infant. Pediat. Radiol. 10 (1981) 233

Seyss, R.: Zu den Verknöcherungen im Bereich des Foramen obturatum. Fortschr. Röntgenstr. 91 (1959) 525

Silverman, F. N.: Caffey's Pediatric X-Ray Diagnosis, 8th ed. Year-Book, London 1984

Smet, A. A., de, J. R. Neff: Pubic and sacral insufficiency fractures. Amer. J. Roentgenol. 145 (1985) 601

Soós, A., E. Balogh: Die aseptische Osteochondronekrose des Tuber ossis ischii als eine Form der Sportverletzung. Fortschr. Röntgenstr. 140 (1984) 740

Tehrandzadeh, J., L. A. Kurth, M. K. Elyaderani et al.: Combined pelvic stress fracture and avulsion of the adductor longus in middle-distance runners. Amer. J. Sports Med. 10 (1982) 108

Teichert, G.: Über Ossifikationsvarianten und Ossifikationsstörungen am Tuber ossis ischii. Arch. orthop. Unfall-Chir. 49 (1957) 169

Tröger, J.: Besonderheiten der Röntgendiagnostik der Synchondrosis ischiopubica und des Femurkopfes beim Kind. Radiologe 23 (1983) 59

Vix, V. A., Ch. Y. Ryu: The adult symphysis pubis, normal and abnormal. Amer. J. Röntgenol. 112 (1971) 517

Voss, A.-C: Kongenitale Aplasie der Symphyse. Fortschr. Röntgenstr. 116 (1972) 837

Walheim, G. G., G. Svelvik: Mobility of the pubic symphysis. Clin. Orthop. 191 (1984) 129

Hip Joint

Normal Findings

 During Growth

The radiographs in Fig. 6.**63** document the basic chronological development of the bony structures of the hip joint from infancy to prepuberty.

The ossification centers for the ilium, ischium, and pubis appear respectively during the 9th, 13th, and 18th week of intrauterine life. They migrate rather uniformly toward the base of the acetabulum around the time of birth. The three bony components of the **acetabulum**—the iliac, ischial, and pubic parts—are separated from one another by a Y-shaped epiphyseal plate, the **triradiate cartilage**. The vertical limb of the triradiate cartilage is between the pubis and ischium, one oblique limb is between the ischium and ilium, and the other is between the ilium and ischium. Only the oblique limbs can be identified on conventional radiographs (Fig. 6.**65**), appearing most clearly in about the 12th year of life (Fig. 6.**65**). At this time the acetabulum may bulge slightly into the interior of the pelvis. In the newborn, the bony acetabulum visible on radiographs is relatively flat. It is not until the 5th year of life that the acetabulum acquires its definitive hemispheric shape, both anatomically and radiographically, through further ossification. One or more ossification centers termed the **os** or **ossa acetabuli** consistently form in the cartilage between the ilium and pubis. They are not clearly distinguishable on conventional radiographs from bony structures located between the limbs of the triradiate cartilage. This can be done only with CT. The triradiate cartilage changes its orientation as growth progresses, the oblique limbs becoming more divergent. The roof of the acetabulum is generally very irregular in the 7- to 12-year-old child, exhibiting a ragged or rippled appearance (Fig. 6.**64**). During this period, various large ossification centers appear along the superior rim of the acetabulum (Figs. 6.**65 b**–6.**67**). These "marginal apophyses" are intracapsular. When located laterally, they can be difficult to distinguish from the apophysis of the anterior inferior iliac spine (compare Fig. 6.**23** with Figs. 6.**65 b**, 6.**66**, and 6.**67**).

The significance of the acetabular teardrop figure is discussed below.

The **first ossification center in the femoral neck** appears in about the 6th month of fetal development. In 25 % of girls and 50 % of boys, the **ossification center for the femoral head** has not yet formed by 12 months of age. The upper end of the femur in the newborn shows a prominent medial projection, the "diaphyseal peak" (Fig. 6.**63 a, b**). Disparities in the shape and size of the capital femoral ossification centers are considered normal variants during the first year of life, especially in infants that show no abnormalities on clinical examination or ultrasonography.

> Multiple ossification centers for the femoral head, especially when bilateral and not accompanied by clinical complaints, are a normal variant and should not be interpreted as Perthes disease.

From 3 to 4 years of age, the capital femoral ossification center assumes its future hemispheric shape. The growth plate between the femoral head and neck is slightly wavy and runs obliquely downward from lateral to medial. Peripheral gapping of the growth plate is normal. The head and neck fuse after 18 years of age.

The **greater trochanter** (Fig. 6.**68**) becomes radiographically visible between the 2nd and 5th years of life, usually between the 3rd and 4th years, and consists of one or more centers.

These centers fuse with each other and with the femur in about the 20th year of life. The epiphyseal line remains faintly visible on radiographs for some time, especially with the leg in external rotation. The center for the lesser trochanter (Fig. 6.**69**) appears in about the 9th year of life and fuses in the 16th–17th year.

On the whole, the range of variation in the ossification centers of the greater and lesser trochanters is relatively large. This also applies to the timing of their appearance. After an ossification center has appeared, one or more accessory centers may follow later.

Fig. 6.**63 a–f**   Development of the bony pelvis, with special ▷ reference to the hip joints.
a Boy 3 weeks of age.
b Boy 3 months of age.
c Girl 6 months of age.
d Boy one year of age, with mild pelvic tilt (p. 813).
e Boy 6 years of age.
f Boy 10 years of age.

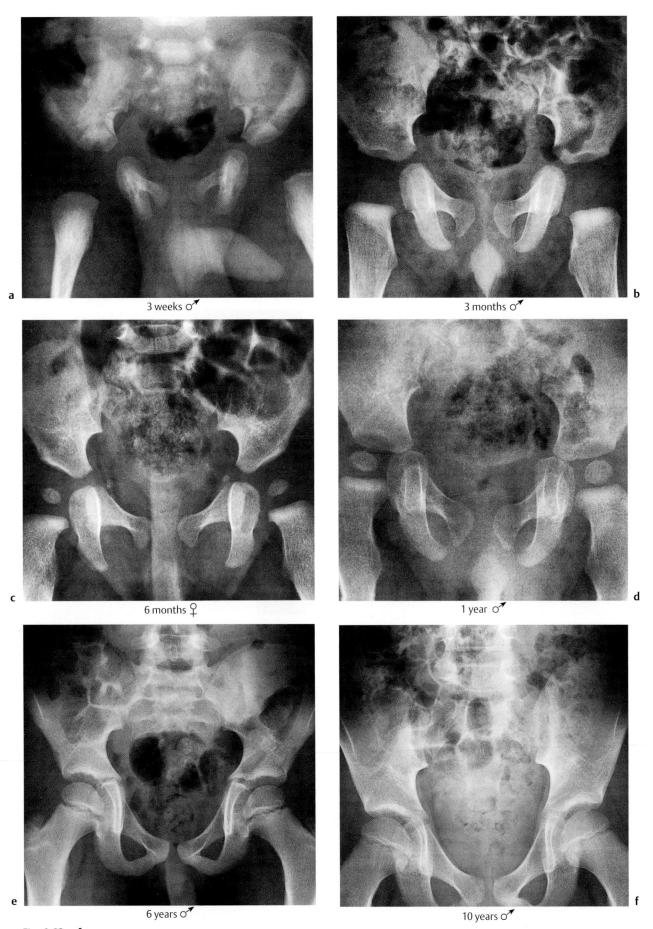

a   3 weeks ♂

b   3 months ♂

c   6 months ♀

d   1 year ♂

e   6 years ♂

f   10 years ♂

Fig. 6.**63 a–f**

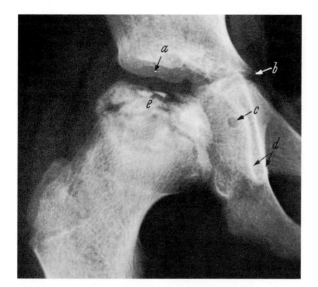

Fig. 6.**64**   Typical appearance of the acetabulum in an 8- to 9-year-old boy, who suffered from Perthes disease. At this stage of the disease the normal anatomy of the acetabulum is not altered.
a Acetabular roof, with typical rippling.
b Triradiate cartilage.
c Nutrient canal.
d Acetabular teardrop figure.
e Femoral head necrosis.

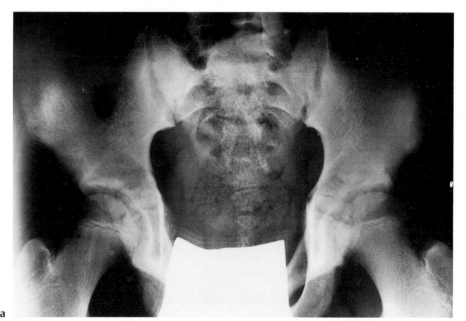

Fig. 6.**65 a–c**   Typical appearance of the acetabula in a 13-year-old boy. Note the numerous, largely asymmetrical lucent lines that represent portions of the intra-acetabular triradiate cartilage. A number of small centers are located between the lucent lines. In the enlarged views in **b** and **c**, note also the marginal epiphyseal centers of the acetabulum, which are particularly distinct on the right side.

a

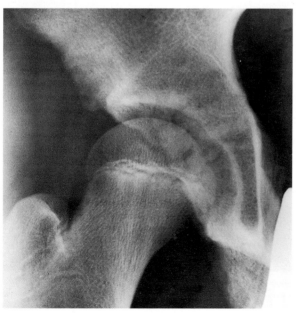

b

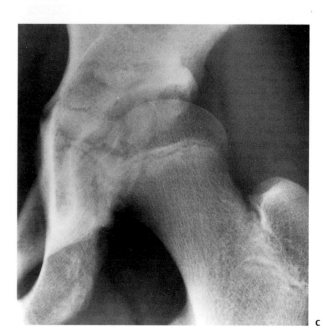

c

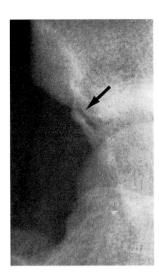

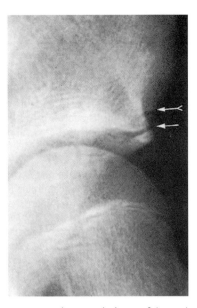

Fig. 6.**66** Lateral apophysis of the acetabular roof ("radiographic os acetabuli" in the old nomenclature) (arrow).

Fig. 6.**67** Ossification center in the acetabular roof (arrow) closely adjacent to the anterior inferior iliac spine (double arrow).

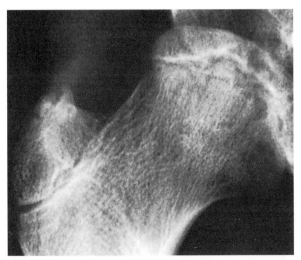

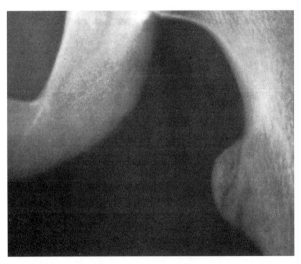

a

Fig. 6.**68** Typical ossification center in the greater trochanter (femoral head shows changes of Legg–Calvé–Perthes disease).

Fig. 6.**69 a–e** Radiographic morphology of the lesser trochanter.
a Apophysis of the lesser trochanter, which first appears in about the 9th year of life.

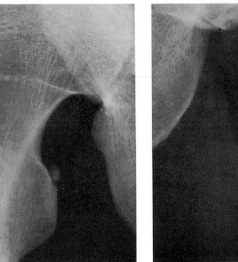

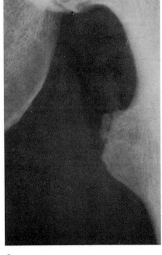

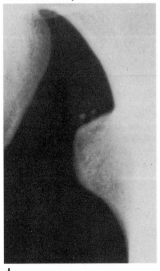

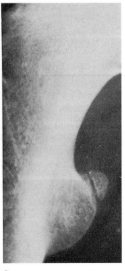

b

c

d

e

Fig. 6.**69 b–e** Persistent accessory apophyseal centers, a normal variant.

In Adulthood

Appearance of the Hip Joint on Conventional Radiographs

The anterior margin of the acetabulum is generally difficult to define on plain radiographs, as it is superimposed on the posterior margin. The latter is more peripheral and easier to identify. The floor of the acetabulum is normally projected as a shallow semicircle, deepened at its center by the acetabular fossa.

A very useful reference line is the **acetabular teardrop figure**. The wall of the acetabular fossa forms the lateral boundary of the teardrop figure, and the cortex of the ischioilial pelvic wall forms its medial boundary (Figs. 6. **70**, 6.**71**).

The teardrop figure, first described by Köhler (the original author of this book), can be seen in its typical configuration only when the central ray is focused on the median plane (Figs. 6.**70**, 6.**72**). It first appears in about the 5th month of life. Variants of the teardrop figure with a normal pelvic position are shown in Fig. 6.**72 a–d**. Degrees of teardrop distortion that exceed the normal variants occur in various forms of hip dysplasia, and fractures about the hip can cause discontinuities in the teardrop (see below).

The subchondral plate of the acetabulum is denser and broader in the pressure-bearing zone than in the floor or margins. On radiographs this creates an eyebrowlike figure in the upper part of the acetabulum. If the pressure load is increased (e.g., due to coxa valga or damage to the shock-absorber function of the articular cartilage), this zone expands and broadens laterally through the acetabular roof (Fig. 6.**73 b**), producing the **eyebrow sign**.

> Thus the **pressure-bearing zone of the acetabulum has a variable shape**, and the eyebrow sign has pathological significance only when accompanied by evidence of osteoarthritis (joint space narrowing, osteophytes, etc.).

The **femoral head** normally appears slightly more than hemispherical on radiographs and presents a uniformly smooth, sharply defined surface. The center of the femoral head opposite the triradiate cartilage bears a small depression, the fovea capitis, where the ligamentum teres is attached. Increased radiolucency in the lower quadrant of the femoral head is a normal finding (Fig. 6.**73 a**).

The radiographic appearance of the **femoral neck** depends entirely on the positioning technique (Fig. 6.**74 a, b**):

- In external rotation, the lesser trochanter appears prominent while the femoral neck angle appears increased and the neck itself is foreshortened (Fig. 6.**74 b**).
- The neck-shaft angle is most accurately measured in slight internal rotation (20° of internal rotation is recommended for standard radiographs). This gives a clear projection of the femoral neck. Only the tip of the lesser trochanter is visible (Fig. 6.**74 a**).

Small tubercles on the medial femoral neck (Fig. 6.**74 c, d**) are still considered a normal variant, especially when coxa valga is present. The presence of coxa valga in itself does not have pathological significance.

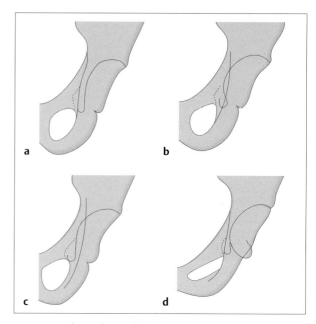

Fig. 6.**70 a–d**   Radiographic variants of the acetabular teardrop figure (original drawings by A. Köhler).

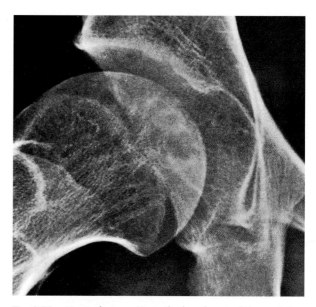

Fig. 6.**71**   Atypical concavity in the basal part of the acetabulum, with narrowing of the teardrop figure.

Fig. 6.**72 a–h** Schematic representation of the variable appearance of the teardrop figure in adults (after Peic).
a–d Variable widths seen with a normal pelvic position.
e–g Crossing of the teardrop figure with different distances of the central ray from the median plane.
h In an oblique projection of the pelvis, the inner margin of the teardrop figure appears as a thin, sclerotic line. The anterior line appears more dense (ilioischial line of Armbruster).

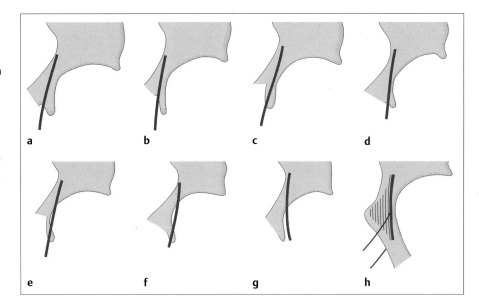

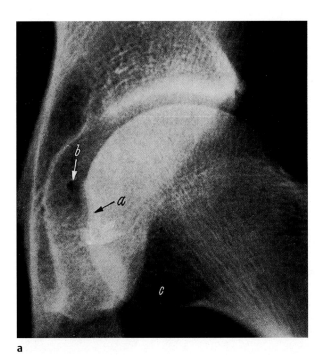

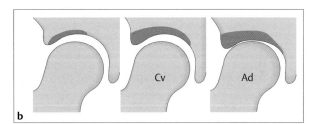

Fig. 6.**73 a, b** On the morphology of the femoral head and acetabulum.
a Fovea capitis (a), nutrient canal in the acetabular floor (b), and "osteolysis" simulated by a normal rarefied area in the lower quadrant of the femoral head (c) in a 35-year-old man.
b Eyebrow sign.
Cv Coxa valga
Ad Degenerative arthritis (osteoarthritis)

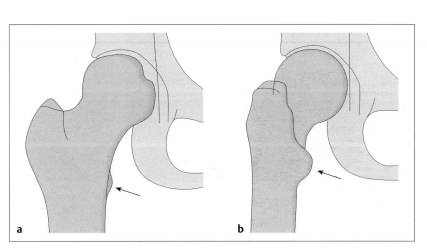

Fig. 6.**74 a–d** Morphology of the femoral neck.
a, b Projection of the femoral neck and lesser trochanter in internal rotation (**a**) and external rotation (**b**).

Fig. 6.**74 c** and **d** ▷

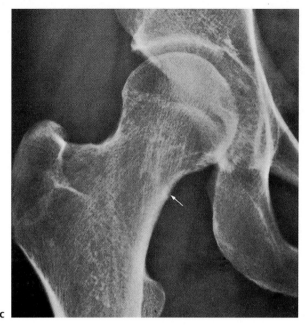

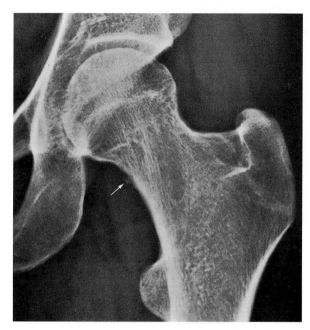

c

d

Fig. 6.**74 c, d**   Bilateral coxa valga in an asymptomatic 30-year-old woman. The small tubercles on the medial aspect of both femoral necks are a normal variant (arrows).

The **width of the hip joint space** averages 4–5 mm in the pressure-transfer zone, with a lower limit of 3 mm. It should be noted that these values are projected widths, since the relatively large object-film distance in hip radiographs causes considerable geometric magnification. The width of the hip joint space in the 45- to 85-year-old population is not gender- or age-dependent and is not affected by overweight (Pogrund et al. 1983). The **maximum width of the capsular structures** of the hip joint (fibrous capsule and synovial membrane) on CT scans is approximately

6 mm. A greater width signifies effusion (with subcapsular fluid, Fig. 6.**128 a**) and/or a proliferative synovial process (synovitis, tumor, or tumorlike lesion).

The bony structures in the lateral portions of the greater trochanter normally show less radiographic density.

Semiaxial views of the hip show linear densities or lucencies that are caused by the groin crease. Lucent lines that are projected over the femoral neck or ischium can mimic fracture lines (Fig. 6.**75 b**). Linear densities or lucencies caused by overlying soft tissues are easy to recognize

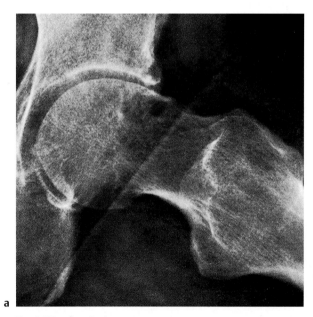

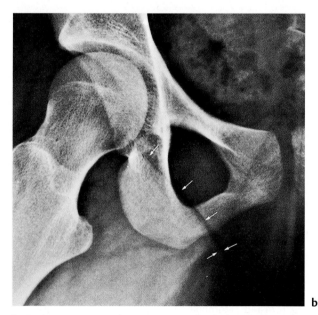

a

b

Fig. 6.**75 a, b**   Groin crease.
a Typical appearance of the groin crease on a Lauenstein projection of the hip. The lucent streak extends past the femoral neck and crosses part of the ischium.

b Groin crease on the opposite side (arrows) (see also Fig. 6.**52**).

as such, however, by noting that they transcend the boundaries of the bony structures.

Linear lucencies in the hip joint space represent a physiological vacuum phenomenon caused by gaseous nitrogen that has been released from body fluids into the joint in response to a low intra-articular pressure (e.g., in recumbency or hip abduction) (Fig. 6.**134 b**).

Imaging the Hip Joint with CT, MRI, and MR Arthrography

The above descriptions of the hip joint were based on conventional radiographs. The various radiographic projections of the hip can be understood, however, only if the normal anatomy is known (Fig. 6.**76**) and is also "reconstructed" on sectional images. Figure 6.**77** shows a series of typical **axial CT scans** through the hip joint.

MRI has become increasingly important in hip examinations, based largely on its ability to define soft-tissue structures like the cartilage, capsule, labrum, etc. It is important to know the **typical signal characteristics**, especially of the femoral head during growth, to avoid misinterpreting MR images of the hip joint. As growth progresses, the signal intensity of the femoral head on SE sequences increases due to the increasing conversion of red marrow to fat marrow.

As a result of this, the femoral epiphyses become increasingly "white" with aging (Fig. 6.**78**).

In adults, the femoral head has a relatively nonhomogeneous MRI signal intensity that includes broad bands of low intensity extending in the posteromedial-to-anterolateral direction (Fig. 6.**78 c, d**). The articular cartilage appears as a halo surrounding the femoral head. Koo et al. (1998) made a very detailed study of age-related bone marrow conversion in the proximal metaphysis of the femur on T1-weighted images. The **acetabular labrum** is among the anatomic structures that are defined particularly well by **MR arthrography**. In current orthopedic practice, MR studies of the labrum play a major role in the investigation of hip pain (e.g., after hip trauma and in hip dysplasia). In the past, arthroscopy was the only tool available for examinations of the labrum. The labrum encircles the entire outer rim of the acetabulum, being attached at the bony acetabular margin (limbus) and the transverse ligament. The transverse ligament bridges the acetabular notch (incisura acetabuli) and the bony margin of the acetabulum (Fig. 6.**76**). The labrum is composed of fibrocartilage and tough connective tissue. It is triangular in cross section and is continuous internally with the lunate surface. The main function of the labrum is to compensate for irregularities in the bony limbus. The joint capsule is attached externally to the limbus at the base of the labrum. This arrangement forms the perilimbic recess, which allows the labrum to project freely into the joint cavity.

Evaluation of the acetabular labrum by MR arthrography requires a great deal of experience. It is important to know the variants and the specific tear patterns identified by Czerny et al. (Fig. 6.**79**) and to understand that the la-

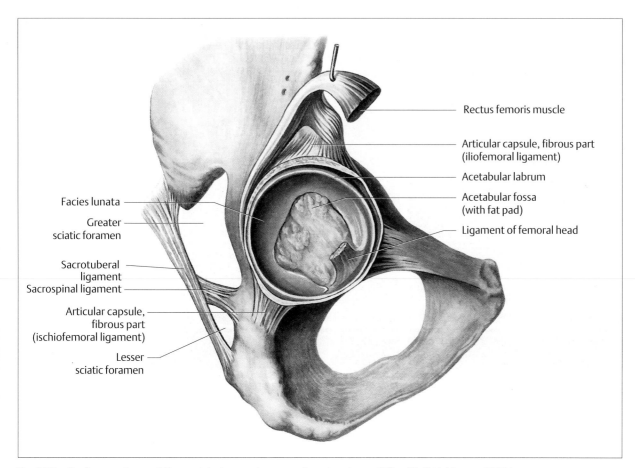

Fig. 6.**76** Surface anatomy of the acetabulum and surrounding structures. (After Wolf-Heidegger 1961.)

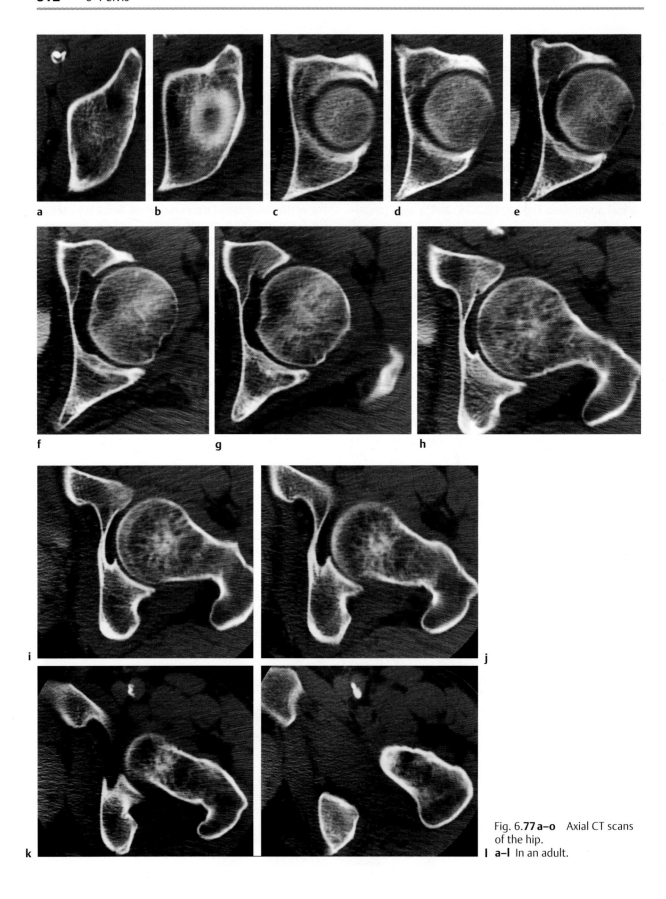

a b c d e

f g h

i j

k l

Fig. 6.**77 a–o** Axial CT scans of the hip.
a–l In an adult.

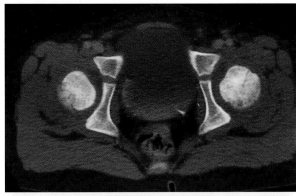

m

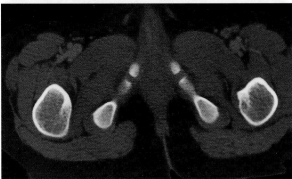

n

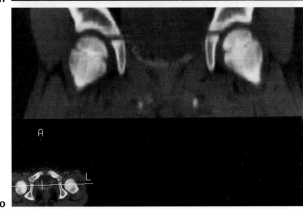

o

Fig. 6.**77 m–o**   In a 5-year-old child. The ischiopubic plate is shown in **m**, and the ilioischial plate is shown in **o** (frontal reconstruction). The perpendicularity of the two plates is readily appreciated. The spaces in **n** represent the ischiopubic synchondrosis.

brum undergoes degenerative changes with aging that do not necessarily have pathological significance (Czerny et al. 1999, Abe et al. 2000, Petersilge 2001).

Figure 6.**80** shows a labral tear and detachment demonstrated by MR arthrography.

Radiographic Measurements of the Hip

Dysplasia of the hip is not uncommon in infants, children, and adults (see below). An experienced radiologist can tell a dysplastic hip from a healthy hip "at first glance," but even so will have to take measurements when findings are borderline. Hip dysplasia is generally considered a pre-osteoarthritic condition, and there are certain patterns of measurements that have therapeutic implications. The measurements are designed to detect abnormalities in the shape of the acetabulum and proximal femur as well as possible faulty positioning of the upper femur in the hip joint.

Criteria for radiographic positioning

➤ The iliac wings and obturator foramina should appear roughly symmetrical on both sides. Angles can be substantially altered if the pelvis is rotated about the longitudinal body axis. For example, the *acetabular angle*, or measurable slope of the acetabular roof, is increased by body rotation toward the opposite side and decreased by rotation toward the same side.

➤ In the supine AP pelvic radiograph, the pubic symphysis appears below the level of the sacral promontory. This results from the physiological inclination of the pelvis, the linea terminalis forming a 50–70° angle with the horizontal in upright stance. In patients with *pelvic tilt* (increased pelvic inclination), the pubic symphysis is projected at a lower level, the measurable acetabular angle is decreased, and the shape of the Kopits rectangle is altered (Fig. 6.**83 a**). With an *upright pelvis* (decreased pelvic inclination), the symphysis is projected at a higher level and the acetabular angle is increased. Pelvic inclination can be evaluated by noting the relationship between the superior borders of the pubis and ischium on the AP radiograph: the upper contours of both bones should align. If pelvic inclination is increased, the upper contour of the ischium extends past that of the pubis (Fig. 6.**63 d**). If pelvic inclination is decreased, the opposite relationship is seen. With a normal pelvic inclination, the *Hilgenreiner line* through the triradiate cartilages lies approximately between the S4 and S5 vertebrae.

➤ The AP pelvic radiograph should be obtained with the legs in *neutral rotation*. This is achieved by flexing the knees 90° over the edge of the x-ray table.

Adduction and *abduction of the thighs* can produce distortions in various measurements (e.g., the β angle).

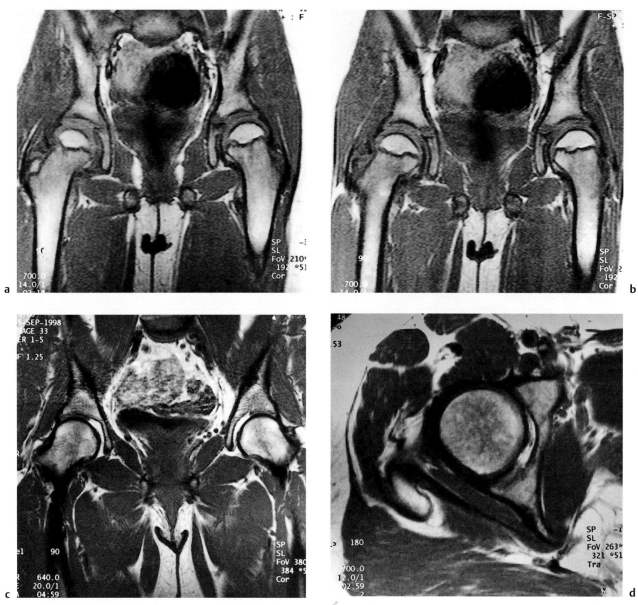

Fig. 6.**78 a–d**   Typical MR images of the hip joint, coronal and axial.
a, b Child 5 years of age.
c, d Adult.

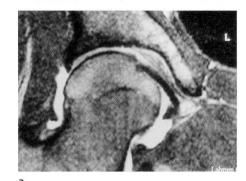 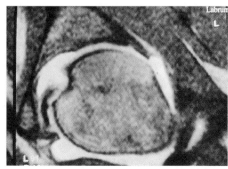

Fig. 6.**79 a–c**   The labrum visualized by MR arthrography.
a, b Normal labrum.
c   ▷

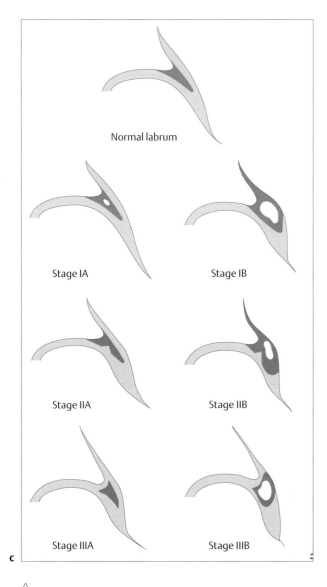

c

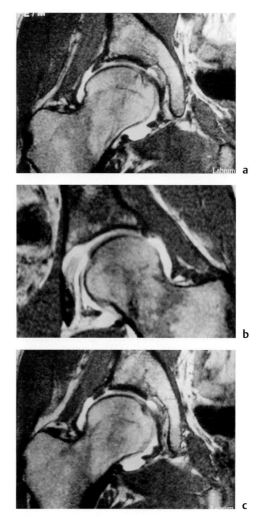

a

b

c

Fig. 6.**80 a–c**   Labral lesion on MR arthrography.
a, b Type IIA labral tears.
c Labral detachment (avulsion).

△
Fig. 6.**79 c**   Classification of lesions of the acetabular labrum.
(After Czerny et al. 1996.)

Stage I: Degeneration.
Stage IA: Circumscribed hyperintensity at the center of the
                   labrum.
Stage IB: Like IA, but the labrum is thickened and there is no
                   visible labral recess.
Stage II: Tear.
Stage IIA: Contrast medium enters the labrum, which is not
                   detached from the acetabulum; it is triangular and
                   has a labral recess.
Stage IIB: Like IIA, but the labrum is thickened and there is no
                   visible labral recess.
Stage III: Avulsion.
Stage IIIA: The labrum is detached from the acetabulum but
                   still has a triangular configuration.
Stage IIIB: The labrum is thickened and detached from the
                   acetabulum.

Measurements of the hip in newborn and children

Andrén View:

The Andrén view (Fig. 6.**81**) is a supine radiograph obtained with both femurs strongly rotated internally and
abducted 45°.

Normally an upward extension of the longitudinal axis
of the femoral shaft will pass through the superior lateral
rim of the acetabulum. In conditions ranging from subluxation to severe hip dysplasia with dislocation, the line
will pass through the pelvis above the acetabulum. Generally this method can be successfully used **in the first
weeks of life** to provoke and detect malalignments of the
hip bones from the subluxation stage onward.

Hilgenreiner Line:

The distance of the femoral metaphysis from the Hilgenreiner line through the triradiate cartilages (Fig. 6.**82**) can
be used to measure proximal migration of the femur.

Ombrédanne Line:

The Ombrédanne line (Fig. 6.**82**) is a line drawn through
the superior acetabular rim, perpendicular to the Hilgenreiner line. If the diaphyseal peak is located above a line
drawn tangent to the superior border of the obturator
foramina and parallel to the Hilgenreiner line, and if it is
lateral to the Ombrédanne line, it is very likely that a subluxation or dislocation is present (left hip in Fig. 6.**82**).

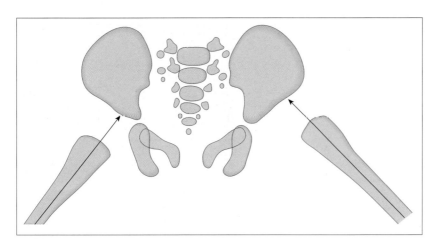

Fig. 6.**81**   Andrén radiograph of the hip joints.

Ménard–Shanton Line:
The Ménard–Shanton line is a smooth, continuous curve that follows the inferior border of the ascending pubic ramus and the inferior contour of the femoral neck. Any discontinuity in this curve signifies a subluxation. One disadvantage of this method is that it is extremely dependent on correct positioning (the femurs must be strictly parallel with no abduction or adduction, etc.).

Acetabular Angle (Acetabular Index, Fig. 6.82):
A line is drawn from the most inferior point of the ilium at the triradiate cartilage to the superior acetabular rim. The angle between that line and the Hilgenreiner line is defined as the acetabular angle. Normal values are as follows: in infants 29° (boys) and 32° (girls); at 18 months 26° (boys) and 28° (girls); and at 12 months 24° (boys) and 26° (girls). The acetabular angle declines with further aging, reaching values as low as 18° (boys) and 19° (girls) by 7 years of age. Since the acetabular roof still has a normal shape in most newborns, the acetabular angle is very rarely abnormal during the first three months of life, cast-

ing doubt on the value of measuring the angle during that period.

Kopits Parallelogram (Fig. 6.83 a, left):
Lines tangent to the acetabular roof and the proximal femoral metaphysis are normally parallel and form a right parallelogram when their end points are connected. In a dysplastic hip, the tangents form a rhomboid (B), or an oblique parallelogram with unequal sides. The capital femoral ossification center is located outside the rhomboid.

Beta Angle of Zsernaviczky and Türk (Fig. 6.83 b, right):
This angle is formed by a tangent to the proximal end of the femur and a line connecting the medial metaphyseal peak to the superior acetabular rim. The normal range is from 35° to 56°. Higher values signify a pathological condition. The Z line that connects the metaphyseal peak to the acetabular rim should pass through the epiphyseal center (if it is visible).

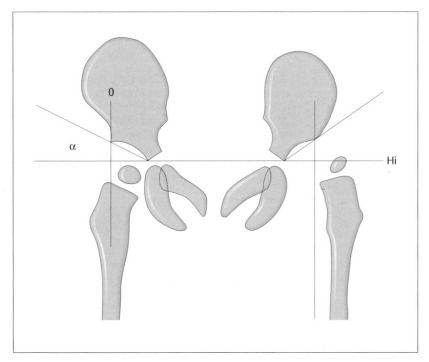

Fig. 6.**82**   Reference lines and angles for detecting (congenital) hip dysplasia. The right hip joint is normal; the left hip joint is dysplastic.
α   Acetabular angle
0   Line through the lateral acetabular rim, perpendicular to the Hilgenreiner line
Hi Hilgenreiner line through the triradiate cartilages

Femur–Iliac Angle of Grossmann (Fig. 6.83 c):
A line is drawn connecting the point at which the Ménard–Shanton line leaves the femoral neck to the point at the superior inner border of the ilium in the triradiate cartilage. The angle formed by this line with the Hilgenreiner line (Hi in Fig. 6.82) is called the gamma angle or femur-iliac angle. The relationship of this angle to the acetabular angle yields a ratio whose numerical value expresses the risk of hip dislocation.

Measurements of the Acetabulum after Puberty

The following methods are recommended for radiographic measurements of the acetabulum after puberty (Delaunay et al. 1997).

- *Center–edge (CE) angle of Wiberg* (Fig. 6.84). The CE angle lies between a vertical line through the center of the femoral head (parallel to the vertical body axis) and a line connecting the center of the femoral head to the superolateral rim of the acetabulum. The CE angle defines the lateral and superior coverage of the femoral head by the bony acetabulum. According to Wiberg, normal values are greater than 25°. Values from 20° to 25° are borderline, and values less than 20° indicate acetabular dysplasia. According to Delaunay et al. (1997), the vertical line through the center of the femoral head should be perpendicular to a line through the centers of both femoral heads. When the CE angle is determined in small children, it should be considered that the angle tends to alter with external rotation of the femur, because the femur then deviates slightly in a lateral position. Care should be taken, therefore, to position the child with the legs extended and both patellae facing precisely forward (upward).
- *HTE angle* ("horizontal toit extern" angle; Fig. 6.85). This angle defines the slope of the acetabular roof in the coronal plane and gives information on the superolateral coverage of the femoral head (Lequesne 1963). An oblique line is drawn from the superior acetabular rim (E) to point T, which is the most medial point of the weight-bearing portion of the acetabulum (i.e., the medial end of the "eyebrow"). The angle between that line and a horizontal line through the centers of the both femoral heads is the HTE angle, which normally measures 10° or less. Values greater than 10° signify acetabular dysplasia.
- *Acetabular depth-to-width index* (Fig. 6.86). The width (*W*) of the acetabulum is measured from the superolateral rim to the lowest point of the acetabulum. Acetabular depth *d* is defined as the length of a line drawn from point T (the medial end of the "eyebrow") perpendicular to line defining *W*. The depth-to-width index is obtained by taking the ratio of depth to width (*d/W*) and multiplying it by 100. The normal value in adults is approximately 60. In a comparison of normal hips and dysplastic hips with secondary osteoarthritis, all of the dysplastic hips had an index of less than 39 (Murphy et al. 1995).
- *False-profile view and VCA angle* (after Lequesne and de Séze 1961; Fig. 6.87). When an acetabular abnormality is detected on the AP pelvic radiograph, especially a deficiency of acetabular roof coverage (CE angle), a false-profile view of the pelvis can be obtained to define the anterior acetabular coverage. This view represents a true lateral projection of the abnormal hip and permits the measurement of anterior acetabular coverage. It

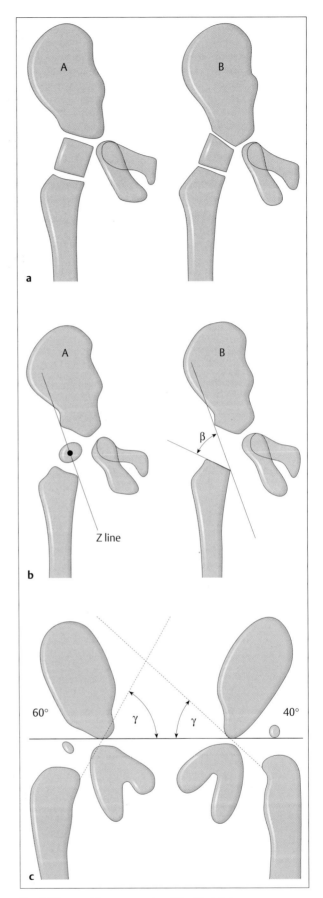

Fig. 6.**83 a–c**   Measurements of the hip joint.
a Kopits parallelogram.
b Z line (A) and β angle (B) of Zsernaviczky and Türk.
c Femur–iliac (gamma) angle of Grossmann.

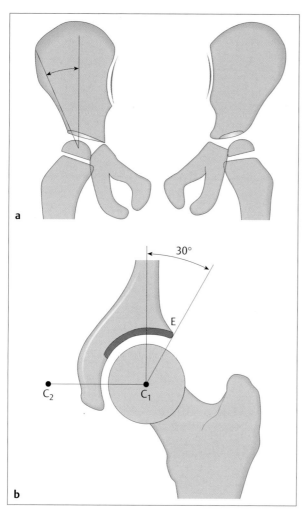

Fig. 6.84 a, b Center–edge (CE) angle of Wiberg.
a In a child.
b In an adult.

also helps to detect early degenerative changes in the anterior portion of the acetabulum. The anterior acetabulum cannot be properly evaluated on AP, semi-axial, or axial radiographs. The false-profile view is obtained with the patient standing ("stress" radiograph of the hip) and the pelvis rotated 65° relative to the cassette. In an accurate projection, the distance between the femoral heads should approximately equal the diameter of one femoral head. Anterior acetabular coverage is measured by determining the VCA angle (vertical-center-anterior angle of Lequesne) on the radiograph. It lies between a vertical line perpendicular to the line connecting the femoral heads and an oblique line from the center of the femoral head to the most anterior point on the acetabular rim (Fig. 6.**87 b**). Values greater than 25° are normal, similar to the CE angle. Lower values signify acetabular dysplasia.

- *Computed tomography.* CT would appear to be an ideal method for defining the acetabular configuration. A good description of the use of CT in acetabular dysplasia can be found in Anda et al. (1991). First a scout view of the pelvis is obtained, followed by axial scans through the center of both femoral heads. Anterior acetabular coverage is defined by the anterior acetabular sector angle (AASA), posterior acetabular coverage by the posterior acetabular sector angle (PASA). Global acetabular coverage can be measured by the horizontal acetabular sector angle (HASA). A line is drawn through the centers of both femoral heads (line C1-C2). Then an oblique line is drawn from the center of each femoral head to the anterior and posterior acetabular rim. The angle between line C1-C2 and the anterior acetabulum (AASA) averages 63° in men and 64° in women. The PASA angle averages 105° for both sexes. Smaller values are measured in patients with hip dysplasia. The HASA values are calculated from the sum of AASA and PASA. Hip dysplasia is most commonly associated with anterior acetabular hypoplasia and deficient coverage of the femoral head (Fig. 6.**88**).

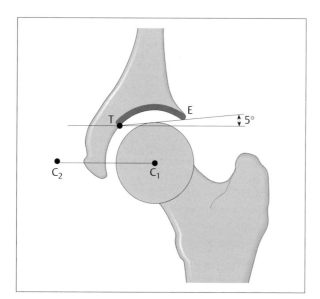

Fig. 6.85 a, b HTE ("horizontal toit extern") angle.

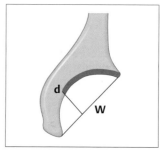

Fig. 6.86 Acetabular depth-to-width index.

Fig. 6.**87 a, b** False profile view.
a Positioning technique.
b VCA angle.

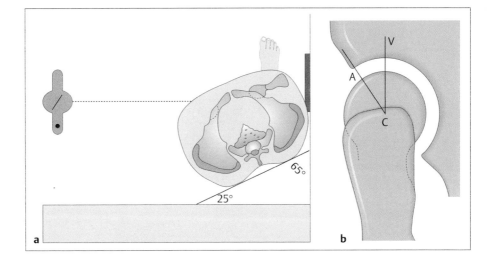

Measurements of the Femoral Head

- *Conventional radiographs.* The shape and position of the femoral head can be evaluated reasonably well on conventional AP radiographs. Normally the femoral head is round and congruent with the acetabulum. In congenital hip dysplasia, the femoral head may be abnormally flat and/or laterally displaced, causing loss of congruence with the acetabulum and predisposing to secondary osteoarthritis.

> The congruence between the femoral head and acetabulum is defined as the percentage of the femoral head that is covered by the acetabulum (Fig. 6.**89**).

This is determined by drawing three vertical lines: line 1 through the most medial part of the joint space, line 2 through the lateral boundary of the acetabulum, and line 3 through the most lateral border of the femoral head. The distance between lines 1 and 2 (*A*) is divided by the distance between lines 1 and 3 (*B*). The ratio *A/B* is multiplied by 100. Values less than 75% are considered abnormal.

- *Computed tomography.* CT is excellent for evaluating the shape of the femoral head, especially when multiplanar reconstructions are used. Apparently, however, no specific CT measurements have been devised for evaluating the shape and position of the femoral head.

Measurements of the Proximal Femur

- *Center–collum–diaphyseal (CCD) angle* (Fig. 6.**90 a**). The CCD angle is formed by lines drawn along the axis of the femoral shaft and along the axis of the femoral neck through the center of the femoral head. The center of the femoral neck is located as follows: A circular arc drawn around the center of the femoral head (C) intersects points on the medial and lateral contours of the femoral neck. A line is drawn connecting these points, and a bisector is constructed. The line connecting the center of the femoral head and the midpoint defined by the bisector is extended to define the line of the femoral neck axis. The femoral shaft axis is drawn through two points obtained by bisecting two transverse diameters of the subtrochanteric femoral shaft. Normal values for

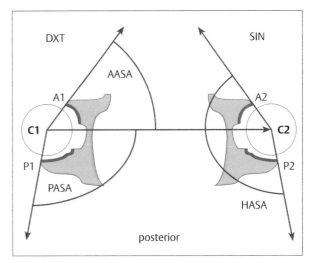

Fig. 6.**88** Determination of acetabular coverage by CT.

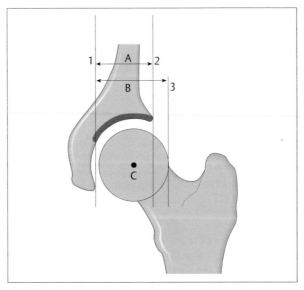

Fig. 6.**89** Percent coverage of the femoral head by the acetabulum: (*A/B*)×100. Values less than 75% are abnormal.

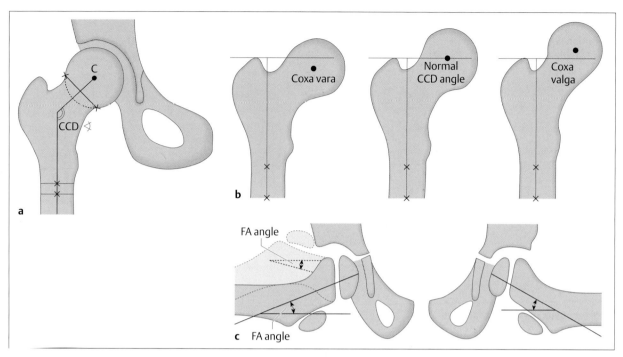

Fig. 6.90 a–c   CCD angle and femoral anteversion angle.
a Determination of the CCD angle.
b Simplified assessment of the CCD angle.

c Determination of the femoral anteversion angle by the method of Rippstein.

the CCD angle range from 125° to 135°. Angles less than 125° signify coxa vara, angles greater than 140° coxa valga. It should be added that in patients with congenital coxa vara, the medial contour of the femoral neck is often not defined. In this case the medial point of intersection with the circular arc is replaced by the point where a perpendicular to the femoral shaft axis intersects the highest point on the inferomedial contour of the femoral neck in defining the center of the femoral neck.

 Femoral anteversion significantly affects the projection of the CCD angle.

For this reason, the radiograph for determining the CCD angle should be obtained with the legs in a position of slight internal rotation (about 20°). In planning surgical procedures, correction tables should be used to determine the true CCD angle and femoral anteversion angle (see below). The simplified drawings in Fig. 6.90 b show a normal CCD angle and its deviations toward coxa vara or coxa valga.

- *Femoral anteversion (FA) angle.* The FA angle is closely related to the CCD angle. Both angles should be determined prior to any corrective surgical procedure, and correction tables should be used when the angles are determined on conventional radiographic films. The method of Rippstein (Fig. 6.90 c) requires two radiographs: an AP pelvic view to measure the CCD angle,

and a second view taken in a positioning device that holds the thighs in 20° abduction with the knees and hips flexed 90°. The crossbar of the device, which appears on the radiograph, forms a posterior tangent to the femoral condyles and defines the bicondylar femoral axis. Reference was made earlier to the correlation between femoral anteversion and CCD angle, which can be obtained from tables. The relationship between anteversion and the transverse axis of the femoral condyles and its abnormalities are shown in Fig. 6.91.

CT has become the current method of choice for determining the FA angle (Weiner et al. 1978, Grote et al. 1980, Mesgarzadeh et al. 1987). Two or three scans are performed through the femoral neck (slice thickness 5–10 mm) to obtain a line through its axis, and two or three scans are acquired through both femoral condyles to obtain a posterior bicondylar tangent. The angle between them is the FA angle. The normal range of femoral anteversion is 12–15° for adults. The examination can be performed with low dose. In recent years the same principle has been applied to MRI.

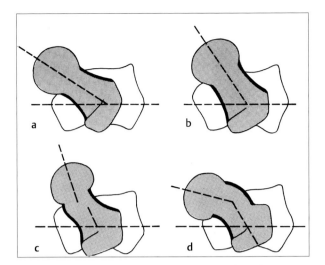

Fig. 6.**91 a–d**   Relationship between femoral neck anteversion and the transverse axis of the femoral condyles.
a Normal anteversion.
b Increased anteversion between the femoral neck and condylar axis.
c Increased anteversion due to anterior angulation of the femoral neck.
d Decreased anteversion due to posterior angulation of the femoral neck.

Pathological Finding?

Normal Variant or Anomaly?

Variants

The triradiate cartilage may persist. **Persistence of the marginal acetabular epiphysis and apophysis is a clinically innocuous variant** (Figs. 6.**92**–6.**94**).

These structures have also been called the "ossa ad acetabuli." The term "os acetabuli" is incorrect, as it is reserved for the ossification centers located in the central part of the acetabulum. The "ossa ad acetabuli" were formerly called the "ossa roentgenologicum," or radiographic ossa. These bony elements are usually located in close proximity to the superior acetabular rim. They may be small and multiple (Fig. 6.**92 a, b**) or assume larger, solid forms (Figs. 6.**92 c**, 6.**93**). It is uncertain whether they actually represent persistent apophyses or epiphyses, foci of metaplastic bone formation (Fig. 6.**95**), or even older bony capsular avulsions that the patient cannot recall, but ultimately there is no practical value in making this distinction. A bony element occurring at a lower level next to the posterior acetabular margin (Fig. 6.**94**) might be interpreted as an accessory bone element in the form of a persistent apophysis. The case shown in Fig. 6.**95**, in which an "os ad acetabulum" disappeared from radiographs over a six-month period, is more consistent with the spontaneous resorption of a metaplastic ossification than a solid accessory bone.

Fig. 6.**92 a–c**   "Ossa ad acetabulum."

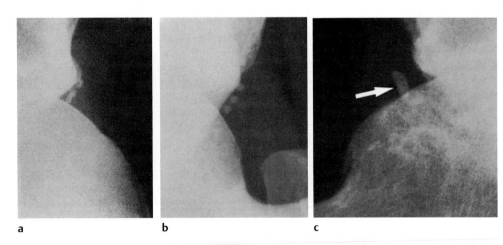

a   b   c

Fig. 6.**93 a–c**   "Ossa ad acetabulum."

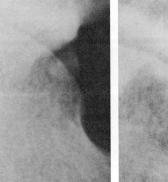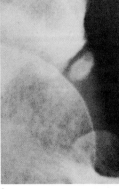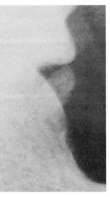

a   b   c

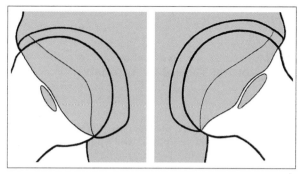

Fig. 6.**94** Bilateral accessory bones located at the approximate center of the posterior acetabular margin (after Heidenblut).

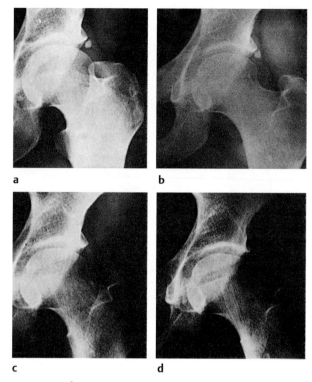

Fig. 6.**95 a–d** Spontaneous resorption of an "os ad acetabulum." It is more likely that the bony element was a metaplastic ossification.
a November 1965.
b February 1966.
c March 1966.
d May 1966.

Larger, very dense bony elements with irregular margins in the region of the "ossa ad acetabuli" are a particularly common finding in osteoarthritis (Fig. 6.**96**).

Their pathogenesis may be based on metaplastic bone formation in the para-articular soft tissues, much as in Heberden arthropathy, or it may involve a detached osteophyte or a preexisting "os ad acetabulum" whose shape changed during the course of the osteoarthritis.

The differential diagnosis of "ossa ad acetabuli" is reviewed in Table 6.**5** and Figs. 6.**97** and 6.**98**.

Fig. 6.**96 a–e** Typical forms of a large, deformed, osteoarthritic "os ad acetabulum."

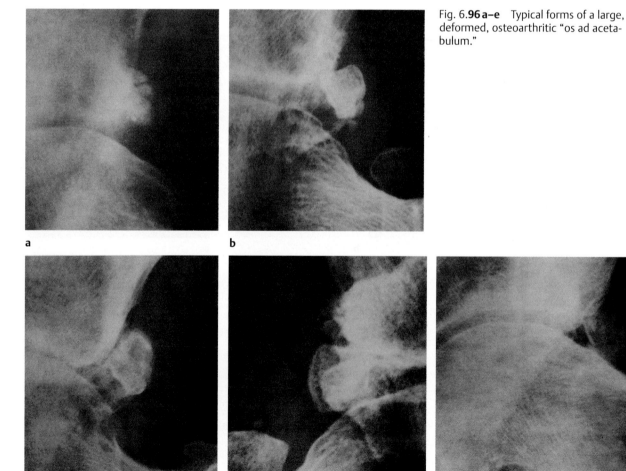

Table 6.**5**   Differential diagnosis of "ossa ad acetabuli"

- Intra-articular loose body due to osteochondritis dissecans (there must be a matching defect in the articular
  surface of the hip)
- Detached osteophyte in osteoarthritis
- Incipient articular chondromatosis
- Heterotopic metaplastic bone formation in the adjacent
  soft tissues, especially the muscles and tendons (Figs.
  6.**97**, 6.**98**)

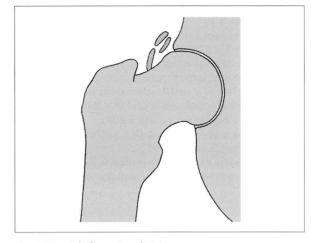

Fig. 6.**97**   Calcific peritendinitis.

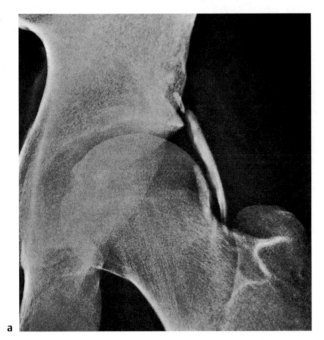

a

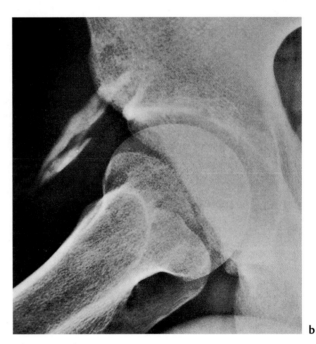

b

Fig. 6.**98**   Heterotopic ossifications in the area of the tensor fasciae latae muscle.

Persistence of the epiphyseal plate between the **femoral head and neck** is believed to occur as a normal variant, like persistence of the apiphyseal plates in the greater and lesser trochanters. It should be noted that, in some individuals, remnants of the former growth plates are still visible as double lines until about 25 years of age, and that this does not mean that the plates are still open or still have growth potential.

It is unclear whether **duplication of the lesser trochanter** should be classified as a normal variant or an abnormality. In the case shown in Fig. 6.**99**, it is necessary to consider whether the "second lesser trochanter" might be a cartilaginous exostosis located at a low, diaphyseal level and displaying only its prominent portion with the anteromedial or posteromedial femoral cortex superimposed.

Fig. 6.**99**   "Duplication" of the lesser trochanter or cartilaginous exostosis. ▷

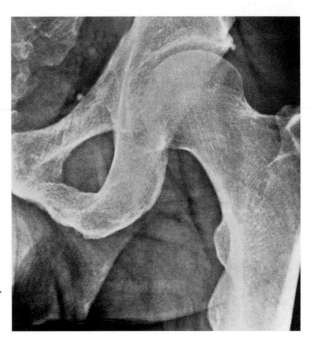

Another possibility, though indeterminate at present, is that the feature is an old ossified subperiosteal hematoma. This case was taken from the previous edition, where it was interpreted as a "duplication of the lesser trochanter." As long as the finding cannot be investigated by a sectional imaging procedure, it must remain indeterminate.

A final variant is a **small, sclerosis-rimmed defect** in the superomedial acetabular border that is continuous superiorly with a kind of sulcus (Fig. 6.**100**).

While it was once felt that this might be a nutrient canal, authors such as Teichert (1956) and Johnstone et al. (1982) believe it is an **accessory fossa** arising from the roof of the acetabulum (**superior acetabular notch**).

Anomalies

The following changes are no longer considered variants but are classified as definite abnormalities.

Primary protrusio acetabuli (Fig. 6.**101**) is a deformity that may be caused by a hormonal disorder during puberty. The radiographic floor of the acetabulum extends past the linea terminalis, and the teardrop figure may disappear. This deformity occurs predominantly in females. Protrusio acetabuli is assumed to be present if the acetabular line (medial cortex of the acetabular floor) in adults is more than 3 mm medial to the ischioiliac line in men or more than 6 mm in women (Armbruster et al. 1978).

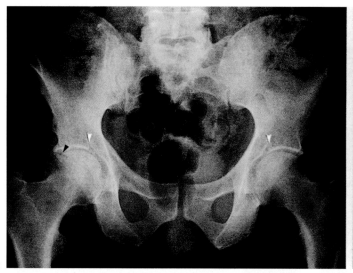

a

b

Fig. 6.**100a, b** Small bony defects in the acetabula as a normal variant.
a Marked with white arrows in the AP radiograph. The black arrow in **a** points to a linear lucency that is not a fracture but a Mach effect produced by the anterior acetabular rim.

b Tomogram.

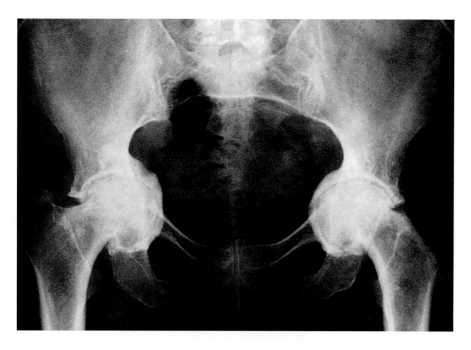

Fig. 6.**101**
Protrusio acetabuli.

Congenital dislocation of the hip is among the most common anomalies of the musculoskeletal system (approximately 1.5 in 1000 live births, Ponseti 1982). Geographic and ethnic factors contribute to regional variations in incidence rates, which range from 1% to 10%. Dislocation (not dysplasia without dislocation and not subluxation) is six times more common in girls than boys. Congenital hip dislocation can also be termed anthropological hip dislocation to distinguish it from teratological dislocation. The latter occurs in the setting of skeletal dysplasias and malformation syndromes and accounts for approximately 2% of all cases.

There is still no consensus on the underlying morphological factors that predispose to hip dislocation. Morphological abnormalities and impaired ossification of the acetabulum, morphological changes in the proximal end of the femur, and intrauterine hormone-induced laxity of the capsule and ligaments of the hip are considered significant etiological factors. A flat acetabulum appears to be a secondary phenomenon. It results from a faulty position of the femoral head that alters the direction of stress transfer across the hip, so that the **femoral head is unable to mold the acetabulum**. Capsular laxity is probably the precipitating factor in constitutionally predisposed individuals (mostly girls). It is believed that this laxity develops at the end of the fetal period in response to maternal hormones. Another factor may be an extreme intrauterine position of the hip joint (e.g., in oligohydramnios and breech presentation). If a prenatal or postnatal dislocation due to capsular laxity persists for some time, progressive changes develop in the cartilaginous and bony acetabulum. If the femoral head is moved to a normal position without undue delay and is maintained in that position, the acetabulum will either remain normal or will regain a normal configuration in response to molding by the femoral head.

A **constitutional flat acetabulum without hip dislocation** and a **flat acetabulum with hip dislocation** are often referred to by the collective term "**hip dysplasia**." But this term expresses only one aspect of the overall concept of congenital hip dislocation.

> **The stages of congenital hip dislocation**
> ➤ Hip dysplasia
> ➤ Subluxation
> ➤ Dislocation

It should be noted that a **predisposition** to hip dislocation can be demonstrated clinically by the **Ortolani maneuver**, in which the femoral head slips palpably or audibly over the limbus or labrum when the femur is passively displaced backward and upward. Screening examinations have shown that an unstable hip joint, or "clicking hip," is detected in 1 out of 100 newborns. Generally, however, these findings normalize during the first weeks of life (Walker 1971, Noble et al. 1978).

The **early diagnosis** of congenital hip dislocation relies on **ultrasonography**, which is outside the scope of this monograph. By the time the child reaches 3 months of age, ossification of the superior acetabular rim and incipient ossification of the capital femoral ossification center have laid the groundwork for the radiographic measurements described on p. 815 ff.

One of the most serious complications of congenital hip dislocation is the development of **aseptic necrosis of the femoral head** ("dislocation Perthes"). This complication may result from a reduction maneuver or from several months of hip splinting to maintain the reduction.

Untreated congenital hip dislocations follow the course that is shown schematically in Fig. 6.102.

The femoral head increasingly dislocates behind the ilium and becomes lodged there, while the lesser trochanter forms a nearthrosis with the bony structures of the acetabulum (Figs. 6.102 a, 6.103).

It is also possible for the femoral head to "excavate" a shallow secondary acetabulum on the posterior surface of the ilium (Fig. 6.102 b). Generally the secondary acetabulum will display very severe degenerative changes. In some cases of untreated congenital hip dislocation, the femoral head comes to rest against the gluteal muscles and has no bony contact at all. In this case the femoral head remains underdeveloped (Fig. 6.102 c), but degenerative changes do not develop as in the other two situations shown in Fig. 6.102 a, b. Possible sequelae in the femoral head and acetabulum despite reduction of the dislocation are shown in Fig. 6.104 a.

Hip dysplasia in adults (Fig. 6.104) can have many causes, the main one being congenital hip dislocation. Other causes are neuromuscular diseases (especially cerebral palsy), prior epiphysiolysis, Perthes disease, and epiphyseal dysplasia. Hip dysplasia in adults is characterized by a steep, shallow acetabulum with a hypoplastic roof (i.e., an underdeveloped superior acetabular rim) and

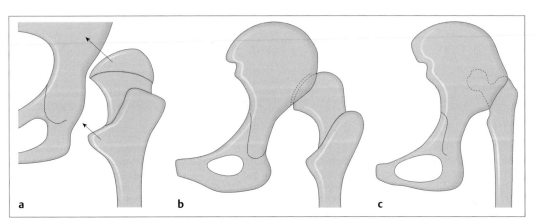

Fig. 6.**102 a–c**   Possible progression of an untreated congenital hip dislocation (after Dihlmann).

a thickened acetabular floor. The femoral head is flattened, and the femoral neck shows coxa valga with increased anteversion (Fig. 6.**104 b**). All of these abnormalities can be readily detected and defined by using the radiographic measurements described above. The Ménard–Shanton line is not disrupted in adult hip dysplasia, thereby distinguishing that condition from the remnants of congenital hip subluxation in adults.

Congenital coxa vara is the mildest form of congenital femoral defect. It occurs in 1 of 25 000 live births and is usually detected only after the child has begun to stand and walk. During the first weeks and months of life, the proximal end of the femur is broadened. More severe cases in infants and small children present with cap-shaped (Perthes-like) fragments at the proximal end of the diaphysis (Fig. 6.**105**).

Varus curvature and pseudarthrosis may develop in the proximal third of the shaft. **Symptomatic coxa vara** is encountered in rickets, in fibrous dysplasia and other tumor-like lesions, Paget disease, trauma, slipped capital femoral epiphysis, Perthes disease, etc.

Coxa valga with anteversion may result from an untreated hip dislocation or from prolonged abduction splinting. Circumscribed osteonecrosis or even Perthes disease may develop from this condition.

Idiopathic coxa valga with anteversion is actually a variant. It does not require special treatment measures, as it is not considered a preosteoarthritic condition.

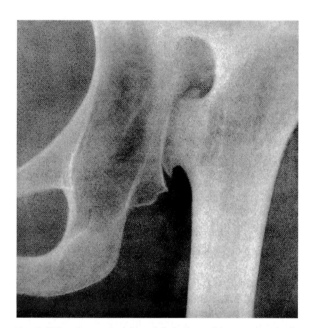

Fig. 6.**103**   Congenital hip dislocation with nearthrosis formation between the lesser trochanter and acetabulum.

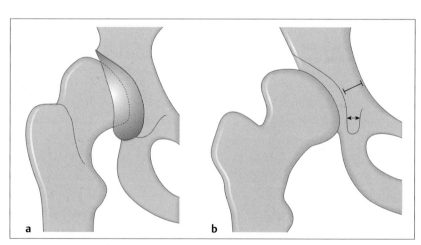

Fig. 6.**104 a, b**   Hip subluxation and hip dysplasia.
a Congenital hip subluxation in an adult. Note that the Ménard–Shanton line is interrupted due to the high, lateral position of the femoral head and its lack of coverage by the shallow, steep, elliptical acetabulum.
b Hip dysplasia in an adult. The acetabulum is steep and shallow with a hypoplastic roof. The femoral head is flattened, there is coxa valga with increased anteversion, and the acetabular floor is thickened (after Dihlmann).

Note that congenital hip subluxation in the adult (**a**) is a secondary phenomenon that is morphologically different from the adult hip dysplasia shown in **b**. In the first case the Ménard–Shanton line is interrupted; in the second case, it is not.

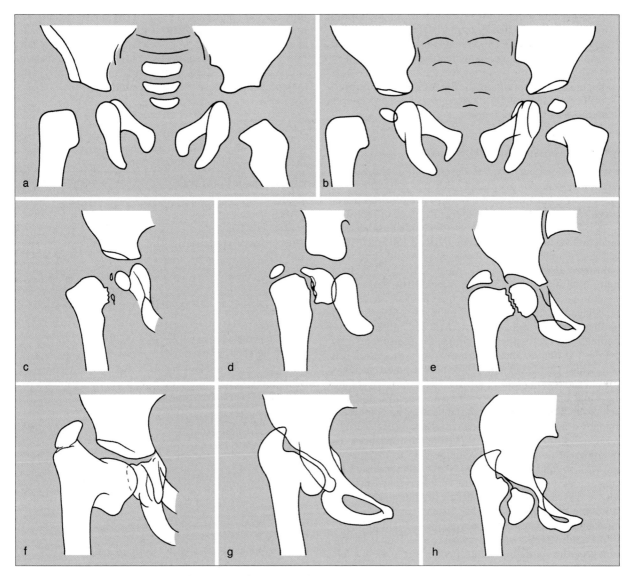

Fig. 6.**105 a–h** Radiographic manifestations of congenital coxa vara (based on radiographs from Kreuz, Leger, Glauner, and Marquardt).

a Child 8 months of age: metaphyseal border on the right side is steep and relatively distant from the acetabulum; thick cortex along the medial border of the proximal shaft.

b Child 14 months of age: femoral ossification centers visible, otherwise similar to **a**.

c Pediatric patient: broad necrotic zone in the metaphyseal part of the femoral neck, incipient downward movement of the epiphysis.

d Girl 6 years of age: broad necrotic zone with shortening of the femoral neck, reactive sclerosis about the lesser trochanter, coxa vara.

e Adolescent patient: bone fragment at the inferior border of the necrotic zone near the epiphysis, coxa vara, rotation of the femoral head. The lucent lines form a Y.

f Boy 12 years of age: repair stage; short femoral neck with a rufflike head, high position of the greater trochanter (shepherd's crook deformity).

g Late stage with shepherd's crook deformity in an adult.

h Late stage with shepherd's crook deformity and pseudarthrosis in an adult: downward rotation of the femoral head, reactive protuberance formation on the medial side of the femoral shaft where it touches the head.

Imaging Strategy for Evaluating Hip Dysplasia in Adults

- First a standing AP pelvic radiograph is obtained to determine the CE angle of Wiberg. A value less than 25° is suspicious for acetabular dysplasia.
- Next a false-profile view is obtained (see above) to evaluate anterior acetabular coverage and check for early osteoarthritic changes not visible on the standard AP film. The detection of early degenerative changes is of major importance, especially in young patients and in selecting patients for corrective osteotomies. The VCA angle measured on the false-profile view is not identical to the AASA determined by CT, because the VCA angle is measured in a sagittal plane and reflects anterosuperior acetabular coverage while the AASA is measured in a horizontal (axial) plane and describes anteromedial coverage (p. 817 f).

- CT is a useful adjunct for investigating congenital hip dysplasia. It is specifically used to determine the AASA and PASA (see above) in patients with neuromuscular dysplasias, etc. An interesting feature of cerebral palsy is hypoplasia of the posterior acetabulum, which is best diagnosed by determining the PASA. CT can also be used for the precise planning of various operative procedures on the acetabulum or femur.

Syndromes Associated with Hip Anomalies

It would exceed our scope to describe all of the various syndromes that are associated with hip anomalies, but **congenital syndromes with a shallow acetabulum or reduced FA angle** (CE angle of Wiberg) are listed in Table 6.**6**.

Two typical examples of severe developmental disturbances of the hip joint are shown in Figs. 6.**106** and 6.**107**.

The case in Fig. 6.**106** involves a 6.5-year-old child with **hypothyroidism**. The severe disturbances of skeletal maturation and growth (which affected the rest of the skeleton and especially the growth zones) are evidenced by delayed ossification of the epiphyses. The femoral epiphysis on the right side is small and appears fragmented, and the ossification center for the greater trochanter has not yet appeared (normally in the 3rd to 5th year of life). On the left side we see only stippled calcifications in the region of the epiphysis. The femoral necks are short and broad, and the acetabula are shallow due to a lack of molding by normal femoral heads. The epiphyseal changes should not be confused with Perthes disease.

Figure 6.**107** shows very severe disturbances of metaphyseal growth and development in a 13-year-old boy with **metaphyseal chondrodysplasia**, manifested by short, broad femoral necks with very irregular calcifications and varus deformity, especially on the right side. Because the child also had celiac disease and associated anomalies, we considered Shwachman–Diamond syndrome and MMN chondrodysplasia (MMN = malabsorption, growth retardation, neutropenia). The patient's left hand was radiographed at 7 years of age to determine skeletal maturity (Fig. 6.**107 d**), and marked growth retardation and dissociation were found (skeletal age 4.5 years

in the distal epiphyses, 3 years in the carpal region). MR images of the hips (Fig. 6.**107 b, c**) clearly demonstrate the severe transformation processes with replacement of normal fatty tissue by a connective tissue of low proton density. Figure 6.**107 c** shows irregular cartilage columns in the metaphysis like those seen in enchondromatosis.

Table 6.**6**   Congenital syndromes that are associated with a shallow acetabulum or reduced FA angle

Type A pelvis (small pelvis with square iliac wings and irregular acetabular roofs)
- Achondrogenesis types I and II
- Achondroplasia
- Asphyxiating thoracic dysplasia (Jeune syndrome)
- Caudal regression syndrome
- Cephaloskeletal dysplasia (Taybi–Linder syndrome)
- Chondrodysplasia punctata (rhizomelic form)
- Chondroectodermal dysplasia (Ellis–van Creveld syndrome)
- Dyggve–Melchior–Clausen syndrome
- Segmental dysplasia
- Hypochondrodysplasia
- Kniest dysplasia
- Metaphyseal chondrodysplasia (advanced)
- Metatrophic dysplasia
- Morquio syndrome
- Short ribs-polydactyly syndrome (Saldino–Noonan type)
- Congenital spondyloepiphyseal dysplasia
- Thanatophoric dysplasia

Type B pelvis (flared iliac wings, less square)
- Acrocephalopolydactyly (Carpenter syndrome)
- Acrocephalosyndactyly (Waardenburg syndrome)
- Aminopterin fetopathy
- Arthrogryposis
- Bladder exstrophy
- Cleidocranial dysplasia
- Cockayne syndrome
- Cornelia de Lange syndrome
- Hypophosphatasia
- Hypothyroidism (cretinism)
- Metaphyseal chondrodysplasia (mild form)
- Mucopolysaccharidoses, mucolipidoses
- Nail–patella syndrome
- Osteodysplasia (Melnick–Needles syndrome)
- Osteogenesis imperfecta
- Popliteal pterygium syndrome
- Prune Belly syndrome
- Rubinstein–Taybi syndrome
- Sacral agenesis
- Trisomy 13 syndrome
- Trisomy 21 syndrome (Down syndrome)

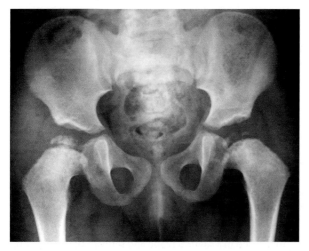

Fig. 6.**106**   Typical hip joint configuration in hypothyroidism in a 6.5-year-old child (compare with Fig. 2.**27 c, d**; also see text).

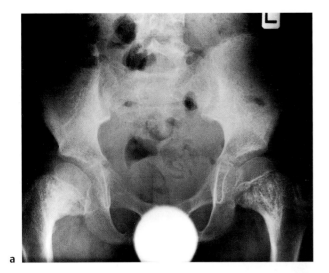

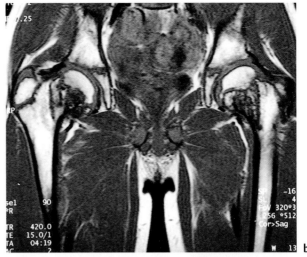

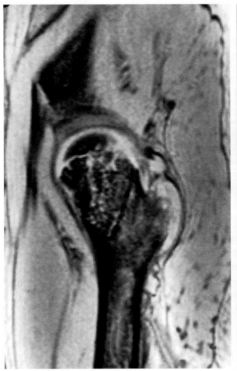

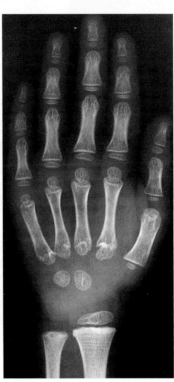

Fig. 6.**107 a–d**   Metaphyseal chondrodysplasia in a 13-year-old boy. The irregularities in the femoral necks appear partly as irregular cartilage columns on MRI (see text for further details).

 Fracture, Subluxation, or Dislocation?

Fractures about the hip joint will be discussed only to the extent that the radiologist must know where the fractures are likely to occur and where they are apt to be confused with persistent epiphyseal plates or other structures.

With an **acetabular fracture**, attention should be given to the following six radiographic lines. The interruption of these lines indicates a fracture.

- Iliopectineal line
- Teardrop figure
- Ilioischial line
- Acetabular roof
- Posterior acetabular rim
- Anterior acetabular rim (if defined)

Judet and Letournel subdivided the acetabular and peri-acetabular bone structures into an anterior and a posterior column.

> **Judet and Letournel classification of acetabular and periacetabular bone structures**
> ➤ Anterior column: anterior half of acetabulum, anterior ilium, pubis
> ➤ Posterior column: posterior half of acetabulum, posteroinferior portions of the ilium, ischium

Acetabular fractures can be classified into basic and combined forms based on the column model, as shown in Fig. 6.**108**.

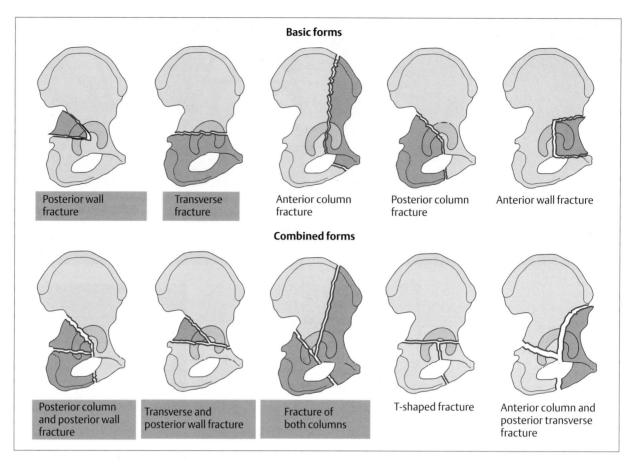

Basic forms

| Posterior wall fracture | Transverse fracture | Anterior column fracture | Posterior column fracture | Anterior wall fracture |

Combined forms

| Posterior column and posterior wall fracture | Transverse and posterior wall fracture | Fracture of both columns | T-shaped fracture | Anterior column and posterior transverse fracture |

Fig. 6.**108**   Judet–Letournel classification of acetabular fractures.

Each of these fracture types may be associated with dislocation of the femoral head. The femur usually dislocates inferiorly in the basic forms, but it may also dislocate centrally in the combined forms. The decision whether to operate is based partly on whether the fracture extends into the load-bearing superomedial portions of the acetabulum.

The Judet and Letournel classification of acetabular fractures is based on conventional radiographs, which include an AP projection as well as obturator and alar views. The latter views permit an extended evaluation of the acetabular roof, especially in the pressure-transfer zone, and help to determine whether incongruence exists between the femoral head and acetabular roof.

Table 6.**7**   Information added by CT in the diagnosis of acetabular fractures

- Detection of fractures in the weight-bearing zone, which extends about 10–12 mm inferiorly from the highest point of the acetabulum (2-mm slice thickness should be used).
- Detection of intra-articular loose fragments, which should be surgically removed if dislocation has occurred.
- Exclusion of femoral head fractures.
- Defining the extent of a dislocation and the size of a posterior wall fragment (these findings guide patient selection for operative treatment).

Today, CT has become an indispensable tool in the diagnosis of acetabular fractures (Fig. 6.**109**). Table 6.**7** outlines the additional information that CT scans can furnish in the diagnosis of these fractures.

Traumatic hip dislocations are classified as follows:

Classification of traumatic hip dislocations
- ➤ Iliac dislocation: posteriorly and superiorly (most common form, Fig. 6.**111 c**)
- ➤ Ischial dislocation: posteriorly and inferiorly
- ➤ Pubic dislocation: anteriorly and superiorly
- ➤ Obturator dislocation: anteriorly and inferiorly
- ➤ Perineal dislocation (extremely rare)
- ➤ Scrotal dislocation (extremely rare)

Dislocations of the hip joint are very often associated with concomitant fractures of the acetabulum and femoral head.

Small acetabular rim fractures require differentiation from an "os ad acetabulum," osteochondritis dissecans, and preexisting soft-tissue calcifications as shown in Figs. 6.**92**–6.**97**.

The **Pipkin classification** is used for **femoral head fractures** (Fig. 6.**110**).

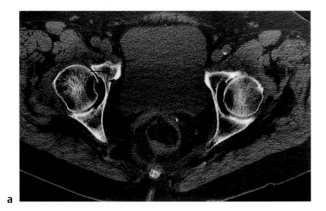

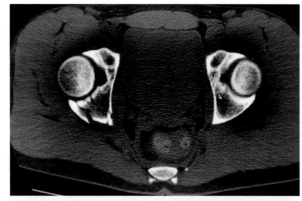

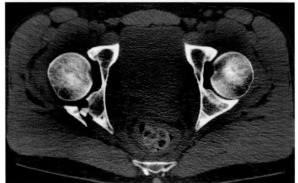

Fig. 6.**109 a–c**   Value of CT scans in hip fractures.
a Extra-articular sagittal anterior column fracture on the right side (black arrows) in an elderly woman, not visible on conventional radiographs.
b, c Comminuted fracture of the posterior column in a young man. The interposed fragment in image **c** cannot be identified as such on conventional radiographs.

Fig. 6.**110**   Pipkin classification of femoral head fractures.

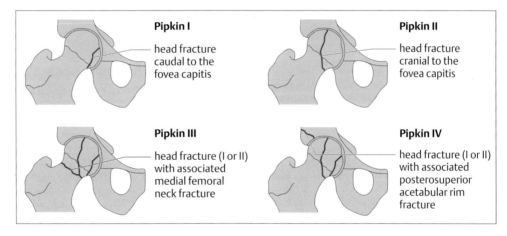

Pipkin I
head fracture caudal to the fovea capitis

Pipkin II
head fracture cranial to the fovea capitis

Pipkin III
head fracture (I or II) with associated medial femoral neck fracture

Pipkin IV
head fracture (I or II) with associated posterosuperior acetabular rim fracture

---

Classification of femoral neck fractures (Fig. 6.111)

➤ *Medial femoral neck fracture:* intracapsular; the most common type of proximal femoral fracture. The relative high complication rate (ischemic femoral head necrosis in 10–20% of cases, delayed union and nonunion in 5–25% of cases, secondary osteoarthritis) correlates with the obliquity of the fracture line relative to the horizontal.

The steeper the fracture line on the radiograph, the greater the likelihood of femoral head slippage.

Pauwels defined three grades: I up to 30°, II 30–70°, and III more than 70°.

The angle of the fracture line is measured in relation to the horizontal plane.

In the *Garden classification* of femoral neck fractures, four types are distinguished according to the pattern of fragment displacement:

Garden I Impacted fracture.

Garden II Complete, nondisplaced fracture with normal trajectorial patterns in the femoral head and neck.

Garden III Displaced fracture with some residual fragmental contact and trajectorial disruption in the femoral head and neck.

Garden IV Complete displacement (the complication rate rises with increasing grade).

➤ *Lateral femoral neck fracture.*

➤ *Pertrochanteric femoral fracture:* The fracture usually runs from the lesser trochanter to the greater trochanter. A reverse pertrochanteric fracture is less common. Multi-part fractures are common, the degree of instability increasing with the degree of involvement of the calcar femorale and lesser trochanter.

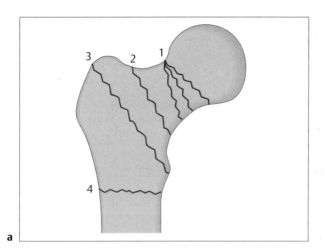

Fig. 6.**111 a–h**   Subcapital femoral fractures.
a Classification of subcapital femoral fractures.
1   Medial femoral neck fracture
2   Lateral femoral neck fracture
3   Pertrochanteric fracture
4   Subtrochanteric fracture
b Mach effect from the posterior rim of the acetabulum mimics a medial femoral neck fracture.
c Classic traumatic hip dislocation with "disappearance" of the joint space (iliac hip dislocation).
d Two different trabecular patterns in the femoral neck, both normal.
e Impacted subcapital femoral neck fracture with a typical trabecular discontinuity and valgus deviation of the femoral head.

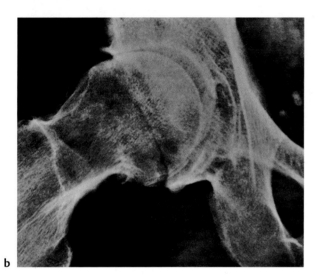

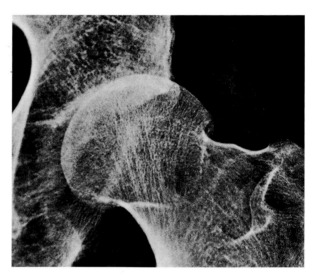

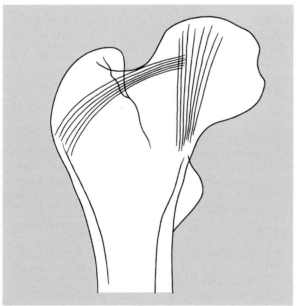

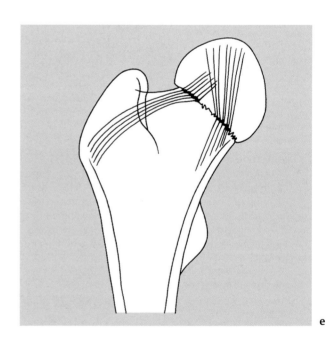

Fig. 6.**111 f–h** Follow-up radiographs of an impacted (**f**) medial femoral neck fracture. Note the increasing angulation of the femoral head.

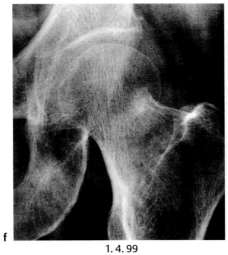

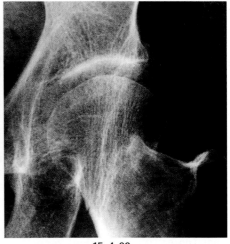

f   1. 4. 99   g

Fractures of the proximal femur may escape radiographic detection, especially in the case of an impacted fracture (slightly increased density in the femoral neck, for example) or a nonorthograde projection of the fracture line.

Because patients with osteoporosis are predisposed to proximal femoral fractures, especially in the femoral neck and pertrochanteric areas, diagnosis is hampered by the fact that fractures are particularly difficult to detect in osteoporotic bone. It can be helpful in these cases to note the trajectorial patterns of trabecular lines in the proximal femoral neck (Fig. 6.**112**). A small transverse density that disrupts the trajectorial pattern, or even a slight interruption, signifies a discontinuity in the bone.

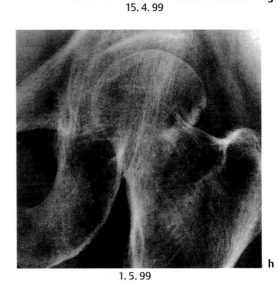

h   1. 5. 99

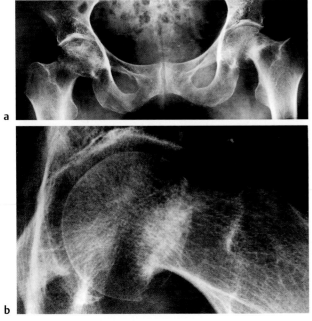

a

b

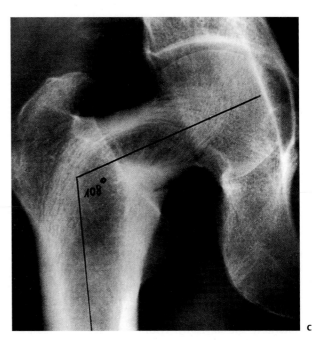

c

Fig. 6.**112 a–c** Stress fractures of the femoral neck.
a, b Insufficiency fractures due to osteoradiodystrophy. Note the densities in both femoral necks in radiograph **a**, which does not give a clear projection of the fracture lines.

c Overweight patient with coxa vara. The lucent fracture line is just visible on the inferomedial aspect of the femoral neck. Note the pronounced trabecular remodeling with marked thickening of the superior and inferior cortex.

If the diagnosis is equivocal based on biplane radiographs, CT or MRI should be used at an early stage. Radionuclide bone scans become positive in about 4–5 days.

Avulsion fractures of the lesser trochanter and its apophysis are common in young persons, especially in connection with athletic activities. They should be differentiated from persistent apophyses and accessory bone elements in this region (Fig. 6.**69**).

Stress fractures, including fatigue fractures and insufficiency fractures, are not uncommon in the acetabulum and proximal femur (Figs. 6.**32**, 6.**112**). Osteoporotic insufficiency fractures predominate in the acetabulum and femoral neck (Fig. 6.**32**), while fatigue fractures occur mainly in the lesser trochanter area and also in the femoral neck.

For semantic reasons, stress fractures are distinguished from **Looser (transformation) zones** (pseudofractures) (Fig. 6.**18 d**). These zones most commonly occur in the femoral neck and lesser trochanter, especially in patients with osteomalacia and renal osteopathy (Fig. 6.**53 b**).

Slipped capital femoral epiphysis is seen most typically between 12 and 15 years of age, generally occurring somewhat earlier in girls than in boys. The slip involves the proximal femoral epiphysis along with the actual cartilage proliferation zone, which is of great (positive) importance in terms of growth potential. If the slip is stopped in time, the proximal femur can continue to grow normally. The principal causes are endocrine disorders such as adiposo-genital dysplasia and gigantism, as well as the adolescent growth spurt. The incidence is estimated at 2 per 100.000 population. Boys are affected more frequently than girls by a 2.5 : 1 ratio. The prognosis depends on early diagnosis, as untreated slippage can lead to gross deformities with coxa vara and secondary osteoarthritis, chondrolysis of the femoral head, Perthes disease, etc. The early clinical symptoms are nonspecific and consist of a dull pain that radiates to the thigh or knee, causing a limp and reducing the range of internal hip rotation and external thigh rotation in flexion. The clinical course of the disease is classified as **acute** if the symptoms last for less than three weeks and **chronic** if they last for more than three weeks. The symptoms associated with a chronic slip are even less specific. The slip is bilateral in up to 40% of patients. Half of all cases are bilateral at the time of diagnosis, and the rest develop contralateral symptoms after a period of several months to five years. Bilateral slippage is particularly common in patients with endocrine disorders (e.g., hypothyroidism, growth hormone deficiency). Younger children (girls 11 and under, boys 12 and under) appear to have a stronger predilection for bilateral involvement. The **preslip** stage is distinguished from the **shear stage** and from an **acute slip**. Preslip is characterized by morphological changes in the metaphysis and epiphyseal plate with no displacement of the epiphysis relative to the metaphysis. As will be explained below, the radiographic diagnosis at this stage is very vague, but MRI can provide early evidence of incipient slippage based on widening of the epiphyseal plate on T1-weighted images (Umans et al. 1998, Fig. 6.**117**).

The direction of the slip is related to the CCD angle. With a CCD angle of approximately 90°, the femoral head slips anteriorly and inferiorly. With a 120° angle it slips posteromedially, with a 140° angle it slips posteriorly and inferiorly, and with a 160° angle it slips posterolaterally and inferiorly. The posteroinferior direction is the most common,

suggesting that a large CCD angle, when combined with other factors, predisposes to slipping.

The **radiographic evaluation of slipped capital femoral epiphysis** should include the following:

- *AP radiograph:* A very accurate projection is required. The anterior surface of the patella should be exactly parallel to the plane of the x-ray table. If necessary, the pelvis on the affected side should be elevated on a cushion.
- *Lauenstein I view:* This view indicates the amount of displacement of the epiphysis in the posteroinferior or anteroinferior direction. The leg should be externally rotated until the lower leg, flexed at the knee, is parallel to the film plane. The measurements taken on these standard views are shown in Fig. 6.**113**.

The degree of displacement can be measured with considerable precision on CT scans.

 A head-neck angle of more than 2° is considered abnormal or at least predisposing when corresponding clinical symptoms are present.

As mentioned above, the preslip stage (Fig. 6.**117**) is diagnosed entirely from morphological changes (if present) seen on plain radiographs and CT scans, but the confidence level is relatively low. The epiphyseal plate appears widened in comparison with the opposite side, and the metaphyseal margin bordering the physis appears indistinct (Fig. 6.**114**).

The **Klein sign** (Klein line) is negative at this stage. This line is drawn along the lateral border of the femoral neck on the AP radiograph and should cut off about 20% of the lateral portion of the femoral head (Fig. 6.**115 a**, left). In the subsequent **tilt stage**, the femoral head gradually tilts posteriorly downward (assuming a CCD angle of 140°).

At this stage there is still no visible stepoff between the femoral neck contour and the base of the femoral head. The subsequent **shear stage** (Fig. 6.**115 b**) is marked by tilting and slipping of the epiphysis, with the Lauenstein I view showing a stepoff between the femoral head and neck. This progresses to an acute slip marked by a complete discontinuity of the epiphyseal plate, the direction of the slip varying with the CCD angle as noted above (Figs. 6.**115 c**, 6.**116**).

The space between the femoral head and neck gapes open, and the femoral head "rides" on the corner of the metaphysis. These changes, visible in the Lauenstein I projection, are associated with increasing separation of the femoral head from the tangent to the femoral neck. Another important sign on AP radiographs is the **"sunset" sign** that occurs when the femoral epiphysis is projected lower on the affected side than on the healthy side.

Finally looser zone, represent a special form of the group of insufficiency fractures, because the bone is damaged with a consecutive reduced weight–fearing.

Fig. 6.**113 a, b**   Radiographic measurements of slipped capital femoral epiphysis.
a AP radiograph. Normally the femoral neck axis forms a 90° angle with the baseline of the femoral epiphysis and divides the epiphysis into two approximately equal parts. Deviations from this scheme may indicate the presence and especially the direction of epiphyseal slippage.
b Lauenstein view (frog-leg projection). The epiphyseal baseline is perpendicular to the longitudinal femoral neck axis, forming a 90° angle (after Dihlmann).

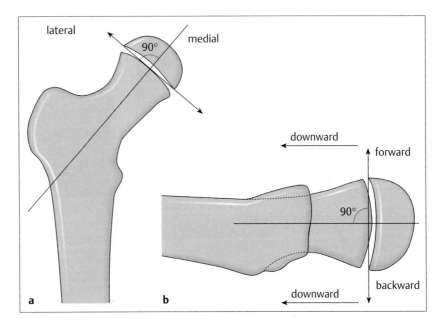

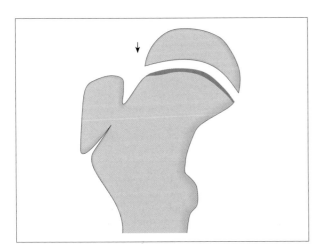

Fig. 6.**114**   Early radiographic sign of slipped capital femoral epiphysis. In the preslip stage, an experienced examiner using good technique may detect slight widening of the epiphyseal plate and an indistinct metaphyseal margin.

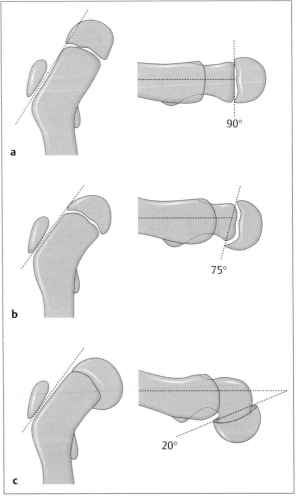

Fig. 6.**115 a–c**   Drawings from radiographs of slipped capital femoral epiphysis. The Klein line is shown on the AP projections in the left half of the figure. This line does not replace the standard reference lines shown in Fig. 6.**113**.
a Preslip stage. Measurements are normal, and the Klein line cuts off approximately 20% of the epiphysis.

b Shear stage. The Klein line bypasses the epiphysis. The angle in the Lauenstein view is reduced to 75°, and both projections show a stepoff on the medial or flexor side.
c Acute slip with complete discontinuity of the epiphyseal plate and posteroinferior slippage of the epiphysis.

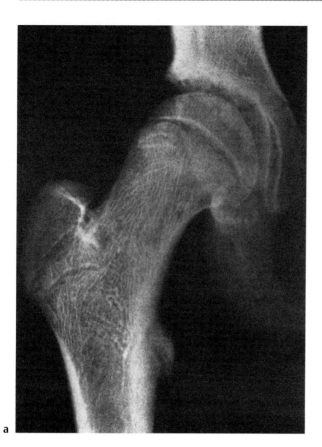

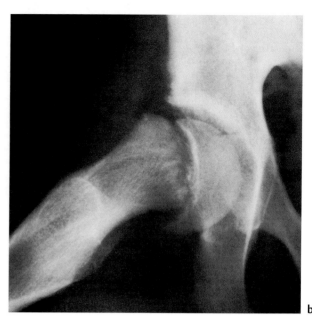

Fig. 6.**116a, b**   Slipped capital femoral epiphysis.
a AP projection.
b Lauenstein projection.

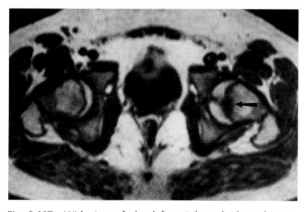

Fig. 6.**117**   Widening of the left epiphyseal plate demonstrated by T1-weighted MRI.

 Necrosis?

The hip region is subject to a great many osteonecrotic changes, all of which cannot be discussed here. We shall focus on a few diseases that can be difficult to distinguish from normal findings and normal variants while still in their initial stages.

Osteonecrotic Changes in Children and Adolescents

Idiopathic Chondrolysis

Histologically, idiopathic chondrolysis of the femoral head is characterized by devitalized chondrocytes, destruction of the upper layer of articular cartilage, and a reactive synovitis. Radiographs show joint space narrowing of sudden onset, erosive changes in the femoral head and acetabulum (probably due to synovitis), and periarticular osteoporosis. The changes may regress, probably because the cartilage in children and adolescents can still regenerate. Ankylosis rarely occurs. If the changes do not regress completely, the disease is considered a preosteoarthritic condition.

Symptomatic Chondrolysis

Not infrequently, symptomatic chondrolysis of the femoral head develops as a sequel to slipped capital femoral epiphysis, occurring on the contralateral side.

Osteochondritis Dissecans

Osteochondritis dissecans may affect the femoral head and the acetabulum. The disease may be idiopathic or symptomatic (e.g., as a result of cretinous femoral head changes or hereditary epiphyseal growth disturbances). Osteochondral fatigue fractures are thought to be an important cause of the idiopathic form, since a large percentage of cases involve weight-bearing epiphyses, especially those with a convex articular surface. **Principally, osteochondritis dissecans corresponds to a subarticular focal avascular necrosis.** Familial cases are not uncommon, leading some authors to postulate a dysplasia of the articular cartilage as the cause, at least for this subgroup (Kozlowski and Middleton 1985). Osteochondritis dissecans is considered a preosteoarthritic condition, especially when the osteochondral fragment separates from the bone and becomes an intra-articular loose body, causing arresting of the hip joint and damaging the cartilage. The initial stage is characterized by the presence of a fine, semicircular, subchondral lucency (subchondral fracture) associated with increasing density of the underlying cancellous bone. The bandlike lucency widens, and finally the affected segment separates and enters the joint cavity as a loose body, leaving behind a crater-shaped defect. We know from osteochondritis dissecans in the knee that the size of the osteochondral fragment determines the prognosis. Early forms that have no radiographic abnormalities can be detected by MRI. T2-weighted images show a bandlike, crescent-shaped hyperintense zone. Further details on the MRI appearance of osteochondritis dissecans are given in the chapter on the knee joint. Dynamic studies after intravenous gadolinium administration provide additional information:

- Rising signal intensity in the fragment indicates its residual viability.
- Rising signal intensity in the boundary zone between the fragment and the epiphysis suggests the presence of a fibrous tissue bridge that is tethering the fragment to its epiphyseal bed and may allow conservative treatment.

Legg–Calvé–Perthes Disease (Juvenile Osteonecrosis of the Hip)

This disease is an aseptic osteonecrosis of the femoral head that predominantly affects boys. It occurs between 3 and 10 years of age and rarely as late as age 15. Bilateral involvement is not uncommon, and the two hips are usually affected successively following an interval of several months. When Perthes-like changes occur simultaneously in both hips, cretinism or a mucopolysaccharidosis should be suspected as the cause. The etiology of Perthes disease is uncertain, but genetic factors appear to play a role. A traumatic etiology has also been proposed.

Early Radiographic Signs of Legg–Calvé–Perthes Disease:

- **Early stage I:** Increased distance between the medial border of the capital epiphysis and the lateral contour of the acetabular teardrop (Fig. 6.**118a**). As the capital epiphysis becomes smaller, the distance also increases between the superior border of the epiphysis and the acetabular roof (Fig. 6.**120a**). Radiographic joint space widening may also be due to the undisturbed or perhaps even increased proliferation of articular cartilage on the femoral head combined with a cessation of enchondral ossification. The joint space widening may amount to several millimeters but is not specific for Perthes disease, as it may also occur in coxitis.
- **Late stage I** (called also the florid stage, Fig. 6.**118b, c**): There is increasing flattening of the femoral head, especially in its upper anterolateral segment. The subchondral femoral head becomes somewhat more dense and shows a slightly indistinct contour, seen best on Lauenstein radiographs. These signs may be accompanied by disuse osteoporosis. Three-phase radionuclide scan shows clear evidence of decreased perfusion in the affected segment.
- **Stage II:** The hallmarks of this stage are patchy densities and fragmentation of the femoral head, metaphyseal defects, and lateral subluxation (Figs. 6.**118d**, 6.**120**, 6.**121a**).
- **Stage III** (called also the repair or remodeling stage): The fragments are resorbed, and a solid bony structure is reconstituted (Figs. 6.**118e**, 6.**121b**).
- **Stage IV, end stage:** As remodeling progresses, the residual femoral head gradually acquires a cylindrical or mushroom shape with widening or shortening of the femoral neck, coxa vara, and a high position of the greater trochanter (Figs. 6.**118f**, 6.**121c**).

It is clear from the description of stage I that the pathoanatomic changes of femoral head necrosis must be relatively far advanced before initial radiographic changes are seen. This has led to a current preference for MRI (Fig. 6.**119**) or radionuclide scanning. Studies by Ranner (1990) indicate that both modalities are equally sensitive in early diagnosis (Table 6.**8**).

In any case, it appears that MRI is more accurate than conventional radiographs in defining the extent of the affected epiphyseal area. It is noteworthy that the prognostic assessment and/or the need for treatment depend on the extent of the altered epiphyseal area. As for radionuclide scanning, it appears to be the best modality for determining the onset of femoral reconstitution.

It can be difficult to distinguish Perthes disease from multiple epiphyseal dysplasia (with or without "superimposed" Perthes disease) (Mandell et al. 1989). Irregularities of the proximal femoral epiphysis are an essential feature of both diseases. The subchondral fracture line on conventional radiographs appears to be typical of necrosis, even with preexisting dysplasia. Some cases will require the additional use of bone scanning (photopenic defect) and/or MRI (low T1-weighted signal intensity) to advance the differential diagnosis in patients with clinical complaints.

The differential diagnosis should also include the femoral abnormalities in cretinism (Fig. 6.**106** and p. 828).

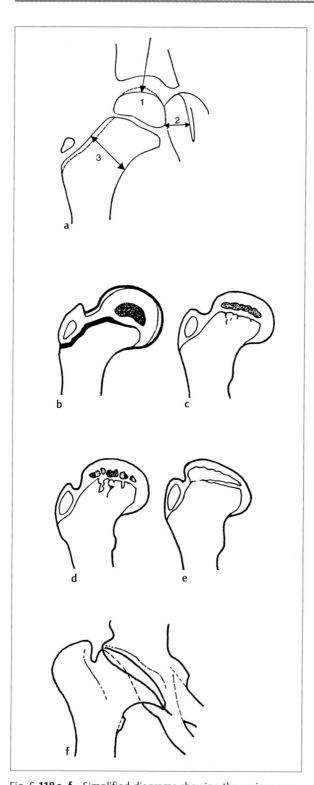

Fig. 6.**118 a–f** Simplified diagrams showing the various possible stages of Perthes disease.
a Early stage I.
b, c Late stage I.
d Fragmentation stage.
e Repair stage.
f Possible end stage.

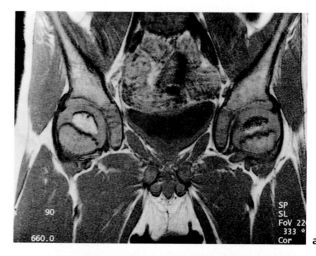

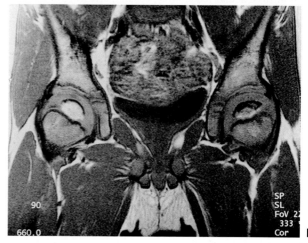

Fig. 6.**119 a, b** T1-weighted MR images of early Perthes disease. On the right side is a normal "white" epiphysis. On the left side, the superior portions of the epiphysis show little or no signal intensity. Note the slightly increased cartilage thickness compared with the contralateral side.

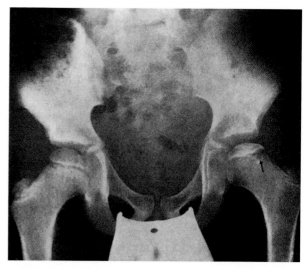

Fig. 6.**120** Perthes disease of the left hip in the early fragmentation stage. Note the marked widening of the left joint space and the flat, dense epiphyseal center with a transverse fragmentation line. The proximal femur shows marked demineralization on the left side.

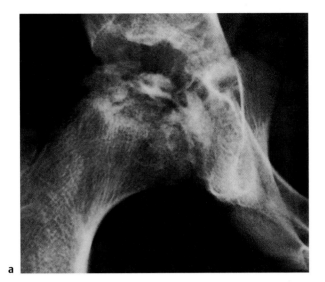

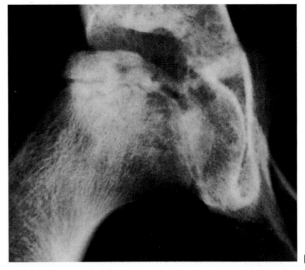

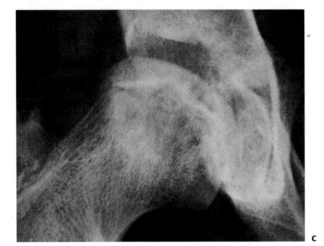

Fig. 6.**121 a–c** Radiographs showing the course of Perthes disease over a 20-month period.
a Advanced fragmentation stage (stage II).
b Repair stage 14 months later (stage III).
c Six months later, remodeling is largely complete with moderate cylindrical deformity of the femoral head, shortening of the femoral neck, and a high position of the greater trochanter.

Table 6.**8** Perthes disease: correlation between conventional radiographs, radionuclide bone scans, MRI, and pathologic anatomy (after Ranner)

Formal pathogenesis	Radiographs	Bone scans	MRI
Initial stage (fresh necrosis)	Normal findings, then joint space widening. "Condensation" of the epiphysis (I)	Cold lesion	Poorly marginated zone of decreased signal intensity
Resorption stage (after onset of revitalization)	Fragmentation of the epiphysis (II)	Disappearance of the cold lesion, then slightly increased uptake	Demarcation of the necrotic area and usually a further decrease in signal intensity[1]
Repair stage	Reossification of the epiphysis (III)	Usually increased uptake	Rise of signal intensity in the necrotic area (initially only noted by comparing sequential images[1])
End stage	Reconstitution completed (IV)	Increased uptake or normal findings	Fat-equivalent signal intensity throughout the epiphysis

[1] Can be clearly appreciated only after early childhood (2–3 years)

Osteonecrotic Changes in Adults

Osteochondritis Dissecans

Osteochondritis dissecans of the acetabulum and femoral head is less common in adults than in adolescents, but the radiographic signs are largely the same.

"Idiopathic" Avascular (Aseptic) Femoral Head Necrosis in Adults

Despite increasing awareness of the pathogenesis of idiopathic avascular femoral head necrosis in adults, its etiology is poorly understood. The disease is known to be associated with:

- Alcoholism
- Diseases of the liver and pancreas
- Primary and secondary metabolic disorders (e.g., hyperlipoproteinemia, antiphospholipid antibody syndrome, renal osteopathy, Gaucher disease, hyperuricemia, collagen diseases, coagulation disorders, hemoglobinopathies)
- Decompression trauma

The vascular (arterial) status of patients with idiopathic femoral head necrosis does not differ significantly from that in healthy individuals. Only traumatic necrosis is necessarily associated with the occlusion of larger arteries that supply the femoral head (e.g., the medial femoral circumflex artery). This has led some authors to postulate a relationship with the premature conversion of hematopoietic (red) marrow to fat marrow in the trochanteric region (Mitchell et al. 1986).

While fat marrow requires relatively little blood, its has a disproportionately scant vascular supply, making it many times more susceptible to osteonecrotic processes. Most osteonecrotic processes take place in the fat marrow. It is conceivable, then, that impaired venous drainage from the medullary cavity can lead to edema, causing a rise of intraosseous pressure that in turn restricts arterial perfusion and sets the stage for osteonecrosis. Impaired venous drainage can result from thrombotic occlusions of the venules, due for example to metabolic disorders or microfractures of the cancellous bone. In any case, the rise of intramedullary pressure (due to edema) is a critical initial factor in the pathogenesis of femoral head necrosis, prompting some orthopedists to treat early forms by core decompression. Other etiological factors, such as the compartment syndrome theory, are beyond our present scope.

The disease predominantly affects middle-aged adults 20–50 years of age, with a peak incidence around age 35. Both hips are affected in approximately 50–70% of cases. Patients present clinically with more or less severe hip pain caused by the elevated intraosseous pressure, concomitant synovitis, and limitation of motion. In some cases these symptoms are absent and the femoral head necrosis is detected incidentally.

Here we are concerned mainly with establishing an early diagnosis of the disease, since early diagnosis is crucial to the fate of the femoral head and potential sequelae such as severe osteoarthritis.

Only MRI and radionuclide scanning can provide the early diagnosis that is necessary for prompt initiation of treatment. This cannot be accomplished with conventional radiographs, although it is important to know the stages of femoral head osteonecrosis that can be recognized on plain radiographs:

> **Cruess stages of femoral head osteonecrosis on conventional radiographs** (Fig. 6.**122**)
> ➤ *Stage I:* Normal findings
> ➤ *Stage II:* Radiolucent area and/or sclerosis in the femoral head
> ➤ *Stage III:* Subchondral bandlike lucency (lucent crescent, Fig. 6.**124a**)
> ➤ *Stage IV:* Collapse of the subchondral bone (Fig. 6.**123b, c**)
> ➤ *Stage V:* Involvement of the entire hip with joint space narrowing, secondary osteoarthritis, etc.

The following are "**early**" **radiographic signs**:

- Sclerosis at the head–neck junction
- Periosteal deposits or thickening along the inferior aspect of the femoral neck

The above classification was developed by Cruess (1986). The classification of Ficat (1985) consists of four stages, with stage 0 defined as the preradiographic and preclinical stage.

In both staging systems, stage III disease or higher indicates definite osteonecrosis of the femoral head.

The **ARCO stages** (Association Research Circulation Osseous) can be used for the **classification of MRI changes** found in femoral head osteonecrosis (Table 6.**9**).

- Very early MRI changes in ARCO stage I show edema-equivalent signal intensity in the perfusion-impaired area (low T1-weighted intensity, high T2-weighted intensity). The process may still be reversible at this stage (Fig. 6.**124**).

Fig. 6.**123 a–c**   Radiographic progression of osteonecrosis of ▷ the left femoral head in a woman who was treated with cortisone and cyclosporine following renal transplantation.
a This radiograph, taken on 23 September 1971, shows a fine subchondral lucent line below the femoral head contour with marked structural irregularities toward the femoral head. This "early" radiographic finding was considered innocuous, and the patient continued to bear weight normally.
b, c These radiographs were taken four months later on 17 January 1972. The true extent of the fragmentation, now advanced, can be seen in the superomedial and superolateral portions of the necrotic area, especially in the axial view.

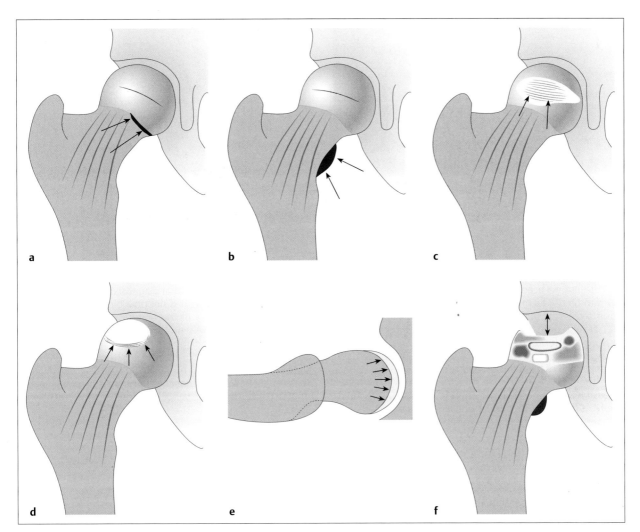

Fig. 6.**122 a–f**   Diagrams showing the principal radiographic signs of idiopathic femoral head osteonecrosis in adults.

a, b "Early" signs are sclerosis at the head-neck junction (**a**) and periosteal thickening on the medial aspect of the femoral neck (**b**). There may also be slight blurring of the trabecular structure (not shown) in the upper, subchondral portion of the femoral head.

c–f Late signs. Panel **c** shows bandlike sclerosis at the center of the femoral head bordering the crescent-shaped antero-superior area that will later become necrotic. Other signs are blurred cancellous trabeculae along with fine lucencies and densities in the higher necrotic area (not shown). These changes and those shown in **a** and **b** correspond to stage II of the Cruess classification described in the text. Panel **d** shows more pronounced, circumscribed trabecular blurring and lucencies in the upper part of the femoral head, surrounded by a sclerotic border. The semiaxial or axial view (**e**) shows the subchondral lucency (crescent sign) that signifies a subchondral fracture. Thus, **d** and **e** correspond to stage III in the Cruess classification. The subchondral fracture is difficult or impossible to find if there is preexisting osteoarthritis with areas of cartilage destruction. Panel **f** shows advanced destruction of the upper femoral head in the pressure-transfer zone with decreased volume and flattening of the femoral head, initially causing an apparent widening of the radiographic joint space. This stage (Cruess IV) is also characterized by fragmentation, which for simplicity is not shown here. Cruess stage V (Ficat stage IV) with secondary osteoarthritis is also omitted from the figure.

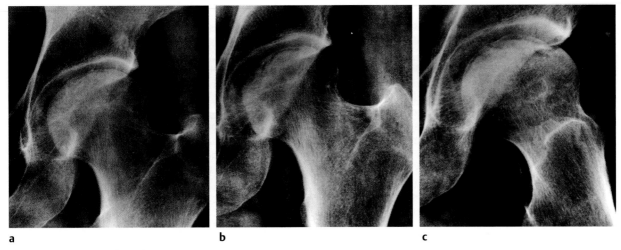

Fig. 6.**123 a–c**   Legend on the opposite page

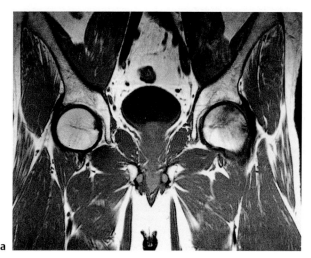

a

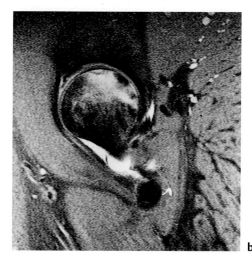

b

Fig. 6.**124a, b**   MRI appearance of an incipient perfusion deficit in the femoral head of a 36-year-old man, otherwise healthy
and with no risk factors. There is a potential for avascular necrosis to develop, but it is not inevitable.
a T1-weighted image shows very low signal intensity in the
pressure-transfer zone.
b T2-weighted sagittal image shows pronounced edema in
the upper half of the femoral head.
Note the small subchondral "fracture" below the upper
convexity and the associated effusion. Conventional radiographs at this stage are normal, and bone scans show slightly
increased uptake in the left femoral head. Following strict im-

mobilization, the edema cleared completely in four months,
raising the possible differential diagnosis of transient edema.
In the pure edema stage, it is not possible to distinguish incipient avascular necrosis of the femoral head (ARCO stage I)
from transient edema. A typical double-line sign must be present before a confident diagnosis of femoral head osteonecrosis can be made. In most cases, however, the process is irreversible by that time. Studies by Van de Berg et al. (1999) indicate
that a subchondral "fracture line" more than 12 mm long and/
or more than 4 mm wide very likely signifies an irreversible lesion.

Table 6.**9**   ARCO stages of avascular necrosis of the femoral head. Correlation with imaging procedures and treatment options

Stage	Histology	Radiographs	CT	Bone scan	MRI	Treatment
0	+	–	–	–		
I (reversible)	+	–	–	?	Edema	Core decom-pression
II	+	Possible osteopenia	Osteopenia	+	Double-line sign	
III	+	Subchondral lucency	Like radiographs; change in asterisk sign	+	Fragmentation[1], etc.	Revasculariza-tion surgery?
IV	+	Fragmentation and altered shape	Like radiographs	+		Osteotomy, prosthesis

[1] Crescent sign, indicating a subchondral fracture.

● Relatively early MRI changes in ARCO stage II consist of a
fat-equivalent area in the periphery of the femoral head
(usually in the pressure-transfer zone) with a surrounding border (see below). Mitchell (1986, 1987) defines
this as class A or "initial" femoral head osteonecrosis, in
which reparative or reactive changes have not yet com-
menced in the necrotic segment, so that the actual
necrotic area contains fat-equivalent signals rimmed by
a reactive border. Recent findings indicate, however,
that this stage is already irreversible. The demarcating
border has a bandlike pattern and is described as the
double-line sign. It is hypointense on T1-weighted images and hyperintense on fat-suppressed T2-weighted
images (e.g., STIR sequence) on the necrotic side (due to

granulation tissue) but hypointense on the healthy
bone side. This pattern is highly specific and is unlike
that associated with neoplastic or coxitic changes in the
femoral head. In class B, the necrotic area (usually the
anterosuperior segment) develops reactive changes
with capillary ingrowth, and bleeding occurs. The affected head segment has high (blood-equivalent) signal
intensity on both T1- and T2-weighted images. Further
stages relate mainly to mechanical factors and need not
be described here. The double-line sign should **not** be
confused with the former epiphyseal plate.

In the early stage of avascular necrosis, the affected avascular area shows decreased tracer uptake on **bone scans**, but this can be accurately documented only by SPECT imaging. This stage is rarely seen in avascular necrosis of the hip, however, because the examination usually is performed too late. It is more common to find intense radionuclide uptake in the affected segment due to reparative processes.

The **CT appearance** of avascular necrosis was described by Dihlmann and Heller (1985; Fig. 6.**125**). On thin contiguous slices 2–3 mm thick, normal trabecular lines in the bone (a combination of pressure and tension trajectories) create a stellate pattern called the asterisk sign. In aseptic necrosis of the femoral head, the stellate pattern appears distorted even in the precollapse stage (Fig. 6.**125 d–g**).

 ## Inflammation?

The causes of inflammatory changes in the hip joint range from bacterial infections and aseptic coxitis (e.g., in seronegative spondylarthritis) to sympathetic arthritis like that caused by an osteoid osteoma. Early inflammatory changes are currently diagnosed based on soft-tissue thickening about the hip, effusion, and the results of joint aspiration (Fig. 6.**128**). Radiographs show absence or blurring of the fat stripe about the hip, and the joint contours and subchondral bone structures become indistinct. In children, it is not uncommon for effusion to cause severe joint distension with subluxation of the femoral head (Fig. 6.**126**).

A special entity called the **irritable hip** (coxitis fugax) can occur between 1 and 14 years of age and produce initial signs similar those of bacterial arthritis (Fig. 6.**127**). This condition, whose etiology is unclear, is an acute to subacute, painful, unilateral coxitis that generally resolves spontaneously within weeks but can occasionally progress to Perthes disease or result in an enlarged femoral head due to an inflammatory growth disturbance. Bone scans in about 50% of cases show increased uptake in the acetabulum and femoral head. MRI shows decreased T1-weighted signal intensity and increased T2-weighted signal intensity in the acetabulum and femoral head combined with effusion. Irritable hip may correspond to the condition in adults known as transient osteoporosis (p. 849).

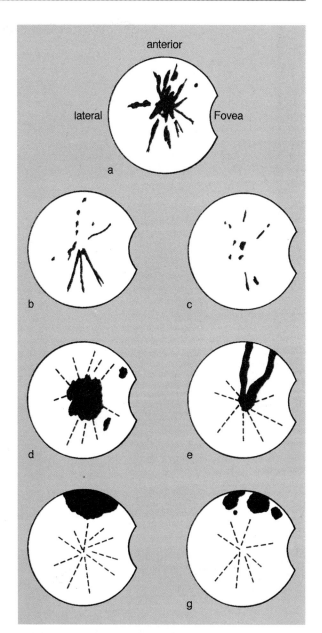

Fig. 6.**125 a–g**   The asterisk sign and its pathological changes in adult ischemic necrosis of the femoral head (individual cases).
a Normal asterisk sign of the femoral head in the foveal region (schematic).
b, c Partial or complete "breakup" of the asterisk sign.
d Central blotch (not yet pathological in itself).
e Centrifugal pseudopodia.
f Peripheral fusion in the form of sector sclerosis (shown here for the anterior part of the femoral head).
g Peripheral blotches.
Any combination of findings **d–g**, such as **d, e, g** or **d, f** or **e, f**, etc., excludes the presence of **b** or **c** (after Dihlmann and Heller).

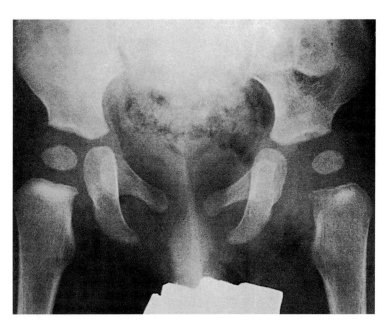

Fig. 6.**126**   Subluxation of the left femoral head secondary to heavy effusion in coxitis.

Fig. 6.**127 a, b**   Irritable hip (left side) in a 10-year-old boy. Note the subtle findings in the AP radiograph. Effusion is manifested by significant widening of the fat strip adjacent to the hip joint (arrows). There is slight demineralization of the acetabulum, femoral head, and femoral neck and slight enlargement of the entire proximal femoral epiphysis and metaphysis. The bone scan (**b**) shows intense uptake in the acetabulum and femoral head.
▽

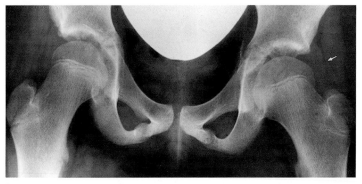

a

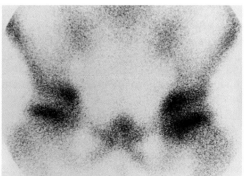

b

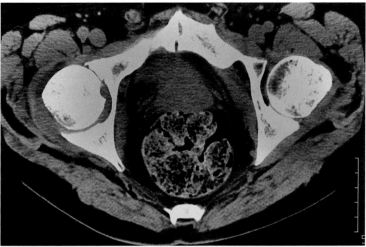

a

Fig. 6.**128 a–c**   Bacterial coxitis.
a Staphylococcal coxitis of the right hip in a man. Conventional radiographs show only slight joint space narrowing and spotty demineralization of the bone structures about the joint (not shown). CT shows marked widening of the periarticular soft-tissue structures on the right side due to effusion, with a thickened and distended joint capsule. The normal width of the periarticular soft-tissue structures on CT is 6 mm, compared with 10 mm in the image.
b, c T2-weighted MRI of tuberculous coxitis shows massive effusion, which in image **b** has spread to the iliopectineal bursa. Note the marked loss of substance in the femoral head and neck, especially in the sagittal image (**c**), with replacement by "white" effusion and inflammatory proliferation of the synovial membrane.

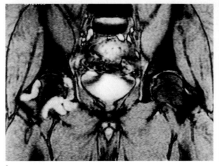

b

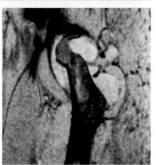

c

Tumor?

Any type of tumor can occur in the bones that comprise the hip, ranging from metastases (in adults) and solitary plasmacytoma to primary tumors (e.g., chondroblastoma, osteoid osteoma, various malignant tumors).

 Figure 6.**129** illustrates how long-standing benign tumors can lead to significant growth disturbances.

Osteoma, Giant Osteoma

The least harmful "tumor" of the hip region, and especially of the femoral neck, is benign osteoma (Fig. 6.**136a**). It probably represents a reactive process and not a true bone tumor. As a rule, it is detected incidentally. **Giant osteomas** may pose difficulties in patients with equivocal clinical symptoms, as they are positive on radionuclide scans, making it virtually impossible to distinguish them noninvasively from a solitary osteonecrotic metastasis in tumor patients.

Villonodular Synovitis

Tumorlike lesions in the hip region also include villonodular synovitis, which may have very characteristic features consisting of erosions in the acetabulum, femoral neck, and femoral head ranging to gross bone destruction (Fig. 6.**130**).

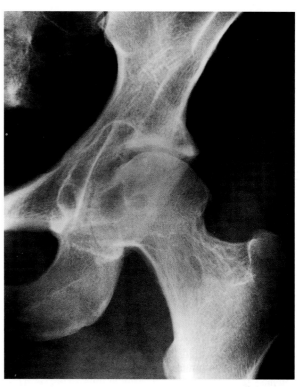

Fig. 6.**130** Typical villonodular synovitis of the left hip joint in a young man. Extensive erosions in and on the acetabulum and the femoral head and neck appear as multicentric lucencies with sclerotic margins. The erosive narrowing of the femoral neck is also called the **apple core sign** (see also Fig. 6.**131**).

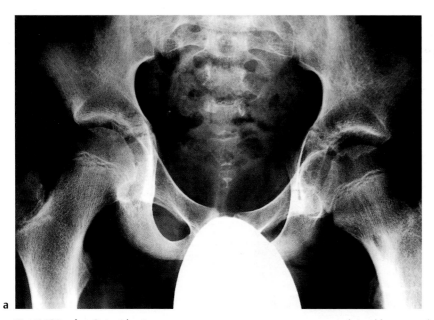

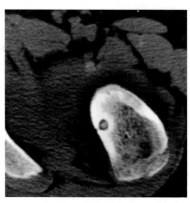

Fig. 6.**129a, b** Osteoid osteoma.
a Osteoid osteoma of the left femoral neck with severe concomitant (sympathetic) coxitis. The left femoral head and neck and acetabular structures show a marked increase in size, and there is joint space widening with marked periarticular demineralization. The hypertrophy of the femoral head and neck is explained by more than a one-year history of tumor-associated coxitis in the 11-year-old boy.
b CT clearly demonstrates the calcified nidus of the osteoid osteoma that was already visible on the plain film. Gross effusion appears as a black border surrounding the femoral neck.

Initial changes are difficult to detect on conventional radiographs (see below). The cystlike lucencies are located more in the upper medial or lower marginal part of the acetabulum—a finding that helps differentiate villonodular synovitis from subchondral cysts, which generally occur in the pressure-transfer zone. In the femur, the cystlike lucencies are located mainly in the femoral neck and in the weight-bearing portions of the femoral head. Because they are located a small distance from the subchondral plate, they can mimic true intraosseous changes in the frontal projection. As a general these changes correspond to the "apple-core sign" (Freyschmidt 2002). It is interesting to note that Cotten et al. (1995) observed the classic form described above in only 36 of 58 patients with pigmented villonodular synovitis. Eight of the cases had arthritic features and nine had osteoarthritic features. Conventional radiographic findings in three cases were normal. These numbers underscore the importance of adding CT and/or MRI when hip findings are equivocal.

Amyloid Arthropathy

Amyloid arthropathy of the hip joint can have features similar to villonodular synovitis (Fig. 6.131).

The erosive changes in the femoral neck (apple core sign), caused in both diseases by proliferative processes in the synovial membrane, can make the conditions indistinguishable on conventional radiographs. This is true, however, only if the patient's prior history (long-term dialysis, etc.) is not taken into account.

Subchondral Synovial Cyst

Another tumorlike lesion is the subchondral synovial cyst (intraosseous ganglion), which appears as a cystic lucency that is typically located in the pressure-transfer zone of the acetabulum (Figs. 6.132, 6.133).

A normal joint-space width serves to distinguish this lesion from a degenerative subchondral cyst in osteoarthritis.

Herniation Pit

The **herniation pit**, located in the proximal anterior quadrant of the femoral neck (Figs. 6.134–6.137), is a radiolucent lesion that is often misinterpreted, especially in patients with "hip symptoms." It is a true variant (Pitt et al.

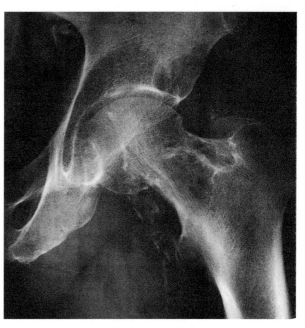

Fig. 6.**131** β_2-Microglobulin arthropathy (amyloid arthropathy) in a long-term dialysis patient. The proliferative processes in the synovial membrane have caused multicentric lucencies to develop in the femoral neck (apple core sign), accompanied by gross lateral supra-acetabular osteolysis below the superolateral rim. Contralateral changes were even more pronounced (not shown here). Compare with Fig. 6.**130**.

1982, Nokes et al. 1989). It develops in the vulnerable "reaction area" in the anterosuperior quadrant of the femoral neck, an area where purely mechanical forces from the contiguous joint capsule can incite circumscribed bone resorption. Physiologically histological sections from this area show the presence of connective tissue, newly formed cartilage, and reactive new bone formation, although these changes do not correlate with changes on radiographs. The prevalence and prominence of the reaction area correlate closely with the thickness and roughness of the apposing joint capsule. In some cases this is sufficient to cause more

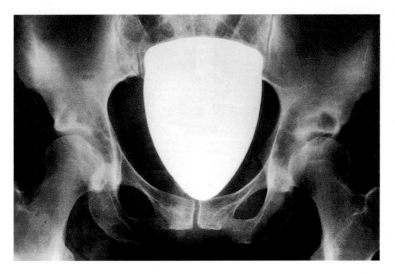

Fig. 6.**132 a–c**   Typical intraosseous ganglion on the left side.
a Fairly large lesion in a young woman. There are no signs of osteoarthritis.

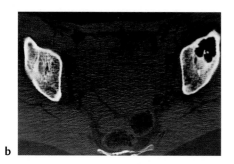

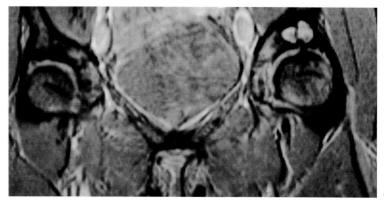

Fig. 6.**132 b, c**   CT and MRI views of the ganglion. The area of very high signal intensity traversed by a "septum" is a typical pattern seen in other skeletal regions as well.

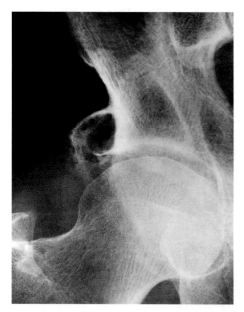

Fig. 6.**133**   Relatively large intraosseous ganglion, which apparently developed at the very margin of the joint or at the subperiosteal level. There are no classic signs of osteoarthritis.

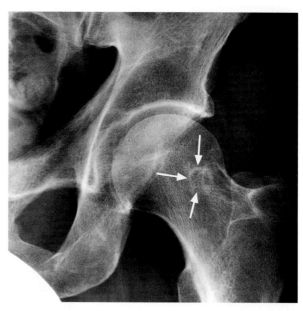

Fig. 6.**134 a**

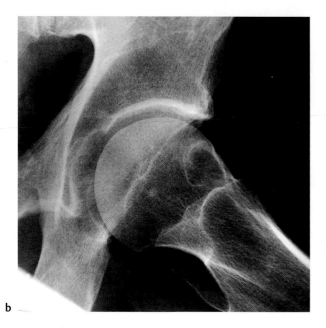

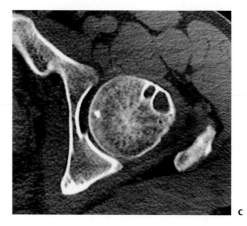

Fig. 6.**134 a–c**   Herniation pit of the left femoral neck, detected incidentally (arrows in **a**). Note the subtle physiological vacuum phenomenon in the joint space of the left hip (in **b**).

pronounced resorptive femoral neck changes that resemble a small bone tumor. Almost all herniation pits
studied to date are asymptomatic lesions that were detected incidentally. The lesion appears to be more common
in cases where the hip is subjected to relatively high mechanical loads, including in overweight individuals. Radiographically, herniation pits correspond to a Lodwick type
IA lesion (osteolysis) rimmed by a solid sclerotic border.
The various imaging appearances are illustrated in
Figs. 6.134–6.137). Individual lesions may be as large as

1 cm, bicentric, and may show significant reactive sclerosis, manifested on bone scans by a slight increase in tracer
uptake. The lesions are hypointense on T1-weighted MR
images but often hyperintense on T2-weighted images,
usually with a peripheral rim of low signal intensity
(Fig. 6.137).

The increased signal intensity is attributable to a higher
fluid content in the connective tissue occupying the defect
(Nokes et al. 1989).

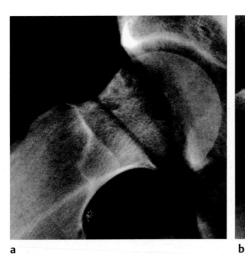
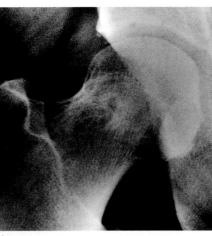

a

b

Fig. 6.**135 a, b** Multicentric
herniation pit of the right
femoral neck.

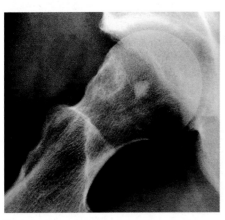
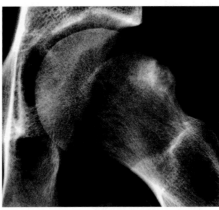

a

b

Fig. 6.**136 a, b** Bilateral
herniation pits in an asymptomatic patient. The pit on the
left side has a fairly prominent
sclerotic border. An osteoma is
noted on the right side as an
incidental finding.

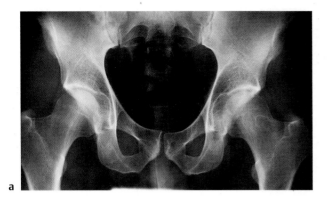

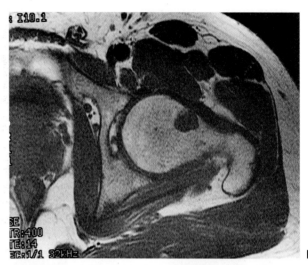

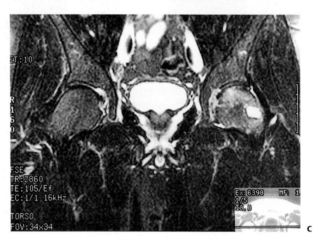

Fig. 6.**137 a–c**   Transient osteoporosis (left) coexisting with a herniation pit (left) in a young man. Note the very slight decrease in the density of the left femoral head and neck. The key diagnostic criterion can also be recognized, even in this reproduction: blurring of the cancellous bone structures in the femoral neck with an absence of trajectorial lines. The herniation pit shows an absence of signal on the T1-weighted image (**b**) and high, fluid-equivalent signal intensity on the T2-weighted image (**c**). Note the pronounced edema throughout the left femoral head. With proper immobilization of the hip and treatment with biophosphonates, the transient osteoporosis resolved completely in six months.

 Other Changes?

Transient Osteoporosis, Transient Edema

Transient osteoporosis is a disease of unknown etiology that bears some resemblance to reflex sympathetic (Sudeck) dystrophy. Transient osteoporosis belongs to the class of algodystrophies, which include Sudeck dystrophy. Transient osteoporosis has a certain affinity for the hip joint. It is generally preceded by **transient edema**, which is marked by severe pain of sudden onset. This edema usually occurs close to the joint, especially on the femoral side, and is accompanied by synovitis with effusion (Figs. 6.**137**, 6.**138**).

T2-weighted MRI shows an area of very high signal intensity encompassing the femoral head and neck. Increased signal intensity is also occasionally seen in the acetabulum. The physiological fat marrow signal is absent on T1-weighted images. This transient bone marrow edema may resolve spontaneously, or it may progress to transient osteoporosis or even to avascular necrosis of the femoral head if stresses continue to be imposed on the joint. On radiographs, transient osteoporosis is associated with **increased density** of the femoral head and neck,

which is sometimes very subtle (Fig. 6.**137**). **Blurring or unsharpness of the trabecular structure** is a key diagnostic criterion, and biopsies often reveal histological changes that resemble osteomalacia.

 The radiographic features, then, are true borderline findings between normal and abnormal and pose a challenge to the eye of the radiologist.

The changes take up to six months to resolve completely. The rate of recovery depends on hip stresses: the sooner non-weight-bearing is enforced, the sooner the disease will regress. Higer et al. (1989) published a good study on the early MRI diagnosis of transient osteoporosis. Radionuclide scans always show increased uptake in the femoral head and neck, often with extension to the acetabulum. Bone scans are already positive in the transient edema stage, but usually they are nonspecific because coxitis can produce the same findings.

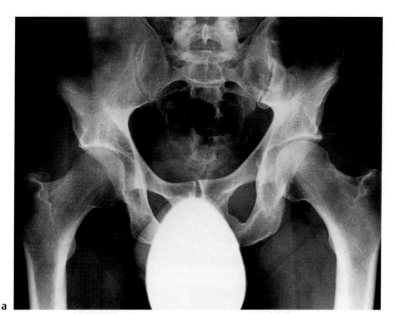

a

Fig. 6.**138 a–c**   Transient osteoporosis of the right hip in a young man. The changes are easy to interprete, because they are somewhat advanced. The marked blurring of trabecular structures in the femoral neck is an essential diagnostic criterion, along with the demineralization. The bone scan shows very intense uptake in the femoral head and neck and, to a lesser degree, in the acetabulum. MRI shows significant edema and mild effusion.

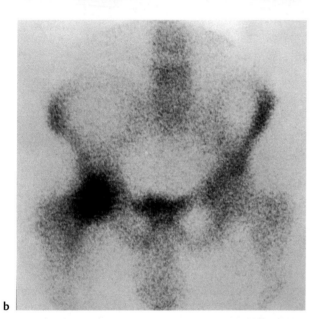

b

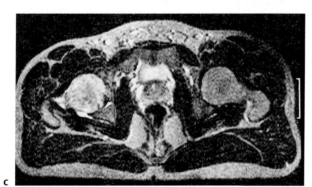

c

Osteoarthritis of the Hip (Coxarthrosis)

There is no need to discuss osteoarthritis and its typical radiographic features in detail, as the morphology of this condition is generally well known. It is important to note the following, however:

> A thickened "eyebrow" (p. 808) and osteophytes on the articular margin of the acetabulum are not conclusive signs of osteoarthritis, especially if the width of the joint space is normal (at least 3 mm on the standing radiograph, 3–5 mm on the supine radiograph).

In particular, marginal osteophytes that are located a slight distance from the capsular insertion are not degenerative osteophytes that develop from regenerative cartilage or fibrocartilage. The latter osteophytes are always intra-articular. Only an osteophyte located at the superior or inferior articular margin of the femoral head may signify osteoarthritis. Another early manifestation of osteoarthritis on conventional radiographs is the **plaque sign** (Fig. 6.**139 b**).

This sign is visible only on Lauenstein views. It reflects cartilage proliferation and subsequent ossification in the "reaction area" on the anterior aspect of the femoral neck (see herniation pit, p. 846). This sign should not be confused with the **physiological articular eminence of the femoral neck** (Dihlmann and Frick 1971)—a convex articular tubercle on the femoral neck that is also covered by cartilage but never shows the density and irregularity of the plaque sign (compare **b** and **d** in Fig. 6.**139**).

Figure 6.**140** illustrates the changes that may be observed in advanced osteoarthritis of the hip.

Degenerative metaplastic bone formation in the anterior or posterior part of the capsule can produce a Mach effect that simulates a fracture (Fig. 6.**111 b**).

Fig. 6.**139 a–d** Osteoarthritis of the hip: early and advanced radiographic signs.
a Typical marginal osteophytes on the fovea capitis and at subcapsular sites on the superior and inferior margins of the femoral head.
b The plaque sign.
c Wiberg sign on the inferior aspect of the femoral neck in advanced osteoarthritis.
d Physiological articular eminence of the femoral neck as described by Dihlmann and Frick. This feature should not be mistaken for the plaque sign (**b**).

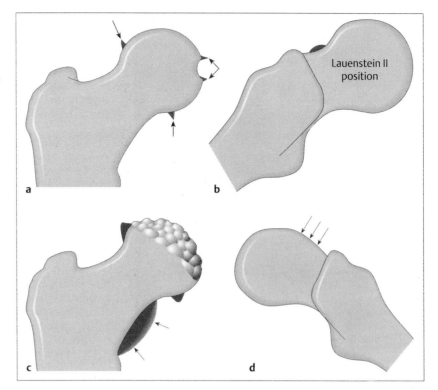

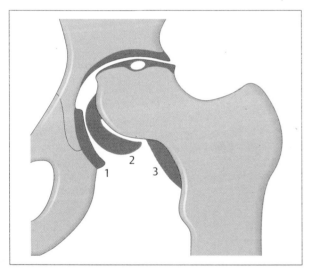
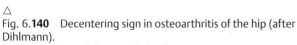

△
Fig. 6.**140** Decentering sign in osteoarthritis of the hip (after Dihlmann).
1 Duplication of the acetabular floor
2 Subfoveal osteophyte
3 "Hammock" sign of Wiberg

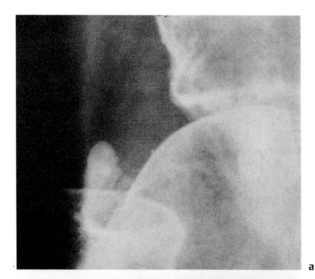
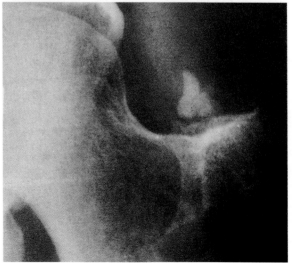

Fig. 6.**141 a, b** Calcific bursitis of the trochanteric bursa. ▷

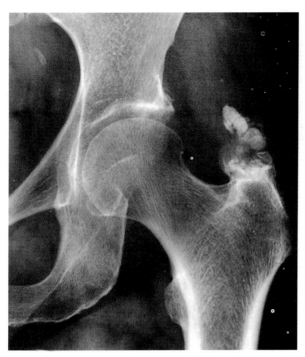

Fig. 6.**142** Unusually pronounced calcific bursitis detected incidentally in an asymptomatic patient.

Rapidly Destructive Hip Disease

Rapidly destructive hip disease is characterized by rapid deterioration of the femoral head in the absence of severe reactive changes. The features are strongly reminiscent of a neuropathic arthropathy. The pathogenesis relates to chondrocalcinotic changes in the cartilage with reactive synovitis, severe drug abuse (analgesic hip), etc.

Calcification of Ligaments, Bursae, and Tendon Sheaths

There are many ligaments, bursae, and tendon sheaths in the hip region that may undergo regressive calcification (calcific tendinitis, calcific peridentinitis, calcific bursitis) resulting in more or less characteristic radiographic changes (Figs. 6.**141**, 6.**142**, 6.**145**).

Localized regressive calcifications, particularly when located around the greater trochanter, should not be mistaken for bony avulsions or persistent apophyses.

Chronic bursitis can occasionally lead to destruction of the underlying bone, such as the lateral border of the greater trochanter (Figs. 6.**144**, 6.**145**), and mimic a tumor arising from the periosteum, cortex, or soft tissues. Heterotopic ossification (due to hemorrhage, etc.) can also contribute to juxtacortical "soft-tissue calcifications" (Fig. 6.**143**).

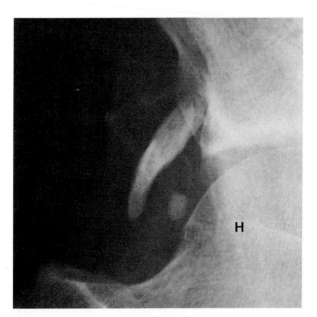

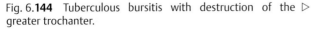

Fig. 6.**143** Myositis ossificans in the area below the anterior inferior iliac spine, which itself appears intact. The myositis ossificans (heterotopic ossification) appears to have occurred in the rectus femoris muscle.

Fig. 6.**144** Tuberculous bursitis with destruction of the ▷ greater trochanter.

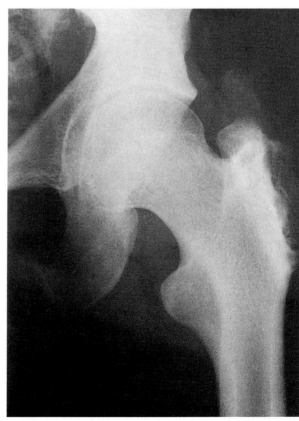

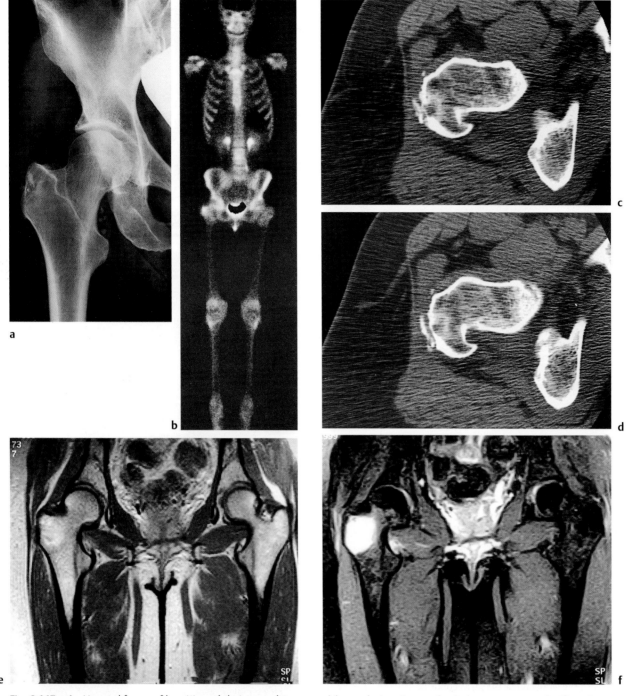

Fig. 6.145 a–j Unusual forms of bursitis and their sequelae. **a–f** Active calcific bursitis on the right greater trochanter with destruction of the trochanteric cortex and underlying cancellous bone (shown most clearly in **c** and **d**). T2-weighted MRI (**f**) shows massive edema that is far more extensive than the actu- al bone destruction and mimics a gross neoplastic process ("much edema about nothing"). The contrast enhancement in the T1-weighted image (**e**) was also interpreted accordingly. Because the woman was a cancer patient (breast carcinoma), the finding was confirmed histologically.

Fig. 6.**145 g–j** ▷

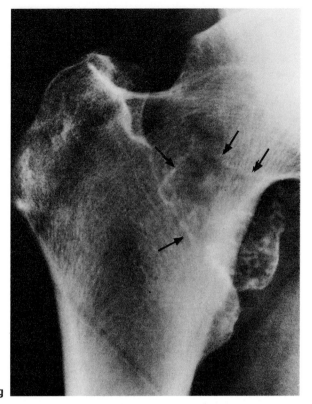

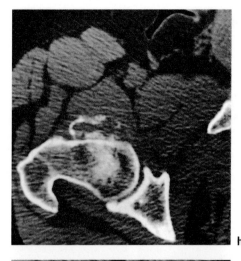

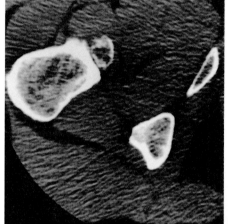

Fig. 6.**145 g–j**   Calcific bursitis of the iliopectineal bursa. The calcific density that is projected over the right femoral neck and extends past it on the medial side corresponds anatomically to the iliopectineal bursa, as confirmed by the CT scans in **h** and **i**. MRI (**j**) demonstrates a small, stalklike connection between the residual, noncalcified, fluid-filled bursa and the joint.

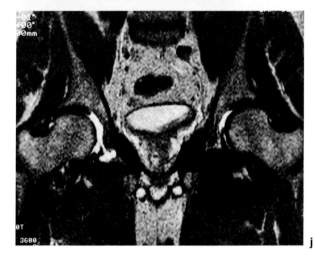

Articular Chondromatosis

Articular chondromatosis (synovial chondromatosis, Reichel disease; Fig. 6.**146**) is classified by some authors as a tumorlike lesion of the joint.

It is more likely, however, that it results from a failure of differentiation of the joint-forming mesenchyma with the transformation of fibroblasts to chondroblasts, which can then lead to tumorlike foci of cartilage proliferation with secondary ossification. The chondromas typically occur in large numbers in the synovial membrane and are arranged in clusters or chains. The individual nodules may be up to 1 cm in size, develop toward the interior of the joint, and are occasionally driven more deeply into the joint by articular motion. Sometimes they remain attached to the synovium by a small pedicle that may rupture, creating an intra-articular loose body. Radiographs show only the larger cartilaginous bodies that have ossified. The smaller nodules ("micronodular chondroma chains") are not visible on conventional radiographs and are clearly defined only by MRI, which shows hyperintense bodies on T2-weighted images. The lesions may show a stippled or speckled calcification pattern on radiographs, and some show homogeneous calcification. We know from our own

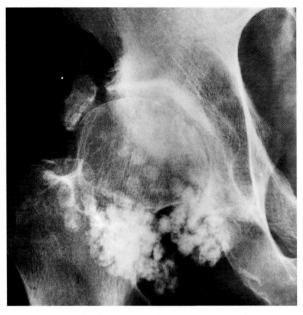

Fig. 6.**146**   Marked articular chondromatosis. The patient presented clinically with recurrent arresting of the hip joint.

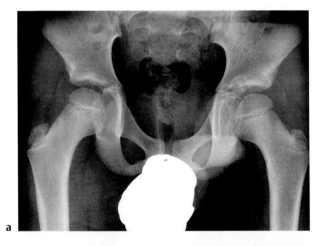

a

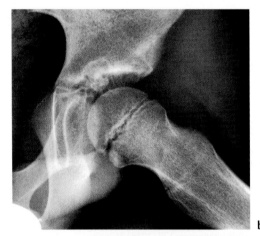

b

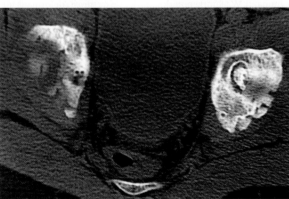

c

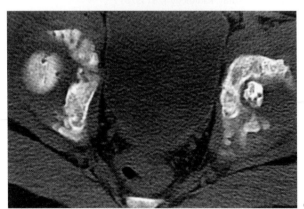

d

Fig. 6.**147 a–f**   Trevor disease (hemimelic epiphyseal dysplasia) in an 8-year-old boy with intermittent pain in the left hip and periodic locking. The Lauenstein view shows a sclerosis-rimmed osteolytic area in the medial part of the acetabulum (**b**). An ossification figure is visible within the osteolytic area. The CT scans (**c–f**) show a ringlike interface between the ossified body and the sclerotic rim, apparently representing a kind

of cartilaginous cap. We believe that the ossification figure in the acetabular lacuna is caused by the proliferation or hyperplasia of one of the many ossification centers of the acetabulum, creating a mechanical pressure that has caused bone resorption in the adjacent acetabulum (a similar mechanism occurs with osteochondroma). The absence of additional ossified bodies in the joint makes it unlikely that the body is an os-

Fig. 6.**147 e–f** ▷

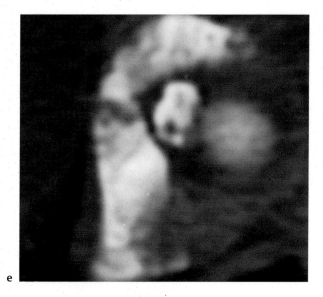

e

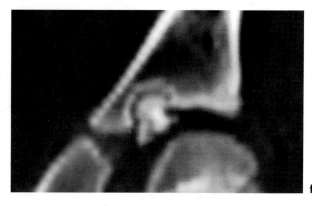

f

sified articular chondroma. The finding is not clinically or radiographically consistent with prior osteochondritis dissecans. Note on the AP radiograph that the left femoral head has already begun to subluxate from the acetabulum.

case material that a secondary chondrosarcoma can develop from articular chondromatosis in the hip (Freyschmidt et al. 1998). Differentiation from intra-articular loose bodies in osteochondritis dissecans relies on the fact that radiographs or CT scans in osteochondritis dissecans will generally show defects in the joint contours from which the loose bodies have separated. An unusual differ-

ential diagnosis is Trevor disease (Fig. 6.**147**). Another MRI differential diagnosis is multiple **rice body formation** in the bursae (rice bodies show low signal nodules in high signal effusion; cartilage-containing masses of synovial chondromatosis are isointense or slightly hyperintense on T1-weighted sequences relative to hypointense skeletal muscle).

References

Abe, J., Y. Harada, K. Oinuma et al.: Acetabular labrum: Abnormal findings at MR imaging in asymptomatic hips. Radiology 216 (2000) 576

Anda, S., T. Terjesen, K. A. Kvistad et al.: Acetabular angles and femoral anteversion in dysplastic hips in adults: CT investigation. J. Comput. assist. Tomogr. 15 (1991) 115

Andrén, L.: Aetiology and diagnosis of congenital dislocation of the hip in newborns. Radiologe 1 (1961) 89

Angel, J. L.: The reaction area of the femoral neck. Clin. Orthop. 32 (1964) 130

Armbruster, Th. G., J. Guerra jr., D. Resnick et al.: The adult hip: an anatomic study. Radiology 128 (1978) 1

Billing, L., O. Eklöf: Slip of the femoral epiphysis: revival of a method of assessment. Pediat. Radiol. 14 (1984) 413

Billenkamp, G., G. Bongartz: Die Osteochondrosis der Hüftgelenkspfanne. Fortschr. Röntgenstr. 143 (1985) 359

Brossmann, J., G. M. G. Plötz, J.-C. Steffens et al.: MR-Arthrographie des Labrum acetabulare — Radiologisch-anatomische Korrelation an 20 Leichenhüften. Fortschr. Röntgenstr. 171 (1999) 143

Chrispin, A. R., N. Harris, G. L. Roberts: A method for calculating acetabular anteversion in children. Pediat. Radiol. 7 (1978) 155

Clarke, N. M. P., H. Th. Harcke, P. McHugh et al.: Real-time ultrasound in the diagnosis of congenital dislocation and dysplasia of the hip. J. Bone Jt Surg. 67-B (1985) 406

Cohen, M. S., R. H. Gelberman, P. P. Griffin et al.: Slipped capital femoral epiphysis: assessment of epiphyseal displacement and angulation. J. pediat. Orthop. 6 (1986) 259

Conn, K. S., R. N. Villar: Die Labrumläsion aus der Sicht eines arthroskopischen Hüftchirurgen. Orthopäde 27 (1998) 699

Cooper, K. L., J. W. Beabout, R. McLeod: Supraacetabular insufficiency fractures. Diagn. Radiol. 157 (1985) 15

Cotten, A., R. M. Flipo, P. Chartanet et al.: Pigmented villonodular synovitis of the hip: Review of radiographic features in 58 patients. Skeletal Radiol 24 (1995) 1

Cruess, R. L.: Osteonecrosis of bone: current concepts as to etiology and pathogenesis. Clin. Orthop 208 (1986) 30

Czerny, C., S. Hofmann, A. Neuhold et al: Lesions of the acetabular labrum: Accuracy of MR imaging and MR arthrography in detection and staging. Radiology 200 (1996) 225

Czerny, C., S. Hofmann, M. Urban et al.: MR arthrography of the adult acetabular–labral complex: correlation with surgery and anatomy. Am J Roentgenol. 173 (1999) 345

Delaunay, S., R. G. Dussault, P. A. Kaplan et al.: Radiographic measurements of dysplastic adult hips. Skelet. Radiol. 26 (1997) 75

Dihlmann, W.: Über ein besonderes Coxarthrosezeichen (Pseudofrakturlinie) im Röntgenbild (Kritik des sogenannten Mach-Effektes). Fortschr. Röntgenstr. 100 (1964) 383

Dihlmann, W.: Röntgenmerkmale der Coxarthrosis deformans und coxaler Präarthrose. Radiologe 14 (1974) 352

Dihlmann, W., W. Frick: Das Plaquezeichen am Hüftgelenk. (Spezielle, weniger beachtete Röntgenbefunde am Stütz- und Gleitgewebe 2). Fortschr. Röntgenstr. 114 (1971) 297

Dihlmann, W., M. Heller: Asterisk-Zeichen und adulte ischämische Femurkopfnekrose. Fortschr. Röntgenstr. 142 (1985) 430

Dihlmann, W., B. Tillmann: Perikoxale Fettstreifen und Hüftgelenkkapsel. Anatomisch-radiologische Korrelation. Fortschr. Röntgenstr. 156 (1992) 411

Dorne, H. L., Ph. H. Lander: Spontaneous stress fractures of the femoral neck. Amer. J. Roentgenol. 144 (1985) 343

Fernbach, S. K., A. K. Poznanski, A.S. Kelikian et al.: Greater trochanteric overgrowth: development and surgical correction. Radiology 154 (1985) 661

Ficat, R. P.: Idiopathic bone osteonecrosis of the femoral head: early diagnosis and treatment. J. Bone Joint Surg (Br) 67 (1985) 3

Freyschmidt, J.: The apple core sign. Eur. Radiol. 12 (2002) 245

Grote, R., H. Elgeti, D. Saure: Bestimmung des Antetorsionswinkel am Femur mit der axialen CT. Röntgen-Bl. 33 (1980) 31

Haag, M., A. Reichelt: Widening of the teardrop distance in early stages of Legg-Calvé-Perthes disease compared with the late fate. Arch. orthop. traum. Surg. 100 (1982) 163

Hackenbruch, W.: Die idiopathische Coxa antetorta (Antetorsionssyndrom). Z. Kinderchir. 38 (1983) 404

Heidenblut, A.: Doppelseitig persistierender Schaltknochen am hinteren Rand des Azetabulum (Os acetabuli posterius bilaterale). Fortschr. Röntgenstr. 99 (1963) 109

Herrlin, K., L. Ekelund: Radiographic measurements of the femoral neck anteversion. Acta orthop. scand. 54 (1983) 141

Hernandez, R. J., A. K. Poznanski: CT evaluation of pediatric hip disorders. Orthop. Clin. N. Amer. 16 (1985) 513

Higer, H. P., J. Grimm, P. Pedrosa et al.: Transitorische Osteoporose oder Femurkopfnekrose? Frühdiagnose mit MRT. Fortschr. Röntgenstr. 150 (1989) 407

Hofmann, S., G. Kramer, K. Leder et al.: Die nichttraumatische Hüftkopfnekrose des Erwachsenen: Pathophysiologie, Klinik und therapeutische Möglichkeiten. Radiologe 34 (1994) 1

Imhof, H., M. Breitenseher, S.Trattnig et al.: Imaging of avascular necrosis of bone. Europ. J. Radiol. 7 (1997) 180

Johnstone, W. H., Th. E. Keats, M. E. Lee: The anatomic basis for superior acetabular roof notch "superior acetabular notch". Skelet. Radiol. 8 (1982) 25

Kölbel, R., H. Golzo: Die Köhler'sche Tränenfigur. Fortschr. Röntgenstr. 127 (1977) 326

Komprda, J.: Beitrag zur Diagnostik der acetabulären Dysplasie im Säuglingsalter. Z. Orthop. 122 (1984)

Koo, K. H., R. Dussault, P. Kaplan et al.: Age-related marrow conversion in the proximal metaphysis of the femur: evaluation with T1-weighted MR imaging. Radiology 206 (1998) 745

Kopits, E.: Ein sicheres Verfahren zur Frühdiagnose der angeborenen Hüftverrenkung. Z. Orthop. 69 (1939) 167

Korovessis, P.: Beidseitige Ermüdungsfraktur des Schenkelhalses bei M. Bechterew. Z. Orthop. 122 (1984) 623

Kozlowski, K., R. Middleton: Familial osteochondritis dissecans: a dysplasia of articular cartilage? Skelet. Radiol. 13 (1985) 207

Kozlowski, K., J. Scougall: Idiopathic chondrolysis — diagnostic difficulties (report of 4 cases). Pediat. Radiol. 14 (1984) 314

Lequesne, M.: Coxometrie. Mesure des angles fondamentaux de la hanche radiographique de l'adulte par un rapporteur combiné. Rev. Rhum. 30 (1963) 479

Lequesne, M., S. de Séze: Le faux-profil du bassin. Rev. Rhum. 28 (1961) 643

Littrup, P. J., A. M. Aisen, E. M. Braunstein et al.: Magnetic resonance imaging of femoral head development in roentgenographically normal patients. Skelet. Radiol. 14 (1985) 159

Mandell, G. A., W. G. McKenzie, C. J. Scott et al.: Identification of avascular necrosis in the dysplastic proximal femoral epiphysis. Skelet. Radiol. 18 (1989) 273

Mesgarzadeh, M., G. Revesz, A. Bonakdarpour: Femoral neck torsion angle measurement by computed tomography. J. Comput. assist. Tomogr. 11 (1987) 799

Meyer, J.: Dysplasia epiphysealis capitis femoris. Acta orthop. scand. 34 (1964) 183

Mitchel, M. D., H. L. Kundel, M. E. Steinberg et al.: Avascular necrosis of the hip: comparison of MR, CT and szintigraphy. Amer. J. Roentgenol. 147 (1986) 67

Mitchell, D. G., V. M. Rao, M. K. Dalinka: Hematopoietic and fatty bone marrow distribution in the normal and ischemic hip: new observations with 1.5 T MR imaging. Radiology 161 (1986) 199

Mitchell, D. G., V. M. Rao, M. K. Dulinka et al.: Femoral head avascular necrosis: correlation of MR imaging, radiographic staging, radionuclide imaging, and clinical findings. Radiology 162 (1987) 709

Murphy, S., R. Ganz, M. Muller: The prognosis of untreated dysplasia of the hip. J. Bone Jt Surg. 77-A (1995) 986

Nicol, R. O., P. F. Williams, D. J. Hill: Transient osteopaenia of the hip in children. J. pediat. Orthop. 4 (1984) 590

Noble, T. C., C. R. Pullan, A. W. Craft et al.: Difficulties in diagnosing and managing congenital dislocation of the hip. Brit. Med. J. 1978/II, 620–623

Nokes, St. R., J. B. Vogler, Ch. E. Spritzer et al.: Herniation pits of the femoral neck: Appearance at MR imaging. Radiology 172 (1989) 231

Orlic, D., I. Ruszkowski: The radiological appearance of appositional new bone on the medial part of the neck of the femur in coxarthrosis. Intern. Orthop. (SICOT) 7 (1983) 11

Peic, St.: Die Köhlersche Tränenfigur und ihre Bedeutung in der Röntgendiagnostik. Fortschr. Röntgenstr. 114 (1971) 305

Pelker, R. R., J. C. Drennan, M. B. Ozonoff: Juvenile synovial chondromatosis of the hip. J. Bone Jt Surg. 65-A (1983) 552

Petersilge, Ch. A.: MR arthrography for evaluation of the acetabular labrum. Skeletal Radiol. 30 (2001) 423

Pitt, M. J., A. R. Graham, J. H. Shipman et al.: Herniation pit of the femoral neck. Amer. J. Roentgenol. 138 (1982) 1115

Pogrund, H., R. Bloom, P. Mogle: The normal width of the adult hip: the relationship to age, sex and obesity. Skelet. Radiol. 10 (1983) 10

Ponseti, I.: Early diagnosis and pathology of congenital dislocation of the hip. Pediat. Ann. 11 (1982) 512

Ranner, G.: Die osteochondrosis deformans coxae juvenilis im MR-Tomogramm: Diagnose und Verlaufsbeurteilung in Korrelation zu Röntgen und Szintigraphie. Fortschr. Röntgenstr. 153 (1990) 124

Reeder, M. M.: Gamuts in Bone, Joint and Spine Radiology. Springer, Berlin 1993

Reikeras, O., J. Bjerkreim, A. Kolbenstoedt: Anteversion of the Azetabulum and femoral neck in normals and in patients with osteoarthritis of the hip. Acta orthop. scand. 54 (1983) 18

Rippstein, J.: Zur Bestimmung der Antetorsion des Schenkelhalses mittels 2 Röntgenaufnahmen. Z. Orthop. 86 (1955) 345

Schmidt, H.: Rückbildung eines Pfannenrandknochens (Os acetabuli). Fortschr. Röntgenstr. 106 (1967) 471

Schmidt, H.: Pfannenrandepiphyse und Pfannenrandknochen der Hüfte (Epiphysis acetabuli und Os ad acetabulum). Zbl. allg. Pathol. pathol. Anat. 92 (1954) 271

Schöneich, R.: Persistierende Epiphyse des rechten Hüftgelenkes. Fortschr. Röntgenstr. 87 (1957) 417

Skinner, H. B., St. D. Cook: Fatigue failure stress fracture of the femoral neck. Amer. J. Sports Med. 10 (1982) 245

Swiontkowski, M. F., R. A. Winquist, S. T. Hansen: Fractures of the femoral neck in patients between the ages of twelve and forty-nine years. J. Bone Jt Surg. 66-A (1984) 837

Teichert, G.: Eigenartiges Strukturbild im Pfannendach der Hüfte. Arch. orthop. Unfall.-Chir. 48 (1956) 297

Tonnis, D.: Normal values of the hip joint for the evaluation of x-rays in children and adults. Clin. Orthop. 119 (1976) 39

Umans, H., M. S. Liebling, L. Moy et al.: Slipped capital femoral epiphysis: a physeal lesion diagnosed by MRI, with radiographic and CT correlation. Skelet. Radiol. 27 (1998) 139

Urban, M., S. Hofmann, C. Tschauner: MR-Arthrographie bei der Labrumläsion des Hüftgelenkes. Orthopäde 27 (1998) 691

Van de Berg, B. C., J. J. Malghem, F. E. Lecouvet et al.: Idiopathic bone marrow edema lesions of the femoral head: predictive value of MR imaging findings. Radiology 212 (1999) 527

Walker, G.: Problems in the early recognition of congenital hip dislocation. Brit. Med. J. 1971/13/I, 147–148

Weiner, D. S., A. J. Cook, W. A. Hoyt jr et al.: Computed tomography in the measurement of femoral anteversion. Orthopedics 1 (1978) 299

Wilson, A. J., W. A. Murphy, D. C. Hardy et al.: Transient osteoporosis: Transient bone marrow edema? Radiology 167 (1980) 757

Wolf-Heidegger, G.: Atlas der systematischen Anatomie des Menschen, 2. Aufl. Karger, Basel 1961

Wolinski, A. P., I. W. McCall, G. Evans et al: Femoral neck growth deformity following the irritable hip syndrome. Brit. J. Radiol. 57 (1984) 773

Wray, D. G., N. M. Bisalahallin: Congenital diclocation of the hip. The high incidence of familial aetiology — a study of 130 cases. Brit. J. clin. Pract. 37 (1983) 299

Ziegler, G.: Partielle Ossifikation des Labrum glenoidale. Fortschr. Röntgenstr. 78 (1953) 222

Zsernaviczky, J., G. Türk: Der β-Winkel. Ein diagnostisches Zeichen für Frühdiagnose der angeborenen Hüftdysplasie. Fortschr. Röntgenstr. 123 (1975) 131

7 Lower Extremity

J. Freyschmidt

Femur

Femoral Shaft

Normal Findings

 #### During Growth

The ossification of the femoral diaphysis beginns in the 8th week of fetal development at the latest. Much as in the humerus, radiographs in newborns and infants show an ill-defined cortex with striation of the surface that apparently relates to the still-incomplete ossification of new osteoid formed by the periosteum and laid down along the cortex. This phenomenon appears to be most pronounced in premature infants (Shopfner 1966).

> It is normal to observe slight varus bowing of the femur in small children. Mild anteversion is also normal.

The femoral shaft contains many nutrient canals, especially in its proximal portion, that show considerable variation in their course (from oblique to horizontal) and their site of entry into the cortex (Fig. 7.**2**).

 #### In Adulthood

The linea aspera of the femoral shaft, shown on the anatomical photograph in Fig. 7.**1**, is an important feature on projection radiographs and CT scans.

> When the **linea aspera** is especially prominent, AP radiographs may show it as a bandlike density in the medullary cavity, especially in the middle third of the shaft, that can mimic a bone marrow infarction, enchondroma, or other intramedullary process (Fig. 7.**3a**).

The nutrient canals are more conspicuous in adults than in children (Fig. 7.**3a–d**).

- When projected end-on, they appear as a hole surrounded by a sclerotic margin.

- In a tangential projection, they form a fine linear lucency whose thin, dense margins distinguish it from a fracture line.

> **High signal intensity of the medullary cavity in MRI** of the femur (see also Fig. 7.**36a–c**) may be an **extreme normal variant**. For this reason, the opposite side should also be imaged in questionable cases. If the opposite femur has the same appearance and the patient shows no clinical signs of a systemic bone marrow process (e.g., no anemia), it is reasonable to assume that the finding is a normal variant.

Pathological Finding?

 #### Normal Variant or Anomaly?

Variants

Except for occasional prominence of the linea aspera (Fig. 7.**3a**) and prominent or irregular nutrient canals, there are no variants in the femur that might be mistaken for true pathological changes.

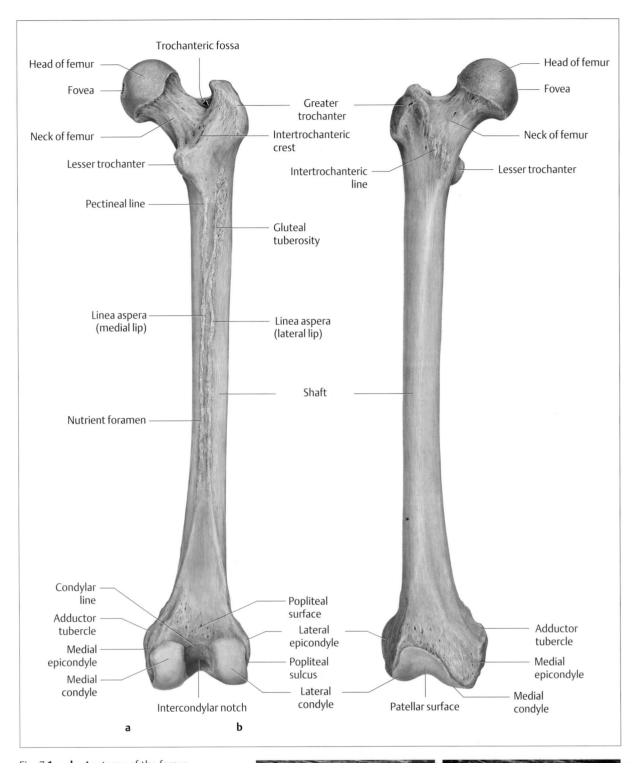

Trochanteric fossa

Head of femur

Fovea

Neck of femur

Lesser trochanter

Pectineal line

Linea aspera
(medial lip)

Nutrient foramen

Condylar
line

Adductor
tubercle

Medial
epicondyle

Medial
condyle

Intercondylar notch

Greater
trochanter

Intertrochanteric
crest

Intertrochanteric
line

Gluteal
tuberosity

Linea aspera
(lateral lip)

Shaft

Popliteal
surface

Lateral
epicondyle

Popliteal
sulcus

Lateral
condyle

Head of femur

Fovea

Neck of femur

Lesser trochanter

Adductor
tubercle

Medial
epicondyle

Medial
condyle

Patellar surface

a   **b**

Fig. 7.**1 a–d**   Anatomy of the femur.
a, b Gross anatomy of the femur, posterior
(**a**) and anterior aspect (**b**). Note particularly
the linea aspera in **a**, which is continuous
proximally with the gluteal tuberosity and
pectineal line (after Wolf-Heidegger).
c, d Axial CT at the level of the lesser trochanter (**c**) and at a slightly more distal level
(**d**). The gluteal tuberosity and linea aspera
normally have a somewhat "rarefied" appearance on CT scans.

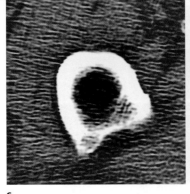

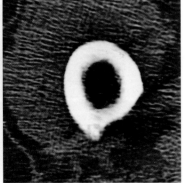

c   **d**

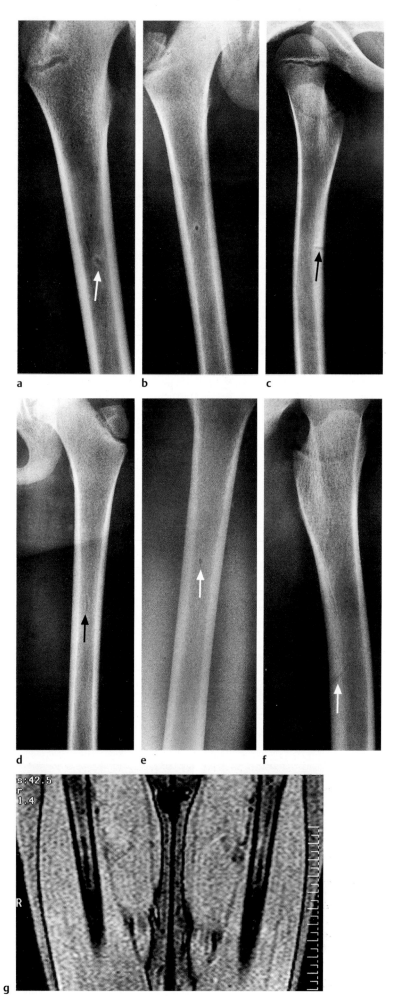

Fig. 7.**2a–g**   Course and projection of nutrient canals in a 6-year-old girl with nonspecific knee pain.

a This finding (arrow) was first interpreted as a small osteoid osteoma.

b, c In fact, the finding in radiograph **a** is an oblique projection of a nutrient canal. This is apparent in radiograph **b**, where the tube is angled slightly downward. The canal enters the posterior side of the bone horizontally, which is somewhat unusual (**c**).

d In the opposite femur, the nutrient canal is projected as a fine radiolucent line (arrow).

e Angling the tube downward gives a projection of the canal similar to that in **b**.

f In the lateral view, we see that the nutrient canal runs obliquely upward and anteriorly as it enters the medullary cavity.

g On MRI, the two larger vessels in the proximal diaphyses appear as bands with little or no central signal intensity (flow voids).

Fig. 7.**3 a–d**   Projection of the linea aspera and nutrient canals.

a Bandlike density in the distal femoral shaft resembles a calcifying process of the medullary cavity. In fact, the density is a prominent linea aspera.

b, c In these specimen radiographs, a long, thin cannula has been inserted to mark the course of a large nutrient canal. The cannula was inserted into a large, distal canal on the posterior aspect of the femur, and we see that it runs for some distance through the cortex (**b**) before entering the medullary cavity. Radiograph **c** is a slightly rotated view compared with **b**.

d Unusually well-defined nutrient canal, not a fracture. Noted incidentally in a patient with a plasmacytoma.

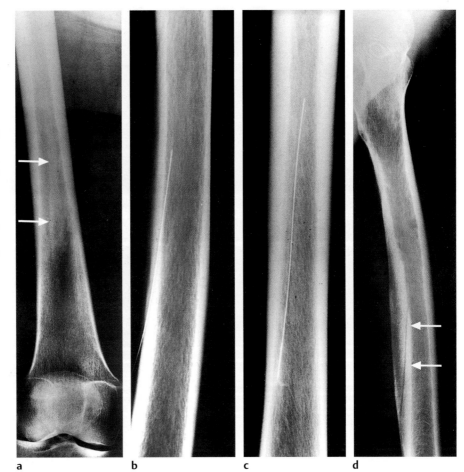

a   b   c   d

True Anomalies

The **femur–fibula–ulna complex** (Fig. 7.4) is a developmental anomaly that chiefly affects the femur and is therefore included in this chapter. It is characterized by a sporadic combination of unilateral hypoplasia or aplasia of the femur and defects of the fibula with variable defects of the ulna or peromelia in one or both arms. Bilateral defects can occur.

The diagnostic criteria for femur-fibula-ulna complex are listed in Table 7.**1**.

The etiology is unknown but may relate to a somatic mutation in early embryonic development. The case in Fig. 7.**4** is a striking example of how acetabular development depends on a normal femoral head and normal weight bearing; otherwise the acetabulum fails to develop. Fibular hypoplasia also results from altered weight-bearing loads, and the same applies to the round obturator foramen that is fairly typical of this disorder.

The most common **congenital** and **acquired deformities** of the femur are listed in Table 7.**2**.

Table 7.**1**   Diagnostic criteria for the femur-fibula-ulna complex

- Proximal femoral hypoplasia, usually unilateral. Four types are defined in the classification of Levinson et al. (1997):
  – Type A: Femur shortened; bony continuity of femur at skeletal maturity; femoral head centered in acetabulum; subtrochanteric varus
  – Type B: Femur shortened; no bony connection between head and shaft; femoral head present, but very shallow acetabulum
  – Type C: Proximal femur shortened; no bony connection between head and shaft; acetabulum flat and barely discernible
  – Type D: Femur shortened; absence of femoral head and acetabulum on radiographs at skeletal maturity
- Fibular hypoplasia or aplasia
- Fibular oligodactyly
- Defects of ulna or ulnar rays
- Peromelia at level of elbow joint or distal humeral hypoplasia; occasional phocomelia of ipsilateral or contralateral arm
- Radiohumeral synostosis with ulnar defect; aplasia of fourth and fifth rays; radial hypoplasia
- Syndactyly of fourth and fifth fingers
- Occasionally, no abnormalities of upper extremities
- No internal malformations
- No familial occurrence

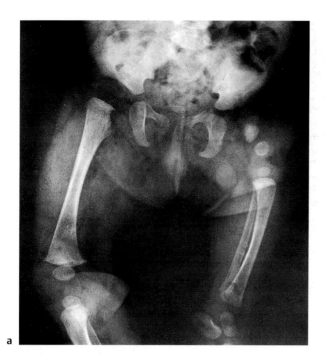

a

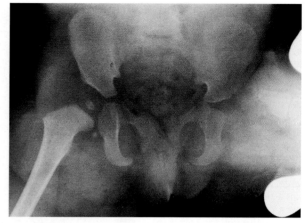

b

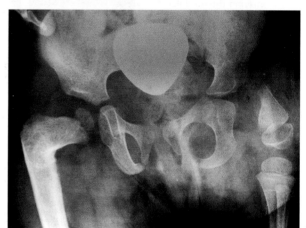

c

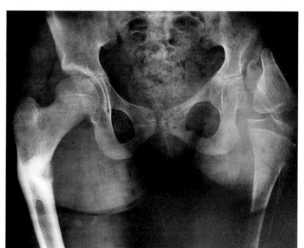

d

Fig. 7.**4a–d**   Unilateral femoral hypoplasia in a girl.
a Age 4 months.
b Age 14 months.
c Age 2 years.
d Age 11 years.
The patient has type C femoral hypoplasia in the left leg (see Table 7.**1**). The left acetabulum in radiograph **a** is barely discernible. Radiograph **c** shows a very small capital femoral ossific center projected over the superolateral part of the ischium. The left acetabulum is poorly developed, lacking the necessary mechanical stimulus. Note the very round obturator foramen on the left side, which is part of the syndrome. The left fibula is hypoplastic. The right side shows a type A femoral deformity with strong varus angulation of the neck. The angle in **c** might also be the result of a stress fracture caused by the patient's compensatory overuse of the right limb. As growth continued, the stress fracture or transformation zone caused by the varus deformity moved distally, appearing in **d** as a very dense area in the proximal shaft.

Table 7.**2**   Congenital and acquired deformities of the femur

- Erlenmeyer flask deformity caused by bone marrow processes (thalassemia, Gaucher disease) or bone transformation processes (Fig. 7.**5**)
- Enchondromatosis (Fig. 7.**6**)
- Cartilaginous exostosis disease (Fig. 7.**7**)
- Fibrous dysplasia (Fig. 7.**8**)
- Paget disease (Fig. 7.**9**)

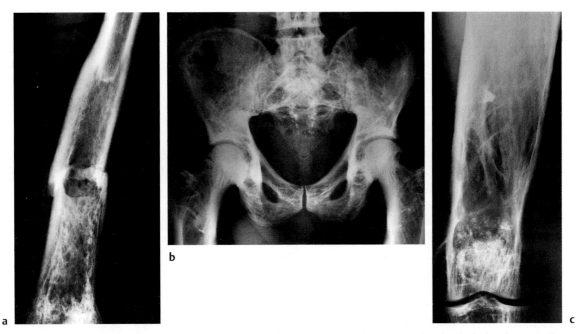

a

b

c

Fig. 7.**5 a–c**   Erlenmeyer flask deformity.

a Gaucher disease. Expansile infiltration of the bone marrow by kerasin-laden cells leads to cancellous bone resorption with coarse and irregular cancellous trabeculae. Cortical thinning occurs, but concomitant periosteal new bone formation leads to relative cortical thickening, giving the bone a straight or convex margin known as the Erlenmeyer flask deformity. Note the spontaneous fracture in the distal shaft. The irregular sclerosis in the distal shaft represents a large bone marrow infarct that has undergone dystrophic calcification.

b, c Buchem disease (endosteal hyperostosis). Again, the femur has lost its normal waisted contour and acquired an Erlenmeyer flask deformity. A detailed description of this case can be found in Freyschmidt (1997).

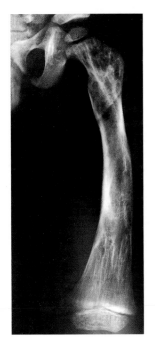

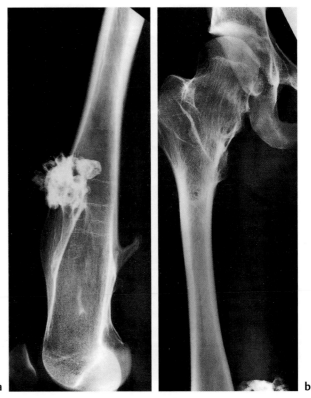

a

b

Fig. 7.**6**   Deformity of the femur with marked varus angulation and metaphyseal enlargement in enchondromatosis. The streaklike features, most prominent at the distal diaphyseal-metaphyseal junction, are cartilage columns. An up-to-date discussion of this disease can be found in Freyschmidt et al. (1998).

Fig. 7.**7 a, b**   Typical multiple (cartilaginous) exostosis disease with marked deformities caused by masses of flat and pointed osteochondromas involving the femoral neck and distal diaphyseal-metaphyseal junction area that represent growing zones. Note the valgus deformity of the femoral neck. The sagittal diameter of the distal femoral shaft and metaphysis is markedly expanded.

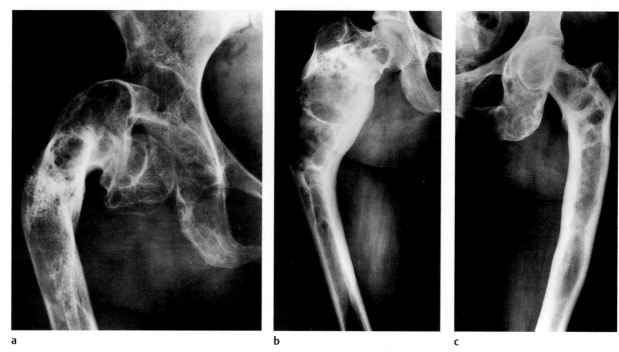

a   b   c

Fig. 7.**8 a–c**   Femoral deformities in fibrous dysplasia.
a Involvement of the acetabulum and the proximal and distal (not shown) femur with shepherd's crook deformity.
b Another example of gross femoral deformity. The massive expansion of the proximal shaft and metaphysis is due partly

to regressive liquefaction with a rise of intramedullary pressure and increasing endosteal bone resorption accompanied by periosteal new bone formation.
c Case showing extensive involvement of the ischium.

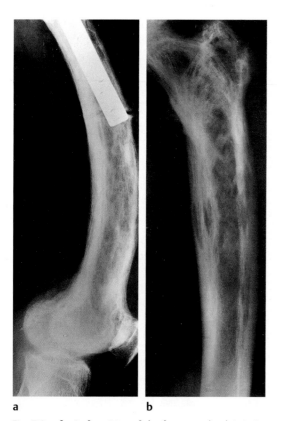

a   b

Fig. 7.**9 a–f**   Deformities of the femur and pelvis in Paget disease.
a, b A long segment of the femur shows typical streaklike bone transformation mainly affecting the cortex, which is thickened. Note also the anterior bowing of the femur. Corrective osteotomies were attempted. A horizontal stress fracture ("banana fracture") has developed at the distal end of the metal plate.

Fig. 7.**9 c–f**   These radiographs show an unusual case of extensive bone transformation involving the entire skeleton in Paget disease. Bone demineralization on the initial radiographs was so advanced that the pelvic structures could hardly be identified, similar to the condition of the distal femur in **e**. Treatment with high doses of a bisphosphonate led to radiographic improvement and a dramatic fall of extremely high alkaline phosphatase levels. The patient, initially confined to a wheelchair, was able to walk again with crutches. Note the impressive reossification that occurred between radiographs **e** (before treatment) and **f** (after treatment). The radiographs in **c** and **d** were taken after seven months of treatment. A detailed description of this case can be found in Freyschmidt (1997).

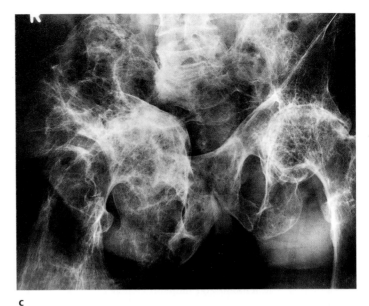

c

d

e

f

Fracture, Subluxation, or Dislocation?

Reference was made earlier to the possibility of confusing nutrient canals with nondisplaced fractures.

Stress fractures of the femoral shaft are relatively rare (6.1% of all stress fractures in military recruits; Muerman and Elfving 1980). The convexity of a bowed femur creates a site of predilection for insufficiency fractures (Fig. 7.**9a**).

An unusual oblique stress fracture of the proximal femur is shown in Fig. 7.**10**.

 ## Necrosis?

Cortical necrosis of the femoral shaft is extremely rare. We have seen one such case with disseminated osteonecrotic lesions of the tubular bones in a 27-year-old woman who had a complicated delivery and gross consumption coagulopathy. The femoral and humeral changes looked like disseminated foci of tumor destruction and resolved almost completely over the next six months (detailed case description in Freyschmidt 1997).

Bone marrow infarctions, which occur predominantly in the distal metaphysis, are discussed in more detail on p. 880 ff.

 ## Inflammation? Tumor?

Osteomyelitis rarely affects the femoral shaft, unlike the distal metaphyseal region (Fig. 7.**11**), and usually occurs only in immunocompromised adults. The radiographic features of these processes are not discussed here in detail.

Any type of primary bone tumor can occur near the growth plates of the proximal and especially the distal femur. These tumors can incite destructive changes, productive processes, and combinations of both. Tumors confined to the medullary cavity of the femoral shaft are less common, and unless they calcify are visible on radiographs only if they cause cortical erosions in the form of small, wavy concavities (scalloping).

Scalloping occurs mainly in association with the following lesions:

- Enchondroma (Fig. 7.**12**)
- Chondrosarcoma
- Slow-growing medullary metastases

 Cortical rarefaction involving a **long segment** of the femoral shaft and showing a fiberous, streaklike pattern occurs in all pathological transformation processes of bone.

This pattern is caused by resorptive widening of the haversian canals. The most common diseases that produce this type of change are primary and secondary **hyperparathyroidism** (Fig. 7.**13**) and **osteomalacia**.

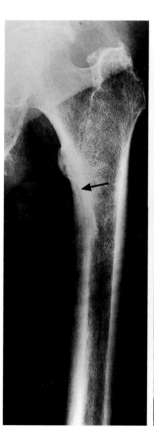

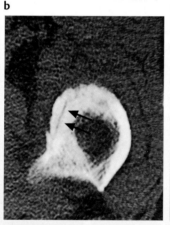

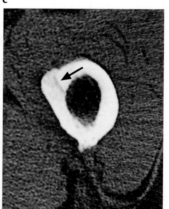

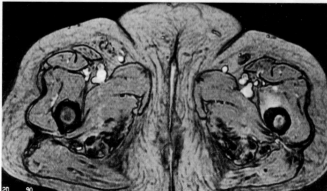

a   b   c   d

Fig. 7.**10 a–d**   Unusual stress fracture extending obliquely downward and laterally from the lesser trochanter region in an elderly overweight woman. The fracture had been missed on prior radiographs of poor technical quality. Subsequent MRI showed perifemoral edema, which was misinterpreted as signifying a neoplastic process. The concomitant marrow edema in **d** was also interpreted as neoplastic. Note the "gray cortex" sign below the lesser trochanter.

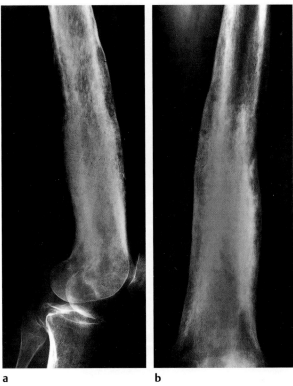

a   b

Fig. 7.**11 a, b** Chronic osteomyelitis in the distal femoral shaft, present for 30 years, apparently originated in the metaphysis and spread up the shaft. Caused by a bacterial infection, this chronic process bears similarities to the abacterial transformation processes that occur in Paget disease, especially in Fig. 7.**9 b**.

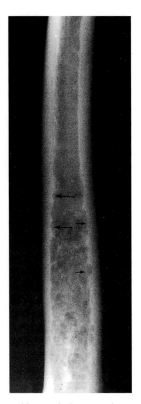

Fig. 7.**12** Endosteal scalloping caused by a calcifying enchondroma. Arrows mark some of the small cortical lacunae that the tumor lobules have "excavated" in the cortex.

Slow-growing bone tumors such as grade I or II chondrosarcoma can also produce a fiberlike appearance of the cortical bone. Especially the proximal femoral cortex below the greater and lesser trochanter is often subject to transformation processes due to various causes (tumors, osteoporosis, osteomalacia). The initial stages of these processes are difficult to detect on radiographs but are clearly demonstrated by radionuclide scans (Fig. 7.**14**).

The tendency for more severe transformation processes to affect the proximal femoral cortex, often including the lesser trochanter, apparently depends on the greater mechanical stresses to which that portion of the femur is subjected.

A **permeative destruction pattern** is one in which small, circumscribed, elliptical lucencies up to 1–2 mm in size are visible in the cortex (Fig. 7.**15**). It occurs in association with highly aggressive, fast-growing tumors of the medullary cavity that have invaded the haversian canals. The phenomenon is very characteristic of small-cell and round-cell tumors such as Ewing sarcoma and is occasionally seen in florid cases of osteomyelitis before periosteal bone formation becomes apparent.

> Permeative destructive lesions, which eventually coalesce to form confluent destruction patterns (Lodwick grades II and III), are often missed initially, especially in osteoporotic bone. They should be distinguished from the fine mottled lucencies in "pseudomalignant" disuse osteoporosis (Figs. 2.**351**, 7.**53**).

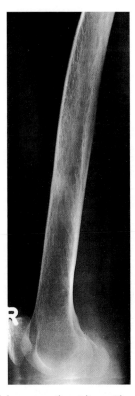

Fig. 7.**13** Typical appearance of hyperparathyroidism. The cortex is sharply defined along its periosteal surface, while its endosteal surface shows streaklike transformation. A small brown tumor is visible in the distal midshaft region.

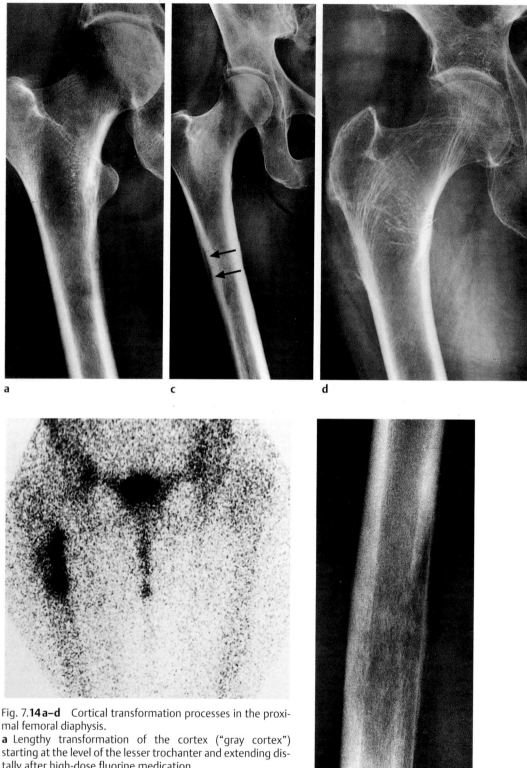

a

c

d

b

Fig. 7.**14 a–d**   Cortical transformation processes in the proximal femoral diaphysis.

a Lengthy transformation of the cortex ("gray cortex") starting at the level of the lesser trochanter and extending distally after high-dose fluorine medication.

b Bone scan shows very intense tracer uptake in that region. Later a spontaneous fracture developed in the proximal femoral shaft.

c Transformation processes in the lateral and proximal femoral cortex due to metastatic breast carcinoma.

d Subperiosteal resorption of the proximal femoral cortex below the greater trochanter in a patient with severe generalized osteoporosis. The patient was asymptomatic, and the finding remained constant for many years. The transformation processes occur at the attachment of the vastus lateralis muscle.

Fig. 7.**15**   Permeative destruction of the femoral shaft by a small-cell aggressive tumor. Confluent, permeative lesions have caused extensive cortical destruction on the flexor side of the bone. The cortex on the extensor side shows very fine osteolytic changes that follow the haversian canals.

Productive cortical changes of the femoral shaft can have the following causes:

- Melorheostosis (Fig. 7.**16a**)
- Osteoid osteoma (Fig. 7.**16b**)
- Periosteal osteosarcoma (Fig. 7.**16c**)
- Reactive changes (e.g., in pustulotic arthro-osteitis, Fig. 7.**16d, e**)
- Ossified subperiosteal hematoma

Generalized increased density of the femur as part of sclerosing bone diseases is most commonly seen in marble bone disease (Fig. 7.**17b**) and osteomyelosclerosis syndrome.

Streaks of increased density in the cancellous bone of the femur are a typical feature of **osteopathia striata** (Fig. 7.**17a**).

Increased density of the medullary cavity of the femoral shaft as an isolated finding can occur in the following conditions:

- Bone marrow infarction (Figs. 7.**37**–7.**39**)
- Calcifying enchondroma (Fig. 7.**18**), osteoid osteoma, osteosarcoma
- Osteosclerotic metastases
- Various storage diseases
- Normal variant due to a prominent linea aspera (Fig. 7.**3a**)

An *increased size of the femur* as well as of other tubular bones can occur in pulmonary hypertrophic osteoarthropathy (Figs. 7.**17c–e**).

Other Changes?

A variety of pathological calcifications can occur in the soft-tissue envelope of the thigh, ranging from ordinary vascular calcifications and heterotopic bone formation to calcifications in parasitic diseases (Fig. 7.**24**).

Circumscribed calcifications located near the linea aspera and its proximal extensions (the gluteal tuberosity and pectineal line) are generally a result of **calcifying tendinitis** (Fig. 7.**19**). The adjacent bony ridge may show structural rarefaction and irregularities that mimic a neoplastic process (Fig. 7.**20**).

Calcifying tendinitis is classified among the productive and destructive changes that can occur at fibro-osseous junctions ("enthesiopathies"). It differs from the more common forms of fibro-osteitis and fibro-ostosis, however, in that we still do not have an understanding of its etiology (Neumann et al. 1996). It is likely that purely regressive processes as well as inflammatory processes in the setting of a seronegative spondylarthritis, for example, contribute to the pathogenesis of calcifying tendinitis.

The diagnosis of calcifying tendinitis at the linea aspera is based on thigh pain in response to weight bearing and on the radiographic detection of calcification or ossification in direct proximity to the linea aspera (Figs. 7.**19**, 7.**20**).

The calcification pattern in the initial phase of the disease is fluffy and indistinct and often can be appreciated only with a magnifying lens. With passage of time, the calcifications become denser, more homogeneous, and more sharply defined and show linear or circular shapes or are spotty. Spontaneous resorption can occur, as in cases with recurrent "superimposed" inflammation. Similar calcific

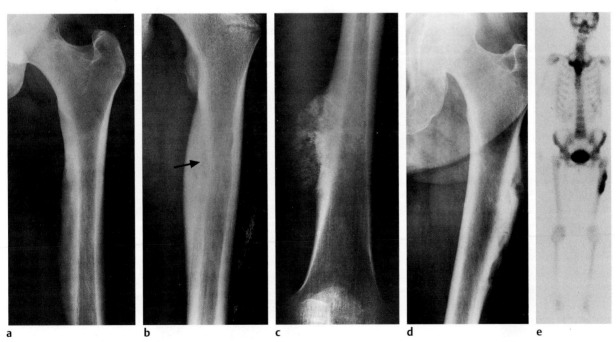

a　　　　b　　　　c　　　　d　　　　e

Fig. 7.**16a–e** Productive changes in the femoral cortex due to various causes.
a Thickening of a long segment of the medial cortex in melorheostosis.
b Osteoid osteoma. The partially calcified nidus is barely visible (arrow).
c Classic periosteal osteosarcoma.

d, e Pustulotic arthro-osteitis with tumorlike hyperostosis along the lateral aspect of the proximal femoral shaft. The radionuclide scan is diagnostic based on the bull's head sign in the sternocostoclavicular region (p. 315 ff.). Clinical inspection revealed palmoplantar pustulosis. These findings made it unnecessary to biopsy the tumorlike lesion of the upper femur.

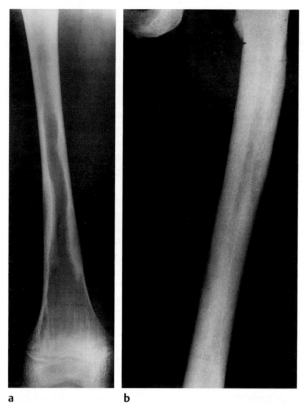

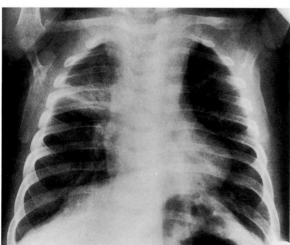

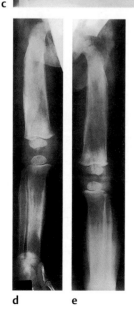

◁ Fig. 7.**17 a–e**   Hyperostosis.

a Mixed sclerosing bone dysplasia. The two components consist of melorheostosis with wavy endosteal hyperostosis of the distal shaft and streaklike cancellous bone densities in the distal femoral metaphysis.

b Typical features of marble bone disease (osteopetrosis). When this type of bone abnormality is seen in a trauma patient, for example, at least one radiographic test region should be examined (e.g., the pelvis or spine) in order to make a prompt, accurate diagnosis and avoid unnecessary clinical and laboratory tests. Often the patients themselves are aware that they have marble bone disease or that it runs in the family.

c–e Pulmonary hypertrophic osteoarthropathy in a 14-month-old child with recurrent pulmonary infiltration of yet unknown origin. (Case courtesy of Dr. O. Sauer, Osnabrück.)

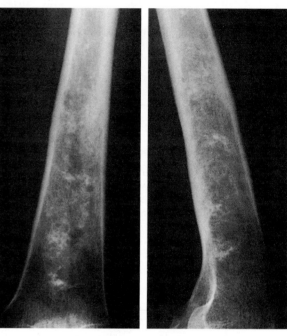

Fig. 7.**18**   Typical calcifying enchondroma in the distal femoral shaft (pp. 880 and 894).

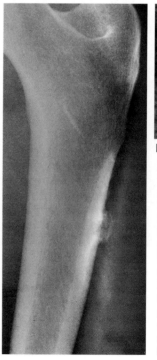

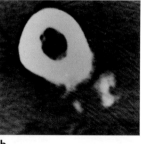

Fig. 7.**19 a, b**   Calcifying tendinitis.

a Typical calcifying tendinitis as one feature of pustulotic arthro-osteitis (PAO, SAPHO) at the insertion of the vastus lateralis muscle.

b CT shows cortical erosion adjacent to sites of dystrophic calcification or metaplastic bone formation. A detailed description of this case can be found in Frey-schmidt (1997) and Kasperczyk et al. (1990).

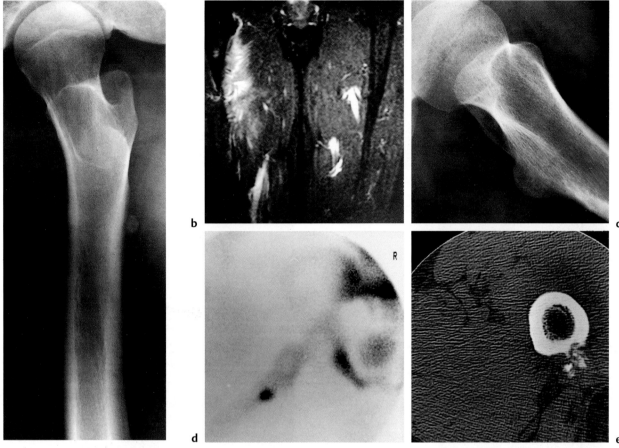

Fig. 7.**20 a–e** Calcifying tendinitis.
a, b Calcifying tendinitis in the region of the gluteal tuberosity. Note the small ossification in the paraosseous soft tissues with rarefaction of the underlying bone structure (gluteal tuberosity). MRI in **b** shows massive perifocal edema that was misinterpreted as a neoplastic process.

c–e Different case of calcifying tendinitis. Axial radiograph (**c**) shows cortical rarefaction in the area of the lesser trochanter and distal to it (on the pectineal line). Bone scan shows intense uptake like that seen in osteoid osteoma (**d**). CT (**e**) shows destruction of the pectineal line and upper linea aspera with calcification at the insertion of the pectineus, gluteus maximus, and/or adductor brevis muscles.

Fig. 7.**21 a, b** Classic myositis ossificans (heterotopic ossification) on the extensor side of the thigh. In contrast to paraosseous and periosteal osteosarcoma, the ossific foci are denser peripherally. This is seen particularly well in the CT scan (**b**) ("reverse trizonal pattern").

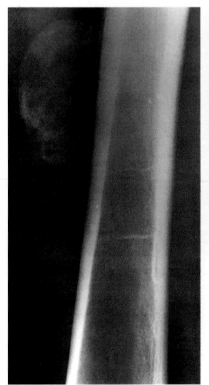

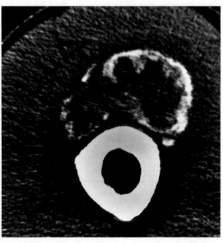

deposits may be found incidentally in patients with no clinical symptoms.

The differential diagnosis includes the following:
- Juxtacortical sarcoma and osteosarcoma of the soft tissues (Fig. 7.**23**)

- Calcified cysticerci (Fig. 7.**24**)
- Myositis ossificans (Figs. 7.**21**, 7.**22**)

We cannot explore the differentiating criteria in detail. The disease is discussed more fully in the article by Neumann et al. (1996).

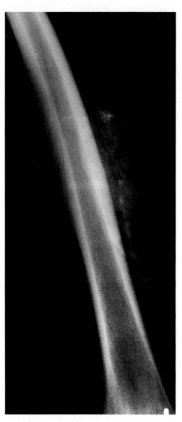

Fig. 7.**22** Myositis ossificans, not a paraosteal osteosarcoma. Note the shell-like paraosseous ossifications.

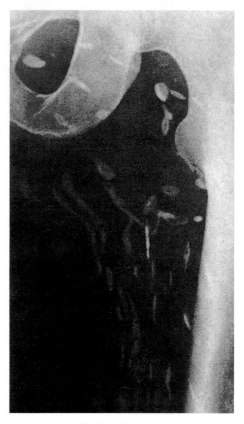

Fig. 7.**24** Calcified cysticerci.

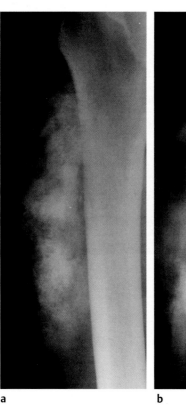 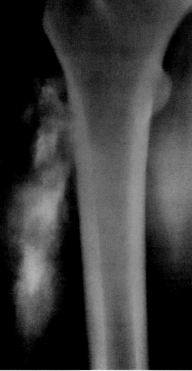

a   b

Fig. 7.**23 a, b** Juxtacortical osteosarcoma. The tumor arose from the proximal lateral cortex below the greater trochanter and spread distally along the lateral surface of the bone (paraosteal osteosarcoma, see tomogram in **b**). The tumor masses are heavily ossified, but more so at the center than peripherally, in contrast to myositis ossificans.

References

Bretagne, M. C.: A propos de périostitifes ou plutô d'apositions périostées en pédiatrie. J. Radiol. Électrol. 58 (1977) 119

Butler, J. E., St. L. Brown, B. G. McConnell: Subtrochanteric stress fractures in runners. Amer. J. Sports Med. 10 (1982) 228

Daffner, R. H.: Stress-fractures. Current concepts. Skelet. Radiol. 2 (1978) 221

Freyschmidt, J.: Skeletterkrankungen, 2. Aufl. Springer, Berlin 1997

Freyschmidt, J., H. Ostertag, G. Jundt: Knochentumoren, 2. Aufl. Springer, Berlin 1998

Iscan, M. Y., P. Miller-Shalvitz: Determination of sex from the femur in blacks and whites. Coll. Antropol. 8 (1984) 169

Kasperczyk, A., J. Freyschmidt, H. Ostertag: Tumorsimulierende Knochenläsionen bei sternokostoklavikulärer Hyperostose und Pustulosis palmoplantaris. Fortschr. Röntgenstr. 152 (1990) 10

Levinson, E. D., M. B. Ozonoff, P. M. Royen: Proximal femoral focal deficiency (PFFD). Radiology 125 (1977) 197

Meurman, K. A. O., S. Elfving: Stress fractures in soldiers: a multifocal bone disorder. Radiology 134 (1980) 483

Neumann, St., J. Freyschmidt, B. R. Holland: Die kalzifizierende Tendinitis am Femur – Diagnose und Differentialdiagnose am Beispiel von 5 Fällen. Z. Rheumatol 55 (1996) 114

Perry, III, H. M., R. S. Weinstein, St. L. Teitelbaum et al: Pseudofractures in the absence of osteomalacia. Skelet. Radiol. 8 (1982) 17

Richter, R., F. J. Krause: Primäre Diaphysentuberkulose der langen Röhrenknochen. Fortschr. Röntgenstr. 139 (1983) 549

Reiner: Über den kongenitalen Femurdefekt. Z. orthop. Chir. 9 (1901) 544

Shopfner, Ch. E.: Periosteal bone growth in normal infants. A preliminary report. Amer. J. Roentgenol. 97 (1966) 154

Vande Berg, B. C.: MR assessment of red marrow distribution and composition in the proximal femur: correlation with clinical and laboratory parameters. Skelet. Radiol. 26 (1997) 589

Distal Femur

▌ Normal Findings

 ### During Growth

The ossification center of the distal femoral epiphysis is normally present in newborns and is considered an important sign of maturity. Its average diameter in the newborn is 5 mm.

This ossification center can be detected sonographically in the fetus between the 28th and 35th weeks of gestation (Mahony et al. 1985).

The distal femoral epiphyseal ossification centers display markedly irregular, frayed, and even spiculated contours, particularly between the 2nd and 6th years of life (Fig. 7.25).

> The ossification centers may also be partially fragmented and multicentric—a finding that should not be confused with osteonecrosis (especially in asymptomatic children) or with the fragmented epiphyses in hypothyroidism or chondrodysplasia punctata (stippled epiphysis, Figs. 2.57, 7.77). Isolated ossification centers can also occur as a normal finding (Maurer and Schreiner 1984).

Accessory ossification centers have also been found in the area of the anterosuperior circumference (Scheller 1965).

The metaphyseal margins of the distal femur show a normal "crumpled" configuration in the 2- to 3-year-old child (Fig. 7.25). This normal finding is different from the "corner sign," or beaklike metaphyseal configuration seen in diseases such as rickets and syphilis.

It is not unusual to find a foramen-like intercondylar lucency in the distal femur of 7- to 11-year-old children. It represents the end-on projection of a nutrient canal (Fig. 7.26). It is also rather common in this age group to find a round or oval area of sparse trabeculae in the lateral femoral epiphysis, which can mimic bone destruction by a tumor (e.g., osteoid osteoma, eosinophilic granuloma) or an osteomyelitic lesion (Fig. 7.25d).

Harcke et al. (1992) investigated the **MRI characteristics of the growth plates of 1- to 20-year-olds** and their possible variants.

Varich et al. (2000) describe the age-associated changes in the normal maturation of the cartilaginous distal part of the femoral epiphysis on MRI (Fig. 7.27).

> It should be noted in this context that the distal epiphyses contribute approximately 70% of the longitudinal growth of the femur (Table 7.3). Consequently, injuries to these plates can have a serious impact on normal longitudinal growth.

Table 7.3 Percentage contribution of various epiphyseal regions to growth (after Freyschmidt et al.)

Epiphyseal region	Proximal	Distal
Humerus	80%	20%
Ulna	20%	80%
Radius	25%	75%
Femur	30%	70%
Tibia	55%	45%
Fibula	60%	40%

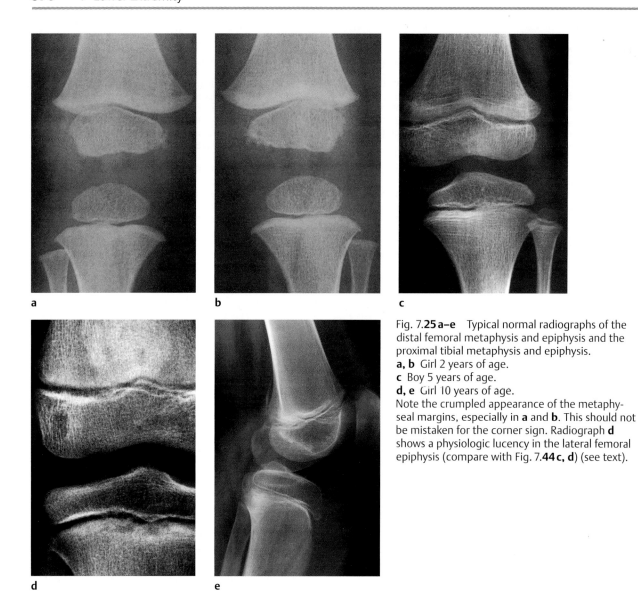

a b c

Fig. 7.**25 a–e** Typical normal radiographs of the distal femoral metaphysis and epiphysis and the proximal tibial metaphysis and epiphysis.
a, b Girl 2 years of age.
c Boy 5 years of age.
d, e Girl 10 years of age.
Note the crumpled appearance of the metaphyseal margins, especially in **a** and **b**. This should not be mistaken for the corner sign. Radiograph **d** shows a physiologic lucency in the lateral femoral epiphysis (compare with Fig. 7.**44 c, d**) (see text).

d e

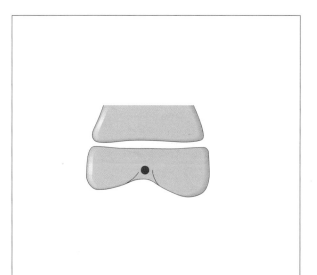

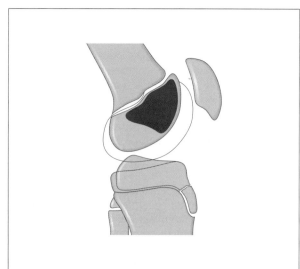

Fig. 7.**26 a, b** Normal structures of the femoral epiphysis.
a Nutrient canal in the distal femoral epiphysis.

b Ludloff's "fleck" (patch, see also Fig. 7.**25 e**).

Lateral radiographs of the knee, both in older children and adults, show a physiological pie-shaped density in the anterior part of the epiphysis (Figs. 7.**26b**, 7.**25e**) known also as Ludloff's fleck or the epiphyseal triangle. It is most conspicuous around 16 years of age.

The anterior and posterior contours of this density outline the cortical borders of the femur between the condyles (compare with Fig. 7.**1**).

In Adulthood

The anatomy of the distal femur is shown in Fig. 7.**1a, b**. In contrast to the elbow, the epicondyles are rudimentary and usually only the lateral can be identified in the AP projection. The **adductor tubercle**, which gives attachment to the adductor magnus muscle, can sometimes be very prominent, especially in enthesiopathy or in response to heavy mechanical stresses. Understanding the radiographic and CT appearance of the distal femur includes a familiarity with the divergent, ridgelike prominences of the linea aspera (Fig. 7.**1a**).

The corners of the condylar articular surfaces become sharper and more distinct with aging, probably as a result of fibrocartilage proliferation. Slight beveling of the lateral joint contour is normal (Fig. 7.**28**).

Both femoral condyles are superimposed in the lateral projection. The condyle away from the film (almost always the medial condyle) appears larger and less distinct. Another feature distinguishes the lateral and medial condyles in this projection: The articular contours along the patellar surface differ in height and shape between the two condyles (Figs. 7.**29**).

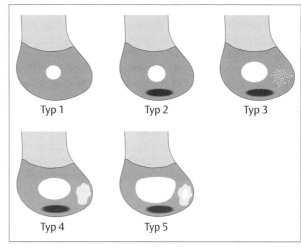

Fig. 7.**27** Age-related signal intensity changes in the distal femoral epiphysis. Five epiphyseal types defined by Varich et al. (2000) in sagittal MRI. (1) Central round or oval white zone, the epiphyseal ossification center, surrounded by a homogeneous gray area, the epiphyseal cartilage. (2) Black zone on the articular side of the epiphyseal center: low signal intensity in the weight-bearing region. The stippled area (3), light gray area (4), and ill-defined gray area around an elliptical white area (5) in the posterior condyles indicate a progression of higher signal intensities. Age association (in months) of types 1–5 (mean value relative to the medial condyle).

- Type 1: 5.9 (1.5–22.0)
- Type 2: 18.8 (4.0–42.0)
- Type 3: 22.5 (8.0–61.0)
- Type 4: 36.8 (13.0–61.0)
- Type 5: 49.8 (45.0–64.0)

Fig. 7.**28** Beveled articular contour of the lateral condyle in a 31-year-old woman.

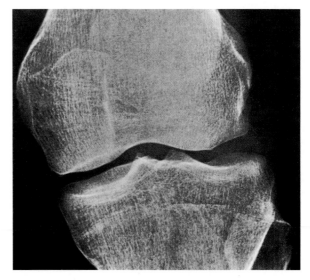

Using a true lateral conventional radiograph of the knee, **femoral trochlear dysplasia** can be diagnosed. Femoral trochlear dysplasia, on the other hand, may be a cause of anterior knee pain (see below).

Femoral trochlear dysplasia is a geometric abnormality of the depth and shape of the trochlear groove, especially in its cranial part (Pfirrmann et al. 2000). The following two criteria can be used for diagnosing trochlear dysplasia:

- The crossing sign: If the floor of the trochlear groove crosses the ventral outline of the lateral femoral condyle, dysplasia is present and the crossing sign positive (Fig. 7.**30b**) (Grelsamer et al. 1992). At the level of this crossing, the trochlea is considered flat.
- Ventral prominence of the trochlear floor: It is measured as the distance between a line drawn through

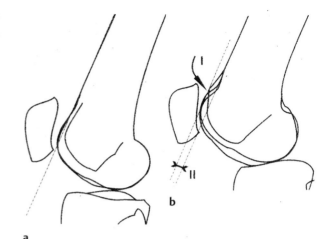

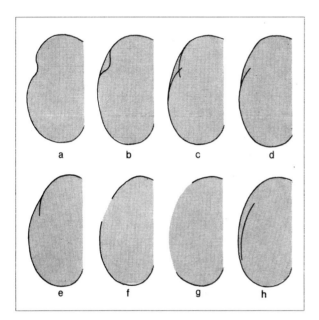

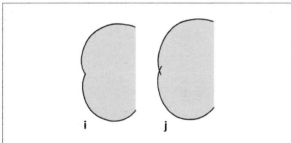

Fig. 7.**29 a–j**
a–h Variations in the contour of the medial femoral condyle in the lateral projection (after Ravelli).
a Medial limiting groove appears as a depression.
b Medial limiting groove appears as a peripheral lucency with a central concave border.
c Peripheral lucency bounded by two convex curves.
d Only the posterior part of the lucency has sharp borders.
e Only the anterior part has sharp borders.
f Indistinct borders.
g Much of the contour of the condyle is indistinct.
h Double contours along the middle third of the condyle.
i, j Contour of the lateral femoral condyle in the lateral projection.
i Lateral limiting groove appears as an indentation.
j Lateral limiting groove is formed by two intersecting arcs.
For the lateral femoral notch sign see Fig. 7.**30c**.

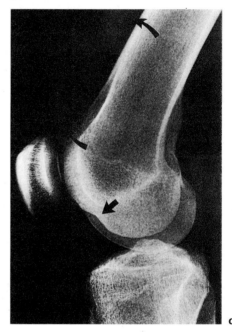

Fig. 7.**30 a–c**   On the diagnostic value of lateral radiographs of the distal femur.
a, b Diagram of a normal knee (from Pfirrmann et al. 2000). The floor of the femoral trochlea does not cross the ventral outlines of the femoral condyles, because it always lies dorsal to the line that parallels the ventral cortical surface of the distal femur. There is no prominence of the trochlear floor (**a**). In the case of trochlear dysplasia (prominence), two signs are positive (**b**). First, the line I, which represents the floor of the femoral trochlea, crosses the ventral outlines of both femoral condyles (positive crossing sign). Second, because of the prominence of the trochlear floor, it is 5 mm ventral to the line that parallels the ventral cortical surface of the distal femur (II, double arrow) (see also text).
(**c**) demonstrates the **lateral femoral notch sign**. According to Pao (2001), this sign is characterized by an abnormally deep depression of the lateral condylopatellar sulcus (straight arrow). The curved arrows in (**c**) indicate a large effusion. An abnormally deep lateral condylopatellar sulcus, also known as the lateral femoral notch, can be attributed to an impacted osteochondral fracture, caused by a torn anterior cruciate ligament (ACL). Disruption of the ACL with valgus stress causes the posterior aspect of the lateral tibial plateau and the middle-to-anterior portion of the lateral femoral condyle to impact forcefully against one another ("kissing contusions"). However, the significance of this sign is limited as it is difficult to distinguish a prominent but normal lateral (condylopatellar sulcus and a shallow impacted fracture at the sulcus) (Pao, 2001). In any case, a depth of greater than 2 mm of the lateral femoral notch is highly suggestive of an ACL injury.

the ventral cortex of the femoral shaft and a parallel line defined as the tangent to the most ventral point of the trochlear floor (Fig. 7.**30 b**) (Pfirrmann et al. 2000, Dejour et al. 1990). For the diagnosis of trochlear dysplasia, the prominence must be more than 3 mm.

A flat or prominent type of trochlear dysplasia may lead to patellar instability with resulting anterior knee pain. For the trochlea configuration on axial views see the patella chapter.

The interior of the intercondylar notch is best demonstrated by the "tunnel view," an AP flexion view of the knee that is perpendicular to the plane of the open joint space (Frik view).

The **popliteal surface** is a triangular area located on the posterior surface of the distal femur between the divergent ridges of the linea aspera and the transverse intercondylar line (which gives attachment to the gastrocnemius and plantaris muscles; see Fig. 7.**1 a**). In many asymptomatic patients this area may appear roughened, irregular, or even spiculated in the lateral projection (Fig. 7.**31**, 7.**46**, 7.**47**). This region may also bear small bony prominences (Fig. 7.**32**) that may result from bone formation in response to mechanical stresses from the attached muscles.

The "Tumor?" section below provides further details on this radiographically important region.

▌ *Pathological Finding?*

Normal Variant or Anomaly?

(On femoral trochlear dysplasia and the lateral femoral notch sign, see above.)

The **distal femoral metaphyses**, like those of the upper tibia and distal radius, may be **very dense** as a normal variant. Occasionally, however, dense metaphyses signify an imbalance between osteoclastic and osteoblastic activity in the provisional calcification zone (too little osteoclastic resorption or too much osteoblastic bone formation).

This type of imbalance can occur in various disorders:

- Rickets
- Hypervitaminosis D
- Renal osteodystrophy
- Severe systemic infections with growth disturbances, congenital hypoparathyroidism and hypothyroidism
- Treated leukemia, etc.

The causal significance of lead poisoning in dense metaphyses ("lead bands") is highly controversial (Schwörer et al. 1983, Freyschmidt 1997).

Morphological variants of the femoral **popliteal surface** were described above (Figs. 7.**31**, 7.**32**). We classify these radiographic patterns as normal findings rather than actual variants.

A true normal variant is an exostosis-like bony outgrowth called a "**coat-hook exostosis**" (Fig. 7.**33**). It is analogous to the supracondylar process of the distal humerus (see Figs. 2.**383**, 2.**384**). Unlike a classic cartilaginous exostosis, the marrow space of the protuberance does not extend into the medullary cavity of the bone. It is purely of academic interest whether the feature is a congenital or early acquired extreme prominence of a proximally displaced adductor tubercle or an insertional tendinopathy that has undergone extensive ossification.

Significant morphological changes in the distal femoral epiphysis, especially widening of the intercondylar notch, are observed in hemophilia (Fig. 7.**34**).

It is beyond our scope to review the many possible dysplasias and deformities of the distal femoral metaphysis and epiphysis. We note, however, that an **enlarged medial femoral condyle** is a cardinal feature of numerous syndromes (Table 7.**4**).

Table 7.**4** Syndromes that may be associated with an enlarged medial femoral condyle

• Chondrodystrophy	• Prader–Willi syndrome
• Blount disease	• Turner syndrome
• Cornelia de Lange syndrome	• Posttraumatic changes
• Dyschondrosteosis	• Vitamin D-resistant rickets

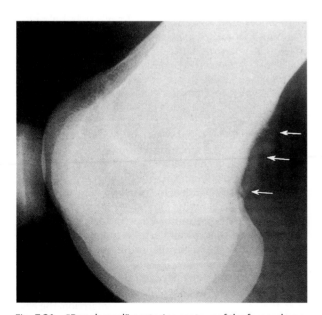

Fig. 7.**31** "Roughened" posterior contour of the femoral popliteal surface (see also Fig. 7.**47**).

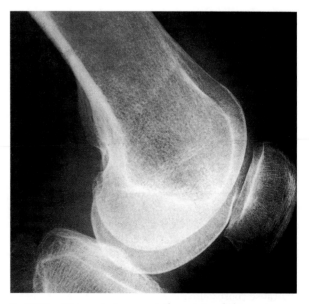

Fig. 7.**32** Bony prominence at the origin of the gastrocnemius medial head (compare with Fig. 7.**47 c, d**).

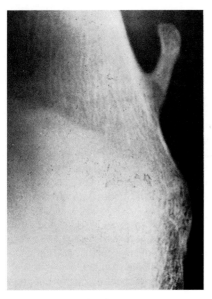

Fig. 7.**33**   "Coat-hook" exostosis.

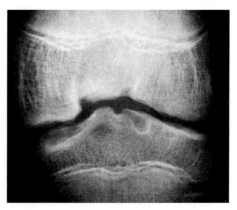

Fig. 7.**34**   Classic signs of hemophilic osteoarthropathy: epiphyseal enlargement, streaklike osteoporosis, incongruities, irregularities and flattening of articular contours, widening of the intercondylar notch, subchondral lucencies.

 ## Fracture?

Fractures of the distal femur during delivery or after a cesarean section have been observed. Early plain films are negative if there is no significant epiphyseal displacement. It takes several days for subperiosteal hemorrhage to incite periosteal bone formation that is visible on radiographs (Rutherford et al. 1983, Banagale and Kuhns 1983). Differentiation is required from septic arthritis, osteomyelitis, and syphilitic periosteitis and is based partly on the clinical presentation.

From 3% to 8% of all pediatric femoral fractures occur in the distal femur (Rumlova et al. 1983). Plain-film diagnosis is aided by noting the course of the various intermuscular fat stripes and the bursal outlines (see also Knee Joint), especially when epiphyseal and metaphyseal injuries cannot be directly visualized. MRI should be added in equivocal cases.

The **classification of distal metaphyseal-epiphyseal femoral fractures** is shown schematically in Fig. 7.**35**.

A knowledge of the basic fracture patterns will make it easier to identify them on radiographs and distinguish them from potential fracture-line mimics such as Mach effects. Because many fracture lines in the lower femur have an oblique sagittal orientation (much as in the upper tibia), we feel that biplane radiographs of the knee should be routinely supplemented by an oblique internal-rotation view in this type of investigation.

 ## Necrosis?

The distal end of the femur is a site of predilection for osteonecrotic changes. Typical examples of these changes are presented below, with special emphasis placed on early forms and their differential diagnosis.

The fat marrow in the distal femoral diaphysis and metaphysis is highly sensitive to perfusion deficits due to any cause (posttraumatic edema, vascular lesions, metabolic disorders, cytostatic agents, steroids, etc.), with the result that **bone marrow infarction** is relatively common

in this region. Early stages that present clinically with nonspecific piercing or drilling pain about the knee can be detected only by MRI or radionuclide scanning (increased uptake). Not infrequently, the infarction is combined with fresh bleeding into the infarcted tissue ("hemorrhagic infarction"). Bone marrow infarcts appear on T1-weighted MRI as an elliptical area in the medullary cavity, usually surrounded by a hypointense scalloped border. This border may appear hyperintense on T2-weighted images, depending on the stage of the infarction. The infarct contains serpiginous areas that have the signal characteristics of fat, blood, and fluid (Fig. 7.**36 d, e**).

Actually the imaging appearance of bone marrow infarction is unmistakable and easily distinguished from enchondroma, which is not uncommon in this region. Differentiation is required, however, from an **atypical reconversion of fat marrow to red marrow**, especially in women (Fig. 7.**36 a–c**). But the areas of red marrow in the yellow fat marrow do not show the scalloped pattern that is so typical of an infarct. Also, there is no sign of the perifocal edema that is invariably seen in association with an acute hemorrhagic bone marrow infarction.

The MRI differential diagnosis should also include bone marrow changes like those in **cachexia** and/or **anorexia nervosa**, which are characterized by a loss of fatty marrow tissue along with a reduction of cellularity and fluid accumulation (e.g., hyaluronic acid) ("serous atrophy" of the marrow; Vande Berg et al. 1994). In similar cases we have personally observed saponification processes in the bone marrow, especially in the femur.

The evolution of a bone marrow infarction is marked by an eventual demarcation of the infarcted marrow from the healthy medullary cavity by a **dystrophic calcification line**. Later the more central infarcted areas also calcify, culminating in the appearance of a more or less heavily ossified area in the distal shaft and metaphysis that resembles a plug (Fig. 7.**37**). Ill-defined patchy densities in the distal femoral medullary cavity and metaphysis are also observed as an intermediate stage (Fig. 7.**38**).

In the end stages of a bone marrow infarction, the central areas in the irregular woven bone again undergo fatty degeneration and are demarcated from healthy marrow in

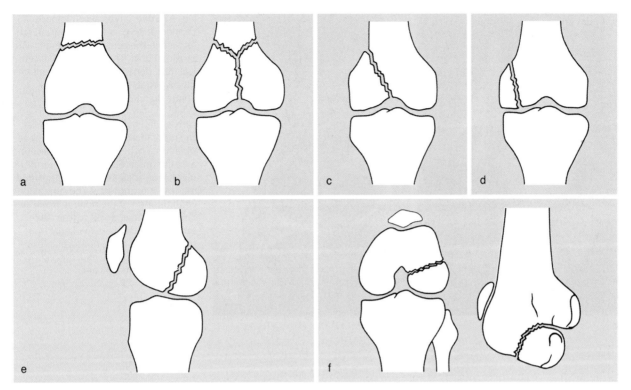

Fig. 7.**35 a–f** Typical fracture patterns encountered in the distal femur (after Rogers).
a Supracondylar.
b Y-shaped intercondylar.

c Oblique through one condyle.
d Sagittal.
e Coronal.
f Oblique coronal.

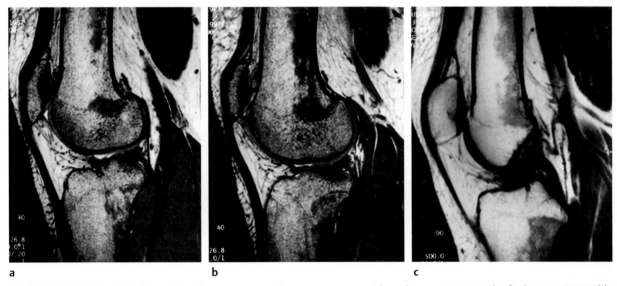

Fig. 7.**36 a–e** Differential diagnosis of bone marrow infarction on MRI.

a–c Atypical bone marrow signal intensities in the distal and posterior femur and also in the proximal and posterior tibia in a woman with no knee symptoms. The findings are caused by the reconversion of fat to red marrow, occurring on both sides and also detectable in the humeri and other bones.

Fig. 7.**36 d, e** ▷

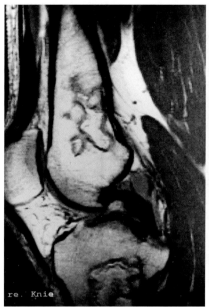

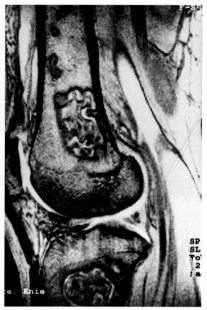

d   e

Fig. 7.**36 d, e**   Typical serpiginous configuration of bone marrow infarcts located in the central distal femur and proximal tibia. They show partial central fatty degeneration or still contain fat (hyperintense in T1-weighted image **d** and T2-weighted image **e**). While the larger femoral infarct in **e** is surrounded by a hypointense border, the bone marrow infarct in the upper tibia has a hyperintense rim, indicating a fresher infarction, i.e., the intermediate zone adjoining the healthy bone marrow is proton-rich. The serpiginous configuration of the bone marrow infarcts in images **d** and **e** (from the same patient) differs markedly from the more eccentric, nonserpiginous configuration of the marrow reconversion areas in images **a–c**.

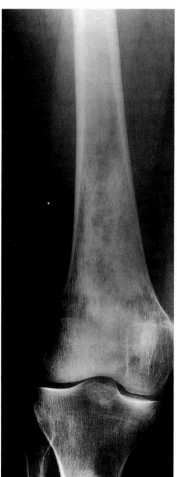

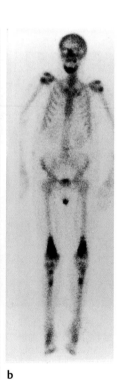

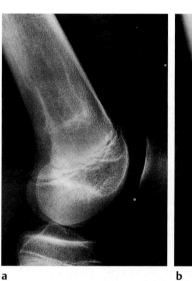

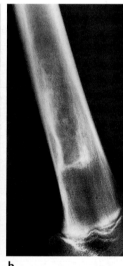

a   b

Fig. 7.**37 a, b**   Intermediate bone marrow infarcts in the distal femur appear on radiographs as sclerotic "plugs" in the shafts of the tubular bones. The central portion of the bone marrow infarct in **b** probably derives its lucency from fatty degeneration.

a

b

◁ Fig. 7.**38 a, b**   Patchy, ill-defined calcifying bone marrow infarction involving the distal femoral metaphysis, epiphysis, and diaphysis and also the proximal tibial diaphysis. The bone scan shows intense uptake in the infarcted areas (**b**).

a scalloped or serpiginous pattern (Fig. 7.**39**). This creates an MRI appearance similar to that of a fresh bone marrow infarction.

Differentiation from a calcified enchondroma (Fig. 7.**18**) can generally be accomplished by noting a continuous sclerotic border that separates the infarct from the rest of the marrow cavity. Also, an infarction does not produce endosteal scalloping of the cortex.

Osteochondritis dissecans (subarticular avascular necrosis) is a limited or focal osteonecrosis with an affinity for the distal femoral epiphysis. Several etiologies have been proposed, including osteochondral stress fractures. Individuals with hemoglobinopathies (e.g., in sickle cell anemia) are predisposed. Also a familial incidence is known, raising the question of whether at least these cases may involve a kind of dysplasia of the articular cartilage, which is often found to be disproportionately thick in the necrotic area of affected individuals. The disease is essentially a preosteoarthritic condition, especially when the osteochondral fragment separates from the articular surface and enters the joint as a loose body, leading to entrapment and other types of cartilage injury.

The earliest clinical symptom is nonspecific knee pain, occasionally combined with a mild effusion. Most patients are in the second to fourth decade of life, and the most common location is the distal femoral epiphysis of the medial condyle. Radiographs in the initial stages are negative. T2-weighted MRI shows a bandlike, crescent-shaped hyperintense zone that grows wider as the fragment loosens. This hyperintense zone apparently represents proton-rich repair tissue, the presence of which also probably accounts for spontaneous recoveries. In dynamic MRI studies with intravenous Gd-DTPA, Adam et al. (1994) noted a rise of signal intensity in the boundary zone indicating the presence of granulation tissue that stabilized the fragment. A concomitant rise of signal intensity in the fragment itself indicates that it is still viable. However, the hyperintense band between the fragment and healthy bone could also be intra-articular fluid, implying that the fragment has already separated. The prognosis of osteochondritis dissecans depends on the size of the necrotic area and the age of the patient. The younger the patient, the greater the likelihood of spontaneous healing (especially if the growth plates are still open). Bohndorf (1998) developed prognostic imaging criteria that could be used to discriminate surgical from nonsurgical lesions. The MRI detection of still-intact articular cartilage (stage I lesion) is relevant in making this distinction.

The earliest sign on conventional radiographs is a thin, crescent-shaped, subchondral lucency (subchondral fracture, Fig. 7.**40e**), below which there is increasing density of the cancellous bone on the articular side. This bandlike lucency becomes wider, and finally the affected segment detaches to form a loose intra-articular fragment, leaving a craterlike osteochondral defect in the articular surface (Fig. 7.**41**).

Larger fragments with a very dense reactive border are at greater risk for detachment. On bone scans, the intensity of the tracer uptake correlates with the risk of detachment.

Detached fragments may become fixed to the joint capsule and later develop into a "capsular osteoma." Spontaneous resorption may also occur.

Figure 7.**40** traces the chronological development of osteochondritis dissecans on MR images and radiographs. An atypical location of osteochondritis dissecans is shown in Fig. 7.**41**.

> Osteochondritis dissecans mainly requires differentiation from transient subchondral lucencies in the femoral condyles of older children and adolescents (Fig. 7.**42**).

We have observed many such cases which did not subsequently develop into osteochondritis dissecans and resolved without treatment, causing no clinical complaints or only relatively mild, nondescript pain. Apparently the lucencies are transient stress-related phenomena with a high potential for spontaneous recovery. Similar findings were described as "lucent articular lesions" in male athletes 14–27 years of age, occurring predominantly on the lateral femoral condyles at the level of the patella (Cayea et al. 1981). Radionuclide bone scans were also positive. Clinically, the patients had symptoms consistent with chondromalacia patellae. Arthrography showed that the overlying articular cartilage was intact. The authors had no follow-up findings to report. Because it cannot be determined in any given case whether such findings may develop into classic osteochondritis dissecans, we recommend non-weight bearing as a routine precaution.

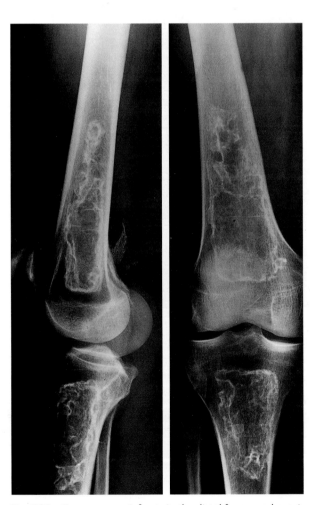

Fig. 7.**39** Bone marrow infarcts in the distal femur and proximal tibia show a classic pattern of peripheral dystrophic calcification, with serpiginous or scalloped sclerotic borders and central lucency, probably due to regressive fatty transformation of the infarcted areas.

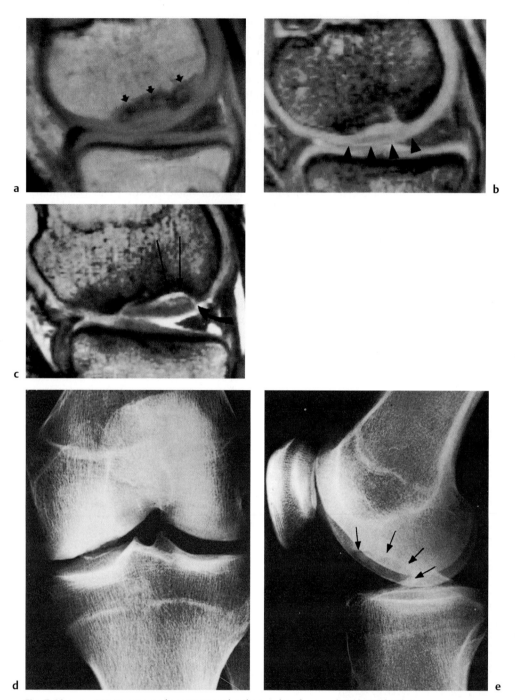

Fig. 7.**40 a–g**   MR images and conventional radiographs of osteochondritis dissecans.
a, b Stage I lesion in a 15-year-old boy. In the T1-weighted image (**a**), the subchondral necrotic bone appears as a hypointense band (arrows). In the T2-weighted image (**b**), completely normal cartilage covers the necrotic bone area.
c Adult patient. In this case a hyperintense (fluid-equivalent) area demarcates the fragment from healthy bone. (From Bohndorf 1998.)
d Irregular contours of the medial condyle with greatly increased density of the underlying bone.
e Arrows indicate the necrotic area. The AP extent of the infarcted osteochondritic area is larger than its mediolateral extent in **d**.

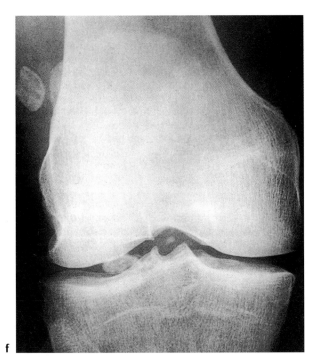

f

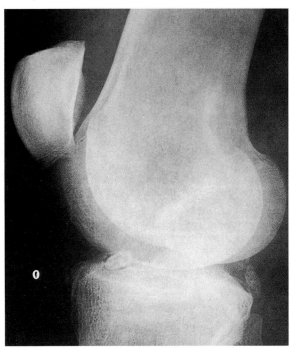

g

Fig. 7.**40f, g** Late sequelae of osteochondritis dissecans, consisting of numerous intra-articular loose bodies, some of which are solid and ossified. Reparative processes have smoothed the articular contours to a degree, especially on the lateral femoral condyle. It is obvious, however, that the con-tours of the lateral condyle are not normal. The ossified loose bodies exhibit some degree of corticocancellous structure, distinguishing them from other diseases such as primary artic-ular chondromatosis (see also Fig. 7.**147**).

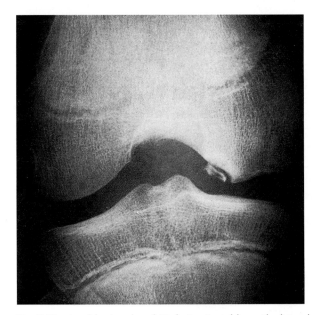

Fig. 7.**41** An old osteochondritic lesion is visible on the lateral femoral condyle, which shows a flattened and irregular joint contour. A fresher lesion with a separating fragment is also visible.

Another important differential diagnosis is **dysplasia epiphysealis multiplex**, which is associated with epiphy-seal deformities affecting many joints in addition to the knee (Fig. 7.**105**).

Ahlbäck disease (spontaneous osteonecrosis of the knee) is a disease that occurs predominantly in the fourth to sixth decades and leads to osteonecrosis of the medial femoral condyle.

Its initial symptom is sudden, severe knee pain, fol-lowed several months later by slight flattening of the me-dial femoral condyle on AP and lateral radiographs (Fig. 7.**43**). Finally, faint densities appear in the affected re-gion, sometimes detectable only with a magnifying lens. Two to three months later, lucencies are found in the sub-chondral bone, and over time a flat contour defect develops that is surrounded by a sclerotic border and often contains a small bone fragment (Fig. 7.**43c**). In contrast to osteo-chondritis dissecans in adolescents, the defect in Ahlbäck disease is located a greater distance from the intercondylar eminence. The early stage, marked by subtle flattening of the medial femoral condyle, is the key differentiating crite-rion.

We know of cases where spontaneous recovery oc-curred in 1–2 years even in patients who already had condylar flattening, subchondral lucency, and severe clinical symptoms.

Today, of course, an early diagnosis can be made with MRI. The findings are basically the same as those seen in classic osteochondritis dissecans.

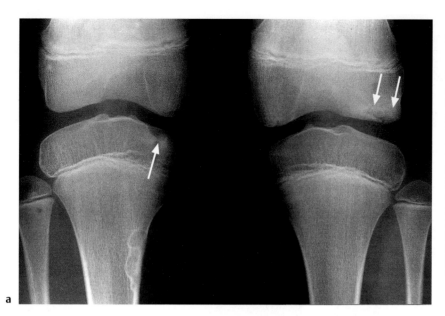

Fig. 7.42 a–g Differential diagnosis of classic osteochondritis dissecans. This case illustrates transient osteochondritis dissecans-like subchondral lucencies that are clinically asymptomatic, disappear in a period of months to years, and probably represent extreme stress-related normal variants (see text).
a Radiograph of a 10-year-old girl with "growing pains" in both knees shows an osteochondritis dissecans-like lucency in the left femoral condyle, a short linear lucency in the medial condyle, and an osteochondritis-like subchondral lucency in the right medial tibial plateau. A fibrous metaphyseal defect (FMD) is noted incidentally in the proximal medial tibial diaphysis and metaphysis.

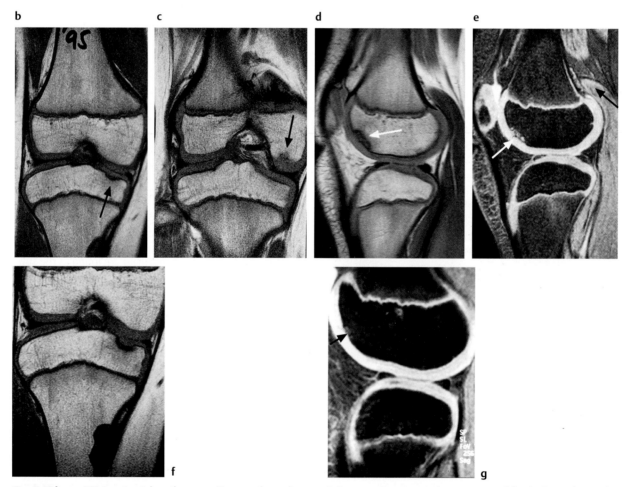

Fig. 7.42 b–e   MR images taken the same time as the radiograph show that the cartilage over the lesions is intact.
f, g Images two years later show that the depression under the still-intact tibial cartilage has deepened, while the femoral defect has become smaller.

Follow-up documented regression of both the radiographic and MRI findings. In image **e** note the impressive view of the attachment of the gastrocnemius medial head on the back of the femur (black arrow).

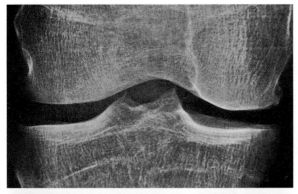

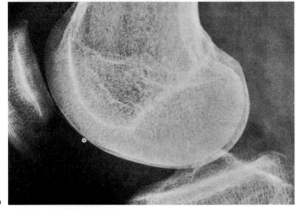

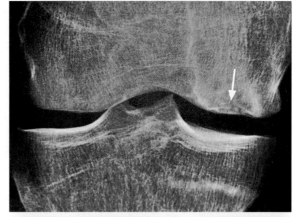

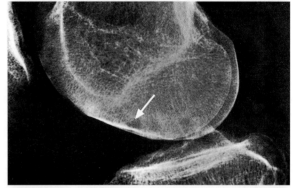

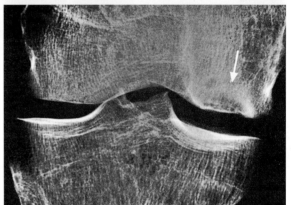

Fig. 7.**43 a–e**   Serial radiographs of spontaneous osteonecrosis of the medial femoral condyle in a 53-year-old man.
a, b 4 May 1972: normal appearance in the AP and lateral projections.
c, d 15 November 1972: typical appearance with fracturing and sclerotic rimming of the "crater." There is marked flattening of the articular contour.
e 7 July 1973: Large fragments are no longer visible in the "crater," and the sclerotic border with healthy bone has broadened.

 Inflammation?

The distal femoral metaphysis is one of the most common sites of occurrence of osteomyelitis due to various causes.

> Early borderline findings with subtle blurring of cancellous trabeculae and incipient periosteal bone formation are difficult to distinguish from normal findings. This is particularly true with chronic recurring multifocal osteomyelitis in children (Figs. 7.**44 b**, 7.**25 d**).

Ultrasound, radionuclide scanning, and/or MRI are generally used today in suspected early cases of osteomyelitis.

Syphilitic metaphyseal and periosteal changes are discussed on p. 929 and illustrated in Figs. 7.**119** and 7.**120**.

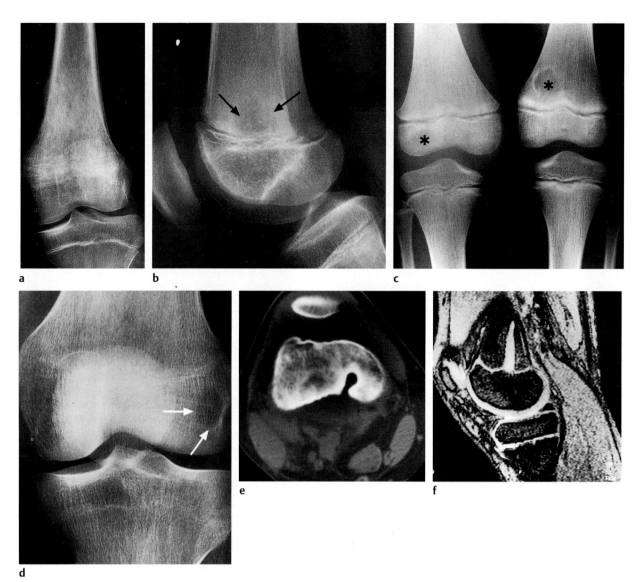

a   b   c

d   e   f

Fig. 7.44 a–f Osteomyelitis of the distal femoral metaphysis.
a Relatively early radiograph shows moth-eaten pattern of destruction, haziness of the trabecular structures, and faint periosteal new bone formation. Prior ultrasound showed marked paraosseous edema with incipient abscess formation.
b Chronic recurring multifocal osteomyelitis. The femoral lesion appears as a relatively subtle lucency bordering directly on the growth plate.

c Two findings: FMD in the left distal femur and a Brodie abscess in the right epiphysis of a 7-year-old boy (see also Fig. 7.**25 d**).
d–f Brodie abscess, appearing as a Lodwick grade IB lesion in radiograph **d**. Note the fine rim of reactive sclerosis. This excludes a physiological lucency, regardless of the clinical presentation (see also Fig. 7.**25 d**). CT (**e**) and sagittal MRI (**f**) in another young patient with Brodie abscess show sinus formation and considerable surrounding sclerosis.

 ## Tumor?

The distal femoral metaphysis and epiphysis are among the most common sites of occurrence of bone tumors in children, adolescents, and young adults (chondroblastoma, chondromyxoid fibroma, osteosarcoma, etc.). The details of these tumors are beyond our scope.

> Our primary concern is early tumors that create true borderline findings and, from the standpoint of differential diagnosis, normal variants that are stress-related in varying degrees.

The attachment of the adductor magnus muscle at the adductor tubercle and the attachments of the medial and lateral gastrocnemius heads (Fig. 7.**42 e**) are sites in the distal femur where stress-induced resorptive changes are most likely to mimic neoplasms. Because these phenomena are relatively common in daily practice and are detected more or less incidentally, we classify them as normal variants.

● **Cortical irregularities** (synonyms: cortical desmoid, paraosseous or juxtacortical desmoid, fibroplastic periosteal reaction, nodular cortical defect) on the medial border of the metaphysis are most commonly found in active children and adolescents (Fig. 7.**45 a, b**). Resorp-

Fig. 7.**45 a–d** Differential diagnosis of cortical irregularities.

a, b Typical appearance of cortical irregularities (arrows) in an 11-year-old asymptomatic boy. Note the roughened, partially spiculated appearance of the femoral metaphyseal borders and the rarefaction of the underlying cancellous structures. The bilaterality and the absence of clinical complaints confirm the diagnosis of benign cortical irregularities. Complete reossification (not shown here) occurred during the following six months.

c, d Development of an early osteosarcoma in the distal femoral metaphysis. The patient presented with significant pain and palpable soft-tissue swelling. Radiograph **c** shows a very subtle cortical lucency that was detectable with a magnifying lens. However, the underlying cancellous bone already shows moth-eaten destructive changes. Faint, initial signs of abnormal periosteal bone formation are evident toward the diaphysis. Radiograph **d**, taken four months later, shows an increase of moth-eaten destruction. The cortex is completely disrupted, and there is an accompanying periosteal reaction on the adjacent proximal cortex.

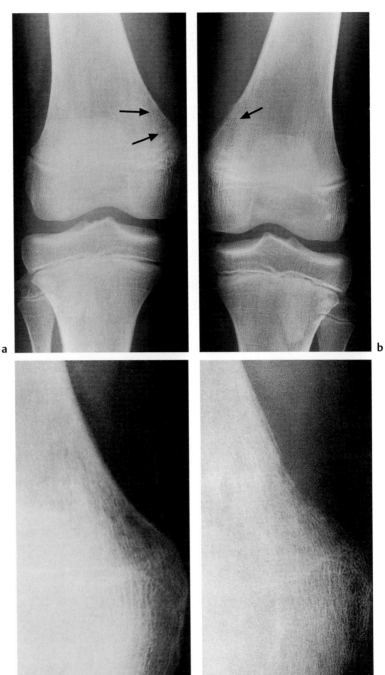

tion of the cortex exposes the underlying cancellous bone, causing irregular or even spiculated transformation of the outer contours. The underlying cancellous bone may also rarefy. But unlike an early osteosarcoma (Fig. 7.**45 c, d**) or early osteomyelitis (Fig. 7.**44 a**), the findings are asymptomatic and negative on bone scans. MRI may show stress-related edema for a relatively long period, prompting an erroneous diagnosis.

- Bone resorption may occur at the **attachment of the gastrocnemius medial and lateral heads** on the femoral metaphysis, just above the medial or lateral condyle. It is clinically asymptomatic and occurs mainly in response to local mechanical stresses. Radiographs show more or less pronounced lacunar defects that may

be surrounded by a wide rim of sclerosis (Fig. 7.**46 d**). The lesions are negative on bone scans (Fig. 7.**46 c**) but may form circumscribed hyperintensities on MRI, since apparently the stressed muscle attachment is a proton-rich area (Fig. 7.**47 k**). The lacunar defects may be very prominent in adults (Fig. 7.**47 a, b**). For the most part, the findings are detected incidentally. The opposite side should always be imaged in doubtful cases; this led to a correct diagnosis in the case shown in Fig. 7.**45**. The resorptive changes can probably evoke an exuberant reparative response (perhaps also triggered by small hemorrhages, Fig. 7.**47 e–j**) that culminates in parosseous ossification (Fig. 7.**47 c, d**).

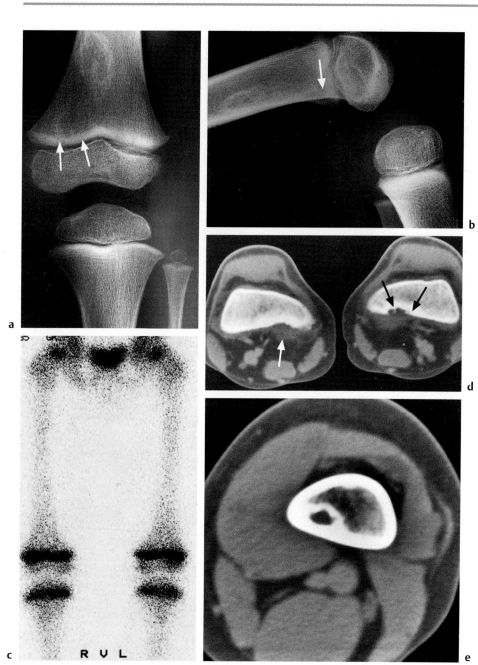

Fig. 7.**46 a–e** Nonossifying fibroma plus cortical irregularities or lacunar resorption at the attachment of the gastrocnemius medial head on both sides. The patient, an athletic boy, complained of nonspecific "growing pains" alternating between the right and left knees. Radiograph **a** shows a vague lucency below the medial metaphyseal calcification line (arrows). The lateral view (**b**) shows that it is located posteriorly and extends past the posterolateral metaphyseal cortex. Correlative CT scan in **d** shows various pits or depressions in the area of the muscle attachment, the muscles themselves appearing as elliptical soft-tissue shadows adjacent to the bone (white arrow, right side). An MRI correlate is shown in Fig. 7.**47 k** (see text). Radionuclide scan is negative (**c**). The same child has a nonossifying fibroma in the distal posteromedial femoral metaphysis. The location is typical, and the lesion corresponds to Lodwick grade IA (nonaggressive). This lesion is shown in the CT scan in **e**. In principle, there was no need for CT or radionuclide documentation in this case. The radiographs are diagnostic, especially considering the bilaterality of the changes.

● We also believe that **fibrous metaphyseal defects (FMD, fibrous cortical defect, nonossifying fibroma)** are the result of local mechanical stresses. More than 80% of these lesions are located about the knee joint. More than 60% occur in the distal femoral metaphysis, showing a predilection for the posteromedial site where the adductor magnus attaches to the bone. As the name implies, the lesion consists of a cortical defect filled with fibrous tissue. Fibrous cortical defect has the potential to enlarge and become a nonossifying fibroma. Apparently, nonossifying fibromas develop when fibrous cortical defects or deep resorption zones at the attachment of the gastrocnemius heads are not

eliminated by modeling of the bone during further growth. More details on this process can be found in Freyschmidt (1997) and Freyschmidt et al. (1998). The lesions always relate closely to the cortex, where they form a 2- to 30-mm defect in the stage of the fibrous cortical defect. Occasionally the defect is covered externally by a thin, slightly bulging shell of calcified periosteum (Fig. 7.**48 a**). Somewhat larger defects have a sclerotic rim that is usually most pronounced on the diaphysis. Nonossifying fibromas may reach 70 mm in their longitudinal diameter. Their major axis is always directed along the femoral axis (Fig. 7.**48 b, c**). They appear as cluster-of-grapes lucencies below the thin,

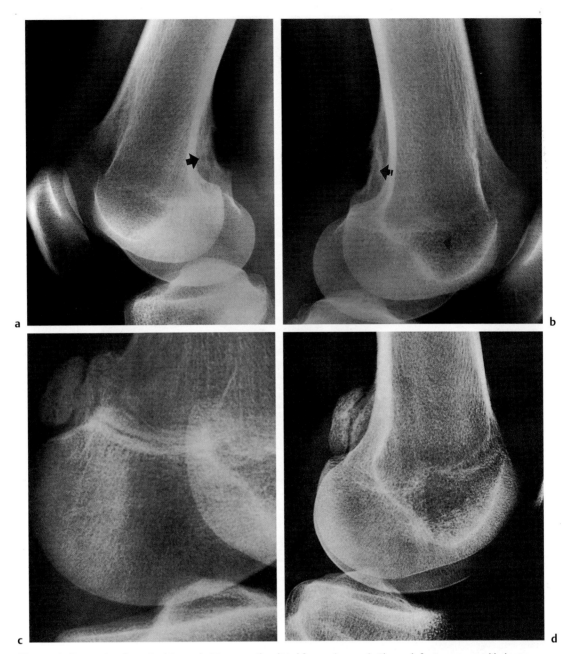

Fig. 7.**47 a–k** Differential diagnosis of cortical irregularities and proliferative changes at the attachment of the gastrocnemius medial head.

a–d Radiographs **a** and **b**, from an active 19-year-old male, show smoothly marginated defects in the popliteal surface of the distal femur (arrows). These defects are most likely stress-induced, and it is quite conceivable that they could develop (perhaps triggered by small hemorrhages) either into a prominence like that shown in Fig. 7.**32** and panels **e–j** or into bony elements abutting the prominence as shown in **c** and **d**.

Fig. 7.**47 e–k** ▷

bulging residual cortex. With older lesions, the overlying cortex is of normal thickness or may even be thickened. The cluster-of-grapes pattern on radiographs is caused by reeflike protrusions in the inner surface. Generally the lesions are surrounded by a dense, scalloped sclerotic border.

The following conditions must be met in order to diagnose a fibrous metaphyseal defect (i.e., fibrous cortical defect or nonossifying fibroma): the patient must be under 25 years of age, the defects must be located in the metaphysis or border the diaphyseal-metaphyseal junction, and they must involve the cortex. Fibrous metaphyseal defects are generally negative on radionuclide scans (e.g., Fig. 7.**46 c**). On MRI, however, they can produce very conspicuous and confusing findings (probably due to trauma) with persistent high signal intensity on T2-weighted images (Summers et al. 1998).

> Avoid confusion by MRI findings such as subtle perifocal edema. The diagnosis is established by conventional radiographic signs, combined if necessary with a negative radionuclide scan.

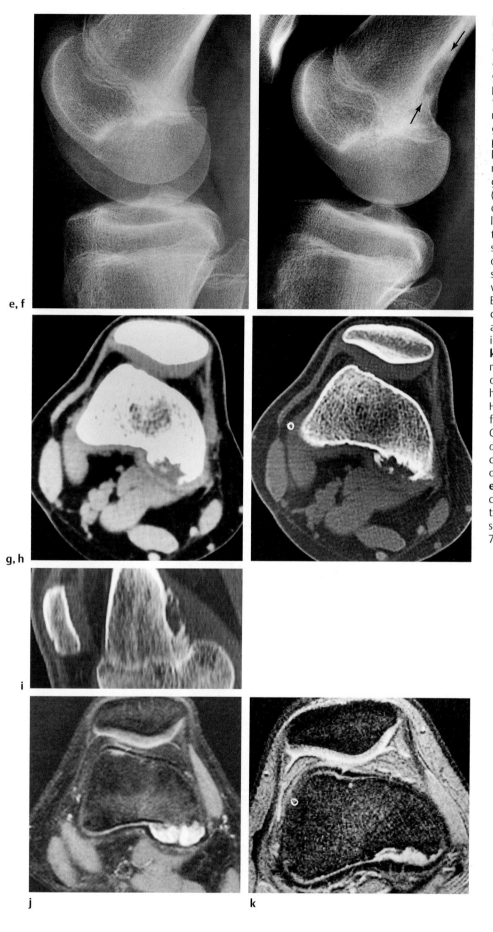

e, f

g, h

i

j

k

Fig. 7.**47 e–j** These images show unusual proliferative changes induced by a chronic avulsion injury in a 16-year-old girl with a six-month history of pain in the popliteal area. Initial radiographs (**e**) were unremarkable. The current radiograph (**f**) shows very subtle paraosseous calcifications behind the eroded cortex (arrows; visible only with a halogen lamp). CT (**g–i**) and MRI (**j**) clearly demonstrate a paraosseous "tumor mass." The location and radiographic features in themselves are consistent with a paraosseous osteosarcoma, but biopsy showed only reactive changes with cartilage proliferation. Both the radiological and clinical features (pain!) in this case are quite different from those in Figs. 7.**46** and 7.**47 a–d**. **k** Stress-induced cortical irregularities at the attachment of the gastrocnemius medial head in a different patient. Hyperintense structures are found *in* the lacuna (see also CT scan in Fig. 7.**46 d**) and *not on* the bone. This raised suspicion of a paraosseous osteosarcoma in the case in **e–j** and prompted an excisional biopsy. Compare also the basic differences in lesion structure in Figs. 7.**46 d** and 7.**47 g–i**.

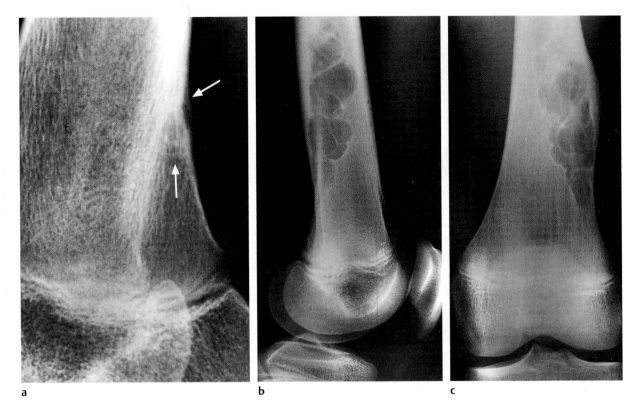

a

b

c

Fig. 7.**48 a–c**   Typical fibrous metaphyseal defect (FMD).
a Stage of fibrous cortical defect.
b, c Stage of nonossifying fibroma.

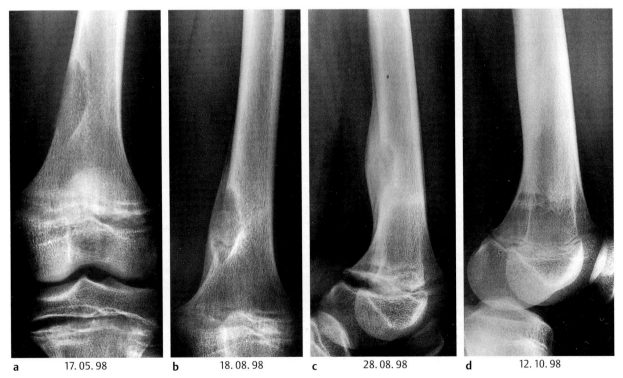

a   17. 05. 98   b   18. 08. 98   c   28. 08. 98   d   12. 10. 98

Fig. 7.**49 a–g**   Differential diagnosis of nonossifying fibroma, which itself is a normal variant, and another tumorlike lesion (brown tumor). The 11-year-old Turkish girl presented with pain in the left distal femur. Radiograph shows an elliptical
Continue p. 894, Fig. 7.**49 e–g** ▷

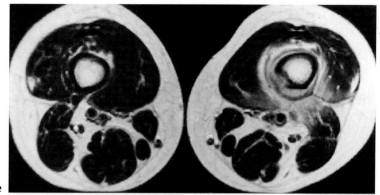

e   17. 05. 98

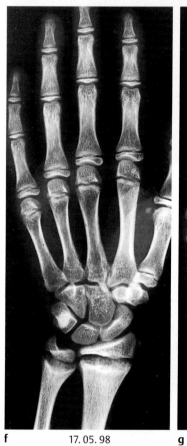

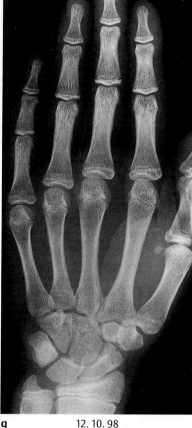

f   17. 05. 98   g   12. 10. 98

Continue Fig. 7.49 e–g
Lucency at the distal, postero medial diaphyseal-metaphyseal junction. If the lesion had been rimmed by sclerosis, it could have been interpreted as a nonossifying fibroma. The very broad epiphyseal plates of the distal femur and proximal tibia appeared abnormal, however. Combined with a slight blurring and rarefaction of the cancellous trabeculae, this finding raised suspicion of "immigrant rickets" with secondary hyperparathyroidism. The MR images in **e** show a massive hemorrhage encircling the tumorlike process and confused the differential diagnosis. A concurrent hand radiograph (**f**) confirmed the suspicion of severe rickets with secondary hyperparathyroidism, and laboratory findings were consistent with this diagnosis. The girl had to cover herself in public, depriving herself of the sun exposure necessary to convert vitamin D precursors into active vitamin D. Vitamin D replacement produced clinical improvement, but the patient developed an insufficiency fracture (**b, c**) with a marked periosteal reaction due to hemorrhage. By five months after initial presentation (**d, g**), the changes resolved completely. Note the accentuated Harris growth lines in radiograph **d**. This case is presented here to demonstrate that the adductor attachment is a relative "weak point." Heavy mechanical stresses in that area can lead to a fibrous metaphyseal defect in children and adolescents with healthy bones. In patients with a disorder of bone metabolism, a transformation zone or brown tumor may develop in
association with primary or secondary hyperparathyroidism.

Our assumption of a traumatic pathogenesis for cortical irregularities and fibrous metaphyseal defects is indirectly supported by case observations like that in Fig. 7.49. This case involves an 11-year-old Turkish girl with "immigrant rickets" and secondary hyperparathyroidism who sought medical attention for pain in the left distal femur. A brown tumor was found at the site where nonossifying fibromas occur, and MRI (Fig. 7.49 e) showed it to be encircled by a large hematoma. Despite massive vitamin D replacement, three months later the patient developed an insufficiency fracture with more bleeding into the lesion. Therapy was continued, however, and complete bony consolidation was achieved after a total of five months. Radiographs of the left hand also documented the positive response.

As described earlier, circumscribed changes located near the center of the distal femoral metaphysis may represent bone marrow infarctions (Figs. 7.36–7.39) or cartilaginous tumors (Fig. 7.12). **Noncalcified central enchondromas of the distal diaphysis and metaphysis** represent a true diagnostic challenge on conventional radiographs (Fig. 7.50).

Circumscribed destructions in the distal femoral metaphysis and epiphysis must be at least 3–4 mm in diameter to be identified as such, especially if there is no perifocal (sclerotic) reaction in the surrounding cancellous bone. We cannot explore the full differential diagnostic spectrum, but we emphasize that an **osteopenic or osteoporotic reduction in bone mass with fatty replacement** can mimic a **radiolucent lesion** (Fig. 7.51).

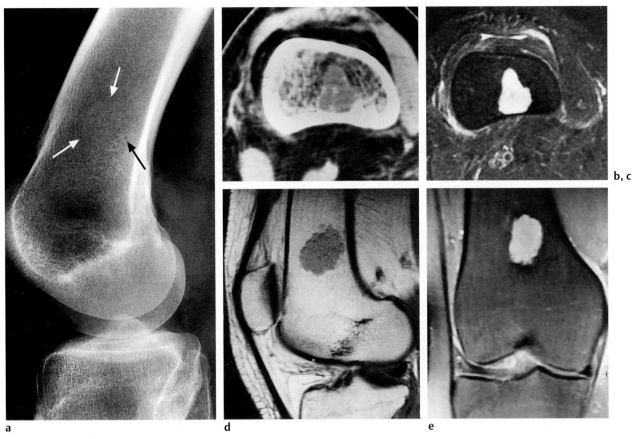

a

d

e

b, c

Fig. 7.**50 a–e**   Subtle enchondroma.
a Noncalcified enchondroma in the distal femoral metaphysis is very difficult to detect on the plain film.
b–e The lesion was discovered incidentally in an MRI examination of the knee for a torn meniscus (**c–e**). The lobular structure of the lesion is clearly visible on the MR images. Low T1 and high T2 signal intensity and a lobular structure are virtually diagnostic of a cartilaginous tumor. The lesion also has a characteristic CT appearance (**b**). CT additionally shows small calcifications that further support the diagnosis. Since the patient was asymptomatic, no further studies were done and one-year follow-up was recommended.

When a patient is examined for unexplained knee symptoms and this type of finding is seen, it should at least be further investigated with several CT scans to check for the presence of fatty tissue in the cancellous bone defects.

Multiple densities in the distal femoral diaphysis, metaphysis, and epiphysis can have a great many causes. The differential diagnostic spectrum ranges from osteoplastic metastases, multiple small featureless infarcts, and reactive sclerosis (e.g., in sarcoidosis) to osteopoikilosis (Fig. 7.**52**), osteopathia striata (Fig. 7.**17 a**), and melorheostosis (Fig. 7.**17 b**).

 ## Other Changes?

After the proximal femur, the distal femoral metaphysis and epiphysis are major sites of predilection for **transient osteoporosis** (Fig. 7.**54**), a special form of algodystrophy. Radiographic changes are usually preceded by (painful) edema on MRI. More patchy demineralization, known also as **pseudomalignant osteoporosis** (Fig. 7.**53**), results from disuse, as in patients with a painful underlying knee disorder. Much like transient osteoporosis, these changes are closely related to the **reflex dystrophies**.

Soft-tissue calcifications, especially when located adjacent to the medial femoral epicondyle, are referred to as **Köhler–Stieda–Pellegrini shadows** (Fig. 7.**55**).

Stieda classification of soft-tissue calcifications

➤ *Stieda I:* Fibro-ostosis or ossified avulsion of the adductor magnus or ossifications in the soft tissues adjacent to that site
➤ *Stieda II:* Paraosseous ossifications near the junction of the shaft with the inner surface of the condyle
➤ *Stieda III:* Ossification in the collateral ligament (after an avulsion). The displaced bone fragment fits a matching defect in the adjacent condyle or epicondyle

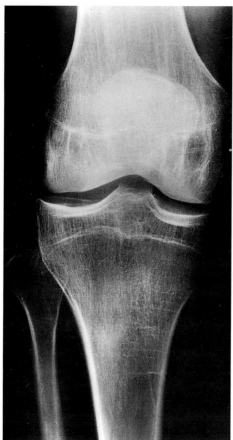

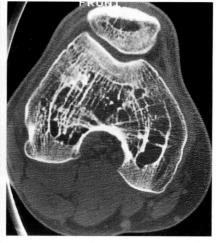

b

a

Fig. 7.**51 a, b**   Circumscribed lucency in the distal femoral epiphysis resulting from prolonged disuse of the right lower extremity during adolescence. CT (**b**) shows accumulations of fatty tissue between the accentuated residual trabeculae and a similar finding in the patella. The CT evidence of fatty tissue in the medial condylar "lesion" on the AP radiograph (**a**) is sufficient proof that it is harmless. Fat (and air) is the radiologist's friend!

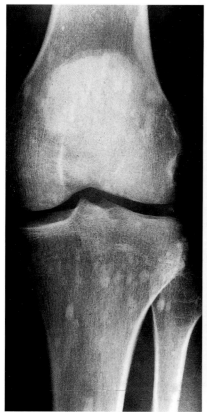

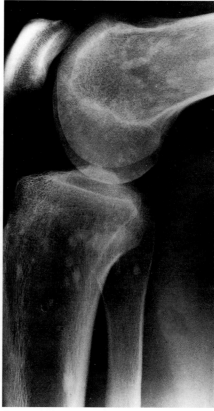

a

b

Fig. 7.**52 a, b**   Typical osteopoikilosis (spotted bones) with very small, sharply circumscribed densities clustered about the knee. The patient was clinically asymptomatic. The oblong density in the lateral cortex of the distal femoral metaphysis may be a "transition" to melorheostosis or osteopathia striata.

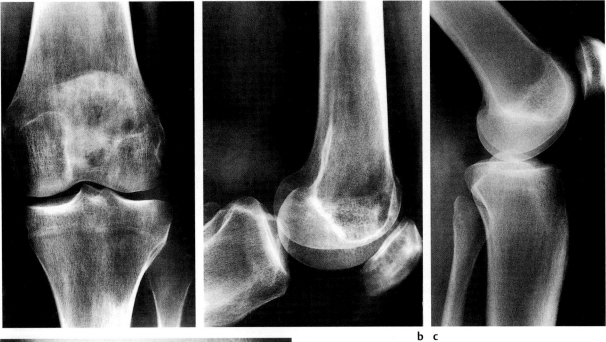

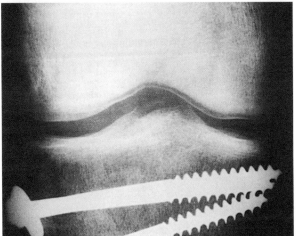

Fig. 7.**53 a–d**   Osteoporotic changes about the knee joint.
a, b "Pseudomalignant" patchy demineralization about the left knee joint in a patient with a painful internal knee derangement and three weeks' immobilization.
c The healthy side for comparison.
d Sharp linear zone of subchondral demineralization in the femur following internal fixation of the upper tibia.

While a Stieda I shadow may represent an adductor magnus avulsion or metaplastic ossification, the Stieda II shadow is unrelated to an avulsion injury. It represents a metaplastic ossification that may have a firm fibrous attachment to the bone. The ossification shown in Fig. 7.**55 d** adjoins the lateral condyle and, if located at a corresponding site on the medial condyle, would be classified as a Stieda II shadow.

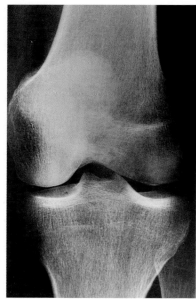

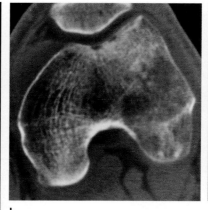

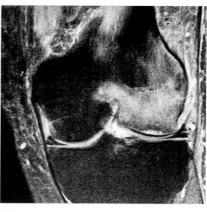

b

c

a

◁ Fig. 7.**54 a–c**   Osteoporosis of the distal femur.
a, b Typical transient osteoporosis in the lateral femoral condyle of a 50-year-old man with significant knee pain and effusion. Note the very pronounced demineralization throughout the lateral condyle in the AP radiograph and the fine lucencies in the CT scan with patchy sclerosis on the anterior side.
c Different patient with the same clinical symptoms but no radiographic abnormalities. The very high T2-weighted signal intensity in the lateral condyle is caused by edema, which may resolve spontaneously (transient edema) or may progress to transient osteoporosis. Such findings are not always easy to classify, especially when differentiating them from circumscribed infiltrative neoplasms such as malignant lymphoma.

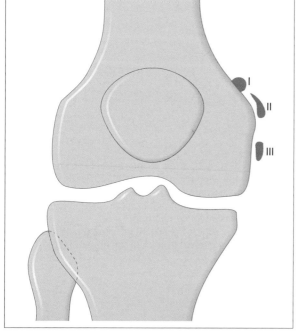

a

Fig. 7.**55 a–d**   Köhler–Stieda–Pellegrini shadows.
a Classification of the individual bony structures adjacent to the medial femoral condyle (see text).
b, c Type II and II/III Stieda shadow. The ossified structure at a somewhat more distal level represents a type III shadow.
d Counterpart to a Stieda II shadow on the proximal lateral femoral condyle.

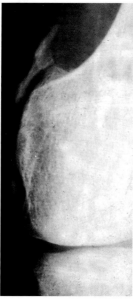

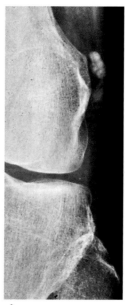

b   **c**   **d**

References

Adam, G., J. Neuerburg, J. Peiß et al.: Magnetresonanztomographie der Osteochondrosis dissecans des Kniegelenkes nach intravenöser Gadolinium-DTPA-Gabe. Fortschr. Röntgenstr. 160 (1994) 459

Ahlbäck, S., G. C. H. Bauer, W. H. Bohne: Spontaneous osteonecrosis of the knee. Arthr. and Rheum. 11 (1968) 705

Albers, W., H. Blümlein, H. Sühler: Die spontane Femurkondylennekrose des Kniegelenks. Zbl. Chir. 110 (1985) 607

Banagale, R. C., L. R. Kuhns: Traumatic separation of the distal femoral epiphysis in the newborn. J. pediat. Orthop. 3 (1983) 396

Barnes, G. R., J. L. Gwinn: Distal irregularities of the femur simulating malignancy. Amer. J. Roentgenol. 122 (1974) 180

Bohndorf, K.: Osteochondritis (Osteochondrosis) dissecans: a review and new MRI classification. Europ. Radiol. 8 (1998) 103

Burt, R. W., T. J. Matthews: Aseptic necrosis of the knee: bone szintigraphy. Amer. J. Roentgenol. 138 (1982) 571

Cayea, P., H. Pavlov, M. R. Sherman et al.: Lucent articular lesion in the lateral femoral condyle. Amer. J. Roentgenol. 137 (1981) 1145

Danzig, L. A., J. D. Newell, J. Guerra et al.: Osseous landmarks of the normal knee. Clin. Orthop. 156 (1981) 201

Dejour, H., G. Walch, L. Nove-Josserand, et al.: Factors of patellar instability: an anatomic radiographic study. Knee Surg. Sports Traumatol. Arthrosc. 2 (1994) 19

Dejour, H., G. Walch, P. Neyret et al.: Dysplasia of the femoral trochlea: Rev. Chir. Orthop. Reparatrice Appar. Mot. 76 (1990) 45

Dunham, K.: Developmental defects of the distal femoral metaphysis. J. Bone Jt Surg. 62-A (1980) 801

Freyschmidt, J.: Skeletterkrankungen. Klinisch-radiologische Diagnose und Differentialdiagnose, 2. Aufl. Springer, Berlin 1997

Freyschmidt, J., D. Saure, S. Dammenheim: Der fibröse metaphysäre Defekt (fibröser Kortikalisdefekt, nicht ossifizierendes Knochenfibrom). Fortschr. Röntgenstr. 134 (1981) 169

Freyschmidt, J., H. Ostertag, G. Jundt: Knochentumoren. Klinik-Radiologie-Pathologie, 2. Aufl. Springer, Berlin 1998

Grelsamer, R. P., J. L. Tedder: The lateral trochlear sign: femoral trochlear dysplasia as seen on a lateral view roentgenograph. Clin. Orthop. 281 (1982) 159

Harcke, H. Th., M. Synder, P. A. Caro et al.: Growth plate of the normal knee: evaluation with MR Imaging. Radiology 183 (1992) 119

Keats, Th. E., J. M. Joyce: Metaphyseal cortical irregularities in children. Skelet. Radiol. 12 (1984) 112

Lagier, R.: Partial algodystrophy of the knee. J. Rheumatol. 10 (1983) 255

Mahony, B. S., P. W. Callen, R. A. Filly: The distal femoral epiphyseal ossification center in the assessment of third-trimester menstrual age: sonography identification and measurement. Radiology 155 (1985) 201

Maurer, H. J., M. Schreiner: Ossifikation der distalen Femurepiphyse. Zur Frage der Osteochondrosis dissecans bei Kindern. Z. Orthop. 122 (1984) 743

Pao, D. G.: The lateral femoral notch sign. Radiology 219 (2001) 800

Pennes, D. R., E. M. Braunstein, G. M. Glazer: Computed tomography of cortical desmoid. Skelet. Radiol. 12 (1984) 40

Pfirrmann, Ch. W. A., M. Zanetti, J. Romero et al.: Femoral trochlear dysplasia: MR findings. Radiology 216 (2000) 858

Rajah, R., J. Young, W. F. Conway: Acute hemorrhagic infarct with edema. Skelet. Radiol. 24 (1995) 158

Rumlova, E., E. Vogel, A. F. Schärli: Frakturen des distalen Femurendes bei Kindern. Ther. Umsch. 40 (1983) 969

Rutherford, Y., A. K. Fomufod, L. J. Gopalakrishnan et al.: Traumatic distal femoral periostitis of the newborn: a breech delivery birth injury. J. nat. med. Ass. 75 (1983) 933

Scheller, S.: Roentgenographic studies on the ossification of the distal femoral epiphysis. Acta radiol. Suppl. 24 (1965)

Schwörer, I., A. Kaul, H. J. Stolpmann et al.: Bleieinlagerung im Knochen – Röntgenaufnahme als Nachweismethode? Fortschr. Röntgenstr. 138 (1983) 84

Summers, R. M., M. Brune, H. S. Kany et al.: Non-ossifying fibroma: characteristics at MR imaging with pathologic correlation. Radiology 209 (1998) 197

Vande Berg, B. C., J. Malghem, O. Devuyst et al.: Anorexia nervosa: correlation between MR appearance of bone marrow and severity of disease. Radiology 193 (1994) 859

Varich, L. J., T. Laor, D. Jaramillo: Normal maturation of the distal femoral epiphyseal cartilage: Age-related changes at MR imaging. Radiology 214 (2000) 705

Patella

▌ Normal Findings

 During Growth

The patella is usually ossified from multiple centers, beginning in the third year of life.

> A 1- to 2-year range of variation in the timing of patellar ossification (earlier or later) is not unusual and is considered a normal variant.

During growth, the patella may have an irregular, fragmented appearance (Figs. 7.**56**, 7.**57**, 7.**59**) that does not signify necrosis or other abnormalities. It is common to find isolated ossification centers at the distal pole of the patella in children 7–11 years of age (Fig. 7.**58**). It is less common to find disk-shaped centers over the anteroinferior patellar surface (Fig. 7.**60**) or shell-like centers over the proximal patellar border (Fig. 7.**61**). Shell-like centers may occasionally cover almost the entire circumference in the craniocaudal direction (Fig. 7.**62**).

> An apophysis on the posterior surface (facing the femur) that resembles an intra-articular loose body has been described and is still considered a normal variant. It is easily mistaken for a loose body.

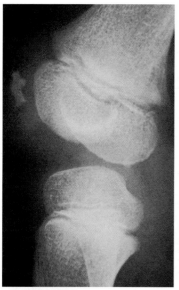 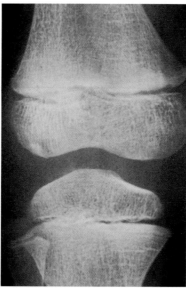

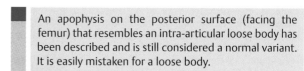
Fig. 7.**56a, b**   Normal "fragmented" appearance of the patella in a 7-year-old boy.

a   b

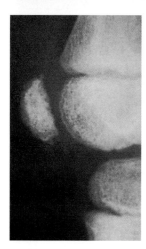 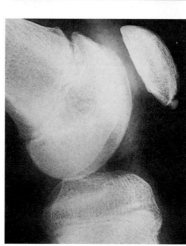

Fig. 7.**57**   Knee joint of a 6-year-old boy. The grainy structure is caused by various small ossification centers.

Fig. 7.**58**   Knee joint of a 10-year-old boy, with a small center at the caudal pole of the patella.

Fig. 7.**57**   Fig. 7.**58**

Fig. 7.**59 a–e** Boy 9 years of age with non-specific "growing pains" alternating between the right and left knee joints.
a–c These patellae have a very irregular, asymmetrical appearance in both the lateral and axial projections. There were no clinical signs of inflammation.
d, e MRI shows abundant cartilage of normal signal intensity around the small ossification center, which appears black on the T2-weighted image (**e**). There are no edematous changes or other abnormalities that might indicate necrosis.

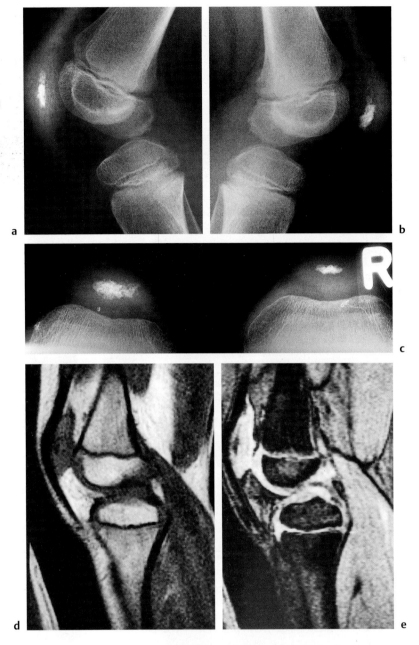

Fig. **7.60** Shell-like ossification center over the distal anterior ▷ surface of the patella.

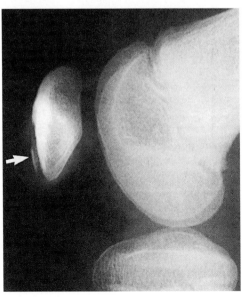

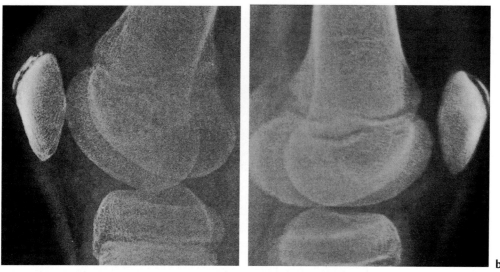

a   b

Fig. 7.**61 a, b**   Bilateral shell-like ossification centers over the proximal part of the anterior patellar surface.

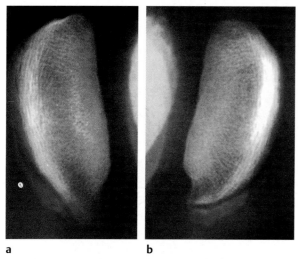

a   b

Fig. 7.**62 a, b**   Shell-like double-centers of the patellae. On the right side, the ossification covers almost the entire anterior circumference. The ossification appears very translucent and indistinct on these images. Asymptomatic 11-year-old child.

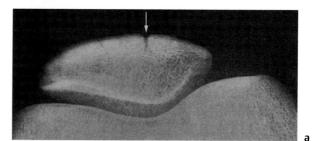

a

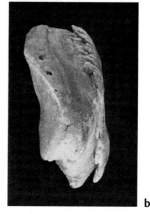

b

Fig. 7.**63 a, b**   Feathery bone proliferation on the anterior patellar surface mimics clefts or fissures on the tangential projection in **a**.

In Adulthood

The anterior surface of the patella may show clefts, especially in the tangential (sunrise) projection, that are caused by physiological bone proliferations (Fig. 7.**63**).

> Flame-shaped spicules on the patellar surface may also be a normal phenomenon, especially when clinical symptoms are absent.

The shape of the patella in adults is subject to a tremendous range of physiological variation.

Classification of morphological variants of the patella Wiberg devised a classification for the various morphological variants of the patella that may be seen in the tangential projection (Fig. 7.**64**). One assumption in this classification is that asymmetries in the femoral trochlea, especially with medial hypoplasia, predispose to the development of chondromalacia patellae. Wiberg (1941) and **Baumgartl** (1964) claimed that a correlation existed between morphological types C–E and the development of chondromalacia, prompting them to classify these types as dysplasia. **Nebel and Lingg** (1981) were able to show, however, that types C–E were more prevalent than the "normal" A and B

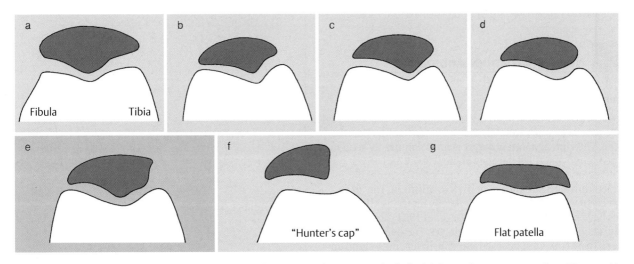

Fig. 7.**64 a–g**   Variable shape of the bony patella in the tangential projection (right leg) (after Wiberg, Baumgartl, and Rau et al.).

types based on autopsy findings. The same authors found no differences among types A–E regarding the frequency of degenerative articular cartilage changes and degenerative osteophytes.

In evaluating the patellar shapes defined by Wiberg, it should be noted that the posterior bony boundary of the patella need not be congruent with the articular cartilage and that the demonstrable transverse configuration of the patella depends entirely on the angle of knee flexion. Only the "hunter's cap" configuration (Fig. 7.**64 f**) appears to create a certain predisposition for chondromalacia and eventual osteoarthritis.

Today, then, the description of patellar shape is mainly of academic interest. We no longer perform this examination, and we obtain tangential radiographs of the knee joint only in trauma cases. MRI is the current method of choice for evaluating the condition of the patellar cartilage and opposing femoral condyles.

Similarly, the morphological variants of the femoral trochlea and condyles (Fig. 7.**65 f, i**) and the classification of

patellar shapes in the Hepp profile view (Fig. 7.**65 a–e**) are no longer considered to have practical importance in the diagnosis of chondromalacia. It should be noted, however, that the trochlea types **g–i** in Fig. 7.**65** predispose to recurrent patellar dislocation (see below).

There is no need to delve further into radiographic methods for measuring **patellofemoral congruency**, especially from an orthopedic standpoint, because many of the methods bear no established relation to the success of corresponding various surgical treatments. McNally (2002) may be consulted for a detailed review of the imaging assessment of anterior knee pain and patellar maltracking.

The **normal height of the patella in the lateral projection** (with the knee flexed 20–70°) is determined by taking the ratio of the patellar diameter to the distance of the inferior pole of the patella to the tibial tuberosity. The normal ratio is between 0.8 and 1.2 (Fig. 7.**66**).

This index is important in answering the question of whether patella alta has causal significance in osteonecrosis and/or chronic avulsion injury of the inferior patellar pole and tibial tuberosity. It can also be helpful in trauma investigations.

Fig. 7.**65 a–i**   Basic patterns of patellar shapes and morphological variants of the femoral trochlea.
a–e Basic patellar shapes seen in the Hepp profile view. The average diagonal diameter is 35–50 mm in women and 40–50 mm in men.
f–i Morphological variants of the femoral trochlea (after Gschwend and Bischofsberger): normal (**f**), medial hypoplasia (**g**), medial aplasia (**h**), flat or convex trochlea (**i**). Types **g–i** predispose to recurrent patellar dislocation. See also p. 878 and 908
a recent paper by Carrillon et al. (2000) about the assessment of patellar instability on MR images by measuring the lateral trochlear inclination.

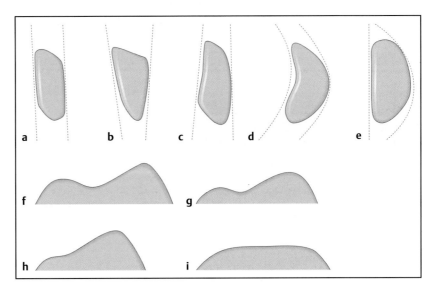

■ *Pathological Finding?*

Normal Variant or Anomaly?

Variants

eA small defect is observed in the superolateral quadrant of the patella in approximately 0.3–1% of the healthy population. This **dorsal patellar defect** is most commonly seen in the second and third decades of life (Fig. 7.**67**).

The etiology of the defect is uncertain. It probably results from a disturbance of normal ossification. The articular cartilage over the defect is generally intact, as MRI studies have proven (e.g., Monu and De Smet 1993). It is usually thickened and projects into the defect. The defects do not tend to progress but heal spontaneously, leaving behind an irregular sclerotic area.

Differentiation is mainly required from a **Brodie abscess**, but this lesion is generally symptomatic in contrast to dorsal patellar defects. The differential diagnosis also includes osteochondritis dissecans, but the overlying cartilage is typically damaged in this condition. Other possibilities are an intraosseous ganglion (uniformly hyperintense on T2-weighted images) and osteoid osteoma (strongly symptomatic).

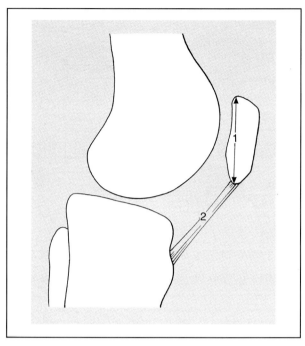

Fig. 7.**66**   Patellar height index in the lateral projection. The normal range is 0.8 to 1.2 (see text).

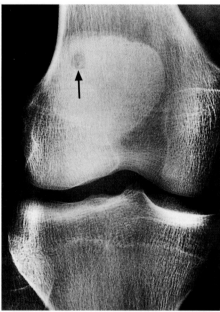

a

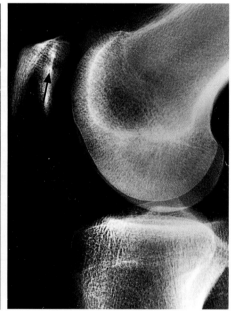

b

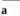

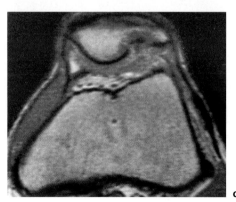

c

Fig. 7.**67 a–c**   Dorsal patellar defect.
a, b The defect appears as a rounded, sharply circumscribed lucency in the superolateral aspect of the patella.
c On MRI, the overlying articular cartilage is intact and extends partly into the defect. The incidental finding was no longer visible on radiographs two years later.

The "**Haglund groove**" in the articular surface of the patella (Fig. 7.**68**) is considered a normal variant. Generally the overlying cartilage is thickened (detectable by MRI).

Another variant consists of comma-shaped or **spurlike bony outgrowths** on the **anterior surface** of the patella (Figs. 7.**69**, 7.**70**). Their etiology is unclear but may relate to stress-induced bone formation at the attachment of the patellar ligament. Asymptomatic bone spurs at **the center of the femoral articular surface** of the patella on lateral radiographs are usually projection effects from lateral osteophyte-like excrescences (probably traction osteophytes, Fig. 7.**71**).

A special variant is the **bipartite, tripartite,** or **multipartite patella**, caused by incomplete fusion of the ossification centers. It is usually bilateral and involves the superolateral quadrant of the bone (Fig. 7.**72**).

The PA projection of the knee is recommended as an aid to conventional differential diagnosis, as it can better define the contour and position of the individual patellar segments. Other special projections are oblique and tangential views (Fig. 7.**74**). The presence of a more or less complete surrounding cortex of the segments helps to differentiate a bipartite patella from an acute fracture. Also, the segments of a bipartite patella generally do not fit together precisely like the pieces of a puzzle (Fig. 7.**73**), as is usually the case with fracture fragments.

Differentiation is also required from **nonunited patellar fractures** (that the patient cannot recall). In cases where pain is felt after a patellar injury and radiographs show definite segmentation of the patella, the differential diagnosis should include the spontaneous rupture of ossification centers bound together by connective tissue. **Double patella** refers to two patellae, one located above the other, that have approximately the same size and shape (Fig. 7.**75**). **Patella emarginata** refers to defects in the patellar contours with no history of trauma (Fig. 7.**76**).

Anomalies and Deformities

Chondrodysplasia punctata (stippled epiphyses, Conradi–Hünermann disease) is not a variant but a **true dysplasia**. It is already apparent in newborns, with radiographs showing punctate calcifications in the patellae (Fig. 7.**77**).

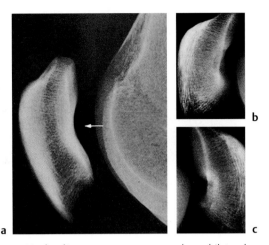

Fig. 7.**68 a–c**   Haglund's groove appears as a deep, bilateral concavity in the patellar articular surface of an 18-year-old (**a**) and a 15-year-old (**b, c**).

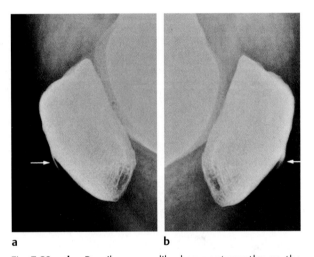

a   b

Fig. 7.**69 a, b**   Pencil- or spur-like bony outgrowths on the anterior patellar surface. Normal variant detected in a 50-year-old man.

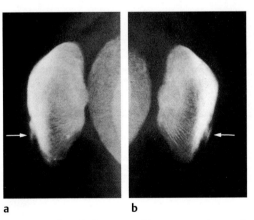

a   b

Fig. 7.**70 a, b**   Shell- or spur-like outgrowths on the anterior surface of both patellae in a 13-year-old boy.

Fig. 7.**71 a, b**   Spur-like "bony excrescence" on the patellar articular surface (arrow in **a**). In the tangential view, the finding is recognized as a projection effect from a medial traction osteophyte.

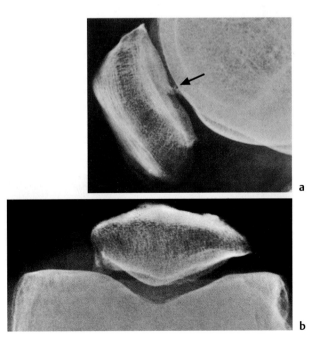

Generally these are not isolated findings, and similar phenomena will be noted in other epiphyses (see Fig. 2.**57**).

In **nail–patella syndrome**, the patellae may be absent or may show atypical configurations (Fig. 7.**78**).

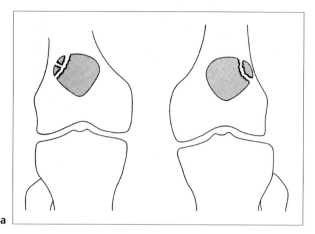

a

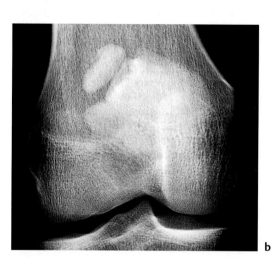

b

Fig. 7.**72 a, b**   Tripartite and bipartite patellae.

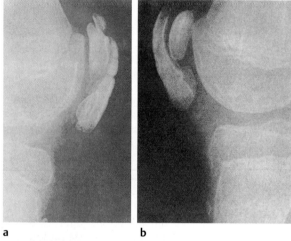

a   b

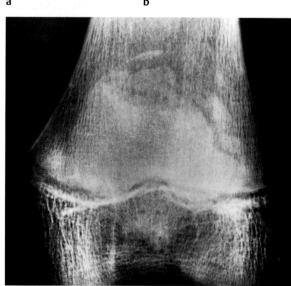

c

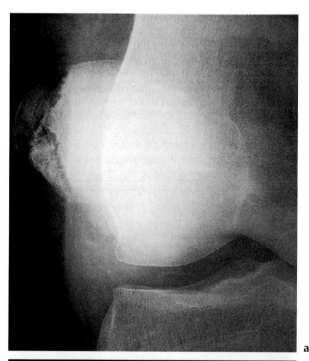

a

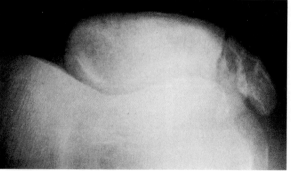

b

Fig. 7.**73 a–c**   Bipartite patella, showing typical division into anterior and posterior parts.
c Multipartite patella or still-unfused ossification centers in an asymptomatic 12-year-old? Contralateral films were not obtained, and there was no follow-up. In either case, the finding is interpreted as a normal variant.

Fig. 7.**74 a, b**   Bipartite patella.
a Special Kuchendorf projection.
b Tangential projection.

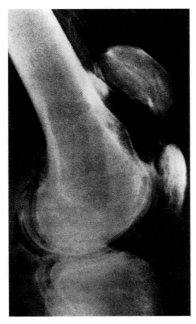

Fig. 7.**75** Arthrogram of a unilateral, congenital double patella.

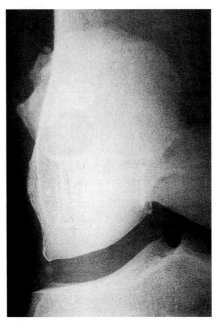

Fig. 7.**76** Patella emarginata.

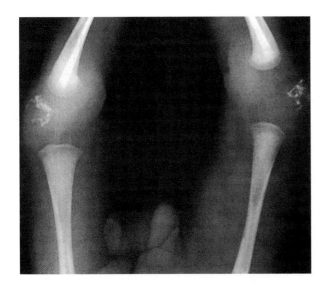

Fig. 7.**77** Chondrodysplasia punctata (stippled epiphyses) involving both patellae.

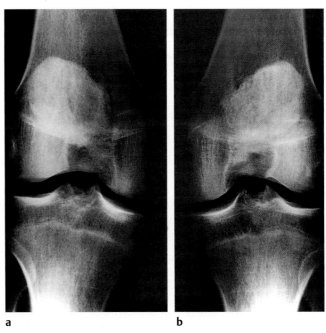

a   b

Fig. 7.**78 a, b** Atypical patellae in nail–patella syndrome. Iliac horns in the same patient are shown in Fig. 6.**26**.

The principal deformities and anomalies of the patellae and their syndromic associations are shown in Table 7.5.

Table 7.5   Deformities and anomalies of the patella and their syndromic associations (after Reeder)

Congenital syndromes associated with absent, hypoplastic, dysplastic bipartite or displaced patella
• Nail-patella syndrome (osteonychodysplasia)
• Acrocephalopolysyndactyly (Carpenter syndrome); the patella is displaced
• Arthrogryposis
• Cerebrohepatorenal syndrome (calcified flecks in the patella)
• Diastrophic dysplasia (displaced, hypoplastic or multipartite patella)
• Familial absence of the patella
• Mesomelic dysplasia (Werner type)
• Multiple epiphyseal dysplasia (displaced or bipartite)
• Neurofibromatosis (absent patella)
• Popliteal pterygium syndrome (absent or bipartite patella)
• Rubinstein–Taybi syndrome (displaced patella)
• Spondyloepimetaphyseal dysplasia
• Spondyloepiphyseal dysplasia
• Trisomy 8 syndrome

Patellar fractures in children can lead to necrosis but also the subsequent presence of two ossification centers if the displaced or avulsed growth cartilage continues to differentiate (Fig. 7.79).

Common **patellar fracture patterns** are shown in Fig. 7.80. It can be seen that most fractures do not involve the superolateral quadrant of the patella where bipartition tends to occur.

> In **Villiger's classification** of patellar fractures, a basic distinction is drawn between subaponeurotic fractures with an intact extensor apparatus and subcutaneous fractures with a ruptured and deficient extensor apparatus (Villiger 1982).

In the normal AP projection, the posterolateral margin of the tibia at the fibular notch appears as a dense vertical line (Fig. 7.184a, b) while the anterolateral margin is projected in the shadow of the fibula (Fig. 7.184a, b). With approximately 30–40 degrees of internal rotation, the posterior tibial margin, and thus the posterior border of the fibular notch, is projected into the fibula and forms the visible bony boundary (Fig. 7.184c).

In the AP projection, the axis of the tibia forms a medially open angle of 92 degrees with the talar axis (the "Johnson angle"). The range of variation is approximately ± 8 degrees.

 Fracture, Subluxation, or Dislocation?

Acquired patella alta (high-riding patella) can occur in association with:

• Chondromalacia
• Neuromuscular diseases (e.g., poliomyelitis)
• Osgood–Schlatter and Sinding–Larsen disease
• Ruptures of the patellar ligament
• Recurrent subluxation

Acquired patella baja (low-riding patella) occurs in association with:

• Quadriceps palsy
• Rheumatoid arthritis, especially the juvenile form
• Ruptures of the quadriceps tendon

Lateral dystopia is usually associated with an underdeveloped lateral condyle and a congenitally small patella, accompanied by genu valgum. These dystopias are usually congenital and predispose to true dislocation or habitual slipping of the patella. Previous injuries can also promote "habitual" or recurrent patellar dislocation.

The following conditions are associated with **recurrent patellar dislocation**:

• Dysplasia of the medial patellar facet
• Flattening of the trochlea groove (see also p. 878)
• Patella alta
• Genu valgum

The **diagnosis of chronic anterior knee pain** is based on patellofemoral tracking, ligament status, etc. We cannot delve into this complex issue here (see also p. 878). A quantitative CT method for detecting possible lateralization of the tibial tuberosity as a cause of anterior knee pain is described on p. 921.

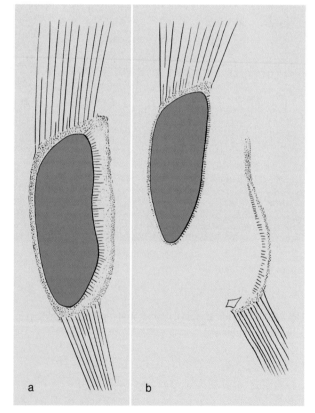

Fig. 7.**79a, b**   Cartilaginous growth plate and avulsion fracture.
a Diagram of the cartilaginous growth plate of the patella.
b Avulsion fracture with significant epiphyseal separation (after Jacquemier et al.).

Fig. 7.**80 a–h** Patellar fracture patterns (after Rogers).
a Transverse.
b Vertical.
c Stellate.
d Transverse with displacement.
e Comminuted with displacement.
f Avulsion of the superior pole.
g, h Traumatic avulsion of the patellar cartilage with displacement of the avulsed fragment into the medial joint space (arrows). The copious effusion aids in clear MRI visualization of the lesion. The arrows in **g** indicate the cartilage defect, which is now occupied by fluid (white). The cartilage fragment in **h** is located in the articular fluid.

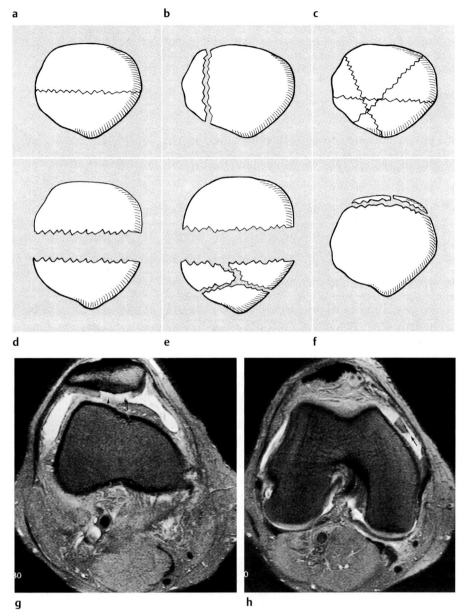

a   b   c

d   e   f

g   h

Fig. 7.**81** Chronic traction injury of the patella with ossification in the quadriceps tendon (arrows). (From Donnelly et al. 1999.) ▷

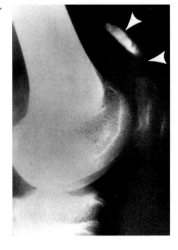

The width of the talocrural joint space is normally about 3–4 mm in adults. The 20 degree internal rotation view is important for evaluating the normal anatomy, as it gives a clear projection of the talar trochlea and the articular surfaces of the malleoli (the "mortise view").

 Necrosis?

The condition known as **patellar chondromalacia** should probably be viewed as a form of necrosis. We cannot explore in detail the problems relating to this condition.

> It is now certain, however, that the higher morphological types in the Wiberg classification do not definitely predispose to the development of cartilage ulcerations.

Besides constitutional factors, it is clear that extreme positions of the patella, genu valgum, recurrent patellar dislocation, etc. can precipitate patellar chondromalacia, which is definitely a preosteoarthritic condition. Today the disease is within the domain of MRI. **Osteochondritis dissecans** of the patella represents an extreme form of patellar chondromalacia (Fig. 7.**82**).

There is disagreement whether the condition known as **Sinding–Larsen–Johansson disease** is a type of primary osteonecrosis involving an **irregularity** or an **accessory bone element** at the inferior pole of the patella. We feel that this disease more likely represents a chronic traction injury. Sinding–Larsen–Johansson disease is most common in adolescents 10–14 years of age and is associated with circumscribed pain and swelling over the inferior pole of the patella. There is a general limitation of knee motion. Radiographs show irregular contours of the lower

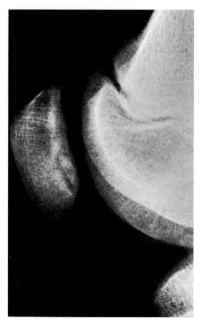

Fig. 7.**82** Osteochondritis dissecans of the patella. The osteochondral lesion is demarcated as a zone of increased density with a lucent rim in the inferior articular part of the patella.

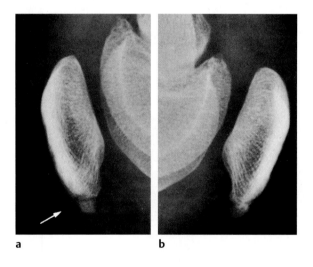

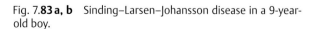

Fig. 7.**83 a, b** Sinding–Larsen–Johansson disease in a 9-year-old boy.

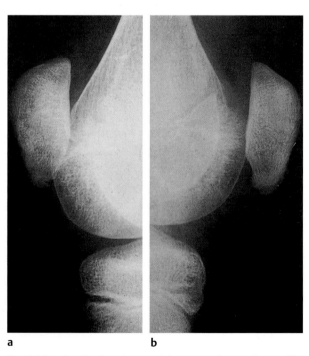

Fig. 7.**84 a, b** Sinding–Larsen–Johansson disease in an 11-year-old girl with positive clinical symptoms, mainly on the left side.

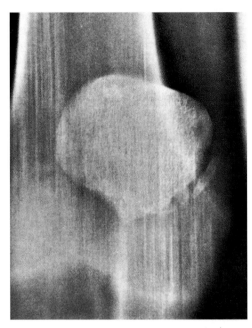

Fig. 7.**85** Late stage of Sinding–Larsen–Johansson disease with shell-like ossification about the inferior pole of the patella.

pole of the patella and bone fragments combined with swelling, thickening, and blurring of the patellar tendon (Figs. 7.**83**, 7.**84**). Late films show shell-like bone fragments about the inferior pole of the patella (Fig. 7.**85**).

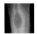 ## Inflammation? Tumor?

Inflammatory processes in the patella are rare. A few authors have described Brodie abscesses and plasma cell osteomyelitis of the patella.

Primary and secondary bone tumors of the patella are also rare. In a series of 48 cases of primary patellar bone tumors published by Kransdorf (1989), 38 were benign lesions (16 chondroblastomas, 8 giant cell tumors, 6 simple bone cysts, 3 hemangiomas, etc.) and only 4 were malignant tumors (3 lymphomas, 1 hemangioendothelioma). In larger statistical series, it has been found that no more than 0.01–0.6% of all bone tumors occur in the patella. The most prevalent benign tumors are **chondroblastoma** and **giant cell tumor**. **Metastases** from a known or unknown primary (CUP syndrome) are extremely rare in the patella. We have personally observed a patellar metastasis of renal cell carcinoma as the initial clinical-radiologic symptom of the tumor (Weber et al. 1999) (Fig. 7.**86**).

Larger defects in the patella may be caused by medullary tophus formation in **gout** (Recht et al. 1994).

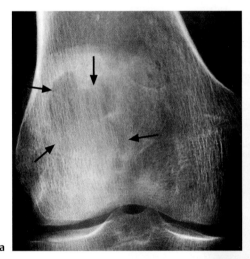

a

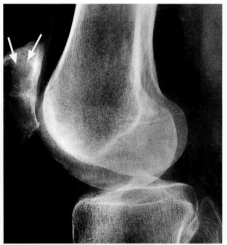

b

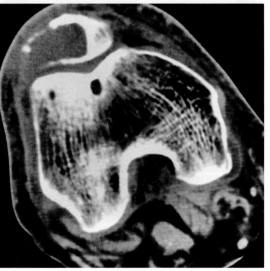

c

Fig. 7.**86 a–c** Metastatic renal cell carcinoma in the patella, noted as the first clinical and imaging manifestation of the disease (CUP [carcinoma unknown primary] or MUP [metastasis unknown primary]).

Other Changes?

The patella, like any other bone, is subject to structural changes that are marked by an increase or decrease in density, depending on the underlying disease. With trophic disturbances, the bone may become extremely demineralized, even showing a pseudomalignant patchy configuration (Fig. 7.**53**). Lagier et al. (1983) described isolated involvement of the patella by **algodystrophy** (reflex sympathetic dystrophy, Sudeck disease).

Patellar involvement in **polyostotic Paget disease** is not unusual, but a solitary pagetic lesion in the patella is extremely rare (Fig. 7.**87**). In this case differentiation is required from a chronic inflammatory process, and generally this can be done entirely from the clinical presentation (Paget disease is usually asymptomatic except for bone enlargement).

As elsewhere in the musculoskeletal system, insertional tendinopathy can affect the quadriceps tendon and patellar ligament. Radiographs may show circumscribed resorption (rarefying fibro-ostitis) or proliferation (productive fibro-ostitis) (Fig. 7.**63b**). These changes are not the same as femoropatellar osteoarthritis, which is characterized by subchondral lucencies, sclerosis, etc. and by the formation of intra-articular osteophytes directly on the patellar articular margins.

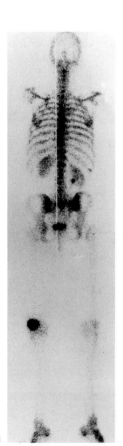

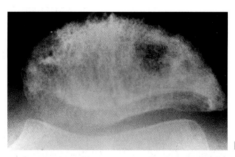

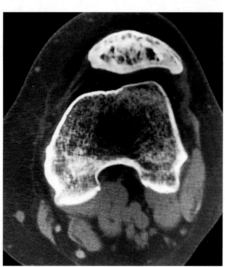

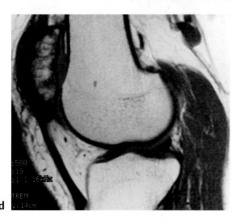

Fig. 7.**87a–d** Unusual solitary pagetic lesion in the left patella of an elderly woman.
a Radionuclide scan shows massive homogeneous uptake in the patella.
b Tangential radiograph shows enlargement of the bone and coarsened trabecular structures.
c, d Both CT (**c**) and MRI (**d**) prove that the altered bone contains fat marrow spaces. This is inconsistent with various diseases including osteosarcoma in Paget disease. (Case courtesy of Professor Lenz, Bremen.)

References

Albert, J., R. Lagier: Enthesopathic erosive lesions of patella and tibial tuberosity in juvenile ankylosing spondylitis. Fortschr. Röntgenstr. 139 (1983) 544

Baumgartl, F.: Das Kniegelenk. Erkrankungen, Verletzungen und ihre Behandlung mit Hinwisen für die Begutachtung. Springer, Berlin 1964

Carrillon, Y., H. Abidi, D. Dejour et al.: Patellar instability: Assessment on MR images by measuring the lateral trochlear inclination–initial experience. Radiology 216 (2000) 582

de Carvalho, A., A. H. Andersen, S. Topp et al.: A method for assessing the height of the patella. Int. Orthop. (SICOT) 9 (1985) 195

Denham, R. H.: Dorsal defect of the patella. J. Bone Jt Surg. 66-A (1984) 116

Donnelly, L. F., G. S. Bisset, C. A. Helms et al.: Chronic avulsive injuries of childhood. Skelet. Radiol. 28 (1999) 138

Evans, D. K.: Osteomyelitis of the patella. J. Bone Jt Surg. 44-B (1962) 319

Ghelman, B., J. C. Hodge: Imaging of the patello-femoral joint. Orthop. Clin. N. Amer. 23 (1992) 523

Goergen, Th. G., D. Resnick, G. Greenway et al.: Dorsal defect of the patella: a characteristic radiographic lesion. Radiology 130 (1979) 333

Greinemann, H.: Zur Bestimmung der vertikalen Kniescheibenposition. Unfallheilkunde 86 (1983) 110

Hanspal, R. S.: Superior dislocation of the patella. Injury 16 (1985) 487

Haswell, D. M., A. S. Berne, C. B. Graham: The dorsal defect of the patella. Pediat. Radiol. 4 (1976) 238

Hepp, W. R.: Die Dysplasie des Femoro-Patellargelenkes als präarthrotische Deformität. In Küsswetter, H., M. Reiser: Der retropatellare Knorpelschaden. Thieme, Stuttgart (1983) 45

Hille, E., K.-P. Schultz: Rotational instability of the patella on radiographic images. Arch. orthop. traum. Surg. 104 (1985) 74

Howie, J. I.: Computed tomography in osteochondritis dissecans of the patella. J. Candad. Ass. Radiol. 36 (1985) 197

Insall, J., E. Salvati: Patella position in the normal knee joint. Radiology 101 (1971) 101

Jakob, R. P., S. v. Gumppenberg, P. Engelhardt: Does Osgood-Schlatter-disease influence the position of the patella? J. Bone Jt Surg. 63-B (1981) 579

Johnson, J. F., B. G. Brodgen: Dorsal defects of the patella. Amer. J. Roentgenol. 139 (1982) 339

Kransdorf, M. J., R. P. Moser, N. Tuyanoa et al.: Primary tumors of the patella. A review of 42 cases. Skelet. Radiol. 18 (1989) 365

Kricun, M. E., D. Resnick: Patellofemoral abnormalities in renal osteodystrophy. Radiology 143 (1982) 667

Lagier, R., I. Boussina, B. Mathies: Algodystrophy of the knee. Anatomico-radiological study of a case. Clin. Rheumatol. 2 (1983) 71

McNally, E. G.: Imaging assessment of anterior knee pain and patellar maltracking. Skeletal Radiol. 30 (2001) 484

Monu, J. U. V., A. A. De Smet: Case report 789 (dorsal defect of the patella). Skelet. Radiol. 22 (1993) 528

Nebel, G., G. Lingg: Sind die Formvarianten der Patella nach Wiberg präarthrogen? Radiologe 21 (1981) 101

Rau, W. S., H.-J. Hehne, M. Schlageter: Die Chondromalacia patellae – Arthrographische Beobachtungen zur Genese und Diagnose. Fortschr. Röntgenstr. 130 (1979) 644

Recht, M. P., F. Seragini, J. Kramer et al.: Isolated or dominant lesions of the patella in gout: a report of seven patients. Skelet. Radiol. 23 (1994) 113

Redlich, F. H.: Osteochondrosis dissecans beider Kniescheiben. Fortschr. Röntgenstr. 111 (1969) 712; 113 (1970) 254

Schäfer, R.: Beitrag zur Osteomyelitis der Patella. Zbl. Chir. 77 (1952) 425

Schutzer, S. F., G. R. Ramsby, J. P. Fulcerson: The evaluation of patello-femoral pain using computerized tomography. Clin. Orthop. 204 (1986) 286

Swaton, S., Z. Huber: Einseitige, angeborene, doppelte Kniescheibe (Patella duplex unilateralis congenita). Zbl. Cir. 85 (1960) 2270

Villiger, K. J.: Patellafrakturen. Schweiz. Rdsch. Med. Prax. 71 (1982) 1708

Weber, J., St. Puschmann, J. Freyschmidt: Patellametastase als klinisch-radiologisches Erstsymptom eines Nierenzellkarzinoms. Fortschr. Röntgenstr. 170 (1999) 228

Wiberg, G.: Roentgenographic and anatomic studies on the femoro-patellar joint with special reference to chondromalacia patellae. Acta orthop. scand. 12 (1941) 319

Proximal Tibia and Fibula

▌ Normal Findings

 During Growth

The **ossification center of the proximal tibial epiphysis** usually appears in the last two months of fetal development and fuses with the shaft in about the 20th year of life. It may consist of two parts (Fig. 7.**88**).

In about the fourth year of life, the anterior cortex of the upper tibia appears relatively thick and wavy. Between 7 and 15 years of age, a beaklike process extends down the anterior surface of the upper tibia from the proximal epiphysis (Fig. 7.**89 b**). In some cases this process is not a coherent structure but consists of isolated centers (Fig. 7.**89 a**) that fuse together at 13–15 years of age and later form the tibial tuberosity (Fig. 7.**89 d**).

The **shape of the tibial tuberosity** shows very great inter- and intraindividual variations in children and adolescents (Figs. 7.**90**–7.**91**, 7.**117**). The spectrum ranges from irregular, fragmented-appearing bony elements to solid, beaklike configurations.

> The cartilaginous gap distal to the bony portions of the tuberosity is also variable in its shape (Fig. 7.**91**). These variations do not necessarily have pathological significance.

The distal, nonossified part of the tuberosity appears as an **oblique lucent line** of variable width on AP radiographs (Fig. 7.**90 a**). It should not be mistaken for a fracture line.

> When the lower leg is slightly rotated externally, the tibial tuberosity may appear as a small lateral prominence in the frontal projection (Fig. 7.**90 c**). This finding is always distinguishable from an abnormal periosteal process by noting that it is directly adjacent to the dense shadow of the tuberosity.

The **ossification center of the proximal fibular epiphysis** becomes visible between the fourth and sixth years of life. Another small center at the tip of the fibular epiphysis generally fuses at 20–25 years of age but may persist.

Mild genu varum is a normal finding in infants, just as mild genu valgum is normal in children.

Harcke et al. (1992) reviewed the MRI characteristics of the physes about the knee, with special emphasis on the proximal tibial and fibular growth plates.

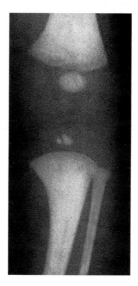

Fig. 7.**88**   Dual ossification centers in the proximal tibial epiphysis of a newborn.

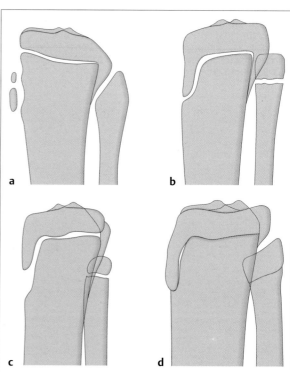

Fig. 7.**89**   Normal variations in the development of the proximal tibial epiphysis and tibial tuberosity (see text).

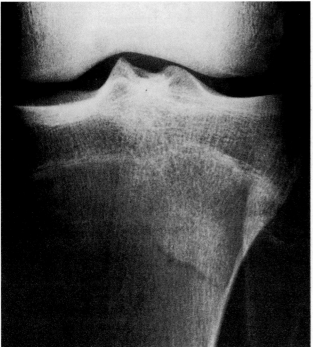

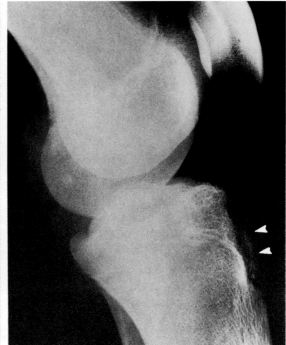

a

b

Fig. 7.**90 a–d** Tibial tuberosity.
a–c Healthy male 17 years of age with no knee symptoms. The oblique lucency in radiograph **a** is caused by the still-cartilaginous distal portion of the tibial tuberosity. The finding in this AP view is explained by the lateral view (**b**) showing the apophysis and the space below it (arrows). Radiograph **c** is a slightly externally rotated view showing the lateral border of the tibial tuberosity, which mimics a periosteal process. Note the dense shadow of the tuberosity in the adjacent tibia. The combination of a dense tuberosity shadow with an adjacent bulge in the lateral tibial contour confirms that the feature is a projection effect from the tuberosity.
d CT scans through the tibial tuberosity of a 28-year-old man. Note the different configurations of the right and left tuberosities. The projection effect in **c** is easily explained by a pointed configuration of the tuberosity, like that shown in **d** (right).

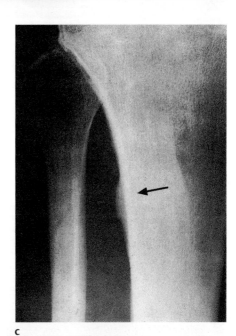

c

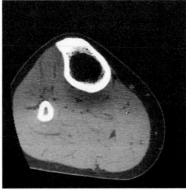

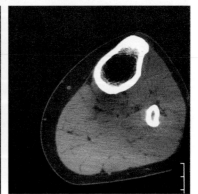

d

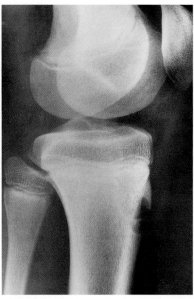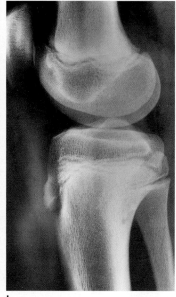

a   **b**

Fig. 7.**91 a–d**   Healthy 14-year-old boy with no knee symptoms. Note the different appearances of the right and left tibial tuberosities, especially regarding the distal portions that are not yet ossified.

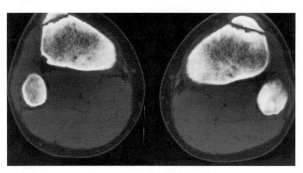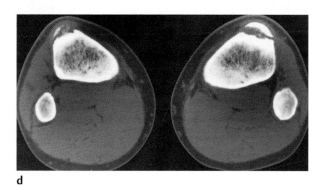

c   **d**

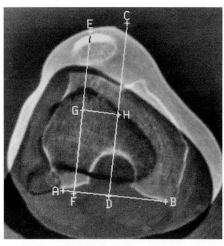

Fig. 7.**92**   Lateralization of the tibial tuberosity as a possible cause of chronic anterior knee pain (after Jones et al.; p. 921).

 In Adulthood

The **medial and lateral articular surfaces of the tibial plateau** slope slightly away from each other.

> The anterior articular margin of the upper tibia forms the proximal contour of the medial articular surface on AP radiographs. This contour may be convex toward the interior of the knee (see also Fig. 7.**90 a**). Less commonly it is slightly concave, and even a straight contour is still considered normal.

The medial joint line often forms a small protuberance just medial to the medial tubercle. It represents the medial border of the medial articular surface, marking the boundary between the surfaces within the knee that are and are not covered by articular cartilage. The radiographic appearance of the upper tibia is best understood by studying the superior aspect of the tibia and its articular structures as shown in Fig. 7.**93**.

A **third intercondylar tubercle** may be located at the insertion of the anterior cruciate ligament in the anterior intercondylar area (Figs. 7.**94**–7.**96**). Data in the literature indicate that this small bony prominence is present in 3% of the population (Ravelli 1955). As a counterpart to the third

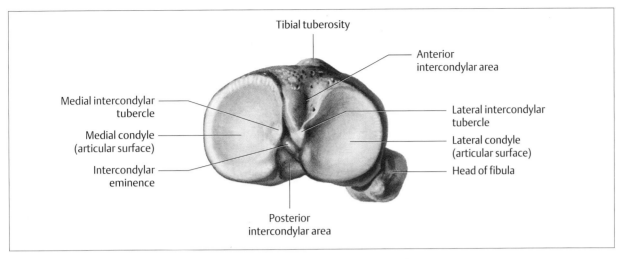

Fig. 7.**93**   Superior aspect of the tibia in an anatomic specimen (after Wolf-Heidegger).

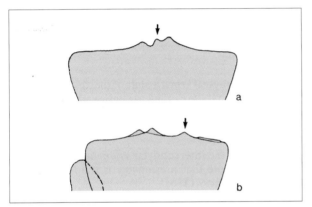

Fig. 7.**94 a, b**   Diagram of a third intercondylar tubercle.
a Normal AP projection.
b Slightly oblique lateral projection.

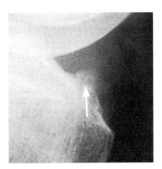

Fig. 7.**95**   Third intercondylar tubercle on the anterior rim of the tibial plateau.

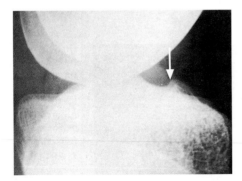

Fig. 7.**96**   Third intercondylar tubercle on the tibial plateau.

tubercle, a **fourth intercondylar tubercle** may occur at the insertion of the posterior cruciate ligament in the posterior intercondylar area. It has been observed in approximately 1% of the population (Ravelli 1955) (Figs. 7.**97**, 7.**98 a**).

Approximately half of individuals with a fourth intercondylar tubercle also have a third intercondylar tubercle. The fourth tubercle is seen most clearly in the lateral projection, as the high anterior margin of the upper tibia may obscure it in the AP projection. Ossification in the posterior cruciate ligament can mimic a fourth intercondylar tubercle.

"**Tubercle avulsions**" can be extremely difficult to distinguish from accessory tubercles on conventional radiographs (Fig. 7.**98 b–f**).

The **intercondylar tubercles** are variable in their size and height, but the medial tubercle is usually taller than the lateral tubercle.

> It is uncertain whether the **tubercle of Gerdy**, located just below the lateral tibial margin, is a normal anatomic variant or a **bony prominence left by a Segond fracture** (Fig. 7.**99 d, e**).

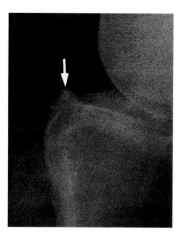

Fig. 7.**97**   Fourth intercondylar tubercle on the posterior rim of the tibial plateau.

We emphasize the importance of taking a thorough history. It is important to know whether a **Segond fracture** has occurred, as this injury has a high association with tears of the anterior cruciate ligament and menisci. The Segond fracture is a small, elliptical bony avulsion from the lateral aspect of the proximal tibia at the site where the middle portion of the lateral capsular ligament complex is attached. This type of avulsion fracture and/or anterior cruciate ligament injury leads to anterolateral rotatory instability (Hughston et al. 1976, Johnson 1979). Bock et al. (1994) examined 129 patients with acute anterior cruciate ligament injuries and found that 3.1% of the patients had Segond fractures. On follow-up radiographic examination, 7 patients exhibited a characteristic bony excrescence arising 3–6 mm below the lateral tibial plateau (Fig. 7.**99**).

Differential diagnosis of the Gerdy tubercle and healed Segond fracture should also include the **Rauber console,** a small area of bony proliferation that may develop on the lateral or medial tibial borders, just below the articular margin, several months after a meniscal tear (Fig. 7.**99 c–e**).

Although a Rauber console resulting from a meniscal tear can, by definition, occur on either the lateral or medial side, a lateral console requires differentiation from the "tubercle of Gerdy" (a possible normal variant) and a healed Segond fracture. To avoid confusion in terminology, it is best to interpret the finding as a "bony excrescence or prominence on the lateral upper tibia" and classify it as a normal variant or a traumatic lesion based on the patient's history, clinical findings, and perhaps MRI findings. Confusion in semantics may occur if we continue to use archaic terms (usually named after the author who first described them) that were coined before the advent of modern imaging procedures and before complex injury patterns were understood. We feel that these terms have become superfluous in the age of functionally oriented diagnostic imaging.

The **fused epiphyseal growth plate** of the tibia may remain visible throughout life as a linear density across the upper tibia. A small cleft may persist at its posterior end and should not be mistaken for an erosion or fissure (Figs. 7.**100**, 7.**101**).

CT scans of the **intercondylar eminence** often show a **small round hole** that presumably is the foramen of a nutrient canal (Fig. 7.**121 b**).

The articular surface of the fibula at the **tibiofibular joint** can exhibit a variety of configurations on radiographs (Fig. 7.**102**).

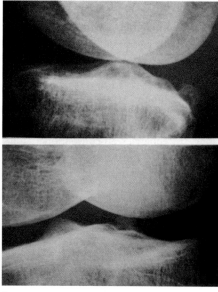

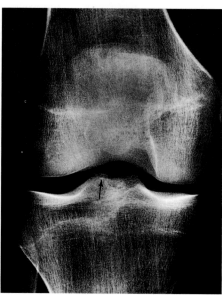

Fig. 7.**98 a–f**   Accessory tubercle or avulsion fracture?
a Radiographs showing a fourth intercondylar tubercle.
b Not an accessory tubercle, but a small bony avulsion (MRI of same case on p. 919).

a   b

Fig. 7.**98 c–f** ▷

Fig. 7.**98 c–f** The AP radiograph (**b**) suggests a bony avulsion of the anterior cruciate ligament, but the MR images show that the ligament is intact (**c, f**). The finding is actually caused by a bony fragment that has separated from a site anterior and lateral to the anterior intercondylar area (lower arrowhead in **d**). Extensive intraosseous edema has developed in the lateral femoral condyle and medial tibial plateau. Apparently the patient suffered a knee sprain in which the distal femur was rotated counterclockwise, pushed forward, and angled inward (valgus), shearing off portions of the anterior mediolateral tibial plateau. The valgus-producing component of the injury is evidenced by the severe disruption of the medial collateral and meniscocapsular ligaments, with subluxation of the medial meniscus. This case demonstrates that conventional radiographs, even when showing a bony lesion, are inadequate for the evaluation of knee trauma and do not tell even a fraction of the "true story." The asterisks indicate sites of intraosseous edema (bone bruise) and the anterior cruciate ligament.

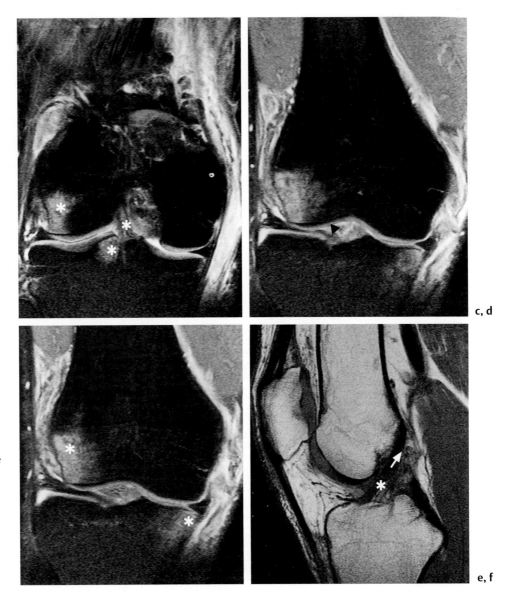

c, d

e, f

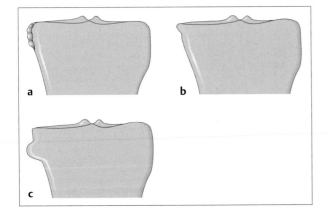

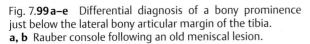

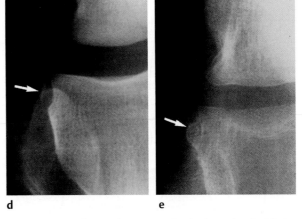

d　　　　　　e

Fig. 7.**99 a–e** Differential diagnosis of a bony prominence just below the lateral bony articular margin of the tibia.
a, b Rauber console following an old meniscal lesion.
c Tubercle of Gerdy.
d, e Healing of a Segond fracture.
A superficial bony avulsion is shown just after the injury in **a** and five years later in **b**. The avulsion has healed, leaving a

10 mm × 10 mm bony excrescence that is almost level with the tibial plateau. No degenerative changes are visible. Comparing radiograph **e** with diagrams **b** and **c**, we can easily see how a "Rauber console" or Gerdy tubercle could result from an old Segond fracture, which is often associated with tears of the anterior cruciate ligament and menisci (from Bock et al. 1994).

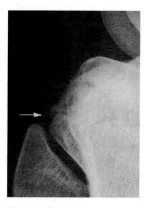

Fig. 7.**100**   Persistent posterior segment of the proximal tibial epiphyseal plate in a 44-year-old man.

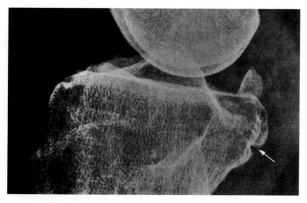

Fig. 7.**101**   Cleft in the posterior border of the upper tibia at the former site of the cartilaginous growth plate (arrow) in a 71-year-old woman. Atypical projection of a fabella in a slightly rotated profile view, not a fourth intercondylar tubercle.

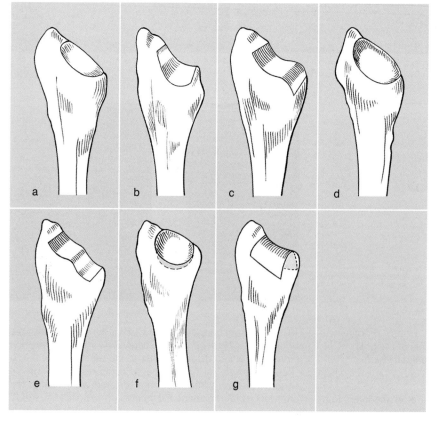

Fig. 7.**102 a–g**   Configurations of the proximal fibular articular surface and their prevalence (after Eichenblatt and Nathan).
a Flat (33.55%).
b Trochoid (29.57%).
c Double trochoid (22.59%).
d Condylar (4.65%).
e Trochlear (0.86%).
f Ball and socket (0.67%).
g Saddle-shaped (2.32%).

Pathological Finding?

Normal Variant or Anomaly?

Variants

In the opinion of various authors (e.g., Jones et al. 1995), **lateralization of the tibial tuberosity** is a potential cause of patellar maltracking that can result in chronic **anterior knee pain**. The above authors have developed a quantitative method for detecting lateralization of the tuberosity: Axial CT scans are obtained through the distal femoral epiphysis, and the scan is selected in which the intercondylar notch is deepest. That scan is superimposed on an axial CT scan at the level of the tibial tuberosity (Fig. 7.**92**). Then a line is drawn between the posterior margins of the femoral condyles (A–B). Two perpendiculars are dropped from line A–B, one passing through the intercondylar notch (C–D) and the other through the tibial tuberosity at the attachment of the patellar tendon (E–F). The distance between the two perpendicular lines (G–H) is measured in millimeters. Values greater than 9 mm indicate lateralization (specificity 95%, sensitivity 85%).

The **proximal fibular epiphysis** may be duplicated, in which case the smaller center frequently persists (Fig. 7.**103**).

> A small **exostosis-like outgrowth** in the area of the pes anserinus (Fig. 7.**104**) is still considered a normal variant.

The causal mechanism of this outgrowth is probably the same as that of a "coat-hook" exostosis (Fig. 7.**33**, p. 879).

Malformations, Deformities

A true deformity of the proximal tibial epiphysis develops from **epiphyseal dysplasia** (dysplasia epiphysealis multiplex). The sequelae of the dysplastic femoral and tibial epiphyses may resemble old idiopathic osteochondronecrosis (Fig. 7.**105**). The diagnosis can always be estab-

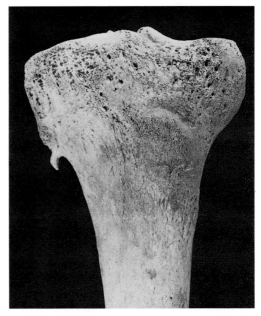

Fig. 7.**104**   Small exostosis-like bony outgrowth in the area of the pes anserinus. A normal variant.

lished by noting additional epiphyseal deformities at other sites in the skeleton.

A typical deformity of the proximal tibia is **Blount disease** (osteochondrosis deformans tibiae, tibia vara). It is a growth disturbance of the medial aspect of the proximal tibial epiphysis that also involves the adjacent epiphysis and metaphysis. As the tibial diaphysis continues to grow normally, a characteristic varus deformity develops in the proximal part of the tibia (Figs. 7.**106**, 7.**107**).

The actual cause of the disease appears to be premature closure of the medial part of the epiphyseal growth plate, leading secondarily to deformities of the epiphysis and metaphysis.

The disease is usually bilateral, occasionally unilateral, and comes to attention in toddler's age, especially in overweight infants (infantile tibia vara). A rare adolescent type can also occur, which is usually unilateral.

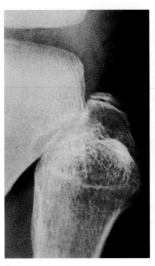 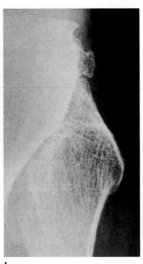 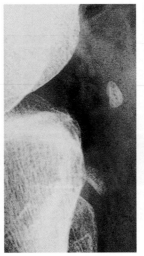 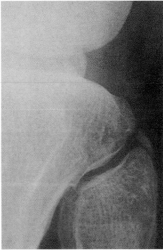

a   b   c   d

Fig. 7.**103 a–d**   Variable appearance of persistent apophyses of the fibular head.

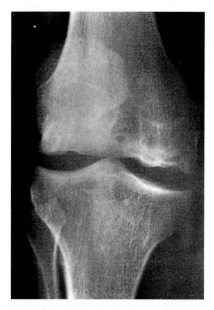

Fig. 7.**105**   Epiphyseal dysplasia with marked flattening and undulation of the femoral articular margins and atypical concavity of the tibial articular margins. Additional epiphyseal deformities were present in other joints—a finding that distinguishes epiphyseal dysplasia from idiopathic osteonecrotic changes. (From Koppers 1982.)

Radiologically metaphyseal irregularity is evident, with enlargement and a beaklike projection pointed medially and distally. The medial aspect of the epiphysis may also be deformed. This is associated with bowing.

Blount disease requires differentiation from **focal fibrocartilaginous dysplasia** (Fig. 7.**108**). This condition involves a well-defined, unilateral defect in the upper metaphyseal portion of the medial tibial cortex combined with marked thickening of the cortex distal to the defect. Focal fibrocartilaginous dysplasia has its onset in small children learning to walk (weight-bearing and ambulation phase), similar to Blount disease, but the varus bowing is noted at a later age.

The first report on this rare disease (about 40 cases described to date) was published by Bell et al. (1985). Histological examination of the defect, which is located at the site of the pes anserinus, shows inactive fibrocytes and connective tissue with interspersed chondrocytes. The key histological criterion is the presence of a collagenous and dense fibrous, tendonlike tissue. The cartilaginous component apparently does not originate from the epiphyseal plate. These histological features led Bell et al. to postulate that a mesenchymal anlage at the tendon insertion fails to differentiate and persists as a focus of fibrocartilage which could interfere with the growth of the medial aspect of the proximal tibia, producing varus deformity.

CT shows attenuation values in the soft-tissue range, while the signal intensities on MRI are consistent with a fi-

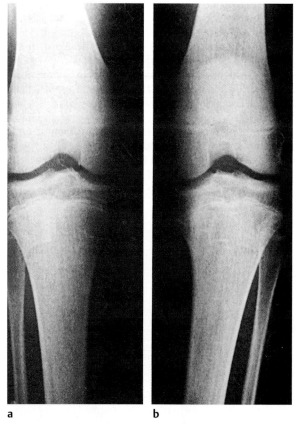

a   b

Fig. 7.**106a, b**   Ossification disturbance on the medial aspect of the proximal tibial epiphysis (Blount disease). Relatively mild grade on the left side compared with the healthy side (adolescent type).

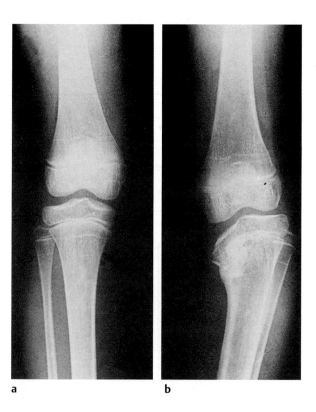

a   b

Fig. 7.**107a, b**   Unilateral Blount disease of the left tibia. The medial epiphyseal plate is no longer defined. The medial portions of the metaphysis are markedly shortened and sclerotic, resulting in genu varum. The metaphysis is generally enlarged. Compare this figure with focal fibrocartilaginous dysplasia in Fig. 7.**108b** and with spondylometaphyseal dysplasia in Fig. 7.**162f**.

brocartilaginous (not purely cartilaginous) tissue showing a mixed, predominantly hypointense pattern. The imaging abnormalities are so typical that there is no need for excisional biopsy. In any case, spontaneous resolution of the deformity occurs in 1–4 years (Fig. 7.**108 c**), making surgery unnecessary. Khanna et al. (2001) published a case of focal fibrocartilagenous dysplasia, which they treated with curretage of the lesion. Resolution of tibia vara and healing of the focal fibrocartilaginous dysplasia was noted at six

months. Another conservatively treated case needed eight years follow-up. Differentiation of focal fibrocartilagenous dysplasia from Blount disease is shown schematically in Fig. 7.**108 h**. As noted above, Blount disease is based on a disturbance of the cartilaginous growth plate, whereas focal fibrocartilaginous dysplasia appears to result from stresses transmitted to the bone through the pes anserinus.

Fig. 7.**108 a–g**   Focal fibrocartilaginous dysplasia in a child one year old when first examined. In marked contrast to Blount disease (Fig. 7.**107**), there is only a metaphyseal defect while the epiphyseal plate is intact. The defect is located precisely at the attachment of the pes anserinus. Note the thickened cortex distal to the defect.
a Radiograph taken in June 1997. The child had no clinical complaints, but the parents noted varus bowing of the leg.
b Radiograph taken in June 1998.
c Radiograph taken in February 2000. The defect has healed, and the varus deformity has mostly resolved. Thickening of the medial tibial cortex distal to the defect has been eliminated by remodeling.

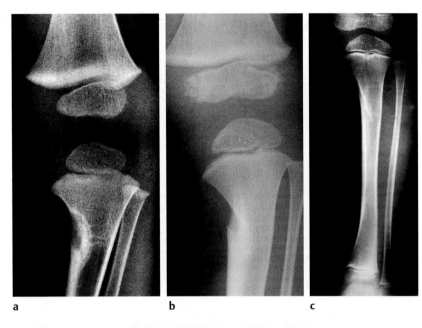

a   b   c

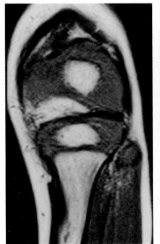 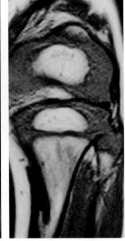 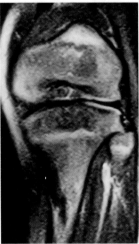 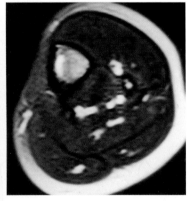

d   e   f   g

d–f On MRI, the structures in the radiographic defect are practically devoid of signal. Only the distal peripheral parts in image **f** show somewhat higher signal intensities, which probably represent more cartilaginous foci.
g Axial MRI shows a bandlike hyperintensity at the edge of the medullary cavity. (Images **a–g** courtesy of Dr. Gross, Hannover.)
h Diagrams of the key radiographic features that distinguish fibrocartilaginous dysplasia (left) from Blount disease (right) (after Cockschott et al.).

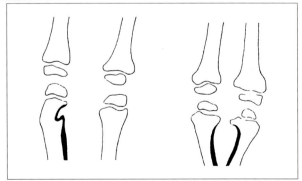

h

Fracture, Subluxation, or Dislocation?

Classification of proximal tibial fractures
➤ Fractures not associated with dislocation (of the knee), tibial plateau fractures
➤ Fracture-dislocations

In many cases fracture-dislocations have reduced spontaneously by the time of the imaging examination and can be recognized only on the basis of typical fracture-line patterns.

The classification of Moore (1981) is currently used for fracture-dislocations of the knee. The advantage of this classification is that it relates a particular fracture type to the ligamentous injuries that may accompany it. We can-

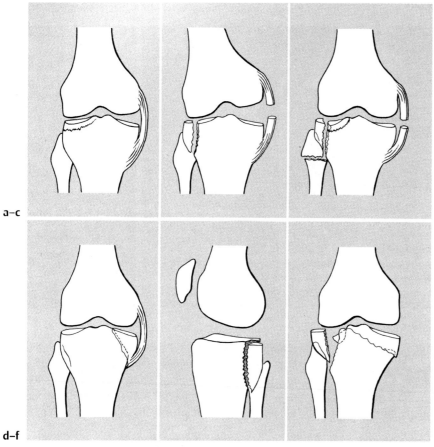

a–c

d–f

Fig. 7.**109 a–f**   Classification and relative frequency of tibial plateau fractures (after Rogers).
a Depressed (26%).
b Split (24%).
c Split and depressed (26%).
d Medial condyle (11%).
e Posterior rim (3%).
f Bicondylar (10%).

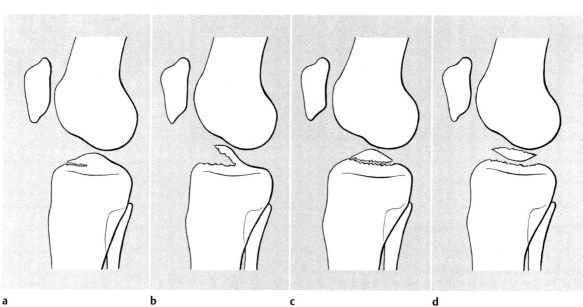

a   b   c   d

Fig. 7.**110 a–d**   Partial and complete avulsions of the intercondylar eminence (after Rogers).
a Nondisplaced partial avulsion.

b Hinged avulsion.
c Complete avulsion.
d Avulsed and inverted fragment.

not give further details within the context of this book, which deals with normal variants. Figures 7.**109** and 7.**110** illustrate common types of proximal tibial fractures and avulsion fractures of the intercondylar eminence as defined by Rogers.

Proximal tibial fractures are easy to miss on conventional radiographs, especially compression fractures (Fig. 7.**111e, f**). Since the tibial plateau has about a 15° downslope from anterior to posterior, it is easy to miss a fracture in the anterior margin and overestimate the extent of a depressed fracture in the posterior margin. Thus, in cases where there is clinical suspicion of a proximal tibial fracture, CT scans should be routinely obtained. If CT is negative and clinical symptoms are present, MRI should also be performed (Figs. 7.**98b–f**, 7.**111**), especially if forensic issues are involved.

By itself, the detection of traumatic edema in the upper tibia (bone bruise) has no therapeutic implications other than resting of the extremity.

As noted earlier, the **nonossified part of the tibial tuberosity appears as a lucent line** that may be mistaken for a fracture (Fig. 7.**90a**).

Fractures of the fibular head and neck rarely occur in isolation and are usually combined with ligamentous injuries or fractures of the lateral tibial plateau or ankle.

Dislocations of the fibular head can occur in any direction. Turco and Spinella (1985) described anterolateral dislocations of the fibular head sustained in athletic injuries.

The typical radiographic features of subluxations and dislocations of the fibular head are shown schematically in Fig. 7.**112**.

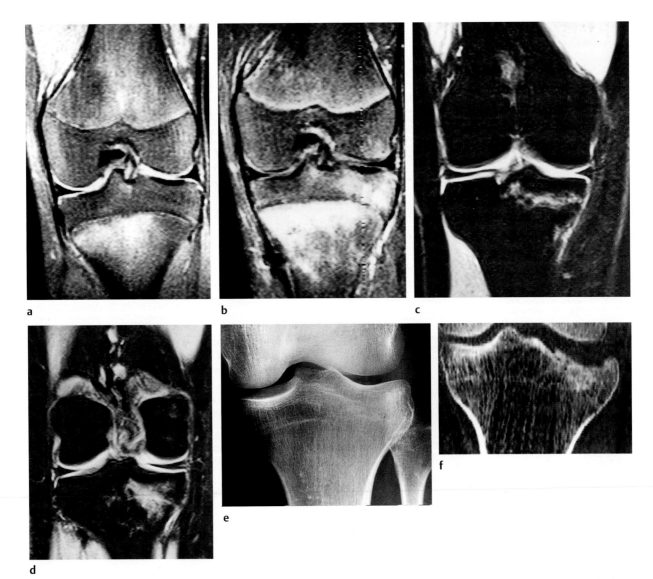

Fig. 7.**111 a–f**   Traumatic lesions of the proximal tibia, negative on conventional radiographs.
a, b Marked traumatic edema of the proximal tibia in a 17-year-old boy with negative radiographic films.
c, d Radiographically occult stress fracture in the medial part of the upper tibia. The fracture occurred at the site of the former growth plate in a young woman who jogged 8 km daily

to prepare for a marathon race. The patient went directly from "0 to 8 km" in her training, and so the bone had no time to adapt gradually to the increased stresses.
e, f Lateral depressed fracture that is easily missed on radiographs. The reformatted CT image clearly defines the true extent of the impacted area.

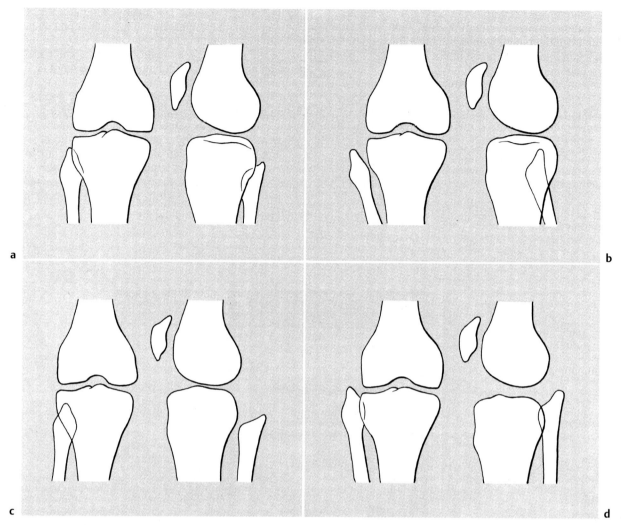

a

b

c

d

Fig. 7.**112a–d** Subluxation and dislocation of the fibular head (after Rogers).
a Normal.

b Anterolateral.
c Posteromedial.
d Superior.

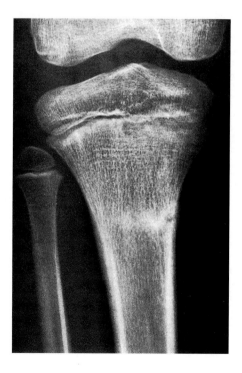

The proximal diaphyseal-metaphyseal junction area of the tibia is a site of predilection for the development of **true stress fractures** (fatigue fractures, Fig. 7.**113**). Apparently this area is subjected to particularly strong loads during walking and all activities performed in an upright position. The pes anserinus is a cofactor.

For this reason, **Looser–Milkman transformation zones** (insufficiency fractures, pseudofractures) occur at that location when the bone has been structurally weakened due to osteomalacia or other disease.

Stress fractures and Looser–Milkman zones are also observed with some frequency in the proximal fibula.

◁ Fig. 7.**113** Typical stress fracture in the area of the pes anserinus in a 9-year-old boy. Clinically, the patient had marked pain and swelling in that area.

Necrosis?

Circumscribed **subchondral necrosis** can affect the proximal tibial epiphysis and may progress toward **osteochondritis dissecans**. This problem was discussed in some detail on p. 883 (see also Fig. 7.**42**).

A condition specific to the proximal tibial metaphysis is the **Osgood–Schlatter lesion** (Osgood–Schlatter disease, aseptic necrosis of the tibial tuberosity). As the alternate term implies, this disease was formerly interpreted as a local apophyseal aseptic necrosis. This was suggested by histological evidence of circumscribed osteonecrotic changes at the tendon insertion on the tibial tuberosity. It was also common to interpret the "fragmented" appearance of the tibial tuberosity in adolescents, with local pain and swelling, as fragmentation due to necrosis, unaware that this is a normal finding also seen in asymptomatic adolescents (Figs. 7.**89**, 7.**91**, 7.**117**). In more recent years, however, views have changed regarding the pathogenesis of Osgood–Schlatter lesions of the tibial tuberosity, and today the disease is classified as **chronic traction trauma (chronic traction tendinitis)** or as a more or less **chronic avulsion fracture of the tibial tuberosity**.

Interestingly, Osgood (1903) assumed in his original work that the disease was caused by a partial avulsion of the tibial tuberosity due to contraction of the quadriceps muscle. This was supported by the fact that symptoms disappeared after callus had formed at the avulsion site, i.e., when the fracture had healed. As a result, immobilization was once considered the standard treatment for adolescents diagnosed with Osgood–Schlatter disease. The chronic traction theory is based on the concept that a localized tendinitis develops at the insertion of the patellar tendon on the tibial tuberosity. This is supported by the fact that the disease affects rapidly growing adolescents whose bones grow faster than the tendons, causing greater tension to be exerted on the tendons, especially during physical exertion. The ossification that occurs at the tendon attachment on the tuberosity would then represent heavy fibroblastic metaplasia in the sense of heterotopic bone formation. Successful local treatment with steroid injections has confirmed the validity of the tendinitis theory.

Rosenberg et al. (1992) used modern imaging techniques to check the accuracy of the fracture or tendinitis hypothesis. But the authors emphasize that the diagnosis can actually be based on the clinical examination alone and seldom requires costly modalities such as CT and MRI. In all of the cases studied (20 patients with 28 lesions), the authors were able to find an objective correlate for the clinical soft-tissue thickening at the tendon attachment on the tibial tuberosity (CT: widening and decreased density of the tendon, Fig. 7.**115**; MRI: enlargement and increased signal intensity of the tendon, Fig. 7.**114**). MRI also detected deep or superficial infrapatellar bursae that do not occur physiologically and presumably reflect bursitis (Fig. 7.**116 b, c**). Tendon thickening and visualization of the bursae disappeared after the regression of clinical symptoms. The authors did not confirm the fragmented appearance of the tibial tuberosity, which was considered a very important sign in the era of plain film radiography (see above). They found an ossicle in only 9 of 28 cases (32%), and in only 6 of these cases did the ossicle fit into a defect in the tibial tuberosity, suggesting a prior bony avulsion (Fig. 7.**115 b**).

In several patients these ossicles became reintegrated into the bone as the symptoms regressed, and in other cases follow-up showed no bony fusion. By the way, in none of the 28 cases did MRI show evidence of a cartilage avulsion, disproving the claim that the disease is based more on—radiographically invisible—cartilage avulsions than bony avulsions (the attachment site is predominantly cartilaginous at the start of the disease). Rosenberg et al. (1992) conclude from their study that the predominance of soft-tissue changes (in 100% of the cases) as opposed to bony changes (in just 32% of the cases) indicate that the trauma in Osgood–Schlatter disease usually occurs at the lower end of the patellar tendon, and that this trauma may sometimes be associated with bony avulsion.

The authors also discuss treatment. Local lidocaine injections into the soft tissues around the tibial tuberosity provided immediate, prolonged relief of pain in most cases (25 of the 28 lesions). Apparently, one benefit of passing a needle into the deep and superficial bursae is to drain the inflammatory exudate and relieve the pressure.

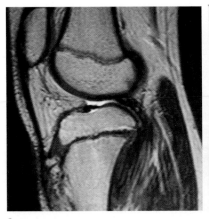
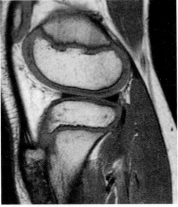
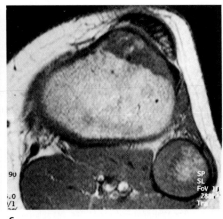

a   b   c

Fig. 7.**114 a–c** Chronic traction tendinitis at the attachment of the patellar ligament on the tibial tuberosity (Osgood–Schlatter disease). Note the marked thickening of the attachment site with patchy hyperintensities in the T2-weighted image (**a**).

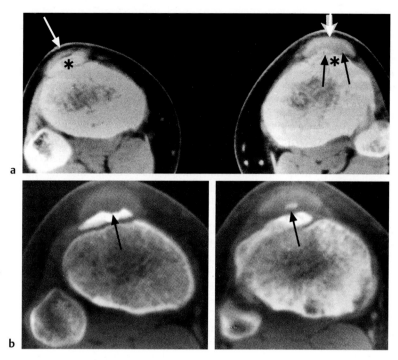

a

b

Fig. 7.**115a, b**   Osgood–Schlatter disease.
(From Rosenberg et al. 1992.)
a Left-sided Osgood–Schlatter lesion in a 13-year-old boy. The patellar tendon (short white arrow) appears thickened and its internal density is decreased (right black arrows). The left arrow points to a small ossicle in front of the tibial tuberosity (asterisk).
b The small bony element (over the arrow in the image on the right) fits into a defect (over the arrow in the left image) shown in the adjacent, more distal scan. Note the marked thickening of the patellar tendon.

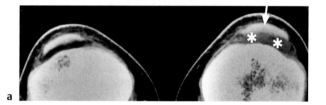

a

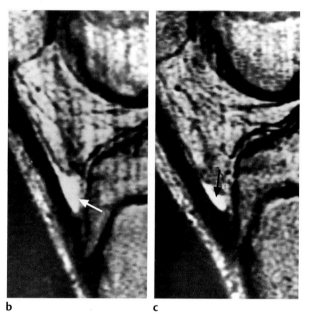

b   c

Fig. 7.**116a–c**   Left-sided Osgood–Schlatter lesion in a 13-year-old boy. (From Rosenberg et al. 1992.)
a Initial CT scan shows a low-density mass behind the patellar tendon, corresponding to an enlarged bursa (asterisks). The opposite side appears normal.
b MR images at the same time show the prominent bursa as an area of very high fluid-equivalent signal intensity (white arrow).
c Following the local injection of lidocaine, the bursa is significantly smaller and symptoms are relieved.

We can summarize the findings of Rosenberg et al. along with known conventional radiographic phenomena as follows:

> The patellar tendon margins at its attachment on the tibial tuberosity are obscured on conventional radiographs, and an "accessory" bony element is occasionally detected. CT and MRI show swelling of the distal patellar tendon at its attachment on the tibial tuberosity. Thickening of the superficial and deep infrapatellar bursae creates soft-tissue masses and obliterates the interstitial fat planes. Fragmentary ossification

> in front of the tibial tuberosity (Figs.7.**117**, 7.**118**) does not confirm the presence of the disease, as it may also be seen in normal individuals. Even when clinical symptoms are present, it cannot be interpreted as a positive roentgen sign. It is better in such cases to rely on the clinical manifestations.

A **white tibial epiphysis** may indicate complete necrosis without fragmentation (idiopathic or posttraumatic), but it may just as well signify a malignant lymphoma with reactive sclerosis (Fig. 7.**127**). This type of finding should be investigated by biopsy.

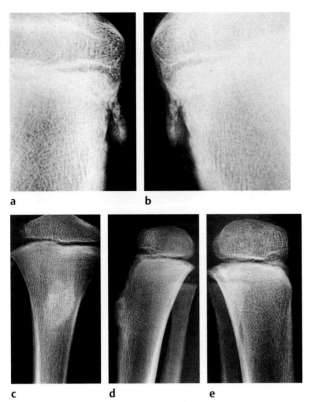

a   b

c   d   e

Fig. 7.**117 a–e**   Variants of the tibial tuberosity.
a, b Irregular ossification of the tibial tuberosity in an asymptomatic child. These radiographic findings do not warrant a diagnosis of an Osgood–Schlatter lesion, even in patients with pain and a palpable swelling.
c–e Very prominent right tuberosity in an asymptomatic 4-year-old child as a normal variant.

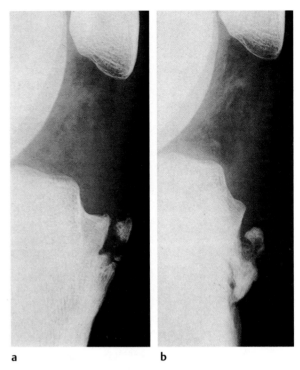

a   b

Fig. 7.**118 a, b**   Bilateral fragmentation of the tibial tuberosities in an adult with no specific history. Either the patient had Osgood–Schlatter disease and was unable to recall it, or the changes reflect chronic traction trauma associated with a relatively high-riding patella. This type of ossification, accompanied by resorptive changes in the tuberosity (**b**), are also seen in occupations that involve prolonged kneeling (e.g., tile layers).

Inflammation? Tumor?

Osteomyelitis of the proximal tibial epiphysis occurs in infants and small children but is very rare in schoolchildren, adolescents, and adults (except for Brodie abscess). This difference in the frequency of epiphyseal involvement by osteomyelitis is related to the blood supply. The capillaries that perforate the epiphyseal plate involute after one year of age, and the epiphysis and metaphysis each have a separate arterial blood supply. As a result, the epiphyseal plate forms a barrier to the spread of infection from the metaphysis to the epiphysis.

Congenital syphilis is typically associated with large erosive lesions in the proximal medial tibial metaphyses (Wimberger sign, Fig. 7.**120**) caused by the infiltrative growth of syphilitic granulation tissue in the metaphyses ("metaphysitis"). There may even be fragmentation of the metaphyses accompanied by heavy periosteal bone formation, similar to that in scurvy (Fig. 7.**119**).

> We mention syphilis in this chapter because far too little is known today about syphilitic changes. As a result, we are unable to show examples of early changes that occupy the borderline range between normal and pathological.

Intraosseous ganglia (subchondral synovial cysts) are not uncommon in the proximal tibia (Figs. 7.**121**–7.**124**). Initially, lesions that are only a few millimeters in size and located just below the subchondral plate may go undetected on conventional radiographs. Nevertheless, even at this stage they can cause considerable pain due most likely to pressure variations in the cysts, which are filled with a viscous, gelatinous fluid.

Intraosseous ganglion requires differentiation from **chondroblastoma**, **giant cell tumor**, and from cancellous bone rarefaction due to severe disuse atrophy with **fatty replacement** (see also Fig. 7.**51**).

The medial aspect of the proximal tibial metaphysis is the second most common site of occurrence (after the distal femoral metaphysis) for **fibrous metaphyseal defects**, whether in the form of a fibrous cortical defect or a nonossifying fibroma (Fig. 7.**125**).

These findings are also normal variants, although they are included under the heading of tumorlike lesions in the WHO classification. They represent harmless growth disturbances that normally migrate toward the diaphysis with growth and are modeled away with normal tubulation of the bone. Fibrous metaphyseal defects that occur relatively late in skeletal growth may persist into adulthood, however (p. 890).

The **insertion of the pes anserinus** is located on the medial aspect of the proximal tibial metaphysis. Significant

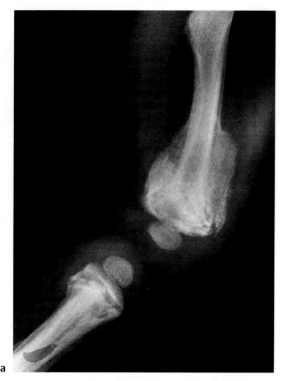

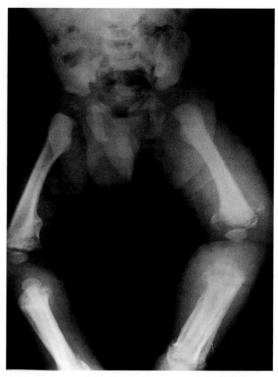

a

b

Fig. 7.**119 a, b**   Extensive periosteal bone formation about the distal femoral diaphysis and metaphysis and the tibial shaft in a 4-month-old child with congenital syphilis. Note the fragmentation of the metaphyses. The fact that the femoral metaphyses are affected more than the diaphyses is inconsistent with Caffey hyperostosis. The differential diagnosis would include severe scurvy with subperiosteal hemorrhages and secondary metaphyseal changes.

traction trauma at that site can incite a variety of resorptive bone changes, ranging in extreme cases to fibrous metaphyseal defects. Especially when bone strength has been compromised due to metabolic disease (e.g., hyperparathyroidism, osteomalacia), considerable resorption can take place at the insertion of the pes anserinus. In severe cases there may be complete destruction of the normal cortex, exposing the cancellous bone and giving the outer contour of the bone a serrated appearance. Focal fibrocartilaginous dysplasia is reviewed on p. 922 and in Fig. 7.**108**.

Fibrous metaphyseal defects can also occur in the proximal metaphysis of the fibula (Fig. 7.**126**).

Cartilaginous exostoses can significantly alter the shape of the proximal tibial metaphysis, producing changes that, at least superficially, resemble those of Blount disease (Fig. 7.**129**).

Malignant bone tumors such as **osteosarcoma** (Fig. 7.**128**) occur predominantly in the proximal tibial metaphysis and not in the epiphysis. The latter is a site of predilection for giant cell tumors and chondroblastoma. Figure 7.**127** shows a **primary malignant non–Hodgkin lymphoma** that is confined entirely to the epiphysis. This tumor was associated with marked reactive sclerosis and initially raised suspicion of nonfragmented osteonecrosis.

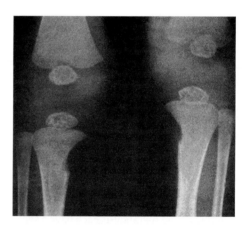

Fig. 7.**120**   Bilateral erosive lesions in the medial aspect of the tibial metaphyses in congenital syphilis (Wimberger sign).

Fig. 7.**121 a–e**   Subchondral synovial cyst (intraosseous ganglion). Radiograph shows an osteolytic area at the center of
the upper tibia (Lodwick grade IA lesion). The lesion has an attenuation of 20–30 Hounsfield units on the CT scans in **d** and
e, which is within the fluid range. Scans **b** and **c** demonstrate a
small nutrient canal (arrow) in the intercondylar eminence.
Formerly we regarded this feature as a kind of pore leading to
the ganglion. But we have become more experienced in interpreting proximal tibial structures on CT scans, and today we
know that it is a small nutrient canal seen in numerous examinations.

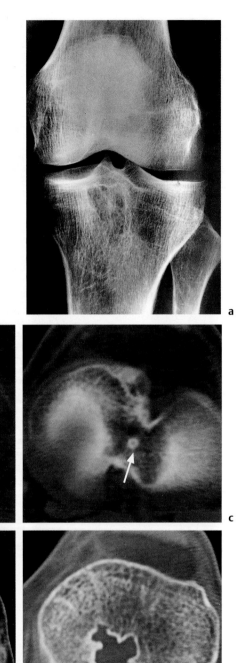

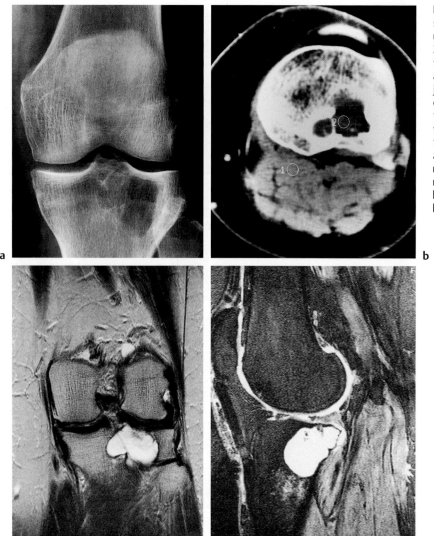

Fig. 7.**122 a–d** Large subchondral synovial cyst in the lateral part of the upper tibia. It has a CT attenuation of 23.5 Hounsfield units (**b**), which is within the fluid range. The absence of any degenerative changes in the knee joint excludes a subchondral degenerative cyst (geode). The attenuation values are also inconsistent with a chondroblastoma or giant cell tumor. The MR images in **c** and **d** are almost pathognomonic, showing homogeneous, fluid-equivalent high signal intensities in the lesion, which may have originated from the posterolateral part of the lateral meniscus.

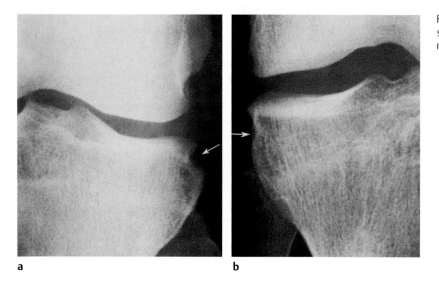

Fig. 7.**123 a, b** Typical proximal erosive lesions with a sclerotic base: meniscal cysts.

Fig. 7.**124** Large subchondral synovial cyst in the medial part ▷ of the upper tibia, possibly arising from a meniscal cyst with intraosseous extension. It is easy to picture this lesion as an advanced form of the lesions shown in Fig. 7.**123**, where there has been sufficient time for the lesion to form a new cortical boundary.

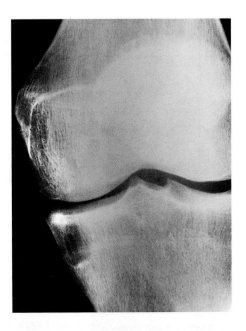

Fig. 7.**125 a–d**   Follow-up of a fibrous metaphyseal defect in the nonossifying fibroma stage. The defect is located in the left proximal tibial metaphysis of an asymptomatic boy 13 years old when first examined. In radiograph **c**, taken two years after **a** and **b**, the osteolytic lesion has enlarged somewhat but shows increasing bony consolidation processes at its periphery. A radiograph taken four years later (**d**) shows almost complete bony consolidation of the defect.

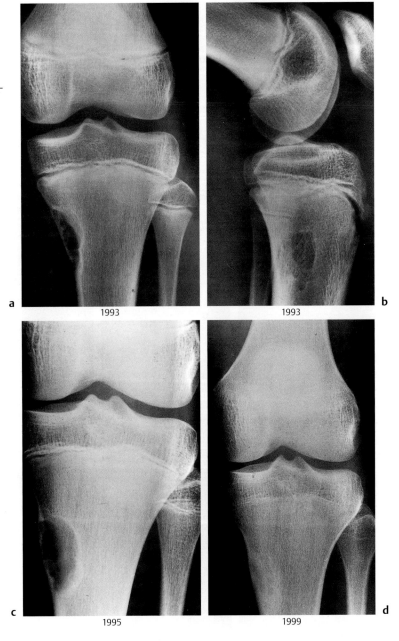

a   1993

b   1993

c   1995

d   1999

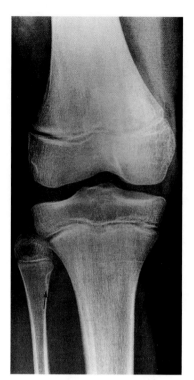

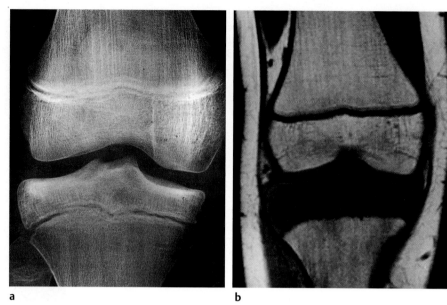

a   b

Fig. 7.**127 a, b**   "White" tibial epiphysis resulting from reactive new bone formation in a 13-year-old boy with a primary non-Hodgkin lymphoma confined to the epiphysis. Note the complete absence of fat signals on MRI (**b**). The lesion does not extend past the epiphyseal plate. Since we had to consider nonfragmented epiphyseal necrosis in our differential diagnosis, we performed a percutaneous biopsy under fluoroscopic guidance and confirmed the lesion as a lymphoma.

Fig. 7.**126**   Small fibrous metaphyseal defect in the fibrous cortical defect stage located in the medial aspect of the proximal fibular metaphysis.

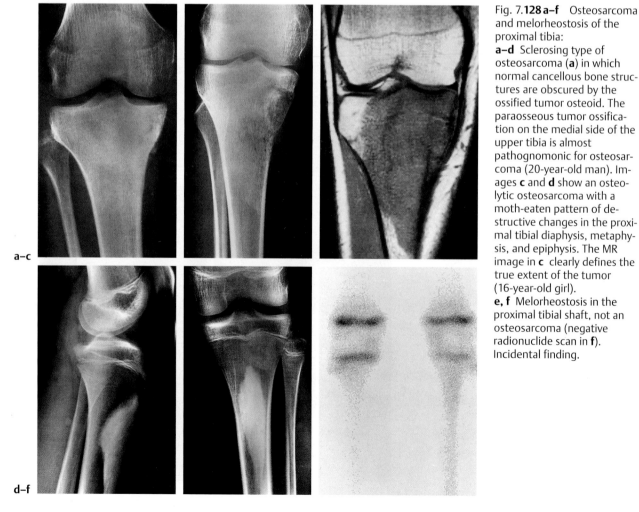

a–c

d–f

Fig. 7.**128 a–f**   Osteosarcoma and melorheostosis of the proximal tibia:
a–d Sclerosing type of osteosarcoma (**a**) in which normal cancellous bone structures are obscured by the ossified tumor osteoid. The paraosseous tumor ossification on the medial side of the upper tibia is almost pathognomonic for osteosarcoma (20-year-old man). Images **c** and **d** show an osteolytic osteosarcoma with a moth-eaten pattern of destructive changes in the proximal tibial diaphysis, metaphysis, and epiphysis. The MR image in **c** clearly defines the true extent of the tumor (16-year-old girl).
e, f Melorheostosis in the proximal tibial shaft, not an osteosarcoma (negative radionuclide scan in **f**). Incidental finding.

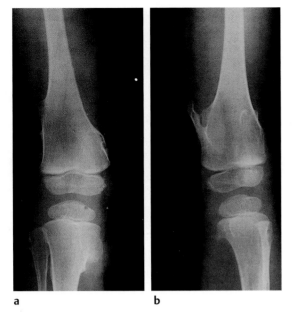

Fig. 7.**129** Cartilaginous exostosis disease with enlargement of the right tibial metaphysis. The impressive exostoses on the distal femoral metaphysis exclude Blount disease (Fig. 7.**107**).

 Other Changes?

Today it is rare to encounter very severe (necrosis-like) rachitic changes about the knee with widening and cupping of the metaphyseal and epiphyseal contours. The case in Fig. 7.**130** is mentioned only because of the valgus deformity that persisted after successful treatment, demonstrating that valgus as well as varus bowing can occur as a residual defect of rickets.

Metaplastic bone formation can occur at the **insertion** and **within the substance of the medial collateral ligament** in response to chronic traction or even a single traumatic event (Figs. 7.**131**, 7.**132**, 7.**134**).

Apparently these changes, which mimic a primary periosteal process, are particularly common in roller skaters, skiers, and soccer players who suffer frequent trauma to the knee.

The **tibiofibular joint** is a **synovial joint** and therefore vulnerable to rheumatic diseases. It is also subject to osteoarthritic changes with joint space narrowing, subchondral sclerosis, and marginal osteophytes. These findings may be detected incidentally in asymptomatic individuals. Posttraumatic capsular ossification should not be mistaken for persistent dual ossification centers of the fibular head (Fig. 7.**133**).

Bony erosions and radiolucencies on or in the fibular head accompanied by similar changes in the opposing tibia should always raise suspicion of villonodular synovitis or a ganglion arising from the joint.

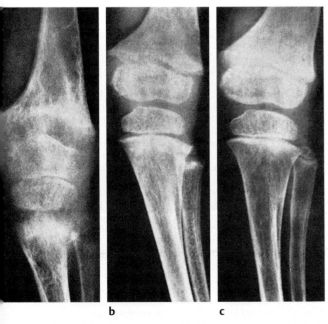

Fig. 7.**130 a–c** Follow-up of a highly acute case of rickets in the bones about the knee joint.
a The radiographic changes are those of a diffuse osteonecrosis, but the widened epiphyseal plates and cupped metaphyses suggest the correct diagnosis.
b After three months of vitamin D replacement.
c The bony structures are again normal after six months of replacement therapy, but there is still some valgus deformity of the knee.

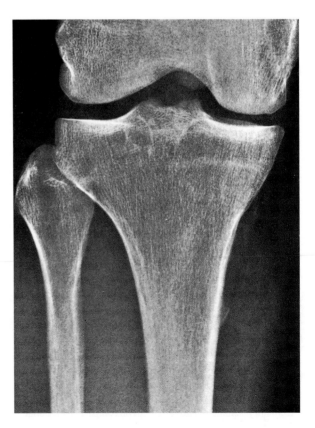

Fig. 7.**131** Small ossification at the insertion of the medial collateral ligament.

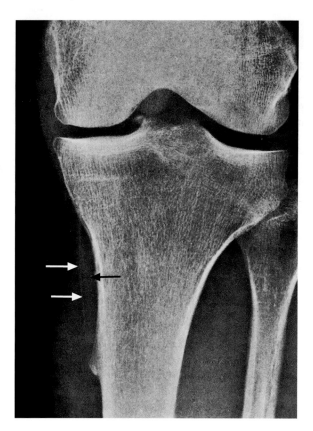

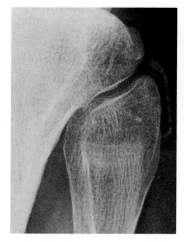

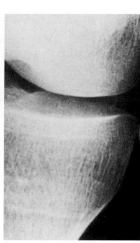

Fig. 7.**133**   Fig. 7.**134**

Fig. 7.**133** Capsular and ligament calcification about the tibiofibular joint.

Fig. 7.**134** Posttraumatic, rounded calcification on the medial side of the proximal tibia in the area of the medial collateral ligament.

◁ Fig. 7.**132** Calcifications in the medial collateral ligament with ossification at the insertion of the ligaments.

References

Baciu, C. C., A. Tudor, I. Olaru: Recurrent luxation of the superior tibio-fibular joint in the adult. Acta orthop. scand. 45 (1974) 772

Bell, S. N., P. E. Camphell, W. G. Cole et al.: Tibia vara caused by fibrocartilaginous dysplasia. J. Bone Jt Surg. 67-B (1985) 780

Blount, W. P.: Osteochondrosis deformans tibiae. J. Bone Jt Surg. 19-A (1937) 1

Bock, G. W., E. Bosch, K. Mishra et al.: The healed Segond fracture: a characteristic residual bone excrescence. Skelet. Radiol 23 (1994) 555

Cockshott, W. P., R. Martin, L. Friedman: Focal fibrocartilaginous dysplasia and tibia vara: a case report. Skelet. Radiol 23 (1994) 333

Currarino, G., D. R. Kirks: Lateral widening of epiphyseal plates in knees of children with bowed legs. Amer. J. Roentgenol. 129 (1977) 309

Eichenblat, M., H. Nathan: The proximal tibio fibular joint. Int. Orthop. (SICOT) 7 (1983) 31

Ghelman, B., J. C. Hodge: Imaging of the patellofemoral joint. Orthop. Clin. N. Amer. 23 (1992) 523

Harcke, H. Th., M. Synder, P. A. Caro et al.: Growth plate of the normal knee: evaluation with MR Imaging. Radiology 183 (1992) 119

Herman, Th. E., M. J. Siegel, W. H. McAlister: Focal fibrocartilaginous dysplasia associated with tibia vara. Radiology 177 (1990) 767

Heuck, F.: Persistierende Apophyse der Tuberositas tibiae, Fortschr. Röntgenstr. 79 (1953) 781

Hughston, J. C., J. R. Andrews, M. J. Cross et al.: Classification of knee ligament instabilities. Part II: The lateral compartment. J. Bone Jt Surg. 58-A (1976) 173

Jakob, R. P., P. Engelhardt: Does Osgood-Schlatter disease influence the position of the patella? J. Bone Jt Surg. 63-B (1981) 579

Janev, St., P. Solakov: Seltener Fall von aseptischer Nekrose im Capitulum beider Fibulae. Fortschr. Röntgenstr. 109 (1968) 675

Johnson, L.: Lateral capsular ligament complex: anatomical and surgical considerations. Amer. J. Sports Med. 7 (1979) 156

Jones, R. B., E. C. Bartlett, J. R. Vainright et al.: CT determination of tibial tubercle lateralization in patients presenting with anterior knee paint. Skelet. Radiol. 24 (1995) 505

Khanna, G., M. Sundaram, G. Y. El-Kloury et al.: Focal fibrocartilaginous dysplasia: curettage as an alternative to conservative management or more radical surgery. Skeletal Radiol. 30 (2001) 418

Koppers, B.: Dysplasia epiphysialis multiplex – szintigraphische, röntgenologische und klinische Korrelation. Fortschr. Röntgenstr. 137 (1982) 291

Kujala, U. M., M. Kvist, O. Heinonen: Osgood-Schlatter's disease in athletes. Amer. J. Sports Med. 13 (1985) 236

Moore, T. M.: Fracture dislocation of the knee. Clin. Orthop. 156 (1981) 129

Ogden, J. A.: Dislocation of the proximal fibula. Radiology 105 (1972) 547

Ogden, J. A.: Radiology of postnatal skeletal development (patella and tibial tuberosity). Skelet. Radiol. 11 (1984) 246

Ravelli, A.: Zum Röntgenbild des proximalen Schienbeindrittels. Fortschr. Röntgenstr. 82 (1955) 48

Resnick, D., J. D. Newell, J. Guerra jr. et al.: Proximal tibio-fibular joint. Anatomic-pathologic-radiographic correlation. Amer. J. Roentgenol. 131 (1978) 133

Rosenberg, Z. S., M. Kawelblum, Y. Y. Cheung et al.: Osgood-Schlatter lesion: fracture or tendinitis? Scintigraphic, CT, and MRT Imaging features. Radiology 185 (1992) 853

Turco, V. I., J. Spinella: Anterolateral dislocation of the head of the fibula in sports. Amer. J. Sports Med. 13 (1985) 209

Knee Joint as a Whole

The bony structures that comprise the knee joint were discussed in the previous chapters. Here we are concerned with soft-tissue structures such as the menisci, articular cartilage, ligaments, etc. that can be imaged with modern techniques (especially MRI), to the extent that these structures can deepen our understanding of the physiological and pathological processes that involve the adjacent bone. It is generally true that changes in osseous structures, such as a small bony avulsion, are merely the tip of an iceberg. The associated soft-tissue injuries that are not visible on conventional radiographs have the greatest clinical importance.

Normal Findings, Variants, Early Pathological Changes

Figure 7.**135** shows the normal anatomy of the knee joint and its principal soft-tissue structures. The radiographic joint space of the knee is approximately 3–5 mm wide.

Faber et al. (2001) measured **gender differences** in knee joint cartilage thickness, volume, and articular surface areas with quantitative three-dimensional MR imaging. Women displayed smaller cartilage volumes than men, the percentage differences ranging from 19.9% in the patella to 46.6% in the medial tibia. The gender differences of the cartilage thickness were smaller, ranging from 2% in the femoral trochlea to 13.3% in the medial tibia for the mean thickness, and from 4.3% in the medial femoral condyle to 18.3% in the medial tibia for the maximal cartilage thickness. The differences between the cartilage surface areas were similar to those of the volumes. Gender differences could be reduced for cartilage volume and surface area when normalized to body weight and body weight x body height. The authors conclude that differences in cartilage volume are primarily due to differences in joint surface areas (epiphyseal bone size), not to differences in cartilage thickness.

Normally the axes of the femur and tibia in the sagittal (AP) projection form a straight line with up to 4° of varus/valgus deviation in women and 5° in men (on standing radiographs).

The standard radiographic views of the knee joint are the AP and lateral projections. A special projection is the Frik tunnel view, which is obtained with the knee flexed 45° and a flexible curved cassette placed behind the popliteal fossa. This gives an excellent view of the intercondylar eminence and also provides information on bony articular surfaces that are not seen in the standard projections (e.g., in suspected cases of osteochondritis dissecans).

Boegård and Jonsson (1999) have published an up-to-date review of the various conventional radiographic techniques for investigating the knee (e.g., flexion weight-bearing radiographs to assess cartilage thickness).

A vacuum phenomenon in the medial or lateral joint space of the knee is essentially normal when seen on supine radiographs. This phenomenon appears as a linear lucency between the menisci and the adjacent articular cartilage of the tibia and femur (Fig. 7.**136**).

The diagram in Fig. 7.**137** shows the anatomy of the normal soft-tissue structures of the knee as they appear on conventional radiographs.

The intermuscular fat planes may be displaced by pathological processes of the knee joint, such as effusion, and they may be completely effaced by extensive inflammatory processes. Although traditional roentgen signs like those in Figs. 7.**138** and 7.**139** have lost most of their practical importance in the age of ultrasonography and MRI, the radiologist should still be familiar with them in the event that sectional images are unavailable.

Fabella

The fabella ("little bean") is a sesamoid bone in the lateral head of the gastrocnemius muscle. It is elliptical or circular in shape, 3.5–13.5 mm long, 2–9 mm wide, and 1.5–10 mm thick. It cannot be identified before 12–15 years of age. A fabella is present in approximately 13–16% of the population. It is generally bilateral (63–85%) and may be duplicated (Fig. 7.**140**). It may enlarge due to osteoproliferative changes (osteoarthritis, diffuse idiopathic skeletal hyperostosis, acromegaly, etc.) (Fig. 7.**141**). Occurrence in the medial head of the gastrocnemius is rare.

Menisci

The menisci can be identified as distinct structures in about the 8th week of fetal development. By about the 10th year of life, the menisci have acquired their definitive shape and histological structure. The surfaces of the menisci are concave superiorly and mostly flat inferiorly (Fig. 7.**142a, b**). The cross section of the menisci is typically triangular or wedge-shaped (Figs. 7.**135a, c**, 7.**142**). The medial meniscus has a crescent shape that is wider posteriorly than anteriorly (Fig. 7.**135c**). It is attached to the medial collateral ligament and peripherally to the joint capsule. Its posterior fibers are continuous with the coronary ligament, which anchors the meniscus to the posterior intercondylar area of the tibia between the insertions of the lateral meniscus and posterior cruciate ligament. The anterior horn of the medial meniscus is firmly attached to the intercondylar area. The transverse meniscal ligament passes through the anterior cruciate ligament, connecting the anterior horn of the medial meniscus to the anterior horn of the lateral meniscus.

The lateral meniscus has a semicircular shape. It covers a larger area of the tibial plateau than the medial meniscus. It is fixed anteriorly to the tibia in front of the intercondylar eminence and posterolateral to the anterior cruciate liga-

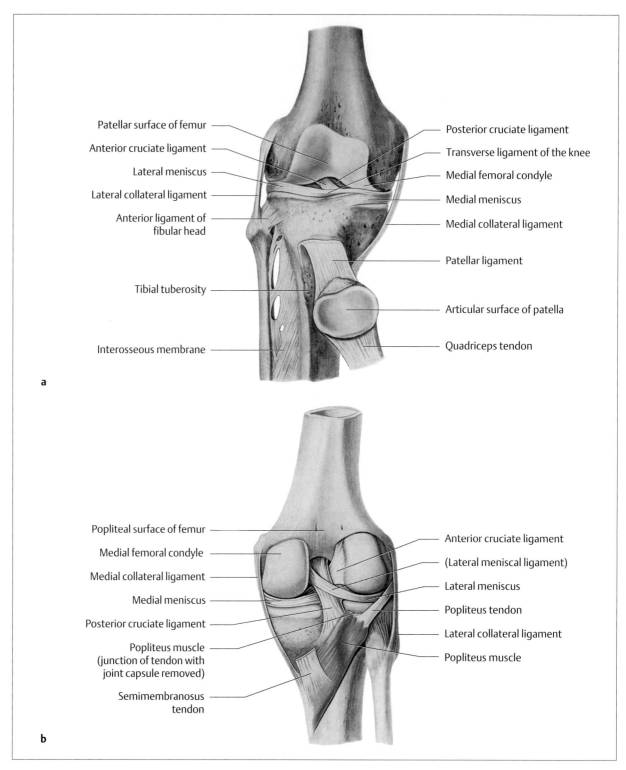

Patellar surface of femur

Anterior cruciate ligament

Lateral meniscus

Lateral collateral ligament

Anterior ligament of
fibular head

Tibial tuberosity

Interosseous membrane

Posterior cruciate ligament

Transverse ligament of the knee

Medial femoral condyle

Medial meniscus

Medial collateral ligament

Patellar ligament

Articular surface of patella

Quadriceps tendon

a

Popliteal surface of femur

Medial femoral condyle

Medial collateral ligament

Medial meniscus

Posterior cruciate ligament

Popliteus muscle
(junction of tendon with
joint capsule removed)

Semimembranosus
tendon

Anterior cruciate ligament

(Lateral meniscal ligament)

Lateral meniscus

Popliteus tendon

Lateral collateral ligament

Popliteus muscle

b

Fig. 7.**135 a–c**   Anatomy of the knee joint (after Wolf-Heidegger).

a Anterior aspect.
b Posterior aspect.

ment, partially blending with its fibers. On the lateral aspect of the medial femoral condyle, the posterior horn of the lateral meniscus is adherent to the meniscofemoral ligaments (lateral meniscal ligaments), which run in front of (Humphrey type) and behind (Wrisberg type) the posterior cruciate ligament (Fig. 7.**135 b, c**; Cho et al. 1999). Also, as Fig. 7.**135** shows, the attachment of the lateral meniscus to the lateral collateral ligament is interrupted posteriorly by the popliteus tendon. The lateral meniscus is more mo-

bile than the medial meniscus because it is not fixed posteriorly to the joint capsule, it is suspended by the meniscal ligaments, and its capsular attachment is interrupted by the popliteus tendon.

The size of the menisci keeps pace with that of the tibial plateau during growth and also in adulthood.

- The medial meniscus covers approximately 65% of the articular surface of the medial tibial plateau. The height of the medial meniscus is approximately 10.6 ± 0.9 mm

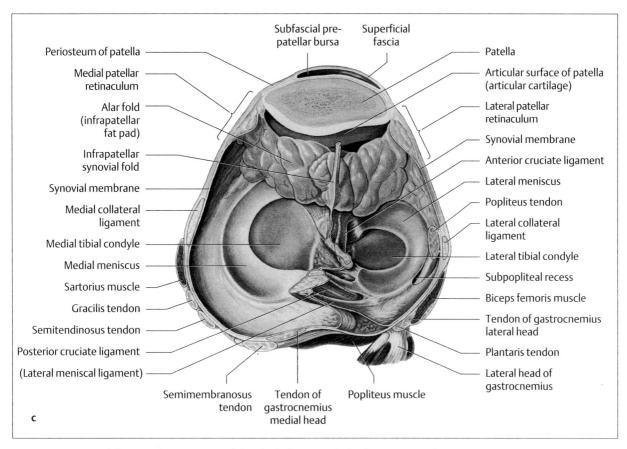

Fig. 7.**135 c**   View of the articular structures of the tibial plateau with the femur removed.

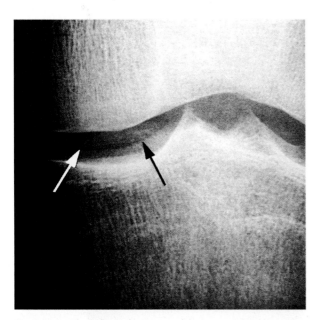

Fig. 7.**136**   Physiological vacuum phenomenon.

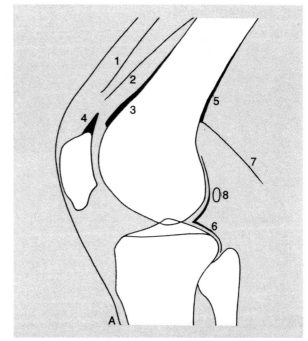

Fig. 7.**137**   Normal soft-tissue structures (after Dihlmann).
1   Fat planes at the rectus femoris muscle
2   Vastus intermedius muscle
3–5 Suprapatellar (4), anterior (3) and posterior (5) femoral metaphyseal fat pad (larger in children than in adults)
6   Physiological fat planes, shaped like the number 3; often invisible unless the joint is distended
7   Border of the gastrocnemius muscle
8   Fabella

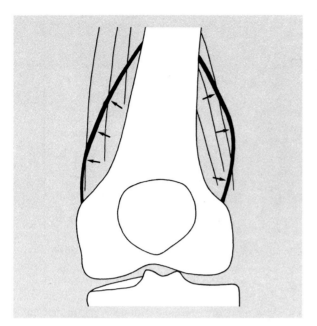

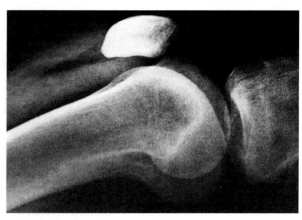

Fig. 7.**139**   Lateral cross-table projection of the extended knee shows a depressed fracture of the lateral tibial plateau. Holmgren sign: fluid level in the suprapatellar pouch (extruded bone marrow fat floating on blood).

Fig. 7.**138**   Suprapatellar bursa, distended by effusion, with a medial and/or lateral convex line (fat plane, arrows) that is superimposed upon, but does not obscure, the lines of the vastus musculature.

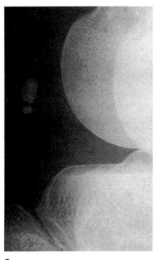

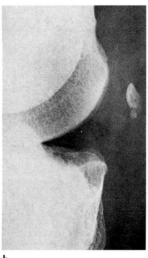

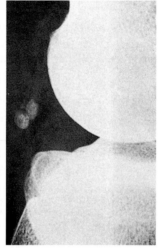

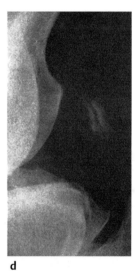

a   b   c   d

Fig. 7.**140 a–d**   Multipartite fabellae.

at the posterior horn, 9.6 ± 0.5 mm in the middle third, and 7.7 ± 1.4 mm at the anterior horn.

- The lateral meniscus covers approximately 85 % of the lateral tibial plateau. The height of the lateral meniscus is almost uniform: 10.2 ± 0.4 mm anteriorly, 11.6 ± 1.4 mm at the center, 10.6 ± 0.9 mm posteriorly.

> The menisci are subject to progressive degenerative changes, regardless of the gender and activity level of the individual.

This degeneration starts in the middle perforating bundle and tends to be symmetrical. Degenerative meniscal changes can be detected *microscopically* in most persons over 40 years of age. On MRI, the degenerative changes appear as hyperintense areas within the meniscus that do not reach the meniscal surface.

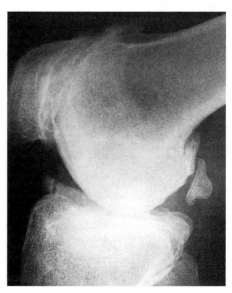

Fig. 7.**141**   Fabella, showing osteoarthritic enlargement.

Fig. 7.**142 a–g**   MR images of the menisci. Note in **b** and **f** the fine intrameniscal foci of increased signal intensity, which represent physiological degenerative changes. The posterior cruciate ligament (asterisks) and anterior cruciate ligament are clearly visualized in **d** and **e** (see text). The diagram in **g** shows the various grades of degenerative meniscal changes (I, II) and meniscal tears (III a and b) in the Stoller classification.

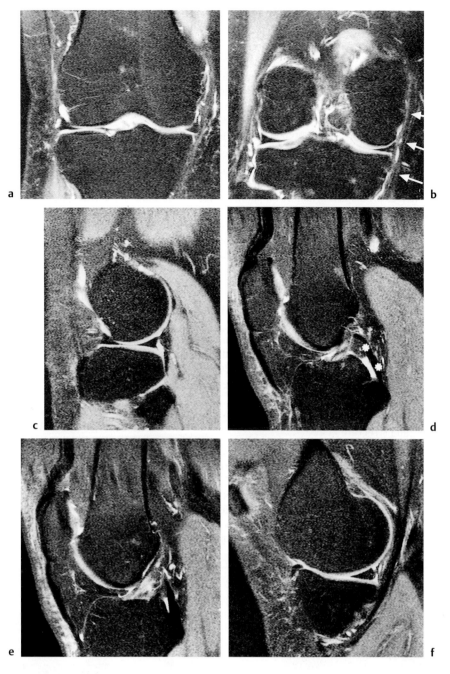

Classification of meniscal degeneration (Fig. 7.**142 g**)
➤ *Type I:* Rounded hyperintensity within the meniscus
➤ *Type II:* Linear hyperintensity within the meniscus
➤ *Type III:* Hyperintensity that reaches the meniscal surface (= meniscal tear)

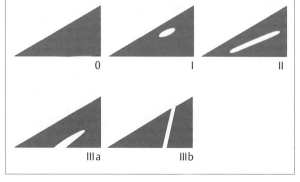

The further subclassification of degenerative meniscal changes (by shape, intensity, and extent) and theories explaining the increased signal intensity in the degenerative area are beyond our scope. As for the interpretation of these MRI changes, however, it is important to note that increased signal intensities can be found in the menisci of at least 25% of all persons 10 to 20 years of age, and that this percentage increases markedly with age. Some 60% of all persons over 60 years of age have a meniscal tear, and nearly one-third of all menisci in this age range contain tears. These "normal" degenerative changes and tears occur predominantly in the posterior horn of the medial meniscus (Fig. 7.**142f**).

Shankman et al. (1997) point out that speckled increased signal intensity (on sagittal proton-density-weighted images) in the anterior horn of the lateral meniscus near its central attachment is practically a normal finding. These data emphasize that one should be cautious in interpreting intrameniscal signal intensity changes on MRI.

At the same time, these same degenerative changes are cited as predisposing factors for spontaneous or traumatic meniscal tears.

The various signal intensity changes in the menisci, including those that extend to the surface, often cannot be detected at arthroscopy, suggesting that the **overinterpretation of MR images** is quite possible. Displaced partial avulsions of the menisci can also lead to misinterpretations, as shown in Fig. 7.**143**.

A true meniscal variant is the **discoid meniscus** (Fig. 7.**144**). This refers to an abnormally enlarged lateral meniscus that has a discoid or semilunar shape. It is found in approximately 1.5 % (4.5 %, Rohren et al. 2001) or more of all knees. Two types may be encountered:

- A complete discoid meniscus that covers the entire tibial plateau
- An incomplete discoid meniscus of variable size, shape, and structure

The **Wrisberg type** of discoid meniscus lacks a posterior capsular attachment. A large percentage of discoid menisci are detected incidentally and are therefore asymptomatic. Reportedly, the type that lacks a posterior attachment is associated with short, thick meniscofemoral ligaments that limit the mobility of the meniscus and thus make it more susceptible to tears. The short, thick meniscal ligaments are also considered responsible for the snapping sound that is occasionally heard.

In some patients with a discoid meniscus, the lateral joint space is widened, the medial femoral condyle may be flattened, and there is cupping of the lateral tibial plateau.

The discoid meniscus is best demonstrated with coronal images on MRI (Fig. 7.**144b**). They show the abnormal meniscus extending into or close to the intercondylar notch. Very posterior coronal images can mimic this finding despite a normal meniscus due to the close proximity of the free posterior end of the meniscus to the meniscofemoral ligaments. On sagittal images, the discoid meniscus appears as a continuous tissue structure in the lateral compartment of the knee, so that it does not exhibit an anterior and posterior horn (Fig. 7.**144c**). In a large MRI study Rohren et al. (2001) found that—compared with the normal semilunar meniscus the discoid lateral meniscus has a higher frequency of meniscal tears (54 % versus 75 %), and solitary tears of the lateral meniscus are more common in the discoid variant (11 % versus 20 %). It appears that discoid menisci predispose to the formation of **meniscal cysts** (meniscal ganglia). In any case, these cysts can be found in up to 20 % of all menisci (Fig. 7.**144d**). They may be associated with pain and swelling, especially when located in the lateral meniscus, but these symptoms are not always present. Many patients give a history of trauma. Erosion of the tibial margin by meniscal cysts (Fig. 7.**144d**) is shown in Fig. 7.**123**.

The **meniscal ossicle** (Yu and Resnick 1994, Tuite et al. 1995) is defined as a solid, intrameniscal bony element that is composed of cortical and cancellous bone with central marrow. Some individuals with a meniscal ossicle are asymptomatic, and some have knee pain. The pain is caused by the space-occupying character of the ossicle and

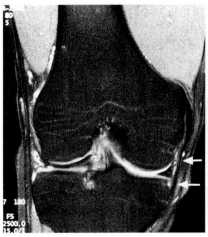 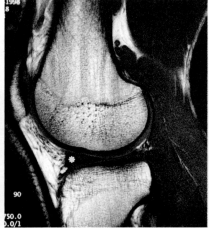 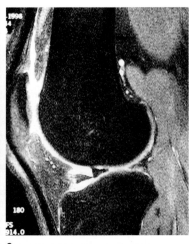

a b c

Fig. 7.**143a–c** Unusual anterior displacement of the avulsed central zone of a lateral meniscus.
a The lateral meniscus appears to be absent in this mid-coronal T2-weighted image.

b, c In the sagittal images, the fragment (asterisk) has been displaced in front of the anterior part of the meniscus. In **b**, the space between the two parts of the meniscus creates the appearance of a meniscal tear. The arrows in **a** point to the normal medial collateral ligament. The fine hyperintense zone below the ligament is fatty tissue.

Fig. 7.**144 a–d**   Discoid meniscus.
a Air arthrography.
b, c MRI.
d Note the small meniscal cyst hanging like a drop over the lateral articular margin of the tibia. There is trauma to the medial collateral ligament.

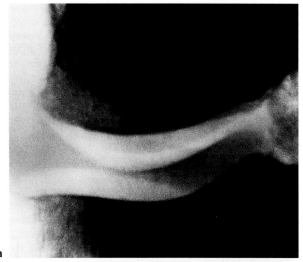

a

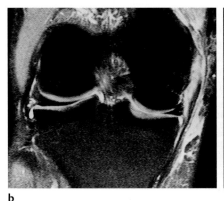

b

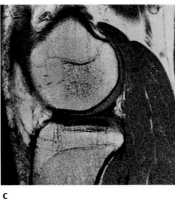

c

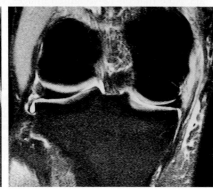

d

perhaps by associated meniscal tears. Meniscal ossicles are most commonly found in the posterior horn of the medial meniscus. Most patients are males between 16 and 40 years of age. Differentiation is mainly required from an osteochondral fragment in osteochondritis dissecans and from a small bony avulsion. The current diagnostic method of choice is MRI, which provides accurate localization of the bony element (Fig. 7.**145**).

Ligaments

The cruciate and collateral ligaments establish the essential ligamentous connections of the knee joint (Fig. 7.**142**). The ligaments are composed of fibrocartilaginous tissue and therefore have low signal intensity in all sequences. Ligamentous injuries are manifested by increased signal intensity within the ligaments, by abnormal morphology, or by the complete absence of a ligament.

The anterior cruciate ligament is particularly susceptible to tears due to knee trauma, especially during sports activities. A torn anterior cruciate ligament is found in more than two-thirds of all surgically treated knee injuries. For the most part, tears of this ligament are associated with tears in the medial meniscus.

The **normal anterior cruciate ligament** arises from the medial aspect of the lateral femoral condyle and runs obliquely forward and medially to insert on the anterior tibia. On MRI, it is most clearly defined by T2-weighted images through the intercondylar notch. It appears as a continu-

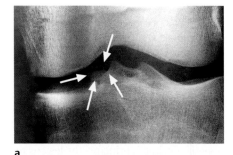

a

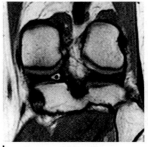

b

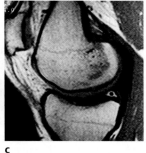

c

Fig. 7.**145 a–c**   Meniscal ossicle.
a The small bony element is marked with arrows.
b, c The MR images (T1-weighted) prove that the fat-marrow-containing element (asterisk) is completely surrounded by meniscal tissue and is therefore located in the medial meniscus.

ous band of low signal intensity, sometimes consisting of two separate fiber bundles (Figs. 7.**142 d, e**, 7.**98 c, f**). Rotating the knee about 10–20° externally provides a very favorable imaging position. The MRI appearance of anterior cruciate ligament tears depends on the age and extent of the lesion. A complete acute tear appears as a discontinuity in the ligament. The gap usually contains fluid. Typically the tears are located in the midsubstance of the ligament near its femoral insertion. A tear in the ligament appears as an irregular soft-tissue feature of moderate signal intensity on T1-weighted images, surrounded by high signal intensity on T2-weighted images due to hemorrhage and edema. With old lesions, imaging may show only small remnants of the original ligament, or the ligament may not be visualized. The origin of the anterior cruciate ligament on the lateral femoral condyle may show intermediate signal intensities on T1-weighted images due to partial volume effects. They should not be mistaken for tears. Note that on T2-weighted images, these effects do not produce the high signal intensity seen with real tears.

Mucoid degeneration of the anterior cruciate ligament should not be mistaken for ligamentous tears (McIntyre et al. 2001).

The **posterior cruciate ligament** arises from the lateral surface of the medial femoral condyle and runs obliquely backward and downward to insert on the medial tibial plateau. It is shorter, thicker, and broader than the anterior cruciate ligament and shows homogeneous low signal intensity in all sequences (Fig. 7.**142 d, e**). It is considerably easier to define and identify than the anterior cruciate ligament. When the knee is extended, the course of the posterior cruciate ligament is convex posteriorly. The ligament normally straightens when the knee is flexed, and this can be used as a test for its integrity.

> Anterior angulation or buckling of the posterior cruciate ligament is always an abnormal sign.

Tears of the posterior cruciate ligament require considerable violence and cause significant instability of the knee. A rupture of the posterior cruciate ligament is generally associated with other serious intra-articular injuries, such as partial detachment of the posterior horn of the medial meniscus, tears of the medial and lateral collateral ligaments, disruption of the posterior medial and lateral capsular ligament, and bony avulsion of its insertion. The morphology of posterior cruciate tears need not be discussed here, but in principle the lesions resemble those of the anterior cruciate ligament.

The **medial** and **lateral collateral ligaments** stabilize the knee joint. The medial ligament consists of a superficial and deep part. The superficial part is the medial collateral ligament proper (Fig. 7.**135 a**). It arises from the medial femoral condyle and inserts on the tibia about 5 cm below its articular margin. The deep part, also called the medial capsular ligament, inserts on the medial meniscus, thus giving it attachment to the femur via the meniscofemoral ligament and to the tibia via the meniscotibial ligament. A severe valgus sprain initially ruptures the deep ligament and then involves the superficial layer (Fig. 7.**98 c–e**). These injuries may be associated with tears of the anterior cruciate ligament and medial meniscus. Lesions of the collateral ligaments are most easily diagnosed on T2-weighted images by noting the hemorrhage and edema that surround the injury.

The normal medial collateral ligament appears as a dark band on coronal MR images (Figs. 7.**142 a, b**, 7.**143 a**). Between the superficial and deep parts is a small bursa surrounded by fatty tissue that is hyperintense on T1-weighted images. This normal finding should not be mistaken for meniscocapsular separation. A tear of the medial collateral ligament appears as an interruption of the normal low signal intensity of the ligament on T1-weighted images. Additionally, the surrounding fat shows high T2-weighted signal intensity due to hemorrhage and edema as mentioned above.

The **lateral collateral ligament** consists of three layers: a capsular layer that is partly adherent to the lateral meniscus and two extracapsular layers composed of a posterior fibular ligament and an anterior iliotibial ligament.

Synovial Plicae

The soft-tissue structures of the knee joint include the **synovial plicae** (Fig. 7.**135 c**), remnants of synovial tissue that divided the joint into three compartments during early development. The three plicae that are most commonly seen are the suprapatellar, medial patellar, and infrapatellar plicae. Rarely, a plica may form a more or less complete septum that can cause transient synovial stasis leading to extremely painful swelling of the joint. This is particularly known to occur with a "transverse suprapatellar plica." Finally, the medial patellar plica may thicken causing a chronic impingement syndrome with erosive changes in the femoropatellar cartilage.

Joint Capsule

The **synovial joint capsule** has two pouches or recesses, one anterior and one posterior:

- The anterior (and superior) recess is actually a bursa (suprapatellar bursa).
- The posterior recess is also formed by a bursa that is located below the popliteus tendon and always communicates with the joint cavity. The volume of this recess is highly variable, as we know from traditional contrast arthrography of the knee.

Pathological Findings

Baker Cyst

A Baker cyst may develop from a posterior synovial protrusion (herniation) through the fibrous membrane of the knee joint due to an inflammatory synovial process. It may also result from the distension of communicating or non-communicating bursae, especially the gastrocnemius-semimembranosus bursa (Fig. 7.**146**). Capsular anomalies have also been discussed as a possible cause fo Baker cysts in children. In rheumatoid arthritis and other chronic forms of knee synovitis, a valve mechanism may be created between the knee cavity and the communicating gastrocnemius-semimembranosus bursa. Synovial fluid enters the bursa from the joint cavity and becomes trapped in the medial popliteal area, gradually producing a Baker

cyst. These cysts may suddenly perforate with fluid extravasation into the muscles of the lower leg, mimicking the symptoms of an acute lower extremity deep venous thrombosis.

Masses in the Knee Joint

The simplest mass in the knee joint is a **traumatic** or **inflammatory effusion**, which was discussed previously (Figs. 7.**137**–7.**139**).

Otherwise the differential diagnostic spectrum of masses about the knee joint ranges from tumorlike lesions such as synovial chondromatosis (Fig. 7.**147**), synovial angiomatosis (Fig. 7.**148**), and villonodular synovitis (Fig. 7.**149**) to true tumors such as hemangioma, lipoma, chondroma, osteoma, synovial sarcoma (Fig. 7.**150**), and chondrosarcoma.

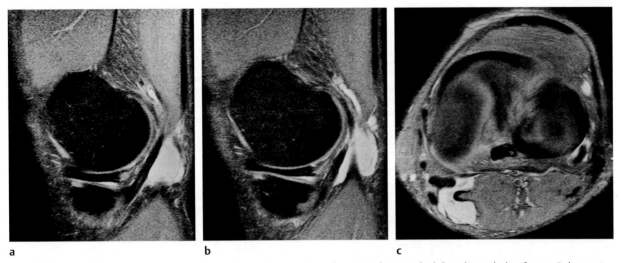

a   b   c

Fig. 7.**146 a–c**   MRI appearance of a large gastrocnemius–semimembranosus bursa, which has distended to form a Baker cyst.

Fig. 7.**147 a, b**   Synovial chondromatosis (compare with Fig. 7.**40 f, g**).

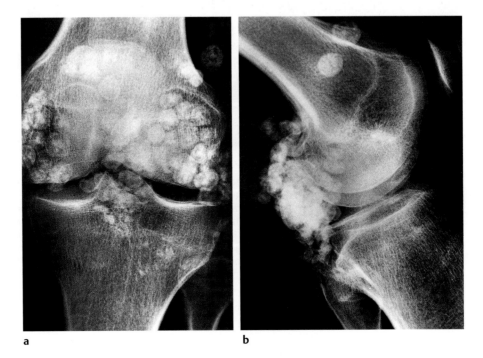

a   b

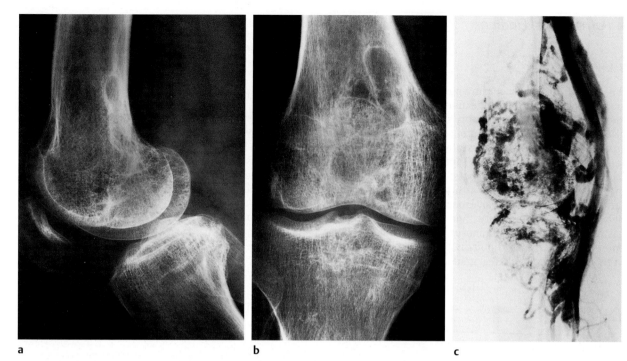

a   b   c

Fig. 7.**148 a–c** Synovial angiomatosis or posttraumatic synovial hemangioma in the right knee joint of a 23-year-old man with a history of knee surgery for a "bloody joint effusion." The surgery was followed by increasing, pulsatile, hyperthermal swelling of the knee joint with recurrent episodes of bloody effusion. Radiographs show considerable erosions in the distal femur and tibia involving the whole circumference of the bones. A subtraction angiogram (**c**) defines the extent of the angiomatous changes. It is reasonable to assume that this is a trauma-induced lesion rather than a true tumor. A detailed description of this case can be found in Freyschmidt (1997).

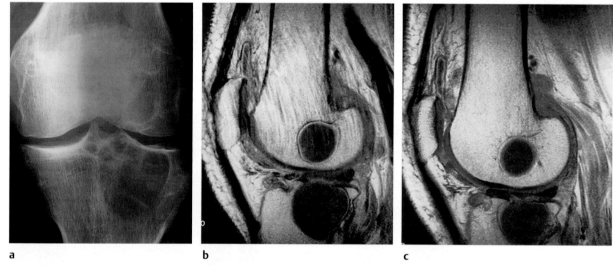

a   b   c

Fig. 7.**149 a–g** Villonodular synovitis of the knee joint.
a–c Man 60 years of age was evaluated for recurrent bloody effusions in the knee. The conventional radiograph is classic, showing deep erosions and lucencies in both the femur and tibia. Smaller erosive changes are seen en face in the medial femoral condyle. Moderate joint space narrowing is apparently caused by cartilage damage from the chronic bloody effusion. The MR images in **b** and **c** (postgadolinium, T1-weighted) show marked synovial thickening in all portions of the joint. The connection between the large intraosseous lesion in the upper tibia and the knee joint is particularly well visualized in **c**. Hemosiderin deposits account for the relatively weak enhancement of the thickened synovial membrane. The intraosseous cavities mostly contain necrotic, liquefied material from the proliferating tumorlike tissue.

Fig. 7.**149 d–g** ▷

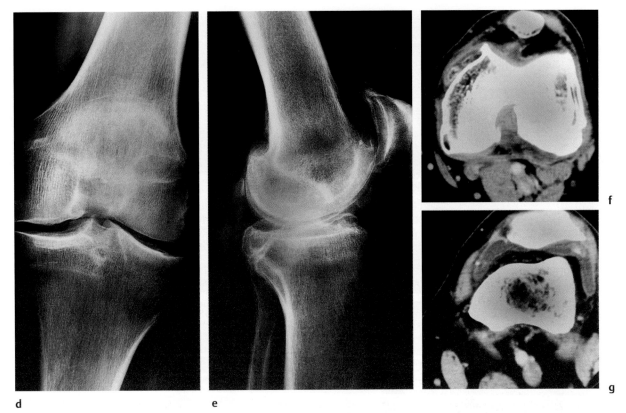

d   e   f   g

Fig. 7.**149 d–g**   Man 52 years of age was evaluated for recurrent bloody knee effusions (**d, g**). This case shows predominantly osteoarthritic changes of villonodular synovitis with subluxation of the patella. The faint subchondral densities and absence of subchondral geodes are not entirely typical of classic (primary) osteoarthritis. The osteoarthritic features are explained by the chronic hemosiderotic cartilage damage caused by the recurrent bloody effusions. In the CT scans in **f** and **g** (after intravenous contrast administration), note the markedly thickened and heavily vascularized synovial membrane, corresponding to the proliferating tumorlike tissue.

CT and MRI are highly effective in discriminating among the different entities and preparing for biopsy and operative procedures.

Melorheostosis is a typical bone disease that may be associated with extensive, tumor-simulating ossifications about the knee joint (Fig. 7.**151**).

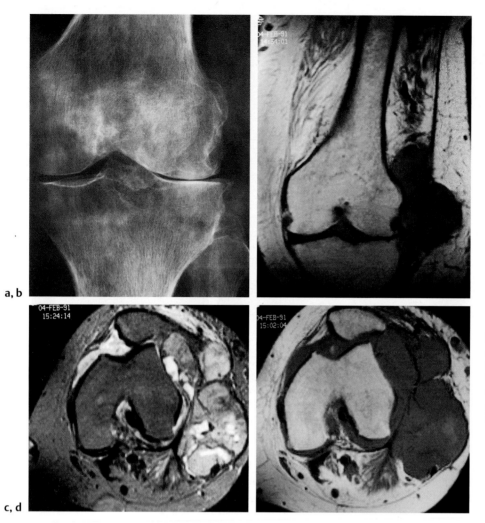

a, b

c, d

Fig. 7.**150 a–d**   Synovial sarcoma in the knee joint of a 64-year-old woman with a 3-month history of pain.
a Conventional radiograph shows relatively coarse, patchy demineralization and erosive changes, particularly in the lateral portions of the distal femur and proximal tibia.
b–d The MR images clearly define the extent of the tumor, which has spread outside the joint, showing conspicuous lateral and superior extension. Intense enhancement occurs after contrast administration (**c**). Comparing the conventional radiograph and MR images, we note that the massive, patchy, dystrophic demineralization in the radiograph, combined with the erosive changes in the bony contours, are unmistakable signs of a proliferative synovial process. The extent of the soft-tissue synovial tumor (synovial sarcoma), however, is accurately appreciated only on MRI (or CT).

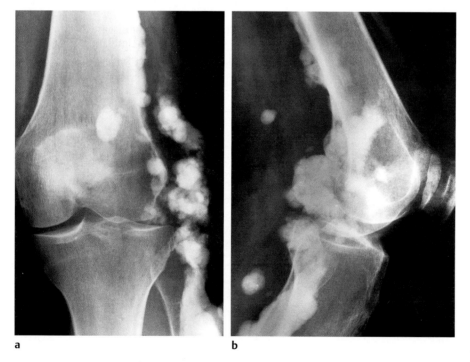

a   b

Fig. 7.**151 a, b**   Extensive melorheostotic changes with ossifications inside and outside the bone. Clinical signs consisted of knee swelling and limited motion. The patient had undergone several operations for a suspected paraosseous osteosarcoma. The biplane radiographs clearly show that the ossifications are located not just outside the distal femur but also within it and especially in the fibula. This lesion distribution is very specific for melorheostosis. The extent of the lesions can be assigned to sclerotomes L5 and S1. Since we have given more attention to this disease in recent years, we have found more or less extensive periarticular and intra-articular soft-tissue ossifications in 5 of 23 patients, occasionally associated with focal atrophic cutaneous changes (morphea) (Freyschmidt 2001).

Trauma to the Knee Joint

A detailed discussion of complex internal knee injuries, whether degenerative or posttraumatic, is outside the scope of this book and is reserved for specialized references. Injuries of the bones that comprise the knee joint (femur, tibia, patella) and their differentiation from normal variants are discussed under the appropriate headings. The information that can be gained by the use of MRI in knee injuries is illustrated in Fig. 7.**98 b–f**.

Soft–Tissue Calcifications

Calcification of the Menisci

An important article on the mechanism of knee trauma and the correlative imaging patterns is Sanders et al. (2000).

Calcification of the menisci is a relatively common incidental finding, especially in older patients. They probably represent purely regressive, dystrophic calcifications in degenerative menisci.

The frequency of meniscal calcifications increases with the extent of other degenerative changes in the knee joint. It is also known that surgery on a meniscus makes it more susceptible to calcification.

The pattern of meniscal calcifications is coarse and plaquelike (fibrocartilage!). Unlike calcifications of the hyaline articular cartilage, meniscal calcifications never extend past the articular margins ("positive meniscogram" sign, Fig. 7.**152**).

Chondrocalcinosis

Regressive meniscal calcifications should be distinguished from calcifications of the hyaline articular cartilage, which are always pathological and are referred to as chondrocalcinosis (pseudogout, Fig. 7.**153**).

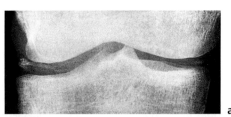
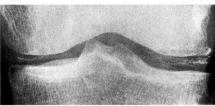

Fig. 7.**152 a, b** Meniscal calcifications in both knee joints, showing a typical flocculent and plaquelike appearance ("positive meniscogram"). There is also some calcification of the hyaline cartilage of the femur and tibia. Note that the meniscal calcifications do not extend past the joint margins as in Fig. 7.**153**.

The hyaline articular cartilage shows a predominantly mixed punctate and coarse pattern of calcification. The calcifications follow the bony articular contours and extend past them.

Chondrocalcinosis can have a variety of causes:

- Primary idiopathic form (pseudogout in the strict sense, CPPD [calcium pyrophosphate deposition disease])
- Symptomatic forms (e.g., in primary and secondary hyperparathyroidism, in hypophosphatasia, hypervitaminosis D, hemochromatosis, ochronosis, etc.)

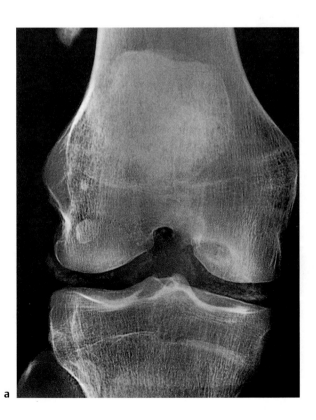
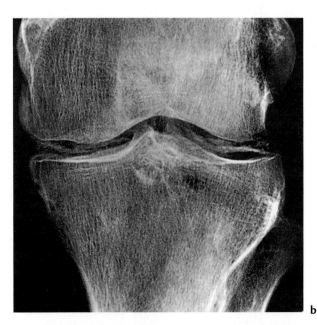

Fig. 7.**153 a, b** Chondrocalcinosis with calcifications predominantly in the hyaline cartilage, mainly affecting the femur in **a** and both the femur and tibia in **b**. The menisci show very little calcification. The calcifications are stippled and flocculent and extend past the joint contours.

The knee joint is considered a radiological test region for primary chondrocalcinosis.

Calcifications in the Bursae of the Knee Joint and Infrapatellar Fat Pad

These calcifications usually have a very dense, coarse appearance. A familiar example of these regressive calcifications in the pre- and infrapatellar bursae is **housemaid's knee** (Fig. 7.**154**).

In principle, all the ligamentous structures of the knee joint can calcify or ossify. Ossification of the oblique popliteal ligament that reinforces the posterior joint capsule is a typical finding (Fig. 7.**155**).

 ## Other Changes?

Traditionally, **marginal osteophytes on the patella, femur, and tibia** with normal joint-space widths have been considered early signs of femoropatellar and femorotibial osteoarthritis (osteoarthritis of the knee). One should be cautious in interpreting these bony excrescences, however (Fig. 7.**156**), as they are found in many asymptomatic individuals over 30 years of age.

They may simply be an expression of **increased traction phenomena**. Osteophytes can also develop in the setting of diffuse idiopathic skeletal hyperostosis (DISH syndrome), in acromegaly, and in other disorders.

 We believe that osteoarthritis should be diagnosed on conventional radiographs only if other signs such as joint space narrowing, subchondral densities, degenerative subchondral cysts, etc. are also present.

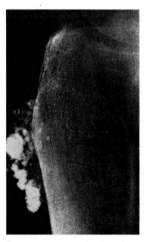

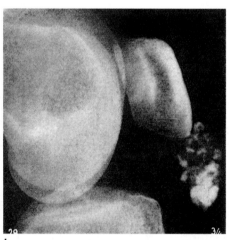

a   b

Fig. 7.**154** Housemaid's knee.

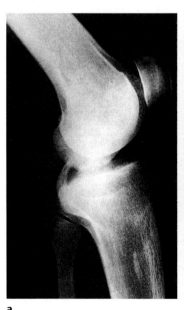

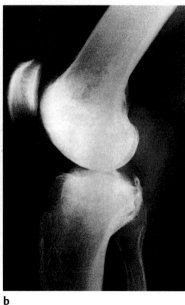

a   b

Fig. 7.**155 a, b** Bilateral calcification of the oblique popliteal ligament.

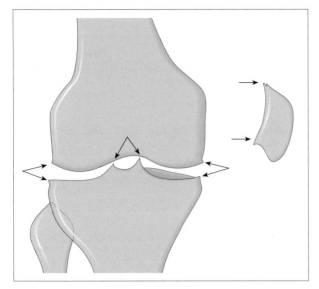

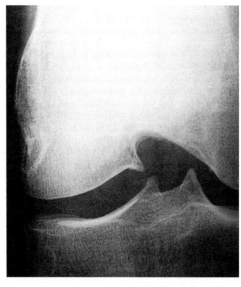

Fig. 7.**156** Typical sites of occurrence of marginal osteophytes in the knee joint. When combined with joint space narrowing, subchondral densities, and more or less pronounced subchondral degenerative cysts, these osteophytes may be taken as a sign of osteoarthritis. But in this case they are always intra-articular and consist of reparative fibrocartilaginous structures that form at the periphery of the degenerative cartilage. If the width of the joint space is normal, the bony excrescences should be interpreted as traction phenomena at the attachments of the capsule and ligaments (after Dihlmann).

Fig. 7.**157**   Knee joint with an old cruciate ligament lesion. There is only slight peaking of the intercondylar tubercles, but a very prominent osteophyte has formed at the lateral articular boundary of the medial femoral condyle with the intercondylar notch.

Fig. 7.**158**   Typical sites where erosions occur in inflammatory knee disease (e.g., rheumatoid arthritis). The arrows mark the most common sites of occurrence; the double arrows indicate circumscribed zones of decalcification and cortical changes (after Dihlmann).

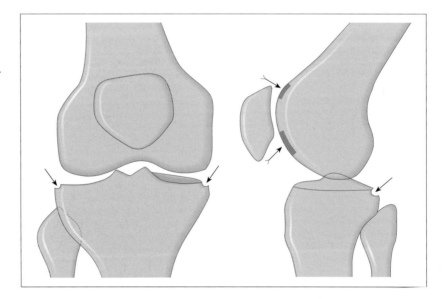

The difference between traction osteophytes and regressive osteophytes was discussed on p. 234. Actually, osteoarthritis should be diagnosed only if cartilage ulcerations are detected, and only MRI can reliably detect these changes at an early stage. Figure 7.**157** shows an example of a traction osteophyte that developed in response to an old ligamentous injury.

Arthritic changes in the knee joint will not be discussed here in greater detail. It is important to note the **typical sites of occurrence of early bone erosions**, however (Fig. 7.**158**), since patients with rheumatoid arthritis, for example, will not always present in the highly acute stage with clinical evidence of effusion.

References

Boegård, T., K. Jonsson: Radiography in osteoarthritis of the knee. Skelet. Radiol. 28 (1999) 605

Buckley, S. L., R. L. Barrack, A. H. Alexander: The natural history of conservatively treated partial anterior cruciate ligament tears. Amer. J. Sports Med. 17 (1989) 221

Carlson, D. H., J. O'Connor: Congenital dislocation of the knee. Amer. J. Roentgenol. 127 (1976) 465

Cho, J. M., J. J. S. Suh, J. B. Na et al.: Variations in menisco-femoral ligaments at anatomical study and MR imaging. Skelet. Radiol 28 (1999) 189

Faber, S. C., F. Eckstein, S. Lukasz et al.: Gender differences in knee joint cartilage thickness, volume and articular surface areas: assessment with quantitative three-dimensional MR imaging. Skeletal Radiol. 30 (2001) 144

Freyer, B: Beobachtung einer Fabella im medialen Gastroknemiuskopf. Fortschr. Röntgenstr. 92 (1960) 469

Freyschmidt, J.: Melorheostosis: a review of 23 cases. Eur. Radiol. 11 (2001) 474

Freyschmidt, J.: Skeletterkrankungen. Springer. 1997 p. 788

Guerra, J., J. D. Newell, D. Resnick et al.: Gastrocnemio-semimembranosus bursal region of the knee. Amer. J. Roentgenol. 136 (1981) 593

Hermann, L. J., J. Beltran: Pitfalls in MR imaging of the knee. Radiology 167 (1988) 775

Johansson, E., Th. Apparisi: Congenital absence of the cruciate ligaments. Clin. Orthop. 162 (1982) 108

Jonasch, E.: Die Verknöcherung des Ligamentum popliteum obliquum. Fortschr. Röntgenstr. 99 (1963) 695

Johnson, R. L., A. A. de Smet: MR visualization of the popliteomeniscal fascicles. Skelet. Radiol. 28 (1999) 561

Kay, St. P., R. H. Gold, L. W. Basset: Meniscal pneumatocele. J. Bone Jt Surg. 67-A (1985) 1117

Kohn, D., B. Moreno: Meniscus insertion anatomy as a basis for meniscus replacement: a morphological cadaveric study. Arthroscopy 11 (1995) 96

Manolakis, P.: Fettkörperverkalkungen des Kniegelenkes beiderseits. Fortschr. Röntgenstr. 99 (1963) 846

McIntyre, J., S. Moelleken, P. Tirman: Mucoid degeneration of the anterior cruciate ligament mistaken for ligamentous tears. Skeletal Radiol. 30 (2001) 312

Mesgarzadeh, M., R. Moyer, D. S. Leder et al.: MR imaging of the knee: expanded classification and pitfalls to interpretation of meniscal tears. Radiographics 13 (1993) 489

Nogi, J., G. D. Mac Ewen: Congenital dislocation of the knee. J. pediat. Orthop. 2 (1983) 509

Peterfy, C. G., D. L. Janzen, P. F. J. Tirmann et al.: "Magic-angle" phenomenon: a cause of increased signal in the normal lateral meniscus on short-TE MR imaging of the knee. Amer. J. Roentgenol. 163 (1994) 149

Rohren, E. M., F. J. Kosarek, C. A. Helms: Discoid lateral meniscus and the frequency of meniscal tears. Skeletal Radiol. 30 (2001) 316

Sanders, T. G., M. A. Medynski, J. F. Feller et al.: Bone contusion patterns of the knee at MRI: footprint of the mechanisms of imaging. Radiographics 20 (2000) 135

Seibert-Daiker, F. M.: Seltene Verknöcherung der Ligamenta decussata. Fortschr. Röntgenstr. 138 (1983) 372

Shankman, St., J. Beltran, E. Melamed et al.: Anterior horn of the lateral meniscus: another potential pitfall in MR imaging of the knee. Radiology 204 (1997) 181

Slanina, J.: Fabella distalis: a new sesamoid bone. Radiol. clin. 25 (1956) 274

Stoller, D. W., C. Martin, J. W. III Crues et al.: Meniscal tears: pathologic correlation with MR imaging. Radiology 163 (1987) 731

Tuite, M. J., A. A. De Smet, J. S. Swan et al.: MR imaging of a meniscal ossicle. Skelet. Radiol. 24 (1995) 543

Tung, G. A., L. M. Davis, M. E. Wiggins et al.: Tears of the anterior cruciate ligament: primary and secondary signs at MR imaging. Radiology 188 (1993) 661

Vahey, T. N., H. T. Bennett, L. E. Arrington et al.: MR imaging of the knee: pseudotear of the lateral meniscus caused by the meniscofemoral ligament. Amer. J. Roentgenol. 154 (1990) 1237

Yao, L., A. Gentili, L. Petrus et al.: Partial ACL rupture: an MR diagnosis? Skelet. Radiol 24 (1995) 247

Yu, J. S., D. Resnick: Meniscal ossicle: MR imaging appearance in three patients. Skelet. Radiol 23 (1994) 637

Shaft of the Tibia and Fibula

Normal Findings

During Growth

The first ossification centers of the tibia and fibula appear between days 40 and 50 of fetal development. Between the 2nd and 6th months of life, the tibia and fibula exhibit double contours, like all the tubular bones, often accompanied by slight cupping and waviness of the metaphyseal contours.

> Cortical irregularities are a normal finding in the proximal and distal metaphyses, especially at the attachment of the pes anserinus (see also pp. 888 and 929). They are identical to the irregularities seen in the distal femur and proximal humerus (q.v.).

Slight **anterior bowing** of the tibia is a normal finding in infants and small children (Fig. 7.**166c**). The normal development of **tibial torsion** was measured by Kristiansen et al. (2001) using CT. The average lateral torsion of the tibia at the age of 4 years is 28° (20–37°). Later the increase in tibial torsion is 1°/year until 10 years of age and, thereafter, 4° until maturity when the mean lateral torsion is 38° (18–47°). This means that tibial torsion in children mainly develops during the first four years of life. After this the increase is of lesser clinical significance.

In Adulthood

To understand the radiographic projection of the tibial and fibular shafts, it is helpful to study anatomic specimens (Fig. 7.**159**).

The anterior and interosseous margins of the tibia form relatively sharp edges, which affect the radiographic contrast. When viewed in a tangential projection, the margins appear somewhat blurred and indistinct in their peripheral portion (toward the soft tissues), since the sharp edge absorbs less x-rays than the underlying bone. This effect can simulate periosteal pathology (Figs. 7.**160**, 7.**161**, 7.**169e**).

When the tibia is rotated slightly externally in the AP projection, the anterior margin is projected over the lateral portions of the tibial shaft. This can mimic a bandlike density in the medullary cavity, much as in the femur (Fig. 7.**3a**). The soleal line of the tibia (insertion line of the soleus muscle) may also appear as a linear density at the

junction of the lateral tibial condyle and tibial shaft in the AP projection (see scout view in Fig. 7.**160**, also 7.**169d**).

The **fibula**, the only non-weight-bearing long tubular bone, has variable margins along its shaft that give attachment to various muscles. In principle, the shaft has three margins: anterior, posterior, and interosseous. The anterior margin can be clearly identified only along the midportion of the shaft, becoming ill-defined proximally and distally. This also applies to the interosseous and posterior margins of the fibula, which follow a slightly spiral course around the shaft. This is particularly evident on axial CT scans (Fig. 7.**160**). Because of this arrangement, the individual margins may overlap or appear closely adjacent on conventional radiographs, mimicking endosteal and periosteal reactions.

>
> The configuration of the fibular head (Fig. 7.**159**) can occasionally mimic an osteochondroma on radiographs.

Both the tibia and the fibula are permeated by **nutrient canals**, which are most numerous in the middle third of the shaft (Figs. 7.**159b, d–j**, 7.**160**, 7.**166**, 7.**168 d**). Lee et al. (2000) investigated the radiographic features of the nutrient canals in the fibula. Imaging of the fibular vessels has assumed great practical importance within the framework of vascularized bone transfers (transfer of the fibula into a femoral defect, for example, using microvascular anastomosis).

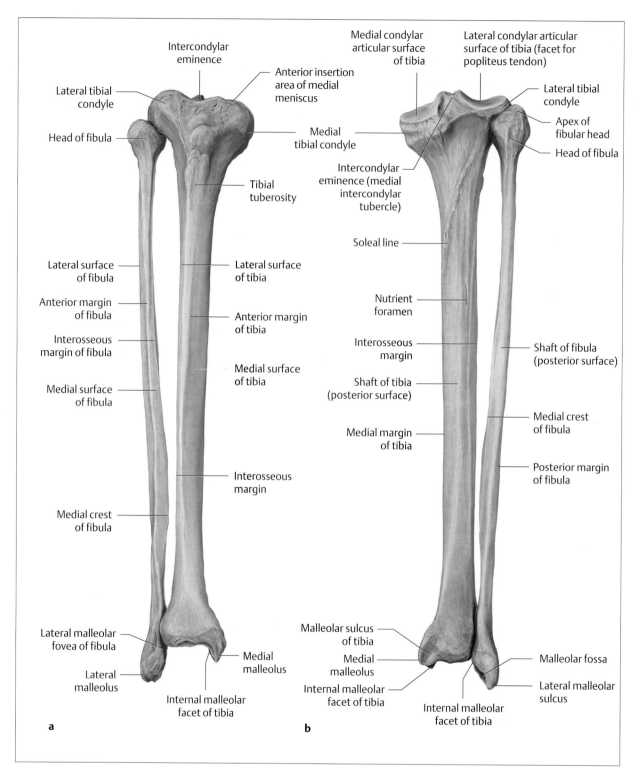

Fig. 7.**159 a–j** Anatomy of the tibia and fibula.
a Anterior aspect.
b Posterior aspect.

Fig. 7.**159 c**　Ligament and tendon attachments (after Wolf-Heidegger).

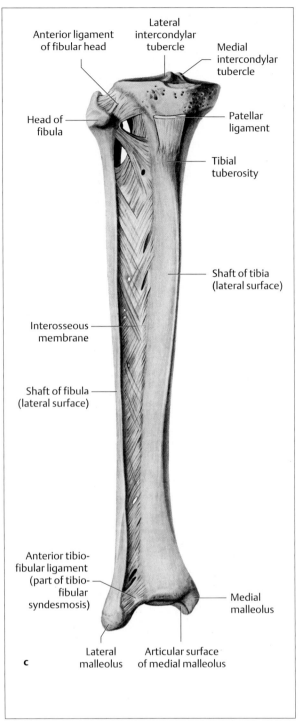

Anterior ligament of fibular head

Lateral intercondylar tubercle

Medial intercondylar tubercle

Head of fibula

Patellar ligament

Tibial tuberosity

Shaft of tibia (lateral surface)

Interosseous membrane

Shaft of fibula (lateral surface)

Anterior tibio-fibular ligament (part of tibio-fibular syndesmosis)

Medial malleolus

Lateral malleolus

Articular surface of medial malleolus

c

Fig. 7.**159 d–j** ▷

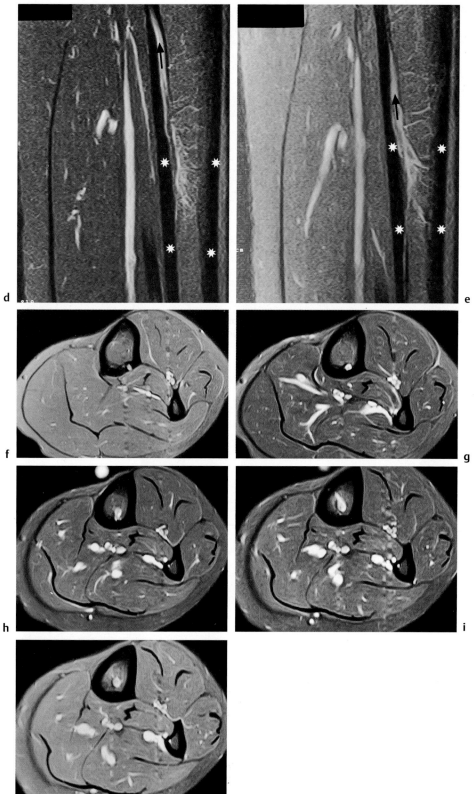

Fig. 7.**159 d–j** Intraosseous blood vessel (vein) on post-contrast MRI. The sagittal images in **d** and **e** show several intramedullary veins joining to form a larger vein that enters the posterior cortex, where it runs a short distance proximally before emerging into the adjacent soft tissues. The vertical black bands (asterisks) represent the tibial cortex. The course of the vessels can also be traced on the axial images in **f–j** . (Case courtesy of Dr. A. Hartmann, Altötting.)

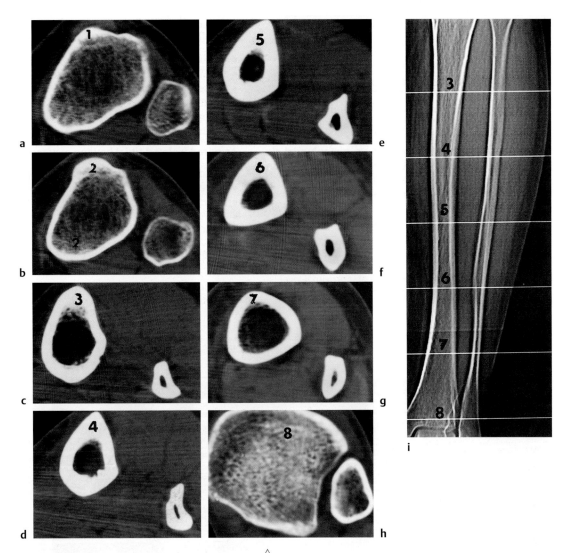

△

Fig. 7.**160a–i**   Representative CT scans through the tibia and fibula. The scout view (**i**) does not show the location of scans 1 and 2 (**a**) through the upper tibia. Note particularly how the shape of the fibula changes along its course. It has four margins in **c–e** and becomes triangular farther distally (scan 7; **g**). Note also the slitlike shape of the fibular medullary cavity in some of the scans (4, 7; **d, g**), and that the medial crest (Fig. 7.**159b**) forms a true crest only along the midportion of the shaft. The anterior margin actually does not begin until the middle third of the shaft (scans 4–6; **d–f**) and then winds toward the lateral side. Note the small osseous prominence on the posterolateral side of the tibial medullary cavity (scan 4; **d**). It represents the bony sheath of a large draining vein.

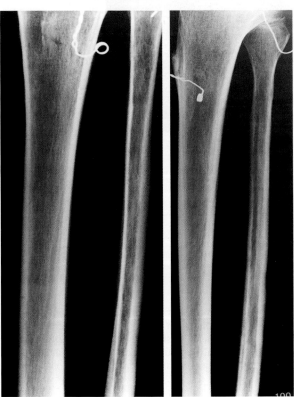

◁ Fig. 7.**161 a, b**   Spot films of an anatomic specimen in different projections. On the internal rotation view in **b**, note particularly the long, bandlike, medial subcortical lucency extending along the proximal and middle thirds of the fibular shaft. It is purely a projection effect caused by the projection of the anterior margin into the middle and posterior medullary cavity, where it produces a linear density. Radiograph **a** also shows slight blurring of the tibial lateral margin in the area where it forms a sharp edge and absorbs less x-rays.

▌*Pathological Finding?*

Normal Variant or Anomaly?

As noted above, the anatomy of the tibia and fibula lead to various projection-related effects that can mimic pathological processes.

Cortical irregularities and **fibrous metaphyseal defects** in the proximal and distal metaphyses are still considered normal variants (p. 929; Figs. 7.**125**, 7.**126**, 7.**170**, 7. **203**). **Transverse linear densities** in the distal tibia are known as **Harris lines** (Figs. 7.**166 e, f**, 7.**182**). They may be the result from a transient growth disturbance due to a fracture, rickets, etc.

> **Synostosis** of the tibia and fibula at a proximal level is definitely pathological (Hippe 1953).

Isolated bowing of the tibia may occur in the following conditions:

- Blount disease (see p. 921)
- Focal fibrocartilaginous dysplasia (see p. 922)
- Absent or hypoplastic fibula
- Elongated fibula
- Klippel–Trenaunay–Weber syndrome
- Neurofibromatosis

Acquired isolated tibial bowing may result from:

- Chronic osteomyelitis, especially in syphilis
- Paget disease
- Trauma, especially with epiphyseal plate injuries
- Fibrous dysplasia
- Rickets

Elongation of the fibula can occur in the following diseases:

- Achondroplasia, hypochondroplasia, mesomelic dysplasia

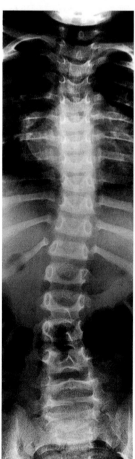

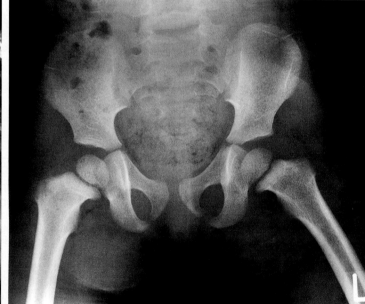

b

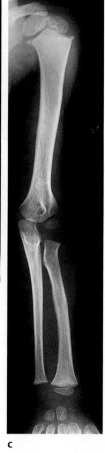

a

c

Fig. 7.**162 a–f** Metaphyseal dysplasia, Schmidt type, with flaring and medial beaking of the metaphyses, especially in the femur and tibia, resulting in varus deformity. The patient has short stature and a waddling gait. The findings should not be mistaken for late rickets. With the slight general flattening of the vertebral bodies and S-shaped scoliosis, the differential di-agnosis should include the Kozlowski type of spondylo-metaphyseal dysplasia, in which there is disproportionate growth retardation with a short trunk. The differential diagnosis should take into account clinical findings, genetics, etc. Sometimes a diagnosis can be made only by following the progression of the disease.

Fig. 7.**162 d–f** ▷

- Metaphyseal chondrodysplasia (Fig. 7.**162**)
- Muscular diseases
- Pseudoachondroplasia
- Spondyloepiphyseal or spondylometaphyseal dysplasia

A **hypoplastic fibula** is observed in the following diseases:

- Seckel syndrome (bird-headed dwarfism)
- Camptomelic dysplasia
- Chondroectodermal dysplasia (Ellis–van Creveld syndrome)
- Chromosome abnormalities
- Chapelle dysplasia

Not infrequently, the cause of a short fibula remains obscure, especially in "historical" cases and other cases lacking clinical data (Fig. 7.**163**).

The longitudinal endosteal or periosteal hyperostosis that occurs in **melorheostosis** is definitely a pathological finding, even though it does not necessarily have pathological significance in all cases (Fig. 7.**164a, b**). Differentiation is required from **bone-matrix-producing tumors** such as osteosarcoma and osteoid osteoma (Fig. 7.**164c, d**) and is often aided by radionuclide scanning. In most cases, bone scans are weakly positive in melorheostosis while the tumors show very intense uptake. The same applies to **reactive periosteal new bone formation** in diseases such as **pustulotic arthro-osteitis** (Fig. 7.**174**).

A rare cause of acquired structural changes in the tibia is **an intraosseous venous drainage in patients with pretibial varices** (Boutin et al. 1997). Similar structural changes may be caused by "**cystic" angiomatosis** or **angiodysplasia** (Fig. 7.**165**).

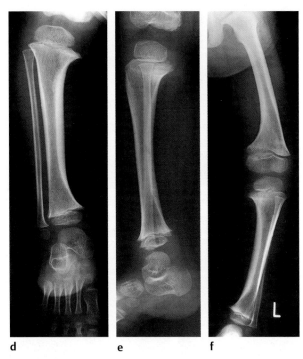

d   **e**   **f**

Fig. 7.**162 d–f**

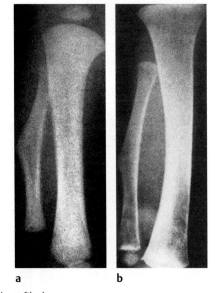

a   **b**

Fig. 7.**163 a, b**   Short fibula.
a Short fibula with slight bowing in a newborn boy. The cause is uncertain. Although Nievergelt syndrome was diagnosed in the previous edition of this book, this seems unlikely because the tibia in that complex syndrome usually shows rhomboid shortening and broadening while the fibula is usually normal and rarely shows severe shortening and deformity.
b Similar fibular changes are noted in the 3-year-old sister of the newborn. These cases underscore the importance of considering clinical-pediatric and genetic findings when interpreting such changes.

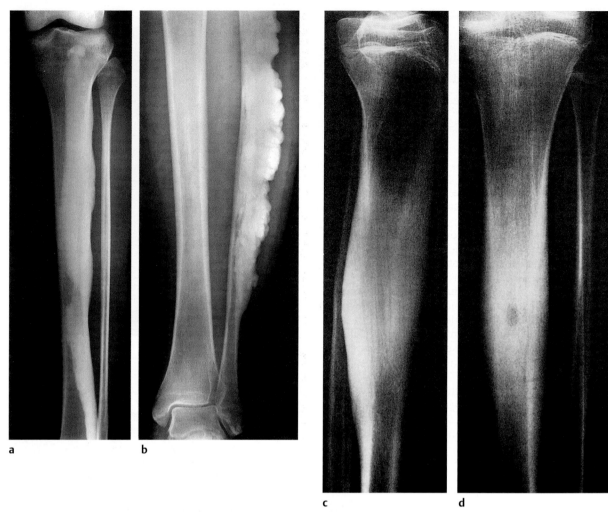

a

b

c

d

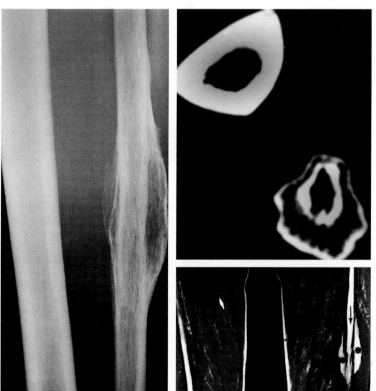

e

f

g

Fig. 7.**164a–g** Differential diagnosis of changes involving long segments of the tibia and fibula.

a, b Typical features of melorheostosis. The hyperostotic changes predominantly affect the endosteal side of the tibia in **a** and the periosteal side of the fibula in **b**. The latter is a dramatic example of the "flowing candle wax" pattern of hyperostoses.

c, d Typical osteoid osteoma with pronounced fusiform hyperostosis in the middle third of the tibial shaft. The small round nidus (the actual tumor) is best demonstrated in the AP projection.

e–g The fibular midshaft lesion is not a tumor but an old subperiosteal hemorrhage that has transformed into cancellous bone. Note that the original fibular cortex in **e** is fully intact. The hemorrhage has elevated the periosteum and later organized and transformed into cancellous bone, as the CT scan (**f**) clearly demonstrates. MRI shows the same (fat) signal intensity in the subperiosteal ossified areas (asterisks) as in the medullary cavity of the fibula itself (arrow). There was actually no need to proceed with CT and MRI in the present case.

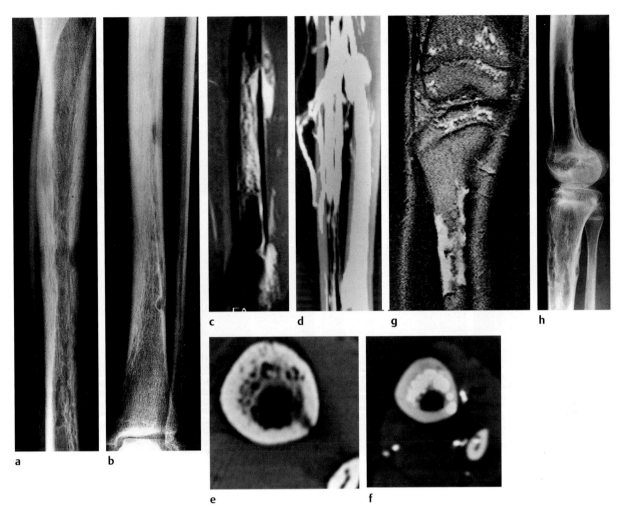

Fig. 7.**165a–h** Longitudinally oriented structural changes in the tibia (and also the distal femur in **g** and **h**) due to vascular disease.

a, b The longitudinal radiolucent grooves in the tibia are typical of vascular dilatation on and within the cortex. The patient is an otherwise healthy 14-year-old girl with mainly nocturnal pain and swelling in the left lower leg.

c–f Both MRI (**c**) and reformatted CT venography (**d**) show extensive venous dilatation in the tibial medullary cavity. Several dilated veins pass through the cortex, especially distally. The axial CT scans in **e** and **f** show hole-shaped and "worm-eaten" defects in the tibial cortex. After contrast administration, the defects are opacified by contrast medium from the ectatic

veins. We classify the case as venous angiodysplasia. Boutin et al. (1997) described similar changes on conventional radiographs in patients with intraosseous venous drainage anomalies due to pretibial varices.

g, h Cystic angiomatosis in the right lower extremity of a 14-year-old boy with diffuse right leg pain, atrophy of the thigh and lower leg muscles, and slight limb shortening. The lucencies, which are partly serpentine and partly vermiform (especially in the anterior and posterior tibia), represent lacunar areas of bone resorption due to malformed vessels. This is clearly demonstrated by T2-weighted MRI (**g**). In other MR images (not shown here), involvement of the synovial membrane was also noted.

 Fracture?

Congenital pseudarthrosis of the tibia is regarded by some orthopedists as an isolated idiopathic disorder. We believe, however, that most cases are caused by neurofibromatosis that has not yet produced dermatological or neurological symptoms when the pseudarthrosis is discovered. Neurofibromatous tissue structures are not found in the area of the tibial pseudarthrosis (Fig. 7.**171c**).

The above-mentioned **nutrient canals in the tibia** (Figs. 7.**166**, 7.**168d**) **and fibula** can mimic **shaft fractures** (Fig. 7.**166**).

Subtle, nondisplaced fractures of the tibial and fibular shaft, especially in children (toddlers' fractures), are often easy to miss on radiographs.

"Acute plastic bowing" is a phenomenon that can affect the tibia and fibula as well as the bones of the forearm (p. 204).

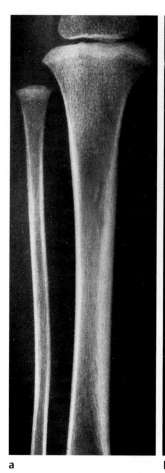

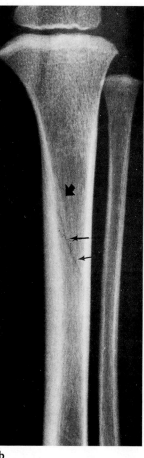

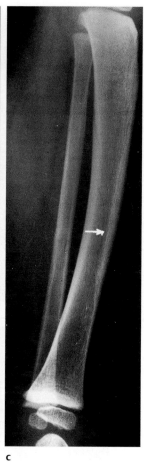

a

b

c

Fig. 7.166 a–f Linear changes in the tibia.

a, b Fracture of the tibial shaft appears as an oblique, sharply defined lucent line (**b**, thin arrows). Broader oblique lucencies proximal to the fracture (thick arrow) and on the opposite side (**a**) are typical nutrient canals that enter the tibia posteriorly and descend along the posterior inner cortex before finally branching in the medullary cavity (Fig. 7.**159 d–j**). This describes the anatomic course of the bony venous canal. The course of the veins themselves would be reversed.

c Lateral radiograph shows a distal hairline fracture (arrow). Note the slight physiological bowing at that location.

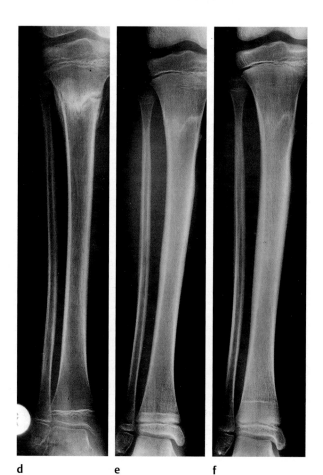

d

e

f

Fig. 7.166 d–f Development of Harris lines in the distal tibia. Radiograph **d** is a follow-up radiograph of a proximal tibial shaft fracture. Note the global demineralization of the bone due to regional acceleratory phenomenon (RAP). The line of provisional metaphyseal calcification is sharply defined. On a follow-up radiograph taken eight months later (**e**), this line has migrated at least 1 cm up the shaft, and the metaphysis shows bandlike increased density extending to the epiphyseal plate. Twelve months later (**f**) the Harris line has migrated several centimeters up the shaft. Harris lines signify a transient growth disturbance with accelerated bone growth, apparently with no opportunity for breakdown and remodeling of the zone of provisional calcification. The accelerated bone growth in the present case is explained by a generalized posttraumatic increase in the blood supply to the lower leg (RAP).

Fig. 7.**167 a, b** Classic stress fracture of the proximal tibia in a 7-year-old boy. Radiographs show a transverse, bandlike density through the upper tibial shaft. A fine transverse fracture line is also faintly visible in the AP projection (large arrow). In the lateral view, the intraosseous density shows a typical triangular configuration. Note the solid periosteal reaction (arrowheads in **a**, arrow in **b**). The detection of a fracture line and the solidity of the periosteal new bone, combined with the clinical presentation (e.g., recent history of very strenuous athletic activities such as soccer and rope jumping), serve to differentiate the stress fracture from inflammatory and neoplastic processes.

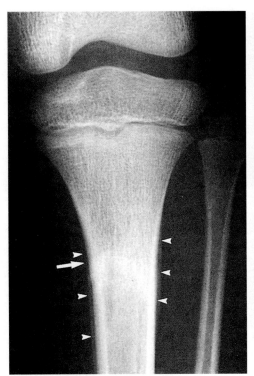

a

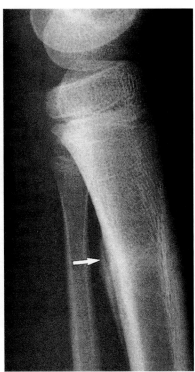

b

The proximal and distal tibia are sites of predilection for **stress fractures** (Figs. 7.**167**, 7.**168**, 7.**173**).

The early features of these injuries are difficult to document, either because they are missed on conventional radiographs despite marked clinical symptoms or because edema is the dominant finding in early MR images. It is our experience, however, that an early stress fracture line can be detected on CT scans, even when the fracture is oblique (Figs. 7.**168**, 7.**173 d**).

Excessive stresses on the anterior tibial margin (e.g., in ballet dancers) can lead to **circumscribed cortical resorption**. This probably results from small microfractures and can mimic the features of a Campanacci-type osteofibrous dysplasia or an inflammatory process (Fig. 7.**169 f**).

Shin splint syndrome can produce dramatic soft-tissue changes on MRI along with severe clinical symptoms. It is a type of compartment syndrome involving the deep muscles of the lower leg in response to excessive mechanical stresses, often combined with periosteal irritation (Anderson et al. 1997).

There are several synonyms for this condition:

- Medial tibial stress syndrome
- Shin soreness
- Soleus syndrome

Periosteal bone formation (Fig. 7.**169 d, e**) can develop as a late sequel to edema and hemorrhage at the insertion of the soleus muscle.

Fig. 7.168 a–d Oblique stress fracture in an overweight 54-year-old woman.

a The oblique lucent line (arrows) was initially overlooked. Early MRI showed massive edema throughout the tibial shaft (not shown here), and bone scans demonstrated a linear zone of increased uptake similar to that shown in Fig. 7.**173 a**. These findings, plus the faint medial and lateral periosteal bone formation in **a**, led the initial examiner to diagnose osteosarcoma.

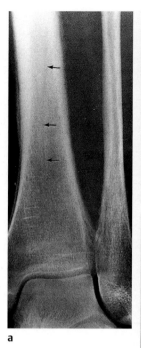

a

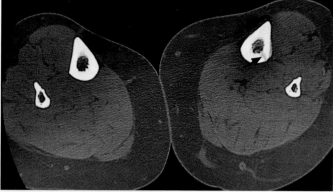

b

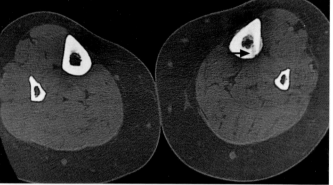

c

b–d The oblique, spiral-shaped fatigue fracture line is unmistakable on the CT scans. Note the sites of irregular periosteal bone formation on the medial side of the tibia, some of which appear spiculated on closer scrutiny and might be misinterpreted as aggressive lesions. (They appear completely solid on the conventional radiograph.) Also note the nutrient canal in **d**, which forms a kind of bony tunnel on the posteromedial inner cortical surface (arrow). The vascular caliber appears larger than on the contralateral side, probably a result of increased blood flow due to a RAP.

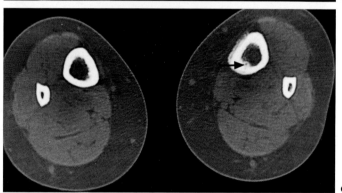

d

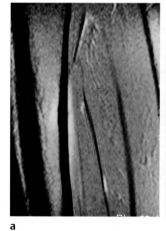

a

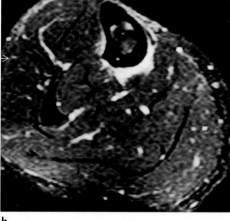

b

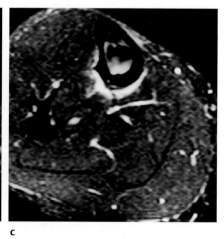

c

Fig. 7.169 a–f Stress-induced changes in the tibia.
a–c Shin splints in an athletically active young woman with severe pain in both lower legs. Conventional radiographs were normal when the patient was first seen. MRI shows extensive edema about the posteromedial and posterolateral circumference of the tibia, including intraosseous edema (see text). (Case courtesy of Dr. Westhaus, Weilheim.)

Fig. 7.**169 d, e**   Periosteal new bone formation along the soleal line (tibial attachment of the soleus muscle). Similar changes were noted on the contralateral side in this middle-aged jogger. It is reasonable to speculate that periosteal changes such as these can develop as a result of previous shin splints with periosteal irritation.
f Stress-induced transverse bandlike lucencies in the tibial anterior margin of a ballet dancer. The same changes were noted on the contralateral side. Similar phenomena can be found in joggers and soccer players.

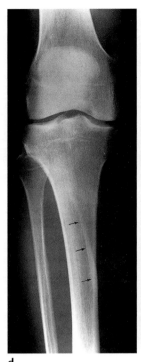 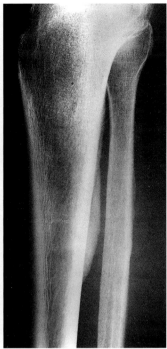 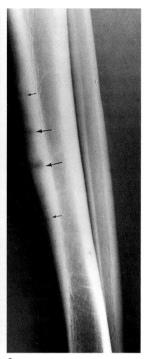

d   e   f

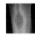 ## Necrosis?

Bone marrow infarction is relatively common in the distal tibial shaft (Fig. 7.**173**). Many of these infarctions are clinically silent and should not be mistaken for calcifying enchondroma. Bilateral occurrence always indicates calcified infarctions.

 ## Inflammation?

The tibia, especially its proximal metaphysis, is a very common site of osteomyelitis in children. The initial changes may be extremely subtle, consisting only of fine intracortical lucencies that correspond to widened vascular channels in the heavily perfused cortex and tiny "moth-eaten" foci of cancellous bone destruction. Another early sign of osteomyelitis is light periosteal bone formation about the site of the inflammation.

Paget disease occurs only in adults and can lead to significant tibial bowing. The lytic stage is characterized by flame-shaped lucent areas that occur mainly in the epiphyses and metaphyses and can mimic bone destruction by a tumor (Fig. 7.**175**). Sometimes the structural changes are extremely subtle, and the lesion is detected incidentally on a radionuclide bone scan obtained for a different reason in an asymptomatic patient.

> Generally the increased tracer uptake in Paget disease, is very homogeneous and involves a long segment of the bone including one fo the epiphyses.

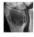 ## Tumor?

The proximal diaphyseal and metaphyseal portions of the tibia are particularly common sites of occurrence of primary bone tumors. Approximately 55% of the longitudinal growth of the lower limb is known to take place in the proximal tibial epiphysis, suggesting that it is a site of predilection for cellular dedifferentiation and tumorigenesis.

We cannot explore the full spectrum of tumors that can occur in the tibia and especially in the tibial shaft. We must limit our attention to special entities that have an affinity for the tibia and are associated with characteristic radiographic findings.

Nonossifying fibromas that migrate toward the shaft (Fig. 7.**170**) can mimic cysts.

Fractures that extend into a nonossifying fibroma rarely show a causal relationship to the lesion (Fig. 7.**170 d**). Nonossifying fibroma is not a true bone tumor but a tumorlike lesion that can be interpreted etiologically as a kind of growth disturbance (p. 890). The anterior tibial margin is typically affected by **Campanacci-type osteofibrous dysplasia**, a special form of fibrous dysplasia with prominent active osteoblasts on the surfaces of the woven bone trabeculae (Freyschmidt et al. 1998). It typically occurs in the tibia, predominantly affects children under 10 years of age, and is usually confined to the cortex, where it produces blisterlike lucencies with sclerotic borders. These lesions are extremely difficult to distinguish from adamantinomas, especially the differentiated forms (Fig. 7.**171 a, d, e, f**; Freyschmidt et al. 1998).

Adamantinoma is a true tumor that affects the tibia almost exclusively and whose radiographic features can resemble Campanacci-type osteofibrous dysplasia when it involves a long segment of the bone (Fig. 7.**171 d**).

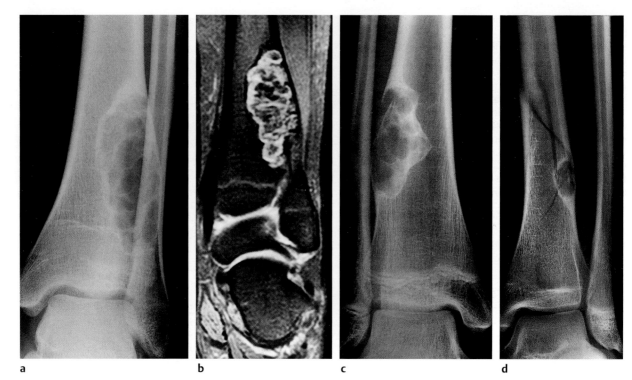

a   b   c   d

Fig. 7.**170 a–d**   Nonossifying fibromas of the distal tibia.
a, b Rather large nonossifying fibroma at a typical location with a very specific radiographic appearance (scalloped sclerotic border, overall Lodwick grade IA lesion). The serpiginous hyperintense structures on MRI (**b**) are a nonspecific finding that might also result from a bone marrow infarction. With a radiographic lesion like that found in **a**, we feel that MRI is unnecessary and will only lead to confusion.
c, d Nonossifying fibromas that have migrated up the shaft. The spiral fracture in **d** was caused by significant trauma, and it is purely coincidental that it extends into the nonossifying fibroma.

Differentiation is also required from syphilitic periostitis (Fig. 7.**171 b**).

Classic fibrous dysplasia (Fig. 7.**172**) also has a predilection for the tibia, which is the second most common site of occurrence (after the proximal femur). Its radiographic features are very diverse and depend on factors that include the "maturity" of the connective tissue that replaces the bone, and on whether the dysplasia is monostotic or polyostotic (the latter often shows more aggressive features).

Accordingly, there are purely lytic lesions that progress through a ground-glass stage to dense sclerotic structures with expansion and bowing of the bone. A highly specific feature is the soap-bubble pattern consisting of multiple lucencies with sclerotic margins (Fig. 7.**172 a, b**).

Periosteal new bone formation in pustulotic arthroosteitis (PAO) can mimic periosteal osteosarcoma (Freyschmidt 1997) (Fig. 7.**174**).

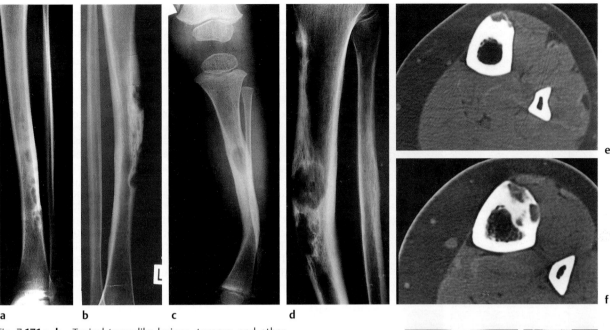

a   b   c   d

e

f

Fig. 7.**171 a–h** Typical tumorlike lesions, tumors, and other lesions that occur predominantly in the tibial diaphysis.

a Classic Campanacci-type osteofibrous dysplasia in a young woman. Because radiographs could not distinguish the lesion from a differentiated adamantinoma and because of the severe clinical symptoms, the anterolateral cortex was "peeled." The surgical specimen is shown in **h**, the corresponding CT scans in **e** and **f**.

b Syphilitic periostitis.

c Bowing of the tibia (tibia vara) in a 2-year-old boy with neurofibromatosis. Note the dense sclerosis of the tibia above the apex of the bow. The cystlike lesion in the proximal sclerotic area was not found to contain neurofibromatous tissue, only fluid and connective tissue. Later a fracture developed at the apex of the bow, followed by nonunion, etc. A number of years passed after initial presentation before the boy developed classic clinical signs of neurofibromatosis.

d Significant structural changes in the tibia with lucencies and irregular sclerotic areas, especially in the midshaft region. This pattern is fairly typical of adamantinoma. But the diagnosis can only be established histologically, especially in terms of differentiating the lesion from marked osteofibrous dysplasia of the Campanacci type.

e, f CT scans corresponding to **a**. The destructive changes are confined to the anterior tibial border. They are well circumscribed with no infiltration of the medullary cavity or soft tissues.

g Differential diagnosis from **c**: osteogenesis imperfecta type IV.

h Surgical specimen corresponding to **a, e, f**.

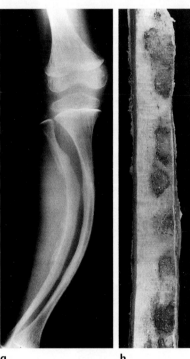

g   h

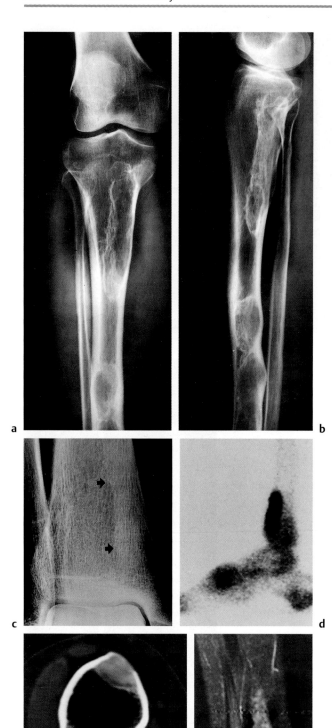

a b c d e f

Fig. 7.**172 a–f** Fibrous dysplasia of the tibia.
a, b Classic longitudinal form with fibrous and osseous structures of varying maturity in place of normal bone. The proximal tibial changes already shows significant sclerosis that includes soap-bubble-like changes. Some ground-glass structural changes are visible in the middle third of the shaft. These findings are pathognomonic, and there is no need for a differential diagnosis.
c–f Ground-glass stage of fibrous dysplasia of the distal tibia. The two arrows in **c** point to the homogeneous sclerotic area. There are no morphological changes (enlargement, deformity, etc.) in the bone. In the lateral view (not shown here), watch-glass-like thinning and bulging were noted in a circumscribed area of the anterior cortex. The bone scan (**d**) shows very intense uptake. The CT scan in **e** is highly specific, showing a ground-glass-like mass formed by moderately mature and calcified fiber bone. The anterior cortex is thinned and almost completely resorbed, but there is no soft-tissue infiltration. The medullary cavity is completely intact. The MR image in **f** was confusing and raised the possibility of enchondroma. This prompted a biopsy (unnecessary in retrospect) for histological confirmation.

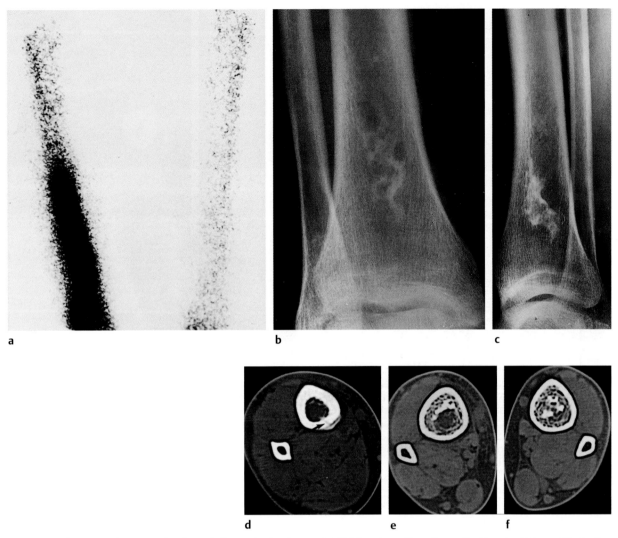

a

b

c

d

e

f

Fig. 7.**173 a–f** Instructive example of a misdiagnosis due to misinterpretation of simple bone marrow infarctions that can occur in the distal tibia. The patient is a 44-year-old man, athletically active, who presented with severe pain in the right distal tibia.

a Radionuclide scan shows a longitudinal area of very intense uptake.

b, c The radiographs show a calcified figure at the center of the tibia, which appears to be localized and shows no lobulation. This pattern indicates a bone marrow infarction. However, the finding was misinterpreted as a calcified enchondroma that had undergone chondrosarcomatous degeneration. The radionuclide findings in particular contributed to this overinterpretation, as it was inconceivable that a harmless calcified enchondroma could produce such an extensive scintigraphic lesion. The latter is derived from periosteal new bone formation along the medial (and posterior, **c**) aspect of the distal tibial cortex. Given the patient's prior history, this finding should actually have raised suspicion of a stress fracture.

d In fact, the CT scan does reveal a definite stress fracture (arrowhead). The fracture appears to be oblique, much like the one in Fig. 7.**168 a**, and this was confirmed by subsequent scans.

e, f CT scans of both lower legs at the level of the central calcified figure show bilateral central bone marrow infarctions. This bilaterality and the normal-appearing areas surrounding the infarcts definitely identify the lesions as calcified bone marrow infarctions. Nevertheless, a biopsy was performed and yielded equivocal results (nonspecific calcifications).

The correct interpretation of the imaging findings is an old calcified (bilateral) bone marrow infarction in the distal tibia accompanied by a stress fracture in the distal tibial shaft. Only the latter produced clinical symptoms.

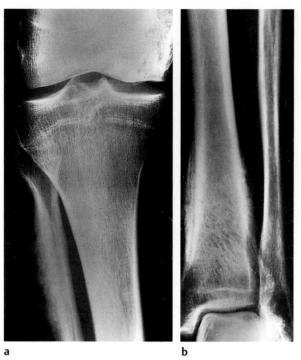

a   b

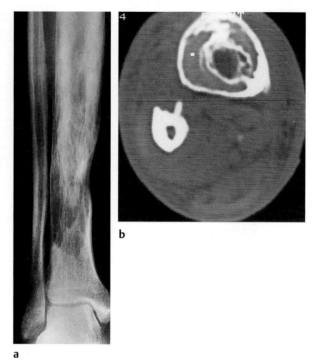

b

a

Fig. 7.**174a, b**   Pustulotic arthro-osteitis (PAO) with unusual, nonspecific, bilateral reactive periosteal new bone formation on the tibia and fibula. A lesion in the right distal fibula (similar to a subsequent proximal lesion, **a**) was interpreted as a periosteal osteosarcoma and was resected. The original radiograph is unavailable. Subsequent radionuclide and radiographic examination showed additional foci in the proximal residual fibula (**a**) and left tibia (**b**). Inspection of the patient's hands and feet revealed palmoplantar pustulosis.

Fig. 7.**175a, b**   Paget disease.
a Typical Paget disease of the tibia in an elderly man. Note the flame-shaped configuration of the osteolytic disease component in the distal tibial shaft. The advanced sclerotic phase is already evident in the middle and proximal shaft. The changes extend into the proximal epiphysis. For an inexperienced examiner, the overall features might suggest a destructive malignant process.
b Axial CT shows a target-like cross section of the tibia with preservation of the central fat-containing marrow cavity. Further details can be found in Freyschmidt et al. (1997).

References

Anderson, M. W., V. Ugalde, M. Batt et al.: Shin splints: MR appearance in a preliminary study. Radiology 204 (1997) 177

Balthasar, D. A., A. Pappas: Acquired valgus deformity of the tibia in children. J. pediat. Orthop. 4 (1984) 538

Boutin, R. D., D. J. Sartoris, St. C. Rose et al.: Intraosseous venous drainage anomaly in patients with pretibial varices. Imaging findings. Radiology 202 (1997) 751

Crivelli, N., J. G. Kundert: Die geschlossenen Frakturen des mittleren und distalen Unterschenkels. Ther. Umsch. 40 (1983) 981

Daffner, R. H.: Anterior tibial striations. Amer. J. Roentgenol. 143 (1984) 651

Daffner, R. H., S. Martinez, J. A. Gehweiler: Stress fractures in runners. J. Amer. med. Ass. 247 (1982) 1038

Ehara, S., Y. Tamakawa, J. Nishida et al.: Cortical defect of the distal fibula: variant of ossification. Radiology 197 (1995) 447

Freyschmidt, J.: Skeletterkrankungen, 2. Aufl. Springer, Berlin 1997

Freyschmidt, J., H. Ostertag, G. Jundt: Knochentumoren, 2. Aufl. Springer, Berlin 1998

Hippe, H.: Seltene proximale tibiofibulare Synostose. Fortschr. Röntgenstr. 78 (1953) 748

Iscan, Y. M., P. Miller-Shaivitz: Determination of sex from the tibia. Amer. J. phys. Anthropol. 64 (1984) 53

Kristiansen L. P., R. B. Gunderson, H. Steen et al.: The normal development of tibial torsion. Skeletal Radiol. 30 (2001) 519

Lee, J-H., S. Ehara, Y. Tamakawa et al.: Nutrient canal of the fibula. Skelet. Radiol. 29 (2000) 22

Rahmanzadeh, R., R. Hahn: Kindliche Tibiaschaftfrakturen. Orthopädie 13 (1984) 293

Schneider, H. J., A. Y. King, J. L. Bronson et al.: Stress injuries and developmental change of lower extremities in ballet dancers. Radiology 113 (1974) 627

Distal Tibia and Fibula

■ Normal Findings

 During Growth

The **ossification center of the distal tibial epiphysis** appears between the 2nd and 8th months of life and fuses with the shaft between 16 and 20 years of age.

The **ossification center of the distal fibular epiphysis** becomes visible on radiographs several months later. It fuses with the shaft at about the same time as the distal tibial epiphysis.

The **epiphyseal plate** of the distal tibia is wavy and irregular. Occasional projections extend from the distal epiphysis into a corresponding notch in the metaphysis (Figs. 7.**176**, 7.**179**, 7.**190**). The distal fibular epiphysis may normally show a slight medial offset in relation to the metaphysis.

A separate ossification center may be found at the tip of the medial and lateral malleolus. This occurs in approximately 30% of medial malleoli (Fig. 7.**177**) and in an even higher percentage of lateral malleoli (Figs. 7.**178**, 7.**179**).

In later stages of ossification, isolated shell-like centers may appear adjacent to the tibial and fibular epiphyses (Fig. 7.**180**).

A typical ossification center also appears lateral to the distal fibular metaphysis, just proximal to the epiphyseal plate, in about the 6th year of life. Known as the **fibular ossicle** (Fig. 7.**181**), this small center fuses with the fibula during puberty.

The former epiphyseal plates of the tibia and fibula can occasionally be seen far into adulthood, appearing as fine, transverse striate densities (lower dense line in Fig. 7.**182**).

Mineralization of the tibial epiphyseal plate begins anteriorly in the area of the medial malleolus and spreads posteriorly and laterally. The anterolateral part of the plate is the last to fuse. A knowledge of this aspect of epiphyseal closure is important in understanding "**transitional fractures**," or fractures occurring at the transitional age between adolescence and adulthood (p. 980).

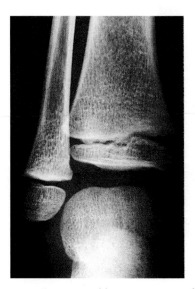

Fig. 7.**176** Normal bony structures of the ankle joint in a 6-year-old boy.

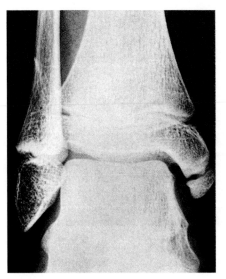

Fig. 7.**177** Large, separate ossification center at the tip of the medial malleolus, present on both sides, in a 10-year-old boy.

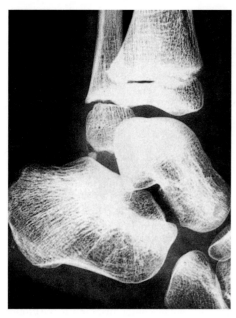

Fig. 7.**178** Separate ossification center in the posterior tip of the lateral malleolus in a 6-year-old boy.

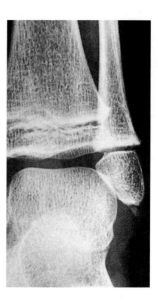

Fig. 7.**179** Separate ossification center below the tip of the lateral malleolus.

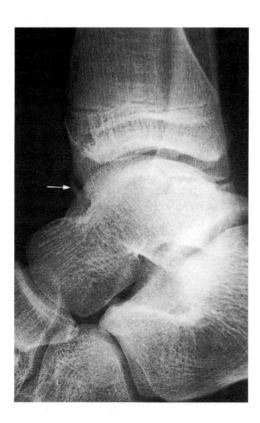

Fig. 7.**180** Shell-like apophysis on the anterior border of the medial malleolus.

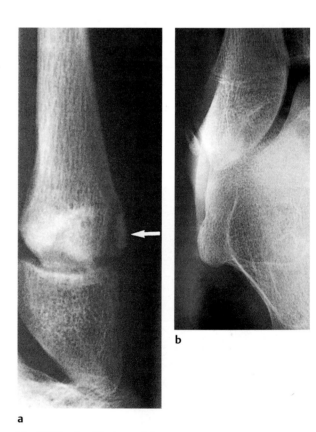

a

b

Fig. 7.**181 a, b** Fibular ossicle.
a Girl 9 years of age.
b Persistence of the ossicle (os retinaculum) in a young adult with otherwise closed epiphyseal plates.

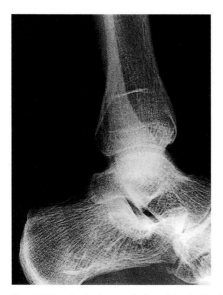

Fig. 7.**182** Typical growth line (Harris line) in the tibia of a patient with a negative history. Compare this figure with Fig. 7.**166 a–c**.

 ## In Adulthood

The Harris lines, or transverse cancellous bone densities at the metaphyseal-diaphyseal junction, were described on p. 958 (Fig. 7.**166**). They usually result from a transient growth disturbance due to various causes but may occur in people without a specific history (Fig. 7.**182**).

The spatial relationship of the tibia and fibula and their appearance on radiographic projections are best appreciated by referring to CT scans (Fig. 7.**183**).

In the former region of the epiphyseal plate, CT occasionally shows a somewhat amorphous cancellous bone structure in the anterior tibia that should not be mistaken for fibrous dysplasia, for example (Fig. 7.**183 a**, right). If the scan cuts the subchondral plate on a tangential plane, it appears as a patchy density (Fig. 7.**183 c, e**).

The lower end of the fibula articulates with the fibular notch of the tibia (Fig. 7.**183**).

An avulsion fracture of the upper pole of the patella is an extracapsular injury, so generally there is no damage to the articular cartilage. In other respects all intra-articular patellar fractures and fractures that involve the cartilage are a potential prelude to osteoarthritis. A special type of injury is the osteochondral "flake fracture." When visible radiographically, it appears as a small, isolated bony shell near the articular surface of the patella. In some cases, however, this very small fragment is only the tip of the ice-

Fig. 7.**183 a–e** Axial CT scans of the distal tibial epiphysis and ▷ fibular metaphysis just above the ankle joint. In **a** note the slightly blurred structures below the anterior tibial surface in the right image. This is completely normal and should not be mistaken for fibrous dysplasia or other pathology. Note also the patchy densities in the CT scans at the level of the subchondral plate (right image in **c**). The CT scans help clarify how the anatomic structures are projected in Fig. 7.**184**, especially with regard to the fibular notch and the anterolateral and posterolateral tibial borders.

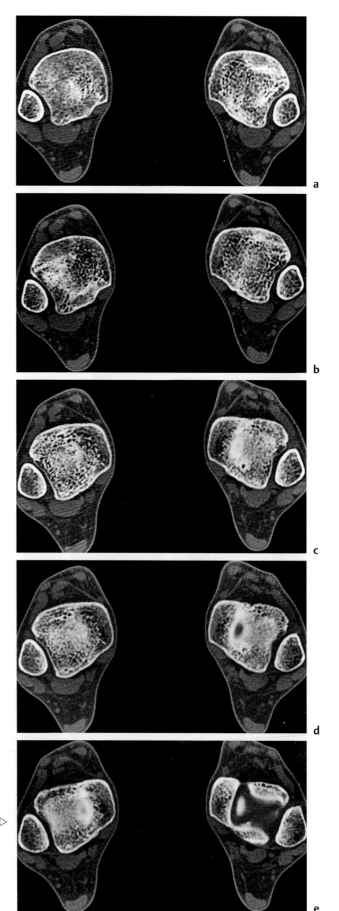

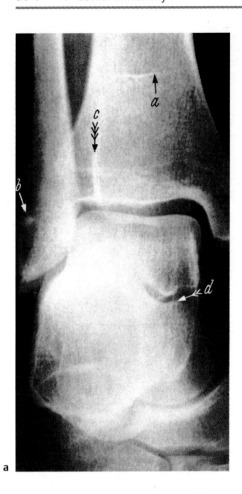

a

◁ Fig. 7.**184a–c** Radiographic projection of the lateral portions of the tibial epiphysis. **a** AP radiograph.
- a   Growth line
- b   Small enostosis (bone island) in the fibula
- c   Posterior rim of fibular notch
- d   Talocalcaneal joint

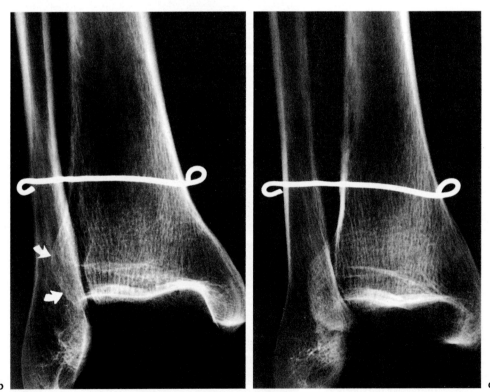

b

c

b Normal AP projection.
Arrows: posterior border of tibia and posterior rim of fibular notch
c Projection with 30° of internal rotation.

Note that the anterior tibial border defines the bony contour in **b**, while the posterior border defines it in **c** and is projected within the fibula.

berg. A pure cartilaginous fracture is a rare lesion that is illustrated in Fig. 7.**80 g, h**.

Chronic traction trauma, either with avulsion of the upper pole of the patella or with metaplastic bone formation in the quadriceps tendon, is illustrated in Fig. 7.**81**.

This type of injury is a counterpart to chronic avulsion fractures of the anterior inferior iliac spine or ischial tuberosity, for example.

Pathological Finding?

 ### Normal Variant or Anomaly?

Various ossifications can occur about the medial and lateral malleoli as normal variants.

- A bone located below the malleolar tip is called either the **os subtibiale** (Figs. 7.**185**, 7.**186**, 7.**198**) or **os subfibulare** (Figs. 7.**186**, 7.**188**, 7.**189**).
- Isolated bony elements located more or less **between** the malleolus and talus (i.e., **paramalleolar** rather than submalleolar) are still referred to as os subtibiale and subfibulare. For the talus secundarius, see p. 1008 and Fig. 7.**248**.
- Paramalleolar accessory **elements** in direct contact with the underlying bone are called **ossa retinaculi** (Fig. 7.**181 b**). They probably represent persistent centers like the fibular ossicle (Fig. 7.**181 a**).

Perimalleolar ossifications can have various causes. The os subtibiale and os subfibulare may be unfused epiphyseal centers, or they may represent supernumerary (true accessory) bones. Another possible cause is ligamentous ossification consisting of small foci of heterotopic bone formation occurring as a sequel to trauma.

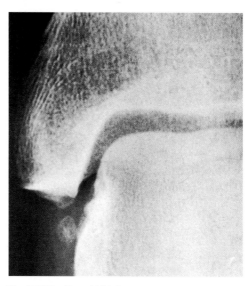

Fig. 7.**185**   Os subtibiale.

The importance of these elements lies in their differentiation from bony avulsions. A useful rule is that if the bony element fits into a defect in the opposing malleolus, it is most likely an avulsed fragment, especially if there is a known trauma history (Fig. 7.**198**).

In any case, accessory bones, unfused centers, old avulsions, and heterotopic ossifications almost always have a complete cortical boundary, whereas fresh avulsion fractures do not have cortical coverage at the fracture site.

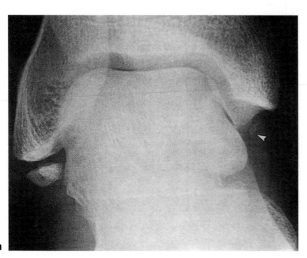 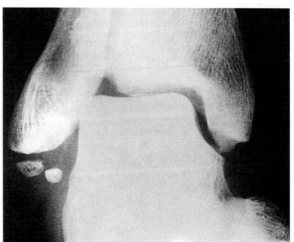

a   b

Fig. 7.**186 a, b**   Os subtibiale and two ossa subfibularia.

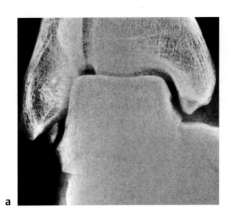

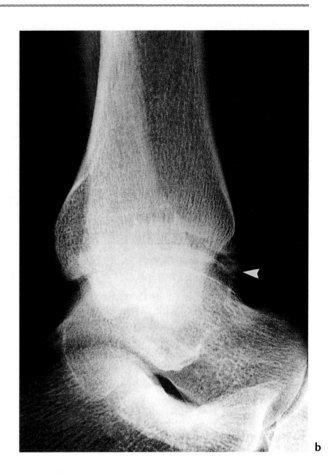

Fig. 7.**187 a, b**   Os subfibulare and os talotibiale.
a Isolated accessory bone element located between the fibular apex and talus, still classified as an os subfibulare.
b Os talotibiale as an accessory bone (p. 1005).

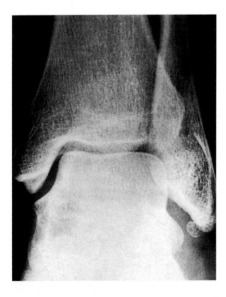

Fig. 7.**188**   Os subfibulare in a 41-year-old woman.

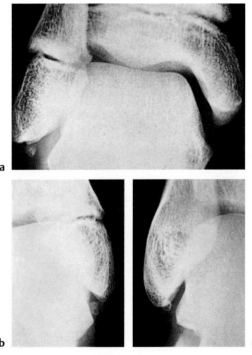

Fig. 7.**189 a–c**   Isolated ossification center or os subfibulare.
a Age 11 years.
b Age 14 years.
c Age 19 years.

In some individuals the **malleolar fossa** (see anatomy in Fig. 7.**159b**) is fairly **pronounced**, a finding that is still considered a normal variant (Figs. 7.**190**–7.**192**).

It is relatively common to find one or more accessory bone element within the fossa.

> Exceptionally large accessory bone elements, as shown in Fig. 7.**193**, may raise the question of whether they are pathological.

Large accessory bones (in this case probably an unusually large os subfibulare) may interfere with ankle motion and can eventually lead to complaints.

A large, exostosis-like protrusion of the distal tibial epiphysis probably also falls within the definition of a circumscribed deformity (Fig. 7.**194**).

If the talar articular surface is angled medially, forming more than about a 100° angle with the axis of the tibial shaft, this creates a valgus deformity in the talocrural joint that is basically considered a **preosteoarthritic deformity**. The inferomedial slant of the ankle joint axis is also known as tibiotalar tilt (Table 7.**6** and Fig. 7.**195**) (Griffiths and Wandtke 1981).

> A radiograph taken with the knee flexed and the foot externally rotated can mimic the presence of tibiotalar tilt.

The many possible epiphyseal and metaphyseal chondrodysplasias need not be reviewed here in detail. Figure 7.**196** illustrates a complex dysplasia that involves both the metaphyses and the epiphyses.

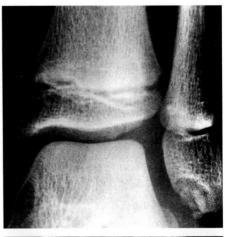

a

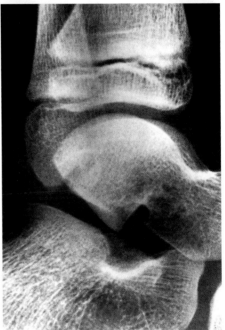

b

Fig. 7.**190 a, b**   Accentuated fossa at the tip of the lateral malleolus, containing a small ossification center, in a 9-year-old boy.

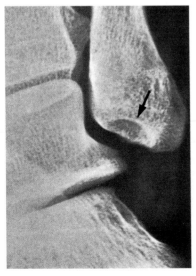

Fig. 7.**191**   Fossa at the tip of the lateral malleolus.

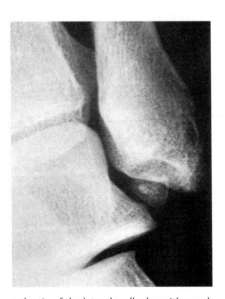

Fig. 7.**192**   Fossa at the tip of the lateral malleolus with an adjacent isolated bony element.

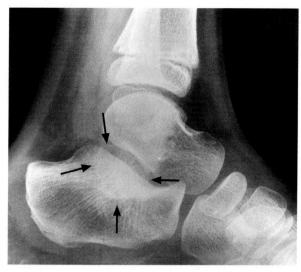

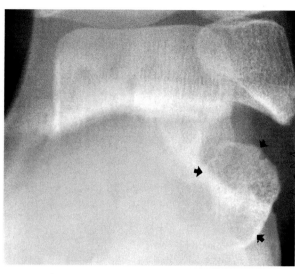

Fig. 7.**193 a, b**   Unusually large accessory bone element adjacent to the talus and calcaneus, precisely below the lateral malleolus in a 7-year-old asymptomatic child. We classify this accessory bone as an unusually large os subfibulare, because it apparently has no relation to the talus and calcaneus. (Case courtesy of Dr. D. Weingard, Freiburg.)

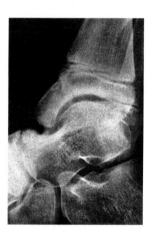

Fig. 7.**194**   Exostosis-like extension of the distal tibial epiphysis.

Table 7.**6**   Conditions that may be associated with tibiotalar tilt

Congenital
- Epiphyseal dysplasia (hemimelic epiphyseal dysplasia, Trevor disease, Fig. 7.**252**)
- Van Buchem endosteal hyperostosis
- Metaphyseal chondrodysplasia
- Multiple epiphyseal dysplasia (Fairbank disease)
- Nail–patella syndrome
- Spondyloepiphyseal dysplasia

Occurring as a deformity during development
- Fibrous dysplasia
- Neurofibromatosis
- Enchondromatosis
- Cartilaginous exostosis disease

Acquired
- Blount disease
- Posttraumatic (e.g., Salter–Harris III or IV fracture of the distal tibia)
- Rheumatoid arthritis
- Hemophilia (Fig. 7.**195 c, d**)
- Cretinism
- Femoral bowing
- Hyperparathyroidism
- Hypophosphatasia
- Poliomyelitis
- Rickets
- Sickle cell disease
- Avascular necrosis

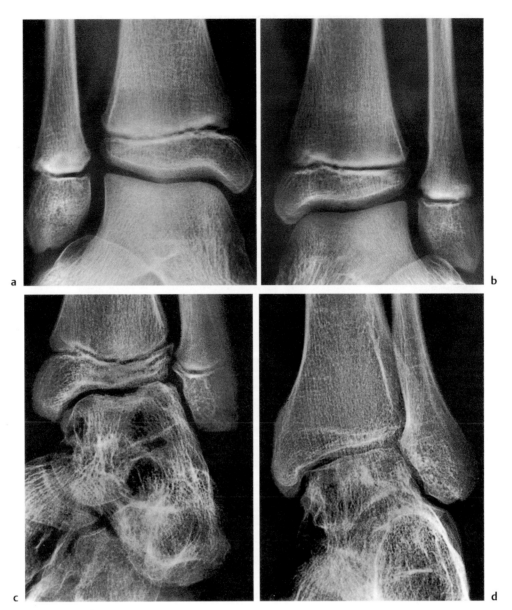

Fig. 7.**195 a–d**   Tibiotalar tilt and hemophiliac joint.
a, b Tibiotalar tilt, i.e., increased medial inclination of the talar articular surface and opposing tibial epiphysis, creating a valgus position in the ankle joint. This 10-year-old asymptomatic child had no other apparent abnormalities, and so the tilt may still represent an extreme normal variant (see text).

c, d Typical hemophiliac joints with a coarsened trabecular pattern. Radiograph **c** is from a 13-year-old patient with hemophilia A. Note the enlarged, deformed tibial epiphysis and the irregular, sunken subchondral plate of the talus, probably due to necrosis. Radiograph **d** is from an adult hemophiliac.

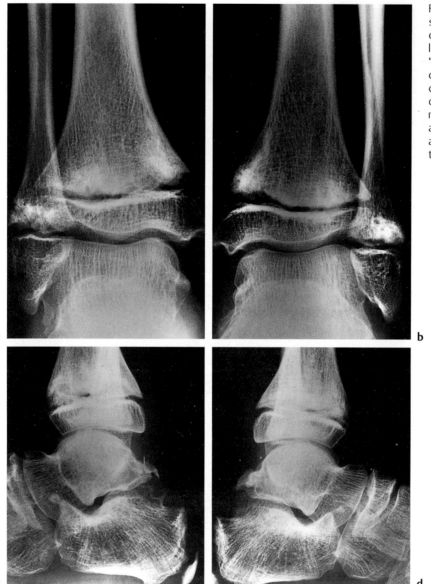

Fig. 7.**196 a–d**   Metaphyseal-epiphyseal chondrodysplasia in a 13-year-old child. Since clinical information was lacking except for the report of "mildly disproportionate growth retardation," there is no way to classify the disorder more precisely. Note the dense and irregular tibial and fibular metaphyses. The epiphyses are unusually flat and irregularly shaped. Note also the spiculated contours of the talus, calcaneus, and navicular bones.

Fracture, Subluxation, or Dislocation?

The nature and extent of injuries to the growth plates of the ankle joint are of major importance during skeletal growth. It is crucial for the radiographic examiner to determine whether the injury is a **pure epiphyseal separation with or without a metaphyseal fragment** (Salter–Harris type I and II) or whether it is an **epiphyseal plate fracture** (Salter–Harris type III–V) (Fig. 7.**197 a**).

With epiphyseal plate injuries, there is always a high risk of secondary growth disturbance if, for example, portions of the epiphyseal plate have been destroyed and can no longer contribute to growth. It is important to note that the distal tibial epiphyseal plates account for approximately 45% of the longitudinal growth of the tibia (Table 7.**3**). Characteristic **triplane fractures (transitional fractures)** can occur shortly before epiphyseal closure. The fracture takes place in the lateral part of the tibial epiphyseal plate, which is the last to ossify, and involves a portion of the posterior tibial metaphysis (Fig. 7.**197 b, c**). Involvement of the epiphysis itself can result in a three-part fracture.

The various **fractures of the malleoli** in both adolescents and adults are associated with **ligament ruptures** in 90% of cases, usually involving the fibular ligaments and less commonly the medial (deltoid) ligament.

The extent of ligamentous injuries can be evaluated on **stress radiographs**. Attention is given to the angulation (especially varus) of the talus in the ankle mortise, the fibulotalar distance, and the anterior displacement of the talus in response to various devices and maneuvers (see also Fröhlich et al. 1984, Jend et al. 1984).

If the distance between a tangent to the posterior talar dome and the posteroinferior corner of the tibia is increased to more than 7 mm, a distortion is present. More than 11 mm indicates a rupture of the anterior fibulotalar ligament. A side-to-side discrepancy of more than 5 mm in the joint space width (on stress radiographs) is very strong evidence of a syndesmotic rupture.

Some 85% of ligamentous lesions can be diagnosed from these values (Jend et al. 1984). Technique: lateral radiograph of the ankle joint after placing a 5-kg sandbag on the distal tibia for five minutes (method of Seiler and Holzrichter).

Fig. 7.**197 a–c** Epiphyseal injuries and triplane fractures.
a Salter–Harris classification of epiphyseal injuries. Types I and II are pure epiphyseal separations, with type II including a metaphyseal fragment. Types III and IV are epiphyseal plate injuries. Type V is a crush injury of the epiphyseal plate.

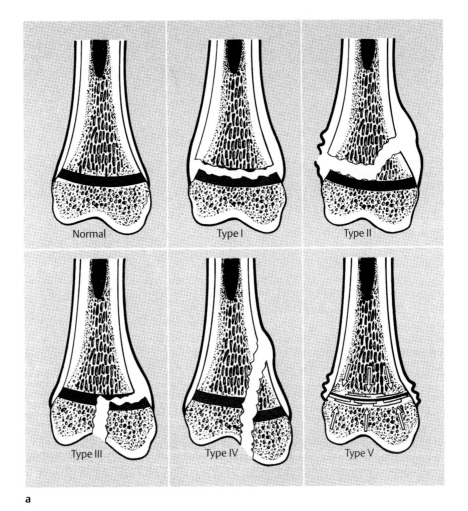

a

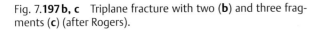

b   c

Fig. 7.**197 b, c** Triplane fracture with two (**b**) and three fragments (**c**) (after Rogers).

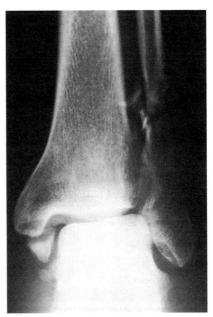

Fig. 7.**198** Nonunited fracture of the medial malleolus. Below it is a small os subtibiale. Fresh gunshot injury of the distal fibula with gross comminution of the bone.

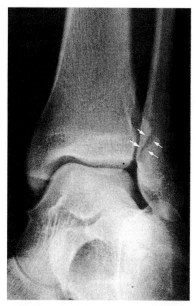

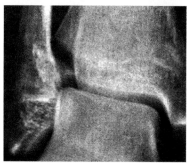

Fig. 7.**199 a, b**   Tubercle of Chaput.
a Isolated accessory bone element next to the anterolateral tibial margin (tubercle of Chaput). The bony element is projected onto the fibula. The arrows indicate a pseudofracture line. Incidental finding with the same phenomenon on the contralateral side (not shown).
b Avulsion of the tubercle of Chaput.

The **Weber** classification is used for **fractures of the fibula and medial malleolus with ligament tears**. It is important to note that the integrity of the tibiofibular syndesmosis (anterior and posterior tibiofibular ligaments, see also Fig. 7.**201**), or the therapeutic restoration of that integrity, is the key criterion for a favorable outcome of malleolar fractures. If this syndesmosis is destroyed by a fracture-dislocation or is inadequately restored by treatment, the likely outcome is talocrural osteoarthritis with valgus deformity.

Weber classification of fractures of the fibula and medial malleolus with ligament tears

> **Weber classification**
> ➤ *Type A:* Fracture of the lateral malleolus below the tibiofibular syndesmosis. Type A may be associated with a medial malleolar fracture but not with injury to the syndesmosis, interosseous membrane, or deltoid ligament.
> ➤ *Type B:* Fracture of the fibula at the syndesmosis. Type B may be associated with a medial malleolar fracture or deltoid ligament tear (in which case the medial malleolus is intact).
> ➤ *Type C:* Fracture of the fibula above the syndesmosis. The fracture can be located proximally until the fibular neck. In type C there may be either a medial malleolar fracture or deltoid ligament tear, and there may be a rupture of the interosseous membrane. The syndesmosis is always ruptured. If a medial malleolar fracture is present, the fibula should be imaged up to the fibular head to exclude a Weber type C fracture. This type of fracture is also called a Maisonneuve fracture.

While nondisplaced Weber type A and B fractures are managed conservatively, type C fractures basically require operative treatment.

A **fracture of the posterior tibial margin** (i.e., a fracture of Volkmann's triangle) and an **anterior tibial fracture** (tubercle of Chaput) may be associated injuries that accompany a Weber type B or C fracture. They rarely occur in isolation, however (Figs. 7.**199 b**, 7.**200**).

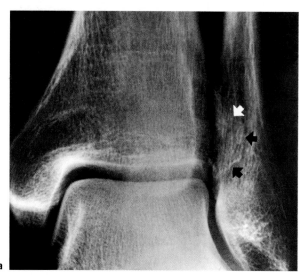

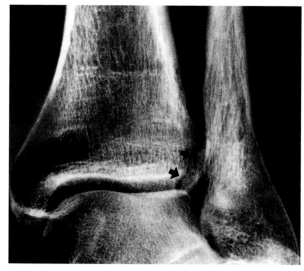

Fig. 7.**200 a, b**   Fracture of the anterolateral tibial triangle (tubercle of Chaput) as an isolated injury. Only the view in strong internal rotation clearly defines the true fracture line (arrows in **b**). The standard view (**a**) shows only the relatively far lateral projection of the bony triangle. The black line bordering the medial aspect of the fibula is a Mach effect, not a fracture line.

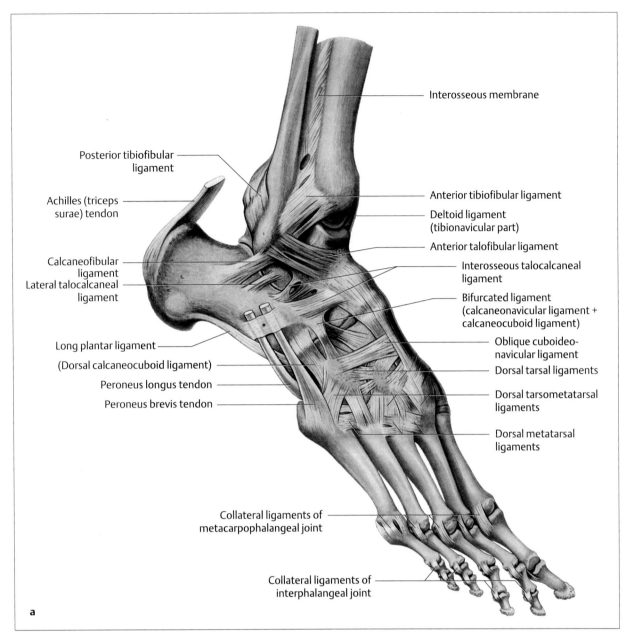

Interosseous membrane

Posterior tibiofibular ligament

Achilles (triceps surae) tendon

Anterior tibiofibular ligament

Deltoid ligament (tibionavicular part)

Anterior talofibular ligament

Calcaneofibular ligament
Lateral talocalcaneal ligament

Interosseous talocalcaneal ligament

Bifurcated ligament (calcaneonavicular ligament + calcaneocuboid ligament)

Long plantar ligament

Oblique cuboideo-navicular ligament

(Dorsal calcaneocuboid ligament)

Dorsal tarsal ligaments

Peroneus longus tendon

Dorsal tarsometatarsal ligaments

Peroneus brevis tendon

Dorsal metatarsal ligaments

Collateral ligaments of metacarpophalangeal joint

Collateral ligaments of interphalangeal joint

a

Fig. 7.**201 a–g**   Talocrural (ankle) joint and talocalcaneal joint.
a–d   Anatomy of the ligaments of the talocrural joint and tarsus (after Wolf-Heidegger).

* in **a**:   inferior peroneal retinaculum
* in **d**:   talar articular surface for calcaneonavicular ligament
** in **d**:   tibialis anterior tendon

Fig. 7.**201 b, c** ▷

All bony injuries mainly require differentiation from accessory bone elements and ossification variants like those shown in Figs. 7.**185**–7.**193** and 7.**198**.

Stress radiographs are not the only important study in the diagnosis of ligamentous ankle injuries. MRI has also become a very valuable tool in equivocal cases (Marder 1994, Breitenseher et al. 1997). This requires a very precise knowledge of the ligamentous anatomy of the ankle region, however (Fig. 7.**201**).

The ligaments have very low signal intensity on both T1- and T2-weighted images. They have smooth margins and contrast sharply with the periligamentous fatty tissue (Fig. 7.**201 f, g**).

Only the posterior fibulotalar ligament, which has a triangular configuration, contains streaks of fatty deposits, and these should not be mistaken for tears on T1-weighted images.

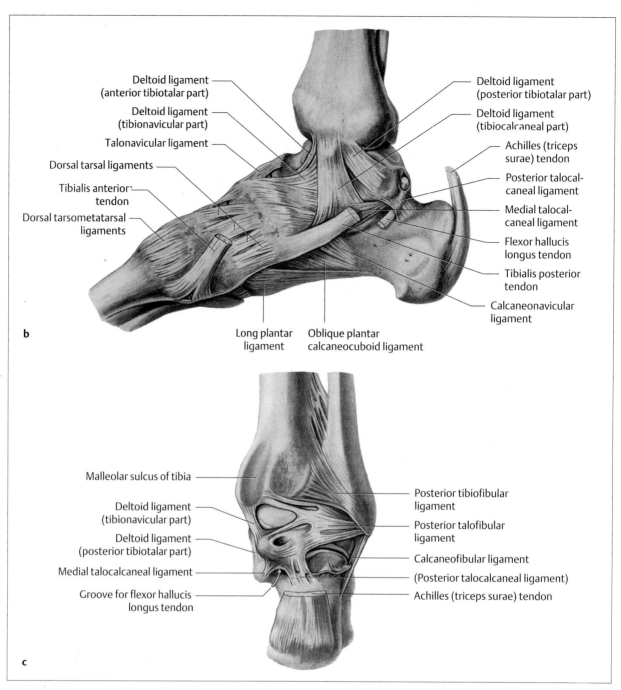

b

Deltoid ligament (anterior tibiotalar part)

Deltoid ligament (tibionavicular part)

Talonavicular ligament

Dorsal tarsal ligaments

Tibialis anterior tendon

Dorsal tarsometatarsal ligaments

Deltoid ligament (posterior tibiotalar part)

Deltoid ligament (tibiocalcaneal part)

Achilles (triceps surae) tendon

Posterior talocalcaneal ligament

Medial talocalcaneal ligament

Flexor hallucis longus tendon

Tibialis posterior tendon

Calcaneonavicular ligament

Long plantar ligament

Oblique plantar calcaneocuboid ligament

c

Malleolar sulcus of tibia

Deltoid ligament (tibionavicular part)

Deltoid ligament (posterior tibiotalar part)

Medial talocalcaneal ligament

Groove for flexor hallucis longus tendon

Posterior tibiofibular ligament

Posterior talofibular ligament

Calcaneofibular ligament

(Posterior talocalcaneal ligament)

Achilles (triceps surae) tendon

Fig. 7.**201 b, c**

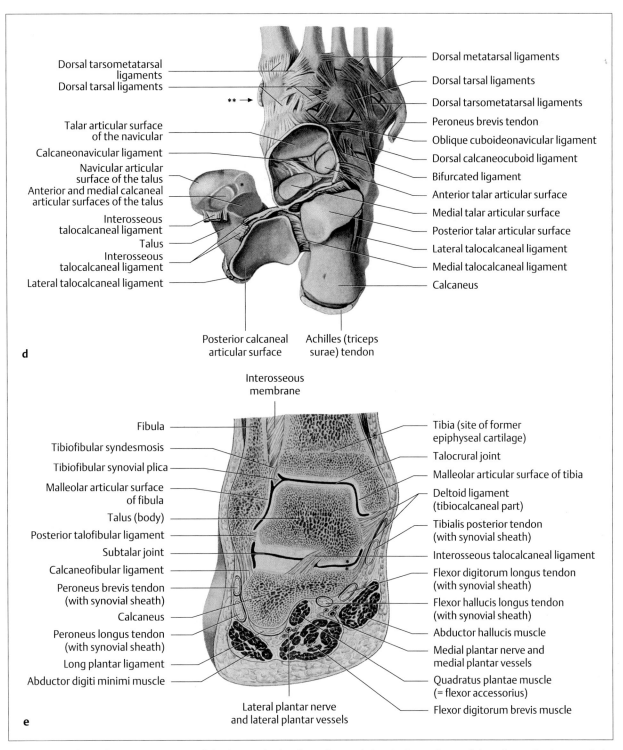

d

Dorsal tarsometatarsal ligaments

Dorsal tarsal ligaments

** →

Talar articular surface of the navicular

Calcaneonavicular ligament

Navicular articular surface of the talus

Anterior and medial calcaneal articular surfaces of the talus

Interosseous talocalcaneal ligament

Talus

Interosseous talocalcaneal ligament

Lateral talocalcaneal ligament

Dorsal metatarsal ligaments

Dorsal tarsal ligaments

Dorsal tarsometatarsal ligaments

Peroneus brevis tendon

Oblique cuboideonavicular ligament

Dorsal calcaneocuboid ligament

Bifurcated ligament

Anterior talar articular surface

Medial talar articular surface

Posterior talar articular surface

Lateral talocalcaneal ligament

Medial talocalcaneal ligament

Calcaneus

Posterior calcaneal articular surface

Achilles (triceps surae) tendon

Interosseous membrane

Fibula

Tibiofibular syndesmosis

Tibiofibular synovial plica

Malleolar articular surface of fibula

Talus (body)

Posterior talofibular ligament

Subtalar joint

Calcaneofibular ligament

Peroneus brevis tendon (with synovial sheath)

Calcaneus

Peroneus longus tendon (with synovial sheath)

Long plantar ligament

Abductor digiti minimi muscle

Tibia (site of former epiphyseal cartilage)

Talocrural joint

Malleolar articular surface of tibia

Deltoid ligament (tibiocalcaneal part)

Tibialis posterior tendon (with synovial sheath)

Interosseous talocalcaneal ligament

Flexor digitorum longus tendon (with synovial sheath)

Flexor hallucis longus tendon (with synovial sheath)

Abductor hallucis muscle

Medial plantar nerve and medial plantar vessels

Quadratus plantae muscle (= flexor accessorius)

Flexor digitorum brevis muscle

Lateral plantar nerve and lateral plantar vessels

e

Fig. 7.**201 e** Coronal anatomic section of the foot at the level of the talocrural joint and both parts of the talocalcaneal joint (subtalar joint and talocalcaneonavicular joint).

* Medial articular surfaces of the talus and calcaneus (talocalcaneonavicular joint).

Fig. 7.**201 f, g** ▷

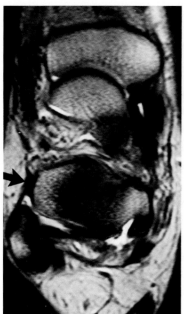
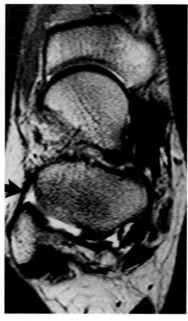

Fig. 7.**201 f, g**   Axial MRI demonstrating the anterior fibulotalar ligament (arrow).

 Inflammation?

Early inflammatory changes in the distal tibial metaphysis due to osteomyelitis are difficult to diagnose on conventional radiographs. The diagnostic strategy is the same as that applied in other metaphyseal regions that are predisposed to osteomyelitis: the early use of ultrasound and MRI. Gross destructive changes and accompanying periosteal reactions, like those shown in Fig. 7.**202**, should no longer occur today. This type of condition usually develops along the lines of chronic osteomyelitis.

The distal tibial metaphysis is not an uncommon site of involvement by chronic recurrent multifocal osteomyelitis.

 Tumor?

Cortical irregularities and **fibrous metaphyseal defects** (fibrous cortical defect and nonossifying fibroma) are relatively common in the distal tibial metaphysis (third most frequent site of occurrence; Figs. 7.**170**, 7.**203**).

They occur predominantly in the posterolateral aspect of the tibial metaphysis, which is subject to the greatest mechanical stresses. These lesions can be confidently identified on radiographs (see also the chapters on the distal femur and proximal tibia, p. 888 ff. and p. 929). **Intraosseous ganglia** (Fig. 7.**204**) typically occur below the medial subchondral plate of the tibia. They correspond to a Lodwick grade IA or IB lesion.

The ganglia have CT attenuation values in the range of 20–30 Hounsfield units, and they show uniform high signal intensity on T2-weighted MRI.

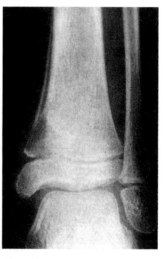

Fig. 7.**202**   Advanced osteomyelitis at an unusual location, with partial destruction of the tibial metaphysis and an accompanying periosteal reaction.

 Other Changes?

Synovial chondromatosis of the talocrural joint is relatively rare. One case is illustrated in Fig. 7.**205**.

Fig. 7.**203a, b** Typical fibrous cortical defect on the posterolateral border of the distal tibia. This is a normal variant, not an aggressive tumor.

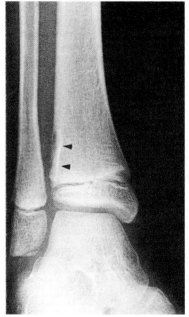

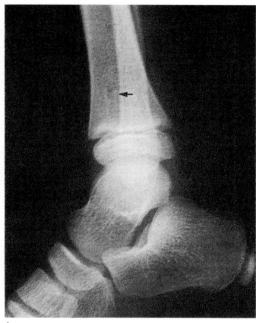

a

b

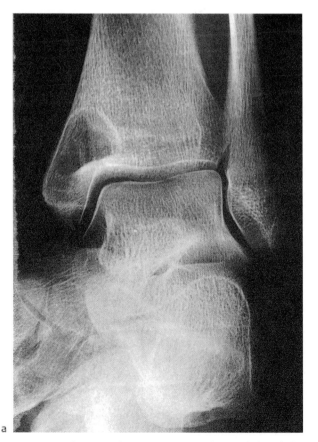

a

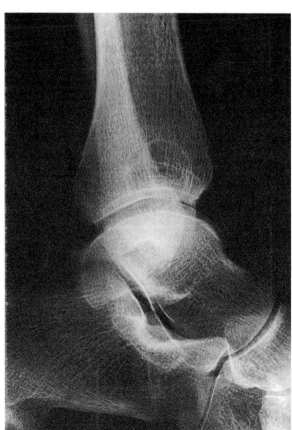

b

Fig. 7.**204a, b** Typical intraosseous ganglion (subchondral synovial cyst) of the distal tibia.

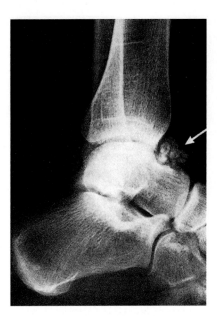

Fig. 7.**205**   Synovial chondromatosis of the talocrural joint.

References

Breitenseher M. J., S. Trattning, C. Kukla et al.: MRI versus lateral stress radiography in acute lateral ankle ligament injuries. J. Comput. assist. Tomogr. 21 (1997) 280

Buschmeyer, R., D. Moschinski: Die isolierte Fraktur der hinteren distalen Tibiakante, des sogenannten hinteren „Volkmann-Dreieckes". Unfallheilkunde 87 (1984) 474

Cone, R. D.: Triplane fractures of the distal tibial epiphysis: radiographic and CT studies. Radiology 153 (1984) 763

Dias, L. S.: Valgus deformity of the ankle joint: pathogenesis of fibular shortening. J. pediat. Orthop. 5 (1985) 176

Dias, L. S., C. R. Giegerich: Fractures of the distal tibial epiphysis in adolescence. J. Bone Jt Surg. 65-A (1983) 438

Ehara, S., Y. Tamakawa, J. Nishida et al.: Cortical defect of the distal fibula: variant of ossification. Radiology 197 (1995) 447

Ehrensberger, J.: Die fibularen Bandverletzungen am Sprunggelenk des Kindes und des Jugendlichen. Ther. Umsch. 40 (1983) 989

Freyschmidt, J., D. Saure, G. Suren et al.: Radiologische Diagnostik von Epiphysenverletzungen im Kindesalter. Röntgen-Bl. 30 (1977) 309

Fröhlich, H., L. Gotzen, U. Adam: Experimentelle Untersuchungen zur Wertigkeit der in zwei Ebenen gehaltenen Aufnahmen des oberen Sprunggelenkes. Unfallheilkunde 87 (1984) 256

Goergen, Th. G., L. A. Danzig, D. Resnick et al.: Roentgenographic evaluation of the tibia-talar joint. J. Bone Jt Surg. 59-A (1977) 874

Griffith, H., G. Wandtke: Tibiotalar tilt — A new slant. Skelet. Radiol. 6 (1981) 193

Jend, H. H., M. Daase, M. Haller et al.: Zur Diagnose von Bandverletzungen des oberen Sprunggelenks mit gedrückten Aufnahmen. Fortschr. Röntgenstr. 139 (1984) 540

Kärrholm, J., L. I. Hansson, K. Svensson: Prediction of growth pattern after ankle-fractures in children. J. pediat. Orthop. 3 (1983) 319

Keats, Th. E., R. B. Harrison: The calcaneal nutrient-foramen: a useful sign in the differentiation of true from simulated cysts. Skelet. Radiol. 3 (1979) 239

Marder, R.: Current methods for the evaluation of ankle ligament injuries. J. Bone Jt Surg. 76-A (1994) 1103

Rumpold, H. J.: Ungewöhnliche Nebenkerne am inneren und äußeren Knöchel. Fortschr. Röntgenstr. 102 (1965) 709

Salter, R. B., W. R. Harris: Injuries involving the epiphyseal plate. J. Bone Jt Surg. 45-A (1963) 587

Synnolt, J.L., O.C. Barry: Bilateral stress fractures of the fused lower fibular epiphysis. Irish J. med. Sci. 153 (1984) 252

Teichert, G.: Os talotibiale. Fortschr. Röntgenstr. 83 (1955) 734

Weber, B., G.: Die Verletzungen des oberen Sprunggelenkes. Huber, Bern 1972

Foot

General Aspects

▌ Normal Findings

Standard plain-film radiography of the foot includes the following views:

- Dorsoplantar view of the forefoot
- Plantodorsal oblique view of the foot
- Tibiofibular lateral view
- AP view of the ankle joint with 20° internal rotation of the leg

CT should be used for all equivocal findings, especially in the tarsal and tarsometatarsal regions.

When radiographs are interpreted, close attention should be given to the relationship of the individual bones of the foot to one another. This interrelationship is of great importance for the load capacity and for any clinical symptoms that may arise. Normally the foot has a **longitudinal arch** and a **transverse arch**.

A tangent to the inferior cortex of the calcaneus forms a 20° angle with the floor. Extending that line to the metatarsus intersects the tangent to the plantar cortex of the first metatarsal. Both tangents together form the **medial longitudinal arch** (Fig. 7.**206**).

The medial longitudinal arch is already present in newborns. Fat pads are present to protect the foot from excessive loads during early walking, but they regress during the first two years of life. Growth of the calcaneus superiorly (and posteriorly) leads to an elevation of the calcaneocuboid joint, the talus, and thus of the talonavicular joint.

The height of the medial longitudinal arch is 2 mm at 3 years of age and increases by 1 mm during the next year. There is a slight further increase until age 6 and an even smaller increase thereafter.

Girls have a higher medial longitudinal arch than boys (Schilling 1985).

The counterpart to the medial longitudinal arch is the **lateral longitudinal arch**. It is flatter and follows the tangent to the cortex of the fifth metatarsal bone (Fig. 7.**206**). This arch has its greatest convexity at the cuboid bone.

The **transverse arch** of the foot is best represented by the line of the metatarsal bones viewed in cross section (Fig. 7.**207**).

The following angles are important:

- **Talocalcaneal angle** (Fig. 7.**208**). Formed by the axes of the talus and calcaneus, it averages approximately 30° in both the dorsoplantar and lateral projections.
- The **tibiocalcaneal angle** (Fig. 7.**209**) averages approximately 18°.
- The **calcaneal-first metatarsal angle** (Fig. 7.**210**) averages 22°.
- The **tibiotalar angle** (Fig. 7.**211**) averages 18° in the AP projection and 110° in the lateral projection.
- The **talar-first metatarsal angle** (Fig. 7.**212**) averages approximately 3°.

These angles are important in the diagnosis of clubfoot. They can also be helpful in other investigations.

The cuboid sign and Y sign of LeNoir are shown in Figs. 7.**213** and 7.**214**.

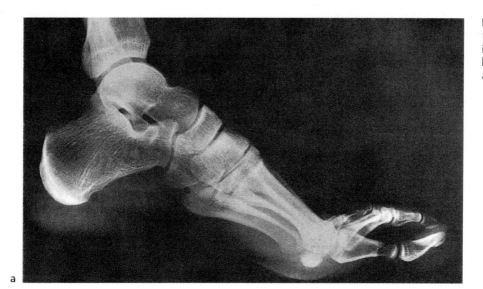

a

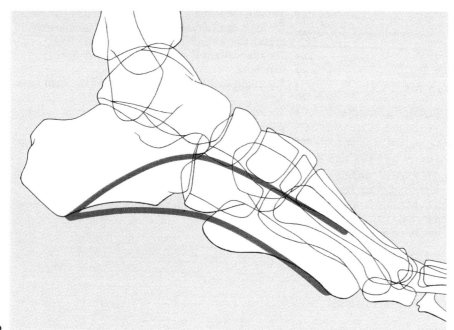

b

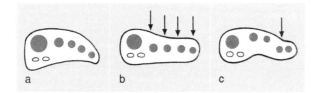

Fig. 7.**207 a–c** Cross section through the metatarsal bones.
a Normal transverse arch.
b Flattened arch in splayfoot.
c Localized plantar position of the fourth metatarsal with consecutive localized depression of the transverse arch.

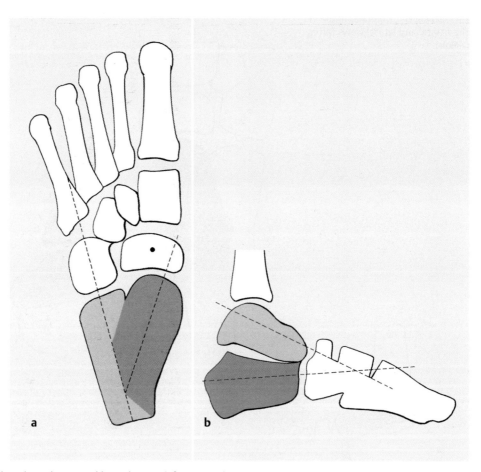

Fig. 7.**208 a, b**   Talocalcaneal angle in the AP and lateral views (after LeNoir).

Fig. 7.**209**   Tibiocalcaneal angle (after LeNoir).

Fig. 7.**210**   Calcaneal-first metatarsal angle (after LeNoir).

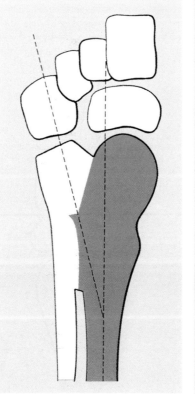

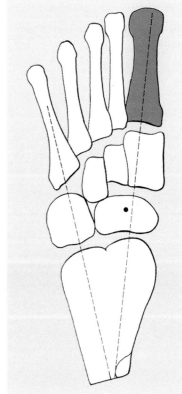

Fig. 7.**209**

Fig. 7.**210**

Fig. 7.**211 a, b**   Tibiotalar angle in the frontal and lateral views (after LeNoir).

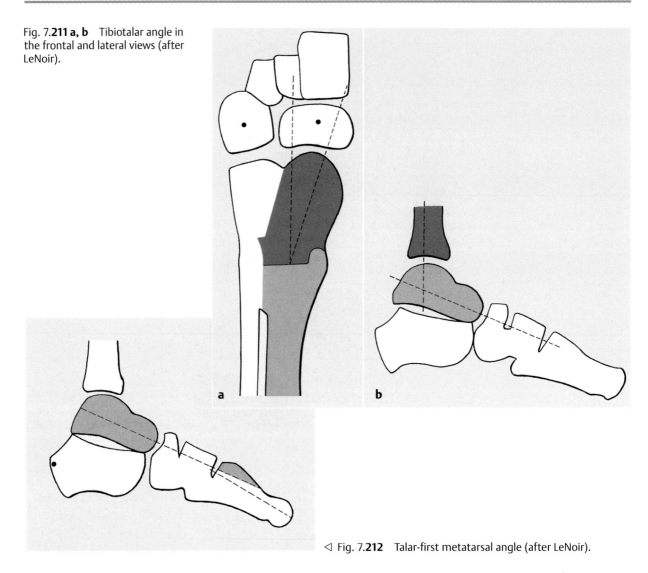

◁ Fig. 7.**212**   Talar-first metatarsal angle (after LeNoir).

Fig. 7.**213 a, b**   Cuboid sign (after LeNoir).

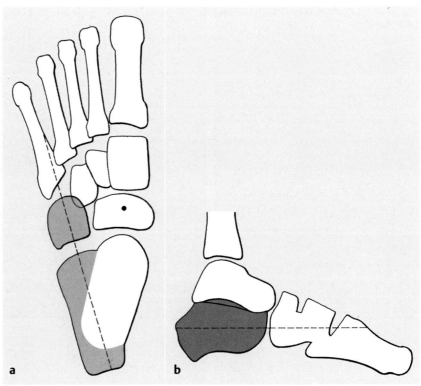

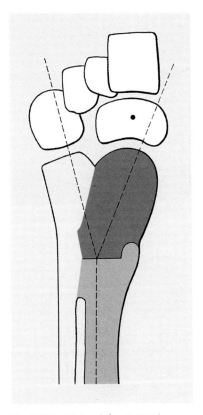

Fig. 7.**214**   Y sign (after LeNoir).

Pathological Finding?

Variants?

The classification of accessory skeletal elements in the foot was first attempted by Pfitzner (1896) (Fig. 7.**215**). Since then it has been modified by numerous authors, including Zimmer, one of the original authors of this book. His classification is shown in Figs. 7.**126**–7.**218**.

Basically, we have the same attitude toward the nomenclature of accessory bones in the foot as in the hand.

> The essential point is this: The reader of the radiograph must be able to recognize an accessory bone as such, regardless of what it is called.

Actually it is enough to give a simple description such as "an accessory bone lateral to the cuboid." As a general rule, an element should be interpreted as an accessory bone if it is asymptomatic and detected incidentally. An accessory bone is generally composed of normal spongiosa surrounded by a thin cortical shell. It does not fit into a matching defect in an adjacent bone. If there is a matching defect, the element may represent an old bony avulsion. With a fresh avulsion, the fracture site lacks coverage by cortical bone. The drawings in Fig. 7.**219** can help differentiate fractures from accessory bones by illustrating bony injuries of the foot that are commonly missed.

It should be noted that accessory bones can have pathological effects on the foot; for example, a bone that interferes with normal pedal motion may incite inflammatory changes in an adjacent tendon. Most such cases involve a local activation of bone turnover in the accessory bore, resulting in focal increased uptake on radionuclide scans. It may be necessary to consider surgical removal of the offending bone. Accessory bones may also become necrotic, again resulting in a positive radionuclide scan. MRI in the early stages reveals edema (Miller et al. 1995).

The following terms and synonyms for accessory bones may be found in the literature:

- About the talus:
  - Os subtibiale = talus accessorius
  - Os trigonum = talus secondarius = talus accessorius = os intermedium
  - Os supratalare = os supertalare = astragalus secondarius (incorrectly called "Pirie's bone")
- About the calcaneus:
  - Os subcalcis = os tuberis calcanei
  - Os subtrochleare calcanei = calcaneus accessorius
  - Calcaneus secondarius = secondary os calcis
- About the navicular:
  - Trochlear process of navicular = dorsal astragaloscaphoid ossicle = intertaloscaphoid = dorsal talonavicular ossicle
  - Os infranaviculare = os naviculocuneiforme I dorsale
  - Os tibiale externum = accessory navicular = os navicular secundarium = sesamoid bone = accessory tarsal scaphoid
- About the cuboid:
  - Os peroneum = cuboideum accessorium

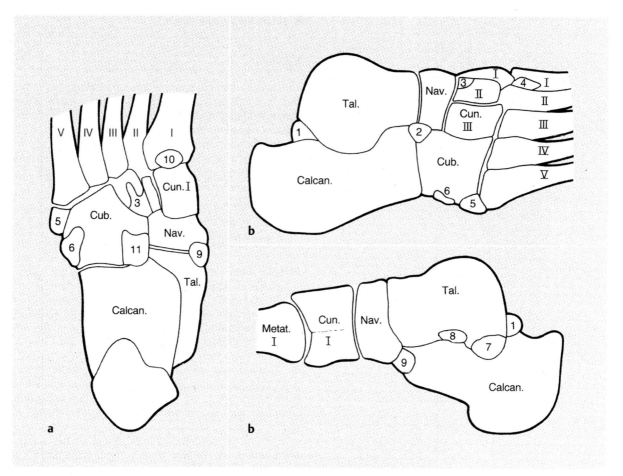

Fig. 7.**215 a–c**   Nomenclature of accessory bones in the foot (after Pfitzner).
a Superior view.
b Lateral view.
c Medial view.
 1 Trigonum (os intermedium cruris)
 2 Calcaneus secondarius
 3 Intercuneiform
 4 Intermetatarsal
 5 Os vesalianum
 6 Os peroneum
 7 Accessory talus
 8 Sustentaculum
 9 Os tibiale externum
10 Pars peronea of first metatarsal
11 Cuboideum secundarium

- About the cuneiforms:
  - Sesamum tibiale anterius = os paracuneiforme = os cuneometatarsale I tibiale = prehallux = pre-cuneiforme
  - Os cuneometatarsale I plantare = pars peronea of first metatarsal
  - Os unci = uncinate process of cuneiform III

Individual accessory bones are discussed under Specific Bones of the Foot.

Fig. 7.**216 a, b** Accessory bony elements of the foot in the lateral projection (after Zimmer).

1 Os talotibiale
2 Os supratalare
3 Avulsion (not an accessory bone)
4 Os supranaviculare
5 Os infranaviculare
6 Os intercuneiforme
7 Os cuneometatarsale II (or possibly os cuneometatarsale I dorsale fibulare)
8 Os intermetatarseum
9 Os unci? Coalition with fourth metatarsal?
10 Accessory bony element on the distal cuboid; migrated os unci?
11 Cuboideum secundarium
12 Calcaneus secundarius
13 Os tibiale externum
14 Trigonum (os talocalcaneare posterius may also be found in this area)
15 Os accessorium supracalcaneum
16 Posterior calcaneal spur (not an accessory bone)
17 Os subcalcis
18 Inferior calcaneal spur (not an accessory bone)
19 Os peroneum
20 Os vesalianum

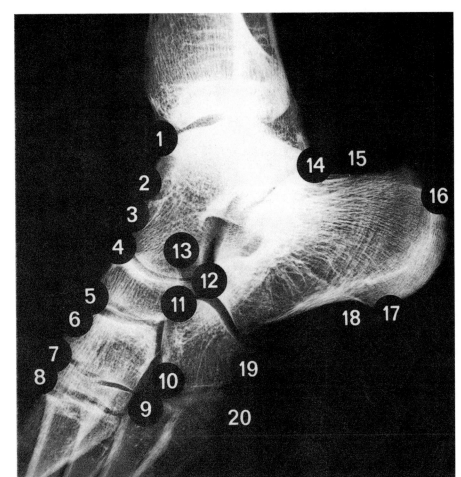

a

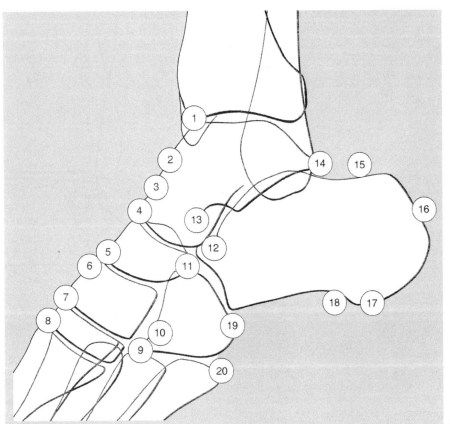

b

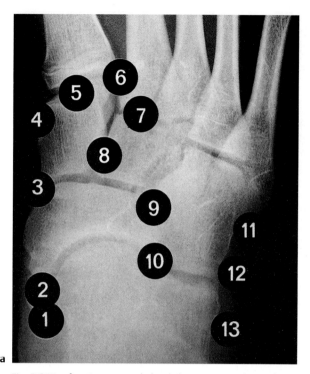
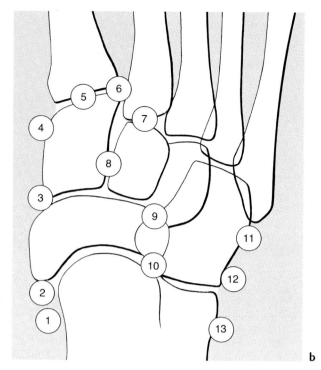

Fig. 7.**217 a, b**   Accessory skeletal elements on a dorsoplantar projection of the tarsus (after Zimmer).

1 Talus accessorius
2 Os tibiale externum
3 Os cuneonaviculare mediale
4 Sesamum tibiale anterius
5 Os cuneometatarseum I plantare
6 Os intermetatarseum
7 Os cuneometatarsale II dorsale
8 Os intercuneiforme
9 Superimposition effect (not an accessory bone)
10 Cuboideum secundarium
11 Os vesalianum
12 Os peroneum
13 Os trochleare calcanei

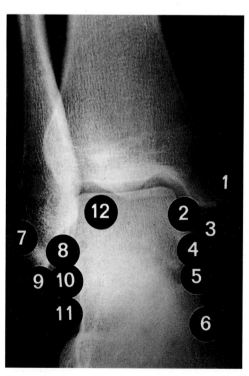
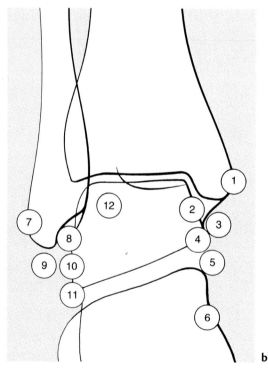

Fig. 7.**218 a, b**   Accessory skeletal elements on an AP projection of the ankle (after Zimmer).

1 Companion shadow on the medial malleolus
2 Sesamoid bone between the medial malleolus and talus
3 Os subtibiale
4 Talus accessorius
5 Os sustentaculi
6 Os tibiale externum
7 Os retinaculi
8 Sesamoid bone between the lateral malleolus and talus
9 Os subfibulare
10 Talus secundarius
11 Os trochleare calcanei
12 Trigonum

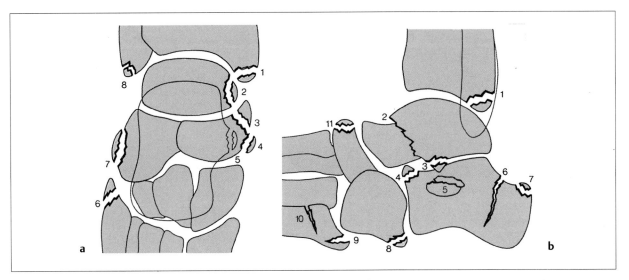

Fig. 7.**219a, b**   Frequently missed bony injuries of the foot (after Zatzkin).
a AP projection.
1   Fracture, tip of medial malleolus
2   Fracture, medial border of talus
3   Os tibiale externum (may be avulsed)
4   Avulsion of medial border of the navicular
5   Fracture, sustentaculum tali
6   Fracture, base of fifth metatarsal
7   Avulsion of lateral border of cuboid
8   Fracture, tip of lateral malleolus

b Lateral projection.
1   Fracture, tip of medial malleolus
2   Fracture, neck of talus
3   Fracture, lateral process of talus
4   Fracture, anterior end of calcaneus
5   Fracture, sustentaculum tali
6   Fracture, body of calcaneus
7   Avulsion fracture, upper part of calcaneus
8   Avulsion fracture, base of cuboid
9   Avulsion of apophysis of fifth metatarsal
10 Transverse fracture, fifth metatarsal
11 Avulsion fracture, dorsum of navicular

 Anomalies?

Synostosis or Coalition of Tarsal Bones

Mild degrees of tarsal synostosis or coalition may still qualify as an extreme normal variant.

In many cases, however, the fusion causes limitation of foot motion and unphysiological loads, resulting in clinical symptoms. This type of anomaly has true pathological significance (O'Rahilley 1953).

The symmetrical occurrence of synostoses is not uncommon. Familial cases have been reported in which tarsal fusions coexisted with symphalangia, short first metacar-

pals, and fusions of the elbow (Fuhrmann et al. 1966, Drawbert et al. 1985). The tarsometatarsal joint and mid-tarsal joint (Lisfranc and Chopart joints) have special significance with regard to foot dislocations and other trauma (Fig. 7.**220b**).

> Tarsal arthritis, which is usually bacterial, can lead to ankylosis. When this type of process occurs during the growth period, the result can be virtually indistinguishable from a congenital coalition.

A coalition in the hindfoot region prevents supination and pronation of the foot. This occurs in talocalcaneal,

Fig. 7.**220a, b**   Synostoses, mediotarsal joint and tarsometatarsal joint.
a Potential sites of synostosis among the tarsal bones (after Mestern).
b Lines of the mediotarsal and tarsometatarsal joints (Chopart and Lisfranc joints).

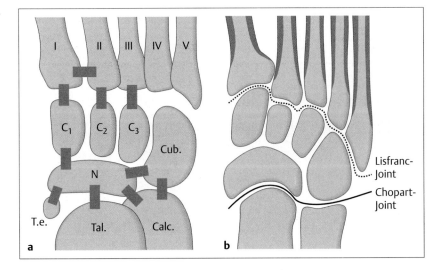

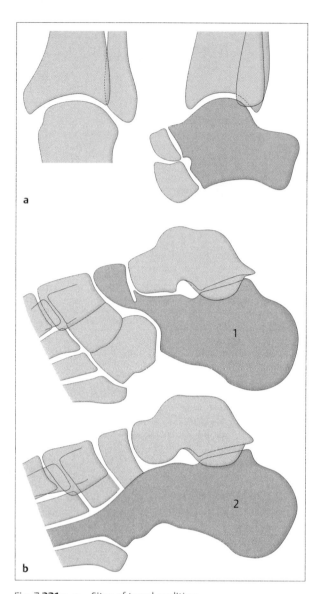

Fig. 7.**221 a–g** Sites of tarsal coalition.
a Talocalcaneal coalition. The fusion has altered the shape of the talocrural joint to a ball-and-socket articulation (see text). **b** Calcaneonavicular coalition (1) and calcaneocuboideal-fourth metatarsal coalition (2). See also calcaneonavicular synostosis, Fig. 7.**295**.

talonavicular, and calcaneocuboid coalitions. One effect of the hindfoot coalition is to transform the **ankle joint** into a **ball-and-socket joint** (Figs. 7.**221 a**, 7.**249**).

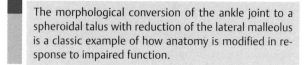

The morphological conversion of the ankle joint to a spheroidal talus with reduction of the lateral malleolus is a classic example of how anatomy is modified in response to impaired function.

Lateur et al. (1994) described a **typical radiographic sign** of **subtalar coalition** in the lateral projection (found in about 1 % of the population). Called the **C sign**, it is an uninterrupted C-shaped line running from the medial border of the talar dome to the inferior outer contour of the sustentaculum tali (Figs. 7.**221 d**, 7.**294**). The authors state that this line may be helpful because classic roentgen signs such as narrowing and subchondral sclerosis of the posterior subtalar joint and absence of the mid-subtalar joint (Fig. 7.**221 e**) and tarsal sinus are often difficult to appreciate on conventional radiographs. Secondary signs such as beaking of the talus (Figs. 7.**230**, 7.**231**), a spheroidal talus (Figs. 7.**221**, 7.**249**), widening of the lateral process of the talus, and a concave inferior surface of the talar neck are known to be nonspecific signs (see p. 1012 for further details). Six years later Brown et al. (2001) found *that the C sign is more specific for flatfoot deformity than subtalar coalition.* They assessed the sensitivity and specifity of the C-sign for patients with both flatfoot deformity and specifically talocalcaneal coalition, using CT as gold-standard method: 10 cases of talocalcaneal coalition were diagnosed, only 4 of which demonstrated a C-sign. Eight cases with a C-sign were encountered, 4 of which had talocalcaneal coalition and 4 did not. All patients with a positive C-sign had a flat foot clinically, while only 8 of 24 flatfooted patients had a C-sign. The authors conclude that *the C-sign is specific, but not sensitive, for flatfoot deformity, and is neither sensitive nor specific for subtalar coalition.* The authors believe that the C-sign is related to a distortion in the normal alignment between the talus and calcaneus, which may or may not be related to the presence of a subtalar bar. Kim (2002) recently commented on the C-sign. More details (classification) about talocalcaneal coalitions are discussed on page 1032.

Calcaneonavicular coalition is of special importance, for when it is associated with a kind of process in the area

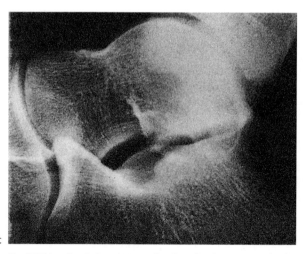

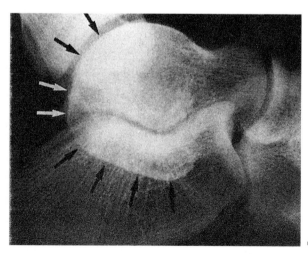

Fig. 7.**221 c, d** C sign. **c** Normal right side. **d** C sign in subtalar coalition on the left side (see text and Fig. 7.**294**). (**c** from Lateur et al. 1994.)

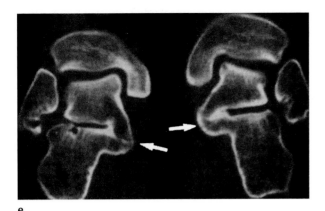

e

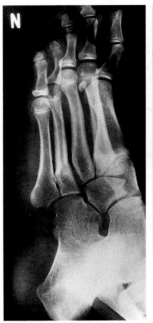 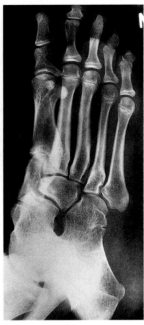

f   g

Fig. 7.**221 e–g**   **e** CT scans of bilateral synostosis of the mid-subtalar joint. Note the horizontal projection of the os sustentaculum and the valgus position of the ossa calcanei. (From Lateur et al. 1994.)
f, g Calcaneocuboid coalition plus fusion of the intermediate and lateral cuneiforms. (Case courtesy of Professor D. Buck-Gramcko, Hamburg; see also Fig. 7.**456**.)

of the calcaneus secondarius or a very well-developed calcaneus secondarius (2 % incidence) and that bone is **fused with the navicular**, it can lead to a planovalgus deformity with limitation of inversion and eversion of the foot. This coalition is clearly visible on oblique radiographs but is best demonstrated by CT (p. 1025 and Fig. 7.**295**).

Hochman and Reed (2000) identified two radiographic features on coronal CT in calcaneonavicular coalition: lateral bridging (an abnormal long mass lateral to the head of the talus) and rounding of the talus.

Talonavicular coalition is very rare (Person and Lembach 1985, Fig. 7.**249**).

Another rare type of fusion is **calcaneocuboid coalition** (Sartoris et al. 1985, Fig. 7.**221 f, g**).

An excellent overview of the CT and MRI features of congenital tarsal coalitions can be found in Newman and Newberg (2000).

Foot Deformities

We cannot detail the great variety of foot deformities that may occur, but the principal deformities are outlined below.

Flatfoot:
Flatfoot (pes planus) results from a congenital or acquired change in the shape of the bony and articular structures combined with ligamentous laxity and muscular insufficiency. It is characterized by a collapse of the plantar vault. Flattening of the longitudinal arch (pes valgus or talipes planus) is often combined with a more horizontal position of the calcaneus and a more vertical position of the talus, as the talar head moves inferiorly and medially. Increased stresses are imposed on the talonavicular joint and surrounding ligaments. Apparently, flatfoot is also associated with a higher frequency of accessory bones such as the os tibiale externum and os supranaviculare. Valgus deformity is also common (Fig. 7.**222**).

Splayfoot (Transverse Flatfoot):
The transverse arch is flattened (Fig. 7.**207**). In some cases the central supports of the transverse arch may sag lower than the two lateral supports. Spreading of the rays is an additional finding, increasing the angle between the longitudinal axes of the calcaneus and first metatarsal bone.

Isolated Sagging of the Head of the Fourth Metatarsal (Fig. 7.**207 c**):
This condition is most easily diagnosed with CT.

Pes cavus:
Pes cavus is the opposite of flatfoot. The calcaneus is tilted steeply upward, the longitudinal arch is heightened, and the forefoot is pronated. In pes calcaneocavus, which results from paralysis of the triceps surae muscle, heel touch-

Fig. 7.**222 a–c**   Pes planovalgus.
a Projecting medial malleolus (1), talar head (2), and navicular tuberosity (3).
b Valgus tilting of the calcaneus.
c Abduction of the forefoot.

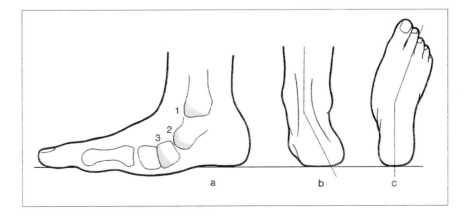

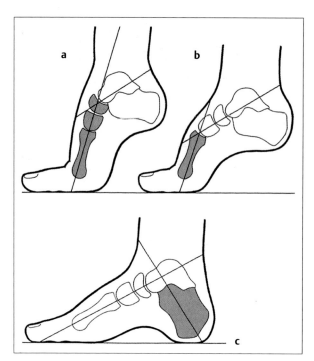

Fig. 7.**223 a–c**   Types of pes cavus.
a, b Anterior pes cavus with a steep first metatarsal and a break at the transverse tarsal joint (**a**) or tarsometatarsal joint (**b**).
c Posterior pes cavus with a steep calcaneus (or occasionally a steep talus).

down occurs on the calcaneal tuberosity (Fig. 7.**223**). Clawing of the toes may also be present. The major cause of pes cavus is muscular paralysis.

Congenital Clubfoot (Congenital Pes equinovarus) (Figs. 7.**224**, 7.**358**):
Congenital clubfoot, the most common foot deformity, has five separate components. Treatment depends on the severity of the components:

- Pes adductus (adduction of the forefoot)
- Pes varus (supination of the heel)
- Pes equinus (due to equinus deformity of the ankle joint)
- Pes cavus (due to equinus deformity in the midtarsal joint)
- External rotation of the ankle mortise

Figure 7.**224** shows the principal lines and angles that are used in evaluating infantile clubfoot on lateral and dorsoplantar stress radiographs with the foot held in a corrected position. The reference lines in the dorsoplantar projection are based on the ossified first metatarsal, as the navicular is not yet ossified in infants.

> But the key factor in determining the extent of clubfoot and assessing the need for surgery is the extent of medial and dorsal subluxation of the navicular bone in relation to the talus.

In particular, if the precise extent of medial subluxation is not recognized and corrected, surgery is likely to have a poor outcome. Simons developed a scoring system based on the relationship between the talus and navicular (Fig. 7.**225**).

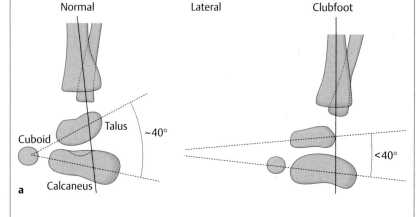

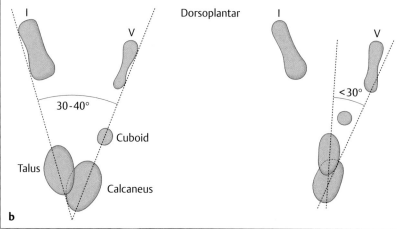

Fig. 7.**224 a, b**   Lines and angles used in the radiographic diagnosis of clubfoot in infants (after Dihlmann). Left = normal, right = clubfoot.
a In the normal lateral radiograph, the longitudinal tibial axis intersects the talus in its posterior third. In clubfoot (right), the talus is anterior to the longitudinal tibial axis. The angle between the longitudinal axes of the talus and calcaneus is approximately 40° in the normal foot and considerably less than 40° in clubfoot. Also, the tarsal sinus cannot be identified in clubfoot.
b In the normal dorsoplantar radiograph, the longitudinal axis of the talus points approximately to the first metatarsal (see also Fig. 7.**225**). In clubfoot (right), this axis is shifted laterally or medially (see also Fig. 7.**225 b**). Moreover, the longitudinal axis of the calcaneus normally passes through the cuboid and runs approximately parallel to the fifth metatarsal. In clubfoot, the axis bypasses the cuboid on the lateral side and intersects the fifth metatarsal. The angle between the longitudinal axis of the talus and calcaneus is normally 30–40°. In clubfoot, it is less than 30°. Additional signs of clubfoot: delayed appearance and reduced size of the ossification centers of the foot. Normally the indentation of the tarsal sinus is visible on lateral radiographs several weeks after birth; it is not visible in clubfoot. Another sign is anterior slipping of the talus over the calcaneus.

Fig. 7.**225 a, b** Simons scoring system for the radiographic grading of clubfoot. Normally the talar axis passes through the center of the base of the first metatarsal (grade 0, see also Fig. 7.**224**). In grade –1 or + 1, the axis is shifted medially or laterally by less than half the width of the base of the first metatarsal; in grade –2 or + 2, by more than half. Grade –1 or + 2 indicates subluxation.
a The navicular is ossified.
b The navicular is not yet ossified.

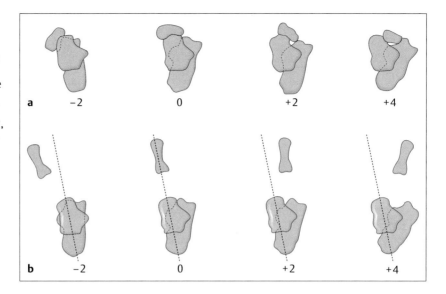

 Simons scoring system: Scores of +2 and –2 denote an axial deviation of the talus by more than half the width of the first metatarsal bone.

This method involves considerable uncertainty, however, including a false-positive rate of 28%. This led O'Connor et al. (1998) to investigate the potential role of MRI, which can demonstrate the unossified navicular. In the 19 clubfeet that were examined, MRI had a sensitivity of 84% in the detection of talonavicular subluxation (vs. 79% for plain radiographs). When used together, both modalities had a sensitivity of 100%.

Soft-Tissue Variants

The **fat triangle (Kager's triangle) in front of the Achilles tendon** may be obscured by inflammatory, traumatic, and neoplastic changes and also by an anatomic variant: the **accessory soleus muscle**. The examiner should be familiar with this variant to avoid errors in diagnosis. MRI is best for establishing the correct diagnosis (Yu and Resnick 1994).

A **low union of the soleus tendon with the gastrocnemius tendon** can mimic an Achilles tendon lesion (Mellado et al. 1998).

References

Azouz, E. M.: Tarsal pseudocoalition. J. Canad. Ass. Radiol. 33 (1982) 105

Brown R. B., Z. S. Rosenberg, B. A. Thornkill: The C sign: more specific for flatfoot deformity than subtalar coalition: Skeletal Radiol. 30 (2001) 84

Dihlmann, W.: Gelenke, Wirbelverbindungen, 2. Aufl. Thieme, Stuttgart 1982

Drawbert, J. P. D. B. Stevens, R. G. Cadle et al.: Tarsal and carpal coalition and symphylangism of the Fuhrmann type. J. Bone Jt Surg. 67-A (1985) 884

Fuhrmann, W., Ch. Steffens, G. Rompe: Dominant erbliche doppelseitige Dysplasie und Synostose des Ellenbogengelenkes. Mit symmetrischer Brachymesophalangie sowie Synostosen im Finger-, Hand- und Fußwurzelbereich. Humangenetik 3 (1966) 64

Hardaker, W. T., S. Margello, L. Goldner: Foot and ankle injuries in theatrical dancers. Foot and Ankle 6 (1985) 59

Hochman, M., M. H. Reed: Features of calcaneonavicular coalition on coronal computed tomography. Skeletal Radiol. 29 (2000) 409

Kim, S. H.: The C-sign. Radiology 223 (2002) 756

Kurz, W., Th. Gündel, H. Hardtmann: Fußwurzelfrakturen im Kindesalter. Zbl. Chir. 109 (1984) 984

Lateur, L. M., L. R. van Hoe, K. V. van Ghillewe et al.: Subtalar coalition: diagnosis with the C sign on lateral radiographs of the ankle. Radiology 193 (1994) 847

Martinez, S., J. E. Herzenberg, J. S. Apple: Computed tomography of the hindfoot. Orthop. Clin. N. Amer. 16 (1985) 481

Mellado, J., Z. S. Rosenberg, J. Beltran: Low incorporation of soleus tendon: a potential diagnostic pitfall on MR imaging. Skelet. Radiol. 27 (1998) 222

Miller, T. T., R. B. Staron, F. Feldman et al.: The symptomatic accessory tarsal navicular bone: assessment with MR imaging. Radiology 195 (1995) 849

Mosier, K. M., M. Asher: Tarsal coalitions and peroneal spastic flatfoot. J. Bone Jt Surg 66-A (1984) 976

Narváez, J. A., J. Narváez, R. Ortega et al.: Painful heel. Radiographics 20 (2000) 333

Newman, J. S., A. H. Newberg: Congenital tarsal coalition: multimodality evaluation with emphasis on CT and MR imaging. Radiographics 20 (2000) 321

O'Connor, P. J., C. F. A. Bos, J. L. Bloem: Tarsal navicular relations in club foot: is there a role for magnetic resonance imaging? Skelet. Radiol 27 (1998) 440

O'Rahilley, R.: A survey of carpal and tarsal anomalies. J. Bone Jt Surg. 35-B (1953) 626

Person, V., L. Lembach: Six cases of tarsal coalition in children aged 4 to 12 years. J. Amer. podiat. med. Ass. 75 (1985) 320

Pfitzner, W.: Beiträge zur Kenntnis des menschlichen Extremitätenskeletts. VII. Die Variationen im Aufbau des Fußskelettes. Schwalbes morphol. Arb. 6 (1896) 245

Resnick, D., C. Pineda, D. Turnell: Widespread osteonecrosis of the foot in systemic lupus erythematosus: Radiographic and gross pathologic correlation. Skelet. Radiol. 13 (1985) 33

Sartoris D. J., D. L. Resnick: Tarsal coalition. Arthr. and Rheuma. 28 (1985) 331

Simons, G. W.: Analytical radiography and the progressive approach in talipes equinovarus. Orthop. Clin. N. Amer. 9 (1978) 187

Simons, G. W.: Complete subtalar release in club feet. J. Bone Jt Surg. 67-A (1985) 1056

Schilling, F. W.: Das mediale Längsgewölbe des Fußes beim Kleinkind. Z. Orthop. 123 (1985) 296

Weber, B.: Multiple symmetrische Synostosen an Hand und Fuß. Arch. orthop. Unfall-Chir. 46 (1954) 277

Yu, J. S., D. Resnick: MR imaging of the accessory soleus muscle appearance in six patients and a review of the literature. Skelet. Radiol 23 (1994) 525

Talus

Normal Findings

 During Growth

The ossification center of the talus becomes visible on radiographs in about the 7th intrauterine month. Occasionally two ossification centers appear. A synonym for the talus is the "astragalus."

A deep notch in the inferior border of the talus, called the subtalar sinus, is commonly found opposite a corresponding groove in the calcaneus in children and adoles-

cents (Fig. 7.**227**). The groove in the calcaneus corresponds anatomically to the **tarsal sinus**. A small pit in the dorsal contour of the pediatric talus, visible in the oblique projection, can mimic a lucent area within the structure of the bone. The posterior process of the talus usually has its own ossification center (Fig. 7.**244c, d**).

 In Adulthood

Figure 7.**226** shows various anatomical views of the talus, demonstrating its complex surface anatomy. It has a total of seven cartilaginous articular surfaces, some of which interconnect.

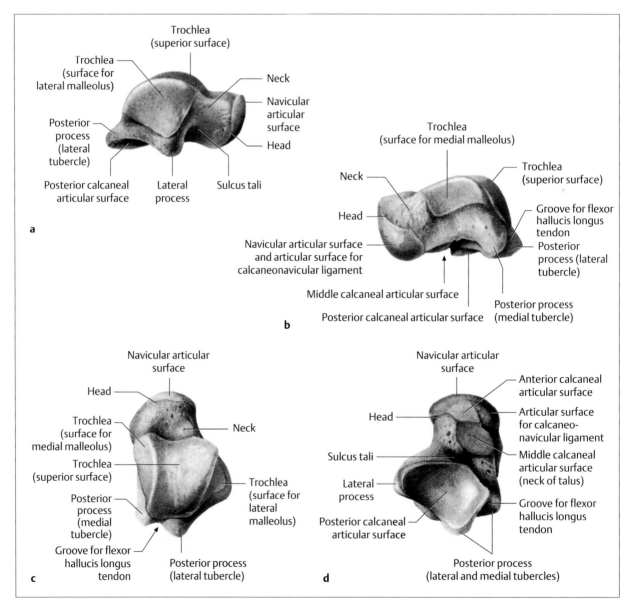

Fig. 7.**226a–d**   Surface anatomy of the talus.
a Lateral aspect.
b Medial aspect.
c Superior (dorsal) aspect.
d Inferior (plantar) aspect.

Two classic radiographic projections of the talus are used:

- AP projection with the lower leg in 20° of internal rotation.
- Lateral projection with the heel raised 20° to compensate for the natural varus position of the calcaneus and to line up the lateral and medial borders of the talar dome.

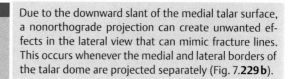

Due to the downward slant of the medial talar surface, a nonorthograde projection can create unwanted effects in the lateral view that can mimic fracture lines. This occurs whenever the medial and lateral borders of the talar dome are projected separately (Fig. 7.**229**b).

The anterior, middle and posterior portions of the subtalar joint are clearly defined in an orthograde projection.

The **curvature of the talar dome** is highly variable in its degree of convexity.

The **neck of the talus** is often quite short, and its dorsal distal portion may appear "crumpled" or beak-shaped (Fig. 7.**230**). The apparent stepoff between the talar neck and the navicular in these cases often disappears on the standing radiograph. As will be explained below in greater detail, a short talar neck with a beak-shaped superior contour can also be a sign of subtalar coalition (Fig. 7.**231**b).

Beaking of the talus should not be confused with a "talar nose," which is a traction osteophyte on the talus (see below and Fig. 7.**231**a).

The inferomedial portion of the talus may appear **rarefied** on AP radiographs, mimicking a pathological finding (Fig. 7.**228**a).

This is a physiological phenomenon based on the normal fatty replacement of cancellous bone, as the CT scans in Fig. 7.**228** clearly demonstrate.

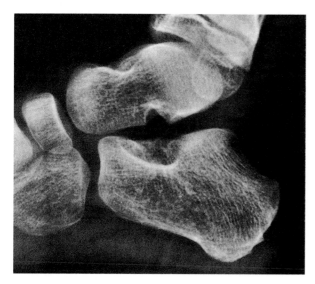

Fig. 7.**227**   Sinus sutalaris.

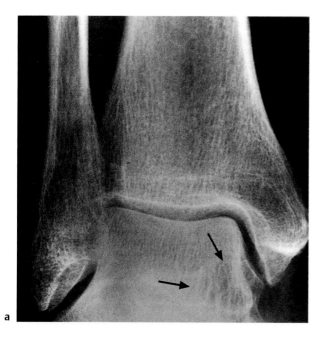

a

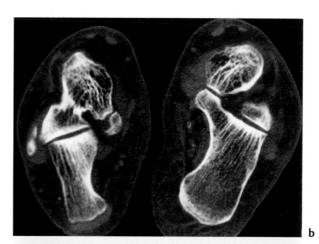

b

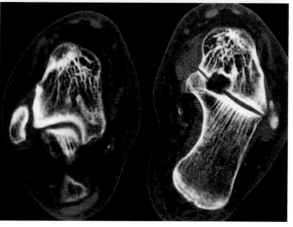

c

Fig. 7.**228**a–c   Rarefied areas of the talus.
a Confusing areas of sparse trabeculae in the medial portion of the talar body, AP projection.
b, c The CT scans show that the trabecular structures in that area are physiologically less dense due to intervening fatty tissue.

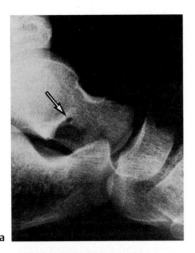

a

A **small nutrient canal** is visible at the junction of the talar dome and neck on lateral radiographs (Fig. 7.**229a**).

On MRI, a **"pseudodefect" in the posterior part of the talus** should not be mistaken for cartilage erosion (Fig. 7.**260a**). It is caused by a normal anatomic groove for the posterior talofibular ligament (Miller et al. 1997).

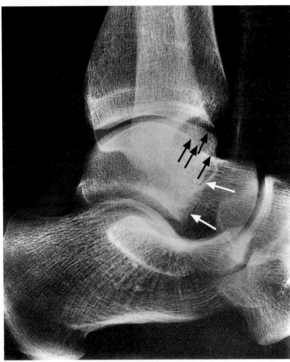

b

Fig. 7.**229a, b**   Radiographic projections of the talus.
a Typical small nutrient canal, viewed end-on, at the center of the talar neck.
b Oblique projection of the trochlear surface of the talus. The borders of the trochlea do not line up as in an orthograde projection, but form double lines with the lateral border uppermost (arrow). The lateral anterior trochlear border appears relatively sharp (white arrows), mimicking a fracture. The three arrows mark the medial border of the trochlea.

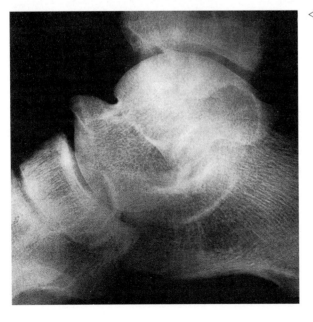

◁ Fig. 7.**230**   Short talar neck with a beak-like anterosuperior configuration (see text).

Pathological Finding?

Normal Variant or Anomaly?

Variants

The **talar nose** mentioned above is an almost physiological feature that we attribute to increased traction on the talus. It does not signify a degenerative process. The talar nose is particularly common in persons who subject the ankle joint to heavy stresses. The talar nose is located on the extensor side of the talus and is more proximal to the distal talar border than the talar beak (Figs. 7.**231**, 7.**232**).

The following accessory bones occur as normal variants about the talus and are not anomalies:

- **Os talotibiale** (Fig. 7.**187 b**).
- **Os supratalare**. This accessory bone is located in the area of the talar nose (Fig. 7.**233**) and may result from metaplastic bone formation in response to the same forces. If the bony shadow has an irregular or shell-like configuration, this usually signifies an avulsion (Fig. 7.**234 a, b**). The talar nose should be distinguished from a degenerative **marginal osteophyte in talonavicular osteoarthritis**. This osteophyte is located directly on the superior articular margin of the talus; it is not separate from it like the talar nose. The presence of an os supratalare may be associated with pain, especially as a result of tight shoes and heavy loads. "**Pirie's bone**" is

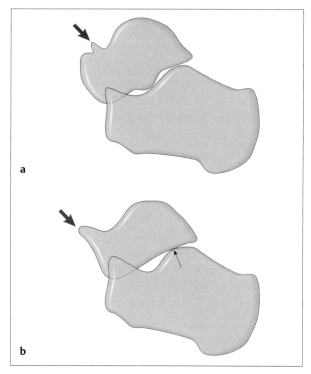

Fig. 7.**231 a, b**   Differentiation of the talar nose (**a**) from beaking of the anterior superior border of the talar neck. The latter configuration is often associated with subtalar coalition (thin arrow in **b**) but is not a definite sign of it. For the C sign of subtalar coalition, see p. 998 and Fig. 7.**221 d**.

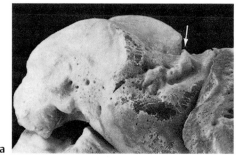

Fig. 7.**232 a–c**   Variable prominence of the talar nose.

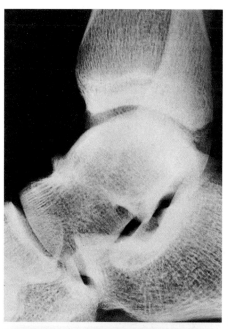

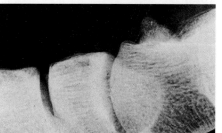

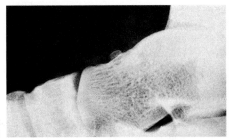

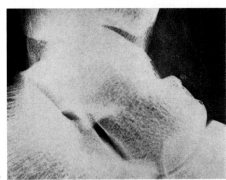

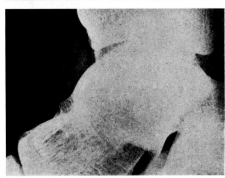

Fig. 7.**233 a–c** Variable prominence of the os supratalare on radiographs. The case shown in **a** presented clinically with pain, probably caused by accompanying tenosynovitis (see text).

sometimes used as a synonym for the os supratalare, but Pirie's bone probably corresponds to the os supranaviculare, as we noted in the previous edition of this book after studying Pirie's original work.

- The **os talocalcaneare posterius** is located at the posterior joint between the talus and calcaneus and is best demonstrated by the Anthonsen view, a projection similar to the oblique view of the ankle mortise. Either this bone is very rare or it is not seen because the Anthonsen projection is very seldom used.

- A common variant is the **os trigonum** (known also by the misleading terms talus secondarius, talus accessorius, and os intermedium tarsi). The anatomic specimens in Fig. 7.**235** clearly demonstrate the location and relationships of this element (see also Fig. 7.**226**). The **posterior process of the talus**, which can vary greatly in prominence among different individuals, consists of a medial tubercle, which is not prominent on radiographs, and a larger lateral tubercle, which is usually more conspicuous. Between the two tubercles is a groove for the flexor hallucis longus tendon. The os trigonum fits into a recess on the fibular side of the lateral tubercle of the posterior process of the talus. It may be duplicated, as the specimen illustrates (labeled Tr and Tc in Fig. 7.**235 a**). The os trigonum also may be fused with the lateral tubercle to form a single process (Fig. 7.**235 b**). Finally, this process may be fused with the talus or may articulate with it. The lateral tubercle and os trigonum vary independently of each other in size and shape. For this reason, the os trigonum cannot be interpreted as an unfused talar posterior process. Figures 7.**236** –7.**238** illustrate the varying radiographic appearance of the os trigonum. The specimen photo in Fig. 7.**235 a** and the radiograph in Fig. 7.**239** show examples of a bipartite or duplicated os trigonum. Less structured bony elements in the area of the os trigonum usually represent heterotopic bone formation due to trauma, as shown in Fig. 7.**240**. Finally, a bony element in this region may be caused by an **avulsion of the talar posterior process**. The fracture mechanism, known also as a Shepherd fracture, involves a pincerlike compression of the posterior process between the posterior tibial border and the calcaneus, which generally is fractured as well. An example is shown in Fig. 7.**241**. The os trigonum may be displaced into the talocrural joint by a hemarthrosis or inflammatory joint effusion (Fig. 7.**242**). Like other accessory bones that interfere

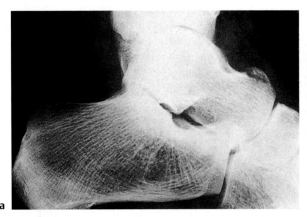

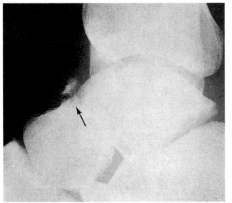

Fig. 7.**234 a, b** Small bony avulsions from the upper talar neck in the area of the talar nose, not to be confused with an accessory bone element (os supratalare).

Fig. 7.**235 a, b**   Specimen photographs illustrate the variable anatomy in the region of the talar posterior process. While a single bony formation is present in **b**, specimen **a** has two separate prominences for the medial tubercle (Tm) and lateral tubercle (Tl) (compare with Fig. 7.**226 b, c**). Between the tubercles is the sulcus for the flexor hallucis longus tendon (S). Two ossa trigoni (Tr, Tc) are seen next to the lateral tubercle.

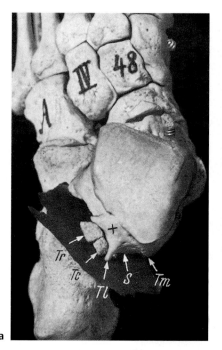
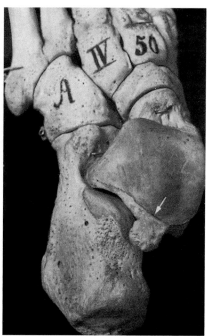

with motion and are themselves affected by that interference, the os trigonum is subject to aseptic necrosis (Fig. 7.**243**). This seems especially likely to occur when the os trigonum rides upon an opposing process arising from the calcaneus (Fig. 7.**244**). The os trigonum also requires differentiation from **articular chondromatosis**, as illustrated in Fig. 7.**245**. The latter condition, however, is usually associated with multiple calcified articular chondromas. The patients are asymptomatic.

Given their "unfortunate" anatomic location, the os trigonum and lateral tubercle may be injured due to heavy mechanical loads (acute forced or repetitive flexion in ballet dancers, soccer players, etc.), resulting in a **posterior ankle impingement syndrome**. Using MRI, Bureau et al. (2000) observed signs of bony contusion in the os trigonum and/or the lateral tubercle, soft-tissue edema, and a number of other changes.

- Another accessory bone is the **os accessorium supracalcaneum**, a unilateral or bilateral bony element located above the calcaneus some distance from the talus (p. 1026, Figs. 7.**280** and 7.**281**).

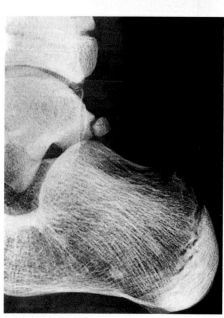

Fig. 7.**236**   Os trigonum in an 8-year-old boy.

Fig. 7.**237 a, b**   Bilateral ossa trigoni, one with two ossification centers, in a 9-year-old boy.

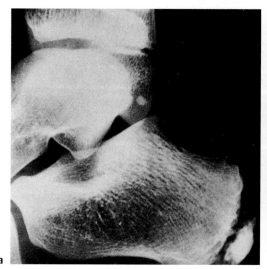
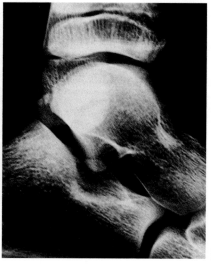

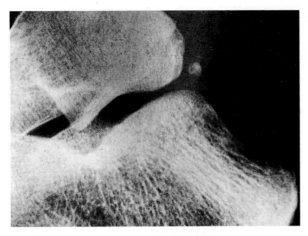

Fig. 7.**238**   Os trigonum in a 14-year-old boy.

- Finally, we call attention to a small bony element located distal to the position of the os tibiale externum. Called the **talus accessorius** by Pfitzner, it is projected next to the inferior border of the medial articular surface of the talus (Fig. 7.**246**). This element may perhaps represent a heterotopic ossification. The radiologist should take time to differentiate this element only in potentially litigious situations. We refer the reader to the unusually large accessory bone in Fig. 7.**247**, which we decided to classify as a talus accessorius. We attribute the partial anterior fusion (see MR image in Fig. 7.**247 b**) to the size of the element. The bony element was detected incidentally (in a posttraumatic examination to rule out a fracture).

- Ossicles similar to the talus accessorius also occur on the lateral side of the talus (**talus secundarius**, Fig. 7.**248**). Differentiation is required from a small avulsion fracture of the fibular process of the talus as well as from an os subfibulare.

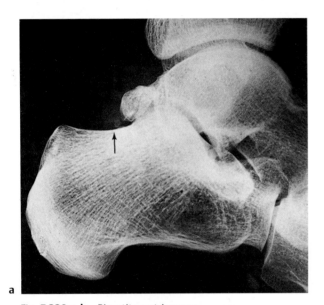
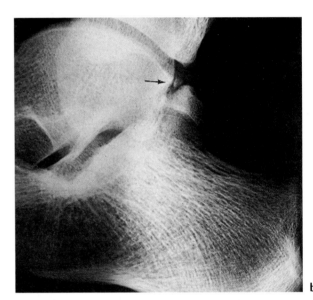

Fig. 7.**239 a, b**   Bipartite os trigonum.

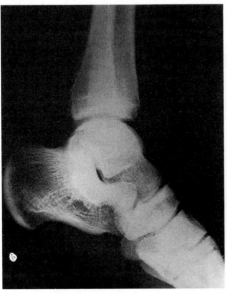
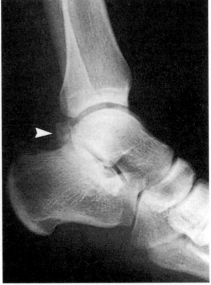

Fig. 7.**240 a, b**   "Acquired" os trigonum.
a Normal-appearing radiograph following a sprain.
b Radiograph two years later after another sprain demonstrates an os trigonum-like heterotopic ossification.

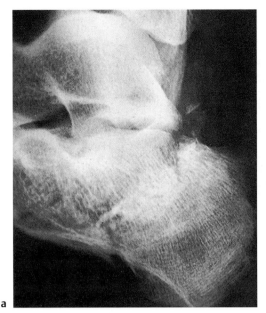
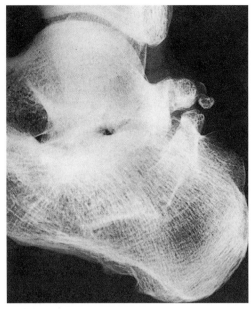

Fig. 7.**241 a, b** Avulsion of the posterior process of the talus with a calcaneal fracture.
a Postinjury radiograph.
b Ten years later.

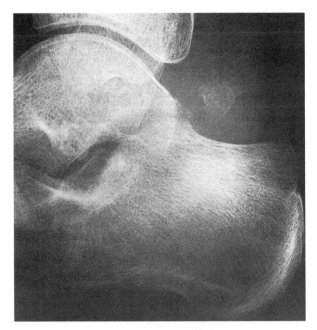

Fig. 7.**242** Tuberculous arthritis in the posterior inferior sub-talar joint. The os trigonum is displaced posteriorly due to effusion.

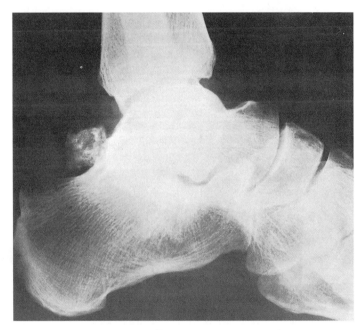

Fig. 7.**243** Aseptic necrosis of an os trigonum. Note the irregular density of the bone and the initial fragmentation.

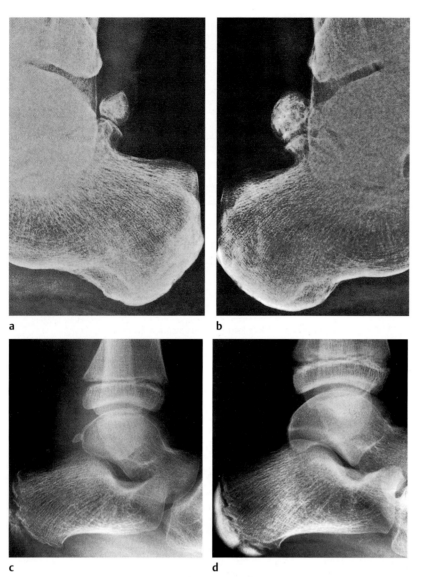

a

b

c

d

Fig. 7.**244 a–d** Bilateral os trigonum and "disappearance" of the os trigonum.
a, b Each accessory bone rides upon an unusual process arising from the calcaneus. Aseptic necrosis of the os trigonum is evident on the left side (**b**).
c, d Disappearance of the os trigonum? These posttraumatic radiographs are from a boy at 10 years of age (**c**) and at 14 years of age (**d**). The small bony element behind the talus is probably an accessory ossification center of the posterior process, which became fully integrated into the talus over the next four years. Another possibility is traumatic necrosis with complete resorption of the necrotic os. (Case courtesy of Dr. C. Füllers, Gevelsberg.)

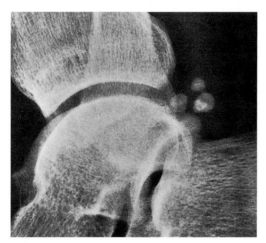

Fig. 7.**245** Synovial chondromatosis with at least three ossified cartilaginous bodies. The element in the angle between the talus and calcaneus may be a fourth cartilaginous body or an os trigonum abutting the bone. Clinically there was pain and swelling on use.

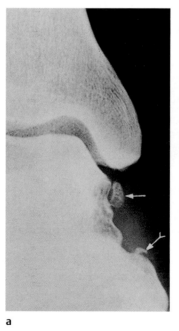

a

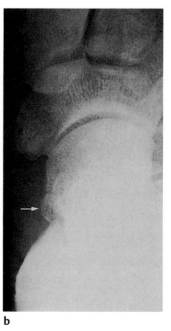

b

Fig. 7.**246 a, b** Talus accessorius (arrow) on the medial border of the talus. Incidental finding: os tibiale externum (double arrow).

Fig. 7.**247 a–c**   Unusually large accessory bone element medial to the right talus in an asymptomatic child. (Case courtesy of Dr. T. Spiro, Bremen.) The accessory bone element, which we classify as a kind of talus accessorius, appears to have both osseous and fibrous contact with the main talus. It is unlikely to be an unusual osteochondroma, because spot films did not show continuous cancellous bone between the talus and the accessory element. Also, the T2-weighted MR images do not show a cartilaginous cap over the accessory bone element. The differential diagnosis also includes an unusual form of Trevor disease (p. 1012).

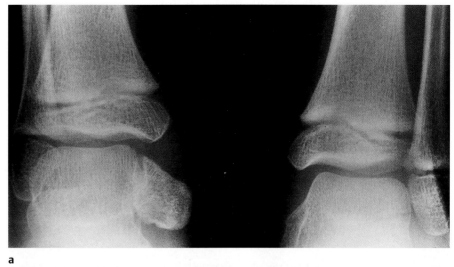

a

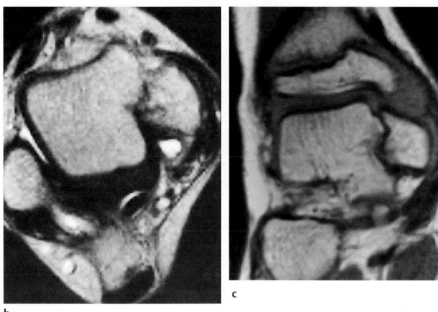

b

c

Deformities

The following are true deformities that can no longer be classified as normal variants:

- Hypoplasia of the talar head and neck with deformity of the navicular, which is sharply tapered on the plantar aspect and prominent on the dorsal and tibial aspects (Bender and Horvath 1961).
- **Congenital vertical talus**, which abuts the navicular on the extensor side, does not appear to be extremely rare. Jacobsen (1983) found 273 cases in the literature and described 11 of his own. The talonavicular joint is displaced downward and medially by the abnormal position of the talus. This creates a planovalgus deformity with a medially convex pedal arch (Robbins 1982).
- A **vertical cleft in the talus** (Fig. 7.**250**) is probably an abortive form of the **classic bipartite talus** (Fig. 7.**251**).
- A **spheroidal talus** must also be considered a true deformity. As explained on p. 998, it can develop as a result of subtalar and talonavicular coalitions (Fig. 7.**249**).

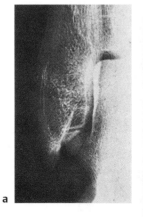

a

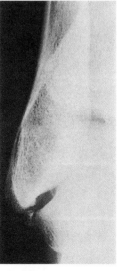

b

Fig. 7.**248 a, b**   Talus secundarius. In theory, the bony element below the fibula could be an os subfibulare, but its proximity to the talus is more consistent with a talus secundarius.

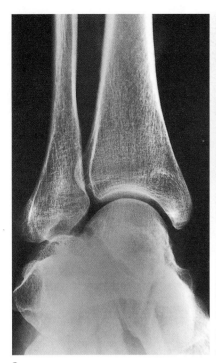
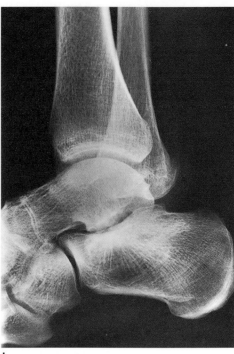

a   b

Fig. 7.**249 a, b**   Spheroidal talus. There is at least partial talonavicular coalition. There appears to be no subtalar coalition, as the C sign is absent (Fig. 7.**221 d**).

- **Dysplasia epiphysealis hemimelica** (Trevor disease) has a certain affinity for the talus (Fig. 7.**252**). It is an symmetrical chondro-osseous hyperplasia associated with pain, swelling, deformity, and synovitis of the affected joint. Other sites of involvement are the epiphyses about the knee and the carpus (Azouz et al. 1985).

- Talonavicular and talocalcaneal **coalitions**, see p. 998 and Figs. 7.**221**, 7.**231**, 7.**294**.

The very rare **posteromedial subtalar coalition** is an incomplete variant of middle facet coalition. McNally (1999) investigated its sectional imaging appearance in three patients.

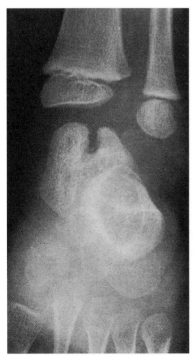

Fig. 7.**250**   Vertical cleft in the talus (see text).

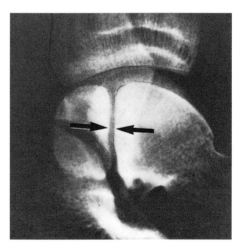

Fig. 7.**251**   Bipartite talus.

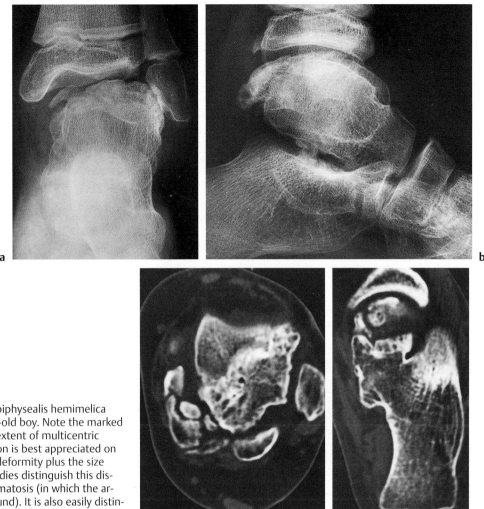

Fig. 7.**252 a–d** Dysplasia epiphysealis hemimelica (Trevor disease) in a 10-year-old boy. Note the marked deformity of the talus. The extent of multicentric chondro-osseous proliferation is best appreciated on CT (**c, d**). The marked talar deformity plus the size and shape of the ossified bodies distinguish this disease from synovial chondromatosis (in which the articular bodies are usually round). It is also easily distinguished from severe osteochondritis dissecans.

Fracture, Subluxation, or Dislocation?

Talar fractures in children are very rare, accounting for just 0.014–0.45% of all fractures. Fracture mechanisms, incidence of necrosis, and treatment of pediatric talar fractures are described fully in Linhart and Höllwarth (1985).

Talar fractures in adults are approximately 10 times more common than in children. About 50% of all talar injuries (fractures, fracture-dislocations, and dislocations) are

fractures, and half of these are avulsion fractures. The rest are vertical or transverse fractures through the body and neck of the talus (Rogers 1982). Vertical fractures more often affect the talar neck than the head. The Hawkins classification is used for talar neck fractures (Fig. 7.**253**).

The mechanism of talar neck fractures was first discovered in World War I pilots who were involved in crash landings. The fracture occurred when the pilot pushed violently on the pedal of the control rudder to avoid a crash. A similar mechanism occurs in automobile accidents when

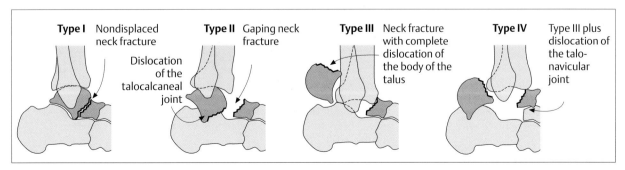

Fig. 7.**253** Hawkins classification of talar neck fractures (after Bohndorf and Imhof).

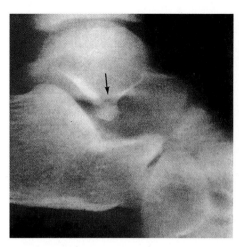

Fig. 7.**254**   Fracture of the fibular process of the talus.

the driver slams his foot on the brake to avoid a head-on collision. With violent dorsiflexion of the foot, the talar neck is caught between the calcaneus and the anterior tibial margin, where it finally fractures.

The main problem with talar neck fractures is **posttraumatic necrosis** (Fig. 7.**257 e**). This results from the vascular supply of the bone. The central and posterior parts of the talus are supplied mainly by plantar vessels from the tarsal sinus and by dorsal vessels that enter the talar neck.

Fractures of the lateral process of the talus account for approximately 24% of all talar fractures. The fibulotalar joint is usually involved (Fig. 7.**254**).

This bony injury has been seen more frequently in recent years due to the growing popularity of **snowboarding**. The mechanism of the fracture involves extreme dorsiflexion and inversion of the talocrural joint. The fracture is easily missed on conventional radiographs, and it may be necessary to utilize CT or MRI (Sanders et al. 1999).

Fractures of the body of the talus include **osteochondral fractures of the talar dome** ("dome fractures"), which are sometimes difficult to detect (Figs. 7.**256**, 7.**277 c**). Often a period of weeks or even months may pass before radio-

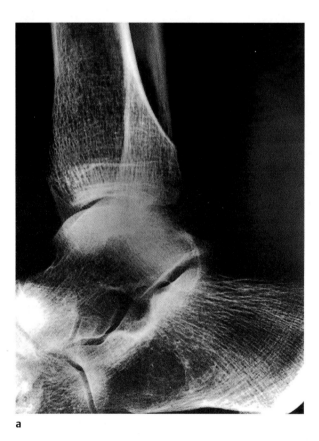

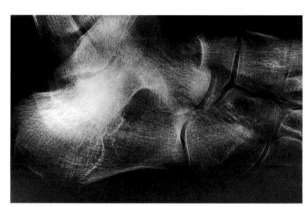

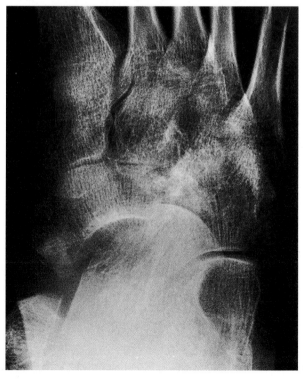

Fig. 7.**255 a–c**   Dislocation of the talonavicular joint missed in the lateral projection (**a**) and oblique projection (**b**). The navicular bone is dislocated medially and shows gross lateral fragmentation.

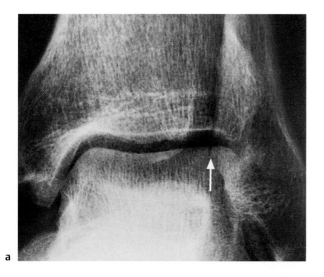

a

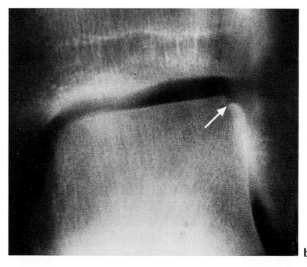

b

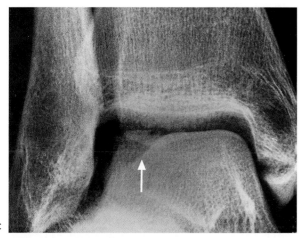

c

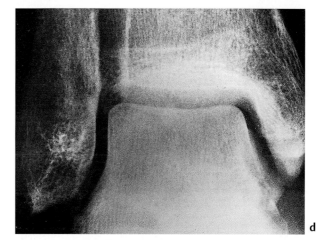

d

Fig. 7.**256 a–d** Osteochondral fractures of the talar dome.
a, b Osteochondral fracture of the lateral talus. The white arrow in **a** (AP radiograph) points to an artifactual black line that passes over the joint space into the distal tibia. The actual fracture is located about 2 mm farther laterally (tomogram in

b). The lateral border of the talar trochlea is displaced inferiorly.
c, d Osteochondral fracture in the lateral talar dome plus a fracture of the medial malleolus. Radiograph **d**, taken one year after **c**, documents complete union of the fractures.

graphic changes appear. This occurs in cases where a kind of osteochondritis dissecans develops from a nondisplaced dome fracture. Osteochondral fractures most often occur on the medial and lateral borders of the talar dome.

A complex fracture-dislocation of the talus is shown in Fig. 7.**255**.

The **tarsal sinus** (sinus tarsi, sinus subtalaris) has special significance in tarsal injuries. The sinus is formed by opposing sulci in the talus and calcaneus (see above) and is traversed by the talocalcanean ligament. Sprains and tears of this ligament can lead to rotatory instability of the posterior subtalar joint (Sharit and Cole 1984). This is characterized on stress radiographs by a combination of anterior displacement, medial offset and slight gaping of the calcaneus relative to the talus, or it can be demonstrated by sectional imaging modalities.

An excellent review of the MRI anatomy of the tarsal sinus and pathologic findings such as tears of the cervical and talocalcaneal ligament can be found in Lektrakul et al. (2001).

Clinical symptoms that are associated with rotatory instability fall under the heading of **tarsal sinus syndrome**. The importance of the tarsal sinus in terms of functional vascular anatomy was mentioned above.

The talar neck is subject to stress fractures, which appear radiographically as vertical zones of increased density. They can be detected much earlier by radionuclide scanning or MRI (though this can be difficult when the dominant finding is edema). Tarsal stress fractures are particularly common in long-distance runners (Campbell and Warnekros 1983).

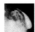 **Necrosis?**

Reference was made earlier to posttraumatic necrosis of the talus (Fig. 7.**257 e**). **Subchondral osteonecrosis** is not particularly rare in the talus (Figs. 7.**257 a–d**, 7.**258**, 7.**259**). The lesions take the form of osteochondritis dissecans (see p. 883 ff. for more details on this disease). Osteochondritis

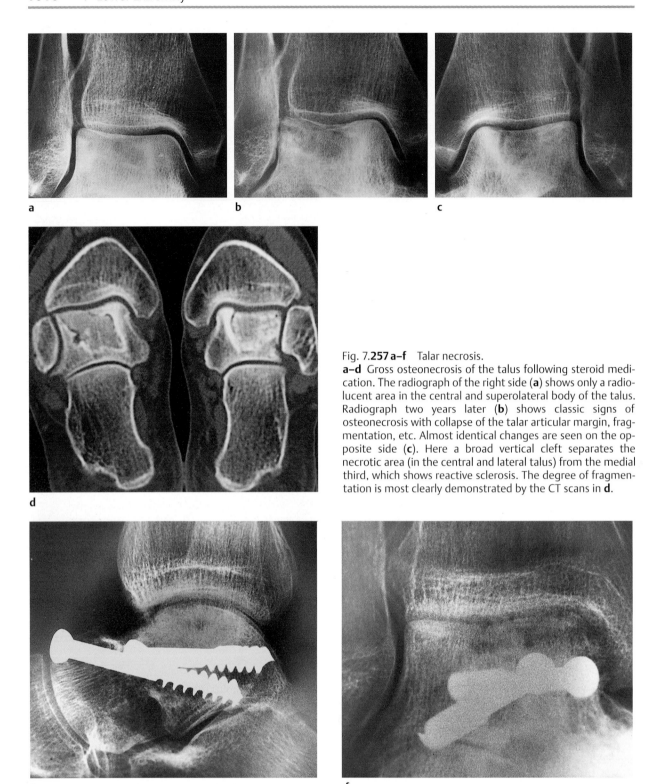

a   b   c

Fig. 7.**257 a–f**   Talar necrosis.
a–d Gross osteonecrosis of the talus following steroid medication. The radiograph of the right side (**a**) shows only a radiolucent area in the central and superolateral body of the talus. Radiograph two years later (**b**) shows classic signs of osteonecrosis with collapse of the talar articular margin, fragmentation, etc. Almost identical changes are seen on the opposite side (**c**). Here a broad vertical cleft separates the necrotic area (in the central and lateral talus) from the medial third, which shows reactive sclerosis. The degree of fragmentation is most clearly demonstrated by the CT scans in **d**.

d

e   f

Fig. 7.**257 e, f**   Complete posttraumatic necrosis of the body of the talus.

dissecans and circumscribed subchondral osteonecrosis are mentioned here only because initial findings may well go undetected on conventional radiographs. In the case shown in Fig. 7.**260**, no bony abnormalities were detected on plain-film examination. It is easy to see how findings like those in Figs. 7.**258** and 7. **259** could develop from these initial changes, that are clearly imaged by MRI.

Fig. 7.**258 a, b** Osteochondritis dissecans of the talus, occurring at a typical site in the medial portion of the bone. The contour over the necrotic area is still intact in **a**, but the later film in **b** shows fragmentation with collapse of the articular margin.

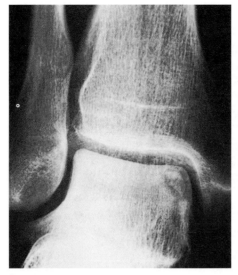
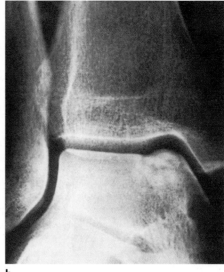

a

b

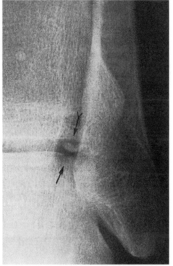
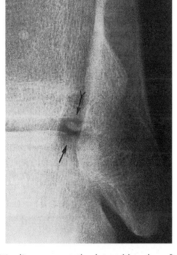

Fig. 7.**259** Osteochondritis dissecans at the lateral border of the talus. (Double arrow points to the osteochondral fragment, single arrow to the "crater.")

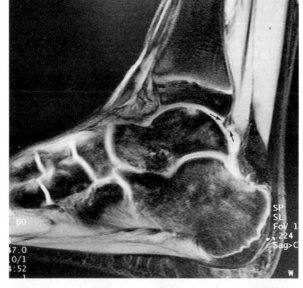

a

Fig. 7.**260 a–c** Subchondral structural change in the talus ▷ with a largely intact subchondral plate and no apparent abnormalities of the overlying articular cartilage (**b, c**) in an 11-year-old child. The mid-talar location of the structural change is somewhat unusual for osteochondritis dissecans. It appears on T2-weighted MRI (**a**) as a circumscribed hyperintense area (edema?). The patient presented with vague ankle pain. The potential for progression to classic osteochondritis dissecans should always be considered in cases of this kind, and the child should be encouraged to rest the affected ankle, preferably by avoiding all sports. This case has another aspect as well: The sagittal image (**a**) reveals a small defect in the talar articular cartilage (between the two arrows). This is a physiological phenomenon caused by the tendon of the posterior talofibular ligament, whose course is easily followed in the images shown here (see text).

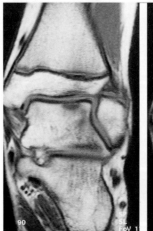
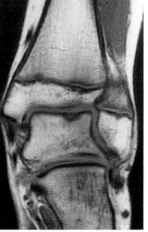

b

c

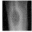 **Inflammation? Tumor?**

Acute hematogenous osteomyelitis in extremely rare in the talus. We have personally observed special forms of osteomyelitis in the talus, such as a **Brodie abscess**.

Osteoid osteoma and **osteoblastoma** are not particularly rare in the talus. In fact, both lesions should be considered at once in the differential diagnosis of talar processes that are associated with new bone formation (Fig. 7.262).

An occasional cause of osteolytic lesions in the talus is a **subchondral synovial cyst** (Fig. 7.261). Also called an intraosseous ganglion, this lesion may develop from small cartilaginous and osseous fissures.

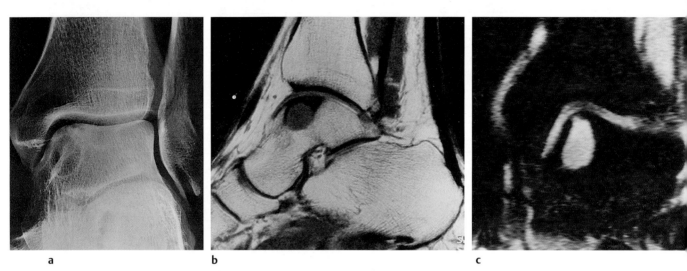

a   b   c

Fig. 7.**261 a–c**   Subchondral synovial cyst (intraosseous ganglion), exhibiting homogeneous high signal intensity on T2-weighted MRI (**c**).

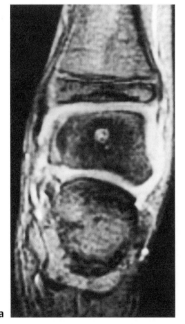
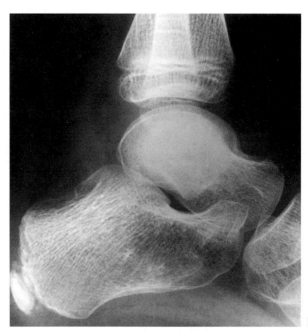

a   b

Fig. 7.**262 a–g**   Osteoid osteoma in the talus.
a, b The nidus is located at the center of the talus in this 10-year-old girl. It is recognized as a round, hyperintense focus in the T2-weighted image (**a**). The dense surrounding sclerosis ("white" talar body in **b**) appears as a signal void on T2-weighted MRI. There is marked concomitant effusion in the talocrural and talocalcaneal joints.

Fig. 7.**262 c–g** ▷

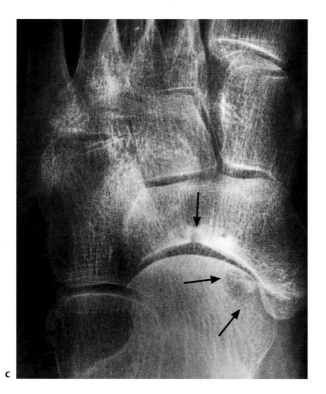

c

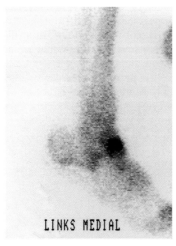

d LINKS MEDIAL

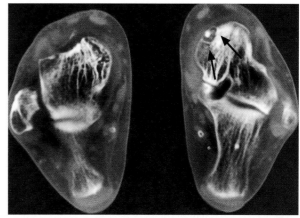

e

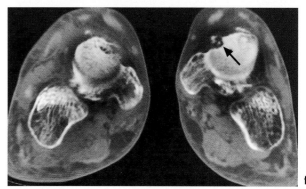

f

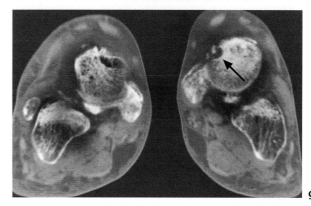

g

Fig. 7.**262 c–g**   Here the nidus appears as a subchondral oste-olytic area bordering the talonavicular joint (paired arrows in **c**). In the CT scans (**e–g**), the nidus shows central ossification. Dense marginal sclerosis is present. The radionuclide scan (**d**) shows intense uptake with a double-density sign (69-year-old woman with severe pain in the left tarsus). Note the broad nutrient canal extending into the talonavicular joint from the center of the navicular bone (vertical arrow in **c**; see also p. 1041).

References

Anderson, I. F., K. J. Chrichton: Osteochondral fractures of the dome of the talus. J Bone Jt Surg. 71-A (1989) 1143

Azouz, E. M., A. M. Slomic, D. Marton et al.: The variable manifestation of dysplasia epiphysealis hemimelica. Pediat. Radiol. 15 (1985) 44

Baron, M., H. Paltiel, Ph. Lander: Aseptic necrosis of the talus and calcaneal insufficiency fractures in a patient with pancreatitis, subcutaneous fat necrosis and arthritis. Arthr. and Rheum. 27 (1984) 1309

Bender, G., F. Horváth: Über eine seltene Entwicklungsanomalie des Talus und des Os naviculare pedis. Fortschr. Röntgenstr. 94 (1961) 281

Bohndorf, U., H. Imhof: Radiologische Diagnostik der Knochen und Gelenke. Thieme, Stuttgart 1998

Borsay, J., G. Kardos: Isolierte Fraktur des Processus posterior tali. Z. Orthop. 82 (1952) 430

Brunner, U., L. Schweiberer: Verletzungen des Talus und Kalkaneus. Unfallchirurg 99 (1996) 136

Bureau, N. J., E. Cardinal, R. Hobden et al.: Posterior ankle impingement syndrome: MR imaging findings in seven patients. Radiology 215 (2000) 497

Campbell, G., W. Warnekros: A tarsal stress fracture in a long-distance runner. J. Amer. podiat. med. Ass. 73 (1983) 532

Cimmino, Ch. V.: Fracture of the lateral process of the talus. Amer. J. Roentgenol. 90 (1963) 1277

Dihlmann, W.: Gelenke, Wirbelverbindungen, 2. Aufl. Thieme, Stuttgart 1982

Flick, A. B., N. Gould: Osteochondritis dissecans of the talus (transchondral fractures of the talus): review of the literature and new surgical approach for medial dome lesions. Foot and Ankle 5 (1985) 165

Grob, D., B. G. Weber, L. A. Simpson: Die traumatisch bedingte Nekrose des Corpus tali. Unfallchirurg. 88 (1985) 175

Haage, H.: Isolierte Fraktur des Processus fibularis tali. Fortschr. Röntgenstr. 95 (1961) 422

Jacobsen, St.,T., A. H. Crawford: Congenital vertical talus. J. pediat. Orthop. 3 (1983) 306

Kavros, St. J., H. D. Schwenhaus: Fracture of the posterior process of the talus. J. Amer. podiat. med. Ass. 73 (1983) 421

Lektrakul, N., Ch. B. Chung, Y. Lai et al.: Tarsal sinus: Arthrographic, MR imaging, MR arthrography, and pathologic findings in cadavers and retrospective study data in patients with sinus tarsi syndrome. Radiology 219 (2001) 802

Linhart, W. E., M. Höllwarth: Talusfrakturen bei Kindern. Unfallchirurg 88 (1985) 168

Mc Nally, E. G.: Posteromedial subtalar coalition: imaging appearances in three cases. Skelet. Radiol. 28 (1999) 691

Maier, K.: Beitrag zur Verschmelzung des Os trigonum mit dem Kalkaneus. Fortschr. Röntgenstr. 98 (1963) 644

Miller, Th. T, J. S. Bucchieri, A. Joshi et al.: Pseudodefect of the talar dome: an anatomic pitfall of ankle MR imaging. Radiology 203 (1997) 857

Mukerjee, S. K., R. M. Pringle, A. D. Baxter: Fracture of the lateral process of the talus. J. Bone Jt Surg. 52-B (1974) 263

Pfitzner, W.: Beiträge zur Kenntnis des menschlichen Extremitätenskelettes VII. Die Variationen im Aufbau des Fußskelettes. Schwalbes morphol. Arb. 6 (1896) 245

Resnick, D.: Talar ridges, osteophytes, and beaks: a radiologic commentary. Radiology 151 (1984) 329

Riedel, K., M. Jobst: Zur Kenntnis und Therapie der Shepherdschen Fraktur. Zbl. Chir. 109 (1984) 746

Robbins, H.: Congenital vertical talus and arthrogryposis. In Jahss, M. H.: Disorders of the Foot. Saunders, Philadelphia 1982 (p. 439)

Rogers, L. F.: Radiology of Skeletal Trauma. Churchill Livingstone, New York 1982 (p. 878)

Sanders, T. G., A. J. Ptaszek, W. B. Morrison: Fracture of the lateral process of the talus: appearance at MR imaging and clinical significance. Skelet. Radiol. 28 (1999) 236

Schreiber, A., P. Differding, H. Zollinger: Talus partitus. J. Bone Jt Surg. 67-B (1985) 430

Schwarz, N., M. Gebauer: Die Fraktur des Sprungbeins beim Kind. Unfallheilkunde 86 (1983) 212

Sharit, F. E., L. F. Cole: Subtalar dislocation. J. Amer. podiat. med. Ass. 74 (1984) 386

Schelton, M. L., W. J. Pedowitz: Injuries to the talus and midfoot. In Jahss, M. H.: Disorders of the Foot. Saunders, Philadelphia 1982 (p. 1485)

Skevis, X. A.: Primary subacute osteomyelitis of the talus. J. Bone Jt Surg. 66-B (1984) 101

Thompson, J. P., R. Loomer: Osteochondral lesions of the talus in a sports medicine clinic. Amer. J. Sports Med. 12 (1984) 460

Zwipp, H., H. Tscherne: Die radiologische Diagnostik der Rotationsinstabilität im hinteren unteren Sprunggelenk. Unfallheilkunde 85 (1982) 494

Calcaneus

Normal Findings

During Growth

The calcaneus ("heel bone," Fig. 7.**263**) is usually ossified from **two centers**.

One center, which is most likely the primordial peroneal trochlea, appears in the 5th month of life. The second center appears in the 7th month of life. Both centers fuse during subsequent months. The site of the union of the ossification centers is occasionally visible as a linear density in early childhood.

The posterior border of the calcaneus, and thus the region of the calcaneal tuberosity, appears wavy and jagged in children, similar to the marginal ridges of the vertebral bodies and the iliac crests. Between 6 and 10 years of age, the **apophyseal centers** appear **posterior to this irregular border** (Fig. 7.**264**), fusing at about age 17 with the rest of the calcaneus. The apophyseal center(s) may be extremely dense (Figs. 7.**265**, 7.**244d**). This can mimic necrosis, especially when conspicuous transverse grooves or clefts are found between the centers (Figs. 7.**264**, 7.**266**), creating the appearance of fragmentation.

The phenomenon of "fluid-filled spaces" in the lucent area below the sustentaculum tali in children is discussed below and illustrated in Fig. 7.**272**.

The **peroneal trochlea** arises from a separate ossification center, as noted above. Also called the peroneal process, it separates the peroneus longus and brevis tendons. It is observed in only about one-third of the population and may be very prominent (Fig. 7.**268**). Very rarely, a large trochlea can apparently cause an **impingement or entrapment syndrome** with peroneus longus tendinitis (Boles et al. 1997).

In Adulthood

The normal anatomy of the calcaneus is shown in Fig. 7.**263**.

The following special projections can be used in plain-film examinations of the calcaneus:

- Axial projection of the calcaneus with passive dorsiflexion of the foot and a 45° oblique central ray (aimed cephalad at a horizontal cassette placed below the heel).
- Double-exposed dorsoplantar projection of the hindfoot with the patient standing on the cassette. The lower leg is angled forward at the ankle for the first exposure and backward for the second exposure.

There are other projections, such as the Broden view, that need not be described here.

The **sustentaculum tali** can occasionally appear **very prominent** in the lateral projection (Fig. 7.**267**).

A **lucent area**, usually triangular in outline, is consistently found **below the sulcus calcanei** (Fig. 7.**269**). This is a physiological area of relatively sparse trabeculae and not a variant.

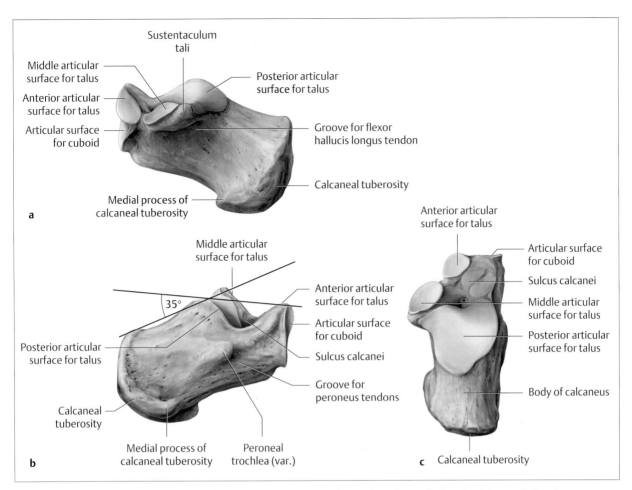

Fig. 7.**263 a–c** Surface anatomy of the calcaneus.
a Medial aspect.
b Lateral aspect.
c Superior aspect.

The angle in **b** is called "tuber-joint-angle" and averages approximately 35° (see also p. 1033).

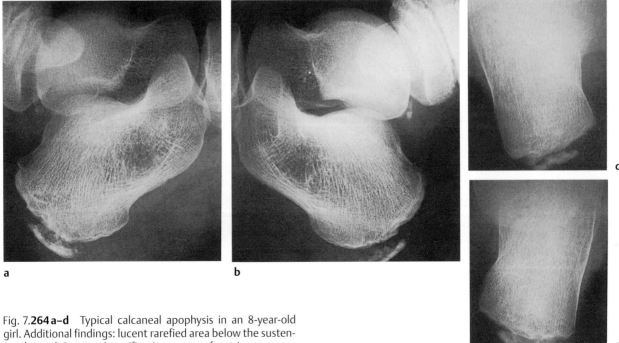

Fig. 7.**264 a–d** Typical calcaneal apophysis in an 8-year-old girl. Additional findings: lucent rarefied area below the sustentaculum tali (see text), ossification center of os trigonum.

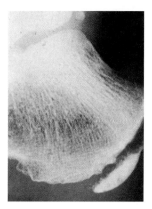

Fig. 7.**265**   Normal density of a calcaneal apophysis.

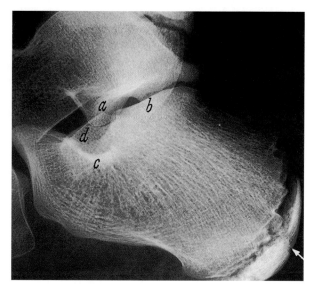

Fig. 7.**266**   Calcaneal apophysis of normal density, located at normal distance from the ribbed body of the calcaneus and showing typical transverse grooves (white arrow).
a   Lateral process of talus
b   Posterior articular surface of calcaneus
c   Cortex
d   Sustentaculum tali

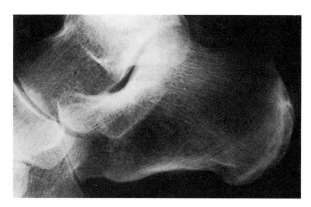

Fig. 7.**267**   Very prominent sustentaculum tali.

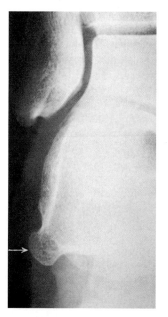

Fig. 7.**268**   Exostosis-like projection of the trochlear process of the calcaneus.

Fig. 7.**269**   Typical area of rarefied trabeculae at the junction ▷ of the anterior process and body of the calcaneus (arrow). Abundant fatty tissue is normally found in this area. The rarefied area has a roughly triangular configuration. The corresponding radiographs are shown in Fig. 7.**270** and 7.**271**.

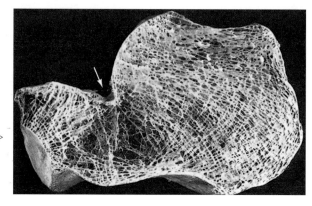

Apparently this area is subjected to much lower functional stresses than the adjacent bony areas. In a series of 1200 normal calcanei, the lucent area was very pronounced in 7.1 % of cases, moderately pronounced in 22.1 %, and faintly visible in 70.8 %. The area normally contains fatty tissue, which is occasionally misinterpreted as evidence of a lipoma (Fig. 7.**302**). The differential diagnosis of this physiological lucency also includes a unilocular bone cyst (Fig. 7.**301**). Conventional radiograph permit an accurate differential diagnosis only if an end-on or oblique projection of a nutrient canal can be seen within the lucent area (Figs. 7.**270**, 7.**271**).

In recent MRI examinations of children, we have observed signal intensity changes in the physiological lucency that are, for the present, difficult to interpret. They appear as signal voids on T1-weighted images and show high signal intensity on T2-weighted images. They may coalesce (Fig. 7.**272 d**) or may have peripheral pseudopod-like extensions (Fig. 7.**272 c**).

We have considered proton-rich residual bone marrow or a transformation of red marrow to fat marrow. We do not regard such findings as intraosseous ganglion-like structures, although this is tempting since the hyperintense foci on T2-weighted images are located just below the tarsal sinus. The phenomenon requires further study, as it was first discovered with MRI and there is no remarkable corresponding finding on plain films or CT (Fig. 7.**272 e–h**).

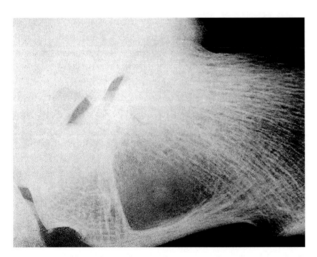

Fig. 7.**270** Physiological area of sparse trabeculae, not a calcaneal cyst. Note the end-on projection of a small nutrient canal at the upper boundary of the lucent area.

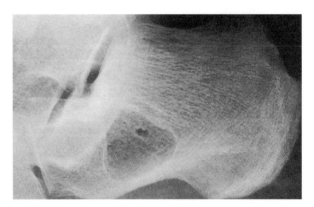

Fig. 7.**271** Physiological triangular lucent area, not a calcaneal cyst. Note the slightly oblique projection of a nutrient canal in the upper part of the lucent area. This sign makes it very unlikely that the area is a true calcaneal cyst or calcaneal lipoma (Figs. 7.**300**–7.**303**).

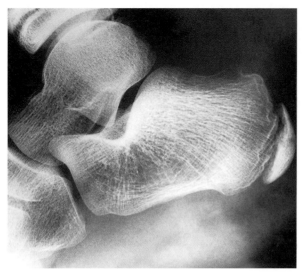

Fig. 7.**272 a–i** Unusual fluid-equivalent structures in the physiological lucent area of the calcaneus (Figs. 7.**269**–7.**271**), detected incidentally in an 11-year-old child.

a An area of trabecular rarefaction is seen at the junction of the anterior process with the body of the calcaneus.

b T1-weighted MR image shows a circumscribed signal void at that location.

c, d This area has high signal intensity on T2-weighted MRI (**d**), appearing isointense to the intra-articular fluid in the tibio-talar joint. Note the pseudopod-like extensions from the hyperintense fluid-equivalent zone (**c**).

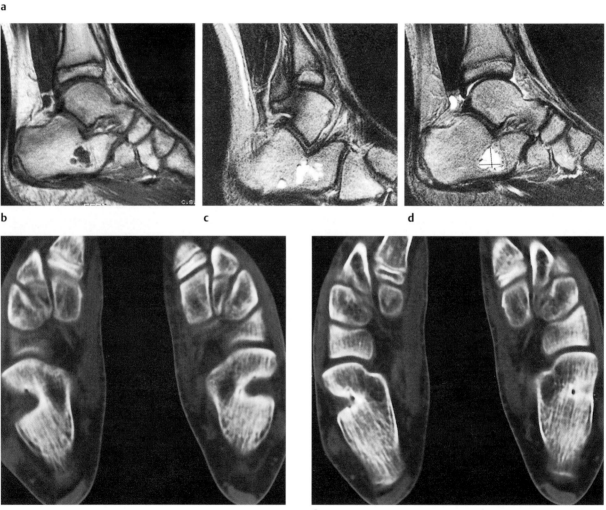

Fig. 7.**272 e–i** The CT scans show no definite abnormalities. The small foramen-like structures in **f** may be the tip of the tarsal sinus or small nutrient canals. Panels **h** and **i** compare axial

CT scans with an axial MR image, showing that the more solid nonosseous structures on CT correspond to the fluid-equivalent multicentric areas on MRI (see text).

Fig. 7.**272 g–i** ▷

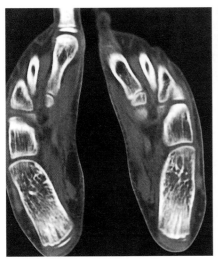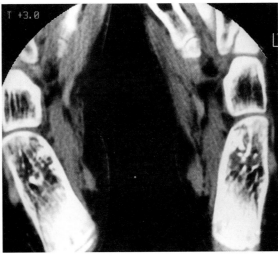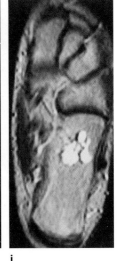

Fig. 7.**272 g**   **h**   **i**

Pathological Finding?

 Normal Variant or Anomaly?

Variants

Bone spurs are occasionally seen on the plantar aspect of the calcaneus in children around one year of age (Robinson 1976). They are located in the posterior half of the calcaneus, are directed toward the tuberosity, and are clinically asymptomatic. They are thought to occur predominantly in boys and usually disappear after one year of age or after 7 years at the latest.

A **spurlike prominence on the posterosuperior border of the calcaneus** is considered a normal variant and is termed a Haglund exostosis (Fig. 7.**273**). When tall shoes are worn, the exostosis may impinge on the adjacent Achilles tendon, producing a condition known as Haglund syndrome or Haglund's heel (p. 1038).

A **spurlike bony excrescence** in the area of the "**anterior calcaneal spur**" may be considered a normal variant in asymptomatic patients (Fig. 7.**274**). It is distinguished from a degenerative heel spur by its internal structure and by the continuity of its own cancellous bone with that of the adjacent calcaneus, similar to an osteochondroma.

Degenerative and inflammatory heel spurs in the strict sense are discussed under Other Changes.

Another variant is a **bony prominence** that may arise from the **superior talonavicular side of the anterior articular surface** of the calcaneus (Figs. 7.**275**, 7.**276**).

> This is the exact location of os calcanei secundarii, suggesting that the os may actually be a nonfused apophysis of this process.

In this sense the calcaneus secundarius would be the "variant of a variant." The pronounced extension of the anterior calcaneus described above points toward the navicular and may form a pseudoarticulation with it (Figs. 7.**277**, 7.**278**), especially if the navicular also has a strong lateral projec-

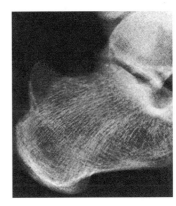

Fig. 7.**273**   Haglund's heel.

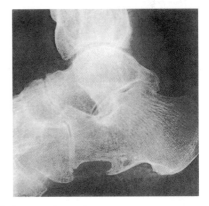

Fig. 7.**274**   Atypical plantar calcaneal spur.

tion. But it should also be discussed whether this "pseudo-articulation" represents a fibrous coalition.

Prominence of the peroneal process of the calcaneus, with possible entrapment of the peroneus longus tendon, is discussed under Normal Findings. Behind the peroneal

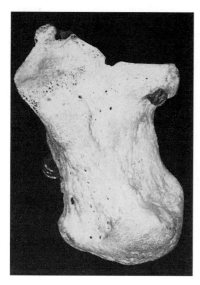

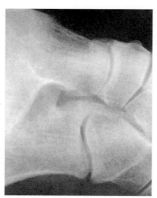

Fig. 7.**275** Specimen showing a kind of process on the anterior articular surface of the calcaneus (compare with Figs. 7.**276**–7.**278**).

Fig. 7.**276** Bony process on the anterosuperior border of the calcaneus, located between the navicular and cuboid bones (Figs. 7.**275**, 7.**277**–7.**278**).

Fig. 7.**276**

Fig. 7.**275**

process is the **retrotrochlear eminence** of the calcaneus. The variable peroneus quarter muscle inserts on the retrotrochlear eminence, and the presence of the muscle is associated with a prominent eminence but with a normal-size peroneal process (Cheung et al. 1997).

The following accessory bones are known to occur about the calcaneus as variants:

- **Os tuberis calcanei** (Fig. 7.**279**). It is located at the posteroinferior border below the calcaneal tuberosity and may occasionally cause complaints.

- **Os accessorium supracalcaneum** (Figs. 7.**280**, 7.**281**). It is located behind the os trigonum (p. 1007).
- **Os trochleare calcanei** (Fig. 7.**282**). This may be an unfused center of the peroneal trochlea (p. 1020) and may cause pain, especially in growing patients.
- **Os sustentaculi** (Figs. 7.**283**–7.**284**). This isolated element is located adjacent or anterior to the sustentaculum tali and sometimes appears to complete it (see CT scans in Fig. 7.**284**). The ossicle may form a fibrous or fibrocartilaginous pseudoarticulation (synchondrosis),

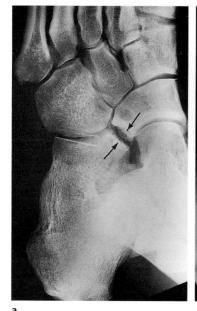

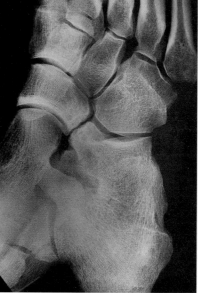

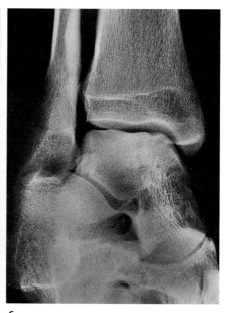

a   b   c

Fig. 7.**277 a–c** Processlike bony structure on the anterior superior calcaneus, directed toward the navicular and apparently forming a pseudoarticulation or synchondrosis or fibrous coalition (compare with Fig. 7.**295**) that shows marked regressive changes on the right side (**a**). The process coincides precisely with the location of a calcaneus secundarius (see text). The oblique tarsal radiographs were obtained during a compensation examination for an old osteochondral fracture of the talus (**c**, medial side). When examined, the patient complained of pain in both calcaneonavicular regions. The pain can be explained in terms of calcaneonavicular anatomy and is unrelated to the old osteochondral fracture of the talus. The patient was also noted to have flat feet.

Fig. 7.**278**

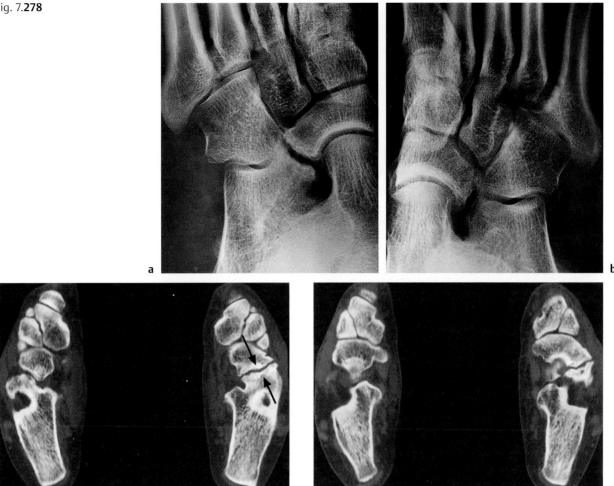

a

b

c

d

Fig. 7.**278 a–d** Pseudoarticulation (synchondrosis? fibrocartilaginous bridge? fibrous coalition?) between the anterior process of the calcaneus and the left navicular (similar to Figs. 7.**275**–7.**277**) in a symptomatic patient. CT vividly demonstrates the pseudoarticulation on the left side (arrows in **c**). It can be imagined that this anterior process corresponds, say, to a calcaneus secundarius that has fused with the calcaneus or even that the calcaneus secundarius (Figs. 7.**285**–7.**290**) corresponds to an unfused accessory apophysis of the variant process. The latter case might be described as a "variant of the variant." In cases where this process forms early, the development of a calcaneonavicular synostosis is also possible (Fig. 7.**295**).

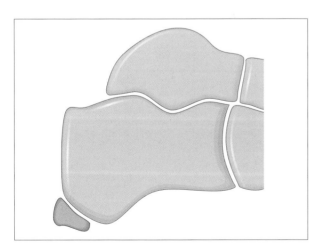

Fig. 7.**279**   Os tuberis calcanei (after Lachapèle).

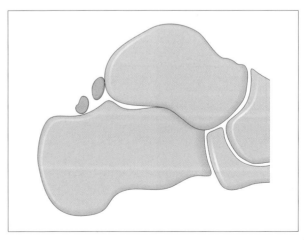

Fig. 7.**280**   Os accessorium supracalcaneum (after Schmitt).

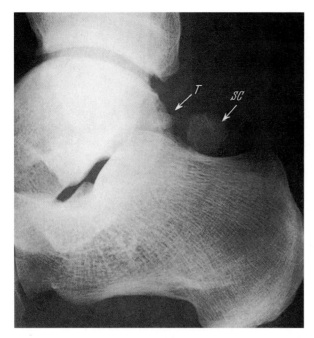

Fig. 7.**281**   Os trigonum (T) and os accessorium supracalcaneum (SC).

fibrocartilaginous bridge) with the sustentaculum tali showing secondary degenerative changes (Figs. 7.**283 b**, 7.**284 a, b**). Bencardino et al. (1997) and Mellado et al. (2002) describe the MRI features of an os sustentaculi in a 14-year old boy respectively in a 49-year old man with medial ankle pain. Mellado et al. (2002) speculate whether their findings (elongated medial tubercle of the talus, hyperintense interfaces between the os sustentaculi and the talus and calcaneus) may be in fact a fibrocartilaginous subtalar coalition with an intercalated accessory bone. Bloom et al. (1986) described an assimilated os sustentaculi.

● **Calcaneus secundarius.** This bone is located in the space between the calcaneus, talus, cuboid, and navicular. It is sometimes round, often triangular, and ranges from a few millimeters to 1 cm in diameter. Figure 7.**285 a, b** shows the anatomic relationships of the calcaneus secundarius; Figs. 7.**185 c–f** and 7.**286**–7.**289** show its various radiographic appearances in different older patients. It was noted earlier that this bone is derived from an unfused apophysis of an atypical bony process of the calcaneus in this region (see also Figs. 7.**277** and 7.**278**). Like other accessory ossicles, the calcaneus secundarius may form pseudoarticulations (synchondrosis or fibrocartilaginous bridge) with the

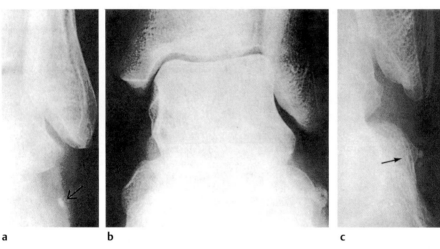

a   b   c

Fig. 7.**282 a–c**   Os trochleare calcanei.
a, b AP projection of the ankle.
c Dorsoplantar projection.

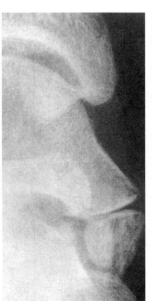

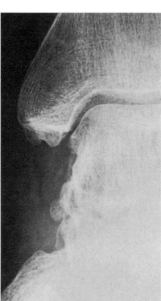

a   b   c

Fig. 7.**283 a–e**   Os sustentaculi tali.
a, b Relatively large elements with a predominantly triangular configuration.
c Relatively small accessory bone with a more rounded shape.

Fig. 7.**283 d, e** ▷

Fig. 7.**283 d, e**
d Anatomic relationships of the os sustentaculi (after Pfitzner).
e The os sustentaculi is apparently displaced, and a small intercalary ossicle is located between it and the calcaneus.

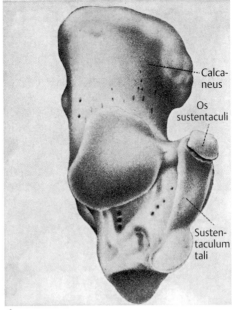

Calca-
neus

Os
sustentaculi

Susten-
taculum
tali

d

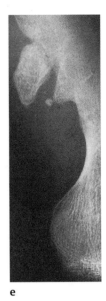

e

adjacent bone, and these connections may show degenerative deformity (Fig. 7.**287 a**). It is conceivable that these bony elements also represent a kind of sesamoid or intercalated bone in growing patients, and that they can be a source of synostosis (coalition), in this case between the calcaneus and navicular (Fig. 7.**295** and p. 998 f.). The calcaneus secundarius should not be mistaken for an isolated chip fracture of the anterior articular surface of the calcaneus (Fig. 7.**290**). A calcaneus secundarius could mimic an os tibiale externum in the oblique projection, but this is easily resolved by obtaining an appropriate dorsoplantar projection (Fig. 7.**291**).

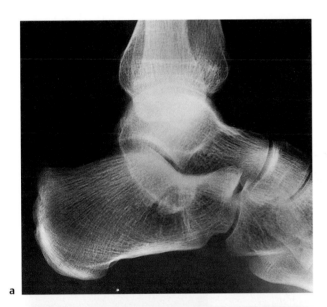

a

Fig. 7.**284 a–c** Os sustentaculi tali forming a pseudoarticulation with the calcaneus. Clinical complaints were probably due to necrotic changes in the inferior portions of the bone. An asterisk marks the location of the accessory bone in **b**, and **c** shows the small bone fragments that most likely represent necrosis.

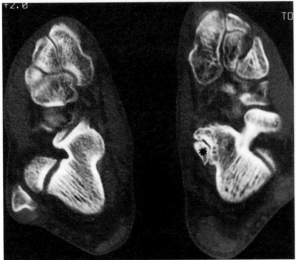

b

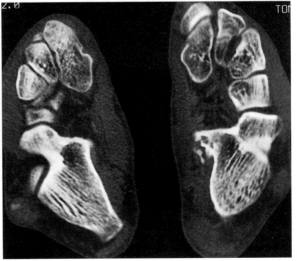

c

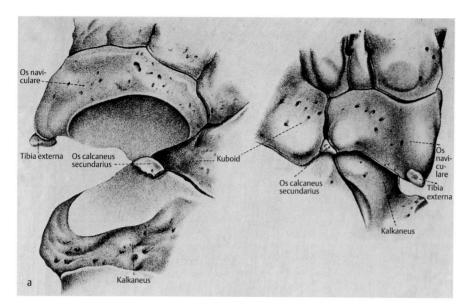

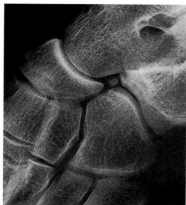

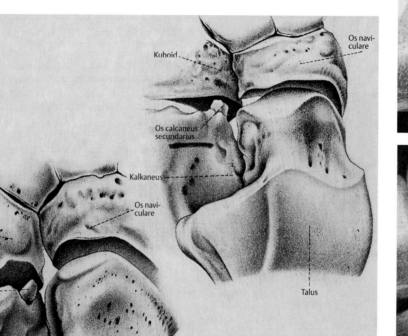

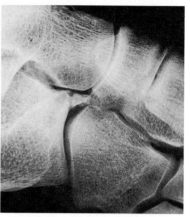

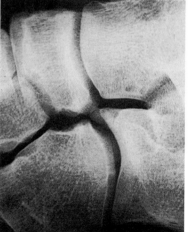

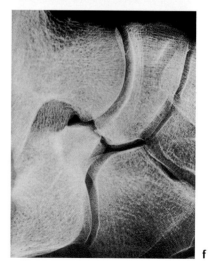

Fig. 7.**285 a–f**   Os calcaneus secundarius.
a, b Anatomic drawings by Pfitzner.
c–f Varying shapes of the accessory bone. In **d** it is shaped like
a kind of process, as illustrated in Figs. 7.**275**–7.**278**.

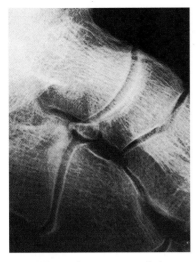

Fig. 7.**286**   Calcaneus secundarius with an atypical shape.

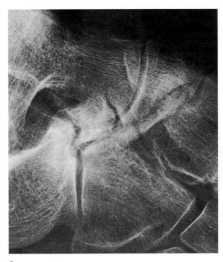

a

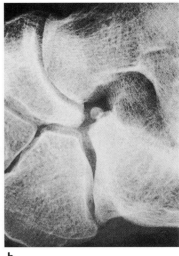

b

Fig. 7.**287 a, b**   Asymmetrical shapes of the calcaneus secundarius.
a On the right side is a large bony element that has formed a pseudoarticulation with the calcaneus, or more specifically with an opposing process on that bone.
b Contralateral radiograph shows a small, round accessory bone.

Fig. 7.**288**   Calcaneus secundarius in a 12-year-old girl.

Fig. 7.**289**   Calcaneus secundarius in a 16-year-old boy.

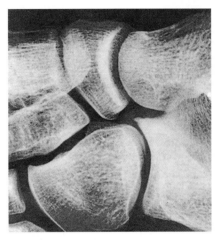

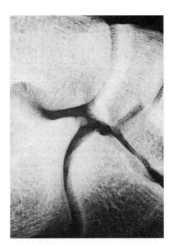

Fig. 7.**288**

Fig. 7.**289**

Fig. 7.**290 a, b**   Chip fracture.
a Chip fracture, not a calcaneus secundarius.
b Healed fracture several months later.

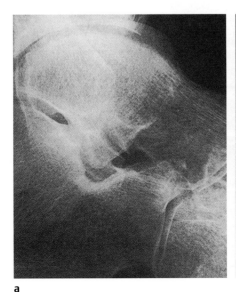

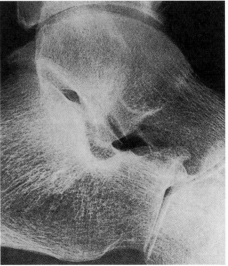

a

b

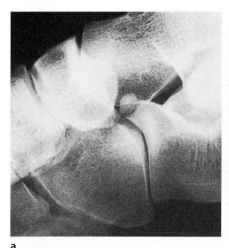

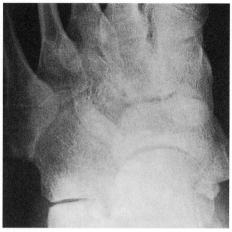

a

b

Fig. 7.**291 a, b**   Os tibiale externum, not a calcaneus secundarius (p. 1044).

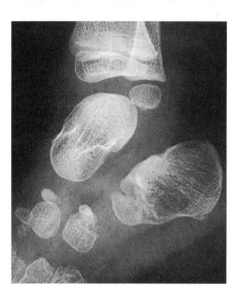

Fig. 7.**292**   Bifid calcaneus and other developmental anomalies in the tarsal bones.

Deformities

A **bifid calcaneus** is considered a true deformity rather than a variant (Figs. 7.**292**, 7.**293**).

Apparently it results from a serious delay or complete failure of fusion of the two ossification centers (larger anterior and smaller posterior). In the case shown in Fig. 7.**293**, the two centers went on to fuse at 5 years of age, leaving behind a sclerotic area. Ogden (1982) investigated an anomalous multifocal ossification of the calcaneus. The literature to date indicates that delayed or absent fusion of the two calcaneal centers is often associated with other foot deformities.

Coalitions of the calcaneus with adjacent bones is also classified as a deformity, as it generally has pathological significance (see under General Aspects, p. 997 ff.). The C sign of talocalcaneal coalition was described on p. 998 (Figs. 7.**220 a**, 7.**221**, 7.**294**).

Harris classification of talocalcaneal synostoses
➤ Complete medial form
➤ Incomplete medial form
➤ Rudimentary medial form with the sustentaculum tali
➤ Rudimentary medial coalition

McNally (1999) described the sectional imaging features of posteromedial subtalar coalition (p. 1012).

Figure 7.**296** illustrates a very rare coalition between the calcaneus, cuboid, and fourth metatarsal.

Synostosis between the calcaneus and navicular is less common. An example is shown in Fig. 7.**295**. Issues relating to the origin of this synostosis or coalition were discussed previously in connection with the calcaneus secundarius.

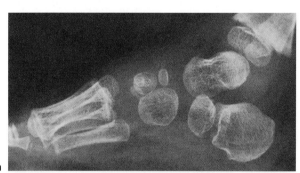

a

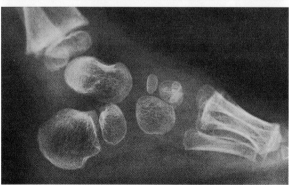

b

◁ Fig. 7.**293 a, b**   Bifid calcaneus in a 21-month-old child.

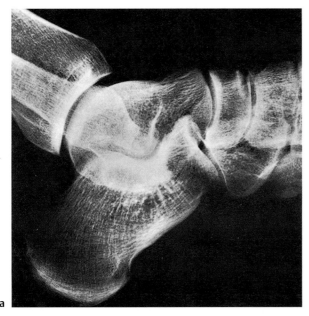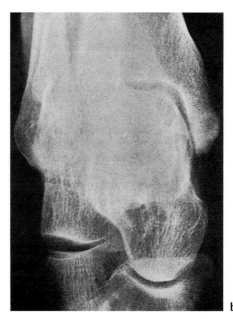

a   b

Fig. 7.**294 a, b**   Talocalcaneal synostosis. Note the "C sign" in radiograph **a** (see text).

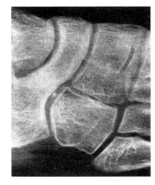

Fig. 7.**295**   Synostosis between the calcaneus and navicular (bilateral).

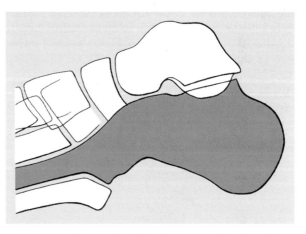

Fig. 7.**296**   Calcaneocuboid-fourth metatarsal coalition (after Dihlmann).

 ### Fracture, Subluxation, or Dislocation?

Pediatric calcaneal fractures are usually compression fractures (Wiley 1984) and are typically caused by jumping from a height. It is difficult to state whether the incidence of calcaneal fractures is lower in children than adults, because clinical symptoms in children often do not appear until 24–48 hours after the injury and also pass more quickly, so that many of these cases do not have a thorough radiographic workup.

> Starshak et al. (1984) found that bone scans become positive just 7 hours after a pediatric calcaneal fracture. A negative bone scan 3 days after the injury excludes a calcaneal fracture.

Calcaneal fractures in adults are the most common type of tarsal fractures. Approximately 75 % are compression fractures caused by falling or jumping from a height. About 10–12 % of calcaneal fractures are bilateral (Rogers 1982). There is an equal incidence of associated compression fractures of the upper tibia and thoracolumbar junction.

Since fractures of the calcaneus are often missed on conventional radiographs, CT should be performed whenever these fractures are suspected clinically. The **tuber joint angle** of Böhler (1935) is important on routine radiographs. This angle normally measures 20–45°, averaging 35.5° in healthy subjects (Fig. 7.**263 b**). Any deviation relative to the opposite side is considered borderline (Rogers 1982). A normal tuber joint angle does not exclude a calcaneal fracture, however.

> Approximately two-thirds of all calcaneal fractures are intra-articular.

This type of fracture occurs when the lateral process of the talus, located above the center of the calcaneus, is driven into the calcaneus by an axial force (e.g., a vertical fall), producing a **primary fracture line** (Fig. 7.**297 a**).

The two main fragments consist of an anteromedial sustentacular fragment and a posterolateral tuberal fragment. In some cases the anterior process is broken from the sustentacular fragment (Fig. 7.**297 a**). More severe compression trauma produces a **secondary fracture line** that separates a posterior facet fragment from the tuberal fragment (Fig. 7.**297 b, c**). Essex–Lopresti distinguishes two types depending on whether the secondary fracture line curves upward around the subtalar articular surface (joint depression type) or runs horizontally back into the tuberosity to create a tongue-shaped posterior facet fragment (tongue type). In both types the posterior facet fragment is impacted into the tuberal fragment, and the facet fragment itself may be fractured. The tuber joint angle is decreased.

The remaining one-third of all calcaneal fractures are extraarticular (Fig. 7.**298**).

Most of these injuries are avulsion fractures, and they are associated with a normal tuber joint angle. The most familiar type is the "duckbill fracture" or "beak fracture" caused by avulsion of the upper part of the calcaneal tuberosity on the Achilles tendon. A fracture that detaches the anterior process of the calcaneus basically requires differentiation from a calcaneus secundarius. This fracture is easily missed in radiographs that are centered on the

mortise joint. The fragment is best visualized on dorso-plantar radiographs.

Stress fractures usually extend vertically through the calcaneus. They are easily missed on conventional radiographs but are reliably detected by bone scanning followed by selective CT. Stress fractures of the calcaneus are particularly common in military recruits ("march fractures") and persons who do high-intensity aerobic workouts (Winfield 1959, Vogel et al. 1985).

Insulin-dependent diabetics are predisposed to insufficiency-type avulsion fractures involving the posterior third of the calcaneus (Kathol et al. 1991).

An **Achilles tendon avulsion** tends to obscure the **Kager triangle** (retromalleolar, supracalcaneal triangular lucency caused by fatty tissue in front of the Achilles tendon) due to edema or blood infiltrating the supracalcaneal area.

 ## Necrosis?

Like other bones, the calcaneus may develop necrotic changes, usually as a result of trauma. A condition specific to the calcaneus is **osteonecrosis (osteochondropathy) of the apophysis of the calcaneal tuberosity** (Fig. 7.**299**).

This condition is named **Sever disease** after the author who first described it. Apparently it is based on a chronic avulsion fracture or chronic traction injury at the tendon insertion, similar to the changes that can occur at the tibial

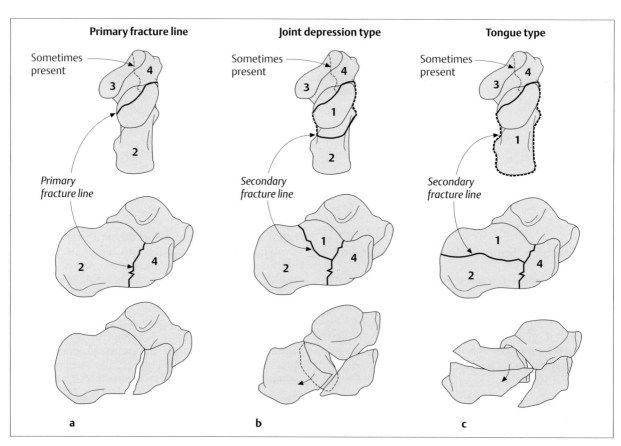

Fig. 7.**297 a–c** Intra-articular calcaneal fractures with involvement of the subtalar articular surface (after Bohndorf and Imhof). The numbers designate the following main fragments:

1   Posterior facet fragment
2   Tuberal fragment
3   Sustentacular fragment
4   Anterior process fragment

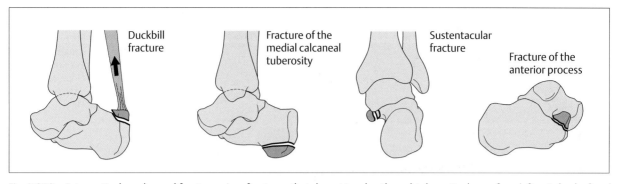

Fig. 7.**298**   Extra-articular calcaneal fractures, i.e., fractures that do not involve the subtalar articular surface (after Bohndorf and Imhof).

tuberosity (q.v.). The terms "chronic avulsion fracture" and "chronic avulsion injury" are used interchangeably in the literature. The phenomenon is particularly common in overweight individuals who perform strenuous physical exertion without proper conditioning. It is also associated with pes planovalgus, pes valgus, and clubfoot. Comparing the cases shown in Figs. 7.**299** and 7.**266**, we see that the former case involves a true pathological process with metaplastic bone formation, whereas the physiologically dense calcaneal apophysis maintains an essentially normal shape.

Involvement of the calcaneus by **diabetic osteoarthropathy** is not uncommon. Insufficiency avulsion fractures of the posterior third of the calcaneus are particularly apt to occur in insulin-dependent diabetes of long duration.

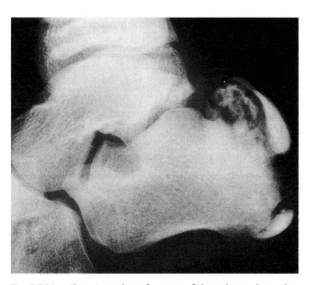

Fig. 7.**299**   Chronic avulsion fracture of the calcaneal apophysis with extensive necrotic changes and metaplastic bone formation in a 21-year-old man (see text).

 Inflammation?

Osteomyelitis can develop in the calcaneus as in any other bones. The calcaneus is most susceptible to primary chronic osteomyelitis, usually in the form of plasma cell osteomyelitis. Initial changes are often difficult to appreciate on conventional radiographs.

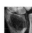 **Tumor?**

Reference was made earlier to the **physiological lucency located below the sustentaculum tali** (Figs. 7.**264**, 7.**269**–7.**271**).

This area can be positively identified as such on radiographs by noting a nutrient canal in an end-on or oblique projection within the lucent area. But if the lucency appears as an actual cavity, perhaps with a dense sclerotic border, and if the inferior border of the calcaneus is bulging, then the differential diagnosis should include a true cyst. These **unicameral bone cysts** occur mainly in adults and less commonly in adolescents (Figs. 7.**300**, 7.**301**).

The physiologic lucency in the calcaneus also requires differentiation from a **calcaneal lipoma**. It was noted earlier that the lucent area in adults normally contains fatty tissue that, in itself, should not be interpreted as a lipoma. A diagnosis of lipoma is justified only if there are larger, confluent spaces filled with fatty tissue that exhibits central necrosis and dystrophic calcification (Fig. 7.**302**).

In equivocal cases where a calcaneal lipoma is suspected, CT or MRI can reliably differentiate normal fatty tissue in the calcaneus from a lipoma.

Osteoblastomas are not uncommon in the calcaneus. Osteosarcomas and a variety of cartilaginous tumors have also been observed. Figure 7.**303** shows a typical **aneurysmal bone cyst** as an example of a tumorlike lesion in the calcaneus.

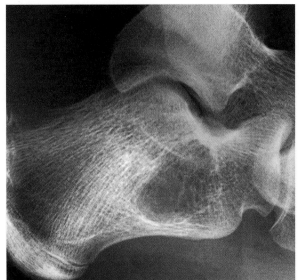

a

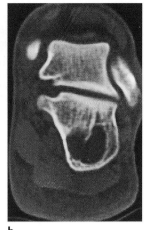

b

Fig. 7.**300 a, b**   True calcaneal cyst. The CT scan (**b**) shows an empty cavity whose attenuation values are consistent with fluid. Contrast this finding with the appearance of the physiological lucent area in Figs. 7.**269**–7.**271**.

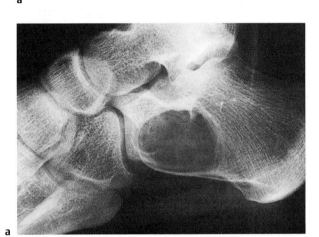

a

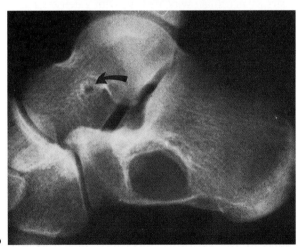

b

Fig. 7.**301 a, b**   Calcaneal cysts. A nutrient canal cannot be seen (see text). Note that the inferior border of the calcaneus is slightly bulging in both cases, confirming the space-occupying nature of the lesion and excluding a physiologic lucency. The arrow in **b** indicates an unusually large nutrient canal in the talus.

Other Changes?

A coarse trabecular pattern, usually involving the entire calcaneus, is observed in **Paget disease** (Fig. 7.**304**).

Rarely is the calcaneus the only site of involvement by this disease, which is more likely to affect the skull, pelvis, etc. Nevertheless, involvement of the calcaneus is not unusual in polyostotic Paget disease.

Spurlike productive bone changes on the posterior and inferior borders of the calcaneus (Fig. 7.**305 a**, 7.**307**), known as **calcaneal spurs**, are a product of regressive changes occurring at fibro-osseous junctions (productive fibro-ostosis or enthesiopathy). When Riepert et al. (1995) studied 1027 lateral radiographs of the heel from a Central European population, they observed a lower spur in 11.2% of the cases and an upper spur in 9.3%. According to this study, the prevalence of both spurs increases markedly with aging, the upper spur appearing somewhat later than the lower spur. The authors also delve into the medicolegal aspects of detecting heel spurs.

> Heel spurs are often asymptomatic. This fact, together with their prevalence, raises the question of whether they should be considered a normal finding in adults.

By contrast, initially **rarefying and later flame-shaped productive changes** about the calcaneus are a manifestation of rheumatoid disease, usually in the form of a seronegative spondylarthritis (Fig. 7.**306**). Occasionally they may be the first objective imaging sign of a Reiter syndrome or other disorder. The productive changes are flame-shaped or sometimes show a bubble like configuration. They are located at the origin of the plantar aponeurosis, flexor digitorum brevis, abductor hallucis, abductor digiti minimi, long plantar ligament, or (as shown in Fig. 7.**305 b**) at the origin of the plantar calcaneocuboid ligament.

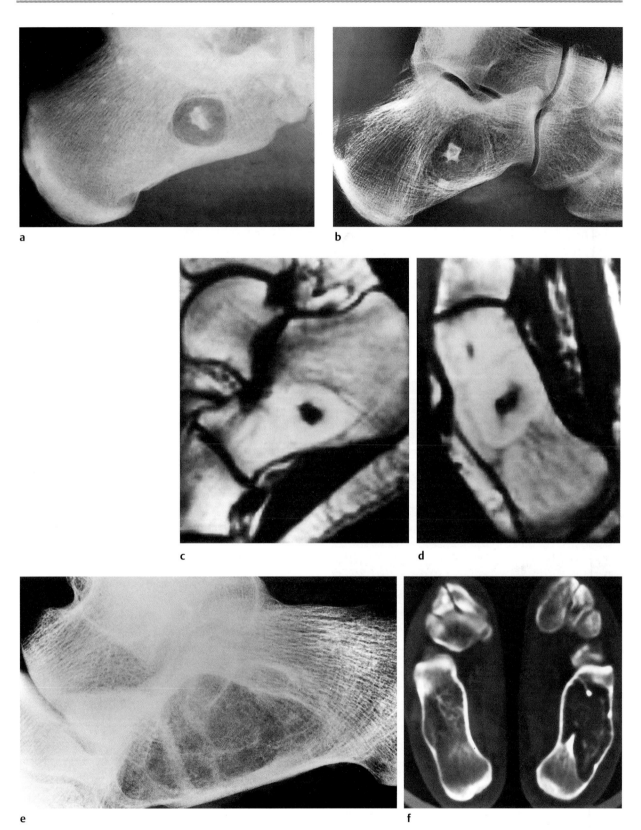

Fig. 7.**302 a–f** Calcaneal lipomas.
a, b Classic radiographic appearance of lipoma: osteolytic area with central dystrophic calcification (the nidus).
c, d T1-weighted MR images demonstrate the fatty nature of the lesion in **b** (surrounding the calcified nidus, which is devoid of signal).

e, f Lipoma without dystrophic calcification. This very extensive lesion is much larger than the physiological lucent area in the calcaneus. The CT scan in **f** shows that it consists almost entirely of fat. The patient was clinically asymptomatic, however.

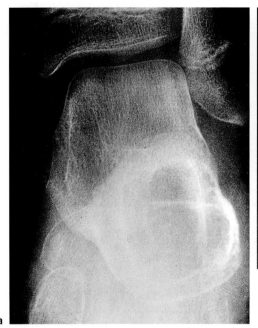

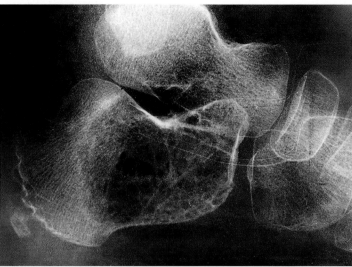

Fig. 7.**303 a, b**   Typical aneurysmal bone cyst in the anterior and central calcaneus. The honeycomb structure in **b** is caused by vessels entering and exiting the bone.

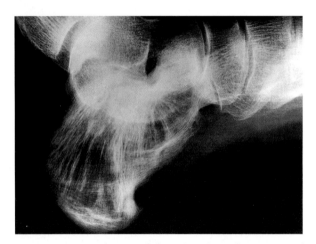

Fig. 7.**304**   Paget disease of the calcaneus with a coarsened trabecular pattern and moderate deformity of the bone.

Often these productive changes are accompanied by lucent areas and especially by areas of increased density in the adjacent cancellous bone. Subachilles bursitis can lead to resorptive changes in the posterior superior border of the calcaneus, creating an **achillobursitis defect** (Fig. 7.**305**, 2, 7.**306b-d**). This defect can also be very specific for an early seronegative spondylarthritis (often combined with signs of periostitis along the adjacent bony contours).

These changes should be differentiated from **reactive inflammatory bursitic changes in the Haglund heel**. The latter is distinguished by an exostosis-like prominence of the posterosuperior border of the calcaneus (p. 1025).

The achillobursitis defect may also occur in rheumatoid arthritis, gout, and other diseases leading to inflammatory tendon changes.

> Calcaneal fibro-osteitis is extremely painful in most cases. Along with the achillobursitis defect, it may initially be missed on conventional radiographs, but radionuclide scans are strongly positive.

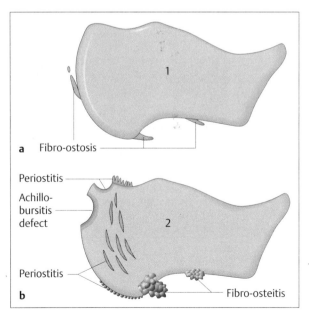

a   Fibro-ostosis

Periostitis
Achillo-
bursitis
defect

Periostitis
b   Fibro-osteitis

◁ Fig. 7.**305 a, b**   Differential diagnosis of degenerative *fibro-ostotic* changes (enthesopathy) (1) and inflammatory *fibro-osteitic* and periostitic changes in "rheumatic" diseases, including an achillobursitis defect (2) (after Dihlmann).

Fig. 7.**306 a–d** Calcaneal changes in ankylosing spondylitis: in (**a**) typical cocks-comb ossifications, an achillobursitis defect, and an inflamed, painful (especially at night) calcaneal spur with sclerosis. In (**b–d**) CT sections of an achillobursitis defect. (**b–d** courtesy of Dr. Dr. Westhaus, Weilheim.)

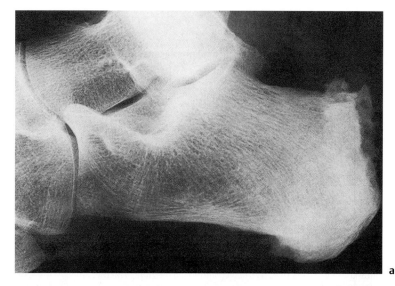

a

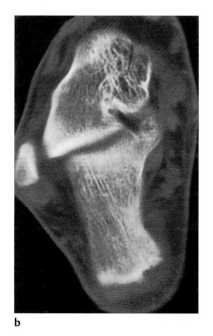

b

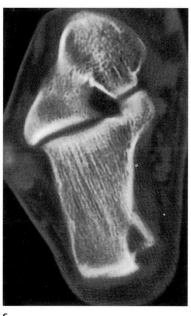

c

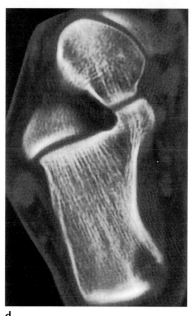

d

Fig. 7.**307 a, b** Follow-up of an activated degenerative fibro-ostosis of the calcaneus. The two radiographs were taken one year apart, during which time the patient developed severe calcaneal pain and palpable swelling. The swelling is due to massive achillobursitis, which has caused significant adjacent bone destruction and reactive sclerosis.

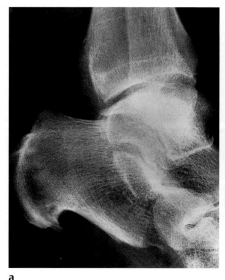

a

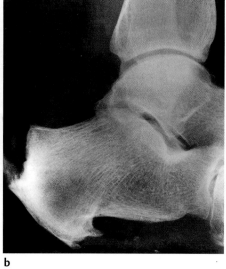

b

References

Azouz, E. M.: Tarsal pseudo-coalition (letter to the editor). J. Canad. Ass. Radiol. 33 (1982) 105

Bencardino J., Z. S. Rosenberg, J. Beltran: Os sustentaculi: depiction on MR images. Skelet. Radiol. 26 (1997) 505

Bohndorf, K., H. Imhof: Radiologische Diagnostik der Knochen und Gelenke. Thieme, Stuttgart 1998

Bloom, R. A., E. Libson, E. Lax et al.: The assimilated os sustentaculi. Skeletal Radiol. 15 (1986) 455

Boles, M. A., L. M. Lomasney, T. C. Demos et al.: Enlarged peroneal process with peroneus longus tendon entrapment. Skelet. Radiol. 26 (1997) 313

Cheung, Y. Y., Z. S. Rosenberg, R. Ramsinghani et al.: Peroneus quartus muscle: MR imaging features. Radiology 202 (1997) 745

de Cuveland, E.: Processus trochlearis oder lateralis tuberis calcanei. Fortschr. Röntgenstr. 84 (1956) 648

Deutsch, A. L., D. Resnick, G. Campbell: Computed tomography and bone scintigraphy in the evaluation of tarsal coalition. Radiology 144 (1982) 137

Dihlmann, W.: Gelenke, Wirbelverbindungen, 2. Aufl. Thieme, Stuttgart 1982

Freund, M., M. Thomsen, B. Hohendorf et al.: Optimized preoperative planning of calcaneal fractures using spiral computed tomography. Europ. Radiol. 9 (1999) 901

Gerster, J. C., P. Piccini: Enthesopathy of the heels in juvenile seronegative B-27 positive Spondylarthropathy. J. Rheumatol. 12 (1985) 310

Gilmer, P. W., J. Herzenberg, J. L. Frank et al.: Computerized tomographic analysis of acute calcaneal fractures. Foot and Ankle 6 (1986) 184

Haglund, P.: Beitrag zur Klinik der Achillessehne. Z. orthop. Chir. 49 (1928) 49

Heneghan, M. A., T. Wallace: Heel pain due to retrocalcaneal bursitis – radiographic diagnosis. Pediat. Radiol. 15 (1985) 119

Keats, Th. E., R. B. Harrison: Hypertrophy of the talar beak. Skelet. Radiol. 4 (1979 a) 37

Keats, Th. E., R. B. Harrison: The calcaneal nutrient foramen: a useful sign in the differentiation of true from simulated cysts. Skelet. Radiol. 3 (1979b) 239

Kathol, M. H. G. Y. El-Khoury, T. E. Moore: Calcaneal insufficiency avulsion fractures in patients with diabetes mellitus. Radiology 180 (1991) 725

Kremser, K.: Os accessorium supracalcaneum. Fortschr. Röntgenstr. 82 (1955) 279

Marti, Th.: Über den Calcaneus secundarius. Fortschr. Röntgenstr. 82 (1955) 124

Mayer, R., K. Wilhem, K. J. Pfeifer: Sonographie der Achillessehnenruptur. Digit. Bilddiagn. 4 (1984) 185

Mellado, J. M., E. Salvado, A. Camins et al.: Painful os sustentaculi: imaging findings of another symptomatic skeletal Vadiant. Skeletal Radiol. 31 (2002) 53

Ogden, J. A.: Anomalous multifocal ossification of the os calcis. Clin. Orthop. 162 (1982) 112

Pavlov, H., M. A. Heneghan, A. Hersh et al.: The Haglund syndrome: initial and differential diagnosis. Radiology 144 (1982) 83

Ravelli, A.: Zur Frage des sogenannten Os accessorium supracalcaneum. Fortschr. Röntgenstr. 83 (1955) 71

Renfrew, D. L., G. Y. El-Khoury: Anterior process fractures of the calcaneus. Skelet. Radiol. 14 (1985) 121

Riepert, T., T. Drechsler, R. Urban et al.: Häufigkeit, Altersabhängigkeit und Geschlechtverteilung des Fersensporns. Fortschr. Röntgenstr. 162,6 (1995) 502

Robinson, H. M.: Symmetrial reversed plantar calcaneal spurs in children. Radiology 119 (1976) 187

Rogers, L. F.: Radiology of Skeletal Trauma. Churchill Livingstone, New York 1982 (p. 864)

Schlefman, B. A., J. A. Ruch: Diagnosis of subtalar joint coalition. J. Amer. podiat. med. Ass. 72 (1982) 166

Schlüter, K.: Ossifikationsanomalien im Kalkaneus, zugleich ein Beitrag zum Auftreten von Ossifikationszentren im Tarsus. Z. Orthop. 87 (1955) 37

Schlüter, K.: Der Calcaneus bifidus, eine Ossifikationsanomalie des Fersenbeins im Hackenplattfuß. Fortschr. Röntgenstr. 85 (1956) 720

Schoen, A.: Aseptische Nekrose akzessorischer Knochen im unteren Sprunggelenk. Fortschr. Röntgenstr. 99 (1963) 843

Smola, E..: Der Calcaneus bifidus. Fortschr. Röntgenstr. 85 (1956) 120

Starshak, R. J., G. W. Simons, J. R. Sty: Occult fracture of the calcancus – another toddler's fracture. Pediat. Radiol. 14 (1984) 37

Vogel, H., D. Pilz, F. Dahms et al.: Ermüdungsbruch des Kalkaneus nach Aerobic-Gymnastik. Z. Orthop. 123 (1985) 69

Wiley, J. J., A. Profitt: Fractures of the os calcis in children. Clin. Orthop. 188 (1984) 131

Winfield, A. C., J. M. Dennis: Stress-fracture of the calcareus. Radiology 72 (1959) 415

Navicular Bone

Normal Findings

 ### During Growth

The ossification center of the navicular (scaphoid) bone is the last ossification center of the tarsal bones to become visible on radiographs, appearing between the third and fifth years of life. It appears one year earlier in girls than in boys. The bone is usually ossified from a single center (Fig. 7.**308**).

But dual ossification centers are still considered normal, in which case the centers are usually located one above the other rather than side by side (Fig. 7.**309**).

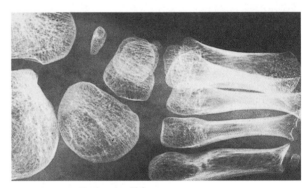

Fig. 7.**308**   Navicular ossification center in a 6-year-old boy.

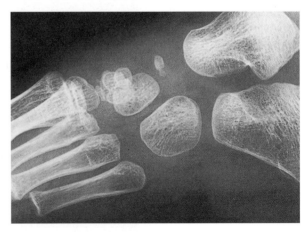

Fig. 7.**309**   A navicular bone ossified from two centers.

Fig. 7.**310 a, b**   Navicular bone of a 7-year-old child.
a Initial radiograph shows narrowing, irregular margins, and increased density of the navicular. The child is clinically asymptomatic.
b Radiograph 20 months later shows a normal-appearing navicular. This confirms that the finding in **a** was a normal variant, not necrosis.

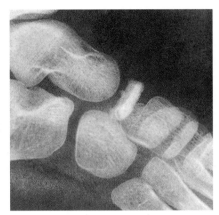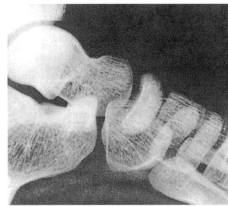

a   b

In the rare instances of multicentric ossification, the centers are flattened and show irregular structure and mineralization (Fig. 7.**357**).

Accessory ossification centers are more common than multiple centers and are also a normal finding. They do not fuse until about 20 years of age (Fig. 7.**311**). The ossification centers are rarely symmetrical between the right and left sides, as illustrated in Fig. 7.**312**.

Very dense (heavily mineralized) ossification centers should not be mistaken for foci of aseptic necrosis, especially in children who have no clinical complaints (Figs. 7.**310**, 7.**311 a**, 7.**312 a**).

Figure 7.**313** shows the purely cartilaginous portion of the navicular in MR images from a 16-month-old girl.

A variant of the navicular ossification is shown in Fig. 7.**342**.

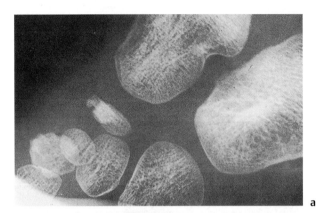

a

 ## In Adulthood

The navicular has one articular surface for the talus and three articular facets for the three cuneiform bones, which together form one joint. The medial surface of the bone is continued downward to form a strong process, the navicular tuberosity (Fig. 7.**314 a, b**).

The term "cornuate navicular" or "hypertrophic navicular" may be used when the tuberosity is exceptionally prominent (Fig. 7.**320**).

Various radiographic projections can give rise to superimposition effects, especially with the cuneiform bones, that occasionally mimic an accessory bone (Fig. 7.**314 c, d**).

The navicular contains nutrient canals of varying prominence. They are distinguished from fractures by the fact that they generally have an inner cortical boundary (Fig. 7.**315**).

Nutrient canals that extend radiographically into the talonavicular joint can produce gaps or defects (Fig. 7.**262 c**).

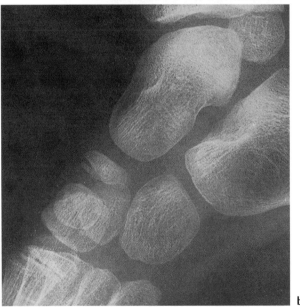

b

Fig. 7.**311 a, b**   Separate ossification center at the dorsal resp. distal dorsal edge of the navicular. Different patients in **a** and **b**.

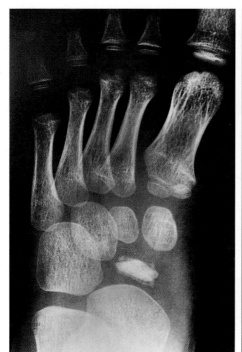
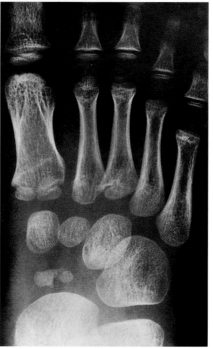

a

b

Fig. 7.**312 a, b** Asymmetry of the ossification centers of the right and left navicular bones. Note that the other tarsal bones are already well formed, including the dual epiphyseal centers of the metatarsals on both sides.

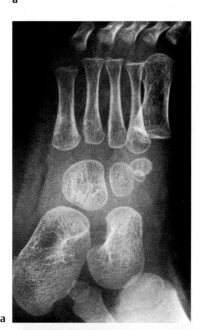

a

Fig. 7.**313 a–f** MR images of the still-unossified navicular in a 16-month-old girl with nonspecific foot pain. The centers of the cuneiform bones and cuboid are well developed. There is still no apparent ossification of the navicular on the plain radiograph. On MRI, the navicular appears only as a cartilaginous structure between the talus and the almost square-shaped medial cuneiform (asterisk in **c**). The "bright" centers of the cuneiform bones and cuboid are clearly visible in the T1-weighted images (**b–d**). In the T2-weighted images (**e, f**), the cartilaginous structures appear as signal voids surrounding the bright ossified areas. (Case courtesy of Dr. Gärtner, Rotenburg/Wümme.)

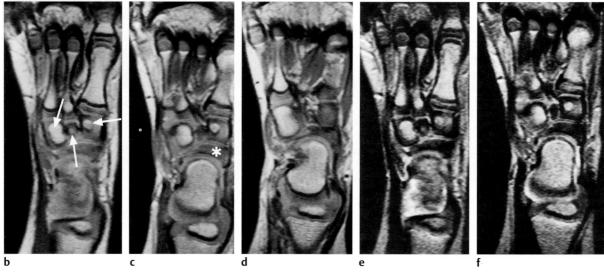

b

c

d

e

f

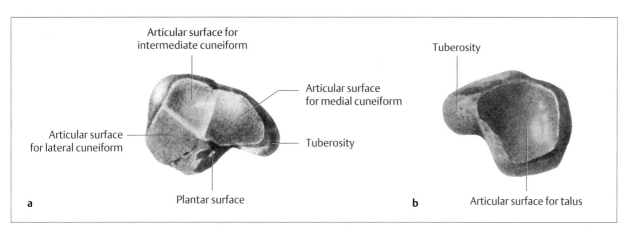

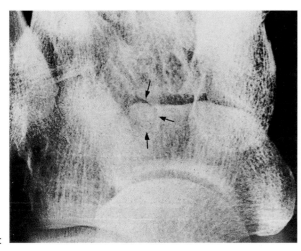

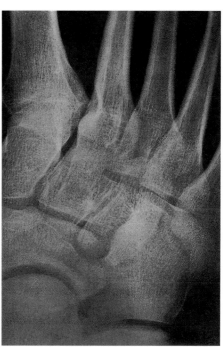

Fig. 7.**314 a–d**   Anatomy of the navicular bone.
a, b Distal (**a**) and proximal (**b**) aspects of the navicular with its articular surfaces (after Wolf-Heidegger).
c, d Superimposition and Mach effects between the lateral cuneiform and navicular, mimicking an accessory bone (arrows).

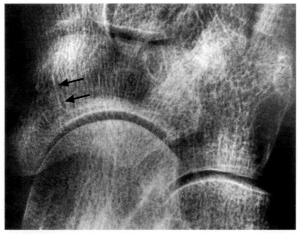

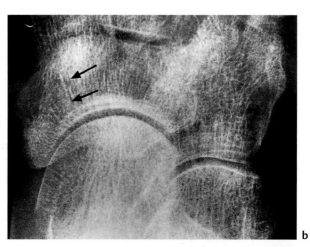

Fig. 7.**315 a, b**   Nutrient canal, not a fracture. Radiograph **a** was taken in June of 1995, radiograph **b** in October. The features marked with arrows are bounded by fine linear densities, which are a typical feature of nutrient canals. Note how the nutrient canal in **a** extends into the proximal articular surface. An extremely broad nutrient canal that disrupts the proximal articular margin is shown in Fig. 7.**262 c**.

Pathological Finding?

 Normal Variant or Anomaly?

Variants

One of the most familiar variants of the navicular is the **os tibiale externum**, known also as the **accessory navicular** (or the os naviculare secondarium or accessorium). Present in 10–16% of the population, it is located posterior to the posteromedial tuberosity and appears during adolescence. According to Mygind, it is more prevalent in women than in men. It is bilateral in 50–90% of cases (Mygind 1953, Romanowski and Barrington 1992).

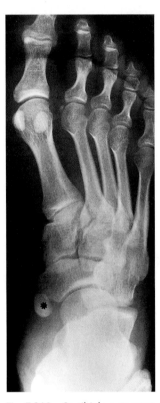

Fig. 7.**316**　Os tibiale externum, type 2.

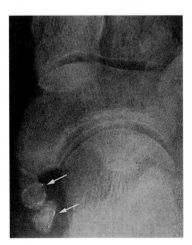

Fig. 7.**317**　Multipartite os tibiale externum in a 45-year-old woman.

Types of os tibiale externum

➤ *Type 1* (os tibiale externum in the strict sense) is a sesamoid bone approximately 2–3 mm in size that is embedded in the distal part of the tibialis posterior tendon (Fig. 7.**319**). It has no cartilaginous connection to the navicular tuberosity and is usually located up to 5 mm from it. Type 1 represents 30% of the total group and generally does not cause complaints (Mygind 1953, Sella et al. 1986, Romanowski and Barrington 1992).

➤ *Type 2* is triangular or heart-shaped and is up to 12 mm in diameter. It accounts for 50–60% of all accessory naviculars (Figs. 7.**316**–7.**318**, 7.**321**–7.**323**). It is interpreted as an accessory ossification center within the cartilage anlage from which the navicular develops (Lawson 1984). As a result, it is connected to the navicular tuberosity by a 1- to 2-mm-thick layer of fibrocartilage or hyaline cartilage (Zadek and Gold 1948, Lawson 1984). Portions of the tibialis posterior tendon may insert on this ossicle. Bony fusion with the tuberosity is relatively common and is clinically asymptomatic in most cases.

➤ *Type 3* denotes an exceptionally prominent navicular tuberosity ("cornuate navicular"). It can be interpreted as a fused version of type 2. Type 3 occasionally becomes symptomatic due to chronic inflammation of the overlying bursa. Figure 7.**320a–e** shows an isolated os tibiale externum combined with a very prominent tuberosity, and Fig. 7.**320f** shows a classic unilateral cornuate navicular. Types 1 and 2 may be duplicated or oligocentric.

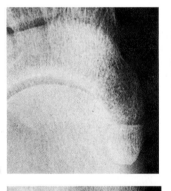
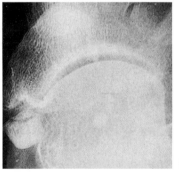
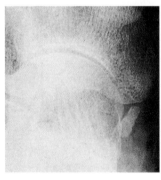
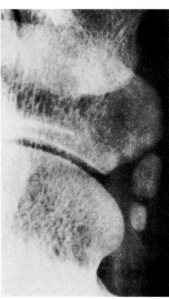

Fig. 7.**318a–d**　Various forms of a type 2 os tibiale externum, which is bipartite in **d**.

Fig. 7.**319 a–c**   Type 1 os tibiale externum. It is duplicated, consisting of a larger and smaller ossicle.

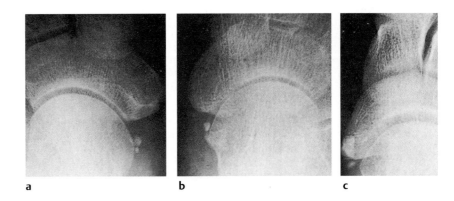

a   b   c

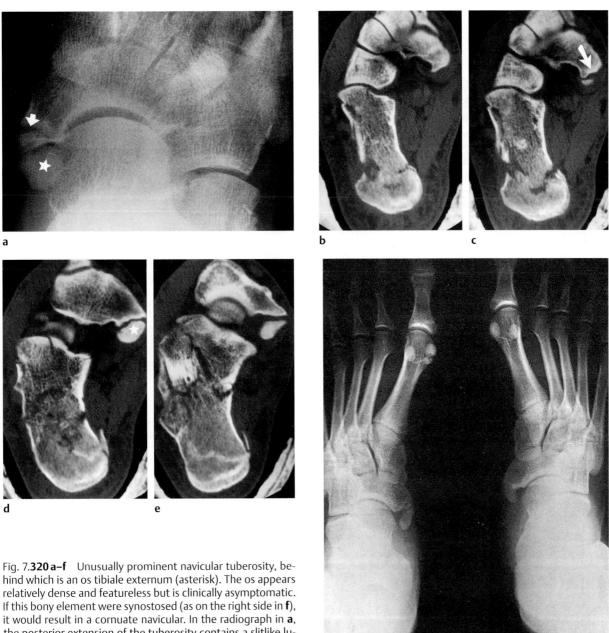

a

b   c

d   e

Fig. 7.**320 a–f**   Unusually prominent navicular tuberosity, behind which is an os tibiale externum (asterisk). The os appears relatively dense and featureless but is clinically asymptomatic. If this bony element were synostosed (as on the right side in **f**), it would result in a cornuate navicular. In the radiograph in **a**, the posterior extension of the tuberosity contains a slitlike lucency (arrow) that mimics a fracture. It is only a superimposition effect from the marked posteromedial extension of the process. There is a complex comminuted fracture of the calcaneus. In **f**, note the os tibiale externum on the left side and the cornuate navicular on the right side.

f

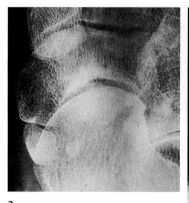
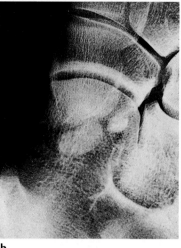

Fig. 7.**321 a, b**   Tilted os tibiale externum (bone island in the talar head).

The fibrocartilaginous or cartilaginous connection of type 2 with the tuberosity is not an articular connection, or at least not a synovial joint. The connection is more accurately described as a synchondrosis. But it is susceptible to regressive changes, which are commonly found in symptomatic patients (Figs. 7.**322**–7.**323**). Symptoms are particularly common following trauma to an os tibiale externum. This can cause displacement and tilting of the accessory

bone, which gives attachment to some of the fibers of the tibialis posterior tendon (Fig. 7.**321**). Uhrmacher (1934) described a situation in which the tibialis posterior tendon—which inserts on the medial navicular surface—had been elevated from its bed (below the sustentaculum tali) by a large os tibiale externum and displaced upward, with a corresponding tilt of the accessory bone.

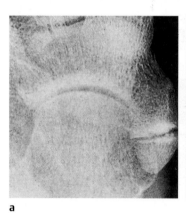
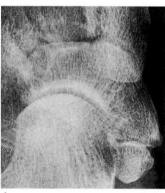
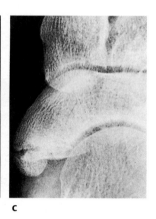

Fig. 7.**322 a–c**   Painful os tibiale externum.
a Woman 18 years of age. Marked subchondral densities are present in the tuberosity and accessory bone.

b Woman 35 years of age with subtle subchondral lucency opposite the os tibiale externum in the navicular.
c Boy 16 years of age with marked structural irregularities in the navicular opposite the accessory bone.

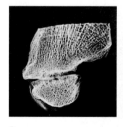
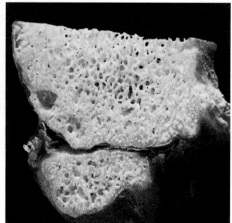

Fig. 7.**323 a, b**   Rarefied areas in the opposing portions of the navicular tuberosity and os tibiale externum (result of regressive changes).
a Specimen radiograph.
b Photograph of a sectioned specimen.

MRI can clearly demonstrate chronic stress on the os tibiale externum (especially type 2) as well as any subsequent necrosis (Miller et al. 1995). An accessory bone under chronic stress appears hypointense on T1-weighted images and hyperintense on T2-weighted images. These phenomena are due entirely to inflammatory edema (Fig. 7.**324**).

Flake fractures of the navicular tuberosity can occasionally be difficult to distinguish from an os tibiale externum on plain radiographs (Figs. 7.**325**, 7.**326**).

Another accessory bone that can occur near the navicular is the **os supranaviculare**. Averaging 6 mm × 5 mm × 6 mm in size, it is located on the dorsal aspect of the talonavicular joint, usually forming a kind of coalition with the navicular bone (Figs. 7.**327**–7.**330**, 7.**338 b**).

Past and present synonyms for the os supranaviculare are the dorsal astragaloscaphoid ossicle, intertaloscaphoid, and dorsal talonavicular ossicle. These terms are cited mainly for historical reasons, but they do emphasize the relationship of the os supranaviculare to the talus. It occurs in about 0.5% of the population and reportedly is more common in individuals with gross foot deformities. This accessory bone mainly requires differentiation from a detached osteophyte, especially in cases where osteophytes are already present on the adjacent articular margins of the talus and navicular (Fig. 7.**328**).

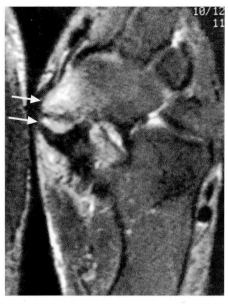

Fig. 7.**324** MRI demonstrates severe edema in the os tibiale externum (arrow) and in the navicular tuberosity (arrowhead). Axial fat-suppressed SE sequence (5300/45). (From Miller et al. 1995.)

Fig. 7.**325 a, b** Fracture of the navicular tuberosity, not an os tibiale externum (**a** 1993, **b** 1999). Radiograph **b** shows a broad callus bridge to the fragment, which shows slight proximal displacement.

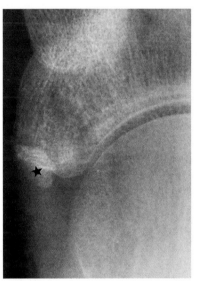

a

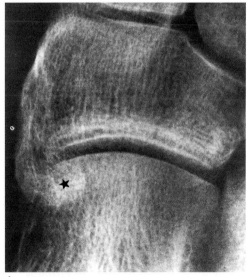

b

Fig. 7.**326** Fresh avulsion fracture of the navicular tuberosity.

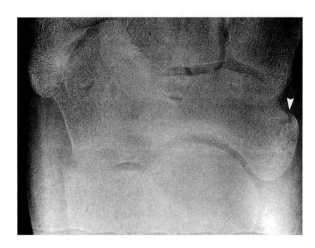

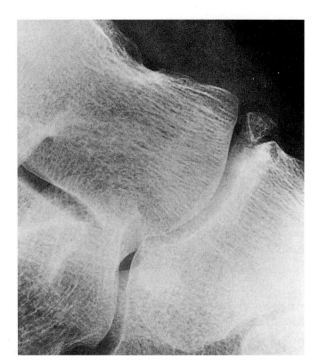

Fig. 7.**327**   Os supranaviculare, probably partially fused with the navicular.

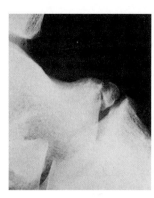

Fig. 7.**328**   Os supranaviculare, probably partially fused with the navicular. Note the conspicuous osteophytes on the superior margins of the talus and navicular.

A final accessory bone that can occur near the navicular is the **os infranaviculare**. This small ossicle is located over the dorsal aspect of the joint between the navicular and intermediate cuneiform bones (Figs. 7.**331**–7.**333**).

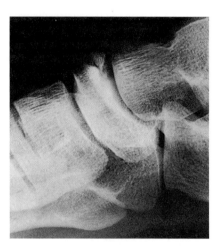

Fig. 7.**329**   Os supranaviculare.

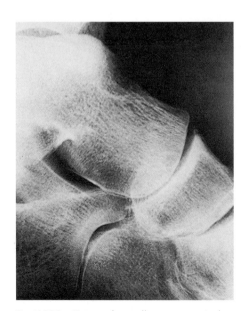

Fig. 7.**330**   Extremely small os supranaviculare.

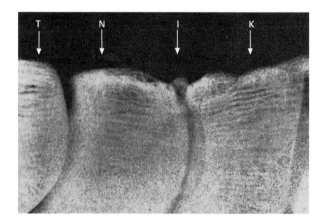

Fig. 7.**331**   Os infranaviculare over the joint between the navicular and intermediate cuneiform bones.
I   Os infranaviculare
K   Cuneiform
N   Navicular
T   Talus

Anomalies

A **bipartite navicular** is probably still a normal variant, despite the fact that it is commonly associated with a painful flatfoot. Of course, this association also suggests that the "variant" may actually be an old fatigue fracture. That would be consistent with the increased density of the lateral component, as shown in Figs. 7.**334** and 7.**335**. In any case, a bipartite navicular is definitely a preosteoarthritic deformity (Figs. 7.**334**–7.**336**).

Figure 7.**338** illustrates a **transverse partition** of the navicular, which probably reflects a deformity.

Multiple ossification centers in the navicular are completely normal during growth and should not be classified as a "partition" (Fig. 7.**337**). On the other hand, a bipartite navicular can result from the failure of two centers to fuse together.

Talonavicular fusion may be unilateral or bilateral (Fig. 7.**249**). Wildervanck et al. (1967) described familial cases that were combined with symphalangia of the fingers.

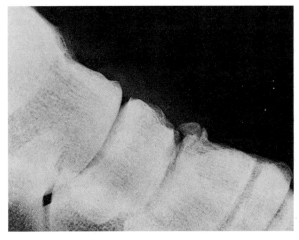

Fig. 7.**332** Example of an os infranaviculare located proximal to a bulge in the cuneiform. In consideration of the regressive changes on the extensor side of the joint, the differential diagnosis should include a fractured and displaced osteophyte and metaplastic bone formation in the tissues that glide over the joint. It is also possible for a primary os infranaviculare to "disrupt" the "physiological harmony" of the dorsal aspect of the joint and induce secondary osteoarthritis.

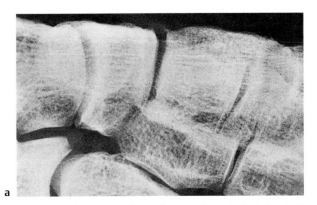
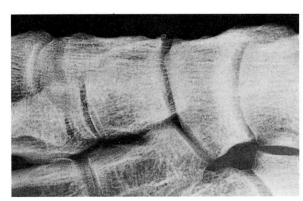

a   b

Fig. 7.**333 a, b** Extremely small ossa infranavicularia bordering the proximal superior rim of the medial cuneiform.

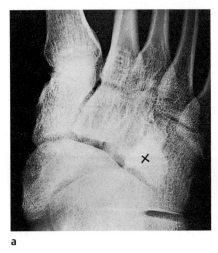
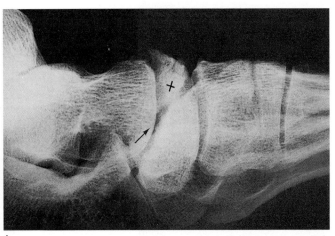

a   b

Fig. 7.**334a, b** Bipartite navicular. The smaller component (×) is relatively dense, raising the question of whether it may result from a stress fracture in a flat foot. The very dense structures clearly indicate at least partial nonfragmented osteonecrosis.

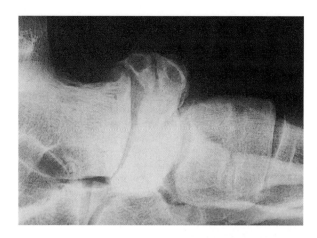

Fusions of the navicular with the calcaneus have been observed in spastic flatfoot (especially due to peroneus muscle spasms). This is particularly understandable in cases where a kind of medial anterior process is present above the calcaneocuboid joint and extends toward the navicular (Figs. 7.**277**, 7.**278** and p. 1028 f.).

◁ Fig. 7.**335** Bipartite navicular projecting well above the dorsal surface of the tarsus. Note the increased density in the plantar part of the navicular and along the adjacent talar head. The dorsal lucencies are also interpreted as regressive phenomena.

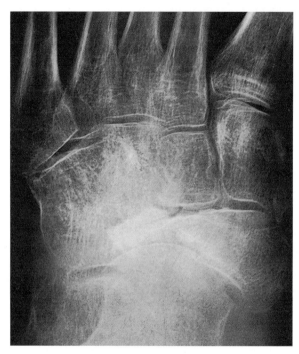

Fig. 7.**336** Bipartite navicular with increased density of the smaller component.

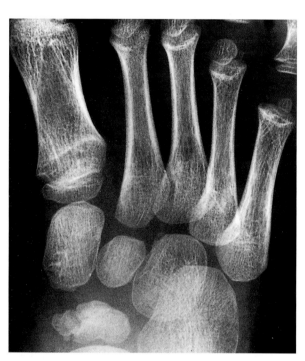

Fig. 7.**337** Not a bipartite navicular, but normal multiple ossification centers.

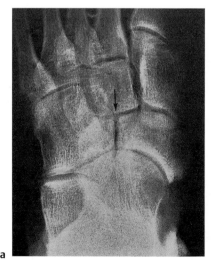

a

Fig. 7.**338a, b** Transverse partition of the navicular bone (unilateral) in a 42-year-old woman. Note the structural irregularities and deformity of the dorsal prominence. The talonavic-

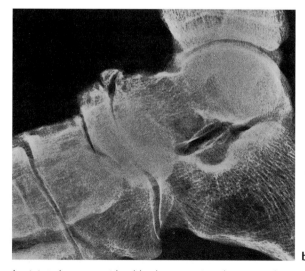

b

ular joint shows considerable degenerative change, with an isolated ossicle having the appearance of an os supranaviculare.

Fracture, Subluxation, or Dislocation?

The most common of the otherwise rare navicular fractures is the **dorsal avulsion fracture**, which may be mistaken for an os supranaviculare (q.v.). The next most common injury is a **fracture of the medial border of the tuberosity** caused by acute eversion with tearing of the tibialis posterior tendon. Usually the fracture is nondisplaced, making it difficult to detect. Differentiation is mainly required from an os tibiale externum (Figs. 7.**325**, 7.**326**).

Injuries of the midtarsal joint may cause **ligament ruptures** with **several millimeters' displacement of the navicular and cuboid**, depending on the direction of the traumatizing force (from the medial side, along the foot axis, or from the lateral or plantar aspect). This type of subluxation is usually caused by a longitudinal impact with the foot in plantar flexion and pressure on the metatarsal bones, causing the navicular to be compressed between the cuneiform and talar head. If the pressure is directed more along the axis of the lateral cuneiform, the forefoot and portions of the bones comprising the midtarsal joint are displaced medially, and the lateral part of the navicular and often the talar head are compressed.

In this type of injury, fragments of the navicular may be extruded dorsally (Fig. 7.**339a**). A flake fracture in the plantar portion of the navicular is shown in Fig. 7.**339b**.

Stress fractures of the navicular generally run longitudinally (Fig. 7.**340a–i**). They are seldom detectable on conventional radiographs (Fig. 7.**340a**) but are strongly positive on bone scans. On MRI, they are generally associated with massive edema that obscures the fracture line. The best modality for defining the fracture line is CT (Fig. 7.**340d–i**).

In the time before advanced imaging modalities (CT, MRI) it was shown that the interval between the onset of complaints and imaging diagnosis may be less than one month or as much as 38 months (Pavlov 1983). Navicular stress fractures occur predominantly in athletes and also in untrained individuals who subject the foot to unaccustomed loads (without prior conditioning of the bone).

 ## Necrosis?

Aseptic necrosis of the navicular is also known as **Köhler disease**. Köhler described it as occurring mainly in "small and asthenic children (especially boys) between 2 and 10 years of age." The main clinical symptom is a painful limp, often with local tenderness over the navicular, a doughy soft-tissue swelling, redness, and warmth. The complaints may subside in a few days or may persist for years. Radiographic healing may take from three months to four years.

> In our own large collection of aseptic necrosis cases, we do not have a single confirmed case of navicular necrosis, although we do not dispute that the condition exists.

Objective documentation of this disease is difficult owing to the natural density and irregularity of the ossification center(s) of the navicular, which are indistinguishable from necrosis by radiographs alone (Figs. 7.**310**–7.**312**, 7.**337**). Earlier descriptions of the radiographic course of the disease suggest that it is actually an ossification variant rather than true necrosis. **Today we require at least MRI abnormality** with a signal void on T1-weighted images and increased signal intensity on T2-weighted images to establish necrosis with reasonable confidence. Köhler's original radiograph from 1908 is shown in Fig. 7.**341**.

Interpreting this radiograph today (and allowing for the poor quality of the time), we would not consider it abnormal. The clinical symptoms may have had a different cause. In the case shown in Fig. 7.**342**, the child had pain on the medial side of the right foot that we could not explain. The roentgen abnormalities, consisting of circumscribed lucencies in the opposing borders of the navicular and medial cuneiform, were at least suspicious for a necrotic process. But the MR images only showed slightly irregular ossification with no signal abnormalities.

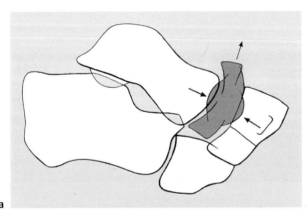

a

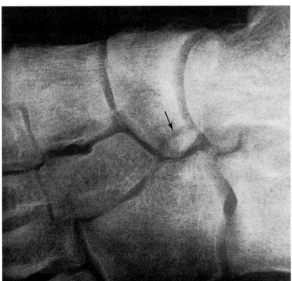

b

Fig. 7.**339a, b** Navicular fractures.
a Compression fracture of the navicular (after Dihlmann).
b Fracture in the plantar portion of the navicular.

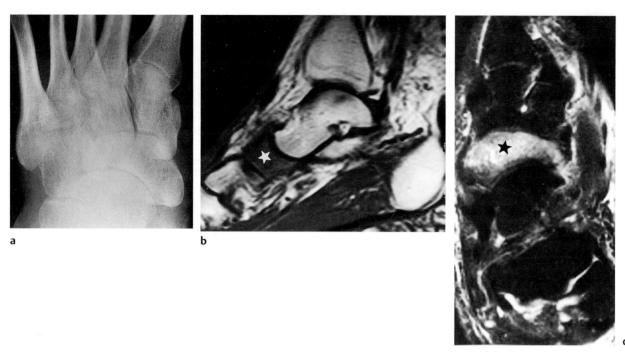

a   b   c

Fig. 7.340 a–i   Incomplete stress fracture in the dorsal part of the navicular.
a Conventional radiograph shows no definite abnormalities. Bone scan showed intense uptake in the navicular (not shown here).

b, c T1-weighted MRI (**b**) shows complete obliteration of the fat signal by edema, which appears in the T2-weighted image (**c**) as a hyperintense area within the navicular (star).

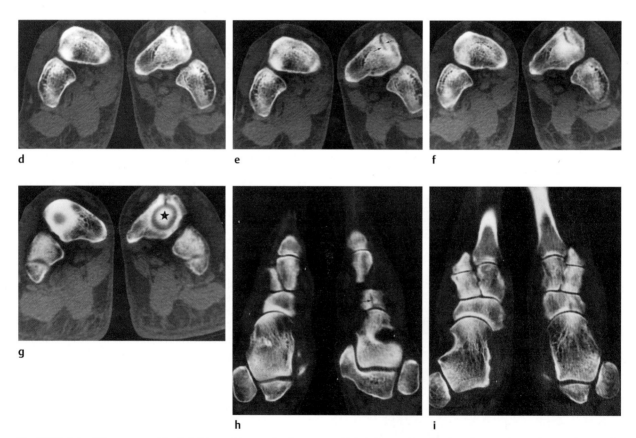

d   e   f

g   h   i

Fig. 7.340 d–i   CT scans provide definitive evidence of a fracture, which is located in the dorsal navicular and extends into the talonavicular joint (**g**). The talar trochlea appears as a spherical density in **g**. Coronal scans (**d–g**), axial scans (**h, i**).

Inflammation? Tumor?

Inflammatory changes in the navicular are rare. Figure 7.**343** shows a case of **articular tuberculosis** that spread to the bone, causing fragmentation.

Osteoid osteoma can occur in the navicular, as well as **chondroblastoma** and other **benign tumors**. Sporadic cases of **osteosarcoma** have also been reported in the navicular.

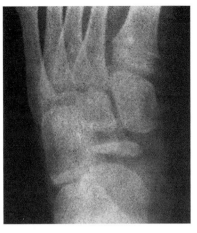

Fig. 7.**341** Köhler's original radiograph taken in 1908 to document "Köhler's disease" (aseptic necrosis of the navicular). Even allowing for the relatively poor image quality, today we would not interpret this finding as abnormal (see text).

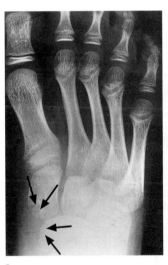
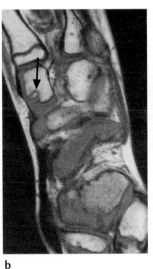
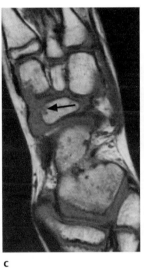
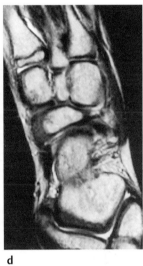

a   b   c   d

Fig. 7.**342 a–d** Clinical suspicion of partial aseptic necrosis of the opposing borders of the navicular and medial cuneiform bones in an 8-year-old boy.
a Dorsoplantar radiograph shows circumscribed lucencies in the opposing medial borders of the two bones.
b–d MR images show normal-appearing cartilage surrounding both bones. On MRI, the radiographic lucencies (arrows) are found to contain a small separate ossification center in the medial cuneiform (**b**) and bone and cartilage in the navicular (**c**). There are no signal abnormalities in the T2-weighted image (**d**). Necrosis was therefore excluded on the basis of MRI findings. (Case courtesy of Dr. L. Baumbach, Rostock.)

Fig. 7.**343 a, b** Navicular bone in a 4-year-old girl.
a The navicular shows increased radiographic density (normal finding?). The borders of the adjacent distal tarsal bones are ill-defined.
b Several months later, bacteriological tests confirmed tuberculosis.

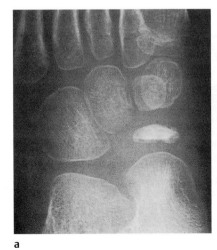
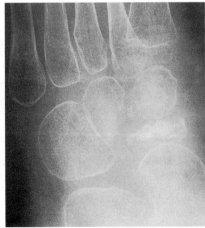

a   b

Other Changes?

The articular surfaces of the navicular are susceptible to **osteoarthritic changes**, especially when the bone occupies an abnormal position (e.g., pes planus with sagging of the navicular due to collapse of the medial arch, Roth et al. 1982).

The imaging features of navicular osteoarthritis are the same as in other joints. Degenerative osteophytes require differentiation from accessory bones (os supranaviculare and os infranaviculare). Marked osteoproliferative changes on the dorsal margins of the navicular and medial cuneiform are particularly common in **gout** (Fig. 7.**344**).

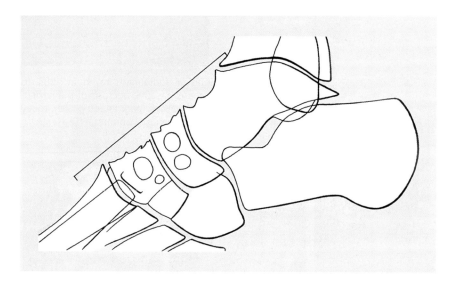

Fig. 7.**344** "Shaggy foot" appearance caused by degenerative osteophytes and fibro-ostosis on the dorsal aspect of the foot (after Dihlmann).

References

Dihlmann, W.: Gelenke, Wirbelverbindungen, 2. Aufl. Thieme, Stuttgart 1982

Gordon, G. M., J. Solar: Tarsal navicular stress fractures. J. Amer. podiat. med. Ass. 75 (1985) 363

Groß, K.: Schmerzhaftes Os naviculare pedis mit histologisch nachgewiesener subchondraler Nekrose. Z. Orthop. 84 (1954) 50

Holmes, C., E. Ronda, J. Vennett et al.: Transverse navicular fracture. J. Amer. podiat. med. Ass. 76 (1986) 43

Köhler, A.: Über eine häufige, bisher anscheinend unbekannte Erkrankung einzelner kindlicher Knochen. Verh. dtsch. Röntg.-Ges. 4 (1908) 110 und Münch. med. Wschr. 37 (1908) 1923

Köhler, A.: Das Köhlersche Knochenbild des Os naviculare pedis bei Kindern — keine Fraktur. Langenbecks Arch. klin. Chir. 101 (1913) 560

Lawson, J. P.: Clinically significant radiologic anatomic variants of the skeleton. Amer. J. Roentgenol. 163 (1994) 249

Lawson, J. P., J. A. Ogden, E. Sella et al.: The painful accessory navicular. Skelet. Radiol. 12 (1984) 250

Mau, H.: Zur Kenntnis des Os naviculare bipartitum pedis. Z. Orthop. 93 (1960) 404

Miller, Th. T., R. B. Staron, F. Feldmann et al.: The symptomatic accessory tarsal navicular bone: assessment with MR imaging. Radiology 195 (1995) 849

Mygind, H. B.: The accessory tarsal scaphoid: clinical features and treatment. Acta orthop. scand 23 (1953) 142

Pavlov, H., J. S. Torg, R. H. Freiberger: Tarsal navicular stress fractures: radiographic evaluation. Radiology 148 (1983) 641

Ravelli, A.: Osteochondritis dissecans am Os naviculare pedis. Z. Orthop. 85 (1954) 485

Reisner, A.: Drei Fälle von Os supranaviculare. Röntgenpraxis 2 (1930) 422

Rogers, L. F.: Radiology of Skeletal Trauma. Churchill Livingstone, New York 1982 (p. 889)

Romanowski, C. A. J., N. A. Barrington: The accessory navicular: an important cause of medial foot pain. Clin. Radiol. 46 (1992) 261

Roth, A., P. Trosko, M. C. Boxer: Osteoarthritis of the tarsal bones of the foot. J. Amer. podiat. med. Ass. 72 (1982) 244

Sella, E. J., J. P. Lawson, J. A. Ogden: The accessory navicular synchondrosis. Clin. Orthop. 209 (1986) 280

Uhrmacher, F.: Varietäten des Fußskeletts als Grundlage von Fußbeschwerden. Z. orthop. Chir. 61 (1934) 180

Wildervanck, L. S., G. Goedhard, S. Mejer: Proximal symphalangism of fingers associated with fusion of naviculare and talus and occurence of two accessory bones in the feet. Acta genet. 17 (1967) 166

Wiley, J., D. E. Brown: The bipartite tarsal scaphoid. J. Bone Jt Surg. 63-B (1981) 583

Zadek, I., A. M. Gold: The accessory tarsal scaphoid. J. Bone Jt Surg. 30-A (1948) 957

Cuboid Bone

Normal Findings

 During Growth

The cuboid bone ossifies at the end of the fetal period or during the first month after birth. It is normally ossified from multiple centers that unite within a short time to form a single center. Figure 7.**313** shows how large the cuboid center may be in a 16-month-old child.

 In Adulthood

Generally, the lateral distal portion of the cuboid is fairly radiolucent because of its relative thinness. On the plantar

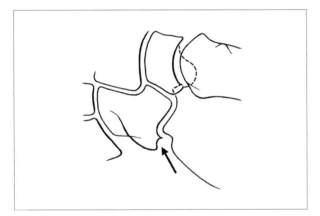

Fig. 7.**345** Notch in the cuboid is the normal groove for the peroneus longus tendon (after Birkner).

side is the relatively broad and solid tuberosity. Between it and the distal articular surface is a deep groove for the peroneus longus tendon, whose extension appears as a notch in the oblique projection (Fig. 7.**345**).

The cuboid articulates proximally with the calcaneus, distally with the third and fourth metatarsals, and medially with the lateral cuneiform.

Pathological Finding?

 Normal Variant or Anomaly?

The most important accessory bone is the **os cuboideum secundarium** (Fig. 7.**346**), which is easily distinguished from the calcaneus secundarius on radiographs (p. 1028). Coalition of an os cuboideum secundarium with the "parent bone" is shown in Fig. 7.**347**.

Another accessory bone is the **os peroneum**, which was first described by Vesalius (synonyms: accessory cuboid, os peroneale, sesamum peroneum). It begins to ossify in the peroneus longus tendon no earlier than the 14th year of life. It is more common in females than in males. The frequency and size of the bone reportedly increase with aging, as does the frequency with which the bone is partitioned (see below). The os peroneum is present in approximately 18 % of the population (Siecke 1964). It is located at the lateral inferior edge of the cuboid in the groove for the peroneus longus tendon. It is both adjacent and distal to the cuboid tuberosity. Generally it has smooth margins, is round to oval, and occasionally forms a pseudoarticulation (or synchondrosis or fibrocartilaginous bridge) with the cuboid (Fig. 7.**348d**).

In a few cases the os peroneum may be located farther dorsally and closer to the calcaneus (Fig. 7.**349a, b**), and it may form a radiographic articulation with the latter bone.

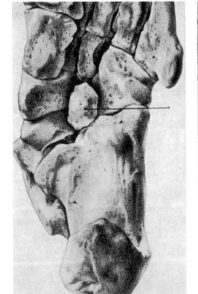
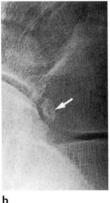

b

a

Fig. 7.**346a, b** Os cuboideum secundarium (arrows in **a** and **b**) (**a** after Dwight).

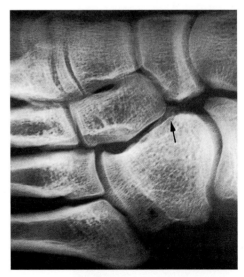

Fig. 7.**347** Prominence on the cuboid bone: most likely an os cuboideum secundarium that has fused with the main cuboid.

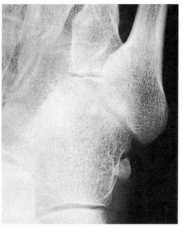
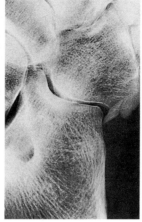
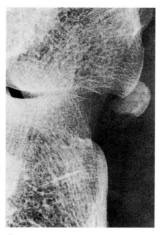

a   b   c

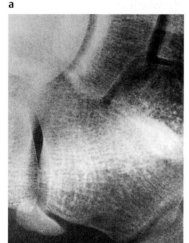

d

◁ Fig. 7.**348 a–d**   Varying shapes of the os peroneum.
a Dorsoplantar projection.
b Lateral projection.
c Large os peroneum with an irregular structure and slightly ill-defined margins (clinically asymptomatic).
d Large os peroneum with a regular structure and sharp cortical delineation.

Regarding the "increased frequency" of the os peroneum with aging mentioned above, the most likely explanation is that the accessory bones that appear in later life are actually a product of metaplastic bone formation. The tendency for partitioning of the ossicle to increase with aging may be a result of necrotic changes with fragmentation (Fig. 7.**350**).

Acute fractures of the os peroneum are rare and are usually combined with fractures of other tarsal bones. Isolated fractures of the os peroneum have been described, however. Most go on to nonunion, but this rarely causes complaints (Fig. 7.**350**). Fractures of the os peroneum may be caused by direct trauma or by vigorous traction on the peroneus longus tendon. The peroneus tendon itself may rupture due to excessive strain, manifested by a **sudden posterior displacement of the os peroneum**, so that it is projected over the center of the calcaneus. Small, fragmentary remnants occupy the original location of the ossicle (Tehranzadeh et al. 1984).

It was noted earlier that the os peroneum may sometimes result from metaplastic bone formation in the region of the plantar aponeurosis or from an old, structured bursal calcification in the peroneus tendon following peritendini-

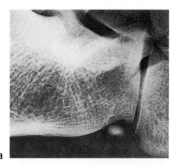

a

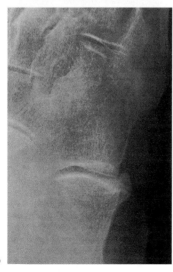

b

◁ Fig. 7.**349 a, b**   Os peroneum.
a Os peroneum below a recess in the calcaneus.
b Os peroneum "articulating" with the calcaneus.

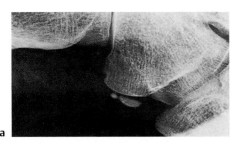

a

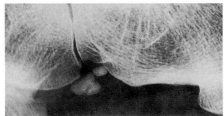

b

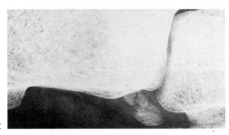

c

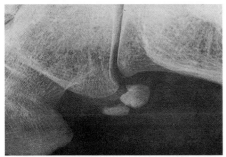

d

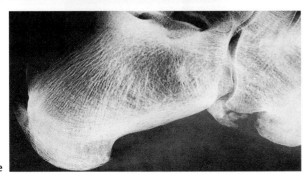

e

Fig. 7.**350 a–e** Partitions and deformities of the os peroneum, probably due to necrosis or fractures. The small bony elements may also be metaplastic ossifications that transformed to lamellar bone over time.

tis (Fig. 7.**351**). The latter condition is especially common in painters who stand on ladders for prolonged periods.

An apparently very rare accessory bone element is located at the distal edge of the cuboid and fills the space between the cuboid, lateral cuneiform, and third and fourth metatarsals (Fig. 7.**354**).

Various types of **synostosis** (coalition) can occur between the cuboid and adjacent bones (see General Aspects, p. 999). **Pes planus** is associated with a large gap between the cuboid, navicular, and talus, visible in the dorsoplantar projection.

 ## Fracture, Subluxation, or Dislocation?

Of primary interest in this context is a lateral avulsion fracture of the cuboid, which should not be mistaken for an os peroneum (Figs. 7.**352**, 7.**353**).

Fractures of the os peroneum are discussed above.

 ## Necrosis?

The literature to date contains very little information on necrotic changes in the cuboid. Early changes are detectable only by MRI in the form of edema.

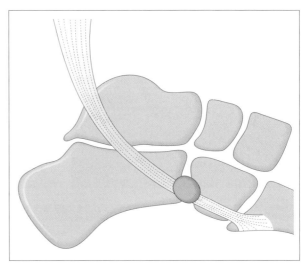

Fig. 7.**351** Calcified bursitis or calcific peritendinitis.

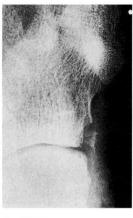

Fig. 7.**352**

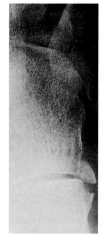

Fig. 7.**353**

 Inflammation? Tumor?

We know of no published reports on circumscribed inflammatory changes in the cuboid. We personally observed a small, subchondral osteoid osteoma located adjacent to the lateral cuneiform (Fig. 7.**355**). This tumor was associated with fairly dramatic symptoms.

Fig. 7.**352**   Lateral avulsion fracture of the cuboid.

Fig. 7.**353**   Calcaneal avulsion resembling an os peroneum.

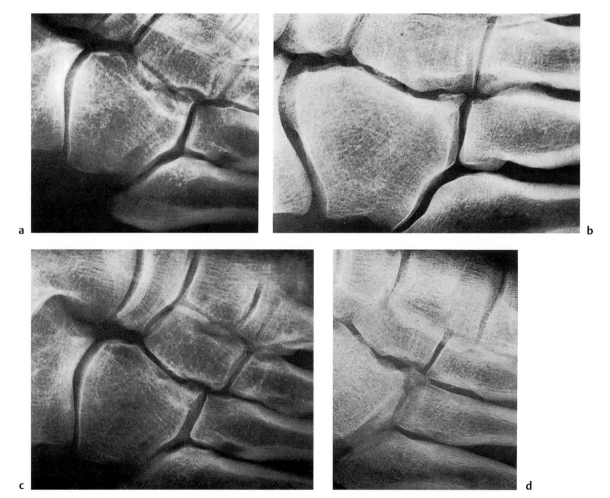

Fig. 7.**354 a–d**   Accessory bone on the medial distal aspect of the cuboid, occupying the space between the cuboid, lateral cuneiform, and third and fourth metatarsals.

Fig. 7.**355a–d**   Small osteoid osteoma located below the cuboid articular facet for the lateral cuneiform.

a On a conventional radiograph hardly discernable (arrows).

b The "dramatic" bone scan, showing intense tracer uptake throughout the tarsus, illustrates the most spectacular feature of this tumor: "small tumor, large reaction". The enormously increased radiotracer uptake results from a "sympathetic" arthritis in the joints of the whole tarsus.

c, d CT scans (in different projections) demonstrate the osteolytic nidus with central calcification (arrows).

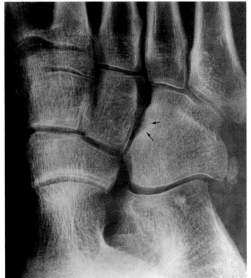

a

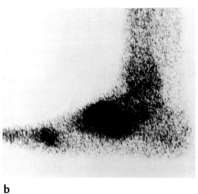

b

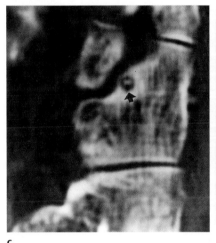

c

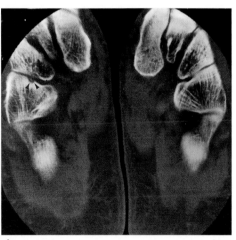

d

References

Hermel, M. B., J. Gershon-Cohen: The nut cracker fracture of the cuboid by indirect violence. Radiology 60 (1953) 850

Miller, C. F.: Occupational calcareous peritendinitis of the feet. Amer. J. Roentgenol. 61 (1939) 506

Nicastro, J. F., H. A. Haupt: Probable stress fracture of the cuboid in an infant. J. Bone Jt Surg. 66-A (1984) 1105

Rogers, L. F.: Radiology of Skeletal Trauma. Churchill Livingstone, New York 1982 (p. 893)

Siecke, H.: Beitrag zur Genese des Os peronaeum. Z. Orthop. 98 (1964) 358

Tehranzadeh, J., D. A. Stoll, O. M. Gabriele: Case report: posterior migration of the os peroneum of the left foot, indicating a tear of the peroneal tendon. Skelet. Radiol. 12 (1984) 44

Medial Cuneiform Bone

▌*Normal Findings*

 ### During Growth

The ossification center for the medial cuneiform bone generally appears between 1 and 4 years of age, but earlier ossification may occur (Fig. 7.**356**). The medial border may exhibit a slightly ragged contour (Fig. 7.**358**). A separate ossification center is often seen at the distal, dorsal corner of the bone (Fig. 7.**358**). Multiple centers are also a normal variant and are apparently related to the development of a bipartite cuneiform (de Cuveland 1957). Multicentric ossification (Fig. 7.**357**) is rare but not abnormal. Occasional circumscribed densities may be found in the distal portions of the medial cuneiform in children without having any pathological implications (Fig. 7.**359**). We have found similar circumscribed densities in other tarsal bones, most notably the navicular.

A small, defect-like gap in the proximal medial circumference of the cuneiform is also considered a normal variant (Fig. 7.**342**).

The medial cuneiform is subject to numerous radiographic superimposition effects involving the base of the first metatarsal and also the intermediate cuneiform, as shown in Fig. 7.**360**.

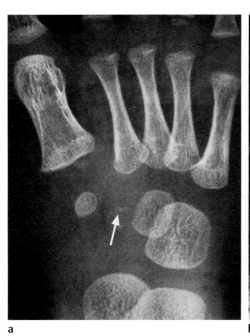

a

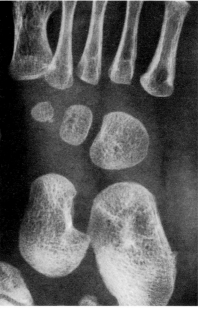

b

Fig. 7.**356a, b** Medial cuneiform bone in the dorsoplantar (**a**) and oblique projection (**b**) in a child 1 year and 7 months of age. Note that the intermediate cuneiform appears as a faint bony shadow in the dorsoplantar view (arrow) and is projected very close to the medial cuneiform in the oblique view (arrow).

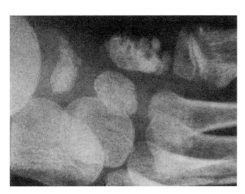

Fig. 7.**357** Multiple ossification centers for the cuneiform and navicular bones.

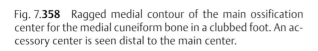

Fig. 7.**358** Ragged medial contour of the main ossification center for the medial cuneiform bone in a clubbed foot. An accessory center is seen distal to the main center.

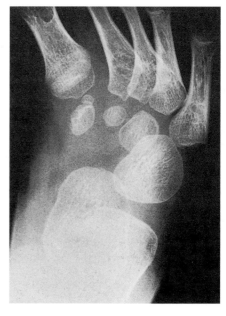

Fig. 7.**359a–d** Small circumscribed density in the distal end of the medial cuneiform (arrow) in a 5-year-old child is a normal variant of cuneiform ossification. Since the child had non-specific complaints in the right foot, the finding was first interpreted as an osteoid osteoma. But the negative bone scan (**d**) excluded this entity. The oblique radiograph (**c**) superimposes much of the medial and intermediate cuneiforms but gives a clear projection of the density, showing its homogeneous continuity with the bone and excluding an accessory center. Similar phenomena of circumscribed densities in an ossification center are also seen in other bones including the navicular (q.v.).

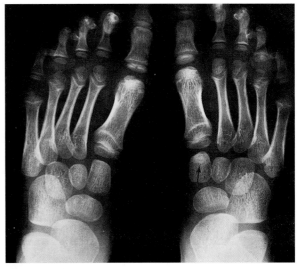

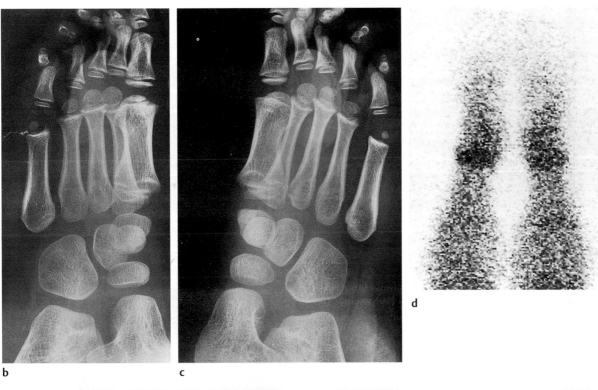

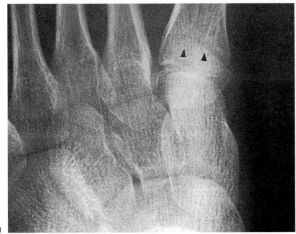

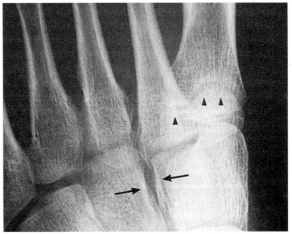

Fig. 7.**360a, b** Superimposition effects from the proximal epiphyseal plate of the first metatarsal in dorsoplantar and oblique radiographs (arrowheads). Apparent gaping of the joint space between the medial and intermediate cuneiform bones (arrows) is a normal finding.

In Adulthood

The medial cuneiform has three articular surfaces that articulate proximally with the navicular, laterally with the intermediate cuneiform, and distally with the first metatarsal. A normal exostosis-like prominence may be found on the medial aspect of the bone (Fig. 7.**361**). Just distal to the prominence is a groove for the tibialis anterior tendon.

Pathological Finding?

Normal Variant or Anomaly?

Variants

Variants in the ossification of the medial cuneiform were discussed above.

A **horizontal cleft in the medial cuneiform (bipartite medial cuneiform)** (Figs. 7.**362**, 7.**363**) is not particularly rare (Zeitler 1959). Whether it is a variant is unknown, as there have been too few follow-up observations. Reportedly, a bipartite medial cuneiform has been found in one-third of patients with a pes adductus deformity. The partition may be incomplete.

> A word of caution for the novice: Radiographic superimposition effects in the foot can mimic an incomplete partition of the medial cuneiform bone where none exists.

The following accessory bones are classified as harmless normal variants:

- The **sesamum tibiale anterius** is a sesamoid bone that occurs in the tibialis anterior tendon (synonyms: os paracuneiforme, os cuneometatarsale I tibiale, Fig. 7.**364**). If this sesamoid is located near the tibialis anterior insertion on the plantar side of the medial cuneiform, it may go undetected on lateral and dorsoplantar radiographs due to superimposition. In patients with flat feet, an accessory bone at this location may be compressed between the medial cuneiform and a shoe insert, stressing the bone and occasionally causing necrosis with clinical complaints. Figure 7.**364 c** shows the unusual case of a large, symptomatic sesamoid bone (with a smaller companion) occurring in the tibialis anterior tendon.
- The **os cuneonavicular mediale** is an accessory bone located somewhat proximal to the sesamum tibiale anterius (Fig. 7.**365**). It is usually quite small and may have an articular connection with the medial cuneiform. Bilateral occurrence is observed (Fig. 7.**367**). These accessory bones should not be confused with fresh avulsion fractures (Fig. 7.**366**).
- The **os cuneometatarsale plantare I** (Fig. 7.**368**) has been described only by anatomists. It may not be visualized on conventional radiographs.
- The **os intercuneiforme** (Fig. 7.**369**) has likewise been documented only in anatomic specimens.

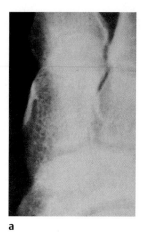
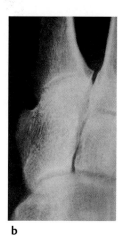

a   b

Fig. 7.**361 a, b** Physiological bony prominence on the medial aspect of the medial cuneiform (**b**). The tibialis anterior tendon lies in the notch or groove distal to the prominence. The tangential projection of the prominence in radiograph **a** accounts for its dense appearance.

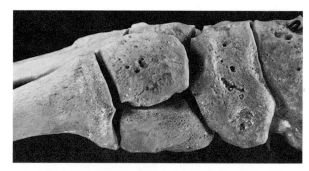

Fig. 7.**362**   Bipartite medial cuneiform in an anatomic specimen.

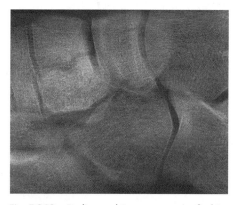

Fig. 7.**363**   Radiographic appearance of a bipartite medial cuneiform.

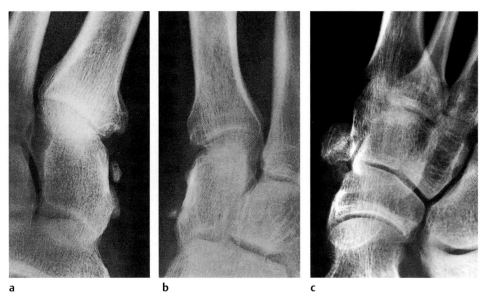

a   **b**   **c**

Fig. 7.**364 a–c**   Sesamoid bone.
a, b Bilateral occurrence of the sesamum tibiale anterius.

c Unusually large sesamoid bone in the tibialis anterior tendon, accompanied by a smaller, more proximal sesamoid.
Clinically the bone was palpable, visible, and very painful.
Complaints were relieved by surgical removal. (Case courtesy
of Dr. G. Puorger, Switzerland; Puorger 1989.)

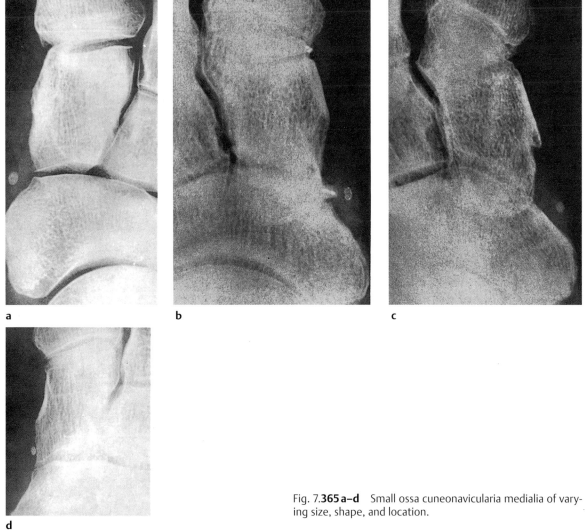

a   **b**   **c**

d

Fig. 7.**365 a–d**   Small ossa cuneonavicularia medialia of varying size, shape, and location.

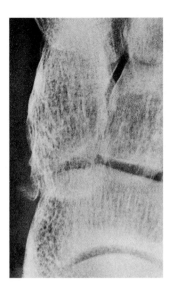

Fig. 7.**366**　Avulsion fracture of the medial cuneiform bone.

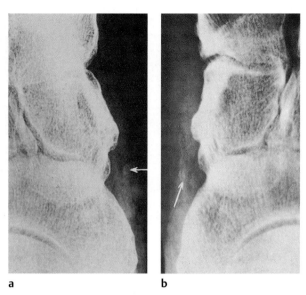

a   b

Fig. 7.**367 a, b**　Bilateral occurrence of the os cuneonavicular mediale (arrows).

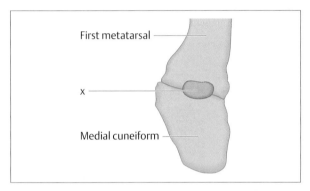

Fig. 7.**368**　Os cuneometatarsale plantare I (×) (after Pfitzner).

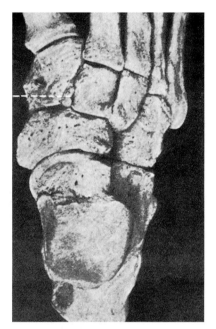

Fig. 7.**369**　Os intercuneiforme (after Dwight).

Anomalies

A definite anomaly is shown schematically in Fig. 7.**370**. It consists of a rudimentary supernumerary phalanx located on the medial side of the medial cuneiform and having a proximal articulation with the navicular.

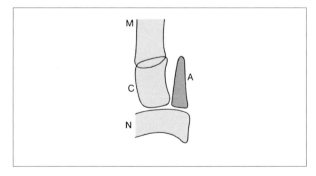

Fig. 7.**370**　Anomaly in which an isolated, phalanx-like bone articulates with the navicular but has no contact with the medial cuneiform (after Babucke).

A　Accessory bone　　　　　M　First metatarsal
C　Medial cuneiform　　　　　N　Navicular

Fracture, Subluxation, or Dislocation?

Isolated cuneiform fractures are most unusual. Distal cuneiform fractures are discussed under the heading of tarsometatarsal dislocations (q.v.).

Reference was made earlier to the potentially important **medial avulsion fracture of the medial cuneiform** and its differentiation from an accessory bone (Fig. 7.**366**).

 Necrosis?

The medial cuneiform is of course susceptible to **aseptic necrosis**, including subchondral involvement (**osteochondritis dissecans**). We have not observed this condition ourselves but presume that the typical radiographic signs of osteonecrosis or osteochondritis dissecans of this bone are the same as elsewhere. Variants in the ossification of the pediatric medial cuneiform were discussed previously (Figs. 7.**342**, 7.**358**, 7.**359**).

 Other Changes?

Osteophytes may occur on the dorsal articular margins of the medial cuneiform and the first metatarsal but do not necessarily signify degenerative joint disease. They are observed in women who frequently wear very high-heeled shoes. They are also found in toe dancers and in patients with valgus foot deformities. Called "wooden shoe knotty excrescence or protuberance" ("Holzschuhknorren") in Sweden (Haglund 1932), these excrescences bear some resemblance to carpal bossing in the upper extremity.

References

de Cuveland, E.: Zur Ossifikation des 1. Keilbeines. Z. Orthop. 89 (1957) 266

Haglund, P.: Die dorsale Tuberosität an der Articulation metatarso-cuneiforme T. Z. orthop. Chir. 56 (1932) 601

Henche, H. J. R.: Die Bedeutung überzähliger Knochenelemente und Exostosen am Fuß. Ther. Umsch. 31 (1974) 29

Leeson, M. C., D. S. Weiner: Osteochondrosis of the tarsal cuneiform. Clin. Orthop. 186 (1985) 260

Morrison, A. B.: The os paracuneiforme (some observations on an example removed). J. Bone Jt Surg. 35-B (1953) 254

Neumann, R.: Das Os praecuneiforme (BAUHIN) am menschlichen Tarsus. Arch. orthop. Unfall.-Chir. 45 (1953) 552

Pfitzner, W.: Die Variationen im Aufbau des Fußskelettes. Schwalbes morphol. Arb. 6 (1896) 245

Puorger, G: Der seltene Fall (2 Sesambeine der Tibialis-anterior-Sehne). Schweiz. Rdsch. Med. Prax. 78 (1989) 18

Rogers, L. F.: Radiology of Skeletal Trauma. Churchill Livingstone, New York 1982 (p. 893)

Zeitler, E.: Multizentrische Ossifikation und Knochendystrophie des Os cuneiforme I bipartitum. Z. Orthop. 92 (1959) 189

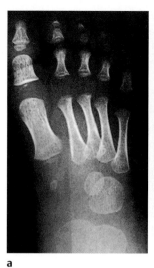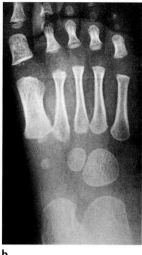

a   b

Fig. 7.**371 a, b**   Radiographs from a 2-year-old girl. The ossification center for the intermediate cuneiform is not yet visible (see also Fig. 7.**356**).

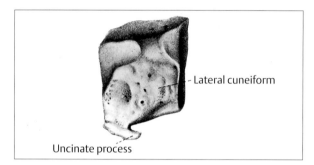

─ Lateral cuneiform

Uncinate process

Fig. 7.**372**   Uncinate process (after Pfitzner).

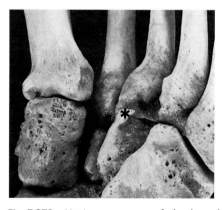

Fig. 7.**373**   Uncinate process of the lateral cuneiform (asterisk) (Department of Anatomy, University of Basel).

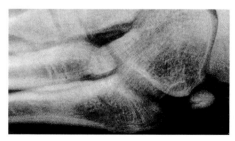

Fig. 7.**374**   Relatively large gap between the lateral cuneiform, cuboid, and base of the fourth metatarsal. The faint densities in that area may represent incipient ossification of the os unci (see text).

Normal Findings

 ### During Growth

The ossification center for the intermediate cuneiform bone appears in the second to fourth year of life, that for the lateral cuneiform bone in the first year of life (Figs. 7.**356**, 7.**371**).

Thus, the ossification center for the intermediate cuneiform is the last of the cuneiform centers to appear on radiographs. Sometimes it appears at about the same time as the center for the navicular, which itself is very late to ossify. Irregularities in the ossification of the intermediate and lateral cuneiforms generally have no pathological significance. They resemble those that have been described for the medial cuneiform.

 ### In Adulthood

It is normal to find notches in the opposing borders of the three cuneiform bones (Figs. 7.**360**, 7.**365 b**). Some are grooves for the interosseous ligaments.

Pathological Finding?

 ### Normal Variant or Anomaly?

The os intercuneiforme was mentioned on p. 1062 (Fig. 7.**369**).

Occasionally an accessory bone element called the **os cuneometatarsale II dorsale** is found close to the intermediate cuneiform. It is interposed dorsally between the intermediate cuneiform and the base of the second metatarsal.

The **uncinate process of the lateral cuneiform** (Figs. 7.**372**, 7.**373**) is also considered a normal variant. It is located on the plantar side by the base of the third metatarsal.

If this process occurs in isolation, it is also termed the **os unci** (Fig. 7.**386**).

Oblique radiographs of the foot often show a gap between the lateral cuneiform, cuboid, and the angled base of the fourth metatarsal. This area could represent the cartilage from which the os unci is derived (Fig. 7.**374**).

Congenital **synostoses** of the two cuneiforms with metatarsal bones have been described. It is unknown whether these fusions have any functional importance.

A case with bilateral synostoses involving the intermediate and lateral cuneiforms in addition to other bones is shown in Fig. 7.**221 f, g**.

Fracture, Subluxation, or Dislocation?

The intermediate and lateral cuneiform bones are susceptible to avulsion fractures, which are usually combined with additional injuries, especially of the tarsometatarsal region. Multiple superimposition effects in this region are occasionally a source of confusion on radiographs (see also Medial Cuneiform Bone).

Necrosis?

Generally the cuneiforms are among the tarsal bones that are affected with some frequency by **osteonecrosis** (**diabetic osteoarthropathy**, Fig. 7.375) in patients with long-standing **insulin-dependent diabetes mellitus**.

Diabetic osteoarthropathy of the foot is found in approximately 2–4% of all long-standing, clinically sympto-

Fig. 7.**375 a–e**   Diabetic osteoarthropathy, follow-up over about a 2-year period.
a Initial radiograph shows only subtle changes: slightly increased density in the medial and intermediate cuneiforms, which are superimposed, and in the base of the first metatarsal.
b Just three months later, gross destructive changes are visible in the intermediate and lateral cuneiforms, with marked derangement of the peripheral intertarsal and tarsometatarsal joints. For comments on the metatarsal changes, see Fig. 7.**410**.
c An oblique view in the same examination shows obvious dislocation of the first metatarsal.
d Radiograph six months after b and c.
e Two years after the initial examination, practically the entire middle and anterior tarsus has been destroyed. The patient had no pain, but there was a perforating ulcer below the medial ball of the foot.

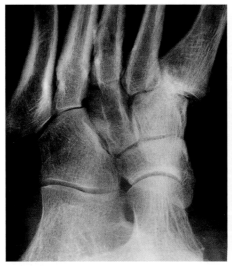

a   15 August 1994

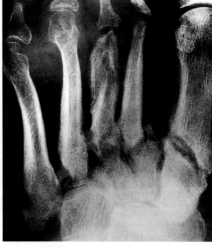

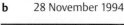

b   28 November 1994

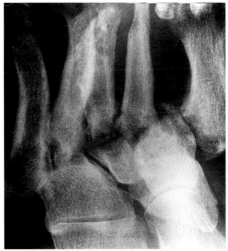

c   28 November 1994

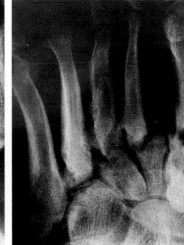

d   28 June 1995

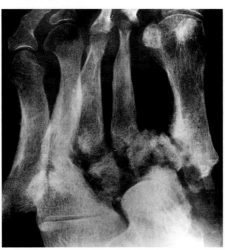

e   31 October 1996

matic cases of diabetes mellitus. The bones and joints of the tarsus are affected in slightly more than one-third of cases, while the tarsometatarsal and metatarsophalangeal joints are each affected in slightly more than one-fourth of cases. This disease is mentioned here because the initial changes are often extremely subtle and consist of subtle foci of increased density in one of the cuneiforms, for example, or at the bases of the metatarsals (Fig. 7.**375 a**). Often these initial changes are succeeded by a painless but rapidly progressive destruction of the articular surfaces accompanied by periosteal new bone formation on the metatarsals, followed later by fragmentation, increasing joint derangement, etc. In extreme cases entire bony segments may be lost. Vascular calcifications can usually be detected at the same time. But the disease is also associated with reparative changes that can reconstitute bone areas that have been lost (see head of third metatarsal in Fig. 7.**375 b, e**).

References

Beltran, J., D. S. Campanini, C. H. Knight et al.: The diabetic foot: magnetic resonance imaging evaluation. Skelet. Radiol. 19 (1990) 37

Geoffroy, J., J. C. Hoeffel, J. P. Pointel et al.: The feet in diabetes. Roentgenologic observations in 1501 cases. Diagn. Imag. 48 (1979) 286

Pfitzner, W.: Die Variationen im Aufbau des Fußskelettes. Schwalbes morphol. Arb. 6 (1896) 245

Sinha, S., S. Munichoodappa, G. T. Kocak: Neuropathy (Charcot joints) in diabetes mellitus. Clinical study of 101 cases. Medicine 51 (1972) 191

Metatarsal Bones

Normal Findings

During Growth

Each metaphyseal shaft has a primary ossification center that appears during the third month of fetal development.

The **epiphyseal centers** of the metatarsal bones have their own bony centers that appear in the third month of life. **Fusion** of the epiphyses with the shafts begins in the 15th year of life.

The metatarsal bones are monoepiphyseal, like the metacarpals. The epiphysis is located at the base of the first metatarsal and at the heads of the remaining four (Figs. 7.**312**, 7.**359**). The **tuberosity of the fifth metatarsal** has a separate apophysis that appears between 10 and 15 years of age (10–14 years in girls, 12–15 years in boys) (Figs. 7.**377**, 7.**378**). It has been known to appear at 6–8 years, but this is unusual. The tuberosity of the fifth metatarsal gives attachment to the peroneus brevis ten-

don. The typically shell-like apophysis borders the lateral plantar edge of the tuberosity. It fuses with the rest of the bone at about 25 years of age. It is normal for the apophysis to have one or multiple centers (Fig. 7.**377 a**).

An **adducted position of the metatarsals** is normal in many infants and will disappear spontaneously after the child begins weightbearing in an upright stance.

In Adulthood

The second metatarsal is generally the longest of the metatarsal bones, and the first metatarsal is the shortest. The shaft of the fifth metatarsal is slightly bowed when viewed in both projections. The second through fourth metatarsals have basically the same length and shape, which is very helpful in the diagnosis of brachymetatarsia. The base of the first metatarsal has a prominence on its lateral plantar angle known also as the tuberosity of the first metatarsal.

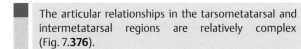

The articular relationships in the tarsometatarsal and intermetatarsal regions are relatively complex (Fig. 7.**376**).

Fig. 7.**376** Longitudinal section through the tarsometatarsal region. Note particularly the course of the various joint spaces (see text).

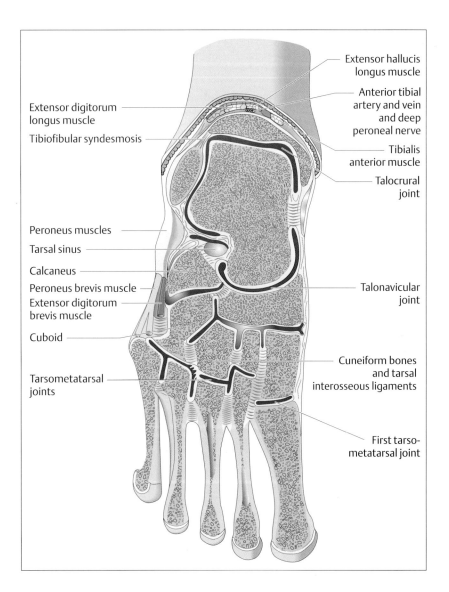

Extensor hallucis longus muscle

Anterior tibial artery and vein and deep peroneal nerve

Tibialis anterior muscle

Talocrural joint

Extensor digitorum longus muscle

Tibiofibular syndesmosis

Peroneus muscles

Tarsal sinus

Calcaneus

Peroneus brevis muscle

Extensor digitorum brevis muscle

Cuboid

Tarsometatarsal joints

Talonavicular joint

Cuneiform bones and tarsal interosseous ligaments

First tarso-metatarsal joint

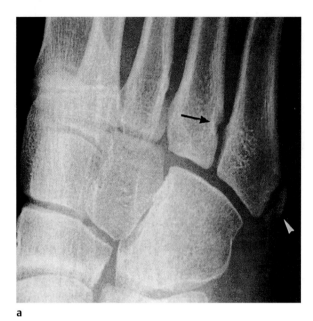

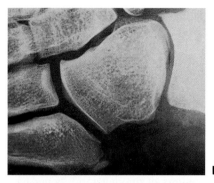

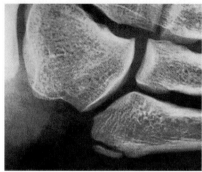

Fig. 7.**377 a–c**   Tuberosity of the fifth metatarsal bone.
a Tuberosity with two apophyseal centers (arrowhead) in an
11-year-old girl. Oblique projection shows a notch, as found in
adults, in the lateral border of the fourth metatarsal bone distal to the fourth and fifth intermetatarsal joint (arrow).

b, c Typical apophysis of the tuberosity of the fifth metatarsal.
Oblique projections in a 12-year-old girl.

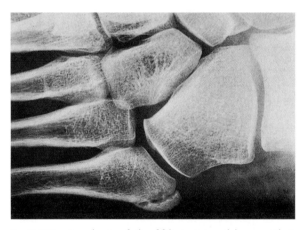

Fig. 7.**378**   Apophysis of the fifth metatarsal bone with irregular lucencies along the cartilaginous plate in a 17-year-old
boy. This is a normal finding, and normal fusion occurred 10
months later.

Three groups of joint spaces are present:

The fourth and fifth metatarsals have a common joint
space with the cuboid bone and between their bases. The
second metatarsal articulates with the intermediate
cuneiform, lateral cuneiform, and third metatarsal. The latter has a synovial joint with the lateral cuneiform. The first
metatarsal has a separate articulation with the medial
cuneiform that does not communicate with any other joint
space. Thus the Lisfranc line, which marks the boundary
between the tarsus and the metatarsal bones, is not a uniform anatomical line. It is discontinuous and makes several
sharp turns. It starts behind the tuberosity of the fifth
metatarsal and runs medially and somewhat distally along
the bases of the fifth, fourth, and third metatarsals. The
second metatarsal is wedged between the lateral and medial cuneiform bones, and so the joint line runs in proximal
direction to its base. The line then returns to a more distal
level at the base of the first metatarsal. The proximal
notches in the lateral aspects of the metatarsals, most conspicuous in the second through fourth bones, are occupied
by cartilage-covered surfaces or ligaments (see above). The
most basal portions of the second through fourth metatarsals are superimposed in the dorsoplantar projection,
giving rise to Mach effects that should not be mistaken for
fracture lines.

The MRI anatomy of the tarsometatarsal joints has been
described by Preidler et al. (1996). The imaging of the intermetatarsal spaces, especially the intermetatarsal
bursae, with MR is reported by Theumann et al. (2001).

The lateral contour of the shaft of the first metatarsal
often appears irregular because the dorsal and plantar
margins of the slightly concave lateral wall are superimposed.

Nutrient canals enter the medial aspect of the metatarsal bones about halfway up the shaft and usually run distally and laterally. Fracture lines that mimic nutrient canals are illustrated in Fig. 7.**404 a, b**.

 Pathological Finding?

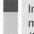 **Normal Variant or Anomaly?**

Variants

The potential variants of the metatarsal bones will be reviewed in brief, as they are strikingly similar to those of the metacarpals.

Accessory epiphyseal centers can occur as variants at the head of the first metatarsal and at the base of the second through fifth metatarsals (Fig. 7.**381**). Reportedly, these variants are particularly common in syndromes such as cleidocranial dysostosis (Maas 1954).

The heads of the second through fifth metatarsals and the epiphysis of the first metatarsal may be duplicated (Figs. 7.**312**, 7.**379**, 7.**380**).

> Irregularity and notching of the distal end of the first metatarsal can still be considered a normal variant (Fig. 7.**312**, 7.**382**).

The following **accessory skeletal elements** may occur about the metatarsals:

- **Os intermetatarseum:** This accessory bone is quite variable in its shape, size, and location, as illustrated in Figs. 7.**383**–7.**385**.
- **Os cuneometatarsale I** plantare (Fig. 7.**368**).
- **Os cuneometatarsale II** dorsale (p. 1066).
- **Os unci** (Fig. 7.**386** and p. 1066).
- **Os vesalianum.** This bone is located in the angle between the cuboid and the fifth metatarsal. It is not identical to the os peroneum, as the latter is located in the peroneus longus tendon while the os vesalianum is located at the insertion of the peroneus brevis. This suggests, of course, that the os vesalianum may well be a sesamoid bone (Fig. 7.**387**). The os vesalianum can oc-

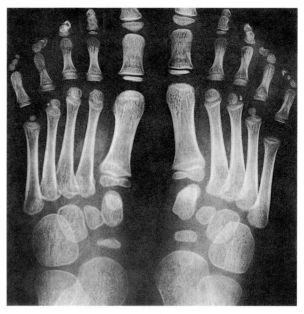

Fig. 7.**379**   Bipartition of the basal epiphyseal centers in both first metatarsals and of the distal centers in the right third metatarsal and left fourth metatarsal.

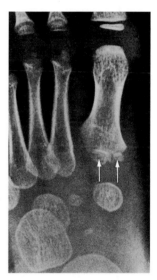

Fig. 7.**380**   Dual centers in the basal epiphysis of the first metatarsal in a 4-year-old boy.

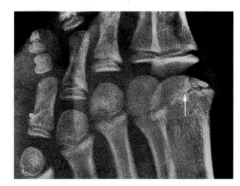

Fig. 7.**381**   Small, bipartite distal epiphysis in a 13-year-old boy.

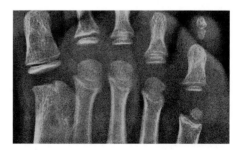

Fig. 7.**382**   The head of the first metatarsal is irregularly shaped and bears a small notch.

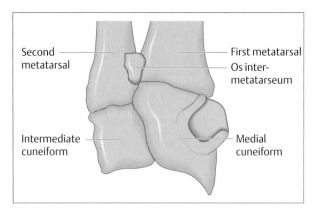

Fig. 7.**383**   Os intermetatarseum (after Pfitzner).

caionally cause clinical complaints that require its extirpation. But before surgery is elected, an effort should be made to determine by bone scanning or MRI whether the ossicle shows any kind of abnormality (increased tracer uptake or increased T2-weighted signal intensity).

● **Persistent apophysis of the tuberosity of the fifth metatarsal.** This is recognized by noting that the accessory bone element "completes" the shape of the tuberosity. The apophysis may become necrotic due to excessive stresses (jogging in tight shoes, ballet dancing, etc.) (Fig. 7.**399**). This can also be considered a form of chronic traction injury like that affecting the ischium, iliac spines, etc.

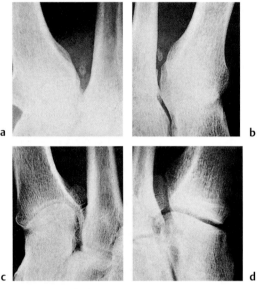

Fig. 7.**384 a–d**   Various forms of the os intermetatarseum.

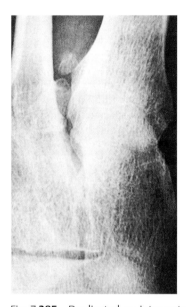

Fig. 7.**385**   Duplicated os intermetatarseum. Differentiation is required from the nonunited fracture of an oversized accessory bone.

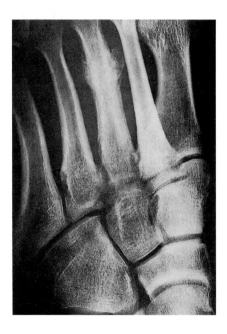

Fig. 7.**386**   Os unci at the medial base of the fourth metatarsal, incidental finding. The radiograph was obtained for a stress fracture in the shaft of the third metatarsal.

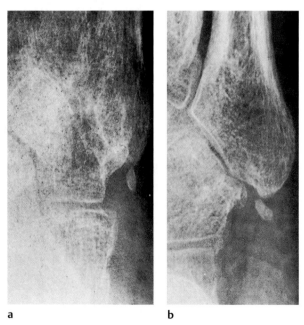

Fig. 7.**387 a, b**   Metaplastic tendon ossification or os vesalianum. Incidental finding.

Deformities

A true deformity is **brachymetatarsia**, which most commonly affects the fourth metatarsal, often bilaterally (ratio of women to men = 25 : 1, Mah et al. 1983). Concomitant shortening of the fourth and fifth metatarsals is also known to occur (Fig. 7.**388**).

The features and significance of brachymetacarpias are discussed on p. 97 ff.

See also Figs. 7.**221f** and 7.**456** regarding the various forms of symphalangia and disproportionate metatarsal bones associated with tarsal coalitions.

Hallux valgus refers to a valgus angulation of the great toe. Usually the head of the first metatarsal is broadened with a plateaulike projection on its medial side, and lateral subluxation of the toe is often present (Fig. 7.**389**).

Hallux valgus may be congenital or acquired, but most cases are an acquired deformity that becomes more frequent with aging and progressive flattening of the longitudinal and transverse pedal arches. The clinical prominence on the medial border of the foot is often caused by the enlargement of a bursa at that location. Concomitant foot deformities are generally present. Hallux valgus is far more common in women than in men (Kelikian 1982) and is exacerbated by improper footwear. It is one of the most common toe deformities and is usually bilateral but affects one side more than the other. It is usually accompanied by metatarsus varus. Hallux valgus also involves a torsional deformity of the great toe with medial rotation of its dorsal border. The great toe crowds the second toe and may ride over it or slip beneath it. Lateral displacement of the sesamoids also occurs, as shown in Fig. 7.**390**.

Metatarsus primus varus is a predisposition to hallux valgus in which the angle between the longitudinal axes of the first two metatarsals is greater than 10°. **Congenital metatarsus varus** (congenital pes adductus) is a deformity in which the first through fourth metatarsals are angled sharply toward the midline while the fifth metatarsal is relatively straight. This condition is associated with a fixed or nonfixed valgus deformity of the calcaneus.

Hallux rigidus, present in 1.5% of children between 10 and 15 years of age, is distinguished by an insidious flexion contracture at the metatarsophalangeal joint of the great toe. This leads to a typical osteoarthritic deformity (Fig. 7.**391**).

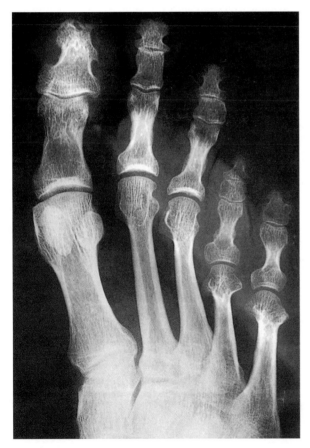

Fig. 7.**388** Brachymetatarsia of the fourth and fifth metatarsals.

Fig. 7.**390** Cross section of the first metatarsal head and ▷ adjacent sesamoids.
a Normal position.
b Lateral subluxation.
c Fixed lateral displacement.

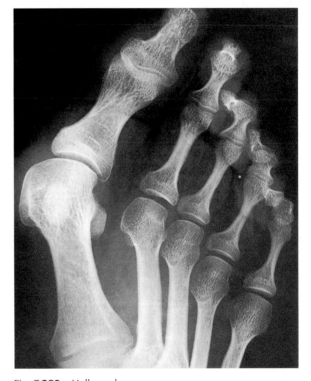

Fig. 7.**389** Hallux valgus.

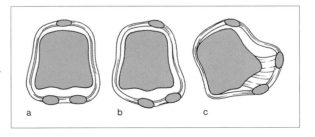

Congenital hallux varus is a rare anomaly that occurs predominantly in the setting of polydactylies and syndactylies. It may also occur in conjunction with partial or complete duplication of the first metatarsal.

 ### Fracture, Subluxation, or Dislocation?

Fractures of the metatarsal shafts need not be discussed here, except to note the possibility of confusing them with nutrient canals. Of greater interest are **tarsometatarsal fracture-dislocations** because they are a challenge to radiographic interpretation, especially in the diagnosis of fractures and deformities located near the tarsometatarsal joints. These fractures are usually the result of excessive plantar flexion. They are classified according to their effect on the two main structural units of the midfoot: the lateral "palette" (formed by the four lateral metatarsals) and the medial "column" (the first ray with its cuneiform). These units may be displaced in the same or different directions, depending on the direction of the traumatizing force (Fig. 7.**392**).

The cornerstone of this process is the base of the second metatarsal, which projects farther proximally than the other metatarsals. It is almost always fractured, but its tight ligamentous attachments keep it from being displaced.

Isolated dislocation of the first metatarsal can occur as a result of direct trauma.

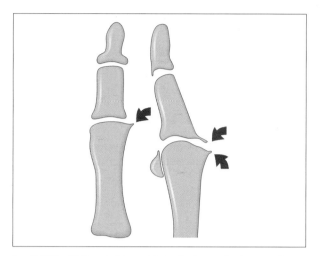

Fig. 7.**391**   Hallux rigidus with typical marginal osteophytes (arrows).

A more common injury is the **transverse fracture through the base of the fifth metatarsal**. Called also the "Jones fracture" after the physician who first described it, it is a typical avulsion fracture caused by excessive traction on the peroneus brevis tendon (Fig. 7.**393**). The fracture can be sustained, for example, by catching a foot and stumbling

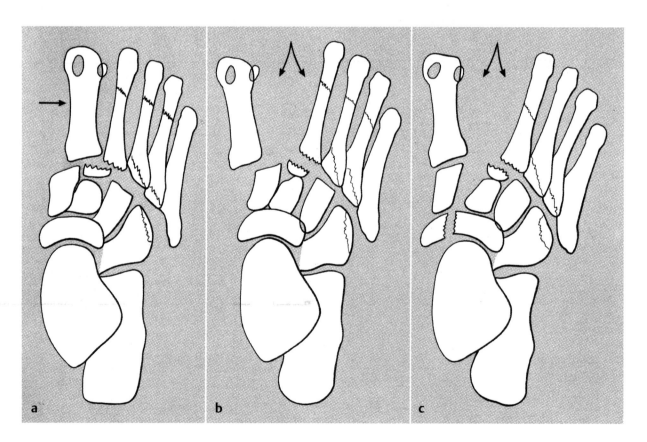

Fig. 7.**392 a–c** Fracture-dislocation of the tarsometatarsal joint (after Aitken and Poulsen).
a Homolateral dislocation.
b Divergent dislocation with disruption of the distal palette.

c Divergent dislocation with disruption of the distal palette and proximal column.

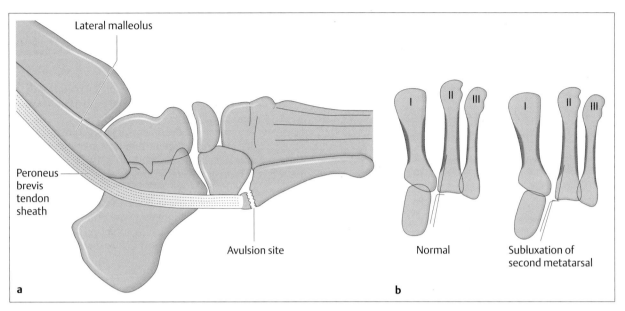

Fig. 7.**393 a, b** Typical injuries involving the fifth metatarsal tuberosity and the second metatarsal bone.

a Avulsion of the fifth metatarsal tuberosity by excessive traction on the peroneus brevis tendon (after Rogers).
b Subluxation of the second metatarsal (after Dihlmann).

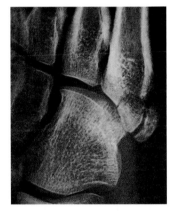

Fig. 7.**394** Apophysis of the fifth metatarsal with a transverse fracture of the fifth metatarsal at the level of the tuberosity. Boy 12 years of age.

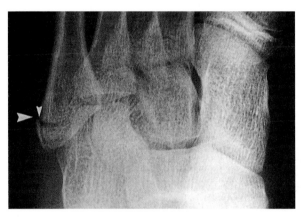

Fig. 7.**395** Transverse fracture of the tuberosity of the fifth metatarsal. Just lateral to the fragment is a small physiological apophysis. Girl 11 years of age.

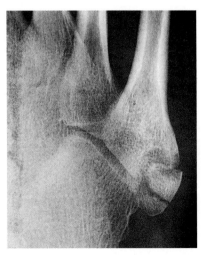

Fig. 7.**396** Two-part avulsion of the tuberosity of the fifth metatarsal. Man 46 years of age.

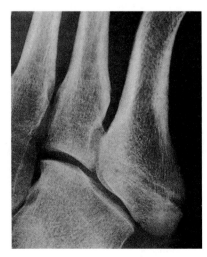

Fig. 7.**397** Old fracture at the base of the fifth metatarsal.

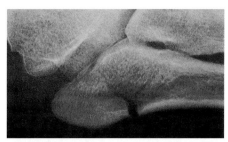

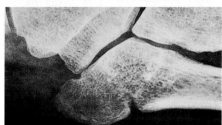

Fig. 7.**398 a, b**   Fracture line through the tuberosity of the fifth metatarsal.
a Minimally displaced fracture of the tuberosity.
b Late follow-up.

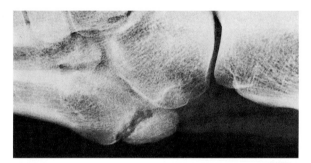

Fig. 7.**399**   Fairly dense-appearing apophysis of the fifth metatarsal in a 30-year-old athlete. This finding and the small ossifications in the apophyseal space suggest necrotic changes in the persistent apophysis.

while descending stairs. This fracture should not be confused with the apophysis of the fifth metatarsal tuberosity, which appears as a longitudinal rather than transverse lucency (Figs. 7.**393 a**–7.**399**).

Figure 7.**400** illustrates how difficult it can be in some instances to diagnose basal fractures of the metatarsals.

The diagrams in Fig. 7.**393 b** demonstrate a **subluxation of the second metatarsal**.

Stress fractures of the metatarsals, known also as "march fractures," occur predominantly in the second and third metatarsals and occasionally in both. Despite severe pain, initial radiographs often show no abnormalities or at most a circumscribed periosteal reaction or subtle lucency in the cortical and cancellous bone (Figs. 7.**401**–7.**404**).

Radionuclide scans can be very helpful in making a diagnosis. If very heavy callus formation occurs over a period of weeks, the finding may be difficult to distinguish from a (periosteal) osteosarcoma, but this tumor is extremely rare in the metatarsal region (Fig. 7.**405**).

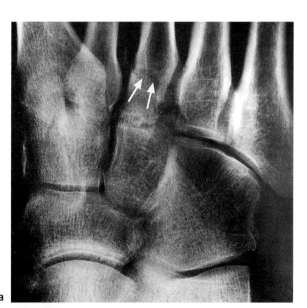

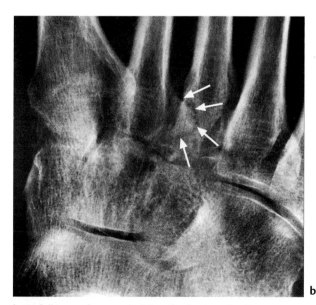

Fig. 7.**400 a, b**   Fracture at the base of the third metatarsal.
a Initial radiograph shows a barely perceptible fracture line (arrows).

b At follow-up four weeks later, the fracture line is more conspicuous. Now the medial fragment is also slightly displaced.

Fig. 7.**401 a–c** Stress fracture
of the second metatarsal.
a Normal finding in a patient
with pain over the second
metatarsal.
b Radiograph two months later
shows a marked periosteal reaction to the stress fracture.
c Radiograph six months later
shows regression of the periosteal callus due to modeling.

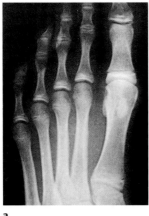
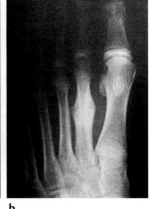
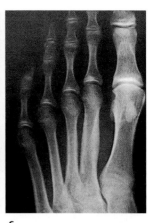

a   b   c

Fig. 7.**402** Stress fracture of the second metatarsal. The
"moth-eaten" appearance of the bone is the result of an excessive RAP (regional acceleratory phenomenon) with marked resorption in the haversian canals.

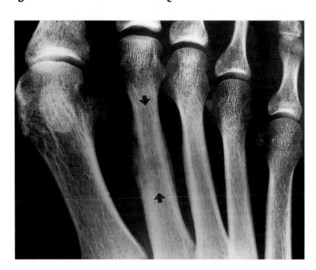

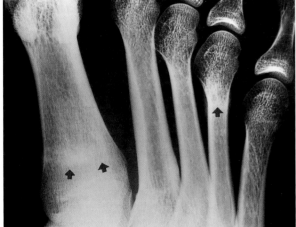

a

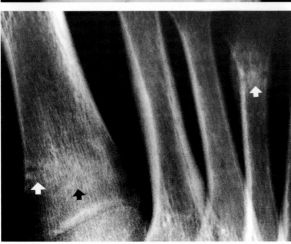

b

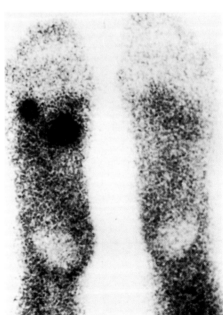

c

Fig. 7.**403 a–c** Stress fracture at the base of the first metatarsal and subcapital fracture of the fourth metatarsal.
a Subtle initial findings with sclerosis (arrows).
b Approximately four weeks later, the fracture lines can be
identified due to structural alterations.
c Bone scan obtained concurrently with radiograph **a** shows
intense uptake in the area of the stress fractures.

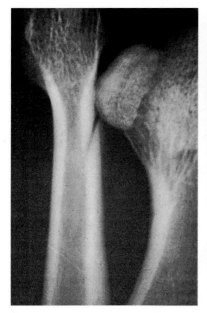

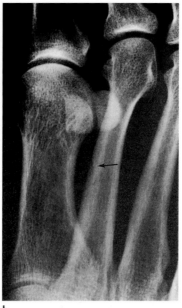

a

b

Fig. 7.**404 a, b** Possible initial findings of stress fractures.

a Incomplete oblique stress fracture of the second metatarsal.

b Barely perceptible incomplete fracture in the shaft of the second metatarsal (arrow). Otherwise typical periosteal changes are not seen (still no RAP?). Radiographs taken just 10 days later showed extensive reparative changes (shown in Fig. 7.**405 b** to contrast with other diseases). Note that the fracture lines in Fig. 7.**404 a** and **b** point *toward* the proximal end of the metatarsal, unlike ordinary nutrient canals, which angle away from the base of the bone as they cross the cortex and enter the medullary cavity.

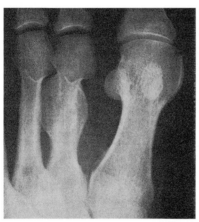

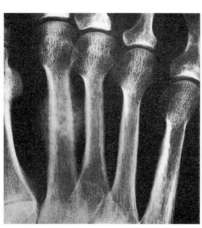

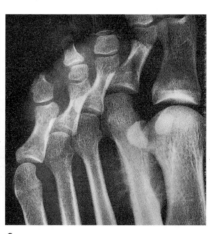

a

b

c

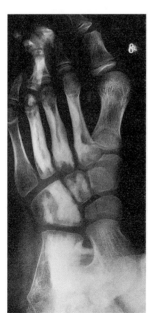

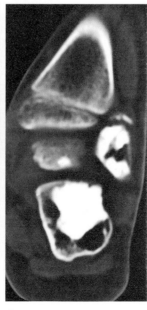

d

e

Fig. 7.**405 a–e** Periosteal and endosteal bone formation on the metatarsals.

a Heavy callus formation in response to a stress fracture.

b Stress fracture with exuberant cotton-wool callus (initial finding in Fig. 7.**404 b**).

c Typical spiculation associated with an osteosarcoma (extremely rare in this location).

d, e Classic melorheostosis of the metatarsals.

Necrosis?

Osteonecrosis of the metatarsal heads is not a rare disorder, especially in the second metatarsal (Fig. 7.**408**). It is also called **Freiberg disease** or **Köhler II disease** after the authors who first described it. Girls and young women are predominantly affected. The disease may relate to improper footwear, but this has not been proven. Any of the

metatarsal heads may be affected including that of the first metatarsal, especially when it has an accessory distal epiphysis. Köhler's original radiographs charting the long-term progression of the disease are shown in Fig. 7.**407**.

In most cases the disease begins with nonspecific pain in the area of the affected metatarsal head. Initial radiographs do not show significant abnormalities (Fig. 7.**409 a**). Some weeks later, however, radiographs show a subchondral lucency accompanied by slight flattening of the

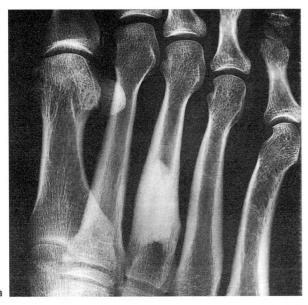

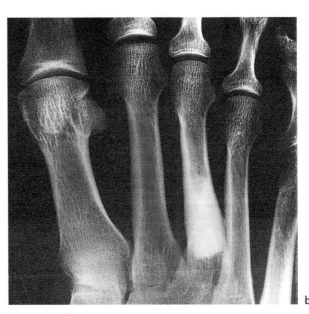

Fig. 7.**406 a, b**   Unusually large osteoma detected incidentally in the proximal shaft of the third metatarsal. Differentiation is required from an osteoma-like pattern of melorheostosis.

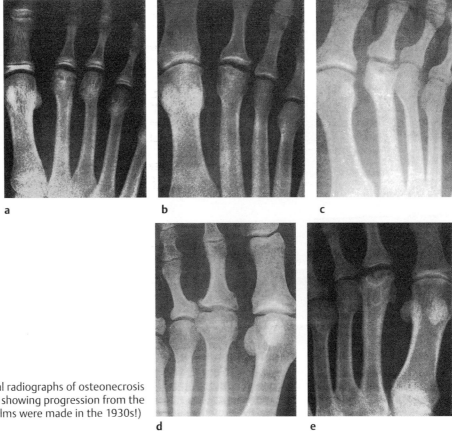

Fig. 7.**407 a–e**   Köhler's original radiographs of osteonecrosis of the second metatarsal head, showing progression from the "initial" to late stages. (These films were made in the 1930s!)

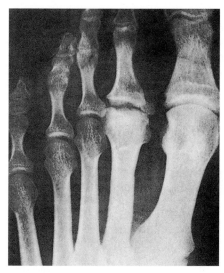

Fig. 7.**408** (Degenerative) osteoarthritis is secondary to necrosis of the second metatarsal head (original radiograph by Köhler).

metatarsal head and widening of the radiographic joint space (Fig. 7.**409 c**). This is followed by increasing fragmentation with a mixed pattern of lucencies and densities. Periosteal new bone formation may occur on the adjacent metatarsal shaft. In the healing stage, the bony contours again become smooth or there may be some residual flattening and deformity of the metatarsal head. In the case of an incidental finding of the end-stage of an osteonecrosis of a metatarsal head, often the patient cannot recall having experienced any symptoms during adolescence. In rare cases, however, the disease may progress to osteoarthritis of the adjacent joint (Fig. 7.**408**).

It should be added that osteonecrosis of the second metatarsal head can also develop as a stress-related condition following the surgical correction of hallux valgus.

After the tarsal bones, the metatarsals are the second most common site of involvement by **diabetic osteoarthropathy** (Fig. 7.**410**). There is gradual destruction of the heads and distal shafts of the affected metatarsals without pain (neuropathy!), the stubs acquiring a tapered "candy stick" appearance. There may finally be a reossification stage in which the original anatomy is reconstituted in varying degrees (Fig. 7.**410 d**).

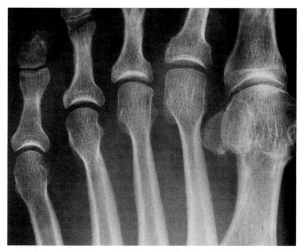

a

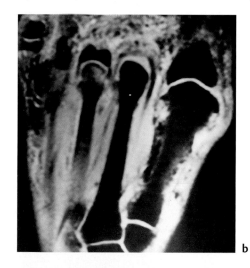

b

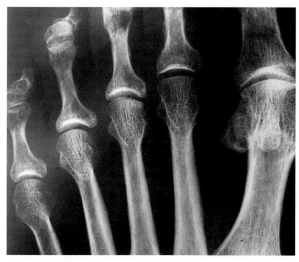

c

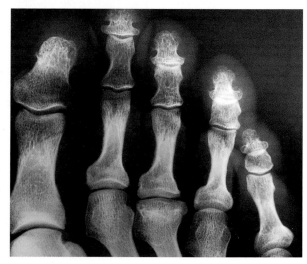

d

Fig. 7.**409 a–d** Osteonecrosis of the third metatarsal.
a–c Woman 55 years of age with moderate aching pain in the left metatarsal region. The radiograph (**a**) appears normal. Concomitant MRI (**b**) shows moderate edema in the head of the third metatarsal. Follow-up radiograph three months later

(**c**) shows slight medial flattening of the metatarsal head at the site where edema was found. No fragmentation was seen on additional follow-ups.
d Marked deformity of the third metatarsal head in a 43-year-old woman with a negative history and no clinical complaints.

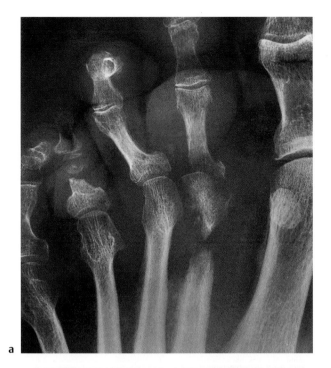

a

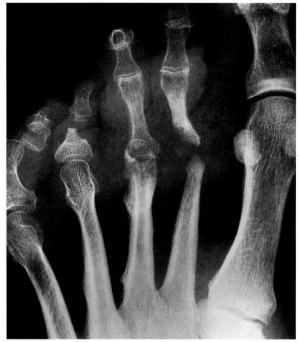

b

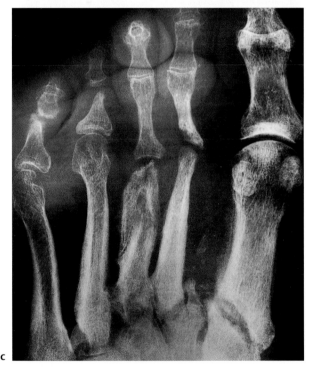

c

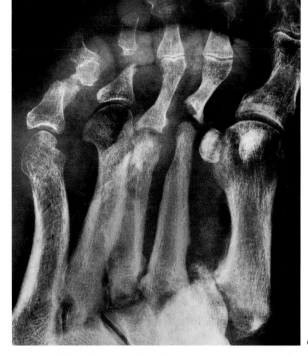

d

Fig. 7.**410 a–d** Follow-up of diabetic osteoarthropathy in a man with a long history of insulin-dependent diabetes mellitus.

a Osteolytic destruction of the second metatarsal head and the base of the opposing proximal phalanx. A marked periosteal reaction is noted on the residual shaft. Other findings are derangement of the third metatarsophalangeal joint and osteolytic destruction or acro-osteolysis of the fourth proximal and middle phalanges.

b Radiograph approximately seven months later also shows severe destructive changes in the head of the third metatarsal, with dislocation of the associated joint. The second metatarsal has been reduced to a tapered stub, and the remnants of the head still visible in **a** have been resorbed. The contours of the stub of the second proximal phalanx have been smoothed. The periosteal reaction on the first and second metatarsals have

regressed while those on the third metatarsal have become more dense and solid. A new periosteal reaction is now seen on the lateral shaft of the fourth metatarsal.

c, d Radiographs four months later show a marked progression of periosteal bone formation on the third metatarsal, whose distal shaft and head have been destroyed. Marked destruction and derangement are noted in the first through fourth tarsometatarsal joints, with fragmentation of the medial and intermediate cuneiform bones. These changes are more clearly visualized in Fig. 7.**375** (same case). The articular structures of the fifth proximal interphalangeal joint have been completely resorbed. The mixed radiographic pattern of bone destruction, resorptive tapering, periosteal reaction, joint derangement, etc. is highly specific for diabetic osteoarthropathy. Note also in **c** the vascular calcification between the first and second metatarsals, which is a consistent feature of the disease.

Diabetic osteoarthropathy (see also p. 1067 f.) is mentioned here because the initial changes may consist only of very subtle lucencies in the metatarsal heads or epimetaphyseal junctions or of subtle periosteal reactions.

 Interestingly, necrotic changes due to trophic disturbances are more likely to develop in the bones of the foot (especially the metatarsal heads) than in the hand, where reflex sympathetic dystrophy is a more common finding.

It is known that osteonecrosis is relatively common after foot reimplantations, whereas hand reimplantations tend to be followed by transient demineralization (see Fig. 2.**47 d–f**).

Inflammation?

Osteomyelitis of the metatarsal bones is rare. Early changes are the same as those in other skeletal regions.

The metatarsophalangeal joints are of particular interest in this book as early indicators of inflammatory rheumatoid disorders:

These joints are considered a radiographic test region for **gouty arthritis**. The great toe is affected with notable frequency. Initial changes consist of subtle osteolytic lesions in the metatarsal heads, usually accompanied by soft-tissue swelling. The osteolytic lesions may grow larger and eventually form a medullary tophus that breaks through the bone and incites a periosteal reaction. The process may culminate in gross destructive changes and mutilation that create an unmistakable picture (Fig. 7.**412 b**). It is essential to recognize the initial changes, however, which consist of fine subchondral lucencies (Figs. 7.**412 a**, 7.**413**) combined with characteristic clinical findings (elevated uric acid level, paroxysmal pain, etc.). Figure 7.**413 a** shows gouty destruction of the base of the right third metatarsal that was detectable only with CT. Conventional radiographs showed no abnormalities. The patient complained of severe pain in that area, and the bone scan (Fig. 7.**413 b**) defined the region of interest for selective CT scanning.

Psoriatic arthritis has a predilection for the distal interphalangeal joints of the foot, but the changes there are typically associated with fine periosteal bone formation on the medial aspect of the first metatarsal head (Fig. 7.**411**).

The **arthritis in Reiter syndrome** typically involves the joints of the lower extremity, including the metatarsophalangeal joints, and shows a nonuniform distribution. If changes are not yet visible in the joints themselves, fine **periosteal new bone formation** will occasionally be seen on the shafts of the affected metatarsals.

The metatarsophalangeal joints are among the radiographic test regions for **rheumatoid arthritis** that should always be included in the primary examination, whether specifically requested or not. In about 10 % of all cases the metatarsophalangeal joints will show unequivocal signs of rheumatoid arthritis, even if the joints themselves are not painful, at a time when radiographs of the painful metacarpophalangeal joints do not yet show definite abnormalities. Initial changes typically consist of rounded subchondral lucencies ("signal cysts"). It is only later that initial erosive changes are seen in the articular margins (Fig. 7.**414**).

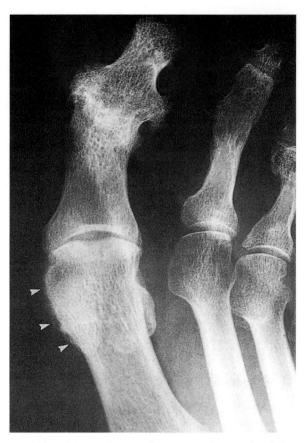

Fig. 7.**411** Advanced stage of psoriatic arthritis with ankylosis of the distal and proximal interphalangeal joints of the first through third rays. Typical periosteal new bone formation is evident along the head of the first metatarsal (arrowheads).

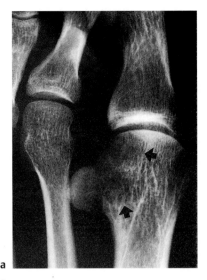

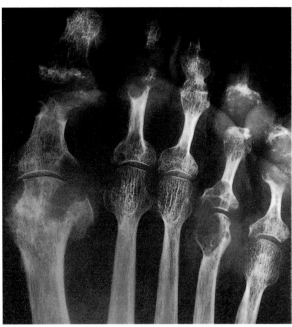

Fig. 7.**412 a, b**   Gout.
a Medullary tophus in the lateral part of the first metatarsal head (arrows).
b Gross destructive changes are evident in all the metatarsal heads and all interphalangeal joints (also in the first tarsometatarsal joint, not shown).

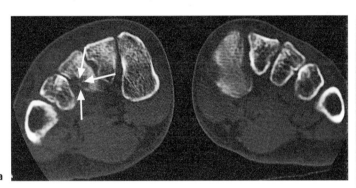

Fig. 7.**413 a, b**   Gouty arthritis with destruction of the lateral base of the right third metatarsal (arrows). No radiographic abnormalities were seen. Clinical findings consisted of severe pain and a moderately high uric acid level. The CT examination (**a**) was directed by a prior radionuclide scan (**b**), which showed a localized increase in metabolic bone activity. Uricosuric therapy was followed by a reduction in pain and repair of the osseous defect.

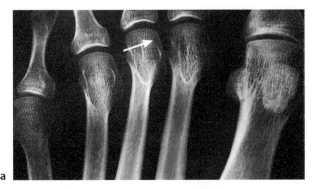

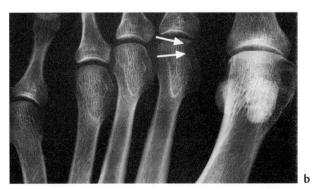

Fig. 7.**414 a, b**   Follow-up of rheumatoid arthritis.
a Small cystic lucencies ("signal cysts") in the metatarsal heads. The arrow indicates a representative cyst. Similar lesions were found on the opposite side (not shown).

b Radiograph three years later shows marked marginal erosions in the metatarsal heads, especially in the second metatarsal (arrows). The bones of the hand showed no significant changes.

Tumor?

Osteochondromas of the metatarsal metaphyses are rare as isolated lesions, and their occurrence there is more common in the setting of a cartilaginous exostosis disease.

Primary bone tumors of the metatarsals are rare.

We have seen **osteoid osteomas** in the metatarsals, particularly in the head area. The initial changes may be extremely subtle despite very severe clinical symptoms. Sometimes the dominant features are those of an accompanying sympathetic arthritis.

With regard to tumorlike lesions, **aneurysmal bone cysts** occasionally occur in the metatarsals. **Osteomas** are not uncommon in the metatarsals, and larger lesions (as shown in Fig. 7.**406**) should not be mistaken for malignant tumors. The same applies to melorheostotic changes (Fig. 7.**405 d, e**).

Other Changes?

Hypertrophic osteoarthropathy occurs most frequently in the bones of the foot, followed by the hand, forearm, and lower leg (Fig. 7.**415**).

Periosteal new bone formation can be extremely subtle initially and shows a marked predilection for the metatarsals. Often, only radionuclide bone scans can detect early changes (increased uptake along the metatarsals) that may correlate clinically with severe pain (as a paraneoplastic disease in bronchial carcinoma, for example).

Reflex sympathetic dystrophy is a subgroup of the **algodystrophies** that also occurs in the foot, where it apparently creates more problems of differential diagnosis than in the hand. The changes may affect the tarsus and particularly the metatarsal and phalangeal regions (Fig. 7.**416**).

It was mentioned under Necrosis (p. 1082) that the algodystrophies are less common in the foot than in the hand and that the foot is a site of predilection for osteonecrosis (e.g., following reimplantation).

Soft-tissue calcifications in the intermetatarsal region, especially between the first and second metatarsals, usually represent vascular calcifications (Fig. 7.**418**). Ossification of the accessory arcuate tendon of the dorsal interosseous muscle (Fig. 7.**417**) appears much more solid, as it usually consists of differentiated cancellous bone. Figure 7.**419** shows a rare type of ossification in the intermetatarsal soft tissues, which we assume to be a supernumerary ray.

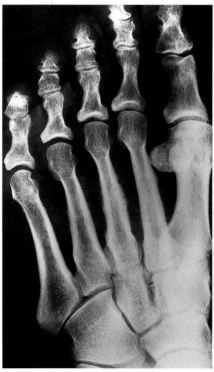 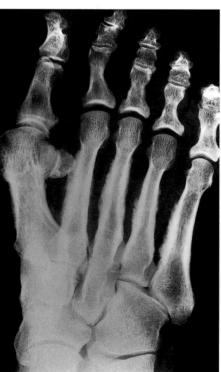

a   b

Fig. 7.**415 a, b** Hypertrophic osteoarthropathy.
a Male patient with bronchial carcinoma (pulmonary form).
b Female patient with Crohn disease (intestinal form).

Fig. 7.**416 a, b** Reflex sympathetic dystrophy.

a The patient presented clinically with marked swelling and livid discoloration of the tarsometatarsal area with severe pain. There was no history of injury. Initial radiograph shows slight demineralization that is most evident in the intermediate cuneiform and third metatarsal.

b Radiograph three months later shows massive progression of patchy demineralization that also involves the metatarsophalangeal region.

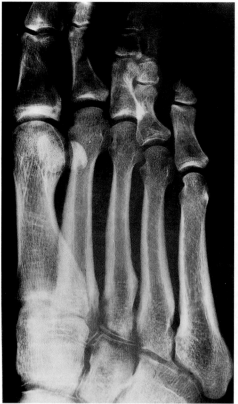
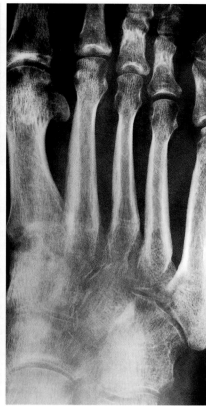

a

b

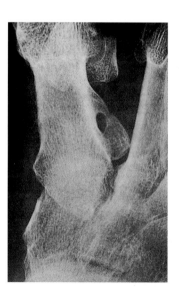

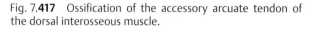

Fig. 7.**417** Ossification of the accessory arcuate tendon of the dorsal interosseous muscle.

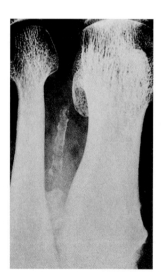
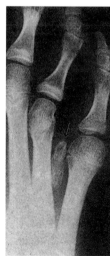

Fig. 7.**418**

Fig. 7.**419**

Fig. 7.**418** Intimal calcification in the first intertarsal artery.

Fig. 7.**419** Supernumerary ray between the fourth and fifth metatarsals.

References

Aitken, A. P., D. Poulson: Dislocations of the tarsometatarsal joint. J. Bone Jt Surg. 45-A (1963) 246

Arangio, G. A.: Proximal diaphyseal fractures of the fifth metatarsal (Jones' fracture): two cases treated by cross-pinnng with review of 106 cases. Foot and Ankle 3 (1983) 293

Bojsen-Mller, F.: Normale und pathologische Anatomie des Vorfußes. Orthopädie 11 (1982) 148

Bonnat, H., H. Bensahel, C. Themar-Noel: Le metatarsus varus congénital. Chir. Pédiat. 22 (1981) 405

de Cuveland, E.: Die Apophyse des Metatarsale V und Os vesalianum. Fortschr. Röntgenstr. 82 (1955) 251

Dihlmann, W.: Gelenke, Wirbelverbindungen, 2. Aufl. Thieme, Stuttgart 1982

Ehrensberger, J.: Frakturen des kindlichen und jugendlichen Fußes. Ther. Umsch. 40 (1983) 996

Erseven, A., A. Garti, K. Weigl: Aneurysmal bone cyst of the first metatarsal bone mimicking malignant tumor. Clin. Orthop. 181 (1983) 171

Foster, S. C, R. R. Foster: Lisfranc's tarsometatarsal fracture-dislocation. Radiology 12 (1976) 79

Freyschmidt, J.: Skeletterkrankungen, 2. Aufl. Springer, Berlin 1997

Gold, R. H., L. W. Bassett: Radiologic evaluation of the arthritic foot. Foot and Ankle 2 (1982) 332

Jonasch, E.: Brachymetatarsie als Folge eines Fremdkörpers in der Wachstumsperiode. Fortschr. Röntgenstr. 89 (1958) 378

Kelikian, H.: The hallux. In Jahss, M. H.: Disorders of the Foot. Saunders, Philadelphia 1982 (p. 545)

Kite, J. H.: Congenital metatarsus varus. J. Bone Jt Surg. 49-A (1967) 388

Köhler, A.: Eine typische Erkrankung des 2. Metatarsophalangealgelenkes. Münch. med. Wschr. 67 (1920) 1289

Lagier, R.: Posttraumatic Sudeck's dystrophy localized in the metatarso-phalangeal region. Fortschr. Röntgenstr. 138 (1983) 496

Lemont, H., J. S. Smith: Subchondral bone cysts of the head of the first metatarsal. J. Amer. podiat. med. Ass. 72 (1982) 233

Lenen, L. P. H., C. van der Werken: Fracture-dislocation of the tarsometatarsal joint, a combined anatomical and computed tomographic study. Injury 23 (1992) 51

Maas, W.: Multiple Pseudepiphysen bei Dysostosis cleidocranialis. Fortschr. Röntgenstr. 80 (1954) 788

Mah, K. K. S., T. R. Beegle, D. W. Falknor: A correction for short fourth metatarsal. J. Amer. podiat. med. Ass. 73 (1983) 196

McKeever, D. C.: Surgical approach for neuroma of plantar digital nerve (Morton's metatarsalgia). J. Bone Jt Surg. 34-A (1952) 490

Norfray, F. J., R. A. Geline, R. I. Steinberg et al.: Subtleties of Lisfranc fracture-dislocations. Amer. J. Roentgenol. 137 (1981) 1151

Preidler, K. W., Y. C. Wang, J. Brossmann et al.: Tarsometatarsal joint: anatomic details on MR images. Radiology 199 (1996) 733

Rana, N. A.: Juvenile rheumatoid arthritis of the foot. Foot and Ankle 3 (1982) 2

Rogers, L. F.: Radiology of Skeletal Trauma. Churchill Livingstone, New York 1982 (p. 23)

Schinz, H. R.: Das Os Vesalianum ist das Tarsale 5. Fortschr. Röntgenstr. 87 (1957) 126

Sedlin, E. D. Early fusion in Freiberg's infraction. Foot and Ankle 3 (1982) 297

Skirving, A. P., J. H. Newman: Elongation of the first metatarsal. J. pediat. Orthop. 3 (1983) 508

Theumann, N. H., C. W. A. Pfirrmann, C. B. Chung et al.: Intermetatarsal spaces: Analysis with MR bursography, anatomic correlation, and histopathology in cadavers. Radiology 221 (2001) 478

Wiley, J. J.: The mechanism of tarso-metatarsal joint injuries. J. Bone Jt Surg. 53-B (1971) 474

Wiley, J. J.: Tarso-metatarsal joint injuries in children. J. pediat. Orthop. 1 (1981) 255

Sesamoid Bones

Normal Findings

During Growth

Sesamoid bones are true bones that develop out of a cartilaginous anlage. Although their cartilaginous centers begin to appear as early as the 12th week of fetal development, ossification does not begin before the 8th year of life and is not complete until the 12th year. Ossification of the lateral sesamoid bone precedes that of the medial sesamoid.

On average, ossification of the sesamoids can be detected radiographically at 11–12 years of age in boys and at 9–10 years of age in girls.

Normally two sesamoids are found on the plantar aspect of the head of the first metatarsal and one each (rarely two) at the heads of the second and fifth metatarsals. Very rarely, a medial sesamoid is present at the head of the third metatarsal (Fig. 7.**420**).

In summary, it is not abnormal to find sesamoid bones below all of the metatarsal heads and at the first and second distal interphalangeal joints (Figs. 7.**421**, 7.**422**).

The sesamoid bones of the great toe are embedded in the strengthened joint capsule of the fibrocartilaginous layer and articulate with hyaline cartilage facets on the head of the first metatarsal. The medial head of the flexor hallucis brevis inserts jointly with the abductor hallucis on the medial sesamoid bone, and the lateral head of the flexor hallucis brevis inserts with the adductor hallucis on the lateral sesamoid bone.

In Adulthood

As noted above, the **metatarsosesamoid articulations** are **true synovial joints**, a fact that can be important in the diagnosis of diseases such as rheumatoid arthritis.

The medial sesamoid is typically larger than the more rounded lateral sesamoid. Figure 7.**423** illustrates normal variations that can occur in the shape of the sesamoid bones of the hallux.

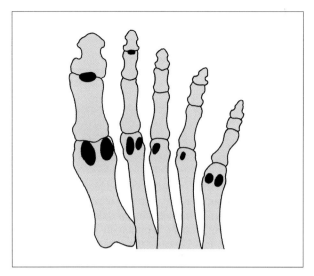

Fig. 7.**420**   Sesamoid bones of the foot (after Köhler).

We cannot fully describe the function of the sesamoid bones within the scope of this book (detailed information may be found in Potter et al. 1992). The topographic relationship of the sesamoids to the metatarsophalangeal joints and to the weight-bearing axis of the foot makes them highly susceptible to trauma.

> It is estimated that the forces acting on the sesamoid bones during normal walking are three times greater than the body weight (McBryde and Anderson 1988).

The medial sesamoid is subject to the greatest stresses because of its direct proximity to the metatarsal head.

The sesamoids of the great toe are separated by a bony ridge on the first metatarsal head that is easily demonstrated by axial radiographs and CT scans (Fig. 7.**441 d**).

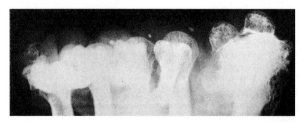

Fig. 7.**422**   Axial radiograph showing numerous sesamoid bones.

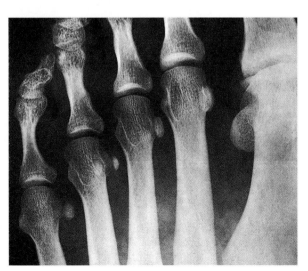

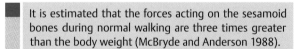
◁ Fig. 7.**421**   Sesamoid bones on all of the metatarsal heads.

▌ *Pathological Finding?*

Variant or Anomaly/Deformity?

> As a rule, the number and distribution of the sesamoid bones are not symmetrical in the same individual. Complete absence of the medial sesamoid is still considered an extreme variant.

Sesamoid partition is found in 10.7–33% of the population. It results from a failure of fusion of multiple ossification centers. Bipartition is seen in approximately 13.5–25% of cases. Partition is more common in the medial than lateral sesamoid, and bipartite sesamoids are reportedly more common in women than in men.

Various types of sesamoid partition are illustrated in Fig. 7.**429**. Figures 7.**424**–7.**428** and 7.**430** show radiographs of bipartite and multipartite sesamoids.

Sesamoid partition or duplication can also occur at other locations, such as the second or fifth metatarsal (Figs. 7.**428**, 7.**432**).

The bony fusion (Fig. 7.**431**) of a sesamoid to the associated metatarsal bone is rare. We still have too little information to decide whether this represents an extreme normal variant or a deformity.

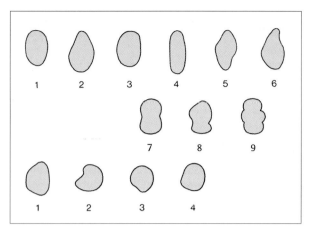

Fig. 7.**423**   Normal variations in the shape of the sesamoid bones of the great toe, arranged in order of frequency.
Top and middle row: medial sesamoid
Bottom row: lateral sesamoid

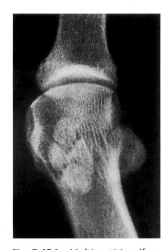

Fig. 7.**424**   Multipartition (four parts) of the medial sesamoid of the great toe. The multipartite medial sesamoid appears considerably larger than the lateral sesamoid, which is not partitioned.

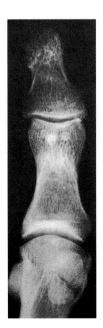

Fig. 7.**425**   Two small sesamoids at the interphalangeal joint of the great toe.

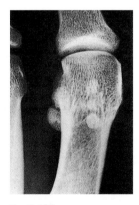

Fig. 7.**426**

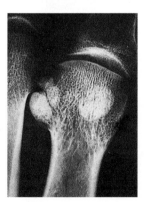

Fig. 7.**427**

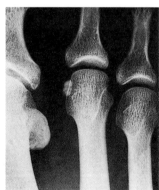

Fig. 7.**428**

Fig. 7.**426**   Partition of both sesamoids of the great toe.

Fig. 7.**427**   Partite lateral sesamoid of the great toe (less common than a partite medial sesamoid).

Fig. 7.**428**   Bipartite sesamoid of the second metatarsal.

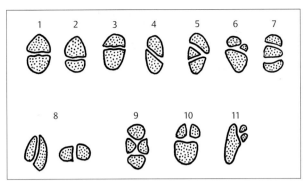

Fig. 7.**429** Various partitions of the sesamoid bones of the great toe, arranged in order of frequency.

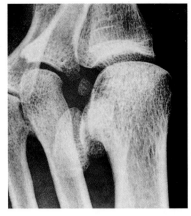

Fig. 7.**430** Duplication of the medial sesamoid of the great toe. The smaller bone is located at an atypically distal level.

 Fracture, Subluxation, or Dislocation?

It can be extremely difficult to distinguish a fractured sesamoid bone (Figs. 7.**434**–7.**436**) from a congenital bipartite or multipartite sesamoid on radiographs. This differentiation is important especially in forensic questions, however, as the clinical manifestations are fairly nonspecific.

Axial radiographs have proven particularly helpful in the diagnosis of sesamoid fractures, and CT can also be used if required. Radionuclide bone scans have proven useful in cases where chronic trauma is suspected. It is important in these cases to place the foot directly on the collimator. MRI is another current option if information on ligamentous injuries is desired.

The radiographic signs listed in Table 7.**7** are indicative of a fracture.

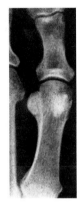
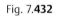

Fig. 7.**431**

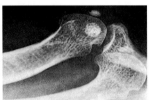

Fig. 7.**432**

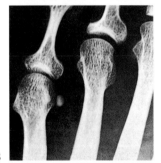

Fig. 7.**433**

Fig. 7.**431** Bony fusion of the lateral sesamoid to the first metatarsal.

Fig. 7.**432** Two sesamoid bones on the fifth metatarsal.

Fig. 7.**433** Small, almost featureless sesamoid on the small toe. Clinically asymptomatic.

Table 7.**7** Radiographic signs indicating the fracture of a sesamoid bone

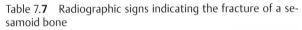

- Irregular, sharp, serrated contours of the opposing elements (Fig. 7.**434**).
- Marked diastasis of the opposing fragments (Fig. 7.**436**)
- Fragmentation
- Callus formation
- Normal sesamoid bone on prior radiographs
- Partite sesamoid bones are normally larger than their intact counterpart and also larger than reassembled fracture fragments (typically the same size or smaller than an intact bone).

It should be added, however, that partite sesamoids may also have sharp, serrated margins and that comparisons with the contralateral side are problematic in that sesamoid partition is bilateral in only 13–25% of cases (although most partitions in these cases show a symmetrical configuration).

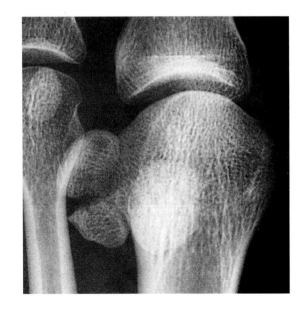

Fig. 7.**434** Fracture of the lateral sesamoid of the great toe. ▷

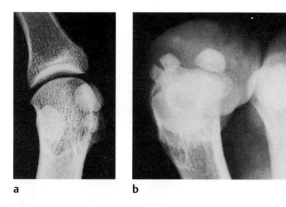

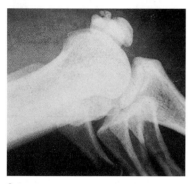

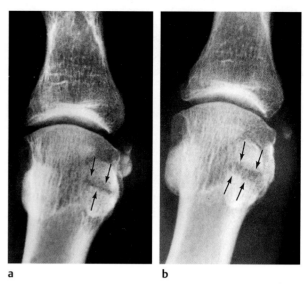

Fig. 7.**436 a, b**   Follow-up of a sesamoid fracture.
a Fresh trauma with a transverse fracture of the largest element of a multipartite medial sesamoid bone. The sharply defined transverse fracture line was not identified as such but was interpreted as a space between two larger partite sesamoid elements.
b Three years later, the marked widening of the space between the two bony elements, together with the history, establishes the prior occurrence of a fracture.
In radiograph **a**, at least two bony elements (one larger and one very small) are visible at the medial border of the metatarsal head. Only the small element is seen on the follow-up radiograph, and even extra projections failed to demonstrate the larger element. We presume that the missing element underwent complete necrosis as a result of the trauma.

Fig. 7.**435 a–c**   Girl 17 years of age with severe pain in the ball of the great toe. Fracture of the medial (tibial) sesamoid examined in three projections.
a Transverse partition of the medial sesamoid.
b Longitudinal fracture on axial examination.
c Other small accessory centers on profile view.

Sesamoid fractures can have several mechanisms:

- Direct trauma due to falling or jumping from a height (especially in ballet dancers)
- Acute hyperextension (e.g., during soccer)
- Repetitive stresses in long-distance runners

Preexisting hallux valgus deformities promote fractures due to the lateral displacement of the sesamoids (Fig. 7.**390**).

In a hyperextension injury of the great toe in which the base of the proximal phalanx dislocates over the head of the metatarsal, the sesamoids may be displaced laterally. If the tendon attachments are disrupted, they can even dislocate toward the neck of the metatarsal. There have been reports of fragments displaced into the metatarsophalangeal joint and of the entrapment of a displaced sesamoid in the interphalangeal joint (Fig. 7.**437**).

 Necrosis?

Osteochondronecrosis of the sesamoids may be idiopathic, occurring in the absence of demonstrable trauma (Ilfed and Rosen 1972, McBryde and Anderson 1988). In most cases, however, osteochondronecrosis (osteochondritis dissecans) is definitely a result of previous chronic trauma. **Primary avascular necrosis** affects either the medial or lateral sesamoid, and bilateral necrosis occurs rarely. Avascular necrosis of the sesamoids is reportedly

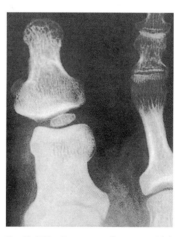

Fig. 7.**437**   Interposed sesamoid bone following dislocation of the interphalangeal joint of the great toe.

more common in women, possibly due to the wearing of high heels.

The typical radiographic features of sesamoid necrosis are as follows (Figs. 7.**438**–7.**440**):

- Patchy demineralization
- Increased density
- Fragmentation

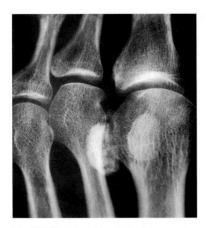

Fig. 7.**438** Typical, clinically symptomatic necrosis of the lateral sesamoid in an elderly woman. All criteria for necrosis are satisfied: areas of increased density plus beginning fragmentation, which appears as small irregular lucencies between the denser areas.

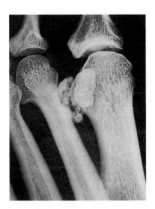

Fig. 7.**439** Necrosis of the lateral sesamoid of the great toe with typical fragmentation.

But since clinical pain may be present for some time before these signs appear, today it is best to proceed with radionuclide scanning (Fig. 7.**440d, e**) or MRI in the earlier stages. Sudden pain, incidentally, may be caused by an acute fragmentation of the perfusion-impaired bone. Persistent complaints due to necrosis are easily relieved by surgical removal of the necrotic bone element.

 ## Inflammation?

Osteomyelitic changes in the sesamoid bones may result from the contiguous or hematogenous spread of infection.

Freund (1989) described sesamoid osteomyelitis in children and adolescents that apparently resulted from blunt trauma to the sesamoids.

Because the sesamoids have synovial articulations, they may be involved by systemic rheumatoid diseases, especially rheumatoid arthritis, leading to erosive changes.

 ## Other Changes?

Since the sesamoid articulations are synovial joints, they are basically susceptible to any diseases that can affect the joints, including **chondrocalcinosis** (Fig. 7.**441**).

In one elderly patient, we were able to make this diagnosis only with the aid of CT.

Osteoarthritic changes may also be encountered in the synovial sesamoid joints (Figs. 7.**442**, 7.**443**).

Moderately severe to advanced cases of **acromegaly** are invariably associated with enlargement of the sesamoids, much as in the skeleton of the hand.

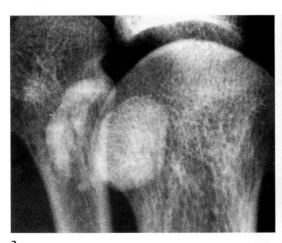
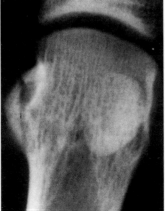
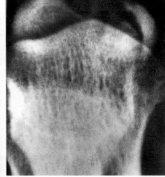

Fig. 7.**440a–e** Middle-aged woman with pain and palpable swelling (bursitis) below the left great toe. The lateral sesamoid shows structural irregularities. Necrosis? Multipartite sesamoid? Extra projections (**b, c**) cannot resolve the problem. Radionuclide scans (**d, e**) show increased uptake in the sesamoid area, proving at least that there is significant pathology to account for the pain. The necrotic sesamoid was surgically removed, relieving the patient's complaints.

Fig. 7.**440d, e** ▷

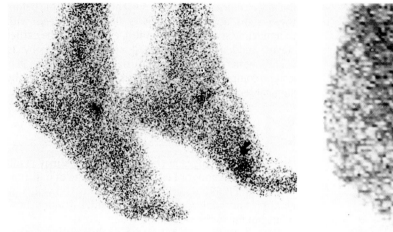

Fig. 7.**440d**

Fig. 7.**440e**

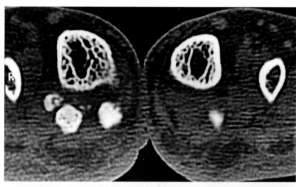

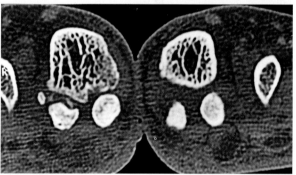

a   b

c

d

Fig. 7.**441 a–d** Curious case of chondrocalcinosis in a multi-partite or former necrotic fragmented lateral sesamoid in a patient who presented with significant pain. CT scans (**c, d**) demonstrate the multipartite sesamoid and also fine calcifications between the sesamoid and metatarsal head, representing calcifications of the hyaline cartilage. All of these findings are consistent with chondrocalcinosis. Regarding the

pathogenesis of this apparently unifocal lesion, we assume that the preexisting or fragmented "multipartite" sesamoid bone caused a disturbance of joint mechanics, leading to secondary chondrocalcinosis (as in the knee joint, for example). Interestingly, the typical radiological signs of osteoarthritis are absent.

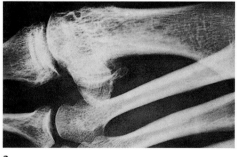

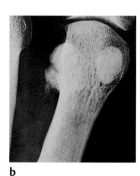

a   b

Fig. 7.**442 a, b** Degenerative arthritis of the first metatarsal sesamoids and first metatarsophalangeal joint.

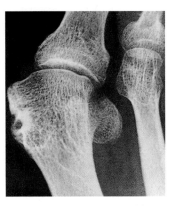

Fig. 7.**443** Lateral dislocation of the eroded sesamoid bone in a pronounced case of hallux valgus.

References

Aseyo, D., H. Nathan: Hallux sesamoid bones. Anatomical observations with special reference to osteoarthritis and hallux valgus. Int. Orthop. (SICOT) 8 (1984) 67

Bowers, K. D., R. B. Martin: Turf-toe: a shoe-surface related football injury. Med. Sci. Sports 8 (1976) 81

Brown, T. I. S.: Avulsion fracture of the fibular sesamoid in association with dorsal dislocation of the metatarsophalangeal joint of the hallux: report of a case and review of the literature. Clin. Orthop. 149 (1980) 229

Browne, T., R. F. McCarron: Pseudomonas osteomyelitis of the metatarsal sesamoid: a case report. Orthop. Rev 17 (1988) 601 ·

Capasso, G., N. Maffulli, V. Testa: Rupture of the intersesamoid ligament of a soccer player's foot. Foot and Ankle 10 (1990) 337

Chillag, K., W. A. Grana: Medial sesamoid stress fracture. Orthopedics 8 (1985) 821

Clanton, T. O., J. E. Butler, A. Eggert: Injuries to the metatarsophalangeal joints in athletes. Foot and Ankle 7 (1986) 162

Collwill, M.: Osteomyelitis of the metatarsal sesamoids. J. Bone Jt Surg. 51-B (1970) 464

Conway, W. F., C. W. Hayes, W. A. Murphy: Case report 568: Total resorption of the lateral sesamoid secondary to Pseudomonas aeruginosa osteomyelitis. Skelet. Radiol. 18 (1989) 483

Feldman, F., R. Pochaczevsky, H. Hecht: The case of the wandering sesamoid and other sesamoid afflictions. Radiology 96 (1970) 275

Freund, K. G.: Haematogenous osteomyelitis of the first metatarsal sesamoid. Arch. orthop. traum. Surg. 108 (1989) 53

Gordon, S. L., C. Evans, R. B. Greer: Pseudomonas osteomyelitis of the metatarsal sesamoid of the great toe. Clin. Orthop. 99 (1974) 188

van Hal, M. E., J. S. Keene, T. A. Lange et al.: Stress fractures of the great toe sesamoid. Amer. J. Sports Med. 10 (1982) 122

Hulkko, A., S. Orava, P. Pellinen et al.: Stress fractures of the sesamoid bones of the first metatarsophalangeal joint in athletes. Arch. orthop. traum. Surg. 104 (1985) 113

Ilfed, F. W., V. Rosen: Osteochondritis of the first metatarsal sesamoid. Clin. Orthop. 85 (1972) 38

Kliman, M. E., A. E. Gross, K.P. Pritzker et al.: Osteochondritis of the hallux sesamoid bones. Foot and Ankle 3 (1983) 220

Lapidus, P. W.: Congenital unilateral absence of the medial sesamoid of the great toe. J. Bone Jt Surg. 21-A (1939) 208

Lemont, H., M. St.Khoury: Subchondral bone cysts of the sesamoid. J. Amer. podiat. med. Ass. 75 (1985) 218

McBryde, A. M., R. B. Anderson: Sesamoid foot problems in the athlete. Clin. Sports Med. 7 (1988) 51

Ogata, K., Y. Sugioka, Y. Urano et al.: Idiopathic osteoonecrosis of the first metatarsal sesamoid. Skelet. Radiol. 15 (1986) 141

Potter, H. G., H. Pavlov, T. G. Abrahams: The hallux sesamoids revisited. Skelet. Radiol. 21 (1992) 437

Resnick, D., G. Niwayama, M. L. Feinagold: The sesamoid bones of the hands and feet: participators in arthritis. Radiology 123 (1977) 57

Stadalnik, R. C., A. B. Dublin: Sesamoid periostitis in the thumb in Reiter's Syndrome. Case report. J. Bone Jt Surg. 57-A (1975) 279

Szucs, R., J. Hurwitz: Traumatic subluxation of the interphalangeal joint of the hallux with interposition of the sesamoid bone (letter). Amer. J. Roentgenol. 152 (1989) 652

Toes

Normal Findings

During Growth

The first ossification center for the toes appears in the distal phalanx of the great toe during the 9th week of fetal development. The centers for the distal phalanges of the second through fifth toes appear in the 11th–12th weeks, those for the proximal phalanges in the 14th week, and those for the middle phalanges at the end of the 4th fetal month.

The epiphyses of the proximal phalanges appear between the 5th month of life and the 2nd year, those of the middle phalanges between the 9th month and 2nd year. The epiphysis of the distal phalanx of the great toe appears during the first two years of life.

The epiphyseal centers fuse with the metaphysis between the 15th and 17th years in females and between the 17th and 23rd years in males.

With less longitudinal growth the diaphysis alone can ossify, i.e. without an epiphyseal ossification center, as for example in the middle phalanx of the small toe.

The axis of the great toe normally deviates 10° laterally at the metatarsophalangeal joint. This angle is already present in infants and subsequently increases through greater growth of the medial half of the epiphyseal center of the distal phalanx.

The basal epiphysis may be bipartite as a normal variant, consisting of two centers separated at the middle (Fig. 7.**444**).

Flat and very dense epiphyses are considered normal findings in the proximal phalanges of the first and fifth toes (Figs. 7.**444**–7.**446**).

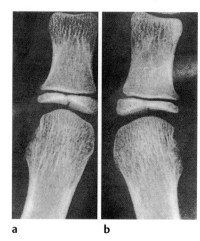

Fig. 7.**444a, b** Bipartite basal epiphyses of the proximal phalanx of the great toe.

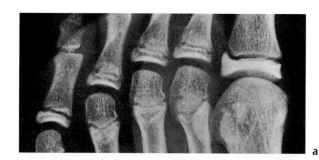

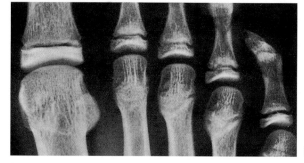

Fig. 7.**445a, b** Dense epiphysis of the proximal phalanx of the great toe and, to a lesser degree, of the small toe.

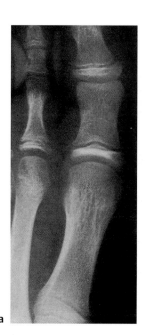

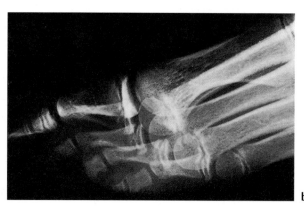

Fig. 7.**446a, b** Dense epiphysis at the metatarsophalangeal joint of the great toe, unilateral, in an 11-year-old girl.
a Dorsoplantar projection.
b Lateral projection.

In Adulthood

The shape of the **proximal phalanges** is more uniform than that of the middle and distal phalanges. The medial half of the base of the second through fifth toes is more prominent than the lateral half—a pattern that is sometimes reversed in the great toe.

> In lateral and oblique radiographs of the toes, a **lamellar bone formation** is often seen along the plantar aspect of the larger phalanges. This is caused by the osseous tendon bed and is not a lamellar periosteal reaction.

A slight spindle-shaped widening is often visible in the shafts of the proximal phalanges near the base (Fig. 7.**447**).

According to Dihlmann (1972), the first toe displays this widening in 20% of cases, the second toe in 90%, the third toe in 85–95%, the fourth toe in 90%, and the fifth toe in 80%. Dihlmann calls this phenomenon the "diaphyseal cuff," claiming that its thickness is inversely proportional to the mineral content and diameter of the diaphysis. We believe that the cause of this phenomenon is the same as in the hand: prominent attachments of the plantar interosseous muscles. Even when solitary, these expansions should not be mistaken for postfracture callus formation or other pathology.

The shape of the **middle phalanges** is extremely variable. Sometimes they lack a waisted contour and appear almost rectangular. The beveled ends of the shafts can give the toes an angled appearance.

> The **middle and distal phalanges of the small toe** are **fused together (synostosed)** in approximately 25–33% of all cases. Hence this is a normal finding rather than a normal variant and is definitely not pathological (Fig. 7.**448**).

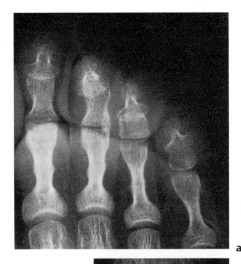

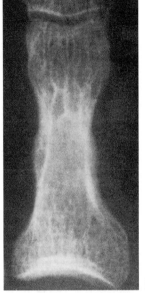

Fig. 7.**447 a, b** Typical ▷ spindle-shaped configuration of the proximal shafts of the basal phalanges. Magnified view on the right. This is not an abnormal periosteal reaction due to a fracture or other pathology. Same findings in Fig. 7.**388**.

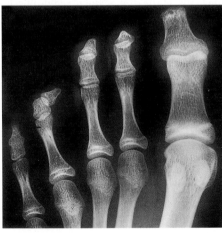

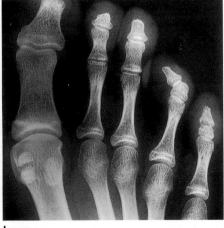

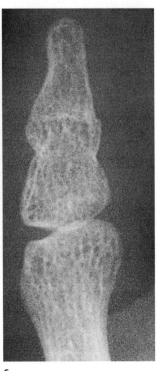

Fig. 7.**448 a–c** A somewhat confusing case. The patient, a 14-year-old girl, sustained trauma to the fifth toe of the right foot eight weeks earlier, followed by pain and swelling. Based on a single radiograph of the right foot, the orthopedist diagnosed arthritis of the fifth interphalangeal joint. When the case was referred to us for consultation, we were struck by the shortened distal phalanges of the second and third toes, which raised the possibility of an acro-osteolysis syndrome with destruction of the interphalangeal structures of the right fifth toe. When the left foot was radiographed, it also showed shortening of the second and third distal phalanges along with varus of the fourth toe (as in the right foot) and synostosis of the middle and distal phalanges of the fifth toe. At this point the diagnosis was clear: a fracture of the synostosis of the right fifth toe and brachytelephalangia of the second and third toes. Symphalangia (magnification view in **c**) is a normal finding in the small toe but anomalous in other toes.

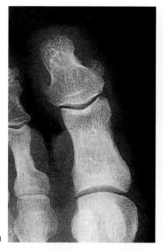
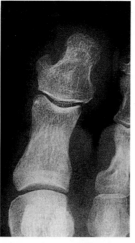

a   b

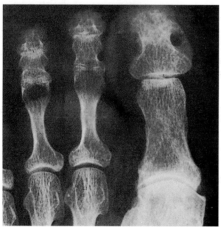
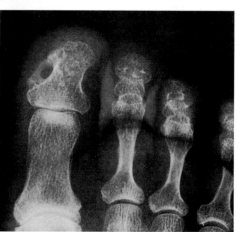

c   d

Fig. 7.**449 a–d**   Distal phalanges of the great toe.
a, b Normal bony excrescences or "protuberances" at the medial base of the first distal phalanges in a 73-year-old man.
c, d Bony bridges have formed between the base and tuberosity of the distal phalanges of the great toes in this 62-year-old woman. This probably represents an extreme form of the reactive excrescences shown in **a** and **b**.

An **exostosis-like bony excrescence** is found at the medial base of the distal phalanx of the great toe in almost all individuals (Fig. 7.**449 a, b**). It develops from the plantar and medial aspects of the base of the distal phalanx, just distal to the medial tuberosity. Lee et al. (1992) investigated this bony excrescence (which they found in 88.5% of 157 dorsoplantar foot radiographs in 117 adults and children), including histological analysis, and found that it consisted mainly of reactive bone, probably induced by repetitive forces occurring during ambulation. The outgrowth appears after closure of the adjacent epiphyseal plate and is rarely symptomatic. The bony bridges that formed between the medial protuberances and terminal tufts in Fig. 7.**449 c, d** may well represent an extreme case of reactive bone formation in response to sustained stresses.

As described under General Aspects in the chapters on the metacarpus and phalanges of the hand (p.24), cone-shaped epiphyses may be based on a developmental disturbance in which the peripheral segments continue to grow while the central segments are arrested in their growth, at least temporarily. Cone-shaped epiphyses are only occasionally associated with clinical symptoms (in the hand Fig. 2.**18 d, e**). Cone-shaped epiphyses are usually bilateral and are most common in the proximal phalanges of the second through fourth toes. They are rare in the middle phalanges and fifth toe.

A **longitudinally bracketed diaphysis** (Figs. 7.**454**, 7.**455**) is a pathological finding that is observed in various skeletal dysplasias (p.26).

Pathological Finding?

   Normal Variant or Anomaly?

Apparently there are accessory bones called the **lateral** and **medial os paraarticulare** (Fig. 7.**450**) that may be harmless or may lead to growth disturbances and necrosis (Fig. 7.**451**).

   Cone-shaped epiphyses in the foot can occur as a variant in individuals who are otherwise completely healthy (Figs. 7.**452**, 7.**453**, 7.**464**).

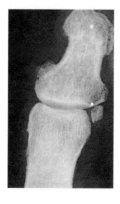

Fig. 7.**450**   Accessory bone (lateral os paraarticulare) at the interphalangeal joint of the great toe. Note also the normal bony excrescence at the medial base of the distal phalanx.

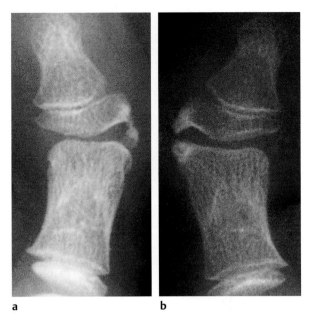

a   b

Fig. 7.**451 a, b**   Partial fusion of the os paraarticulare.
a Medial os paraarticulare partially fused with the epiphysis in
a 12-year-old girl.
b Radiograph of the right side in the same patient shows apparently circumscribed necrotic changes at the fusion site. In
this case, furnished by Holthusen (Hamburg), it is unclear
whether the valgus position of the distal phalanges is related
to the foregoing anatomic peculiarities. The observation that
the epiphysis is broader medially than laterally is still a normal
finding.

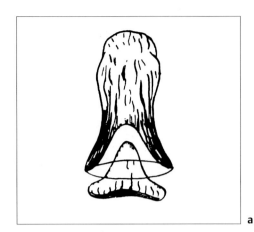

a

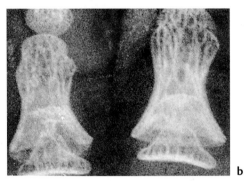

b

Fig. 7.**452 a, b**   Cone-shaped epiphyses.

Fig. 7.**453**   Cone-shaped epiphyses of the proximal phalanges of the second through fourth toes, and probably of the
middle phalanx of the second toe, in an 8-year-old girl.

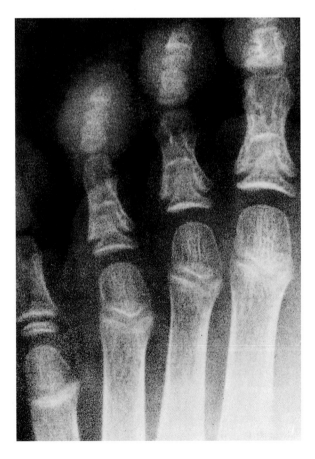

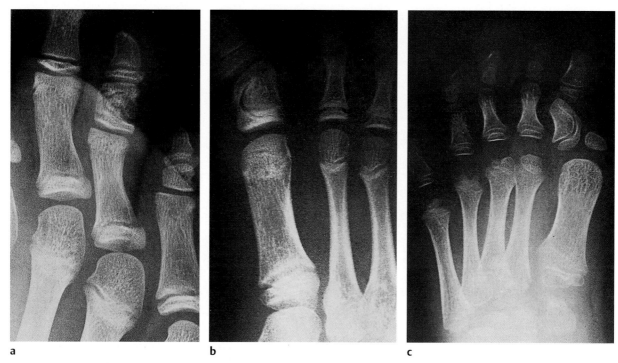

a   b   c

Fig. 7.**454 a–c**   Bracketed diaphyses (in different patients).

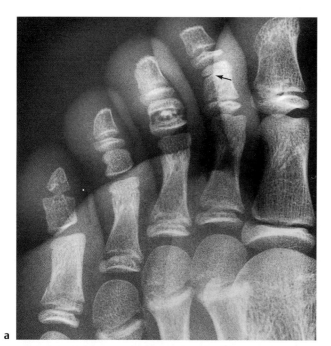

a

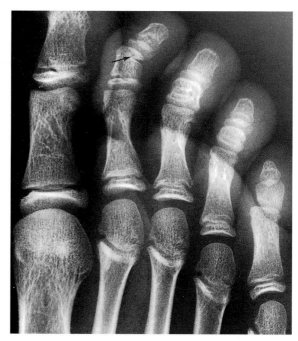

b

Fig. 7.**455 a, b**   Bilateral bracketed diaphyses in the middle phalanges of an 8-year-old girl. Other unusual findings: small pseudoepiphyses on the second middle phalanges (arrows) and, to a degree, on the third and fourth proximal phalanges of the right foot. All of the second and third middle phalanges are too short. Note also the valgus deformity of the second distal phalanx in the right foot. (Case courtesy of Dr. H. Bartel, Düsseldorf.)

This condition, named for the "bracketing" of the diaphysis by the epiphysis, apparently leads to brachyphalangias.

> **Symphalangias** (Fig. 7.**456**) are also definitely pathological (hereditary dysplasia), except in the small toe.

Brachydactylies are usually an hereditary anomaly (Fig. 7.**458 a**).

The bones of the foot are susceptible to the same types of deformities that are found in the hand. They include:

- Supernumerary rays (Fig. 7.**458 b**)
- Supernumerary phalangeal bones (four short phalanges instead of three, etc.)

- Syndactylies
- Transverse partitions (Fig. 7.**457**)

Hallux abductus interphalangeus refers to a solitary valgus deformity of the distal phalanx relative to the middle phalanx at the interphalangeal joint. It is inversely related to hallux abductovalgus: the greater the degree of hallux abductovalgus, the less the degree of hallux abductus interphalangeus, and vice versa. Even in severe cases, the angular deformity is not caused by lateral slippage on the head of the proximal phalanx (as in hallux valgus) but by disproportionate growth of the medial half of the epiphyseal center of the distal phalanx (phalanx unguicularis hallucis valgus).

Fig. 7.**456 a–f** Follow-up of symphalangia. The patient is the mother of a child with similar changes (shown in Fig. 7.**221 f, g**).
a, b Radiographs at 15 years of age show complete symphalangia of all three phalanges in the third ray of the right foot. The middle phalanges are absent in the second through fifth toes on both sides. The middle phalanx of the great toe on the right side is brachyphalangic.
c, d Radiographs seven years later.
e, f Hand radiographs of the same patient in 1981 (**e**) and 1990 (**f**) show pronounced symphalangia of the second through fifth rays. This case is also discussed in the chapter on the hand and is the same patient whose tarsal coalitions are shown in Fig. 7.**221 f, g**. (Case courtesy of Professor D. Buck-Gramcko, Hamburg.)

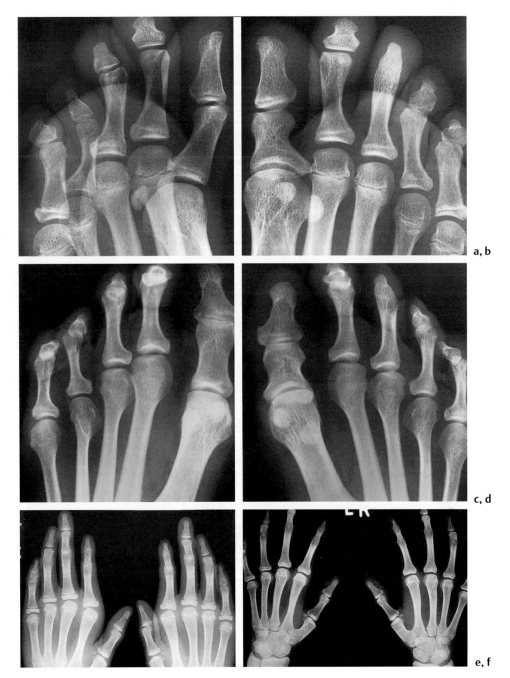

a, b

c, d

e, f

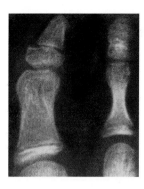

Fig. 7.**457** Transverse partition of the distal phalanx of the great toe, not an abnormally wide distal epiphysis.

Congenital or acquired **hammer toe** generally involves almost 90° contractures with subluxation and dislocation of the metatarsophalangeal joints, usually affecting the second and fifth toes (Fig. 7.**459**).

The hammer deformity of the fifth toe can be seen as a developmental involution of the metatarsophalangeal joint. Any of three different deformities can develop (Fig. 7.**459**) as a result of congenital or acquired foot deformities, or as a result of nerve palsies or failed corrective surgery for hallux valgus. In the pathogenesis of these deformities a flexor-extensor imbalance with excessive loading of the forefoot plays an important role.

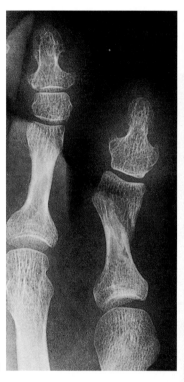

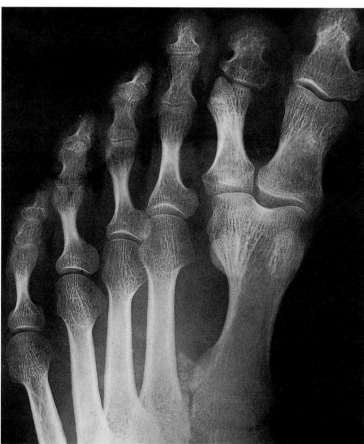

Fig. 7.**458 a, b** Foot deformities.
a Radiograph taken to evaluate an oblique fracture of the small toe in a 39-year-old man. The middle and distal phalanges of the small toe are synostosed, producing a single stout bone. Viewed in isolation, the fused phalanges of the small toe would still be considered normal, but brachyme-sophalangia is also noted in the third toe (not shown) and fourth toe.
b Supernumerary great toe. The head of the first metatarsal is splayed and broadened, as if to accommodate its articulation with both proximal phalanges.

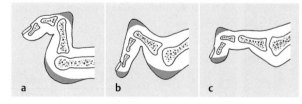

Fig. 7.**459 a–c** Toe deformities.
a Claw toe.
b Hammer toe.
c Mallet toe.

Fracture, Subluxation, or Dislocation?

Fractures of the toes are most often caused by falling objects. Fifty percent of these fractures affect the great toe, usually the distal phalanx, and the first metatarsal bone; 25% affect the fifth ray; and the remaining 25% affect the other bones. Dislocations of the toes are usually associated with the avulsion of small bone fragments. Diagnosis is challenging due to projection-related difficulties, especially if there is age-associated clawing of the toes.

Epiphyseal injuries can also be difficult to diagnose. A stumbling type of injury can cause traumatic epiphyseal separation at the distal interphalangeal joint that is very difficult to detect on radiographs unless there is significant displacement. This injury is of no consequence, however, as it does not involve the epiphyseal plate and does not damage the growth cartilage. Epiphyseal plate injuries are sometimes difficult to distinguish from a duplicated ossifi-

cation center (Fig. 7.**444**). Like all other bones, the toes and especially the proximal phalanges are susceptible to **stress fractures** ("march fractures").

 ## Necrosis?

Small, often peripheral osteolytic lesions with sclerotic margins are not an uncommon finding in the proximal phalanges, especially in young men. They are detected incidentally and, according to Keats et al. (1989), are probably a result of stress-induced osteonecrosis.

Many diseases from the **acroosteolysis** group can cause bone resorption that predominantly affects the distal phalanges (see also Tables 2.**6** and 2.**9**). The changes are very similar to those seen at the hand (q. v.). One of the most frequent causes of acroosteolysis of the toes is diabetic osteoarthropathy (Fig. 7.**460**, see p. 1067 f).

Fig. 7.**460 a–d**
Acroosteolysis of the toes.
a, b Acroosteolysis or osteonecrosis in diabetic osteoarthropathy. This case (same as that shown in Figs. 7.**375** and 7.**410**) involves extensive tarsal and metatarsal necrotic changes.
a Radiograph taken in May 1993. The patient presented with a perforating ulcer on the anterolateral sole of the foot. The film shows subluxation of the fourth proximal interphalangeal joint (due to ligament destruction).
b Three months later, the distal portion of the fourth proximal phalanx has been resorbed. Incipient osteolytic changes are also seen in the opposing middle phalanx, which shows central resorption. Complete documentation on this case can be found in Freyschmidt (1997).
c, d Hereditary palmo-plantar Keratosis (same case as in Fig. 2.**100**). Note the acroosteolysis in the distal phalanges with pencil-like configuration especially of the 4th and 5th toes.

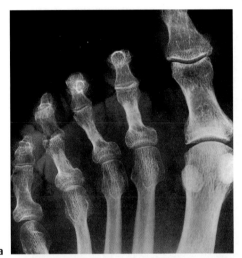
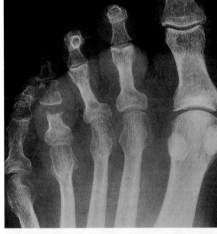
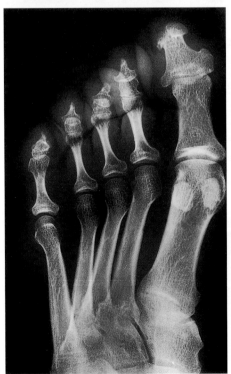
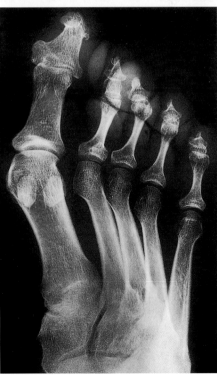

a

b

c

d

Ainhum syndrome (spontaneous dactylolysis) typically affects the toes. Hyperkeratotic changes lead to a constriction of the soft-tissue mantle, causing circulatory impairment and interrupting blood flow to the acral parts of the toes, which undergo resorption. The disease is most common in persons who habitually go barefoot, such as the dark-skinned population of Western Africa and other warm climatic zones. In Nigeria, for example, 2% of the population have Ainhum syndrome. The diagnosis is established by noting the clinical presence of acral hyperkeratosis and atrophy.

 Inflammation? Tumor?

Osteomyelitis of the phalanges is usually the result of an open injury and need not be discussed here in detail.

Of course, the interphalangeal joints may also be involved by inflammatory rheumatic processes, but often this is extremely difficult to diagnose due to preexisting foot deformities.

The distal phalanges are important in the diagnosis of **psoriatic arthritis** (Fig. 7.**461**). As in the hand, these bones show more or less pronounced and characteristic protuberances. A radionuclide scan can accurately document the pattern of involvement in most cases (Fig. 7.**461 c**).

Bone tumors and tumorlike lesions of the toes are rare. Reactive changes such as **subungual exostoses** (Figs. 7.**462**, 7.**463**) are not uncommon in daily practice, however. They apparently result from a reactive proliferative process that belongs in the category of **proliferative changes in the**

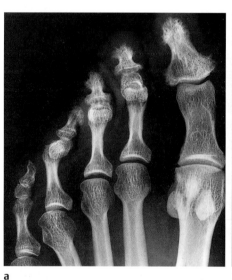

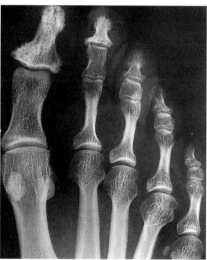

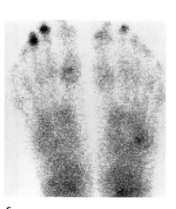

a   b   c

Fig. 7.**461 a–c**   Psoriatic osteoarthropathy.
a, b Typical psoriatic osteoarthropathy with spiculated proliferation on the terminal tufts of the first through fourth phalanges of the left foot, the second phalanx of the right foot, and at the bases of the first through third distal phalanges on both sides.

c Bone scan shows a predominantly transverse pattern of involvement with very intense uptake in the second and third distal phalanges of the right foot and increased uptake in the first through third phalanges of the left foot.

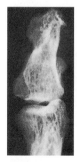

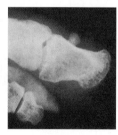

Fig. 7.**463**

Fig. 7.**462**

Fig. 7.**462**   Subungual exostosis of the great toe (symptomatic).

Fig. 7.**463**   Subungual exostosis of the great toe in a 38-year-old woman.

hands and feet (e.g., florid reactive periostitis, bizarre paraosseous osteochondromatous proliferation, etc.).

The radiographic features of these changes are influenced by local anatomy, especially in the distal phalanges of the foot. Exostoses on the distal phalanges are consistently located on the extensor or dorsal side, and further modifications can result from the nail bed itself. If the nail is lost, the lesion is called a **turret exostosis**.

True and **solitary osteochondromas** are extremely rare in the skeleton of the foot (Fig. 7.**464**). When they occur, it is near the metaphysis and almost always in a setting of cartilaginous exostosis disease.

Approximately 5% of all enchondromas occur in the phalanges. Radiographs show a smoothly marginated, more or less centrally located osteolytic lesion, occasionally with fine matrix calcifications. This pattern may change, however, if a spontaneous fracture occurs (Fig. 7.**465**).

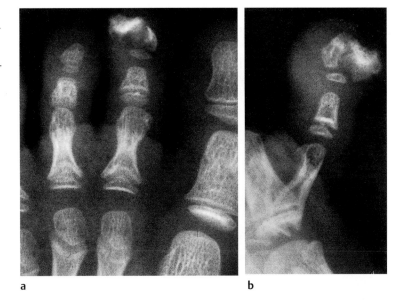

Fig. 7.**464 a, b** Unusual osteochondroma on the second distal phalanx of a 5-year-old child. Clublike enlargement of the second distal phalanx was noted clinically. The diagnosis was confirmed histologically by a bone pathologist. Incidental finding: cone-shaped epiphyses in the second and third toes.

a

b

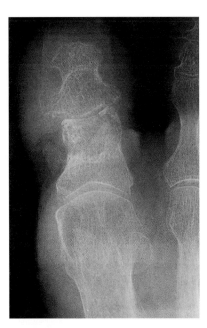

Fig. 7.**465** Enchondroma in the proximal phalanx of the great ▷ toe, with an associated spontaneous fracture. The differential diagnosis should include a large gouty tophus and even a metastatic lesion (e.g., from bronchial carcinoma).

References

Blodgett, W. H.: Injuries of the forefoot and toes. In Jahss, M. H.: Disorders of the Foot. Saunders, Philadelphia 1982 (chapter 23)

Brahms, M. A.: The small toes. In Jahss, M. H.: Disorders of the Foot. Saunders, Philadelphia 1982 (p. 622)

de Cuveland, E.: Zur Herkunft des Os pararticulare am interphalangealen Großzehengrundgelenk. Fortschr. Röntgenstr. 105 (1966) 591

Dihlmann, W., M. Cen, W. Sturm: Über die Diaphysenmanschette an den Grundphalangen der Zehen. Fortschr. Röntgenstr. 117 (1972) 350

Duke, H., L. M. Newman, B. L. Bruskoff et al.: Hallux abductus interphalangeus and its relationships to hallux abductovalgus. J. Amer. podiat. med. Ass. 72 (1982) 625

Endler, F., K. Fochem, U. H. Weil: Orthopädische Röntgendiagnostik. Thieme, Stuttgart 1984

Fischer, E.: Zur Ätiologie der knöchernen Brücken an den Seiten des Großzehenendglieds. Radiologe 27 (1987) 279

Freyschmidt, J.: Skeletterkrankungen. Springer 1997 (p. 772–774)

Keats, T., R. R. Johnson, R. E. Fechner: Idiopathic punctate necrosis of the phalanges of the feet. Skelet. Radiol. 18 (1989) 25

Lee, M., J. Hodler, P. Haghighi et al.: Bone excrescence at the medial base of the distal phalanx of the first toe: normal variant, reactive change, or neoplasia? Skelet. Radiol. 21 (1992) 161

Mozena, J. D., L. R. Kroepel: Digital fractures in children. J. Amer. podiat. med. Ass. 75 (1985) 288

Ogden, J. A., T. R. Light, G. J. Conlogue: Correlative roentgenography of the longitudinal epiphyseal bracket. Skelet. Radiol. 6 (1981) 109

Rausher, H., R. B. Birrer, M. R. Camiel et al.: Ainhum-dactylolysis spontanea. N. Y. St. J. Med. 12 (1981) 1779

Ravelli, A.: Zapfenepiphysen an den Mittelphalangen der Zehen. Fortschr. Röntgenstr. 84 (1956) 498

Rosenfeld, S. L., P. T. Slowik: Osteochondritis dissecans traumatically induced in the hallux interphalangeal joint. J. Amer. podiat. med. Ass. 72 (1982) 261

Index

A

Abt–Letterer–Siwe disease 400
accessory bones 4
acetabular index 816
 depth-to-width 817, 818
acetabulum
 accessory bones 821–2, 823
 accessory fossa 824
 anatomy 811, 813, 814
 apophyses
  marginal 804, 806–7
  persistence 821–2
  persistent accessory 807
 bony defect 824
 center–edge angle of Wiberg 817, 818
 components 804
 congenital dislocation of hip 825, 826
 constitutional flat 825
 CT imaging 818, 819
 epiphysis persistence 821–2
 eyebrow sign 808, 809
 false-profile view and VCA angle 817–18, 819
 fractures 829–30, 831
  stress 834
 growth 804–7
 HTE angle 817, 818
 labrum 811, 813, 814
  lesion classification 815
  tears 811, 813, 815
 measurements after puberty 817–18
 ossification centers 804, 807
 osteochondritis dissecans 837, 840
 pressure-bearing zone 808
 primary protrusio acetabuli 824
 rim fractures 830
 secondary 825
 subchondral synovial cyst 846, 847
 tear drop figure 804, 808, 809
 variants 821–4
 villonodular synovitis 845
Achilles tendon
 calcaneal tuberosity avulsion 1034
 fat triangle 1001
achillobursitis defect 1038, 1039
achondrogenesis 6
achondroplasia 6
 axial deviations 28, 37
 cervical spine 621
 foramen magnum 438
 humerus varus 253
 lumbar canal narrowing 698, 699
 nasal bone congenital hypoplasia 513
 short ulna 194
acoustic neurinoma 484, 489
acro/acro-mesomelic dysplasias 8
acro-osteolysis 44, 56–7, 73, 77, 78
 clavicle 289
 distal phalanges (finger) 76, 77, 80, 81
 hyperparathyroidism 81, 88
 middle phalanges (finger) 88
 ribs 350
 scapula 281
 syndrome 289
 thumb 93
 toes 1101
acrocephalosyndactyly 468, 506
 delta phalanges (finger) 26
 thumb 91
acrocephaly 391
acromegaly 70
 distal phalanges (finger) 78
 intervertebral disk calcification 639
 lumbar canal narrowing 698
 lumbar vertebrae 710
 mandible 547

 osteophytes 950
 productive bone changes 69
 sesamoid bones 1091
acromioclavicular joint 287–91
 anomalies 287–8
 calcification 287, 290
 degenerative change 290
 dislocation 280, 288, 289
 fractures 288, 289
 inflammation 290
 joint space widening 290, 302
 necrosis 289–90
 normal variants 287–8
 osteoarthritis 290, 291
 posttraumatic ossification 289
 pseudodislocation 288, 289
 rheumatic disorders 290
 subluxation 288, 289
 Tossy classification of dislocations 288
 tumors 290
acromioclavicular ligament 287
acromion 264, 265, 270, 273
 arch shape variation 272, 273–4
 isolated bony element 2–3, 277–8
 morphological types 272–4
 ossification centers 264, 278, 287
  persistence 276, 277
 stress fracture 277, 278
actinomycosis
 cervical spine 629
 mandible 545
 skull base 442
adamantinoma, tibial 965, 967
agger nasi 520, 531
Ahlbäck disease 885, 887
Ainhum syndrome 1102
air cells 464–77
 clouding 471, 472
 maxillary sinus 520–1
 osteomyelitis 475
 sigmoid sinus 465
Albers–Schönberg marble bone disease see osteopetrosis
algodystrophy 1084, 1085
alkaptonuria 639
 ochronosis 721, 758
allocephaly 368
alveolar canal
 mandible 547
 posterior superior 521
ameloblastoma, mandible 545–6, 547
amyloid deposits, β2-microglobulin 64, 65, 846
amyloidosis, intervertebral disk calcification 639
anal atresia 653
anatomic snuffbox, scaphoid contusion 154
Andersson lesions 702
anemia
 congenital 36, 38
 hair-on-end appearance 379, 380
 skull 369
 see also sickle cell disease
angel wing syndrome 453
angiodysplasia
 hypertrophic osteoarthropathy 81
 Klippel–Trenaunay type 34, 36
 Servelle–Martorell-type 36
 tibia 959, 961
 Weber-type 34, 35, 36
angioma, orbital 508
ankle impingement syndrome, posterior 1007
ankle joint see talocrural joint
ankylosing hyperostosis see DISH syndrome
ankylosing spondylitis 317
 bamboo spine 704, 705
 calcaneus 1039

 cervical spinous processes 631
 cervical vertebrae 599, 626, 629, 631, 632
 double trolley back 704
 lumbar vertebrae 702–6
 occipitoatlantoaxial joints 600
 sacroiliitis 755–6
 thoracic vertebrae 662, 663
 triple trolley back 704
ankylosis
 acquired bony 27–8
 apophyseal joint spaces 612, 613
 carpal inflammatory 131
 cervical spine 629, 630
 sacroiliac joint 758
 thoracic vertebrae 662–3
annulus fibrosus 558
 calcification 721, 722, 723
anorexia nervosa 880
anotia 468
AO classification of spinal injuries 659
aorta
 coarctation 348
 ectasia 668
aortic aneurysm 668, 710
Apert syndrome see acrocephalosyndactyly
apical ligament of dens 558
aplasia, hereditary 27
apophyseal joints
 ankylosis 631
 spaces in cervical spine 612, 613
apophyseal ring 562
apple core sign 845, 846
arachnodactyly 34
arachnoid cysts 428–9
arachnoid villi 371
arhinencephaly 524
arm see forearm
arm, upper
 diaphysis 238–44
 see also humerus; humerus, distal; humerus, proximal
Arnold–Chiari malformation 438
arthritis
 bacterial
  acromioclavicular joint 290
  joint erosions 57, 58
  manubrioclavicular joint 313
 carpal 130, 131
 proximal phalanges (finger) 90
 psoriatic 57, 59, 60, 61
  bamboo spine 706
  carpal 131
  cervical spine 631
  distal phalanges (finger) 83
  distal phalanges (toe) 1102
  lumbar vertebrae 704, 705
  metacarpal 101
  metatarsal bones 1082
  occipitoatlantoaxial abnormalities 600
  sacroiliac joint 756–7
 sympathetic 130, 131
  carpal 163
 tarsal bones 997
 temporomandibular joint 551, 552
 uncovertebral joints 624
 see also osteoarthritis; rheumatoid arthritis
arthrography
 three-compartment 111
arthro-osteitis
 scapula 281–2
 see also pustulotic arthro-osteitis
arytenoid cartilage 493
aspergillosis
 calcification 517
 nasal cavity 515, 516, 517
asterion/asterion process 407
astragalus see talus

atelosteogenesis 6
atheroma, calcified of calvarium 405
athyrosis, sella turcica 453
atlanto-occipital joint 572
 arthritis 599
 dislocation 596, 597
 dysplasia 622
 motion 573
 osteoarthritis 601
 synostosis 435, 588–9
atlanto-occipital membrane, anterior 603
atlantoaxial joint
 fusions 589
 osteoarthritis 601, 602
 rotational analysis 574
atlantoaxial segmentation, irregular 590
atlantoaxial subluxation 597–8, 599, 600, 631
 rotary 597, 598
atlantodental distance 567
atlantodental joint, osteoarthritis 602
atlas 558, 564–604
 accessory joint 575, 576
 accessory ossicles 590–2
 anatomy 564, 566
 anomalies 575–83
 anterior displacement 597
 anterior tubercle fracture 592
 arch 567–8, 569
  anterior 575, 576, 577, 579–83
  aplasia 577, 578
  clefts 579, 593
  hemiaplasia 577, 578
  posterior 575–8, 592, 593
  pseudofractures 569
 arcuate foramen 581
 assimilation 435, 588–90
 bipartite 579
 burst fracture 592
 cleft
  paramedian 593
  posterior arch 575, 576, 577
 duplication of anterior arch 580
 epitransverse process 581, 582, 583
 fractures 592–8
 infratransverse process 582, 583
 Jefferson fracture 592, 593
 Kimmerle variant 580
 lateral bending 573
 lateral displacement 597
 lateral ponticulus 580
 line 573
 notch-shaped lucencies 568, 570
 os suboccipitale 591
 ossification 565
 paracondylar mass 582
 paracondylar process 581, 582, 583
 plane 572
 pneumatization 580
 ponticulus 581
  posterior 580, 581
 posterior arch
  cleft 575–8, 576, 577
  fracture 592, 593
 pseudo-Jefferson fracture 593
 pseudodislocation 597
 pseudotumor 579
 rotary subluxation 597, 598
 rotation 573–5
 spina bifida 575, 576, 577
 spinous process
  frictional sclerosis 603
  joint formation with axis 584
 split 579
 stenosis 575, 576
 styloid process 582, 583
 transverse foramen
  absence 580
  asymmetry 568, 570

transverse process anomalies 580–3
tumors 600–1
unilateral irregular segmentation 590
auditory canal, external 459, 464–77
aneurysmal bone cyst 476
atresia 468
bleeding 470
foreign bodies 476
growth 478
auditory canal, internal 459–64, 479, 480
growth 478
transverse crest 479, 482
auditory ossicles 360, 457, 468
dislocation 470
petrous bone fracture 469
rupture 470
auricle 459
avascular necrosis
coccygodynia 743
femoral head 840, 841–3
humerus head 253, 256
sesamoid bones 1090–1
axis 558, 564–604
accessory ossicles 590–2
anatomy 564–5, 566
anomalies 584–8
assimilation 589
cartilaginous disk persistence 571
dens 564–5, 570–1
aplasia 587
bicornuate 586, 595
crowned 602
curvature determination 588
dysplasia 587
elongated 587
fracture 586, 587, 594–5, 595
fracture nonunion 586, 595
hyperlordosis 587, 588
hypoplasia 585, 587
lateral tilting 588
necrosis 598
ossification 565, 567
ossification centers 571, 572
persistent synchondrosis remnant 595
recurvatus 587, 595
rheumatoid arthritis 599
tertiary condyle 591
vertical subluxation 599
dislocations 596–8
dolichodens 587
fractures 592–5
lateral bending 573
os odontoideum 585, 586, 595
ossiculum terminale of Bergmann 584, 585, 591
ossification 565, 567
ossification centers 571, 572
plane 572
rotation 573–5
malalignment 575
scalloping of inferior end plate 588
spina bifida 584
spinous process 574
frictional sclerosis 603
joint formation with atlas 584
spondylolysis 584
subluxation 596–8
rotary 597
synchondrosis 567
tertiary condyle 591
transverse processes anomalies 584
tumors 600–1
unilateral irregular segmentation 590
vertebral arch 584
vertebral body anomalies 584–8

B

Baastrup phenomenon 603
Baastrup syndrome 718–19
Baker cyst 945
bamboo spine 704, 705
Reiter syndrome 706
Bankart lesion 297, 298
Barnett—Nordin index 18, 20, 47
metacarpus 94
basal angle 431, 432
basal ganglia calcification 386, 387
basilar impression 422, 430–3

craniometric measurements 431, 432
basilar processes 434, 435
bathrocephaly 368, 394
battered child syndrome 206, 207
Bergmann ossicle see terminal ossicle
Bernageau view 299
bilharzial arthropathy, sacroiliac joint 757
Binder syndrome 524
birth trauma
clavicular fractures 310
distal femoral fractures 880
bite abnormalities 550
blastomycosis, nasal cavity 516
Blount disease 921–3, 930, 935
Boeck disease 515
bone 67, 68
cortex 5
cystic tuberculosis 60
density 4, 18, 20–1
acquired generalized increase 38, 39, 40
generalized loss 47
pelvis 773, 774, 775
periosteal processes 44
detached fragment 4
felon 59, 62, 84
formation of periosteal new 46
inflammation 59–60, 63
lucency within 4
necrosis during growth 52–6
Parisian Nomenclature of diseases 5, 11–13
trauma 62
bone cyst
aneurysmal 476, 477
calcaneus 1035, 1038
cervical spine 600, 632, 633
ischium 801
lumbar vertebrae 711
pubis 801
idiopathic of hand 64
simple 712
unicameral of calcaneus 1035, 1036
bone-in-bone appearance
carpal bones 123
hand 38, 39
bone islands 67, 117
bone marrow
cavity loss of differentiation with cortex 5
infarction 36, 38
femur 871, 880, 881, 882, 883
tibia 965, 969
necrosis 258
bony arch fusion 562
bony structure, unusual shape/size 5
Boogaard angle 431
Boogaard line 432
Bourneville—Pringle disease see tuberous sclerosis
boxer's nose 514
brachycephaly 368, 392
brachydactyly
fingers 34, 86
toes 1099, 1100
brachymesophalangia 24, 85, 86
brachymetacarpia 96, 97
disproportional 34
brachyphalangia 89
toes 1099
brachytelephalangia 91
breast cancer radiotherapy 281, 282, 350
bregma 405
Brodie abscess 350, 351, 888, 904
patella 911
talus 1018
brucellosis
lumbar vertebrae 702
sacroiliitis 754
Buchem disease see endosteal hyperostosis
bursae, calcinosis circumscripta 71, 72–3
button sequestrum 397–8
calvarium 405

C

C sign 998, 1032, 1033
cachexia 880

Caffey syndrome 206
calcaneal-first metatarsal angle 989, 991
calcaneocuboid coalition 999
calcaneocuboid—fourth metatarsal coalition 1032, 1033
calcaneonavicular coalition 998–9
calcaneus 985, 1020–39
accessory bones 1026, 1028–32
anatomy 1020–5
ankylosing spondylitis 1039
apophysis 1020, 1021, 1022
bifid 1032
bone cyst 1035, 1036, 1038
bone spurs 1025
bony process on anterior articular side 1025, 1026, 1027
coalitions 1032, 1033
deformities 1032–3
diabetic osteoarthropathy 1035
dislocation 1033–4
fibro-ostosis 1038, 1039
fracture 1033–4, 1035
chip 1031
stress 1034
inflammation 1035
lucent area 1020, 1022, 1023–5, 1035
necrosis 1034–5
ossification centers 1020
osteoarthritis 1035
osteomyelitis 1035
osteonecrosis 1034–5
Paget disease 1036, 1038
peroneal process prominence 1025–6
pseudoarticulation 1027, 1028–9
retrotrochlear eminence 1026
secundarius 1027, 1028–31
seronegative spondylarthritis 1036–7, 1039
spurs 1036, 1038, 1039
subluxation 1033–4
synostosis with navicular 1032, 1033
trochlear process 1020, 1021, 1022
tuber joint angle 1033
tuberosity avulsion 1034
tumors 1035–6, 1037, 1038
valgus deformity 999
variants 1025–32
calcific bursitis
hip joint 852–4
peroneus tendon 1056–7
calcification
acromioclavicular joint 287, 290
annulus fibrosus 721, 722, 723
aspergillosis 517
basal ganglia 386, 387
cervical soft tissues 498, 638–41
choroid plexus 381–2
costal cartilage 354
costochondral 324
craniopharyngioma 455
cysticerci 874
diaphysis 242, 243–4
distal femur 895, 897, 898
dystrophic line in bone marrow infarction 880
elbow joint 234, 235
falx 382–3
globe 507
habenulae 381
hip joint ligaments/bursae/tendon sheaths 852–4
hyoid bone 491
iliolumbar ligament 725, 758, 759
infectious intracranial 384–7
intermetatarsal region soft-tissue 1084, 1085
internal carotid artery 384, 451, 455
intra-articular 71, 75
intracerebral tumors 385
intracranial 374
intracranial hemorrhage 385, 386
intratumoral 455
ischium soft tissue 803
knee joint soft-tissue 949–50
lacrimal glands 510
lens 507, 510
lumbar vertebrae 720–5
lunate bone 169
meningeal 382
middle meningeal artery 412
mucormycosis 517

neurocysticercosis 384–5
nuchal ligament 626, 638, 639
nucleus pulposus 640, 668, 721, 722
occipitoatlantoaxial region 603
parahippocampal gyrus 453
pectineal ligament 771
pelvic soft tissues 768, 770–2
petrosellar ligament 449, 482
pineal 380–1
retina 510
sacrococcygeal intervertebral disk 745
sacroiliac ligaments 755–6, 758, 759
sacrospinal ligament 745, 746
sacrotuberal ligament 745
sagittal sinus 382
shoulder joint 299–302
bursae 299, 300, 301
soft-tissue 71–5
Sturge—Weber disease 384, 385
stylohyoid ligament 496
supraspinous ligament 638, 639
tentorial 382, 383
thyroid cartilage 493, 611, 612
trapezium 135
triangular fibrocartilage 132
triquetrum 179
tuberculosis 384
tuberous sclerosis 386
vascular of skull 384
calcifying tendinitis, thigh 871, 872, 873, 874
calcinosis, interstitial 71
shoulder girdle 301, 302
universal 71, 73
calcinosis circumscripta 71
calcium phosphate 71
precipitation 71, 74–5
calcium pyrophosphate deposition disease see pseudogout
calcium specks 21, 22
Caldwell—Luc operation defect 527
calvarial bone 367
thickening/thinning 407
calvarium 358, 359, 361
blood vessels 369–73, 397
bone flap 397
button sequestrum 397–8, 405
calcified atheroma 405
cerebral ridges 373–4
convolutional markings 373–4
increased 389, 392
decalcification 376, 377, 378
density 373–4, 376, 377
increased 398–9
depression 393
dermoid cysts 399, 400
emissary vein canals 371
eosinophilic granuloma 400
epidermoid cysts 399
fibrolipoma 403, 404
fibrous dysplasia 402–3
fracture 392–6
adult 393–6
children 393
ping-pong 393
hemangioma 400, 401
hyperparathyroidism 376, 378, 405
Langerhans cell histiocytosis 397, 400, 547
meningioma en plaque 403, 404
metastases 373, 400, 402
mixed lytic/sclerotic changes 401–2
necrosis 397
neurofibromatosis 403, 405
nutrient canals 369–73
occipital spur 373
osteolysis 399–402
osteoma 398
osteomalacia 376
osteomyelitis 397, 441–2
osteopetrosis 398–9
osteoporosis 376
Paget disease 373, 400, 401–2, 403
parietal foramina 373
pathological findings 375–80
pitting atrophy 378
plasmacytoma 400
pneumocephalus 395, 396
radiation necrosis 397
sarcoidosis 400
sarcomatous transformation 402

sclerosis 398–9
syphilis 398
thickness 373–4, 376, 377
thinning 392
trauma 393
tuberculous lesions 397
tumors 398–419
vascular grooves/markings 369–73
Calvé disease 628, 712
camptodactyly 28, 29
Camurati–Engelmann disease 442, 443, 507
candidiasis, nasal cavity 515
capitate bone 140–3
  bipartite 141
  fractures 141, 142
  fusion to hamate 140, 144
  necrosis 141, 142
capitolunate angle 108
capitulum
  dislocation 229
  ossification center 213
  osteochondritis dissecans 230
carcinoma, mandible 547
carotid artery 423
  external 397
  internal
    aneurysms 455, 510
    calcification 384, 451, 455
    vascular grooves in sphenoid sinus 535
carotid canals 423, 424, 442, 482
  tumors 444
carotid tubercle 611
carotid–cavernous fistula 510
carpal angles 106–8
carpal anomaly 30
carpal bones
  arcs 106
  bipartite 122–3
  duplicated 123
  fusions 122
  ossification centers 123
carpal bossing 138, 139, 141, 142, 143
carpal height index 108, 109
carpal instabilities 127–8
  classification 127
carpal joint 109
  compartments 109–11
carpal ligaments 111–14
carpal translation 108, 109
  index 108
carpal tunnel 144
carpometacarpal dislocation 129
carpometacarpal fracture–dislocation 129
carpometacarpal line, M-shaped 106
carpus 104–83
  accessory bones 117–22, 138, 139, 141, 145–7
    lunate 167–8
    scaphoid 155–7
    triquetral 175–6, 179
  angles of radial articular surface 105
  anomalies 117–25
  bone islands 117
  capitate bone 140–3
  CT scans 111, 114–16
  cysts 131
  diagnostic methods 104–5
  dislocation 125–9
  fractures 125–9
  fracture-dislocation 127
  hamate 144–8
  imaging 104–5
  inflammation 130–1
  intercarpal dislocations 127
  ligament ruptures 127
  lunate bone 164–73
  morphometry 105–17
  necrosis 130
  normal 104–17
  normal variants 117–25
  nutrient canals 118
  pisiform 180–3
  rheumatoid arthritis 117
  scaphoid bone 148–63
  subluxation 125–9
  trapezium 132–7
  trapezoid 137–40
  triangular fibrocartilage complex 111, 114

triquetrum 174–80
tumor 131–2
zigzag deformity 128
cartilage calcification 71, 75
cartilaginous multiple exostosis in femur 864, 865
Catel–Manzke syndrome 26
caudal regression syndrome 740, 741
cavernous hemangioma 510
cementum 540
cephalhematoma 375
cephalocele 387–8, 410, 416, 428
  frontoethmoid 508
ceratohyal bones 492
cerebellar meningoencephalocele 488
cerebellar suture, median 438
cerebellopontine angle 459–64, 478, 479
  tumors 488
cerebral hemiatrophy 429, 430
  frontal sinus 530
cerebral veins, cortical 397
cerebrospinal fluid (CSF)
  posttraumatic leak 533
  rhinorrhea 470
cervical flexion 574, 596
cervical lymph nodes 494
cervical ribs 616, 617, 622
cervical soft tissue calcification 498
cervical spinal canal stenosis 636
cervical vertebrae (C1–C2) 564–604
  ankylosing spondylitis 599
  assimilation 588
  clefts 595
  dislocations 596–8
  fibrous dysplasia 601
  fractures 592–5
  hypermobility syndrome 596
  origin of segments 561
  Paget disease 601
  pseudodislocation 596
  range of motion 596
  rheumatoid arthritis 599
  rotary fixation 597
  seronegative spondylarthritis 599
  spondylolysis 594
  subluxations 596–8
  transverse process persistent apophysis 595
  tuberculous spondylitis 598–9
  tumors 600–1
  see also atlas; axis
cervical vertebrae (C3–C7) 608–41
  accessory bone 635, 636
  achondroplasia 621
  actinomycosis 629
  ankylosing spondylitis 626, 629, 631, 632
  ankylosis 629, 630
  anomalies 620–4
  apophyseal joints 612, 613
    ankylosis 631
    facets 617
    fractures 626
    indentation 626
  block vertebrae 620, 621, 623
  bone spurs 618, 619
  bony septum 610, 611
  calcification 638–41
  carotid tubercle 611
  degenerative changes 634–8
  diastematomyelia 621
  dislocations 627–8
  epiphyses 618, 626
  erosions 601, 633
  fibrous dysplasia 633, 634
  flexion–extension 627, 628
  fractures 624–7
    ankylosing spondylitis 631
    hyperextension 626
    vertical split 625
  gout 629
  hemispheric spondylosclerosis 635
  hemivertebrae 622, 624
  hemodialysis 629
  hyperflexion 624
  hypoplasia 621
  inflammation 628–32
  instability 631
    criteria 628
  interspinous distance
    decrease 627
    widening 625, 627

intervertebral disk
  calcification 639–41
  spaces 612, 635
intervertebral foramina narrowing 636
intervertebral osteochondrosis 634–5
juvenile rheumatoid arthritis 629, 630
Klippel–Feil syndrome 621, 622, 623
kyphosis 627
lateral bending 615
lordosis 612, 627
marginal ridges 608–9, 610
melorheostosis 639, 640
myositis ossificans 638–9
necrosis 628
neurocentral synchondrosis fusion 608
normal variants 615–20
notochord remnant persistence 624
nuchal ligament calcification 626, 639
ossification 610, 638–41
  foci 616
  paravertebral 631
ossification centers 608, 615, 624
  accessory 619
osteoblastic diathesis 635
osteochondrosis 634–5, 636, 637
osteomyelitis 628
osteosclerosis 632
Paget disease 639, 640
pediatric 608, 609, 624
pedicles 610, 611
piriform recess 611
platyspondyly 621
pseudodislocation 614, 627
pseudofractures 635, 637
pseudogaping 625
pseudospondylolisthesis 636
range of motion 614–15
retrolisthesis 636, 637
rheumatoid arthritis 629, 630, 636
rima glottidis 611, 612
rotation 615
scoliosis 636, 638
seronegative spondylarthropathies 629
spinal canal 612, 613
  stenosis 621–2, 623
spinal nerve groove 610, 611, 612, 613
spinous processes 611, 613
  accessory bone elements 620, 626
  ankylosing spondylitis 631
  anomalies 618, 619, 620
  avulsion fractures 626, 627
  chronic overuse injury 626, 629
  clefts 621, 622
  double 626, 627
  rheumatoid arthritis 631
  sharp tapering 629
spondylarthrosis 634, 635, 636
spondylitis 628, 629
spondylodiscitis 628
spondylolisthesis 621, 622
spondylophytes
  hyperostotic 635, 636
  marginal 634
  submarginal 635, 636
spondylosis deformans 635, 636
stepladder effect 614
sternocostoclavicular hyperostosis 629
subluxations 627–8, 629, 630
synostosis 628
syphilis 629
transverse processes 610, 611, 612
  accessory processes 616
  apophyses 609, 610, 616
  elongation 616
  persistent apophyses 616
  tubercles 616
trauma 636
tuberculous spondylitis 628
tumors 632–4
uncinate processes 610, 611
  accessory ossicles 615, 626
uncovertebral joints 610
  arthrosis 634, 635, 637

degenerative arthritis 624
  fractures 626
  vacuum phenomenon 634, 637
vertebra plana 621, 624, 628
  eosinophilic granuloma 633
vertebra prominens 611
vertebral arch
  clefts 621, 622, 623, 625, 626
  lateral dysplasia 621
vertebral artery
  compression 636
  elongation 601, 633
vertebral bodies 609, 612
  burst fractures 624
  clefts 622, 623
  compression fractures 624
  eosinophilic granuloma 633
  fusion 620, 621, 629
  persistent epiphyseal centers 615
  split fractures 624, 625
  teardrop fracture 624, 625
vertebral end plate
  erosion 631
  sclerosis 635
whiplash injuries 627
cervicothoracic junction 610, 614
  caudal/cranial variants 616
  transitional vertebrae 617
Chance fracture 659
cherubism 545
chest
  funnel 331, 333
  see also ribs; sternum
choanal atresia 512
choanal polyp 516
choanal stenosis 512
cholesteatoma
  labyrinthitis 486, 487
  middle ear 473, 474
  petrous bone 473
cholesterol cyst, petrous apex 489–90
chondral centers 560
chondroblastoma
  lumbar vertebrae 711
  navicular bone 1053
  patella 911
  proximal tibia 929, 930
chondrocalcinosis 71, 74, 75
  distal radius 198
  distal ulna 198
  elbow 234
  knee joint 949–50
  metacarpals 95, 100
  metacarpophalangeal 59, 62
  proximal phalanges (fingers) 91
  sacroiliac joint 758
  sesamoid bones 1091, 1092
  triquetrum 178
chondrocranium 358, 421
  see also skull base
chondrodysplasia
  metaphyseal 828, 829
  metaphyseal–epiphyseal of tibia/fibula 977, 980
chondrodysplasia punctata 8, 54
  carpal ossification centers 123, 130
  patella 905, 907
  segmentation anomalies 657
chondrodystrophia calcificans 721
chondroectodermal dysplasia 29
chondrolysis of femoral head 836
chondroma
  articular 220, 223
  cervical vertebrae 601
  hand 63
  proximal humerus 251, 252, 259
  ribs 351, 352
  triquetrum 176
chondromalacia
  lunate bone 165, 173
  patellae 883, 910
  ulna 190
chondromatosis
  articular 223, 230, 231–2
  hip 855–6
  os trigonum 1008
  knee joint 945
  shoulder joint 301, 304
  synovial 201, 230, 231–2, 552
  talocrural joint 986, 988
chondrosarcoma
  femoral shaft 868, 869
  larynx 498

lumbar vertebrae 711
proximal humerus 251, 259
ribs 351, 352
scapula 282–3
sternum 337
chordal canal, persistent 452–3, 655,
686
chordoma
cervical vertebrae 600, 633, 634
clivus 455
dorsum sellae 455
lumbar vertebrae 712
sacrococcygeal region 743–4
skull base 444
choroid plexus calcifications 381–2
CIC 127
CID 127
CIND 127
Citelli angle 466
clavicle 305–18
acro-osteolysis 289
aging 305, 306
anomalies 309
aseptic necrosis 311, 312
chronic recurring multifocal osteomyelitis 312, 313
complete absence 309
connection with coracoid process
271, 272
curvature 305, 306
dislocations 310–11
duplication 309
fractures 310
infantile cortical hyperostosis 312
inflammation 312–17
lateral hook 309
ligament attachments 306, 307, 308
medial epiphysis 309
necrosis 311–12
nerve canal defect 307
normal variants 309
nutrient canals 307, 314
ossification 305, 306
ossification center 305
osteitis condensans 311, 313, 314
osteolysis 289
osteomyelitis 313
Paget disease 313, 314
pseudotumors 317
regressive change 310, 311
subluxations 310–11
syphilis 313, 314
tumors 317
unilateral hyperplasia 309
see also sternoclavicular joint
clay shoveler's fracture 626, 627
cleft lip and palate 524
cleidocranial dysostosis 23, 389, 390
mandible anomaly 542
clinodactyly 24, 28, 29
phalanges (finger)
distal 77
middle 85, 87
clinoid processes
anterior 447, 448, 450, 506
air cells 449
pneumatization 532
medial 449, 450
pneumatization 534
clivus
angle 431
basilar processes 434, 435
chordoma 455
transverse basilar clefts 438, 439
clubbing, fingers 44, 80–1
thumb 91
clubfoot, congenital 1000–1
coarctation of aorta 348
coccidiomycosis, nasal cavity 516
coccygeal vertebrae 733, 734
coccygodynia 743, 745
coccyx 558, 731–46
agenesis 740
anatomy 733–6
anomalies 738, 740–1
dislocations 743
fractures 742–3
growth 731–3
ossification 733
osteomyelitis 743
sacral apex attachment 734
tumors 743–5
variants 736–8

cochlea 478, 484
cochlear aqueduct 478
cochlear ganglion 479
cochlear nerve 464
Cockayne syndrome 781
collagen disease
acro-osteolysis 57, 73
interstitial calcinosis 71
collateral ligament 943
lateral 944
medial 935, 944
complex carpal instabilities 127
computed tomography (CT) image
interpretation 2
concha bullosa 512, 531, 532
condylar angle 431, 432
condylar canal 424, 425, 427
condylar emissary vein 424, 427
condyle, tertiary 435, 437–8
condylopatellar sulcus, lateral 878
connective tissue diseases of sacroiliac joint 758
Conradi–Hünermann disease 53, 54
carpal ossification centers 123, 130
iliac wing hypoplasia 781
metacarpal necrosis 98
contour defects of phalanges (finger)
52, 57, 83
coracoacromial arch 272
coracoclavicular bursa 295
coracoclavicular joint 271, 272
coracoclavicular ligament 287
ossification 271, 272, 301
coracoid center, apical 263, 264
coracoid process 263, 264, 270, 271
accessory bones 279
apophyseal separation 280
connection with clavicle 271, 272
epiphyseal separation 280
fractures 277, 280
coracoid tubercle 307
coronal synostosis with plagiocephaly
506
coronoid fossa 220
coronoid process 218
persistent ossification center 218
costal arch 355
costal cartilage
calcification 354
chondritis-perichondritis 335
parasternal 335, 337
fusiform broadening 331, 332,
338
costochondral calcification 324
costoclavicular joint 309
costoclavicular ligament 306, 307,
308
costotransverse joints 341
coxa valga 809, 810, 826
coxa vara
congenital 826, 827
femoral neck fracture 833
coxitis 843, 844, 845
cranial fossae 365–6
anomalies 428–39
compensatory changes 429
growth 421
mass effects 429
normal variants 428–39
cranial index 367
cranial trabeculae 360
cranial vault 358–9, 363, 367–419
growth 367–8
measurement 368–74
sinus grooves 369
vascular grooves 369
craniocervical dysplasia 577
craniodiaphyseal dysplasia 38, 442,
443, 507
craniofacial dysostosis 392, 468, 506
craniolacunia 389
craniometaphyseal dysplasia 38, 442,
507
craniopharyngeal canal 446, 451
craniopharyngioma 455
craniosynostosis 390–2
craniovertebral developmental
anomalies 434–3
craniovertebral joints 558
osteoarthritis 601
range of motion 572
cranium bifidum occultum 387, 405,
410

crankshaft phenomenon 778
cretinism
carpal bone duplication 123
scaphoid fragmentary ossification
159
cricoarytenoid joint 497
cricoid cartilage 493
chondrosarcoma 498
cricothyroid joint 497
crista galli 532
Crohn disease
enteropathic spondylarthropathies
706
hypertrophic osteoarthropathy 45
osteomyelitis of sacrum/coccyx 743
sacroiliac joint 757
Cronqvist index 367, 375
Crouzon syndrome see craniofacial
dysostosis
cruciate ligament, anterior 941, 943–4
injury 878
cruciate ligament, posterior 941, 943,
944
cryptococcosis of nasal cavity 516
crystal synovitis 71
cubital fat pad sign 227, 228
cuboid bone 1055–9
accessory bones 1055–6, 1058
anatomy 1055
anomalies 1055–7
fractures 1057, 1058
inflammation 1058
necrosis 1057
notch 1055
ossification 1055
synostosis 1057
tumors 1057, 1059
variants 1055–7
cuboid sign 989, 992
cuneiform bone, intermediate 1061,
1066–8
accessory bones 1066–8
fractures 1067
ossification centers 1060, 1066
synostosis with lateral cuneiform
998, 1066
cuneiform bone, lateral 1066–8
fractures 1067
ossification centers 1066
synostosis with intermediate
cuneiform 998, 1066
uncinate process 1066
cuneiform bone, medial 1060–5
accessory bones 1062–4
anomalies 1064
aseptic necrosis 1065
bipartite 1062
bony prominence 1062
fractures 1064, 1065
joint gape 1061
ossification centers 1060–1
osteochondritis dissecans 1065
osteophytes 1065
variants 1062–4
Cupid's bow contour 678
cushion epiphysis 187, 188
cystic angiomatosis, tibial 959, 961
cystic fibrosis 528
cysticerci, calcified 874
cysts
congenital 745
primordial 527
sentinel 64
see also specific types of cysts

D

dactylitis, tuberculous 60
dactylolysis, spontaneous of toes 1102
delta phalanx 87
deltoid tendinitis, calcifying 243–4
demineralization, patchy periarticular
47–51
dens apex 432, 433
dental cysts 527
dental fractures 543
dentin 540
dermatomyositis 71
dermoid cysts
calvarium 399, 400
cerebellopontine angle 488
middle ear 476

nasal cavity 513
orbit 510
skull base 455, 456
diabetes mellitus, insulin-dependent
calcaneal fractures 1034, 1035
osteoarthropathy 1035
cuneiform bones 1067–8
metatarsal bones 1080–2
toes 1101
dialysis, long-term 71, 846
diaphyseal dysplasia 442, 443, 507
diaphysis see humerus, diaphysis
diastematomyelia
cervical spine 621
lumbar vertebrae 688, 689
thoracic spine 657, 658
diastrophic dysplasia 6
Dieterich disease 53, 54
metacarpal necrosis 98
diffuse idiopathic skeletal hyperostosis see DISH syndrome
digastric line 431
Dihlmann syndrome 714
diploe 364, 368
lacunae 370–1
nutrient canals 369, 370–1
vascular supply 441
diploic veins 370–1
diplomyelia, lumbar vertebrae 688
discitis, calcifying 640, 641, 668
lumbar spine 721
DISI 108
DISH syndrome 635, 636, 663–4, 719,
720, 722
osteophytes 950
pelvic ligament ossification 768
sacrotuberal/sacrospinal ligament
calcification 745, 746
dissociative carpal instabilities 127
dolichocephaly 368, 391, 392
Dorello's canal 449
Dorsal intercalated segmental instability 108
dorsum sellae 447, 448
chordoma 455
elongatum 452
fractures 537
ossification center 446
osteophytes 449
pneumatization 534
double-density sign 67
double spinous process sign 626, 627
Down syndrome
accessory epiphyses 96
atlantoaxial displacement 598
brachymesophalangia 85
clinodactyly 77
delta phalanges (finger) 26
frontal sinus 528
lumbar vertebral bodies 686
pseudoepiphyses 23, 24
suture abnormalities 389
drug addicts, sacroiliac joint 743, 753,
754
dura 366
dural sinuses 397
grooves 370, 392
pacchionian granulations 373
dwarfism/dwarfism syndrome
mandible 543
osteodysplastic primordial 8
dyskinetic cilia syndrome 528
dysmelia, supracondylar process 224
dysmesophalangia 24
dysostoses
cleidocranial 23
Parisian Nomenclature 12
dysostosis multiplex group 7
dysplasia
bent bone 8
bone density decrease/increase 9
congenita 7
craniodiaphyseal 38
craniometaphyseal 38, 442, 507
defective mineralization 9
diaphyseal 442, 443, 507
diastrophic 6
dystrophic with lumbar canal narrowing 698
fibrous 38, 39
frontal 507
frontometaphyseal 507
hand 36–8

hereditary 27
Kniest—Stickler 6
with membranous bone involvement 8
mixed sclerosing 38, 42, 43–4
multiple dislocations 8
multiple epiphyseal 53
osteofibrous of tibia 965, 967
spondylocostal of thoracic vertebrae 658
spondylometaphyseal 7
see also metaphyseal dysplasia; osteodysplasia
dysplasia epiphysealis hemimelica *see* Trevor disease
dystelephalangia *see* Kirner deformity

E

Eagle syndrome 495
ear 457, 459, 460–4
see also inner ear; middle ear
edema, transient 849, 850
Edgren—Vaino sign 666, 667, 668
elbow 210–36
accessory bones 220, 222
anomalies 217–26
apophyseal center 211, 229
bony fossa 214
calcification 234, 235
chondrocalcinosis 234
dislocation 227–9
epicondyles 211, 213, 218, 219, 220
ossifications 234, 235
epiphyseal center 211, 229
fractures 227–9
inflammation 234–6
loose bodies 232
myositis ossificans 235, 236
necrosis 229–32
normal variants 217–26
ossification centers 211–13, 229
multiple 227
osteochondritis dissecans 230, 231
osteoid osteoma 232, 233
osteonecrosis 230, 231
osteophytes 234, 235
osteopoikilosis 232, 233
radial tuberosity 214–15
subluxation 227–9
supinator fat line 227, 228
tumors 232–3
ulnar clubhand 205
Ellis—van Creveld syndrome *see* chondroectodermal dysplasia
Elsberg—Dyke sign 709, 710
emissary cells 465
emissary vein canals 371
EMO syndrome 44
empty sella 454, 455
enamel 540
encephalocele 410, 428
enchondral ossification disorders 123
enchondroma 91
femur
distal 883, 894, 895
shaft 868, 869, 871, 872
lumbar vertebrae 711
proximal humerus 258, 259, 260
ribs 351
toes 1103
enchondromatosis
femur 864, 865
neck 828
Madelung deformity 124
multiple 64, 65
proximal humerus 258
endochondral ossification of skull 358
endocrine disorders 34
endosteal hyperostosis 38, 40
femur 865
pelvis 773
van Buchem type 442
enostoma 67, 76, 91
enostoses 67
lumbar vertebrae 710
entrapment syndrome, calcaneal trochlea 1020
eosinophilic granuloma 283
calvarium 400
cervical spine 633
lumbar vertebrae 710, 712

mandible 547
thoracic vertebrae 662
ependymoma, sacral 745
epicondyle
humerus 220
inflammation 234, 235
ossification center 211, 213
persistence 218, 219
ossifications 234, 235
ulnar 220
traumatic displacement 227
epidermoid cysts 66
calvarium 399
cerebellopontine angle 488
middle ear 476
petrous bone 488
skull base 455, 456
epidural space 365
mastoiditis 473
epiphyseal dysplasia 7
multiple 53
tibia 921, 922
see also Trevor disease
epiphyses
accessory 96
cone-shaped 24–6
middle phalanges (finger) 85
toes 1096, 1097
hand 22, 23
ivory 52, 53, 76
slipped capital 834, 835–6
stippled 53, 54
very dense 26
white 80
Epipyramis 176
epitrapezium 157, 158
epulis, mandible 547
Erdheim—Chester lipoid granulomatosis 400
Erlenmeyer flask deformity 38, 864, 865
esophageal atresia 653
ethmoid bone 511
aplasia 533
fractures 533
mucocele 533–4
perpendicular plate 531
pyocele 533–4
ethmoid bulla 520, 521
ethmoid cells 520–1, 531–4
anomalies 533
ballooning 535
pneumatization 531–2
size change 533
tumor 534
variants 533
ethmoid labyrinth 518, 531–2
inflammation 533–4
Ewing sarcoma
femoral shaft 869
ilium 787
lumbar vertebrae 708, 712
ribs 351, 352
exophthalmos + myxedema pretibialis + osteopathy 44
external ear 459
eyebrow sign 808, 809
eyelid, conjunctival calcification 510

F

fabella 937, 940
osteoarthritis 940
facial canal 459, 482
facial nerve 457, 459, 464, 478–9
neurinoma 489
palsy 470, 487
petrous bone fracture 469
facial skeleton 363, 502–52
ethmoid cells 531–4
fibrous dysplasia 402–3
frontal sinus 528–31
mandible 539–47
maxillary sinus 519–27
nasal cavity 511–17
orbit 502–10
paranasal sinuses 517–19
sphenoid sinus 534–8
temporomandibular joint 548–52
zygomatic arch 538–47
Fairbank disease 53, 123
fallopian canal *see* facial canal

falx 382–3
Fanconi anemia 226
fat strip of subdeltoid bursa 294
feet *see* foot
femoral anteversion angle 820, 821
femoral head
anatomy 808, 809
aseptic necrosis 825
avascular necrosis 840, 841–3
chondrolysis 836
congenital dislocation of hip 825, 826
CT imaging 819
diaphyseal peak 804, 805
epiphysis persistence 823
fractures 830, 831
idiopathic osteonecrosis 840, 841–3
imaging 811
measurements 819–20
ossification center 804
osteochondritis dissecans 837, 840
percentage covered by acetabulum 819
Perthes disease 253, 256
rapidly destructive hip disease 852
villonodular synovitis 845
femoral neck
anatomy 808, 809
epiphysis persistence 823
femoral anteversion angle 820, 821
fractures 831, 832–3
stress 833
herniation pit 847, 848–9
Looser zones 834
metaphyseal chondrodysplasia 828, 829
neck—shaft angle 808, 809
ossification center 804
physiological articular eminence 850, 851
trabecular structure blurring 849, 850
tubercles 808, 810, 850, 851
valgus deformity 865
villonodular synovitis 845
Wiberg sign 851
femoral notch sign, lateral 878
femur 804, 860–98
acquired deformities 864
anatomy 860, 861
bone marrow infarction 871, 881, 882, 883
cartilaginous multiple exostosis 864, 865
center—collum—diaphyseal angle 819–20
coat-hook exostosis 879, 880
condyles 877, 878
medial 878, 879, 885, 887
spontaneous osteonecrosis 885, 887
congenital deformities 864
density increase 871
diaphysis ossification 860
distal 875–98
anatomy 861, 877
anomalies 879–80
bone marrow infarction 880, 881, 882, 883
bone resorption at gastrocnemius head attachment 889, 890, 891–2
calcification 895, 897, 898
cortical irregularities 888–9
epiphysis 875, 876, 877, 879, 880
fatty replacement 894, 896
fibrous metaphyseal defects 890–1, 893–4
fractures 880, 881
growth plates 875
inflammation 887, 888
melorheostosis 895
metaphyseal—epiphyseal fractures 880, 881
metaphysis 875, 876, 879
multiple densities 895, 896
necrosis 880, 881, 882, 883–7
ossification 875, 876
osteochondritis dissecans 883, 884–5, 886
osteomyelitis 887, 888, 889
osteopathia striata 895
osteopenia 894

osteopoikilosis 895, 896
osteoporosis 894, 895, 897, 898
osteosarcoma 889
popliteal surface 879
tumors 888–95
variants 879–80
enchondromatosis 864, 865
endosteal hyperostosis 865
Erlenmeyer flask deformity 38, 864, 865
fibrous dysplasia 864, 866
fractures 868
pediatric 880
stress 866, 868
Gaucher disease 865
hyperostosis 871, 872
hypoplasia 863–4
Paget disease 864, 866–7
popliteal surface 879
proximal
fractures 833
measurements 819–20, 821
osteoporosis 833
stress fractures 833, 834
shaft 860–76
anomalies 863–7
Ewing sarcoma 869
fractures 868
hyperparathyroidism 868, 869
inflammation 868–71
linea aspera 860, 863, 871
necrosis 868
nutrient canals 860, 862, 863
osteomalacia 868, 869
osteomyelitis 868, 869
osteoporosis 869
permeative destruction 869, 870
productive cortical changes 871
scalloping 868, 869
transformation processes 869, 870
tumors 868–71
variants 861, 863
slipped capital epiphysis 834, 835–6
trochlear dysplasia 878–9
trochlear groove 878
varus angulation 865
see also femoral head; femoral neck
femur—fibula—ulna complex 863–4
fibro-ostosis
calcaneal 1038, 1039
ilium 788
navicular bone 1054
pubic symphysis 801
fibrocartilaginous dysplasia 922, 923
fibrolipoma of calvarium 403, 404
fibrolipomatous hamartoma 34
fibrolipomatous nerve enlargement 34
fibroma, nonossifying
distal femur 890–1, 893–4
tibia 965, 966
proximal 929, 933
fibromatosis, juvenile 545
fibrous dysplasia 38, 39
calvarium 402–3
cervical vertebrae 601, 633, 634
clavicle 317
facial bones 402–3
femur 864, 866
hand 38
lumbar vertebrae 708, 711
mandible 545
maxillary sinus 527
ribs 353
skull base 443, 444
temporal bone 475
tibia 966, 968
fibrous metaphyseal defects
distal femur 890–1, 893–4
fibula 930, 934
tibia 986, 987
proximal 929, 933
shaft 958
fibula
acute plastic bowing 961
anomalies 958–61
articular surface 918, 920
dislocation 925, 926, 980–6
distal 971–88
anatomy 973–4
inflammation 986

ossification center 971–2
elongation 958–9
fibrous metaphyseal defects 930, 934
fractures 925, 961–5, 980–6
head 925, 926, 935, 936
hypoplastic 959
metaphyseal–epiphyseal chondrodysplasia 977, 980
notch 973
nutrient canals 953, 954–7, 961, 962, 964
ossicle 971, 972
osteomyelitis 986
persistent apophyses 921
proximal 914–36
epiphysis 915, 921
ossification 935, 936
villonodular synovitis 935
pustulotic arthro-osteitis 959, 966, 970
shaft 953–70
anatomy 953, 954–7
ossification centers 953
subluxation 925, 926, 980–6
synostosis 958
tumors 986, 987
variants 921, 958–61, 975–80
fibulotalar ligament
anterior 986
posterior 983
fingers
axial deviations 28–9
clubbing 44, 80–1
disproportionately long/short 34
see also clubbing, fingers; phalanges (finger)
fissula ante fenestrum 488
flatfoot deformity 998, 999, 1057
fluorosis 38, 709
pelvic ligament ossification 768
pelvis 773
fontanelles 359, 364, 368
glabellar 405
mastoid 411
metopic 405
sphenoidal 411
fonticular bones 369
foot 989–1103
accessory bones 993–6, 999
anatomy 989–93
anomalies 997–1001
arches 989, 990
bony injuries 997
calcaneus 1020–39
cuboid bone 1055–9
cuneiform bone
intermediate 1060, 1061, 1066–8
lateral 1066–8
medial 1060–5
deformities 999–1001, 1099, 1100
navicular bone 1011, 1032, 1033, 1041–54
proliferative changes 1102–3
shaggy 1054
talus 1002–19
toes 1094–103
variants 993–7
soft-tissue 1001
see also metatarsal bones; phalanges (toe); sesamoid bones; talocrural joint
foramen lacerum 423, 442
foramen magnum 359, 363
anomalies 438
clivus angle 431
line 432, 572, 573
os suboccipitale 592
foramen ovale 422–3
foramen rotundum 522
forearm
acute plastic bowing 204
anomalies 204–5
deformities 205
diaphysis 202–3
fractures 205
greenstick 204
inflammation 206–7
necrosis 206
normal variants 204–5
see also elbow; radius; radius, distal; ulna; ulna, distal
Forestier disease see DISH syndrome

foveolae granulares 365, 371, 373
fractures
atlas 592–5
axis 592–5
dens 586, 587, 594–5, 595
bone lucency 4
calcaneus 1031, 1033–4, 1035
calvarium 392–6
capitate bone 141, 142
carpus 125–9
cervical vertebrae (C1–C2) 592–5
cervical vertebrae (C3–C7) 624–7, 631
Chance 659
clavicle 310
coccyx 742–3
coracoid process 277, 280
cuboid bone 1057, 1058
cuneiform bone
intermediate 1067
lateral 1067
medial 1064, 1065
dental 543
diaphysis 242
dorsum sellae 537
elbow 227–9
ethmoid bone 533
femur 868
distal 880, 881
pediatric 880
stress 866, 868
fibula 925, 961–5, 980–6
forearm 204, 205
frontal sinus 530
Frykman classification 126, 196
glenoid fossa 550
hamate 144–7
hand 52
hangman 593–4
humerus 242
distal 227, 228
head 254
proximal 254, 255, 256
hyoid bone 497
ilium 781–4
ischium 796–7
Jones 1074, 1075, 1076
larynx 497
lesser trochanter 834
lumbar vertebrae 699, 710
lunate bone 166, 167–9
malleolus 980, 981, 982
mandible 543
mandibular condyle 550
manubriosternal synchondrosis 334
maxilla 525
maxillary sinus 524–5
metacarpals 97–8
metatarsal bones 1074–8
midfacial Le Fort classification 508, 509, 514, 533
nasal bone 514
navicular bone 1051, 1052
occipital bone 440–1
occipital condyles 440, 441
orbit 508–9
os peroneum 1056, 1057
palatoalveolar 524
patella 905, 908–9
petrous bone 469–70, 486
phalanges (finger)
distal 78–9
middle 87
proximal 90
ping-pong 393
pisiform 182–3
pubic symphysis 796–7
pubis 796–7
radius 205
distal 194–7
ribs 348–9
sacroiliac joint 751, 752, 767
sacrum 741–3, 767
scaphoid bone 152–8, 159, 160
scapula 276–80
sella turcica 453, 537
sesamoid bones 52, 93, 94, 1089–90
hallux valgus 1073, 1090
skull 392–6
base 440–1
sphenoid sinus 453, 537
sternum 334, 335
talus 1006, 1009, 1013–15

tarsometatarsal joints 1074
temporal bone 469, 470
temporomandibular joint 550, 551
thoracic spine 658–62
thumb 93
tibia 918, 919, 924–6, 961–5, 971, 980–6
toes 1101
trapezium 132–6
trapezoid 138–40
tripod 524–5
triquetrum 174–9
ulna 205
distal 177, 194–7
head 197
uncovertebral joints 626
zygomatic arch 538
zygomaticomaxillary 524–5
Franceschetti–Zwahlen syndrome 542
Freiberg disease 1079–80
Friedrich disease 311, 312
frontal bone 405–7
dysplasia 507
ossification 405
osteomyelitis 442
frontal emissary vein 405, 407
frontal notch 502
frontal sinus 518, 528–31
anomalies 528, 530
cerebral hemiatrophy 530
development 528
fractures 530
hyperpneumatization 530
inflammation 530
mucocele 530
normal variants 528, 529
osteoma 511
osteomyelitis 531
pneumosinus dilatans 528, 529
polypous densities 531
pyocele 530
septa 528, 529
supraorbital recess 528
tumor 531
frontal sinusitis 530
frontal squama 528, 529
frontal suture, premature closure 405
frontoethmoid, cephalocele 508
frontometaphyseal dysplasia 507
frontonasal suture 405, 406
frostbite 80
hand 54, 55
fungal infections
intraspinal abscesses 599
nasal cavity 515–16
funnel chest 331, 333

G

Galeazzi fracture–dislocation 126, 205
Gamut lists 5
ganglion cyst, shoulder joint 283, 284
gastrocnemius muscle, bone resorption at attachment of heads 889, 890, 891–2
Gaucher disease 545
femur 865
lumbar vertebrae 678
genu valgum 915
genu varum 915
giant cell granuloma, reparative 66
giant cell tumor 64, 91
cervical spine 633
lumbar vertebrae 711
patella 911
proximal humerus 251, 259
proximal tibia 929, 930
ribs 352
sacrum 744
gigantism 34
Gilula lines 127
glenohumeral joint
capsule openings 296
dislocation 297, 298
osteoarthritis 299
glenohumeral ligament 292, 293, 295
glenoid
dysplasia 274, 276
humeral head relationship 248
labrum 292, 293, 295

osteochondritis dissecans 281
glenoid cavity 262, 263
glenoid fossa 548
fractures 550
glenoid rim, posterior 274, 275
globe
calcification 507
posterior margin 519
glomus tumors 66
carotid canals 444
coccyx 745
distal phalanges (finger) 84
middle ear 475–6
gout 64
achillobursitis defect 1038
cervical spine 629
interphalangeal joint 1083
metatarsal bones 1082, 1083
navicular bone 1054
patella 911
pseudotumorous 66
temporomandibular joint 551
gracilis syndrome 798, 801, 802
gracilis tubercles 794, 801
Gradenigo syndrome 471–2
gray cortex 5, 21
Grisel syndrome 598
groin crease 810
ground-glass phenomenon 47
Gruber ossicle 141
guitar-player's fingers 82

H

habenular calcification 381
Haglund groove 905
Haglund heel 1038
Hahn cleft 645, 649, 675
remnants 675, 677
Haller cells 520–1
hallux abductus interphalangeus 1099
hallux rigidus 1073, 1074
hallux valgus 1073
deformity 3
sesamoid dislocation 1093
sesamoid fractures 1073, 1090
hallux varus, congenital 1074
hamate 144–8
aneurysmal bone cyst 148
coalition with capitate 140, 144
fractures 144–7
hook 144, 145, 146
hamatolunate impaction syndrome 165
hand 16–104
anomalies 22–51
bone density increase 38, 39
cyst-like lucencies 64
degenerative changes 69–70
dysplastic structural changes 36–8
epiphyseal plates 23
epiphyses 22, 23
Fanconi anemia 226
fibrous dysplasia 38, 39
fractures 52
frostbite 54, 55
gigantism 34
hyperostosis 38, 39
joint inflammation 57–9, 60, 61–2
linear lucencies 21–2
metacarpus 16–75
normal radiographic appearance 16, 18–19
normal variants 22–51
ossification 16, 17
phalanges 16–75
polydactyly 29–34
proliferative changes 1102–3
pseudoepiphyses 23–4
radiographic technique 91
sarcoidosis 40, 41, 42
skeletal malformations 22–51
soft-tissue calcification 71–5
syndactyly 28
tumors 63–9
see also clubbing, fingers; fingers; phalanges (finger)
Hand–Schüller–Christian disease 400
Harris lines 958, 962, 973
Hart syndrome 507

Haversian canals 21
head, flexion–extension 572, 573
hemangioma
  calvarium 400, 401
  cavernous 510
  cervical vertebrae 633
  knee joint 946
  lumbar vertebrae 707, 711–12
  mandible 546
  nasal cavity 516
hemangiomatosis
  Gorham–Stout 546
  lumbar vertebrae 712
  mandible 546
hematoma
  calcified 725
  subperiosteal of femoral shaft 871
hemifacial–microsomia syndrome
  468, 542
hemimetameric segmentation
  anomaly 656
hemivertebrae
  cervical 622, 624
  sacral 740
hemochromatosis 71
  intervertebral disk calcification 639
  metacarpals 100, 102
hemodialysis 66
  cervical spine 629
  interstitial calcinosis 772
  β2-microglobulin amyloid deposits
    131
hemophilia
  distal femoral epiphysis 879, 880
  periarticular epiphysis deformity
    225, 226
  tibiotalar tilt 979
hemopoietic hyperplasia of ribs 352
hemosiderosis 71
hemotympanum 470
hereditary optic atrophy 507
herniation pit 846, 847, 848–9
herpes zoster oticus 487
heterotopic ossification see myositis
  ossificans
Hill–Sachs lesion 254, 255, 297, 298
hindfoot coalition 997–8
hip joint 804–56
  acetabular angle 816
  anatomy 806–15
  Andrén view 815, 816
  anomalies 824–9
    syndrome association 828
  articular chondromatosis 855–6
  beta angle of Zsernaviczky and Türk
    816, 817
  calcific bursitis 852–4
  calcification of ligaments/bursae/
    tendon sheaths 852–4
  capsular structures 810
  congenital dislocation 825, 826
  decentering sign 851
  dislocation 825, 826, 829–36
    traumatic 830, 831–3
  dysplasia 813
    adults 825, 826, 827–8
  femur–iliac angle of Grossman 817
  fractures 829–36
  herniation pit 846, 847, 848–9
  Hilgrenreiner line 815, 816
  inflammation 843–4
  irritable 843, 844
  Kopits parallelogram 816, 817
  linear lucencies 810, 811
  loose bodies 855, 856
  measurements
    after puberty 817–18
    children 815–17
  Ménard–Shanton line 816
  β2-microglobulin arthropathy 846
  myositis ossificans 852
  necrosis 836–43
  Ombrédanne line 815, 816
  osteoarthritis 809, 850–1
  osteonecrosis
    adults 839–43
    children/adolescents 836–9
  Perthes disease 837–9
  plaque sign 850, 851
  rapidly destructive disease 852
  space width 810
  subluxation 825, 826, 829–36
  transient edema 849, 850

transient osteoporosis 843, 849–50
Trevor disease 855–6
tumors 845–9
variants 821–4
Wiberg sign 851
see also acetabulum; femoral head;
  femoral neck
Hirschsprung disease 653
histoplasmosis, nasal cavity 516
Holt–Oram syndrome 26
  forearm 204
  lateral clavicle hook 309
  os centrale carpi 157
housemaid's knee 950
humeral notch, upper 238, 258
humeroradial joint 215, 217
humeroscapular periarthritis 299
humeroulnar joint 215
humerus
  deltoid tuberosity 239–40, 241
  diaphysis 238–44
    fracture 242
    inflammation 242, 243
    longitudinally bracketed 26
    nutrient canal 239
    soft-tissue calcifications 242,
      243–4
    tumors 242
  distal
    fractures 227, 228
    lateral border 217
    shape 215, 216
  endosteal cortical notch 239, 242
  epicondyle 220
  greater tuberosity 4
  head 245
    avascular necrosis 253, 256
    deformity 253
    fractures 254
    glenoid relationship 248
    metaphyseal calcifications 248
    necrosis 253, 254, 256–8, 303
    osteoarthritis 258
    osteochondritis dissecans 258
    radiographic morphology 245,
      249
    retroversion 254
    syringomyelia 254, 258
    trabecular architecture 250
  hypoplasia of trochlea 225
  lucencies 239, 241
  medial epicondyle 217
  metaphyseal cortical irregularities
    238
  nutrient canals 242
  osteomyelitis 243
  proximal 245–60
    anomalies 253–4
    bone marrow necrosis 248, 258
    cortical irregularities 258, 259
    fracture patterns 254, 255, 256
    fracture–dislocations 256
    greater tuberosity 245, 248, 249,
      256
    growth plate 245, 246–7
    inflammation 249, 259
    intertubercular sulcus 249
    juvenile bone cysts 259
    lesser tuberosity 245, 248, 249,
      256
    lucent area 250–1, 258
    necrosis 253, 258
    Neer classification for fractures
      254, 256
    normal variants 253–4
    ossification center 245
    osteolysis 251
    rarefaction area 250–1, 258
    shape 254
    tumors 251–2, 258–9, 260
  proximal diaphyseal–metaphyseal
    junction 238
  structural irregularities 240, 241
  surface anatomy 239–40, 241
  trauma 242
  varus 253
    congenital 253, 254
hyoid bone 490–8
  anatomy 492, 493
  calcification 491
  development 490–1
  fractures 497
  greater cornu 496, 497

lesser cornu 492, 493
  necrosis 497
hyperlordosis
  axis dens 587, 588
  lumbar vertebrae 719
hypermobility syndrome 596
hyperostosis
  calvaria diffusa 378
  frontalis interna 20, 378, 379
  hand 38, 39
  infantile cortical 542–3
  multiple 759
  triangularis ilii 785, 786
hyperparathyroidism 20, 71
  acro-osteolysis 81, 88
  bone mineral density loss 47, 48
  bone resorption 208
  brown tumors 64, 65, 88
  calvarium 376, 378, 405
  femoral shaft changes 868, 869
  intervertebral disk calcification 639
  mandible 547
  middle phalanges (finger) 88
  sacroiliac joint 758
  secondary 48
hypertelorism 391–2, 506
hyperthyroidism 78
hypervitaminosis A 603
hypervitaminosis D 772
  dense distal femoral metaphyses
    879
hypochondroplasia 698
hypoglossal canal 424, 425, 426
  subdivision 435
hypoglossal nerve foramen 423–4,
  425, 426
hypoparathyroidism 879
hypophosphatasia 390
hypoplasia, hereditary 27
hypothyroidism 828
  accessory epiphyses 96
  congenital osteopenia 47
  dense distal femoral metaphyses
    879
  pseudoepiphyses 23
  sella turcica 453
hypotonia 686

I

iliac crest 778
  spiny contour 780
iliac horns 780–1
iliac spine
  anterior inferior 778–9
  avulsion fractures 781, 782, 783
iliac wing hypoplasia 781
ilioischial plate 813
iliolumbar ligament
  calcification 725, 758, 759
  ossification 722, 759, 770
ilium 778–88
  acetabula 780
  anomalies 780–1
  apophyses 778
  fibro-ostosis 788
  fractures 781–4
  growth 778–80
  hyperostosis triangularis ilii 785,
    786
  inflammation 785–6
  insufficiency fractures 782, 784
  intraosseous pneumocysts 787
  Looser zones 775, 782, 784
  melorheostosis 785
  necrosis 785
  normal variants 780–1
  nutrient canal 779, 780, 782, 784
  ossification center 778
  osteomalacia 782, 784
  osteoporosis 784
  Paget disease 786
  paraglenoid sulcus 781
  preauricular notch 781
  pseudotumors 787
  radiation necrosis 785
  reactive sclerosis 776, 785
  tumors 787
impingement syndrome 245
  calcaneal trochlea 1020
  rotator cuff 272, 276, 296–7
  shoulder dislocation differential di-
    agnosis 299

supraspinatus 278
inca bone 365
incisive canal 513
incus 457
infantile cortical hyperostosis of
  clavicle 312
inflammation
  bone 59–60, 63
  joint 57–9, 60, 61–2
infraorbital canal 506
infraorbital foramen 502, 505, 506
infraorbital recess 519
inner ear 457, 459–64, 477–90
  aplasia 484
  dysplasia 485
  malformations 484
  vestibule 478
innominate line 502
intercalary bones 364–5, 369
intermetatarsal region 1069
  soft-tissue calcification 1084, 1085
  spaces 1070
International Classification of Osteochondrodysplasia (1992) 5,
  6–10
interparietal bone 414, 415, 421
interphalangeal joint
  aplasia 27–8
  dislocation 1090
  distal 76, 77
  gout 1083
  hypoplasia 27–8
  proximal 79
intersphenoidal synchondrosis 446, 451
intervertebral disks 558
  calcification 639–41
    lumbar vertebrae 720–2, 723, 724
    sacrococcygeal region 745
  cervical vertebrae (C3–C7)
    calcification 639–41
    spaces 612, 635
  lumbar vertebrae
    calcification 720–2, 722, 723, 724
    height 701, 710
    narrowing 700
    ossification 722
    space 674
  sacral vertebrae 732–3
  sacrococcygeal 745
  spaces
    in cervical spine 612, 635
    in sacrum 732
intervertebral foramen 558
intracranial hemorrhage, calcification
  385, 386
intracranial pressure 429
  orbital tumors 510
  skull base tumors 442
intraosseous ganglion 66, 67
  see also synovial cyst, subchondral
intrasegmental gaps 559
intrauterine lie, abnormal 410
ischiopubic osteochondrosis 798
ischiopubic plate 813
ischiopubic synchondrosis 789
  anomalies 791, 792–4
  persistent open 794, 796
  pseudotumors 801
  variants 791, 792–4
ischium 789–803
  anomalies 791, 794–5
  apophyses 790
    atypias 798, 799
  bony processes 794
  calcific bursitis 803
  fractures 796–7
  inflammation 799, 801
  melorheostosis 801, 802
  multicentric bony elements 791, 794
  ossification centers 790
  osteomalacia 797
  soft tissue calcification 803
  traumatic apophysiolysis 796
  tumors 801, 802
  unilateral hypoplasia 795
  variants 791, 794–5

J

Jaffe–Lichtenstein disease see fibrous
  dysplasia
joints
  erosion in hand 57, 58

inflammation 57–9, 60, 61–2
Jones fracture 1074, 1075, 1076
jugular bulb, high 465, 466, 467, 468, 484
jugular tubercles 444
jugum sphenoidale 445
junction cells 536, 537

K

Kager triangle 1001, 1034
Kartagener syndrome 528
Kashin–Beck disease 54, 56, 80
  metacarpal necrosis 98
  wrist 130
keratoderma, mutilating palmoplantar 81
Kerckring process 435, 437
Kienböck disease see lunate bone, necrosis
Kirner deformity 77, 78
Klaus height index 432
Klein sign 834, 835
Klinefelter syndrome 47
Klippel–Feil syndrome
  cervical spine 621, 622, 623, 629
  lumbar canal narrowing 698
  split atlas 579
  Sprengel deformity 274
  thoracic spine 657
knee joint 900, 901, 937–51
  anatomy 937–40
  arthritic change 951
  Baker cyst 945
  bursae 950
  chondrocalcinosis 949–50
  chronic anterior pain 908, 916, 921
  fabella 937, 940
  fracture–dislocations 924–5
  gender differences 937
  increased traction phenomena 950–1
  infrapatellar fat pad 950
  ligaments 943–4
  masses 945–8
  melorheostosis 947, 948
  meniscal cysts 942, 943
  meniscal ossicle 942–3
  menisci 937–8, 940–3
    calcification 949
    degenerative changes 940–4
    discoid 942, 943
    tears 941, 942
    Wrisberg type 942
  normal 878
  osteoarthritis 950, 951
  osteonecrosis 885, 887
  osteophytes 950, 951
  pain
    meniscal ossicle 942–3
    nonspecific in child 4
  pseudogout 949
  rheumatoid arthritis 951
  soft-tissue calcifications 949–50
  synovial joint capsule 944
  synovial plicae 944
  transient cortical irregularity 4
  trauma 919, 949
  tumors 945, 948
  vacuum phenomenon 937, 939
  valgus deformity 935
  villonodular synovitis 945, 946, 947
Kniest–Stickler dysplasia 6
Knutsson sign 665
Köhler disease 1051, 1053
Köhler II disease 1079–80
Köhler–Stieda–Pellegrini shadows 895, 898
Kosowicz method for metacarpal length 17, 20, 96
Kümmel–Verneuil disease 628, 662, 710
kyphosis
  cervical vertebrae (C3-C7) 627
  thoracic vertebrae 651, 652, 656, 663, 664, 666

L

labyrinthine capsule 360
  anatomy 478–82
  aplasia 484
development 477
inflammation 486–7
ossification 478
vestibule 478, 479
labyrinthitis 486–7
  cholesteatoma 486, 487
  end-stage 487
  hematogenous 486, 487
  meningogenic 486–7
  ossificans 487
  posttraumatic 486, 487
  tympanogenic 486
lacrimal fossa 502
lacrimal gland calcification 510
Langerhans cell histiocytosis 283
  calvarium 397, 400, 547
  clavicle 317
  mandible 547
  petrous bone 489, 490
  ribs 354
  sella turcica 454
large vestibular aqueduct syndrome 485
Larssen syndrome 598
larynx 490–8
  air 625
  development 490–1
  fractures 497
  inflammation 497
  necrosis 497
  polychondritis 497
  tuberculosis 497
  tumors 498
lead poisoning, dense distal femoral metaphyses 879
Leber disease 507
Legg–Calvé–Perthes disease see Perthes disease
lens calcification 507, 510
leprosy, acro-osteolysis 82
leptomeninges 366
Leri–Weill syndrome 124
leukemia 879
ligamentum flavum ossification 680
limbus vertebra 717
linea aspera 4
  femoral shaft 871
linear lucencies, hand 21–2
lipoid proteinosis 453
lipoma
  calcaneus 1035, 1037
  lumbar vertebrae 712
  nasal cavity 516
longitudinal ligament
  anterior 635, 636, 664
  posterior 631, 638, 664, 666, 722
longus colli muscle, calcifying tendinitis 603, 604
Looser zones 205
  femoral neck 834
  ilium 775, 782, 784
  lesser trochanter 834
  pubis 796
  scapula 280
  tibia 926
lordosis
  cervical vertebrae (C3-C7) 612, 627
  see also hyperlordosis
lower extremity see femur; fibula; foot; patella; talocrural joint; tibia
Ludloff's fleck 876, 877
lumbar ribs 653, 654, 673, 680–1
  pelvic digit differential diagnosis 770
lumbar sympathetic blockade 700
lumbar vertebrae 558, 671–725
  accessory processes 672, 680
  accessory ribs 680–1
  anatomy 671–2, 673–6
  ankylosing spondylitis 702
  anomalies 684–99
    congenital 679
  apophyseal joints 671–2
    ankylosing spondylitis 702, 704
    asymmetry 708
    malalignment 697
    spaces 673, 675
  articular processes 672
    accessory ossicles 680, 683
    aplasia 697, 698, 708
    clefts 680, 693
    duplicated superior 680
dysplasia 697
frictional sclerosis 718, 719
hypoplasia 697, 708
notches 680, 683
persistence of apophyses 680
biconvex 687
blocking 685, 701–2, 723
bone-in-bone appearance 675
bony exostoses 680, 681
brucellosis 702
calcification 720–5
cartilaginous exostoses 680, 681
chordal canal
  narrowing 697–8, 699
  persistent 655, 686
coronal cleft 684–6
costal processes 672, 673
  bony bridges 678, 679
costotransverse foramina 679
costovertebral joints 702
degenerative changes 713–25
diastematomyelia 688, 689
diplomyelia 688
dislocation 699
dysraphism 688
enostosis 710
eosinophilic granuloma 710, 712
epiphyseal ring 675
fibrous dysplasia 708, 711
fifth 672
fish vertebrae 661
flexion–extension 677
foraminal spur 680
fractures 699
  pathological 710
gouty osteoarthropathy 702
growth 672–3
  recovery lines 675
hematogenous infection 700
hemispheric spondylosclerosis 714
hemivertebrae 685
hyperlordosis 719
inflammation 700–6
interspinous distance narrowing 718–19
intervertebral bony bars 680
intervertebral disks
  calcification 720–2, 722, 723, 724
  height 701, 710
  narrowing 700
  ossification 722
  space 674
intervertebral foramina 674, 675
joint space asymmetries 694, 697
lateral bending 677
limbus vertebra 717
lumbar ribs 673
meningocele 688
metastases 709, 710
multiple myeloma 709, 712
myelomeningocele 688
necrosis 700
neurocentral synchondrosis 672
normal variants 677–84
origin of segments 561
ossification 720–5
osteochondrosis 701, 713–14, 724
osteomyelitis 702
osteopetrosis 707
osteophytes 704
osteoporosis 709
Paget disease 708, 709
paravertebral calcification 722, 725
paravertebral ossification 704–6
pedicles 671
  destruction 709, 710
persistent apophyses 699
posture 676–7, 720
promontory angle 676
pseudoretrolisthesis 675
pseudospondylolisthesis 694, 695, 696, 715–16
pseudospondylolysis 675, 692
psoriatic arthritis 704, 705
rachischisis 688
range of motion 676–7
renal osteodystrophy 707
rheumatoid arthritis 702
riblike processes 679
ribs 653, 654
rotatory slippage 720
salmonellosis 702
sarcoidosis 708
Scheuermann disease 710, 716
Schmorl nodes 716–17
scoliosis 688, 710, 720, 725
scotty dog sign of Lachapel 676, 691–2
segmental instability 696
seronegative spondylarthritis 702
spina bifida 688, 689, 708
spinal canal width 673–4
spinous processes 674
  ankylosing spondylitis 702
  apophyses 673
spondylarthrosis deformans 714–15
spondylitis 701–6
spondylodiscitis 700–1, 710
spondylolisthesis 691, 694–6
spondylolysis 680, 683, 690–1, 692, 693, 694
  vertebral arch sclerosis 708
spondyloretrolisthesis 694, 715, 716
styloid process 680
subluxation 699
supernumerary ossicles 680, 682
transverse processes 675
  costotransverse foramina 679
trauma 678, 679
tuberculosis 700, 702
tuberous sclerosis 708
tumors 706–12
underdevelopment 686
vacuum phenomenon 710, 714, 715
vertebra plana 710, 712
vertebral arches 674
  ankylosing spondylitis 702
  anomalies 687–90
  clefts 688–90, 691
  dysplasia 683, 692, 693, 694, 697
  pars interarticularis 690, 691
vertebral bodies 674, 675
  Andersson lesions 702
  anomalies 684–7
  cortical thickening 709
  Cupid's bow contour 678
  end plate concavity 678
  end plate thinning 700, 701
  enlargement 710
  Hahn cleft 675, 677
  height variation 686, 709, 723
  malignant collapse 710
  notches 678
  notochordal remnants 686
  osteosclerosis 706
  persistent apophyses 677, 678
  scalloping 687, 688, 710
  sclerosis 701–2, 706–9
  vertical trabeculation 709
lumbosacral angle 676
lumbosacral junction 676
  assimilation tendency 681, 683
  lumbarization 681, 684
  sacralization 681, 684
  transitional vertebrae 681, 683, 684
  variants 680–1, 683–4
lunate bone 164–73
  anomalies 165–6
  aplasia 150
  bipartite 164
  calcification 169
  chondromalacia 165, 173
  dislocations 167–9
  enlarged bulky 30
  fractures 166, 167–9
  fusion with triquetrum 174
  inflammation 173
  necrosis 169–73
    radiological stages 170, 171
    regression 171
  normal variants 165–6
  nutrient canals 164
  ossification center 164
  osteonecrosis 164
  separate articulation with hamate bone 165
  separate joint facet 144
  subchondral changes 173
  tumors 173
  ulnar impaction syndrome 191
lunatomalacia see lunate bone, necrosis
lunotriquetral dissociation 129
lunotriquetral fusion 122, 165
lymphangioma, lumbar vertebrae 712
lymphangiomatosis, lumbar vertebrae 712

lymphoma
  hair-on-end appearance 380
  ilium 787
  lumbar vertebrae 708, 712
  orbit 510
  proximal tibia 930, 934
  ribs 351, 352
  white tibial epiphysis 928

M

Mach band phenomenon 2, 4, 79, 202
  dens fractures 595
  femoral fractures 880
  hip osteoarthritis 850
  lumbar vertebrae 675
  ribs 348, 349
  scapula 276
macrocephaly 375
macrocranium 375
macrodactylia lipomatosa 34
Madelung deformity 37, 124, 125
  lunate 165, 169
  negative ulnar variance 190
  pseudo-Madelung deformity differ-
    ential diagnosis 194
magnetic resonance imaging (MRI)
  bony element on end of acromion 3
  normal variants 2
malignant fibrous histiocytoma 712
malleolus
  accessory elements 975, 978
  apophysis 972
  fossa 977
  fractures 980, 981, 982
  ossification 975, 976
  ossification centers 971, 972
mallet finger 78–9
malleus 457
malum suboccipitale 598
mamillary process 680
  anomalous development 653
mandible 360–1, 539–47
  alveolar crest atrophy 539
  alveolar process fracture 543
  anatomy 540
  anomalies 541–3
  bite abnormalities 550
  coronoid process widening 547
  development 539
  duplication of condylar process 549
  dwarfism syndrome 543
  eosinophilic granuloma 547
  fibrous dysplasia 545
  follicular cyst 546
  fractures 543
  hypoplasia 542, 549
  inflammation 544–5
  juvenile fibromatosis 545
  melorheostosis 545
  necrosis 544
  normal variants 541–3
  nutrient canals 541
  odontoma 546
  osteitis 544, 545
  osteoma 546–7, 550
  osteomyelitis 544, 545
  osteopetrosis 543, 545
  Paget disease 545
  rickets 547
  tumor 545–7
mandibular canal 540
  bifid 541
mandibular condyle 548
  articular disk displacement 550
  fractures 550
  hyperplasia 552
  hypoplasia 549
  osteophytes 552
mandibular tori 546–7
mandibulofacial dysostosis 468, 542
manubrioclavicular joint
  bacterial arthritis 313
  osteoarthritis 311
manubriosternal synchondrosis 324,
    329
  accessory bone elements 330
  arthritis 335, 336
  degenerative changes 338
  fracture 334
  inflammation 335–6
  necrosis 334

osteophytes 338
physiological sclerosis 338
manubrium 321–2
  examination techniques 323–6
  ossification centers 320
  Srb anomaly 343, 345
marble bone disease see osteopetrosis
Marfan syndrome
  arachnodactyly 34
  frontal sinus 528
  funnel chest 331
marginal cells 465
Maroteaux—Lamy syndrome 543
mastoid emissary vein 467
mastoid process 457, 464
  avulsion 470
  pneumatization 464, 465
  see also air cells
mastoiditis 471, 473
maxilla 360–1
  alveolar recess 522
  fractures 525
  hypoplasia 506
maxillary antrum 521
maxillary sinus 518, 519–27
  air cells 520–1
  anomalies 524
  chronic inflammatory processes
    527
  development 519
  fibrous dysplasia 527
  fractures 524–5
  hypoplasia 523
  inflammation 525–7
  mucocele 526
  mucormycosis 515
  normal variants 523–4
  ostium 521
  polyps 526
  pyocele 526
  reactive sclerosis 527
  septa 523
  tumors 527
  Wegener granulomatosis 515, 527
maxillary sinusitis 525–6
maxillonasal dysplasia 524
McGregor line 431
McRae line 432
Meckel cartilage 360
melorheostosis 44
  cervical spine 639, 640
  distal femur 895
  femoral shaft 871, 872
  ilium 785
  ischium 801, 802
  knee joint 947, 948
  mandible 545
  metatarsal bones 1078, 1084
  proximal tibia 934
  ribs 350, 351
  tibia 959, 960
Ménière disease 485
meningeal artery, middle, groove 412,
    414
meningeal calcification 382
meningeal vessels 397
  grooves 370, 412, 414
meningioma 476
  cerebellopontine 488
  en plaque 388, 403, 404
  frontal sinus 531
  nasal cavity 516
  optic sheath 455, 510
  orbit 510
meningitis, tuberculous 384
meningo-orbital foramen 506
meningocele 428
  lumbar vertebrae 688
meningoencephalocele 387, 388, 474
  cerebellar 488
  nasal cavity 513
  orbit 508
  transsphenoidal 451
mental foramen 540, 541
mental spine 540, 541
mental tubercle 540
mermaid syndrome 740
mesomelic dysplasias 8
metacarpal sign 20
metacarpals 94–102
  anomalies 96–7
  calcium specks 21, 22
  chondrocalcinosis 95

exostoses 95
fractures 97–8
inflammation 100–2
necrosis 98–9
normal variants 96–7
nutrient canals 21, 95–6
pathological conditions 16, 20
shortening 38
tumors 100
metacarpus 16–75, 94–102
  adulthood 16–22
  growth 16
  ossification 16
metaphyseal dysplasia 38, 443, 507
  axial deviations 29
  brachyrachia 8
metaphyseal ring 187
metaphyses 23
metastases
  calvarium 373, 400, 402
  carcinoma in distal phalanx 84
  cervical vertebrae 601, 633
  clavicle 317
  femoral shaft 868, 869, 871
  hip joint 845
  ilium 787
  ischium 801
  lumbar vertebrae 708, 709, 710, 712
  mandible 547
  orbit 510
  ossification 52
  osteolytic 64, 400
  osteosclerotic 706
  patella 911
  pubis 801
  sacrum 745
  scaphoid bone 163
  sternum 338
metastyloid bone 138
metatarsal bones 1069–85
  accessory 1071–2
  adducted position 1069
  anatomy 1069–71
  brachymetatarsia 1073
  deformities 1073–4
  diabetic osteoarthropathy 1080–2
  dislocation 1074–8
  endosteal bone formation 1078
  epiphyseal centers 1069, 1071
  epiphyseal fusion 1069
  first
    dislocation 1074
    stress fractures 1077
  fourth
    calcaneocuboid coalition 1032,
      1033
    fractures 1077
    sagging of head 999
  fifth
    persistent apophysis of tuberos-
      ity 1072, 1076
    transverse fracture 1074, 1075,
      1076
    tuberosity 1069, 1070
  fractures 1074–8
    stress 1076, 1077–8
  gout 1082, 1083
  hallux valgus 1073
  hallux varus 1074
  hypertrophic osteoarthropathy
    1084
  inflammation 1082–3
  joint spaces 1070
  melorheostosis 1078, 1084
  nutrient canals 1071, 1078
  ossification centers 1069
  osteoarthritis 1080, 1082, 1083
  osteonecrosis 1079–82
  periosteal bone formation 1078,
    1082
  reflex sympathetic dystrophy 1084,
    1085
  Reiter syndrome 1082
  rheumatoid arthritis 1082, 1083
  second
    stress fractures 1077, 1078
    subluxation 1075, 1076
  sesamoid bony fusion 1088, 1089
  shortening 38
  subluxation 1074–8
  synostosis 33
  tarsal coalitions 999, 1073, 1099
  third 1076

tumors 1084
variants 1071–2
metatarsophalangeal joint
  dislocation 1100
  involution 1100
  pain 3–4
  rheumatoid arthritis 1082, 1083
  subluxation 1100
metatarsosesamoid articulations 1087
metatarsus primus varus 1073
metatarsus varus, congenital 1073
metatropic dysplasia 6
Michel deformity 484
microcephaly 375
microcranium 375
β_2-microglobulin deposits
  amyloid 64, 65
  hemodialysis 131
  hip joint 846
  scaphoid bone 65, 162
microphalangia 26
microsella 453
microtia 468
mid-subtalar joint coalition 998, 999
midcarpal instability 129
middle ear 457, 464–77
  cavity absence 468
  cholesteatoma 473, 474
  dermoids 476
  epidermoids 476
  glomus tumors 475–6
  inflammation 471–2
  malignancy 475
  mucosal changes 471
  mucosal tears 470
  septa 468
  tumors 476
midtarsal joint injuries 1051
Milwaukee shoulder 258
modiolus 478
Mondini malformation 484
Morgagni syndrome 20, 76
Morgagni—Stewart—Morel syndrome
    378
mucocele
  ethmoid bone 533–4
  frontal sinus 530
  maxillary sinus 526
  sphenoid sinus 455, 537
mucolipidosis 96
mucopolysaccharidosis 96, 124
  atlantoaxial displacement 598
  nasal bone congenital hypoplasia
    513
  short ulna 194
  type VI 543
mucormycosis
  calcification 517
  maxillary sinus 515
  nasal cavity 515, 517, 527
Müller sign 664, 666
multiple exostosis disease of femur
    864, 865
multiple myeloma
  lumbar vertebrae 709, 712
  sternum 337
  thoracic vertebrae 660
myeloma, lumbar vertebrae 708
myelomeningocele
  lumbar vertebrae 688
  thoracic spine 657
mylohyoid line 540
myositis ossificans 4, 301
  elbow 235, 236
  femoral shaft 873, 874
  hip joint 852
  lumbar vertebrae 678, 722, 725
  progressiva 639
  traumatica 638–9

N

nail—patella syndrome 225, 906, 907
  iliac horns 780–1
nails, watchglass 44
nasal alae 522
nasal bone
  congenital hypoplasia 513
  fractures 514
nasal cavity 511–17
  anomalies 512–13
  dermoid cysts 513

foreign body 512, 517
fungal infections 515–16
inflammation 514–16
meningoencephalocele 513
normal variants 512, 513
tumor 516–17
nasal polyposis 514, 526
nasal septum 511
deviation 511, 512, 513
necrosis 514
sarcoidosis 515
Wegener granulomatosis 515
nasal spine, avulsion fracture 514
nasal turbinates 511–12
bullous 512, 513
nasolacrimal duct 502
nasopalatine cyst 513
nasopharyngeal angiofibroma,
juvenile 516
navicular bone 1041–54
accessory bone 1041, 1044
anatomy 1041, 1043
anomalies 1049–50
aseptic necrosis 1051, 1053
bipartite 1049, 1050
cornuate 1041, 1045
deformity 1011
dislocation 1051
fibro-ostosis 1054
fractures 1051, 1052
gout 1054
hypertrophic 1041, 1045
inflammation 1053
nutrient canals 1041, 1043
ossification centers 1040–2
accessory 1041
variant 1041, 1053
osteoarthritis 1054
osteophytes 1054
prominent 1041, 1045
subluxation 1051
synostosis with calcaneus 1032,
1033
transverse partition 1049, 1050
tuberculosis 1053
tuberosity 1041, 1043, 1044, 1046
edema 1047
fractures 1047, 1051
tumor 1053
variants 1044–8
navicular fat stripe 152, 153
nebula frontalis 378, 379
necrosis
local 71
see also avascular necrosis;
osteonecrosis
necrotizing otitis externa see otitis,
externa maligna
necrotizing vasculitis, cocaine-
induced 514
neurinoma
acoustic 484, 489
cervical vertebrae 633, 634
facial nerve 489
lumbar vertebrae 712
multiple 489
trigeminal 442, 443, 489
zygomatic arch 539
neurocentral synchondroses 562
neurocranium 358, 364
neurocysticercosis 384–5
neurofibroma
lumbar vertebrae 712
nasal cavity 516
sacrum 745
neurofibromatosis 430, 489
atlantoaxial displacement 598
calvarium 403, 405
pelvic deformity 773, 775
ribs 347
tibia 961, 967
neurogenic arthropathy, humeral
head 258
neurogenic cysts, sacral 745
neurolipoma 34
Nievergelt syndrome, forearm 204
Nondissociative carpal instabilities
127
notochord
development 558, 559
regression failure 588
nuchal ligament calcification 626,
638, 639

nucleus pulposus 558
calcification 640, 668, 721, 722
precursors 560

O

occipital bone 359, 363, 414–19, 424–
5
asymmetry 433, 434
basal part 422
crest 424
dysplasia 588
fractures 440–1
lateral part 422
ossification 414, 421
osteolysis 417
thinning 373, 374
transverse sinuses 416, 418
variants 434–9
occipital condyles 424
fractures 440, 441
occipital crest 424, 428
occipital dysplasia 438
occipital emissary veins 424, 428
occipital incisure, posterior 435, 437
occipital protruberances 416, 418
occipital spur 416, 419
occipital vertebra 424–5
occipitoatlantoaxial region
calcification 603
fusion 600
ossification 603
occipitocervical dysplasia 588
occiput 558
occupational stresses, thumb 94
ochronosis 71
alkaptonuria 721
odontoma, mandible 546
olecranon
fossa 220, 222
lucency 227
ossification center 210–11
persistent 217, 220, 221, 222
spurs 217, 218
Ollier disease 65
omarthritis 259
Onodi cells 520, 521, 535
optic atrophy, hereditary 507
optic canal
narrowing 507
variants 506
optic glioma 510
sella turcica 455
optic nerve compression 535
optic neuroma 510
optic sheath meningioma 510
sella turcica 455
orbit 502–10
anatomy 502–6
angioma 508
anomalies 506–8
blow-out fractures 508, 509
dermoid cysts 510
empty 428
enlargement 508
fat pad 505
foreign bodies 510
fractures 508–9
inflammation 509
meningoencephalocele 508
normal variants 506
ossification 502
osteitis 509
Paget disease 509
periostitis 509
small 508
tumors 510
Ortolani maneuver 825
os accessorium supracalcaneum 1007,
1026, 1027, 1028
os acetabuli 804
os acromiale 276, 277, 278
os apicis 405
os centrale carpi 155–7
os cuboideum secundarium 1055
os cuneometatarsale
I plantare 1062, 1064, 1071
II dorsale 1066, 1071
os cuneonavicular mediale 1062,
1063, 1064
os daubentonii 175, 179
os epilunatum 167, 168

os epipyramis 175, 178
os epitriquetrum 175
os hamuli proprium 145, 146
os hypolunatum 167
os incae 405, 1064
os infracoracoideum 263
os infranaviculare 1048, 1049
os infrascapulare 262, 263
os intercuneiforme 1062, 1064
os intermetatarseum 1071, 1072
os interzygomaticum 538
os metopicum 405
os odontoideum 585, 586, 595
os omovertebrale 622, 623
os paraarticulare 1096, 1097
os peroneum 1055–6, 1057
fractures 1056, 1057
posterior displacement 1056
os radiale externum 157, 158
os retinaculum 972, 975
os styloideum 138, 142, 143
os subfibulare 975, 976, 978
os suboccipitale 591, 592
os subtibiale 975
os supranaviculare 1047, 1048
os supratalare 1005–6
os supratrochleare 220, 222, 223
os sustentaculi 1026, 1028, 1029
os talocalcaneare posterius 1006
os talotibiale 976, 1005
os tibiale externum 1044, 1045
edema 1047
necrosis 1047
regressive changes 1046
stress 1047
tilted 1046
os triangulare 175, 177
os trigonum 1006, 1007, 1008, 1009,
1028
acquired 1008HNL
aseptic necrosis 1007, 1009
bilateral 1007, 1010
os trochleare calcanei 1026, 1028
os tuberis calcanei 1026, 1027
os ulnare externum 147
os unci 1066, 1071, 1072
os vesalianum 145, 146, 1071–2
Osgood–Schlatter disease 927, 928,
929
ossa ad acetabulum 821, 823
osseous bridge, metaphysis to epiphysis 23, 24
ossiculum terminale of Bergmann
584
ossification
enchondral 69
hand 16, 17
metastatic 52
ossified tissue matrix 4
osteitis
condensans of clavicle 311, 313, 314
mandible 544, 545
orbit 509
pubis 799, 801
syphilitic 207, 313, 314
zygomatic arch 539
osteitis deformans see Paget disease
osteoarthritis
acromioclavicular joint 290, 291
atlantoaxial joint 602
atlantodental joint 602
atlanto-occipital joint 601
Bouchard type 57
calcaneus 1035
craniovertebral joints 601
decentering sign 851
destructive of distal phalanges (finger) 83
fabella 940
first carpometacarpal 132, 135, 136,
137, 140
glenohumeral joint 299
Heberden type 57
hip joint 809, 850–1
humeral head 258
knee joint 950, 951
manubrioclavicular 311
metatarsal bones 1082, 1083
metatarsal head 1080
navicular bone 1054
plaque sign 850, 851
polyarticular 57, 59, 61, 64
distal phalanges (finger) 83

radioulnar joint 200, 201
ribs 354
sacroiliac joint 758
sesamoid bones 1091, 1092, 1093
sternoclavicular 318
talonavicular joint 1005
temporomandibular joint 552
tibiofibular joint 935
trapezium 135
see also diabetes mellitus, insulin-
dependent, osteoarthropathy
osteoarthropathy
diabetic 1035, 1067–8
familial idiopathic hypertrophic 390
gouty 702, 722
hypertrophic 44, 45, 81
metatarsal bones 1084
pulmonary hypertrophic 872
osteoblastoma 63
calcaneus 1035
carpal bone 132
cervical vertebrae 601, 632
lumbar vertebrae 708
talus 1018
osteochondritis dissecans 221, 231
acetabulum 837, 840
distal femur 883, 884–5, 886
elbow 230, 231
femoral head 837, 840
humeral head 258
loose body differential diagnosis 856
medial cuneiform bone 1065
patella 910
scapula 281
talus 1015–16, 1017
tibia 927
ulnar head 198
osteochondrodysplasias
International Classification of
Osteochondrodysplasia (1992)
5, 6–10
Parisian Nomeclature 11–12
osteochondroma 63, 69
cervical vertebrae 601, 633
differential diagnosis 95, 100
lumbar vertebrae 711
metatarsal bones 1084
nasal cavity 516
pubis 801
ribs 351
scaphoid bone 163
scapula 282, 283, 284, 285
temporomandibular joint 551
toes 1103
zygomatic arch 539
osteochondromatosis, hereditary 801
osteochondronecrosis
pubic symphysis 801
sesamoid bones 1090
osteochondrosis
cervical spine 634–5, 636, 637
ischiopubic 798
lumbar spine 701, 713–14, 724
sacral 758
thoracic spine 663, 664
see also Blount disease
osteodysplasia
lateral clavicle hook 309
polycystic lipomembranous 64
osteodysplastic primordial dwarfism 8
osteofibrous dysplasia, tibial 965, 967
osteogenesis
imperfecta 488, 967
spinal column 560
osteoid osteoma 63, 67, 68
capitate bone 141
carpal bone 130, 131, 132
cervical vertebrae 601, 632
elbow 232, 233
femoral head 845
femoral shaft 871
fibula 959, 960
lateral cuneiform 1058, 1059
lumbar vertebrae 708, 710
metatarsal bones 1084
navicular bone 1053
osteolysis 84
proximal phalanges (finger) 91
scaphoid bone 163
talus 1018
tibia 959, 960
osteolysis
calvarium 399–402

clavicle 289
idiopathic 10, 13
occipital bone 417
proximal humerus 251
osteoma
calvarium 398
ethmoid cells 534
falx 382
frontal sinus 511, 531
giant 845
hip joint 845, 848
ischium 801, 802
lumbar vertebrae 708, 711
mandible 546–7, 550
maxillary sinus 527
metatarsal bones 1084
pelvis 777
rib 350, 351
sphenoid sinus 538
temporal bone 475
trapezoid 140
triquetrum 176
zygomatic arch 539
osteomalacia 47
calvarium 376
femoral shaft changes 868, 869
ilium fractures 782, 784
ischium 797
Looser zones 205
pelvis 773, 775
pubis 797
scapula 280
osteomyelitis
air cells 475
calcaneus 1035
calvarium 397, 441–2
cervical spine 628
clavicle 313
chronic recurring multifocal 312, 313
femur
distal 887, 888, 889
shaft 868, 869
fibula 986
frontal bone 442
frontal sinus 531
humerus 243
lumbar vertebrae 702
mandible 544, 545
patella 911
ribs 350, 351
sesamoid bones 1091
skull base 441–2
tibia 986
proximal 929
toes 1102
osteomyelosclerosis 38, 39
femoral shaft 871
pelvis 773
osteonecrosis
adulthood 56–7
calcaneus 1034–5
distal femur 880, 881, 882, 883–7
elbow 230, 231
extreme mechanical stress 51, 55
femoral head 840, 841–3
fragmented 4
frostbite 54, 55
during growth 52–6
hip joint 836–43
humerus head 256–7
lunate bone 164
metatarsal bones 1079–82
phalanges (toes) 1101
pubis 798
scaphoid bone 160
scapula 281
skull base 441
talus 1015, 1016
thoracic vertebrae 662
see also Perthes disease
osteopathia striata
distal femur 895
femoral shaft 871, 872
osteopenia
bone thinning 18
congenital 47
distal femur 894
pseudohypoparathyroidism 37
osteopetrosis 123, 124
calvarium 398, 399
femoral shaft 871, 872
foramen ovale 442, 443

hand 38, 39
lumbar vertebrae 707
mandible 543, 545
pelvis 773, 775
sternum 338
osteophytes
dorsum sellae 449
drooping 59, 95, 100
elbow 234, 235
knee joint 950, 951
lumbar vertebrae 704, 724
mandibular condyle 552
manubriosternal synchondrosis 338
marginal 69
medial cuneiform bone 1065
navicular bone 1054
patella 912
phalangeal 57, 60
sacroiliac joint 758
talonavicular osteoarthritis 1005
temporomandibular joint 552
osteopoikilosis 40, 42–3
distal femur 895, 896
elbow 232, 233
pelvis 774, 776
sacrum 745, 746
osteoporosis 47, 51
acetabular fractures 833, 834
calvarium 376
circumscripta 402
disuse 49
femur
distal 894, 895, 898
fractures 833, 834
shaft 869
ilium stress fractures 784
lumbar vertebrae 709
pelvis 773
pubis 796
radius 208
rib cough fractures 349
scleroderma 82
senile 408, 409
sternal fractures 334, 335
stress fractures 349, 350
thoracic spine fractures 661
transient 843, 849–50
distal femur 895, 897, 898
ulna 208
osteoradiodystrophy
femoral neck stress fractures 833
mandible 544
pubis 798
ribs 350
scapula 281, 282
see also radiation necrosis
osteosarcoma
calcaneus 1035
femur
distal 889
shaft 871, 874
fibula 959
lumbar vertebrae 708, 710
metatarsal bones 1076, 1078
navicular bone 1053
petrous bone 476, 477
temporomandibular joint 551
tibia 959
proximal 930, 934
osteosclerosis
cervical vertebrae 632
diffuse 442–3
distal phalanges (finger) 20, 76
ostiomeatal complex 521
otic capsule ossification 477
otitis
externa maligna 475, 486
neonatal 471
otocraniofacial syndromes 468
otomastoiditis 471, 473
otosclerosis 487–8
fenestral 468, 469
oval window 468, 469, 477
fissula ante fenestrum 488
oxycephaly 391, 392

P

pacchionian granulations 369, 371–3
occipital bone 416, 417, 418
pachydermoperiostosis 44, 46, 81

acro-osteolysis 57
pachymeningitis, hemorrhagic 385, 386
Paget disease
bone demineralization 867
calcaneus 1036, 1038
calvarium 373, 400, 401–2, 403
cervical vertebrae 601, 639, 640
clavicle 313, 314
femur 864, 866–7
forearm 208
ilium 786
lumbar vertebrae 708, 709
mandible 545
metacarpals 63, 100
orbit 509
patella 912
pelvis 774, 776
polyostotic 60, 63
pubis 799
sacrum 743, 745
scapula 282
skull base 443, 444
tibia 965, 970
palatal clefts 524
palato-occipital line 431
palatoalveolar fractures 524
palmar intercalated segmental instability 108
palmoplantar keratosis, hereditary 44
pancreatitis, metacarpal necrosis 98, 99
Panner disease 230
papilloma, nasal cavity 516, 517
paracondylar process 435, 436
parahippocampal gyrus calcifications 453
paranasal sinuses 517–19
aplasia 533
development 517
dilatation 429
foreign body 517
fungal infections 515
imaging 517–18
pneumatization 364, 449
polyps/polyposis 514, 526
retention cysts 537
surgical defects 527
transverse basilar clefts in clivus 438, 439
paraosseous cartilaginous formation 4
paraplegics, sacroiliac joint 759
parasternal ossicles 330, 331
parastyloid bone 138
parasyndesmophytes 704, 705
parietal bone 407–10
parasagittal ossification disturbance 408
thinning 408, 409, 410
parietal emissary veins 408, 409, 410
parietal foramina 408, 409, 410
defects 378
giant 378, 409–10
Parisian Nomenclature of constitutional bone diseases 5, 11–13
patella 900–12
accessory bone element 910
algodystrophy 912
alta 903, 908
anomalies 905–8
baja 908
bipartite 905, 906
bony outgrowths 905
Brodie abscess 911
chondromalacia 883, 910
clefts 902
congenital syndromes 908
dislocation 908–9
dorsal defect 904
double 905
dysplasia 225
emarginata 905
fractures 908–9
nonunited 905
pediatric 908
gout 911
Haglund groove 905
height 903, 904
inflammation 911
lateral dystopia 908
multipartite 905, 906
necrosis 910–11

ossification centers 900, 901–2
osteochondritis dissecans 910
osteomyelitis 911
osteophytes 912
Paget disease 912
shape 903
spicules 902
subluxation 908–9
Sudeck syndrome 912
traction injury 909
tripartite 905, 906
tumors 911
variants 902–3, 904–7
patellar tendon 928
traction tendinitis 927
patellofemoral congruency 903
pattern recognition 2
pectineal ligament calcification 771
pelvic digit 736, 770
pelvic instability 764, 766
pelvic ligament ossification 768, 770
pelvic rigidity 759, 764, 765
diagnosis 766
ossification 768, 769
pelvic ring 750, 764, 766
fractures 769
injuries 767
instability 699
laxity 750, 802
pelvis 764–77
anatomic diameters 766
anatomy 764, 765, 766
anomalies 773–4
bone density 773, 774, 775
congenital syndromes 773–4
deformities 773, 775
endosteal hyperostosis 773
examination 764–7
fluorosis 773
ilium 778–88
injury classification 767–8
ischium 789–803
ligamentous attachments 764, 765
osteomalacia 773, 775
osteomyelosclerosis 773
osteopetrosis 773, 775
osteopoikilosis 774, 776
osteoporosis 773
Paget disease 774, 776
pubic symphysis 789–803
pubis 789–803
soft-tissue ossification/calcification 768, 769, 770–2
trauma 767–8
tumors 777
see also hip joint
periarthropathia calcificans 299
peribulbar cells 465
perichordal septum 559, 560
pericranial sinuses 407
perilunate–transscaphoid–transcapitate fracture–dislocation 127
perilymph fistula 487
perimalleolar ossification 975
periodontal infection 544–5
periodontium 540
periosteal bone 359
new bone formation 46
periostitis
florid reactive 67, 68, 69
orbit 509
syphilitic 398
periostoses, congenital 44
peritubal cells 465
peroneus tendon, peritendinitis 1056–7
Perthes disease 253, 256, 807, 837–9
pes anserinus 926, 953
insertion 929–30
pes cavus 999–1000
pes equinovarus see clubfoot
pes planovalgus 999
pes planus see flatfoot deformity
petromastoid canal 486
petrosal sinuses 458, 467–8, 480, 481
petrosellar ligament 382
calcifications 449, 482
petrosphenobasilar ossicles 482, 483
petrosquamous fissure 412, 413
petrotympanic fissure 412, 413, 469
petrous apex 480, 481
cholesterol cyst 489–90
petrous apicitis 471–2

petrous bone 412, 414, 457, 460–4, 477–90
  air cells 471–2
  cholesteatoma 473
  epidermoids 488
  fractures 469–70, 486
  jugular notch 482
  Langerhans cell histiocytosis 489, 490
  necrosis 486
  osteosarcoma 476, 477
  pneumatization 482, 483
  transverse crest 482
  trauma 470
  tumors 488–90
petrous pyramid 457–9
  high 482
petrous ridge 480, 518, 522
phalangeal microgeodic syndrome 55, 87
phalangeal sign of Kosowicz 17, 20, 96
phalanges (finger) 16–75
  adulthood 16–22
  calcium specks 21, 22
  contour defects 52, 57, 83
  delta 26, 87
  distal 76–84
    acro-osteolysis 82
    anomalies 77–8
    deformities 80
    developmental disorders 80
    fractures 78–9
    inflammation 83–4
    necrosis 80–2
    normal variants 77–8
    osteosclerosis 20, 76
    terminal tuft 76, 78, 82
    tuft fractures 78, 79
    tumor 84
  growth 16
  length 17, 20
  middle 85–8
    anomalies 85–7
    fractures 87
    inflammation 88
    necrosis 87
    normal variants 85, 87
    tumors 88
  ossification 16
  proximal 89–91
    fractures 90
    inflammation 90–1
    tumors 91
    vascular (nutrient) canals 89
  shortening 38
phalanges (toe)
  bony exostosis 1096
  brachyphalangia 1099
  bracketed diaphysis 1096, 1098, 1099
  distal 1096
  epiphysis 1094
    cone-shaped 1096, 1097
  exostoses 1103
  hallux abductus interphalangeus 1099
  middle 1095
  osteolytic lesions 1101
  osteonecrosis 1101
  proximal 1095
  psoriatic arthritis 1102
  supernumerary 1099
  symphalangia 1099
  synostosis 1095
  transverse partitions 1099, 1100
  turret exostosis 1103
pharyngeal tubercle 451
pharynx tumors 498
phleboliths 71
  eyelid 510
phosphatase deficiency, congenital 390
phosphorus, occupational exposure 544
Pierre–Robin syndrome 542
pigmented villonodular synovitis 552
pineal calcification 380–1
pipetter's thumb 94
Pirie's bone 1005–6
piriform recess 611
PISI 108
pisiform 180–3
  bipartite 180

fractures 182–3
hyperplasia 180
inflammation 183
necrosis 183
ossification 181
ossification center 180, 181
pisotriquetral joint, ligamentous injuries 182
pituitary cartilage 360
pituitary dwarfism 453
pituitary tumors
  adenoma 69
  sphenoid bone 538
plagiocephaly 392
  coronal synostosis 506
planum ethmoidale 534
planum sphenoidale 445, 535, 536
  hyperostosis 534
plaque sign 850, 851
plasmacytoma
  calvarium 400
  ilium 787
  lumbar vertebrae 706, 712
  orbit 510
  ribs 354
  sacrum 745
  sternum 337
platybasia 430–3
pneumatocysts, intraosseous 787
pneumatosinus dilatans 465, 466, 483, 523
  frontal sinus 528, 529
pneumocephalus 395, 396
POEMS syndrome 712
poliomyelitis, intervertebral disk calcification 639
polychondritis 497
polydactyly 29–34
  classification 29, 31–2
  delta phalanges (finger) 26
  thumb 93
polyphalangia 30, 34
ponticle formation on C1 435
popliteal ligament, oblique 950
portal hypertension 678
Pott's puffy tumor 530
prechiasmatic sulcus 445
pregnancy, sacroiliac joint 781
preinterfrontal bone 405, 406
preinterparietal bone 414, 415
preoccipital synchondrosis 482
pressure sella 454
pretibial varices 959, 961
primordial cysts 527
processus asteriacus 434
prostaglandin E$_2$ 389
pseudarthrosis, congenital 205, 961
pseudo-Madelung deformity 125, 194
pseudoachondroplasia, lumbar canal narrowing 698
pseudoepiphyses
  frequency 24
  hand 23–4, 96
pseudogout 71, 603
  intervertebral disk calcification 639
  knee joint 949
pseudohypoparathyroidism 16, 34, 37
  basal ganglia calcification 387
  congenital osteopenia 47
  metacarpals 96
Pseudomonas aeruginosa, otitis externa maligna 475
pseudoretrolisthesis 675, 716
pseudospondylolisthesis, lumbar spine 694, 695, 696, 715–16
pseudospondylosis, lumbar vertebrae 675, 692
pseudotumours 64, 65, 66
  ilieum 787
  inflammatory 66
  ischiopubic synchondrosis 801
  psoriasis 311, 315
    cervical spine 631
  see also arthritis, psoriatic
pterotympanic fissure 412, 413
pterygoid canal 522, 523
pterygoid process 423
pterygoid recess 535
pubic symphysis 764, 789–803
  absence 795
  anatomy 791
  anomalies 791, 794–5
  comma-shaped ossifications 791

congenital fusion 795
examination 765, 767
fibro-ostosis 801
fractures 796–7
gracilis syndrome 801, 802
inflammation 799, 801
instability 765
ossification centers 789, 790
osteochondronecrosis 801
reactive sclerosis 802
ruptures 794, 796
tumors 801, 802
variants 791, 794–5
widening 795
pubis 789–803
  anatomy 791
  anomalies 791, 794–5
  fractures 796–7
  inflammation 799, 801
  Looser zones 796
  nutrient canal 791
  ossification centers 789, 790
  ossification delay/defect 795
  osteitis 799, 801
  osteomalacia 797
  osteonecrosis 798
  osteoporosis 796
  osteoradiodystrophy 798
  Paget disease 799
  stress fractures 796, 797
  tumors 801, 802
  unilateral hypoplasia 795
  variants 791, 794–5
pustulosis palmoplantaris 311, 312, 315
pustulotic arthro-osteitis 315–17
  femoral shaft 871, 872
  fibula 959, 966, 970
  sternum 335, 336
  tibia 959, 966, 970
pyknodysostosis 543
Pyle disease see metaphyseal dysplasia
pyocele
  ethmoid bone 533–4
  frontal sinus 530
  maxillary sinus 526
  sphenoid sinus 537

Q

quadriceps tendon ossification 909

R

rachischisis, lumbar vertebrae 688
radial annular ligament, heterotopic ossification 234, 235
radial clubhand 204–5
radial head
  anterior subluxation 227
  dislocation 225
  fractures 228, 229
radial tuberosity 214–15
radiation necrosis
  calvarium 397
  hyoid bone 497
  ilium 785
  larynx 497
  mandible 544
  ribs 350
  sacrum 743
  see also osteoradiodystrophy
radiation therapy, sacral insufficiency fractures 742–3
radicular cysts 527
radiocarpal instability 129
radiography 2
radiolunate angle 108
radionuclide bone scan 2
radioscaphoid angle 108
radioulnar joint
  distal 111, 117
  osteoarthritis 200, 201
  subluxation 111, 117, 126, 196
  synostosis 225, 226
  synovial chondromatosis 201
radioulnar line method, modification 111, 117
radius
  aplasia 204, 205

bowing 204
fracture 205
hypoplasia 204, 205
inflammation 206–7
interosseous crest 202, 203
necrosis 206
nutrient canal 202
tumor 208
radius, distal 186–201
  accessory bones 189
  anomalies 189–94
  Barton fracture 196, 197
  bony column 186, 187
  chondrocalcinosis 198
  Colles fracture 196
  epiphyseal center 186
  epiphyseolysis 194, 195
  epiphysis 189
  fractures 194–7
  Frykman fracture classification 126, 196
  hyperextension trauma 196, 197
  hyperflexion trauma 196
  inflammation 198
  necrosis 197–8
  normal variants 189–94
  ossification center 186, 189
    persistent accessory 196
    ulnar border 190, 191
  reverse Barton fracture 196
  rickets 200, 201
  Smith fracture 196
  stress-induced widening of physis 194–6
  styloid process 189–90, 198
    avulsion fracture 196
  subperiosteal ganglion 188, 189
  transverse striations in cancellous bone 200
  traumatic epiphyseal separation 194
  tumors 198
radius, proximal
  epiphyseal center 210
  fusion with ulna 225
Ramsey–Hunt syndrome 487
RAP 47, 206
Raynaud disease 71
Recklinghausen disease see neurofibromatosis
reflex sympathetic dystrophy 1084, 1085
regional acceleratory phenomenon 47, 51
  pediatric fractures 206
Reichert cartilage 360
Reiter syndrome
  bamboo spine 706
  calcaneus 1036
  cervical spine 631
  metatarsal bones 1082
  occipitoatlantoaxial abnormalities 600
  parasyndesmophytes 705
  sacroiliac joint 757
  syndesmophytes 706
renal osteodystrophy 71, 77, 78
  dense distal femoral metaphyses 879
  elbow calcification 236
  hyperparathyroidism 208
  Looser zones 205
  lumbar vertebrae 707
  middle phalanges (finger) 88
  rugger jersey spine 707
  shoulder girdle interstitial calcinosis 301, 302
repetitive stress injury, triquetrum necrosis 180
reticulohisticytosis
  multicentric 59, 90, 91
  proximal humerus 249
retina, calcification 510
retinoblastoma 510
retrofacial cells 465
retrolenticular fibroplasia 510
retrolisthesis, cervical spine 636, 637
retromastoid process 434
rhabdomyosarcoma
  embryonic 476
  orbit 510
  zygomatic arch 539
rheumatic disorders, acromioclavicular joint 290
rheumatoid arthritis 61

achillobursitis defect 1038
acromioclavicular joint 290, 302
atlantoaxial subluxation 599, 600
carpus 117, 131
cervical spine 599, 629, 630, 636
cervical spinous processes 631
cricoarytenoid joint 497
cricothyroid joint 497
dens 599
distal ulna 198, 199
erosive changes 83
joint erosions 57, 58
juvenile 599, 629, 630, 754
knee joint 951
lumbar vertebrae 702
metacarpals 100
metatarsal bones 1082, 1083
metatarsophalangeal joint 1082, 1083
proximal humerus 249
proximal phalanges (finger) 90
rice bodies 301, 302
sacral insufficiency fractures 742–3
sacroiliac joint 754
sentinel cysts 64
sesamoid bones 1091
temporomandibular joint 551
thoracic vertebrae 662
rhinolith 517
rhinosporidiosis, nasal cavity 516
ribs 340–55
  accessory 736
  acro-osteolysis 350
  anomalies 342–8
  articulation of twelfth 349
  asymmetries in twelfth 343
  bifid 343, 344
  bifid head 343, 346
  bony portion 340, 341
  cartilaginous part 340
  cervical 342
  chondrosarcoma 351, 352
  coarctation of aorta 348
  cough fractures 349
  deformities 343, 344–8
  degenerative changes 354–5
  dislocation 349
  dysplasias 343, 344–8
  epiphyseal centers 340
  fatigue fractures 349
  fibro-osseous lesions 350
  fibrous dysplasia 353
  first
    asymmetrical development 342
    discontinuities 342–3
    fractures 348–9
  fractures 348–9
  fusions 343, 345, 346
  hyperostosis of head 663
  inflammation 350
  intermediary osseous bridges 343,
    344
  intrathoracic 343, 344
  Langerhans cell histiocytosis 354
  melorheostosis 350, 351
  nearthrosis 343, 345, 346
  necrosis 350
  neurofibromatosis 347
  normal variants 342–8
  ossification centers 340
  ossification patterns 340
  osteoarthritis 354
  osteoma 350, 351
  osteomyelitis 350, 351
  osteoradiodystrophy 350
  pelvic 736
  plasmacytoma 354
  radiation necrosis 350
  scleroderma 347
  Srb anomaly 343, 345
  subluxation 349
  thalassemia 347
  tumors 350–4
  twelfth 343, 349
  union to vertebrae/sternum 340–1
  Wien 344
  see also lumbar ribs
rice bodies, rheumatoid arthritis 301,
  302
rickets
  dense distal femoral metaphyses 879
  distal radius/ulna 200, 201
  Looser zones 205
  mandible 547

proximal tibia 935
rima glottidis 611, 612
ring sign 128
Risser sign 778–9
rotary fixation 597
rotator cuff 293, 294, 295
  impingement syndrome 272, 276,
    296–7
  tears 296–7
    shoulder dislocation differential
    diagnosis 299
round window 468
rubella syndrome 686
Rubinstein–Taybi syndrome 91
  delta phalanges (finger) 26
  foramen magnum 438
rucksack sella 446
rugger jersey spine 707

S

saccule 478
sacral canal 738
sacral crests 733, 734
sacral foramina 733, 734
sacral hiatus 733
sacral index 736
sacral vertebrae 731–2
  epiphyses 732
  fusion 732
  intervertebral disk ossification
    732–3
  origin of segments 561
  osteochondrosis 758
sacrocaudal region, transitional vertebrae 733, 734, 738, 742
sacrococcygeal region
  agenesis 740, 741
  intervertebral disk calcification 745
  variants 736–8
sacroiliac joint 749–59
  accessory joint spaces 742, 750–1
  alkaptonuric ochronosis 758
  anatomy 750
  ankylosis 758
  anomalies 750–1
  bilateral fusion 795
  bilharzial arthropathy 757
  bony bridge 751
  capsule ossification 768, 769
  chondrocalcinosis 758
  connective tissue diseases 758
  dislocation 751
  drug addicts 743, 753, 754
  enteropathic spondylarthropathies
    757
  examination 765, 767
  fractures 751, 752, 767
  growth 749
  hyperparathyroidism 758
  injuries 751, 753
  instability 765
  joint space
    narrowing 758
    widening 751, 752
  laxity 759
  ligamentous injuries 767
  multiple hyperostosis 759
  necrosis 752
  osteoarthritis 758
  osteophytes 758
  pneumatocele 758
  pregnancy 781
  pseudoerosions 749, 752
  psoriatic arthritis 756–7
  Reiter syndrome 757
  retroauricular space 750
  rheumatoid arthritis 754
  sacral protruberance 751
  seronegative spondyloar-
    thropathies 755–7
  sickle cell disease 743, 752, 759
  space 732
  stepoff 751, 752
  subchondral synovial cysts 787
  subluxation 751
  syphilis 754
  trauma 751, 752
  uric arthropathy 758
  vacuum phenomenon 758
  variations 750–1
sacroiliac ligaments 749

calcification 755–6, 758, 759
  ossification 754, 755–6, 759
sacroiliitis 753
  ankylosing spondylitis 755–6
  brucellosis 754
  infantile infectious 753
  Reiter syndrome 757
  tuberculous 753–4
sacrolisthesis 759
sacrospinal ligament
  calcification 745, 746
  ossification 770, 771
sacrotuberal ligament 745, 770
sacrum 558, 731–46
  acute 676
  agenesis 740, 741
  anatomy 733–6
  anomalies 738, 740–1
  arched 676–7
  asymmetry 738
  clefts 735, 738, 740
  curvature 736
  dislocations 743
  foramina 735, 767
  fractures 741–3, 767
    insufficiency 742–3
  fusion 732
  growth 731–3
  hemivertebra 740
  hiatus 740, 742
  intervertebral canals 733, 734
  intervertebral disk spaces 732
  intervertebral foramina 734
  ossification centers 731
    persistent 742
  osteomyelitis 743
  osteopoikilosis 745, 746
  Paget disease 743, 745
  pseudocysts 735, 738, 739, 743
  radiation necrosis 743
  tumors 743–5
  variants 736–8
  vertebral arch defect 739
sagittal sinus
  calcification 382
  lateral lacunae 407, 408
salivary stones 547
salmonellosis, lumbar vertebrae 702
salt-and-pepper skull 405
SAPHO syndrome 315, 754
sarcoidosis
  calvarium 400
  hand 40, 41, 42, 60
  larynx 497
  lumbar vertebrae 708
  nasal septum 515
  skeletal 60
SATHO see arthro-osteitis; pustulotic
  arthro-osteitis
scalenus anticus syndrome 342
scaphocephaly 391, 392
scaphoid bone 148–63
  accessory bony element 158
  anomalies 150–1
  aplasias 150–1
  bipartite 153, 159
    asymmetric 157
  contusion 154
  deformity 123
  duplication 122, 151
  fibrous nonunion 159
  fractures 152–8
    complication rate 152
    nonunion 158, 159, 160
    tubercle 154, 155, 157
  fragmentation 159, 160
  hypoplasia 150, 151
  inflammation 162
  intraosseous ganglion 162
  metastases 163
  β_2-microglobulin amyloid deposits
    65, 162
  morphological variation 149
  necrosis 159–61
  normal variants 150–1
  nutrient canals 152, 153
  ossification center 164
    duplication 148, 149, 150, 154
    unfused 155
    unfused accessory 157
  osteonecrosis 160
  protruberances 149, 150
  Trevor disease 161, 163

tubercle fracture 154, 155, 157
  tumors 162–3
scaphoid fat stripe 152, 153
scapholunate
  angle 108
  dissociation 128–9, 166, 170, 178
  fusion 150, 151
scapula 262–85
  accessory bones 279, 280
  acro-osteolysis 281
  angles 262, 266
  anomalies 271–6
  apophyseal center 262
  arthro-osteitis 281–2
  congenital syndromes 274, 276
  deformities 274–6
  dislocation 276–80
  fractures 276–80
  glenoid cavity 270
  inflammation 281–2
  lateral border ossification 271
  lucency 271, 282
  necrosis 281
  normal variants 271–6
  nutrient canals 270
  ossification center 262, 263
  osteochondritis dissecans 281
  osteochondroma 282, 284
  osteomalacia 280
  osteoradiodystrophy 281, 282
  Paget disease 282
  persistent apophyses 276, 277–8
  posttraumatic clefts/gaps 283, 285
  pustulotic arthro-osteitis 281
  radiographic techniques 265, 267–9
  scaphoid 271
  subchondral synovial cyst 282, 283,
    284
  subluxation 276–80
  tumors 282–5
scapular ligament, superior transverse 271
  ossification 271
Scheuermann disease 636, 638, 666
  lumbar vertebrae 710, 716
  thoracic spine 664–7
Scheuthauer–Marie–Sainton syndrome see cleidocranial dysostosis
Schmitt disease 626, 627
Schmorl nodes 634, 650, 665, 666,
  667, 668
  communicating 717
  lumbar spine 716–17
schwannoma, zygomatic arch 539
scintigram, whole-body 2
scleroderma 81, 82
  calcinosis circumscripta 71
  mandible 547
  ribs 347
scoliosis
  cervical spine 636, 638
  lumbar vertebrae 688, 710, 720, 725
  thoracic spine 651, 652, 664
scotty dog sign of Lachapel 676, 691–2
sella turcica 445–56
  configurations 447–8
  deformities 449–53
  fractures 453, 537
  growth 446–7
  J-shaped 455
  Langerhans cell histiocytosis 454
  normal variants 449–53
  ossification 450
  tumors 454–6, 538
sellar bridge 450, 451
sellar diaphragm 382
sellar spine 452
semicircular canals 478
sentinel cysts 64
sesamoid bones 17–18, 1062, 1064,
  1087–93
  acromegaly 1091
  avascular necrosis 1090–1
  bipartite lateral 3–4
  bony fusion to metatarsal 1088, 1089
  chondrocalcinosis 1091, 1092
  deformities 1088–9
  dislocation 1089–90, 1093
  distal interphalangeal joints 76, 77
  duplication 52, 1088, 1089
  fabella 937, 940
  fractures 52, 93, 94, 1089–90

hallux valgus 1073, 1090
growth 1087
hallux valgus 1073, 1090
inflammation 1091
interphalangeal joint dislocation 1090
multiple 21
necrosis 56
ossification 1087
osteoarthritis 1091, 1092, 1093
osteochondronecrosis 1090
osteomyelitis 1091
partitions 1088, 1089
rheumatoid arthritis 1091
small 52
subluxation 1089–90
supernumerary 18
variants 1088–9
sesamum tibiale anterius 1062, 1064
Sever disease 1034–5
Sharp syndrome 71, 81
Shepherd fracture 1006
shin splint syndrome 963, 964
short rib dysplasia 6
shoulder girdle
acromioclavicular joint 287–91
interstitial calcinosis 301, 302
ligament ossification 301
radiograph interpretation 265
transscapular Y view 270
see also acromion; clavicle; scapula;
sternoclavicular joint; sternum
shoulder joint 292–304
anatomy 249, 292, 293
anterior capsular complex 292, 293
Bankert lesion 297, 298
bursae 293, 294, 295, 296, 299, 302–4
calcification 299, 300, 301
calcification 299–302
chondromatosis 301, 304
congenital dysplasia 274, 275
dislocation 254, 255, 297–9
ganglion cyst 283, 284
glenoid labrum 292, 293, 295
impingement 296–7
Neer stages 296
instability 297–9
loose bodies 301, 303
shoulder dislocation differential
diagnosis 299
ossification 299–303
soft-tissue anatomy 292–6
tendon calcification 300
see also Hill–Sachs lesion; rotator
cuff
sialoliths 547
sickle cell disease 547
inflammation 752–7
mandible 547
sacroiliac joint 743, 752, 759
thoracic spine 667, 668
sigmoid sinus 466, 467
Sindig–Larsen–Johansson disease
910, 911
single photon emission computed
tomography (SPECT) 2
sinolith 517
sinusitis
cystic fibrosis 528
frontal 530
maxillary 525–6
sphenoid 537
skeleton
disorganized development 10
see also facial skeleton
SKIBO diseases 81
skull
anemia 369
anomalies 375–92
arterial grooves 365
asymmetries 375–6
calcification 380–7
embryology 358–61
endochondral ossification 358
flat membranous bones 359
fontanelles 359, 364, 368
fractures 392–6
growing 393
intercalary bones 364–5, 369
intracranial calcifications 374
lacunar 389
membranous ossification 358–9
necrosis 397
normal variants 375–92

ossification center 358–9
shape development 361, 363–4
short 392
sutural bones 364–5, 369
sutures 364, 368, 369
fractures 393, 395, 396
mendosal 414, 415
metopic 405
occipital squama 414, 415, 416
premature closure of frontal 405
premature fusion 374, 390–2
sphenosquamous 412, 414
variants 369
widening 389–90
thalassemia 348, 369
tower 391, 392
traumatic depression 393, 394
triangular 392
vascular calcifications 384
see also calvarium; cranial vault; facial skeleton; orbit
skull base 360, 362, 365, 421–98
actinomycosis 442
architecture 421–7
asymmetry 429–30, 433
basilar impression 422
bony thickening 429
hordoma 444
dermoid 455, 456
development 359–60, 363
epidermoid 455, 456
fibrous dysplasia 443, 444
fractures 440–1
hyoid bone 490–8
inflammation 441–4
larynx 490–8
osteomyelitis 441–2
osteonecrosis 441
Paget disease 443, 444
platybasia 430–3
posterior fossa 423–4, 433, 434–9
jugular tubercles 444
sella turcica 445–56, 538
sphenoid angle 422
styloid process 490–8
support columns 421, 422
syphilis 442
temporal bone 457–64
tuberculous lesions 442
tumors 442–4, 538
epipharyngeal 455
vidian canal 423
see also air cells; auditory canal, external; basilar impression;
cranial fossae; middle ear;
petrous bone; temporal bone
slipping rib syndrome 349
snowcap sign 256, 257
soft-tissue necrosis 71
soleus muscle 1001
somatotropin 69
spastic torticollis, atlantoaxial displacement 598
spheno-occipital synchondrosis 421,
439
sphenoid angle 422, 431
sphenoid bone
air cells 423
growth 421
pituitary tumors 538
styloid processes 571
sphenoid sinus 445, 518, 534–8
anomalies 535–6
asymmetry 536
ballooned 535
cysts 537
fractures 453, 537
inflammation 537
mucocele 455, 537
normal variation 535–6
optic nerve compression 535
pneumatization 506, 534, 535, 536
pyocele 537
septa 536, 537
tumor 538
vascular grooves 535
very small 536, 537
sphenoid sinusitis 537
sphenoid wings 360
sphenoparietal sulcus 405
sphenopetrosal ligament 449
sphenosquamous suture 412, 414, 481
spina bifida

atlas 575, 576, 577
axis 584
lumbar vertebrae 688, 689, 708
spina ventosa 60
spinal canal, cervical 612, 613
spinal column 558–62
chondrification 560
curves 558
development 558–62
ossification centers 562
ossification stage 560
osteogenesis 560
see also atlas; axis; cervical vertebrae (C1-C2); cervical vertebrae (C3-C7); lumbar vertebrae; sacral vertebrae; thoracic
vertebrae
spinal fusion 721, 778
spinal ligaments 558
spinal nerve groove in cervical spine
610, 611, 612, 613
spiral organ of Corti 479
splayfoot 999
spondylarthritis, seronegative 315, 317
calcaneus 1036–7, 1039
cervical vertebrae 599, 629
lumbar vertebrae 702
pelvic ligament ossification 768
sacroiliac joint 755–7
sternum 335, 336
temporomandibular joint 551
spondylarthropathies, enteropathic
706
sacroiliac joint 757
spondylarthrosis
cervical spine 634, 635, 636
deformans 636, 714–15
spondylitis
cervical spine 628, 629
lumbar vertebrae 701–6
spondylocostal dysplasia of thoracic
vertebrae 658
spondylodiscitis
cervical spine 628
lumbar spine 700–1, 710
spondylodysplasia 6
spondyloepiphyseal dysplasia congenita 7
spondylolisthesis
cervical spine 621, 622
lumbar vertebrae 691, 694–6
spondylolysis
axis 584
cervical vertebrae 594
lumbar vertebrae 680, 683, 690–1,
692, 693, 694
vertebral arch sclerosis 708
spondylometaphyseal dysplasia 7
spondylophytes
hyperostotic 635, 636
marginal 634, 724
submarginal 635, 636
spondyloretrolisthesis, lumbar spine
694, 715, 716
spondylosclerosis, hemispheric 635,
714
spondylosis deformans 635, 636
thoracic vertebrae 663
spondylosis hyperostotica see DISH
syndrome
Sprengel deformity 274, 622
squamous cell carcinoma, nasal cavity
516
Stafne cyst 541–2
stapes 457
staphylococcal coxitis 844
Steinberg sign 34
step sign 94
sternal angle 322
sternal foramen 329, 330
sternal symphysis 322
sternoclavicular joint 305–18
articular disk 308
capsule 308
epiphyseal separation 310
hyperostosis 311
intra-articular vacuum phenomenon 308, 318
osteoarthritis 318
traumatic dislocation 310
sternocostal joint degenerative
changes 355
sternocostoclavicular hyperostosis
313, 315–17, 336

cervical spine 629
sternum 320–38
anatomy 321
anomalies 326–33
CT dimensions 308
dislocation 334
examination techniques 323–6
fissure 328, 329
fractures 334, 335
inflammation 335–7
multipartite 328
necrosis 334
normal dimensions 323
normal variants 326–33
ossification 320, 321
disturbances 326, 327–8
ossification centers 326, 327
asymmetrical development 326
osteopetrosis 338
osteoporosis 334
parasternal ossicles 330, 331
position 331, 332
posterior displacement 333
premature synostosis 330
pustulotic arthro-osteitis 335, 336
rib union 340–1
segmentation 320
failure 330
persistent 327
seronegative spondylarthritis 335,
336
subluxation 334
suprasternal ossicles 330, 331
tumors 337–8
see also sternoclavicular joint
steroid necrosis 628
sacral insufficiency fractures 742–3
thoracic vertebrae 662
Sturge–Weber disease 384, 385
stylohyoid complex ossification
495–6
stylohyoid ligament 492
calcification 496
ossification 491, 495–6
styloid ligament ossification 492
styloid process 490–8
anatomy 492
elongation 495
styloid process syndrome 495
subacromial–subdeltoid bursa 294,
295, 297
subarachnoid pneumocephalus 473
subarcuate fossa 458, 480, 481
subchondral sclerosis, circumscribed
172
subcoracoid bursa 295
subdural pneumocephalus 473
sublingual fossa 540
submandibular abscess 545
submandibular fossa 540
suboccipital dysplasia 588
suboccipital process 434, 435
subperiosteal ganglion, radius 188, 189
subperiosteal hemorrhage 206
subtalar joint 985
coalition 998, 999
posteromedial 1012
subtalar sinus 1002, 1003
subungual exostoses 1102–3
subungual keratoacanthoma 84
Sudeck syndrome 47, 49–50
forearm 208
patella 912
transient osteoporosis 849
sulcus calcanei 1020, 1022
sulcus calcanei 1020, 1022
supinator fat line 227, 228
supra-acromial bursa 296
supracondylar process 221, 223, 224
trauma 221, 224
supraorbital foramen 502, 505
suprapatellar bursa 940
suprasellar craniopharyngioma 455
supraspinatus impingement syndrome 278
supraspinous ligament calcification
638, 639
suprasternal ossicles 330, 331
supratrochlear foramen 220–1, 222
sustentaculum tali 1020, 1022
sutura mendosa 369
sutural bones 364–5, 369, 407
sutural hyperostosis 369
swan-neck deformity 79

swayback syndrome 719
symphalangia 26, 27–8
  toes 1099
symphysis menti 539
syndactyly
  fingers 26, 28
  toes 1099
syndesmophytes 663, 702, 704
  Reiter syndrome 706
synostosis
  cervical spine 628
  metatarsal 33
synovial angiomatosis, knee joint 945, 946
synovial cyst, subchondral 66, 67, 282, 283, 284
  acetabulum 846, 847
  proximal tibia 929, 931–3
  sacroiliac joint 787
  talus 1018
  tibia 986, 987
synovial sarcoma, knee joint 945, 948
syphilis
  calvarium 398
  cervical spine 629
  clavicle involvement 313, 314
  gummatous 398
  labyrinthitis 487
  mandible 545
  nasal bone congenital hypoplasia 513
  osteolytic changes 206, 207
  proximal tibia 929, 930
  sacroiliac joint 754
  skull base 442
syphilitic periostitis, tibial 966, 967
syringomyelia, humeral head 254, 258

T

talar dome
  curvature 1003
  osteochondral fractures 1014–15, 1026
talar-first metatarsal angle 989, 992
talocalcaneal angle 989, 991
talocalcaneal joint 983–5
  coalition 1012, 1033
talocalcaneonavicular joint 985
talocrural joint 983–5
  chondromatosis 986, 988
  morphological conversion 998
  valgus deformity 977
  see also tibiotalar tilt
talofibular ligament 1003
talonavicular joint 1041
  fusion 999, 1012, 1049–50
  osteoarthritis 1005
  subchondral osteolysis 1019
talus 985, 1002–19
  accessorius 1008, 1010, 1011
  accessory bones 1005
  anatomy 1002–4
  beaking 1003, 1005
  bipartite 1011, 1012
  Brodie abscess 1018
  congenital vertical 1011
  deformities 1011–13
  dislocation 1013–15
  fracture 1006, 1009, 1013–15
  fracture–dislocation 1014, 1015
  hypoplasia 1011
  inflammation 1018–19
  lateral process fractures 1014
  neck 1003
    fractures 1013–14
  nose 1003, 1005
  nutrient canal 1003
  ossification center 1002
  osteochondritis dissecans 1015–16, 1017
  osteonecrosis 1015, 1016
  posterior process 1006, 1007
    avulsion 1006, 1009
  secundarius 1008, 1010, 1011
  spheroidal 1011, 1012
  subchondral synovial cyst 1018
  subluxation 1013–15
  talofibular ligament groove 1003
  Trevor disease 1012, 1013
  tumors 1018–19
  variants 1005–11
  vertical cleft 1011, 1012

tarsal bones
  arthritis 997
  coalition 997–9
  necrosis 1015–17
  synostosis 997–9
tarsal sinus 1002, 1015
tarsal sinus syndrome 1015
tarsometatarsal joints 1069, 1070
  fracture–dislocations 1074
teeth
  displaced with maxillary fracture 525
  ectopic intraorbital 510
  heterotopic buds in maxillary sinus 524
  malposition 542
  mandibular fracture 543
  root resorption 546
  structure 540
  wisdom 543
tegmen tympani 457, 466, 468
temporal bone 424, 457–64
  air cells 429
  anatomy 457–64
  development 457–64
  exostoses 475
  fibrous dysplasia 475
  fractures 469, 470
  growth 421
  osteoma 475
  pneumatization 465, 466, 471–2
  radiographic projections 459–64
  squamous 411–14, 457
    fontanelles 411
    petrosquamous fissure 412, 413
    petrotympanic fissure 412, 413
    senile atrophy 412
    sutures 412, 414
    vascular grooves 394, 395, 412
  temporomandibular joint 548
  trigeminal impression 482, 483
  tumors 475–7
  tympanic part 457
  vascular channel 395
  zygomatic process 457, 465
  see also petrous bone
temporomandibular joint 361, 364, 548–52
  anatomy 548
  anomalies 549–50
  arthritis 551, 552
  development 548
  dislocation 550
  distance to arch of atlas 432
  fractures 550, 551
  function 548
  inflammation 551
  microfractures 550
  necrosis 551
  normal variants 549–50
  osteoarthritis 552
  osteophytes 552
  pigmented villonodular synovitis 552
  subchondral degenerative cysts 552
  synovial chondromatosis 552
  tumors 551
temporozygomatic suture 506
tendinitis, calcifying 603, 604
tendinopathy, insertional 912
tendon sheath, calcinosis circumscripta 71, 72–3
tentorium calcification 382, 383
teratoma, sacrococcygeal region 745
terminal ossicle 435, 438
thalassemia 38
  hair-on-end appearance 379
  lumbar vertebrae 678
  ribs 347
  skull 348, 369
thalidomide embryopathy 657
Thibiérge–Weissenbach syndrome 71
  interstitial calcinosis 301
Thiemann disease 52, 53, 54, 87
thoracic vertebrae 558, 645–68
  accessory diarthrosis 653
  anatomy 648–51
  ankylosing spondylitis 662, 663
  ankylosis 662–3
  anomalies 653–8
  apophyseal ring 647
  block vertebrae 656, 657, 661
  butterfly 653, 654, 655
  calcifying discitis 668

costotransverse joints 649, 662–3
  degenerative disease 663–8
diastematomyelia 657, 658
DISH syndrome 663–4
dislocations 658–62
  Edgren–Vaino sign 666, 667, 668
  eosinophilic granuloma 662
  facet joints 650
  flat 658
  fractures 658–62
    pathological 660–2
  Hahn clefts 645, 649
  hemimetameric segmentation anomaly 656
  hemivertebrae 655–6, 657
  hyperextension–shear injuries 659
  infections 662
  inflammation 662–3
  injuries
    classification 659
    with rotation 659–60
  interpedicular distance 649
  intervertebral osteochondrosis 663
  kyphosis 651, 652, 663, 664, 666
    angular 666
  limbus vertebra 667
  necrosis 662
  normal variants 653
  origin of segments 561
  ossification centers 645
  osteochondrosis 664
  pedicle thinning 653
  perivertebral hyperostosis 663
  persistent chordal canal 653, 655
  physiological wedging 648
  posture 651–2
  progressive fusion 657
  radiate ligament calcification 663
  range of motion 651–2
  rheumatoid arthritis 662
  Schmorl nodes 650, 665, 666, 667, 668
  scoliosis 651, 652, 664
  segmentation anomalies 656–7
  segmentation shift 653
  sickle cell disease 667, 668
  spinous processes 649
    aplasia 658
    fatigue fracture 664
  spondylocostal dysplasia 658
  spondylosis deformans 663
  subluxations 658–62
  synostosis 656, 657
  transverse processes 649
  tuberculous spondylitis 662
  tumors 663
  vacuum phenomenon 662, 665
  vertebra plana 662
  vertebral arch clefts 658
  vertebral bodies 648–9
    anomalies 653, 654, 655
    aplasia 655
    calcification 664
    clefts 653, 655
    compression injuries 659
    coronal clefts 655
    DISH syndrome 664, 665
    Knutsson's sign 665
    marginal ridge 645, 646, 647, 665, 666, 667
    notches 645
    nutrient canals 645, 646, 648
    ossification 664
    ossification centers 645, 647
    partial defects 655–6
    pathological fractures 660–1
    pediatric 645, 646
    persistent notochord 653
  vertebral end plates 650
  wedge 661, 666
  whiplash injuries 659
thoracolumbar junction
  injuries with distraction 659
  wedge-shaped deformity 653, 654
thorax see ribs; sternum
thrombophlebitis, chronic adhesive retrobulbar 510
thumb 91–4
  acro-osteolysis 93
  anomalies 91–3
  clubbed 91
  delta configuration of proximal phalanx 91, 93
  double biphalangism 33

duplication 93, 121
  fracture 93
  gamekeeper's 93
  inflammation 93
  murderer's 91
  necrosis 93
  normal variants 91–3
  occupational stresses 94
  radial clubhand 204
  triphalangeal 91
  tubular bones 17
thyrohyoid ligament 495
thyroid cartilage 491
  calcification 493, 611, 612
tibia
  angiodysplasia 959, 961
  anomalies 958–61
  anterolateral triangle 982
  Blount disease 921–2, 923, 930, 935
  bone marrow infarction 965, 969
  bony prominence 919
  bowing 922–3, 958, 967
    acute plastic 961
  cleft 920
  cortical irregularities 958, 986, 987
  cystic angiomatosis 959, 961
  dislocation 924–6, 980–6
  distal 971–88
    anatomy 973–4
    epiphyseal plate 971
    epiphyseal plate fractures 980, 981
    epiphysis exostosis 978
    inflammation 986
    ossification center 971–2
    triplane fractures 980, 981
  epiphyseal dysplasia 921, 922
  fibrous dysplasia 966, 968
  fibrous metaphyseal defects 986, 987
  focal fibrocartilaginous dysplasia 922, 923
  fractures 924–6, 961–5, 980–6
    Segond 918, 919
    stress 926, 963, 964, 969
    transitional 971
  growth plate
    cleft 920
    fused epiphyseal 918, 920
  Harris lines 973
  inflammation 965
  intercondylar tubercles 916–17, 918
  Looser zones 926
  melorheostosis 959, 960
  metaphyseal–epiphyseal chondrodysplasia 977, 980
  necrosis 927–9
  neurofibromatosis 961, 967
  nutrient canals 953, 954–7, 961, 962, 964
  Osgood–Schlatter disease 927, 928, 929
  osteofibrous dysplasia 965, 967
  osteomyelitis 986
  Paget disease 965, 970
  periosteal bone formation 963, 965
  plateau 916, 917
  pretibial varices 959, 961
  proximal 914–36
    cartilaginous exostoses 930, 935
    congenital syphilis 929, 930
    deformities 921–3
    epiphysis 876, 914, 920
    fatty replacement 929
    fibrous metaphyseal defects 929, 933
    inflammation 929–35
    melorheostosis 934
    metaphysis 876
    osteomyelitis 929
    rickets 935
    subchondral synovial cysts 929, 931–3
    tumors 929–35
    white epiphysis 928–34
  pustulotic arthro-osteitis 959, 966, 970
  Rauber console 918, 919
  shaft 953–70
    anatomy 953, 954–7
    bowing 953, 962
    fibrous metaphyseal defects 958
    Harris lines 958, 962
    necrosis 965, 969
    ossification centers 953

shin splint syndrome 963, 964
stress-induced lucencies 965
subluxation 924–6, 980–6
synostosis 958
syphilitic periostitis 966, 967
traction tendinitis/trauma 927
tuberosity 914, 915–16, 925
    avulsion fracture 927
    lateralization 921
    patellar tendon 928
tumors 965–6, 986, 987
valgus deformity 977
variants 921, 929, 958–61, 975–80
varus deformity 922–3, 958, 961, 967
tibiocalcaneal angle 989, 991
tibiofibular joint 918, 920, 935, 936
tibiotalar angle 989, 992
tibiotalar tilt 977, 978
    hemophilia 979
Tietze syndrome 335
toe, great 1096
    transverse partitions 1099, 1100
toes 1094–103
    accessory bones 1096, 1097
    acro-osteolysis 1101
    brachydactyly 1099, 1100
    brachyphalangias 1099
    bracketed diaphysis 1096, 1098, 1099
    claw 1100
    diabetic osteoarthropathy 1101
    epiphyses 1094
        cone-shaped 1096, 1097
        duplicated 1094, 1101
        injuries 1101
    fractures 1101
    hammer 1100
    mallet 1100
    necrosis 1101–2
    ossification centers 1094
    osteomyelitis 1102
    spontaneous dactylolysis 1102
    subungual exostoses 1102–3
    symphalangia 1099
    syndactyly 1099
    synostosis 1100
    tumors 1103
    see also phalanges (toe)
tonsils 423, 442
tooth see teeth
torticollis
    congenital 435
    muscular 598
    nasopharyngeal 598
tracheal rings 493, 494
tracheobronchopathia calcarea 493
transscaphoid–perilunate dislocation 127
transsphenoidal meningoencephalo-
    cele 451
transverse ligament
    calcification 604
    ossification 603
trapezium 132–7
    anomalies 132
    calcification 135
    dislocation 132–6
    fracture 132–6
    necrosis 136
    normal variants 132
    periarticular ossification 132
    synostoses 132, 133
    tendon sheath tumors 137
    tubercle 132
    tumors 137
trapezoid 137–40
    bipartite 137
    fractures 138–40
    osteoma 140
    pathological findings 137–40
    secondary 138, 139
    synostosis 137
trauma
    bone 62
    calvarium 393, 394
    cervical spine 636
    CSF leak 533
    distal phalanges (finger) 78–9
    knee joint 919, 949
    labyrinthitis 486, 487
    lumbar vertebrae 678, 679
    pelvic ring instability 699
    petrous bone 470
    proximal phalanges (finger) 90

sacroiliac joint 751, 752, 753
sacrotuberal/sacrospinal ligament
    calcification 745, 746
    skull 393, 394
Treacher–Collins syndrome 468, 542
Trevor disease 123–4
    hip joint 855–6
    scaphoid bone 151, 161, 163
    talus 1012, 1013
triangular fibrocartilage complex 173
    cartilage calcification 198
    damage 169, 173
    degenerative changes 192
    ulnar impaction syndrome 191, 192, 193
trigeminal bridge 449
trigeminal impression 482, 483
trigeminal nerve 489
trigeminal neurinoma 442, 443, 489
trigeminal notch 482, 483
trigonocephaly 392, 405
tripod fracture 524–5
triquetrum 174–80
    bony elements 177, 179
    calcification 179
    chondrocalcinosis 178
    chondroma 176
    dislocation 174–9
    fracture 174–9
    fusion with lunate 174
    heterotopic ossification 177
    necrosis 180
    ossification center 174
    osteoma 176
    targetoid ossification 178
    ulnar impaction syndrome 191
triradiate cartilage 804
    persistence 821
trisomy 17 28
trisomy 18 309
trisomy 21 see Down syndrome
triticeal cartilage 495
trochanter
    greater 804, 807
    lesser 804, 808, 809
        avulsion fractures 834
        duplication 823–4
        Looser zones 834
        ossification center 804, 807
        transformation processes 869
trochlea
    hypoplasia 225
    ossification center 211, 213
    osteochondritis dissecans 230
trochlear process 221
trochlear process 221
Troell–Junet syndrome 378
Trummerfeld zones 206
tubercle of Chaput 982
tuberculosis/tuberculous lesions
    calcification 384
    calvarium 397
    coxitis 844
    cystic of bone 60
    larynx 497
    lumbar vertebrae 700, 702
    mandible 545
    navicular bone 1053
    sacroiliitis 753–4
    skull base 442
    subtalar joint arthritis 1009
    zygomatic arch 539
tuberculous spondylitis
    cervical vertebrae 598–9, 628
    lumbar vertebrae 700
    thoracic vertebrae 662
tuberous sclerosis 40, 41
    calcification 386
    lumbar vertebrae 708
turbinate cycle 512
Turner syndrome 124, 781
turricephaly 391
    facial deformity 392
tympanic bone 466
tympanic membrane rupture 470
tympanosclerosis 488
ulcerative colitis
    enteropathic spondylarthropathies 706
    sacroiliac joint 757

bowing 204
congenital pseudarthrosis 205
epicondyle 220
    traumatic displacement 227
fractures 205
groove 215, 216
head
    fractures 197
    osteochondritis dissecans 198
    inflammation 206–7
    length 186–7, 190
        discrepancy 173
    necrosis 206
    notch 215, 216
    nutrient canal 202
    polydactylia differential diagnosis 95, 100
    posttraumatic lengthening 190
    short 194
    translocation 129
    tumor 208
ulna, distal 186–201
    accessory bones 189
    anomalies 189–94
    chondrocalcinosis 198
    chondromalacia 190
    contour ridge 188, 189
    epiphyseal center 186
    epiphyseal plate 186, 187
    epiphyseolysis 194, 195
    epiphysis 189
    fractures 177, 194–7
    inflammation 198
    necrosis 197–8
    normal variants 189–94
    ossification center 186, 189
        persistent accessory 196
    rickets 200, 201
    stress-induced widening of physis 194–5
    styloid process 189–90
        avulsion fracture 196
        erosions 198, 199
        fracture 177
        morphology variation 198, 199
        necrosis 197, 198
    transverse striations in cancellous bone 200
    traumatic epiphyseal separation 194
    tumors 198
ulna, proximal
    fusion with radius 225
    lucency 215
    ossification center 210–11
ulnar clubhand 205
ulnar impaction 173
ulnar impaction syndrome 172–3, 190–4, 225
ulnar impingement 173
ulnar styloid impaction syndrome 190
ulnar styloid process index (USPI) 190
ulnar variance
    measurement 187
    negative 169, 190, 192
    positive 190, 191, 193
ulnocarpal impaction 173
ulnolunate impaction 173
ulnoradial impingement 173
ultrasonography 3
uncinate process 532
uncovertebral joints 610
    arthrosis 634, 635, 637
    degenerative arthritis 624
    fractures 626
Urbach–Wiethe syndrome 453
uric arthropathy, sacroiliac joint 758
utricle 478
uvula 423, 442

symptomatic 2, 3
venous lacunae 371
vertebrae 558
    anatomy 558
    block
        cervical 600, 620, 621, 623
        thoracic 656
    fish 661, 709
    ivory 701, 706
    occipital 424–5
    ossification centers 560, 561
    rib union 340–1
    transitional
        lumbosacral 681, 683, 684
        sacrocaudal 733, 734, 738, 742
    wedge 661
    see also atlas; axis; cervical verte-
        brae (C1-C2); cervical verte-
        brae (C3-C7); lumbar verte-
        brae; sacral vertebrae; thoracic
        vertebrae
vertebral arch 558
    articular process 558
    chondrification 560
    development 559, 560
    spinous process 558
vertebral artery
    compression 636
    elongation/ectasia 601, 633
vertebral bodies 558
    cartilaginous end plate 558, 562
    cartilaginous marginal ridge 562
    cervical 609, 612
        fusion 620, 621
    ossification centers 560
    transverse processes 558
vertebral canal 558
vertebral foramen 558
vestibular aqueduct narrowing 485
vestibular ganglion 479
vestibulocochlear nerve 464, 478, 479
Vidian canal 423, 522, 523
villonodular synovitis
    hip joint 845–6
    knee joint 945, 946, 947
    proximal fibula 935
violin-player's fingers 82
virole see metaphyseal ring
visterocranium 358, 360–1, 363–4
vitamin A excess 603
vitamin C deficiency 206
vitamin D overdose 772
    dense distal femoral metaphyses 879

W

Wegener granulomatosis 497
    maxillary sinus 515, 527
    nasal septum 515
Whipple disease 706
    sacroiliac joint 757
Wiberg sign 851
Wien rib 344
Wilson disease 71
wormian bones 369
wrist see carpus

X

xiphoid process 322, 324
    morphological variations 323
    ossification 320
xiphosternal synchondrosis 322, 331
    degenerative changes 338

Y

Y sign 989, 993
Yune soft tissue index 81

Z

zygoma, bipartite 538
zygomatic arch 538–9
zygomatic recess 519
zygomaticocoronoid ankylosis 549
zygomaticomaxillary fractures 524–5

U

Ullrich–Turner syndrome 616
ulna

V

vacuum phenomenon
    cervical spine 634, 637
    knee joint 937, 939
    lumbar vertebrae 710, 714, 715
    sacroiliac joint 758
    sternoclavicular joint 308, 318
    thoracic vertebrae 662, 665
variants, normal 2–5
    abnormality mimicking 2
    identification 4–5